Community Health Nursing
Concepts and Practice

. . . .

Community Health Nursing
Concepts and Practice

· ·

FOURTH EDITION

Barbara Walton Spradley, RN, MN
Associate Professor
School of Public Health
University of Minnesota
Minneapolis, Minnesota

Judith Ann Allender, RN, C, EdD
Associate Professor
Department of Nursing
School of Health and Social Work
California State University
Fresno, California

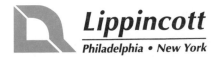

Lippincott
Philadelphia • New York

Sponsoring Editor: Susan M. Glover, RN, MSN
Coordinating Editorial Assistants: Susan M. Keneally and Gene Bender
Production Editor: Virginia Barishek
Production Manager: Janet Greenwood
Production: Textbook Writers Associates
Design: William T. Donnelly
Compositor: Circle Graphics
Printer/Binder: Courier Book Company/Westford
Cover Printer: Lehigh Press

Fourth Edition

Library of Congress Cataloging-in-Publication Data

Spradley, Barbara Walton.
    Community health nursing : concepts and practice / Barbara Walton
Spradley, Judith Ann Allender. — 4th ed.
        p.   cm.
    Includes bibliographical references and index.
    ISBN 0-397-54984-9
1. Community health nursing.   2. Public health nursing.
I. Allender, Judith Ann.   II. Title.
    [DNLM: 1. Community Health Nursing.   WY 106 S766c 1996]
RT98.S68   1996
610.73′43—dc20
DNLM/DLC
for Library of Congress   95-40259
                                                              CIP

The material contained in this volume was submitted as previously unpublished material, except in the instances in which credit has been given to the source from which some of the illustrative material was derived.
Photo credits appear on p. 680.

Any procedure or practice described in this book should be applied by the health-care practitioner under
appropriate supervision in accordance with professional standards of care used with regard to the unique circumstances that apply in each practice situation. Care has been taken to confirm the accuracy of information
presented and to describe generally accepted practices. However, the authors, editors, and publishers cannot accept any responsibility for errors or omissions or for any consequences from application of the information in
this book and make no warranty, express or implied, with respect to the contents of the book.

The authors and publisher have exerted every effort to ensure that drug selection and dosage set forth in
this text are in accordance with current recommendations and practice at the time of publication. However, in
view of ongoing research, changes in government regulations, and the constant flow of information relating to
drug therapy and drug reactions, the reader is urged to check the package insert for each drug for any change in
indications and dosage and for added warnings and precautions. This is particularly important when the recommended agent is a new or infrequently employed drug.

Materials appearing in this book prepared by individuals as part of their official duties as U.S. Government
employees are not covered by the above-mentioned copyright.

9   8   7   6   5   4   3   2   1

To our husbands, Neil and Gil, with love and thanks

Contributors

· ·

Dorothy Brockopp, PhD, RN
> Nurse Researcher
> Department of Nursing
> University of Kentucky
> Lexington, Kentucky
>
> *CHAPTER 26 Research in Community Health Nursing*

Kathy Karsting, RN, MPH
> Director of Nursing
> Northeast Colorado Health Department
> Sterling, Colorado
>
> *CHAPTER 23 Protecting Community Health Through*
> *Control of Communicable Diseases*

Terry Miller, MSN, PHN, PhD
> Associate Dean
> College of Applied Sciences and Arts
> California State University, San Jose
> San Jose, California
>
> *CHAPTER 28 Health Policy, Politics, and*
> *Community Health Advocacy*

Contributors to Previous Editions

Sara T. Fry, RN, PhD

Michele Hadeka, RN, MS

Laura N. Garris, BA

Pamela Thul-Immler, RN, C, MPH

Elaine Richard, RN, MS

Reviewers

. . . .

H. Terri Brower, RN, FNP, EdD
Professor
School of Nursing
Auburn University
Auburn, Alabama

Sharon Davis Burt, MSN, PhDc, PHN
Lecturer
School of Nursing
San Diego State University
San Diego, California

Imelda Clements, RN, PhD
Professor
Lansing School of Nursing
Bellarmine College
Louisville, Kentucky

Mary Louise Jewell, RN, PhD
Associate Professor and Chair
The Nursing Department
Immaculata College
Immaculata, Pennsylvania

Mary D. Jerrett, RN, EdD
Associate Professor
School of Nursing
Queen's University
Kingston, Ontario
Canada

Barbara Leonard, RN, PhD
Associate Professor
University of Minnesota
Minneapolis, Minnesota

M. Peggy MacLeod, RN, MN
Assistant Professor
College of Nursing
University of Saskatchewan
Saskatoon, Saskatchewan
Canada

Melanie McEwan, RN, CS, PhD
Assistant Professor
School of Nursing
Baylor University
Dallas, Texas

Marilyn Morton, RN C, MPH, MS
Associate Professor
Department of Nursing
State University of New York College at
    Plattsburgh
Plattsburgh, New York

Catherine Paradiso, RN, CCRN, MS
Clinical Nurse Specialist
Mobile Health Unit Coordinator
The Visiting Nurse Association
Home Care of Staten Island
Lake Avenue Office
Staten Island, New York

Olive Santavenere, RN, PhD
Associate Professor
Department of Nursing
Southern Connecticut State University
Haven, Connecticut

Preface

. . . .

The fourth edition of *Community Health Nursing: Concepts and Practice* represents a continuing effort to capture the essence and clarify the practice of community health nursing. It is written to share the authors' enthusiasm for a field whose dynamic nature calls for nursing creativity, leadership, and innovation. The potential for community health nurses to protect and enhance the health of at-risk populations and to influence the quality of health services poses an exciting challenge.

As a basic text, the fourth edition, like the other three, is designed to give undergraduate nursing students a comprehensive introduction to the field of community health nursing. It is also designed to be a professional resource in order to enlarge the vision and enhance the impact of practicing community health nurses.

With an escalating demand for nurses to practice in the community, it is important that the meaning of community health nursing as a specialized field of nursing practice be clearly understood. The challenge for the nurse who wishes to practice community health nursing lies in incorporating public health principles with nursing knowledge and skills to offer preventive, health-promoting, and protective services that benefit aggregates. As beginning practitioners, nurses in this field may have limited impact on aggregates, but an aggregate orientation must be germane to their practice. At advanced levels of practice, with advanced preparation in public health, nurses can become specialists in public or community health.

The fourth edition of this text continues to use the term *community health nurse* to describe a practitioner in the community whose work incorporates public health philosophy, theory, and skills with an emphasis on aggregates.

Organization of the Text

In this edition the text is organized into five units. Unit titles as well as most chapter titles have been reworded to include more descriptive language and provide greater continuity for the reader.

Unit I, Understanding the Foundations for Community Health Nursing Practice, introduces the student to the conceptual and historical bases for practice in this field. Eight chapters comprise this unit providing the background of community and health (Chapter 1), the structure and function of community health services (Chapter 2), and health care

(Chapter 3), as the context in which to understand the nature of community health nursing (Chapter 4), and its roles and settings for practice (Chapter 5). The unit ends with three chapters on foundational topics that influence community health nursing practice: health and safety issues in the environment (Chapter 6), cultural influences on health (Chapter 7), and values and ethical decision making in community health nursing (Chapter 8).

Unit II, **Applying the Tools of Community Health Nursing Practice**, provides the student with an understanding of the tools needed for practice in this field and how to use them. The unit opens with two chapters emphasizing the aggregate approach: how to assess and intervene with communities as clients (Chapter 9) and how to work with populations and groups (Chapter 10). The remaining five chapters describe specific tools: the nursing process applied to aggregates (Chapter 11), epidemiological assessment (Chapter 12), communication and collaboration in community health (Chapter 13), educational interventions to promote community health (Chapter 14) and crisis prevention and intervention in the community (Chapter 15).

Unit III, **Promoting and Protecting the Health of Families**, is new and provides the student with background on theoretical bases for promoting family health (Chapter 16), and nursing assessment and practice with families (Chapter 17). These chapters were organized under different units in previous editions. While nurses work with individual families in the community, this text also supports the need to view clusters of families as aggregates for community health nursing intervention.

Unit IV, **Promoting and Protecting the Health of Populations**, helps students to understand the needs of and how to intervene with specific population groups. The first four chapters in this unit emphasize promoting and protecting the health of populations in each major life cycle stage: maternal, prenatal, and newborn populations (Chapter 18), Toddler, preschool, school age, and adolescent populations (Chapter 19), adults and the working population (Chapter 20), and the elderly population (Chapter 21). The remaining three chapters focus on specific at-risk groups: those needing home care (Chapter 22), those at-risk for communicable diseases (Chapter 23), and those who are vulnerable because of socioeconomic, cultural, or behavioral factors (Chapter 24). These last two chapters are entirely new in the fourth edition.

Unit V, **Expanding the Community Health Nurse's Influence**, emphasizes for students the ways in which community health nurses can influence the health care system. The opening chapter (Chapter 25) describes leadership, power, and how nurses can effect change in community health. Next, the need for research in community health nursing (Chapter 26) is stressed with examples of nursing research and discussion of practicing nurses' involvement in and use of research. Promoting quality in health services is the focus of Chapter 27. The text concludes with a clearly presented overview (Chapter 28) of the political process, how health policy is developed, and how the nurse can be involved as an advocate for the health of the community.

New Chapters

To keep abreast of changes in health needs, services, and financing, this edition introduces new topics and expands on many others. Four new chapters have been added. A new chapter on health economics (Chapter 3) incorporates earlier material on health care financing with extensive discussion of the issues and concepts involved in health care reform. Another new chapter, Chapter 13, expands earlier content to emphasize effective communication and collaborative relationships in community health. An entirely new chapter, Chapter 23, deals with communicable diseases, including sexually transmitted diseases, HIV/AIDS, and tuberculosis, that pose serious threats to public health. The fourth, Chapter 24, is also an entirely new chapter that focuses on at-risk populations. This chapter provides a model for understanding the causes of vulnerability and discusses needs and interventions with three specific at-risk populations: homeless persons, substance abusers, and the mentally ill and disabled. The remaining chapters have all been revised, updated, and in some cases expanded to reflect the most recent information on issues affecting community health and the practice of community health nursing.

Key Features

The fourth edition of *Community Health Nursing: Concepts and Practice* includes key features from previous editions as well as new features.

Features continued from previous editions include:

- **An emphasis on aggregate-level nursing** and the community health nurse's opportunity and responsibility to serve not only individuals and families but also to promote and protect the health of communities and populations.
- **An emphasis on health promotion, health protection, and illness prevention.** This, in addition to the aggregate emphasis, reflects the view set forth in this text that community health nursing is the amalgamation of nursing science with public health science. Public health philosophy, values, knowledge, and skills are an essential part of community health nursing practice.
- **A balance of theory with application to nursing practice.** The fourth edition continues the presentation of theoretical and conceptual knowledge to provide students with an understanding of human needs and a rationale for nursing actions. At the same time the text presents practical information on how the nurse can use theory to undergird practice.
- **A summary of highlights** at the end of each chapter provides students with an overview of material covered and serves as a review for study.
- **References and Selected Readings** at the end of each chapter provide students with classic sources, current research, and a broad base of authoritative information for furthering knowledge on the chapter's subject matter.
- **A student-friendly writing style** has been a hallmark of this text since the first edition. Topics are expressed and concepts explained to enhance students' understanding and capture their interest. Writing style remains consistent throughout the text (including contributed chapters) to promote an uninterrupted flow of ideas for students' learning.

Features new to this edition include:

- **Learning Objectives** and **Key Terms** sharpen students' focus and provide a guide for learning the chapter content.
- **Critical Thinking Activities** at the close of each chapter are designed to challenge students, promote critical thinking skills, and encourage their active involvement in solving community health problems.
- **Recurring Boxed Displays** throughout the text highlight important content and create points of interest for student learning. The recurring displays are:
  - **Research Boxes** describe a nursing research study related to the chapter subject matter.

- ■ **Issues Boxes** explore issues affecting community health nursing practice.
- ■ **Levels of Prevention Boxes** address a chapter topic and describe nursing actions at each of the three levels of prevention.
- ■ **World Watch Boxes** emphasize an international perspective on chapter topics.
- ■ **New Photographs and Art** have been added throughout the text to clarify important concepts and enhance students' interest in and understanding of material.
- ■ **Glossary and Appendices** provide definitions of all key terms highlighted throughout the text plus other important resources for student learning and community health nursing practice.

Barabara Walton Spradley, RN, MN

Judith Ann Allender, RN, C, EdD

Acknowledgments

. . . .

We are grateful to many individuals for their assistance in completing this fourth edition. To acknowledge them all would be impossible, given the limitations of space and memory. Many have unwittingly enriched the writing by sharing their experiences and expertise. Others have directly provided ideas, criticism, encouragement, and support. To all we offer our sincere gratitude.

Three individuals have made important new contributions to this fourth edition. Kathy Karsting wrote most of the new chapter on communicable diseases. Dorothy Brockopp and Terry Miller made substantial revisions in their respective chapters on community health nursing research and on politics, policy, and community health advocacy. We are grateful to each of them.

We wish to thank our faculty colleagues for their ideas and encouragement. In particular, we are grateful to Mila Aroskar, Les Block, and Bob Veninga at the University of Minnesota and Joan Heron and Cherie Rector at California State University, Fresno.

Others have made a variety of contributions to this fourth edition. First, we want to thank our respective students for assistance with research, stimulation, and support. We are also grateful to the many community colleagues in both nursing and other fields who have supported and contributed to our efforts.

We would like to thank the many people who provided their suggestions and assistance as reviewers throughout the revision process.

Many people at Lippincott–Raven have provided invaluable assistance. We are grateful to Donna Hilton, our editor for most of the revision, for her support and patience as well as to Sue Glover who took over as editor during the crucial production stage. Special thanks also go to Susan Keneally for outstanding editorial assistance, Carole Wonsiewicz for invaluable critique, and Virginia Barishek and Marty Tenney for excellent production editing. We are grateful to all the other helpful people at Lippincott–Raven, especially designer Bill Donnelly, photo researcher Andrea Champlin, and textbook representative, Ginger Heil.

Finally, we are grateful to the many friends and family members who provided essential encouragement. We especially wish to thank Janet Hagberg, Lois Yellowthunder, and Sr. Ann Wylder for their unfailing friendship. Thanks to our families for encouragement and inspiration, especially Elizabeth Schuepp, Ruth Firth, John Van Doren, James van Doren, Beth Allender, and Zachary Couch. Most importantly, we are grateful to our husbands, Neil Kittlesen and Gil Allender, for their unflagging support, interest, and encouragement. Their contributions are immeasurable.

Contents

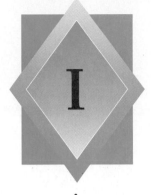

UNIT

I

Understanding the Foundations for Community Health Nursing Practice

1 Conceptual Bases for Community Health Practice

LEARNING OBJECTIVES

Upon completion of this chapter, readers should be able to:

- Discuss the concept of community.
- Identify three types of communities.
- Explain the wellness-illness continuum of health.
- Describe three distinguishing features about health.
- Differentiate between the three levels of prevention.
- Analyze six components of community health practice.
- Describe four characteristics of community health practice.

KEY TERMS

- Aggregate
- Common-interest community
- Community
- Community health
- Community of solution
- Evaluation
- Geographic community
- Health
- Health continuum
- Health promotion
- Illness
- Population
- Primary prevention
- Public health
- Rehabilitation
- Research
- Secondary prevention
- Tertiary prevention
- Wellness

Barbara Walton Spradley and Judith Ann Allender
COMMUNITY HEALTH NURSING: CONCEPTS AND PRACTICE, 4th ed.
© 1996 Barbara Walton Spradley and Judith Ann Allender

Human beings are social creatures. All of us, with rare exceptions, live out our lives in the company of other people. An Eskimo lives in a small, tightly knit community of close relatives; a rural Mexican lives in a small village with hardly more than two hundred members. In complex societies most people find their lives influenced by many overlapping communities such as their professional societies, political parties, religious groups, neighborhoods, and cities. Even those who try to escape community membership always begin their lives in some type of group and usually continue to depend on groups for material and emotional support. Communities are an essential and permanent feature of human experience.

The communities in which people live and work have a profound influence on their collective health and well-being. Research has established, for example, that both smoking and passive exposure to tobacco smoke are directly associated with negative health effects (Brownson, et al, 1992). An increasing number of states, communities and organizations (hospitals, schools, and airlines included) have developed regulatory approaches to smoking. They include removing cigarette vending machines and television commercials, making hospitals and schools no-smoking areas, increasing cigarette taxes, and restricting smoking in public places. Such "community" rules protect nonsmokers, promote the potential for reduced heart and lung disease on a community-wide basis, and have contributed to the downward trend in cigarette smoking in the past 25 years (CDC, 1989; Shea, 1992). Community-wide interventions to reduce cardiovascular disease risk factors have proven successful in a number of cities (Blackburn, 1987; Farquhar, Fortman, Flora, et al, 1990; Shea and Basch, 1990). In recent years Kimberly-Clark instituted a screening and exercise program to reduce coronary heart disease among its employees. More than 90% of the salaried employees were screened, and 25% used the company-furnished exercise facilities. Follow-up tests showed "significant reductions in blood pressure and triglyceride levels and increased treadmill capacity" (Knobel, 1983, p. 19). In this instance, collective health was influenced by the community in which these people worked. On a larger scale, state laws that require seat belt use and child restraints and severely penalize the combination of drinking and driving, protect motorists and reduce the risk of accidents, injuries, and death. Once again, people's health is influenced by the community of which they are a part.

Although many people tend to think of health and illness as individual issues, we know from established evidence that they are also community issues. Spread of the HIV (human immunodeficiency virus) pandemic, nationally and internationally, is a dramatic and tragic case in point (Ehrhardt, 1992). Other problems of community and national concern are the rising incidence and prevalence of sexually transmitted diseases, alcohol and drug abuse, tuberculosis, teen pregnancies, family violence, and pollution-driven environmental hazards. Communities can influence the spread of disease, provide barriers to protect members from health hazards, organize in ways to combat outbreaks of infectious disease, and promote practices that contribute to individual and collective health (Flynn, Rider, and Bailey, 1992; Freudenberg, 1987).

Nursing and Community Health

The relationship between community conditions and people's health is the basis for a challenging field of practice—community health. Many different professionals work in community health to form a complex team. The city planner designing an urban renewal project necessarily becomes involved in community health. The social worker counseling on child abuse or the use of chemical substances among adolescents is involved in community health. A physician treating patients affected by a sudden outbreak of hepatitis and seeking to find the source is engaged in community health practice. Prenatal clinics, meals for the elderly, genetic counseling centers, educational programs for the early detection of cancer, and hundreds of other activities are all part of the community health effort.

Professional nurses are an integral part of community health practice. Their roles and activities are so varied that it is impossible to describe the "typical" community health nurse. They work in every conceivable kind of community health agency from state public health departments to community-based advocacy groups. Their duties range from examining infants in a well-baby clinic or teaching elderly stroke victims in their homes, to carrying out epidemiologic research or engaging in health policy analysis and decision making. Community health nursing is a specialized practice. It combines all the basic elements of professional, clinical nursing with public health and community practice.

This book examines the unique contribution that community health nursing makes to our health care system. Our discussion of the concepts and theories that make community health nursing an important speciality within nursing begins with the broader field of community health, which provides the context as well as essential content for community health nursing practice.

Community health practice, a part of public health, is sometimes misunderstood. Even many health professionals think of community health practice in limiting terms such as sanitation programs, poverty area clinics, or massive campaigns to prevent infectious disease. Although these are a part of its ever-broadening focus, community health practice is much more. In order to understand the nature and significance of this field, it is necessary to look more closely at concepts of community and health.

The Concept Of Community

Broadly defined, a community is a collection of people who share some important feature or features of their lives in common. In this text the term **community** refers to a collection of people who interact with one another and whose common interests or characteristics form the basis for a sense of unity or belonging. It can be a society of people holding common rights and privileges, as citizens of a town, or sharing common interest, as a community of farmers, or living under the same laws and regulations, as a prison community. The function of any community includes its members' sense of belonging and shared identity, values, norms, communication, and supporting behavior (Green and Kreuter, 1991). Some communities, such as a tiny village in Appalachia, are composed of people who share almost everything. They live in the same location, work at a limited number of jobs, attend the same churches, and make use of the single health clinic with its visiting physician and nurse. Other communities, such as Mothers Against Drunk Drivers (MADD) or the community of professional nurses, are large, scattered, and composed of individuals who may share only their common interest and involvement in certain goals. Although most communities of people share many aspects of their experience, the following criteria provide a useful framework for identifying three types

of communities that have relevance to community health practice: geography, common interest, and health problem.

GEOGRAPHIC COMMUNITY

A community is often defined by its geographic boundaries and is thus called a **geographic community**. Green and Kreuter refer to these boundaries as its "structure" (Green and Kreuter, 1991, p. 262). A city, town, or neighborhood is a geographic community. Consider the community of Hayward, Wisconsin. Located in northwestern Wisconsin, it is set in the north woods environment, far removed from any urban center and in a climatic zone characterized by extremely harsh winters. With a population of approximately two thousand people, it is considered a rural community. The population has certain identifiable characteristics such as age and sex ratios, and its size fluctuates with the seasons; summers bring hundreds of tourists and seasonal residents. Hayward is a social system as well as a geographic location. The families, schools, hospital, churches, stores, and government institutions are linked in a complex network. This community, like others, has an informal power structure. It has a communication system that includes gossip, the newspaper, the co-op store bulletin board, and the radio station. In one sense, then, a community consists of a collection of people located in a specific place and is made up of institutions organized into a social system.

Local communities such as Hayward vary in size. A few miles south of Hayward lie several other communities, including Northwoods Beach and Round Lake; these three, along with other towns and isolated farms, form a larger community called Sawyer County. If you worked for a health agency serving only Hayward, that community would be of primary concern; however, if you worked for the Sawyer County Health Department, you would focus on this larger community. A community health nurse employed by the State Health Department in Madison, Wisconsin, would have an interest in Sawyer County and Hayward, but only as one small part of the larger community of Wisconsin.

Frequently, a single part of a city can be treated as a community. In Seattle, for example, the skid row district near the waterfront forms a community of many transients. In New York the section of Manhattan called Harlem is a community as is the Haight-Ashbury district of San Francisco.

For certain purposes in community health, it is useful to identify a geographic area as a community. A community demarcated by geographic boundaries, such as a city or county, becomes a clear target for analysis of health needs. Available data, such as morbidity and mortality figures, can augment assessment studies to form the basis for planning health programs. Media campaigns and other health education efforts can readily reach intended audiences. Examples include information on safe sex, the dangers of drug abuse, or self protection and where to seek shelter from abuse and violence. A geographic community is easily mobilized for action. Groups can be formed to carry out intervention and prevention efforts that address needs specific to that community. Such efforts might include more stringent policies on day care, shelters for battered women, work-site safety programs in local hazardous industries, or improved sex education in the schools. Furthermore, health actions can be enhanced through support of politically powerful individuals and resources present in a geographic community.

COMMON-INTEREST COMMUNITY

A community can also be identified by a common interest or goal. A collection of people, although they are widely scattered geographically, can have an interest or goal that binds the members together. This is called a **common-interest community**. The members of a church in a large metropolitan area, the members of a national professional organization, or women who have had mastectomies, are all common-interest communities. Sometimes within a certain geographic area, a group of people become a community by promoting their common interest. Disabled individuals scattered throughout a large city may emerge as a community through a common interest in their need for improved wheelchair access or other handicapped facilities. The residents in an industrial community may develop a common interest in air or water pollution issues, while others who work but do not live there may not share that interest. Communities form to protect the rights of children, stop violence against women, clean up the environment, promote the arts, preserve historical sites, protect endangered species, develop a smoke-free environment, provide support following some crisis, and many more. The kinds of shared interests that lead to the formation of communities are widely varied.

Common-interest communities whose focus is on a health related issue become a useful medium for

change. The group's single-minded commitment serves as a mobilizing force for action. Many successful prevention and health promotion efforts, including improved services and increased community awareness of specific problems, have resulted from the work of common-interest communities.

COMMUNITY OF SOLUTION

Frequently in community health practice a community is a group of people who come together to solve a problem that affects all of them. The shape of this community varies with the nature of the problem, the size of the geographic area affected, and the number of resources needed to address the problem. Such a community has been called a **community of solution** (National Commission on Community Health Services, 1967). A water pollution problem may involve several counties whose agencies and personnel must work together to control upstream water supply, industrial waste disposal, and city water treatment. This group of counties forms a community of solution around a health problem. In another instance, several schools may collaborate with law enforcement and health agencies as well as legislators and policy makers to study patterns of students' drug use and design possible preventive approaches. The boundaries of this community of solution form around the schools, agencies, and political figures involved. Figure 1.1 depicts some communities of solution related to one city.

In recent years communities of solution have formed in many cities to attack the spread of HIV infection. Public health agencies, social service groups, schools, media personnel and many others have banded together to create public awareness of the dangers present and to promote preventive behaviors. A community of solution is an important medium for change in community health.

Population and Aggregate Concepts

The three types of communities just discussed underscore the meaning of the concept of community: in each instance a collection of people were joined to and interacted with one another around common interests or characteristics. The concept of population has a

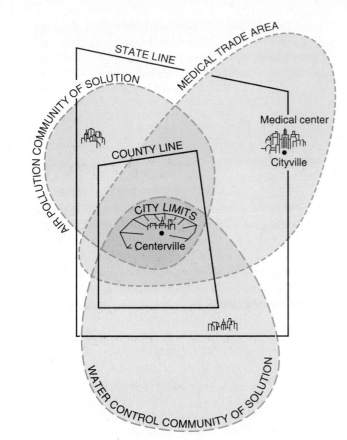

FIGURE 1.1. A city's communities of solution. State, county, and city boundaries (shown in solid lines) may have little or no bearing on health solution boundaries.

somewhat different meaning. In this text the term **population** refers to all the people occupying an area or all those making up a whole, based on having one or more characteristics in common. A population, in contrast to a community, is made up of people who do not necessarily interact with one another and who do not necessarily share a sense of belonging to that group. A population may be defined geographically, such as the population of the United States or a city's population. This designation of a population is useful in community health for epidemiologic study and for collecting demographic data for health planning and other purposes. A population may also be defined by common qualities or characteristics, such as the elderly population or the homeless population. For community health purposes this meaning of the term becomes useful when targeting intervention with a specific group of people, such as the homeless, whose common characteristics, such as their

homelessness with its health-related problems, become a major focus of the intervention.

In this text an **aggregate** refers to a mass or grouping of distinct individuals who are considered as a whole. It is a broader term that encompasses many different sized groups of people. Both communities and populations are types of aggregates. Thus the aggregate focus, or a concern for groupings of people, becomes a distinguishing feature of community health practice in contrast to individual health care.

The recent shift away from hospitals as the focus of the health care system, to community-based services, along with a rising emphasis on "managed care of populations," only serves to underscore the importance of community health nursing's aggregate focus. In fact, "it validates the focus of community health nursing over many decades" (Hegyvary, 1990, p.7). With community as central to the health care model, it becomes all the more essential for nurses to understand the meaning of community health and to assume leadership in aggregate level health care.

Community health workers, including the community health nurse, need to be able to define the community targeted for study and intervention. That is, who are the people that compose the community? Where are they located and what are their characteristics? A clear delineation of the community or population must be established before one can assess needs and design interventions (Shamansky and Pesznecker, 1981). One also needs to understand the complex nature of communities. What are the characteristics of the people in terms of age, sex, race, socioeconomic level, and health status? How does the community interact with other communities? What is its past history? What are its resources? Is the community undergoing rapid change and, if so, what are the changes? These questions and more, as well as the tools needed to assess a community for health purposes, are discussed in detail in Chapter 9, The Community as Client: Assessment and Planning.

The Concept of Health

Health in the abstract refers to a person's physical, mental, and spiritual state; it can be positive (as being in good health) or negative (as being in poor health). The World Health Organization defines health positively as "a state of complete physical, mental, and social well-being and not merely the absence of disease or infirmity" (Pickett and Hanlon, 1990, p.4). Our understanding of the concept of health builds on this classic definition. **Health** in this text refers to a state of well-being which includes soundness of mind, body, and spirit. Community health practitioners value a strong emphasis on **wellness** which includes the above definition of health and is the presence of a positive capacity to develop one's potential and to lead an energetic, fulfilling, and productive life (Smith, 1983). They are growing to understand health broadly through holistic perspectives that recognize the relationship of health to environment. J.M. Last partially defines health as "a state of equilibrium between humans and the physical, biologic, and social environment. . . ."(Last, 1987, p. 5).

Although health is widely accepted as desirable, the exact nature of health is often unclear and ambiguous. Consumers and providers often define health and wellness in different ways. (See Research in Community Health Nursing display.) In order to clarify the concept for nursing's use in considering community health practice, the distinguishing features of health shall be briefly characterized; then the implications of this concept for the activities of professionals in the field can be examined more fully.

THE HEALTH CONTINUUM: WELLNESS–ILLNESS

Health is a relative, not an absolute, concept. Society tends to suggest a polarized or black-and-white way of thinking about health; people are either well or ill. **Illness** is a state of being relatively unhealthy. There are many levels and degrees of wellness and illness. A person with terminal cancer or end-stage renal disease may be classified as very ill. Someone else recovering from pneumonia may be less ill, yet another person with infectious mononucleosis may be mildly ill.

Health, according to the definition used in this text, always involves many levels. From a mildly well teenage boy with limitations in functioning because of episodic depression to a robust 70-year-old woman who is fully active and functioning at an optimal level of wellness, there are variations in degrees of health. Pickett and Hanlon (1990) describe health as a continuum. Health always involves a range of degrees from optimal health at one end to total disability or death at the other (see Figs. 1.2A and B); it is known as a **health continuum**. This continuum of health applies not only to individuals but to families and communities of people. A nurse

Research in Community Health Nursing
DEFINING HEALTH AND HEALTH GOALS

Folden, S. L. (1993). Definitions of health and health goals of participants in a community-based pulmonary rehabilitation program. *Public Health Nursing*, 10(1): 31–35.

Improving health is generally a shared goal between providers and consumers of health services. However, providers and consumers may vary in their conceptions of health which can interfere with communication, lead to disparate goals, and cause dissatisfaction with unmet goals.

This study compared consumer and provider definitions of health and health goals in a nurse-managed, community pulmonary rehabilitation program. The study sample consisted of 132 adults whose charts were reviewed retrospectively. In addition to nursing assessment, health history, and demographic data, participants were asked, "What does the word health mean to you? and, What do you hope to gain from this program; in short, what is your goal?" (p.32). Participants defined health as "being free of disease and its symptoms . . . evidenced by being able to function in the community, and . . . having a general sense of well-being" (p.33). Their most frequently stated goals related to improved functional ability and lessened respiratory symptoms.

Study findings showed that participants had a narrower view of health and health goals than the providers. Implications from this research were that community-based programs targeting specific populations need to learn how those populations define health, what are their health goals, and what brings them to the program. Populations with chronic illnesses could benefit from expanded goals targeting the maintenance of a satisfying lifestyle despite functional disabilities. Providers need to work for congruency of goals with clients to maximize service outcomes.

might speak of a dysfunctional family meaning they are experiencing a relative degree of illness. The nurse might describe a healthy family as one that exhibits many wellness characteristics, such as effective communication, conflict resolution, ability to work together, use of appropriate resources, etc. Likewise a

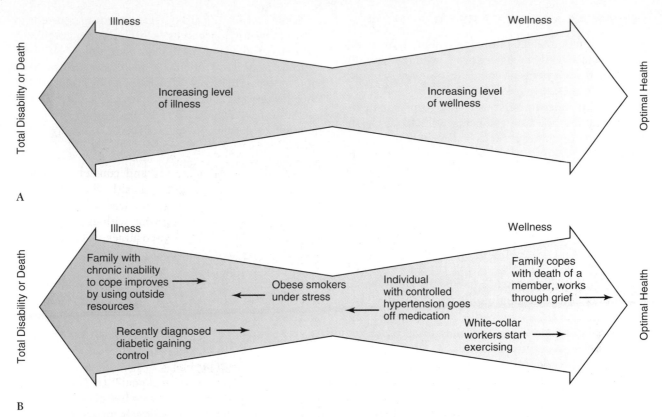

FIGURE 1.2. **A.** The wellness-illness continuum. The level (degree) of illness increases as one moves toward total disability or death; the level of wellness increases as one moves toward optimal health. This continuum shows the relative nature of health. At any given time a person can be placed at some point along the continuum. **B.** Dynamic nature of the wellness-illness continuum. A person's relative health is usually in a state of flux,either improving or deteriorating. This diagram of the wellness-illness continuum shows several examples of people in changing states of health.

community, as a collection of people, may be described in terms of degrees of wellness or illness. A healthy community, first described by Cottrell (1976) as a competent community, is one in which the various organizations, groups, and aggregates of people making up the community do at least four things:

Healthy Communities:

1. "are able to collaborate effectively in identifying the problems and needs of the community;
2. can achieve a working concensus on goals and priorities;
3. can agree on ways and means to implement the agreed-on goals;
4. and can collaborate effectively in the required actions" (Cottrell, 1976, p. 197).

The health of an individual, family, group, or community moves back and forth along this continuum throughout life.

By thinking of health relatively, as a matter of degree, one can help broaden the scope of nursing practice to focus on prevention of illness or disability and promotion of wellness. Traditionally, the majority of health care has been focused on treatment of acute and chronic conditions at the illness end of the continuum. Gradually the emphasis is shifting to focus attention on the wellness end of the continuum (*U.S. Department of Health and Human Services*, 1991). Community health practice ranges over the entire continuum; it always works to improve the degree of health in individuals, families, groups, and communities. In particular, community health practice emphasizes the promotion and preservation of positive health and the prevention of illness or disability (Green and Anderson, 1986).

HEALTH AS A STATE OF BEING

Health refers to a state of being including many different qualities and characteristics. One might describe a person in such terms as energetic, outgoing, enthusiastic, beautiful, caring, loving, and intense. Together, these qualities become the essence of a person's existence; they describe a state of being. Similarly, a specific geographic community, such as a neighborhood, has many characteristics. It might be characterized by the terms congested, deteriorating, unattractive, dirty, and disorganized. These characteristics suggest diminishing degrees of vitality. A third example might be a population, such as workers involved in a massive lay off who band together to provide support and share resources to effectively seek new employment. This community shows signs of healthy and positive coping.

Health involves the total person or the total community. All the dimensions of life affecting everyday functioning determine an individual's or a community's health including physical, psychological, spiritual, economic, and sociocultural experiences. All these factors must be considered when dealing with an individual's or community's health. It should be a holistic approach. Thus, clients' placement on the wellness-illness continuum can only be known if one considers all facets of their lives including not only physical status but status of home, family and work. See Figure 1.3.

When considering an aggregate or group of people in terms of health, it becomes useful for intervention purposes to speak of the "health of a community." With aggregates as well as individuals, health as a state of being does not merely involve that group's physical state but includes psychological, spiritual, and socioeconomic factors as well. The health of South Central Los Angeles following the riots a few years ago is an example. Extensive damage from interracial fighting, burning, and looting left the community totally devastated. This community's health was at a dangerously low point and in need of healing and restoration.

SUBJECTIVE AND OBJECTIVE DIMENSIONS OF HEALTH

Health involves both subjective and objective dimensions. That is, it involves both how a person feels (subjective) and how well a person can function in her or his environment (objective). Subjectively, a healthy person is one who feels well, who experiences the sensation of a vital, positive state. Healthy people are full of life and vigor, capable of physical and mental productivity. They feel minimal discomfort and displeasure with the world around them. Again, people experience varying degrees of vitality and well-being. The state of feeling well fluctuates. Some mornings we wake up feel-

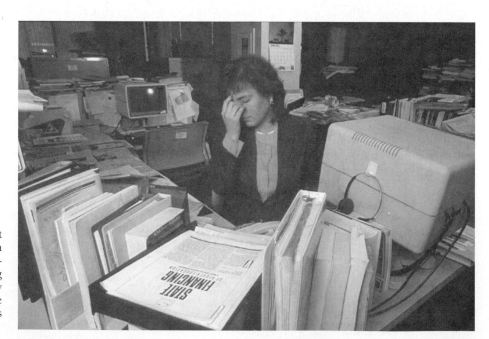

FIGURE 1.3. Pressured to get her work completed between interruptions, this administrative assistant is experiencing work stress and an unhealthy life-style that is likely to move her health state to the illness end of the continuum.

ing more energetic and enthusiastic than we do on other mornings. How people feel varies day by day, even hour by hour; nonetheless, how they feel overall is a strong indicator of their state of health.

Health also involves the objective dimension of ability to function. A healthy individual or community carries out necessary activities and achieves enriching goals. Unhealthy people not only feel ill but are limited, to some degree, in their ability to carry out daily activities. Indeed, levels of illness or wellness are largely measured in terms of ability to function (Stokes et al., 1982). A person confined to bed is labeled sicker than an ill person managing self-care. A family that meets its members' needs is healthier than one that has poor communication patterns and is unable to provide adequate physical and emotional resources. A community actively engaged in crime prevention, or policing industrial wastes shows signs of healthy functioning. Degree of functioning is directly related to state of health.

The ability to function can be observed. A man dresses and feeds himself and goes to work. Despite financial exigencies, a family nourishes its members through a supportive emotional climate. A community provides adequate resources and services for its members. These performances, to some degree, can be regarded as indicators of health status. Some community health agencies assess clients' ability to function as a measure of client progress and nursing care effectiveness (Choi et al., 1983; Martin and Scheet, 1992).

An individual's, family's, or community's actions are motivated by their values. Some activities such as walking and taking care of personal needs are functions almost everyone values. Other actions (for example, bird watching, volunteering to help a charity, or running) have more limited appeal. In assessing the health of individuals and communities, the community health nurse can observe people's ability to function but must also know their values, which may contrast sharply with those of the professional. The influence of values on health is examined more closely in Chapter 8, Values and Ethical Decision Making in Community Health.

Subjective (feeling well or ill) and objective (functioning) dimensions together provide us with a clearer picture of people's health. When they feel well and demonstrate functional ability, they are close to the wellness end of the wellness-illness continuum. Even those with a disease such as arthritis or diabetes may feel well and perform well within their capacity. These people can be considered healthy or closer to the wellness end of the continuum. Figure 1.4 depicts the relationships between the subjective and objective views of health.

Health and Community

Health can be viewed as an important resource, both of individuals and communities. The relationship between health and community has been summarized in Henkel's (1970, p.2) classic work:

1. The physical, emotional, and social health and well-being of individuals is one of their most important assets.
2. Through judicious use of this asset they will be able more effectively to achieve their goals in life.
3. Developing this asset to the greatest possible level requires the concerted and cooperative efforts of many people.
4. Society as a whole will ultimately benefit from healthy citizens.

Reinforcing this view, the document, *Healthy People 2000: National Health Promotion and Disease Prevention Objectives*, provides vision and an agenda for significantly reducing preventable death and disability nationwide, enhancing quality of life, and greatly reducing disparities in the health status of populations. It emphasizes the need for every individual to assume personal responsibility for controlling and improving her or his own health destiny. It challenges society to find ways to make good health available to vulnerable populations whose disadvantaged state places them at greater risk for health problems. And it calls for a shift in focus from treating preventable illness and functional impairment to concentrating resources and targeting efforts that promote health and prevent disease and disability (*U.S. Department of Health and Human Services*, 1991). Healthy people make healthy communities and a healthy society.

The implications of this view of health have far-reaching consequences for persons engaged in health care. No longer can health professionals justify concentrating the majority of their efforts exclusively on treating the sick and injured. For centuries health care has focused on the illness end of the wellness-illness continuum. We now live in an age when it is not only possible to promote health and prevent disease and disability but our mandate and responsibility to do so (*U.S. Department of Health and Human Services*, 1991).

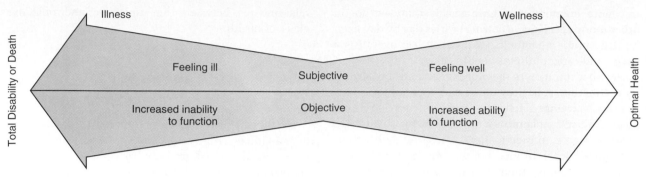

FIGURE 1.4. Subjective and objective views of the wellness-illness continuum.

An important function accompanying health promotion and disease prevention is health assessment. When one considers health status from the perspective just discussed, its measurement becomes more feasible as well as necessary. Health status assessment, health promotion, and disease and disability prevention are all essential aspects of community health nursing and are discussed in detail in later chapters.

Components of Community Health Practice

The discussion thus far has focused on community and on health. Together, these concepts provide the foundation for understanding community health. In acute care the health of an individual is the primary focus. Community health broadens that focus to concentrate on families, populations, and the community at large. The community becomes the recipient of service, and health becomes the product. Viewed from another perspective, community health is concerned with the interchange between population groups and their total environment, and with the impact of that interchange on collective health.

Just as a whole is greater than the sum of its parts, the health of a community is more than the sum of the health of its individual citizens. A community that achieves high-level wellness is composed of healthy citizens, functioning in an environment that protects and promotes health. Community health, as a field of practice, seeks to provide organizational structure, a broad set of resources, and the collaborative activities needed to accomplish the goal of an optimally healthy community.

Community health and public health share many features in common. Both are organized community efforts aimed at the promotion, protection, and preservation of the public's health. Historically, as a field of practice, public health has been associated most often with official or government efforts, such as federal, state, or local tax-supported health agencies that target the whole range of health issues. In contrast, private health efforts, such as the American Lung Association or the American Cancer Society, work toward solving selected health problems. The latter augments the former. Public health practice today encompasses both and works collaboratively with all health agencies and efforts, public or private, concerned with the public's health. In this text, community health practice refers to a focus on specific designated communities. It is thus a part of the larger public health effort and recognizes the fundamental concepts and principles of public health as its birthright and foundation for practice.

Winslow's classic 1920 definition of public health still holds true and forms the basis for our understanding of community health in this text.

> "**Public health** is the science and art of preventing disease, prolonging life, and promoting health and efficiency through organized community efforts for the sanitation of the environment, the control of communicable infections, the education of the individual in personal hygiene, the organization of medical and nursing services for the early diagnosis and preventive treatment of disease, and the development of the social machinery to insure everyone a standard of living adequate for the maintenance of health, so organizing these benefits as to enable every citizen to realize his birthright of health and longevity" (cited in Pickett and Hanlon, 1990, p. 5).

Given this understanding of public health, the concept of community health can be defined. **Community health** is the identification of needs and the protection and improvement of collective health within a geographically defined area.

One of the challenges community health practice faces is to remain responsive to the community's health needs. As a result, its structure is complex; numerous health services and programs are currently available or will be developed in the future. Examples include health education, family planning, accident prevention, environmental protection, immunization, nutrition, early periodic screening and developmental testing, school programs, mental health, and occupational health.

Community health practice can best be understood by examining six basic components, which when combined encompass its services and programs: (1) promotion of healthful living, (2) prevention of health problems, (3) treatment of disorders, (4) rehabilitation, (5) evaluation, and (6) research.

PROMOTION OF HEALTH

Promotion of health is now recognized as one of the most important components of public health and community health practice (*U.S. Department of Health and Human Services*, 1991; Green and Kreuter, 1991). **Health promotion** includes all efforts that seek to move people closer to optimal well-being or higher levels of wellness. Nursing, in particular, has a social mandate for engaging in health promotion (Novak, 1988; Pender, et al, 1992). Health promotion programs and activities include many forms of health education such as teaching the danger of drug use, demonstrating healthful practices like regular exercise, and providing a greater number of health-promoting options like heart-healthy menu selections. Community health promotion, then, "is the combination of educational and environmental supports for actions and conditions of living conducive to health" (Green and Kreuter, 1991, p. 4) of the community. Wellness programs in business and industry are an example (Sciacca, et al, 1990). Health education is a useful tool when accompanied by desire, opportunity, and resources that encourage more healthful practices (Farquhar, Fortman and Flora, 1990; Green and Kreuter, 1991; Pencak, 1991). Demonstration of such healthful practices as eating more nutritious foods (see Fig. 1.5) and exercising more regularly is often performed and promoted by individual health workers. In addition, groups and health agencies that support a smoke-free environment, encourage physical fitness programs for all ages, or demand that food prod-

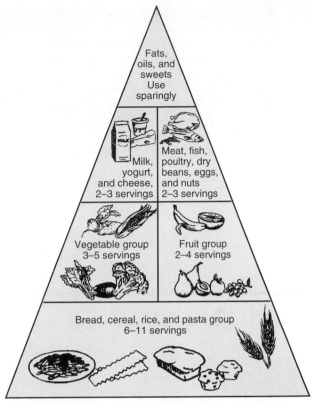

FIGURE 1.5. The Food Pyramid. In April of 1992, the U.S. Department of Agriculture replaced the old four food groups, in use since 1946, with the food pyramid. It emphasizes grains, fruits, and vegetables as the basis of a healthy diet. Recommended daily servings in each group are noted.

ucts be properly labeled underscore the importance of these practices and create public awareness.

The goal of health promotion is to raise individuals', families', populations', and communities' levels of wellness (Moore and Williamson, 1984). Community health seeks to accomplish this goal through a three-pronged effort:

1. to increase the span of healthy life for all citizens,
2. to reduce health disparities among population groups, and
3. to achieve access to necessary preventive services for everyone.

More specifically, the U.S. Public Health Service has outlined 22 priority areas for intervention in its publication, *Healthy People 2000*, 1991. They are listed in the Issues in Community Health Nursing display in this

Issues in Community Health Nursing
PRIORITY AREAS FOR NATIONAL HEALTH PROMOTION AND DISEASE PREVENTION

Determining priorities for health services' intervention is a continuing issue for health planners and decision makers. What areas should rank highest as targets? After extensive and comprehensive study, the U. S. Public Health Service established a list of priorities and goals for the nation's health. Its report, *Healthy People 2000*, states three broad goals: to "(1) increase the span of healthy life for Americans, (2) reduce health disparities among Americans, and (3) achieve access to preventive services for Americans" (1991, p.6). To accomplish these goals, measurable objectives were established under each of the following 22 priority areas.

HEALTH PROMOTION

1. Physical activity and fitness
2. Nutrition
3. Tobacco
4. Alcohol and other drugs
5. Family planning
6. Mental health and mental disorders
7. Violent and abusive behavior
8. Educational and community-based programs

HEALTH PROTECTION

9. Unintentional injuries
10. Occupational safety and health
11. Environmental health
12. Food and drug safety
13. Oral health

PREVENTIVE SERVICES

14. Maternal and Infant Health
15. Heart disease and stroke
16. Cancer
17. Diabetes and chronic disabling conditions
18. HIV infection
19. Sexually transmitted diseases
20. Immunization and infectious diseases
21. Clinical preventive services

SURVEILLANCE AND DATA SYSTEMS

22. Surveillance and data systems

This national listing serves as a guide to policy makers and health planners at all levels. It provides a framework for prioritizing and addressing specific health needs in designated communities.

chapter. Under each of the 22 areas *Healthy People 2000* outlines a number of objectives stated in measurable terms, that specify targeted incidence and prevalence changes and that address age, gender, and culturally vulnerable groups.

It is difficult to provide health-promoting options—that is, opportunities to make more healthful choices—without reexamining and, in many instances, restructuring organizational patterns and policies as well as increasing personal and societal resources. At the local level, many health agencies are offering services at hours more convenient to their clientele and, in some cases, are providing transportation or other means of easier access to service. Furthermore, community residents are forming stronger bonds of partnership with health workers in order to understand and solve their own health problems as well as to assume greater responsibility for achieving positive health for themselves and their communities.

LEVELS OF PREVENTION OF HEALTH PROBLEMS

Prevention of health problems constitutes a major part of community health practice. Prevention means anticipating and averting problems or discovering them as early as possible in order to minimize possible disability and impairment. It is practiced on three levels (see the Levels of Prevention display) in community health: (1) primary prevention, (2) secondary prevention, and (3) tertiary prevention (Moore and Williamson, 1984; Pickett and Hanlon, 1990).

Primary prevention obviates the occurrence of a health problem; it includes measures taken to keep illness or injuries from ever occurring. "It precedes disease or dysfunction and is applied to a generally healthy population" (Shamansky and Clausen, 1980, p. 106). For example, a community health nurse who encourages elderly people to install and use safety devices,

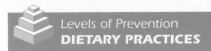

Levels of Prevention
DIETARY PRACTICES

GOAL

To avoid nutritional deficiencies and enhance community nutritional status through healthy dietary practices.

PRIMARY PREVENTION

Provide educational programs, literature, posters of the food pyramid, in schools, work sites, food stores, and other public places to promote awareness. Encourage restaurants to offer healthy menu items.

SECONDARY PREVENTION

Conduct community screening programs for early detection of individuals with poor eating habits among groups such as adolescents, young female workers, and the elderly. Initiate educational and incentive programs to improve dietary practices.

TERTIARY PREVENTION

Case finding in schools, work sites, etc, to determine people with eating disorders, addictions (such as alcoholism), or other life style patterns that inhibit positive dietary practices and initiate treatment.

Secondary prevention involves efforts which seek to detect and treat existing health problems at the earliest possible stage when disease or impairment already exist. Hypertension screening centers in many communities help identify a high-risk group and encourage early treatment to prevent heart attacks or stroke. Other examples are breast and testicular self-examination practices and regular use of mammograms and Pap smears for early detection of possible cancer. Secondary prevention attempts to discover a health problem at a point when intervention may lead to its control or eradication. This is the goal behind water and soil testing for contaminants and hazardous chemicals in community environmental health. It also prompts community health nurses to watch for early signs of child abuse in a family, emotional disturbances in a group of widows, or alcohol and drug abuse among adolescents.

Tertiary prevention attempts to reduce the extent and severity of a health problem to its lowest possible level so as to minimize disability and restore or preserve function. Treatment and rehabilitation of persons following a stroke to reduce impairment, postmastectomy exercise programs to restore functioning, and early treatment and management of diabetes to reduce problems or at least slow their rate of progress are examples. The persons involved have an existing illness or disability whose impact on their lives is lessened through tertiary prevention. In broader community health practice we use tertiary prevention to minimize the effects of an existing unhealthy community condition. Examples of such prevention are insisting that wheelchair access be adhered to or warning urban residents about the dangers of a chemical spill and recalling a contaminated food or drug product.

Health assessment of individuals, families, and communities is an important part of all three levels of preventive practice. One must determine health status in order to anticipate problems and select appropriate preventive measures. Community health nurses working with young parents who themselves have been victims of child abuse can institute early treatment for the parents to prevent abuse and foster adequate parenting of their children. If assessment of a community reveals inadequate facilities and activities to meet the future needs of its growing senior population, agencies and groups can collaborate to develop the needed resources.

Health problems are most effectively prevented by maintaining healthy life-styles and healthy environments. To these ends, community health practice directs many of its efforts to providing safe and satisfying living and working conditions, nutritious food, and

such as grab bars by bathtubs or hand rails on steps, is preventing injuries from falls. Local health departments help control and prevent communicable diseases such as rubeola or poliomyelitis by providing regular immunization programs. Primary prevention involves anticipatory planning and action on the part of community health professionals who must project themselves into the future, envision potential needs and problems, and then design programs to counteract them so that they never occur. A community health nurse who instructs a group of overweight individuals on how to follow a well-balanced diet during weight loss is preventing the possibility of nutritional deficiency. Educational programs that teach safe sex practices or the dangers of smoking and substance abuse are another example of primary prevention. The concepts of primary prevention and planning for the future are foreign to many social groups who may resist on the basis of conflicting values. The "Parable of the Dangerous Cliff" illustrates such a value conflict.

Parable of the Dangerous Cliff

Twas a dangerous cliff, as they freely confessed,
   Though to walk near its crest was so pleasant;
But over its terrible edge there has slipped
   A duke, and full many a peasant.
The people said something would have to be done
   But their projects did not at all tally.
Some said, "Put a fence around the edge of the
      cliff";
   Some, "an ambulance down in the valley."
The lament of the crowd was profound and was
      loud,
   As their hearts overflowed with their pity;
But the cry of the ambulance carried the day
   As it spread through the neighboring city.
A collection was made, to accumulate aid,
   And the dwellers in highway and alley,
Gave dollars or cents.
Not to furnish a fence
But "An ambulance down in the valley."
"For the cliff is all right if you're careful," they said.
"And if folks ever slip and are dropping,
   It isn't the slipping that hurts them so much
As the shock down below when they're stopping."
So for years (we have heard), as these mishaps
      occurred,
   Quick forth the rescuers sally,
To pick up the victims who fell from the cliff,
   With the ambulance down in the valley.

Said one in his plea, "It's a marvel to me
   That you'd give so much greater attention
To repairing results than to cure the cause;
You had much better aim at prevention.
   For the mischief, of course, should be stopped at
      its source,
Come neighbors and friends, let us rally.
   It is far better sense to rely on a fence
Than an ambulance down in the valley."
"He is wrong in his head," the majority said;
   "He would end all our earnest endeavor.
He's a man who would shirk this responsible work,
   But we will support it forever.
Aren't we picking up all, just as fast as they fall,
   and giving them care liberally?
A superfluous fence is of no consequence,
If the ambulance works in the valley."
The story looks queer as we've written it here,
   But things oft occur that are stranger.
More humane, we assert, than to take care of the
      hurt,
   Is the plan of removing the danger.
The very best plan is to safeguard the man,
   And attend to the thing rationally;
To build up the fence and try to dispense
   With the ambulance down in the valley.
Better still! Cut down the hill!

—Author Unknown

---

clean air and water. This area of practice includes the field of preventive medicine, which is a population-focused, or community-oriented, branch of medical practice that incorporates public health sciences and principles (Last, 1987).

TREATMENT OF DISORDERS

The third component of community health practice is treatment of disorders. It focuses on the illness end of the continuum and is the remedial aspect of community health practice. This occurs by three methods: (1) direct service to people with health problems (2) indirect service which helps people obtain treatment and (3) development of programs to correct unhealthy conditions. Examples of direct service include the following: a nursing center serving a homeless population may provide health screening, education, and referral services.

Elderly persons confined to home with disabling chronic illness can obtain home visits from a nursing agency for assistance with treatment regimens, supervision of medications, and personal care. A neighborhood health center can provide an educational program and support group for people wanting to stop smoking or lose weight. Many kinds of community agencies provide direct health care or health-related sevices.

The second method of treating disorders is indirect service by assisting people with health problems to obtain treatment. In many instances a community agency may not be able to provide needed care and will refer the individuals or groups concerned to a more appropriate resource. A young woman with postpartum bleeding, assisted by the community health nurse, can obtain an immediate appointment with a physician at the local clinic. A social worker can help a family that is plagued by personal and economic problems to enter a family therapy and counseling program. A number of community agencies provide information and referral services.

The third method of treatment of disorders is the development of programs to correct unhealthy conditions. One community with a high incidence of alcoholism and drug abuse initiated a chemical dependency counseling and treatment center. In another community, the health department developed new regulations for industrial waste disposal as a result of increased pollution of the water supply. Individual community members and health workers also take corrective action to remedy situations such as a case of apparent child abuse, poor nutrition in a school lunch program, or inhumane conditions and treatment in a nursing home.

REHABILITATION

Rehabilitation, the fourth component of community health practice, involves efforts which seek to reduce disability and, as much as possible, restore function. People whose handicaps are congenital or acquired through illness or accident such as stroke, heart condition, amputation, or mental illness can be helped to regain some measure of lost function or to develop new compensating skills. For example, a factory worker who lost his leg in an industrial accident received good medical and nursing care, prosthetic fittings, and physical and occupational therapy; he thus retrained to assume an office job.

In community health, the need to reduce disability and restore function applies equally to families, groups, and communities as well as to individuals. (See Fig. 1.6) Many groups form for rehabilitative purposes and offer support and guidance for those recuperating from some physical or mental disability. Examples include Alcoholics Anonymous, halfway houses for discharged psychiatric patients, ostomy clubs, or drug rehabilitation programs. Rehabilitation services are often needed and sought by whole communities, as when an inner city area desires to provide decent, safe playgrounds for its children.

As an element of community health practice, rehabilitation becomes increasingly significant when disease trends and changes in life expectancy are considered. Chronic diseases, such as cancer, heart disease, diabetes, and mental illness are major cripplers. So too are accidents and injuries from many causes, including violence. Abuse of drugs, alcohol and tobacco further adds to the list of disabling conditions. As a result, the

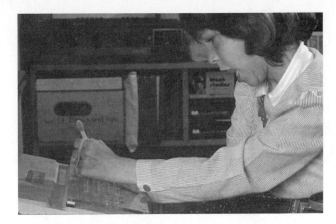

FIGURE 1.6. This retarded young person, functioning well within her capacity, demonstrates that community health efforts can enable people to achieve a high level of health despite disability.

need for rehabilitation services and long-term care has increased, stimulated further by the rising number of elderly persons in the population with chronic health problems.

EVALUATION

Evaluation, the fifth component of community health practice, is the process by which that practice is analyzed, judged, and improved according to established goals and standards. Evaluation of health and health care should be an integral part of every kind of health service from individual practice to national and international programs. Whether done on a single case basis or at the program level, evaluation helps solve problems and provides direction for future health care efforts. Its goals are to determine needs and the success of present activities as well as to develop improved services (Veney and Kaluzny, 1984). In one community, evaluation of mental health services revealed a need for more comprehensive psychiatric emergency care on a 24-hour basis. If a psychiatric crisis occurred during the night, police were the only persons available to help, and jail the only place where the mentally ill could be taken. The deficiency was corrected by providing 24-hour psychiatric emergency service in the community mental health center. In other instances, evaluation of community-wide education programs targeting cardiovascular disease showed a reduction in risk factors (Farquhar, Fortman, and Flora, et al, 1990; Shea and Basch,

1990; Shea, 1992) and evaluation of worksite health promotion programs showed their effect on program goals (Sciacca, et al, 1990; Weisbrod, et al, 1991). Evaluation studies of many types of community health interventions exist in the literature and provide insights and direction for further community health planning.

A comprehensive discussion of evaluation is provided in Chapter 11, Using The Nursing Process to Promote the Health of Communities.

RESEARCH

Research, the sixth component of community health practice, is the systematic investigation which helps discover facts affecting community health and community health practice, solve problems, and explore improved methods of health service. Community health practitioners conduct and utilize scientific investigations at all levels from federal agencies such as the U.S. Public Health Service to state and local groups conducting research. Epidemiology (the study of health and disease determinants and distribution in populations) and biostatistics (the science of statistically measuring population health conditions) are the primary public health measurement and analytic sciences underlying community health practice. Chapter 12, Epidemiological Assessment of Community Health Status, addresses these sciences more extensively.

Researchers in community health investigate the characteristics and patterns of illness and health. Conditions such as food poisoning, trauma, alcoholism, lung cancer, child abuse, drug dependency, and suicide are studied for possible causes and means of prevention. Health and healthful behavior are analyzed, for example, in nutrition projects and studies of normal human growth and behavior, for better understanding of ways to promote healthful living.

Community health researchers explore ways to improve health care. For example, an experimental program of foster home care for the frail elderly proved to be more beneficial and less costly than nursing home care (Oktay and Volland, 1987). A study of school children in Berkeley, California, demonstrated that after screening, public health nursing follow-up increased dental care utilization (Oda, Fine, and Heilbron, 1986). Other research projects might focus on the effectiveness of drug treatment programs, long-term stroke rehabilitation, or improved treatment approaches to obesity.

Community health researchers also examine the impact of social and environmental factors on health and health services provision. For example, one study of work schedules revealed that people working variable shifts are at much greater risk for health problems (Gordon et al., 1986), while another identified social and psychological as well as environmental factors contributing to the poor health of homeless families (Bassuk, Rubin, and Lauriat, 1986; Francis, 1991). A growing number of studies center around needs and care of the elderly and other age-specific groups. Others investigate ways to improve health services planning and policy development through such efforts as studies of community needs and program utilization.

Characteristics of Community Health Practice

Several characteristics of community health practice deserve special emphasis. First, community health practice, unlike the individualized focus of acute health care, is *population-focused*. It is concerned with the health status of people in the aggregate, people who, as a group, form a distinct population. These groups and communities, in turn, are multiple and overlapping. Thus, community health must deal with a complex set of interacting physical, psychological, socioeconomic, cultural, and biological variables that influence human behavior and affect aggregate health (Williams, 1977). Community health as a part of public health is fundamentally concerned with the collective good; it focuses on community and on the values of life, health, and security shared by the community (Forster, 1982; Shea, 1992).

Second, in community health practice the *promotion of health and prevention of illness* are of first-order priority. There is less emphasis on curative care. Some corrective actions are always needed, such as cleanup of a toxic waste dump site, stricter enforcement of day care standards, or home care of the disabled; however, community health best serves its constituents through preventive and health-promoting actions (Beauchamp, 1984; *U.S. Department of Health and Human Services* 1991). These include services to mothers and infants, prevention of environmental pollution, school health programs, senior citizens' fitness classes, "workers-right-to-know" legislation that warns against hazards in the workplace, and numerous other activities (see World Watch display).

World Watch
DEMOCRATIZING HEALTH WORLDWIDE

Inequalities in health and health care between various nations has been a continuing problem for many decades. Developing countries bear the brunt of this inequality with fewer resources to address the problems. To promote health worldwide is one of society's greatest challenges. For some years the World Health Organization (WHO) has responded to this challenge with a goal of health for all by the year 2000. Part of WHO's plan of action has been broadening concepts of health, refocusing on health, renewing resources for health, and democratizing health and health services (Hudson-Rodd, 1994).

The emphasis on democratizing health has become crucial to the success of equality in health at a global level. Involving the active participation of citizens along with professionals is key to understanding health, indigenous health needs, developing common health goals, and creating and sustaining healthier communities world wide (WHO, 1991).

Third, community health practice uses *aggregate measurement and analysis*. The need to collect and examine data on the entire population under study before making intervention decisions is fundamental to community health practice. Analysis of health states, environmental factors, health-related services, economic patterns, and social policy are among the many foci of community health evaluation and research, described further in Chapters 11 and 26, Using the Nursing Process, and Research in Community Health Nursing, respectively.

Finally, community health practice uses principles from *management and organization theory* to provide effective administration of health care services. Public health has long been defined as the protection and improvement of community health "through organized community efforts" (Pickett and Hanlon, 1990, p.5). It is the organization and administration of such services that enables practitioners to ultimately address community needs. Chapter 2, Structure and Function of Community Health Services, elaborates on this subject.

Summary

Community health is much more than environmental programs and large-scale efforts to control communicable disease. To comprehend the nature and significance of community health and to clarify its meaning for the specialty practice of community health nursing, one must understand the concepts of community and of health.

A community, broadly defined, is a collection of people who share some common interest or goal. There are three types of communities: geographic, common-interest, and health-problem-solving. Sometimes a community, such as a city, county, or neighborhood, is formed by geographic boundaries. At other times a community may be identified by its common interest; examples are a religious community, a group of migrant workers, or citizens concerned about air pollution. A community may also be defined by a pooling of efforts by people and agencies toward solving some health-related problem.

Health is an abstract concept that can be understood more clearly by examining its distinguishing features. First, health is a relative, not an absolute, concept. People are not either sick or well in an absolute sense but have levels of illness or wellness. These levels may be plotted along a continuum ranging from optimal health to total disability or death. This is known as the wellness-illness continuum. Thus, a person's state of health is dynamic, varying from day to day and even hour to hour.

Second, health is a state of being that includes all the many characteristics of a person, family, or community, not just physical status. These characteristics often indiciate how well or ill an individual or community is and suggest the presence or absence of vitality and well-being. Health also involves the total person including all the dimensions of life—physical, psychological, social, and spiritual.

Third, health has both subjective and objective dimensions. The subjective involves how well people feel; the objective refers to how well they are able to function. Both are indications of the people's wellness and may be plotted along the wellness-illness continuum. The ability to function, which is observable and often used to measure health status, may also occur anywhere along the continuum. Most often, functional performance diminishes dramatically toward the illness end.

Community health practice, a part of the larger public health effort, is concerned with preserving and promoting the health of specific populations and communities. It incorporates six basic elements: (1) promotion of healthful living, (2) prevention of health problems, (3) treatment of disorders, (4) rehabilitation, (5) evaluation, and (6) research.

Important characteristics of community health practice include its emphasis on populations, promotion of health and prevention of illness, use of measurement and analysis of aggregates, and effective management and organization of health services.

Activities to Promote Critical Thinking

1. Identify a community of people about whom you have some knowledge. What makes it a community? What characteristics does this group of people share?

2. Select a population for whom you have some concern and place that group on the wellness-illness continuum. What factors influenced your decision?

3. Describe three preventive actions (one primary, one secondary, and one tertiary) that might be taken to move the population you selected closer to optimal wellness.

4. Discuss how you might implement one health promotion effort with the population you selected.

5. Place yourself on the wellness-illness continuum. What factors influenced your decision?

REFERENCES

Bassuk, E.L., Rubin, L., & Lauriat, A.S. (1986). Characteristics of sheltered homeless families. *American Journal of Public Health, 76*(9), 1097–1101.

Beauchamp, D. (1984). What is public about public health? *Health Affairs, 2*(4), 76–87.

Blackburn, H. (1987). Research and demonstration projects in community cardiovascular disease prevention. *Journal of Public Health Policy, 4*, 398–421.

Brownson, R., Alvanja, M., Hock, E., & Loy, T. (1992). Passive smoking and lung cancer in nonsmoking women. *American Journal of Public Health, 82*(11), 1525–1530.

Centers for Disease Control. (1989). *Reducing the Health Consequences of Smoking: 25 Years of Progress.* A report of the Surgeon General. Washington, DC: U.S.Department of Health and Human Services, Public Health Service, Centers for Disease Control, Center for Chronic Disease and Health Promotion. Office on Smoking and Health, 259–378. DHHS publication CDC 89-8411.

Choi, T., Josten, L.V. & Christensen, M. (1983). Health-specific family coping index for non-institutional care. *American Journal of Public Health, 73*(11), 1275–77.

Cottrell, L.S., Jr. (1976). The competent community. In B. H. Kaplan, R. N. Wilson, & A. H. Leighton (Eds.). *Further Explorations in Social Psychiatry.* New York: Basic Books.

Ehrhardt, A. (1992). Trends in sexual behavior and the HIV pandemic. *American Journal of Public Health, 82*(11), 1459–61.

Farquhar, J., Fortman, S., Flora, J., et al. (1990). Effects of community-wide education on cardiovascular disease risk factors—The Stanford 5-city Project. *Journal of the American Medical Association, 264*, 359–65.

Flynn, B., Rider, M., & Bailey, W. (1992). Developing community leadership in healthy cities: The Indiana model. *Nursing Outlook, 40*(3), 121–126.

Folden, S.L. (1993). Definitions of health and health goals of participants in a community-based pulmonary rehabilitation program. *Public Health Nursing, 10*(1), 31–35.

Forster, J. (1982). A communitarian ethical model for public health interventions: An alternative to individual behavior change strategies. *Journal of Public Health Policy, 3*, 150–63.

Francis, M.B. (1991). Homeless families: Rebuilding connections. *Public Health Nursing, 8*(2), 90–96.

Freudenberg, N. (1987). Reassessing communities. *Health/PAC Bulletin, 17*(5), 30.

Gordon, N. P., Clearly, P.D., Parker, C.E., & Czeisler, C.A. (1986). The prevalence and health impact of shiftwork. *American Journal of Public Health, 76*(10), 1225–28.

Green, L.W. & Anderson, C.L. (1986). *Community Health.* St. Louis: Times Mirror/Mosby.

Green, L.W. & Kreuter, M. (1991). *Health Promotion Planning: An Educational and Environmental Approach* (2nd ed.). Mt. View, CA: Mayfield Publishing Company.

Hegyvary, S.T. (1990). Redefining community as the center of our health care model. *Journal of Professional Nursing, 6*(1), 7.

Henkel, B. (1970). *Community Health* (2nd ed.). Boston: Allyn and Bacon.

Hudson-Rodd, N. (1994). Public Health: People participating in the creating of healthy places. *Public Health Nursing, 11*(2), 119–126.

Knobel, R.J. (1983). Health promotion and disease prevention: Improving health while conserving resources. *Family and Community Health, 5*(4), 16–27.

Last, J.M. (1987). *Public Health and Human Ecology.* East Norwalk, CT: Appleton and Lange.

Martin, K. & Scheet, N. (1992). *The Omaha System: Applications for Community Health Nursing.* Philadelphia: W.B. Saunders.

Moore, P. V., & Williamson, G.C. (1984). Health promotion: Evolution of a concept. *Nursing Clinics of North America, 19*(2), 195–206.

National Commission on Community Health Services. (1967). *Health Is a Community Affair.* Cambridge: Harvard University Press.

Novak, J.C. (1988). The social mandate and historical basis for nursing's role in health promotion. *Journal of Professional Nursing, 4*(2), 80–87.

Oda, D.S., Fine, J.I., & Heilbron, D.C. (1986). Impact and cost of public health nurse telephone follow-up of school dental referrals. *American Journal of Public Health, 76*(11), 1348–49.

Oktay, J.S., & Volland, P.J. (1987). Foster home care for the frail elderly as an alternative to nursing home care: An experimental evaluation. *American Journal of Public Health, 77*(12), 1505–10.

Pencak, M. (1991). Workplace health promotion programs: an overview. *Nursing Clinics of North America, 26*(1), 233–40.

Pender, N., Barkauskas, V., Hayman, L., Rice, V., & Anderson, E. (1992). Health promotion and disease prevention: Toward excellence in nursing practice and education. *Nursing Outlook, 40*(3), 106–112.

Pickett, G. E. & Hanlon, J.J. (1990). *Public Health Administration and Practice.* (9th ed.). St. Louis: Times Mirror/Mosby.

Sciacca, J., et al. (1990). Evaluating worksite health promotion programs. *Health Education, 21*(3), 17–22.

Shamansky, S., & Clausen, C. (1980). Levels of prevention: Examination of the concept. *Nursing Outlook, 28*, 104–8.

Shamansky, S., & Pesznecker, B. (1981). A community is . . . *Nursing Outlook, 29*(3), 182-85.

Shea, S. (1992). Community health, community risks, community action. *American Journal of Public Health, 82*(6), 785–7.

Shea, S. & Basch, C. (1990). A review of five major community-based cardiovascular disease prevention programs. Part I: Rationale, design, and theoretical framework. *American Journal of Health Promotion, 4*, 203–213.

Smith, J. A. (1983). *The Idea of Health: Implications for the Nursing Professional.* New York: Teachers College Press, Columbia University.

Stokes, J., III, Noren, J.J., & Shindell, S. (1982). Definition of terms and concepts applicable to clinical preventive medicine. *Journal of Community Health, 8*, 33–41.

U.S. Department of Health and Human Services. (1991). *Healthy People 2000: National Health Promotion and Disease Prevention Objectives.* DHHS publication, PHS 91-50213. Washington, DC: U.S. Government Printing Office.

Veney, J.E. & Kaluzny, A.D. (1984). *Evaluation and Decision Making for Health Services Programs.* Englewood Cliffs, NJ: Prentice-Hall.

Weisbrod, R.R., et al. (1991). Current status of health promotion activities in four Midwest cities. *Public Health Reports, 106*(3), 310–317.

Williams, C. A. (1977). Community health nursing—What is it? *Nursing Outlook, 25*, 250–54.

Williams, C. A. (1992). Community-based population-focused practice: The foundation of specialization in public health nursing. In M. Stanhope & J. Lancaster (Eds.). *Community Health Nursing: Process and Practice for Promoting Health.* (3rd ed.). St. Louis: Mosby Year Book.

World Health Organization Study Group. (1991). Community involvement in health development: Challenging health services. WHO Technical Report no. 809. Geneva: Author.

SELECTED READINGS

Anderson, J. & Yuhos, R. (1993). Health promotion in rural settings. A nursing challenge. *Nursing Clinics of North America, 28*(1), 145–155, 157.

Barsky, A.J. (1988). The paradox of health. *The New England Journal of Medicine, 318*(7), 414–18.

Birmingham, J.J. (1987). The wellness frontier: The community. *Nursing Administration Quarterly, 11*(3), 14–18.

Clark, J.M., et al. (1990). Helping people to stop smoking: a study of the nurse's role. *Journal of Advanced Nursing, 15*(3), 357–63.

Collado, C.B. (1992). Primary health care: A continuing challenge. *Nursing and Health Care, 13*(8), 408–413.

Dever, G.E.A. (1991). *Community Health Analysis: Global Awareness at the Local Level* (2nd ed.). Gaithersburg, MD: Aspen.

Erben, R. (1991). Health challenges for the year 2000: health promotion and AIDS. *Health Education Quarterly, 18*(1), 29–37.

Evans, R.G., Barer, M.L., & Marmor, T.R. (Eds.). (1994). Why are some people healthy and others not? The determinants of health of populations. Hawthorne, NY: Aldine de Gruyter.

Hall, B. & Allan, J. (1986). Sharpening nursing's focus by focusing on health. *Nursing and Health Care, 7*, 314–321.

Harper, A.C. & Lambert, L. (1993). *The Health of Populations* (2nd ed.). New York: Springer.

Higginbotham, J.C. (1992). Necessities for evaluating behavior change in health promotion/disease prevention programs: knowledge, skill, and attitude. *Family and Community Health, 15*(1), 41–56.

Houk, V.N., et al. (1989). The Centers for Disease Control program to prevent primary and secondary disabilities in the U.S. *Public Health Reports, 104*(3), 226–31.

Hudson-Rodd, N. (1994). Public health: People participating in the creation of healthy places. *Public Health Nursing, 11*(2), 119–126.

Institute of Medicine Committee for the Study of the Future of Public Health. (1988). *The Future of Public Health.* Washington, DC: National Academy Press.

Lauzon, R. (1977). An epidemiological approach to health promotion. *Canadian Journal of Public Health, 68,* 311–17.

Light, L., et al. (1989). Eat for health: A nutrition and cancer control supermarket intervention. *Public Health Reports, 104*(5), 443–50.

Milio, N. (1976). A framework for prevention: Changing health-damaging to health-generating life patterns. *American Journal of Public Health, 66,* 435–39.

Norman, S.A., et al. (1990). A process evaluation of a two-year community cardiovascular risk reduction program: What was done and who knew about it? *Health Education Research, 5*(1), 87–97.

Parcel, G.S., et al. (1989). Translating theory into practice: Intervention strategies for the diffusion of a health promotion innovation. Minnesota Smoking Prevention Program. *Family and Community Health, 12*(3), 1–13.

Roberts, M. (1990). Little towns that could: Making health a community concern produces dramatic payoffs. *U.S.News and World Report, 108*(24), 74–5.

Rose-Colley, M., et al. (1989). Relapse prevention: implications for health promotion professionals. *Health Values, 13*(5), 8–13.

Swinford, P. & Webster, J. (1989). *Promoting Wellness: A Nurse's Handbook.* Rockville, MD: Aspen.

Travis, J.W. (1990). *Wellness For Helping Professionals.* Sebastopol, CA: Wellness Associates.

Tripp, S. & Stachowiak, B. (1992). Health maintenance, health promotion: Is there a difference? *Public Health Nursing, 9*(3), 155–61.

CHAPTER

2

Structure and Function of Community Health Services

LEARNING OBJECTIVES

Upon completion of this chapter, readers should be able to:

- Trace historic events and philosophy leading to today's health services delivery.
- Outline the current organizational structure of the public health care system.
- Describe the three core functions of public health.
- Differentiate between the functions of public versus private sector health care agencies.
- Explain the influence of selected legislative acts in the United States on shaping current health services policy and practice.

KEY TERMS

- Assessment
- Assurance
- Core public health functions
- Department of Health and Human Services
- Edwin Chadwick
- Hebrew hygienic code
- Medically indigent
- Official health agencies
- Pan American Health Organization
- Policy development
- Proprietary health services
- Public Health Service
- Quarantine
- Sanitation
- Shattuck Report
- Voluntary health agencies
- World Health Organization

Barbara Walton Spradley and Judith Ann Allender
COMMUNITY HEALTH NURSING: CONCEPTS AND PRACTICE, 4th ed.
© 1996 Barbara Walton Spradley and Judith Ann Allender

Nurses preparing for population-based practice need to be familiar with how the health care system is organized and operates because it is through this system that community health services are delivered. This system forms an organizing framework for the design and implementation of programs aimed at improving the health of communities and vulnerable groups. It is within this system or framework that community health nurses work. Furthermore, through the vehicle of this system, community health nurses have the opportunity to shape the future of health services and develop innovative and more effective means of improving community health.

Service delivery systems directed at restoring or promoting the public's health have evolved over centuries. The structure, function, and financing of health care systems has changed dramatically during that time. These changes have come about in response to evolving societal needs and demands, scientific advancements, the development of more effective methods of service delivery, new technology, and varying approaches to resource acquisition and allocation (Pickett and Hanlon, 1990). Considerable progress has been made toward a healthier global society. At the same time many problems remain, particularly those of escalating health care costs, equitable distribution and effectiveness of health services, and assuring the quality of and access to those services (*U.S. Department of Health and Human Services*, 1991; WHO, 1991).

This chapter examines the current structure and functions of community health services in the United States and reviews historical and legislative events that have influenced the planning for and the delivery of those services.

Historical Influences on Health Care

Health care as it is known today has changed dramatically from previous centuries. Yet there is reason to believe that personal and community hygiene and health care were practiced from the beginning of time. Many primitive tribes engaged in sanitary practices, such as burial of excreta, removal of the dead, and isolation of members with certain illnesses. In addition, treatment of the sick included use of a variety of therapeutic agents administered by a "healer." Whether these activities were purely superstitious, derived from sur-

vival needs, or primarily tied to religious beliefs is unknown. Nonetheless, records show that in Egypt and the Middle East, as early as 3000 B.C., people were building drainage systems, using toilets and water flushing systems, and practicing personal cleanliness (Pickett and Hanlon, 1990). The **Hebrew hygienic code**, described in the *Bible* in Leviticus circa 1500 B.C., was probably the first written code in the world and served as a prototype for personal and community sanitation. It emphasized "cleanliness of the body, protection against the spread of contagious diseases, isolation of lepers, disinfection of dwellings after illness, sanitation of campsites, disposal of excreta and refuse, protection of water and food supplies, and the hygiene of maternity" (Pickett & Hanlon, 1990, p.21). Even more advanced were the Athenians, circa 1000–400 B.C., who emphasized personal hygiene, diet, and exercise in addition to a sanitary environment, albeit for the benefit of the wealthy. Their successors, the Romans, added many more community health measures such as laws regulating environmental sanitation and nuisances, and construction of paved streets, aqueducts, and a subsurface drainage system.

The Middle Ages (from about A.D. 500 to 1500) marked a distinct change in health beliefs and practices based on the philosophy that to pamper the body was evil. Neglected personal hygiene, improper diets, and accumulation of refuse and body wastes soon led to widespread epidemics and pandemics of disease including cholera, plague and leprosy (Hecker, 1839). Increased trade between Europe and Asia, military conquests, and Christian crusades to the Middle East only furthered the spread of disease. Bubonic plague, known as the Black Death, in the mid-1300s was the most devastating of pandemics, reportedly killing over 60 million people, half the population of the known world (Hecker, 1839). In response to this, in 1348 Venice banned entry of infected ships and travelers—a form of quarantine. **Quarantine** is a period of enforced isolation of persons exposed to a communicable disease during the incubation period to prevent spread of the disease should infection occur. The first known official quarantine measure was instituted in 1377 at the port of Ragusa (now Dubrovnik in Croatia, formerly, Yugoslavia) where travelers from plague areas were required to wait two months and be free of disease before entry was allowed. Marseilles, in 1383, passed the first quarantine law (Pickett and Hanlon, 1990). During this regressed period in history, health care was scarce, private, and reserved for the wealthy few, while public health problems were rampant but only minimally and ineffectively addressed.

By the end of the Middle Ages, more enlightened European thinkers began to challenge the prevailing beliefs and conditions. They no longer believed that disease was a punishment for sin. However, traces of stigma regarding such conditions as leprosy and tuberculosis can be found yet today, and sexually transmitted diseases, as well as AIDS, are still regarded by some as punishment for immoral conduct. During the late eighteenth century new efforts at reform were influenced by a growing emphasis on human dignity, human rights, and on the search for scientific truth. These efforts continued through the nineteenth and twentieth centuries.

Despite such signs of improvement, during the seventeenth and eighteenth centuries many serious problems persisted and new ones developed. Industrialization, masses of people moving to cities, and low regard for human life all contributed to deplorable living and working conditions. Hundreds of pauper children died in England's abusive but socially approved workhouses and apprentice slavery system. Most of Europe continued in unspeakable misery and filth. Many householders dumped their refuse out windows or doors into the streets. Stinking rivers and water supplies were seriously contaminated. Numerous diseases, including cholera, typhus, typhoid, smallpox, and tuberculosis, took a tremendous toll on human life.

Around the turn of the nineteenth century, England's leaders became increasingly concerned about social and sanitary reform. **Sanitation** referred to the promotion of hygiene and prevention of disease by maintaining health enhancing (sanitary) conditions. The first sanitary legislation, passed in 1837, established vaccination stations in London. One of the most notable reformers, **Edwin Chadwick**, published his *"Report on an Inquiry into the Sanitary Conditions of the Laboring Population of Great Britain"* in 1842 (Richardson, 1887). Chadwick, the father of modern public health, believed that disease and poverty were related and could be changed. His efforts resulted in passage of the English Public Health Act and establishment of a General Board of Health for England in 1848 (Lewis, 1952). Conditions improved and scientific study advanced in England and concurrently in France, Germany, Scandinavia, and other European countries. England, however, set the pace for application of research, particularly with reference to public health measures, through steadily improved legislation. British laws subsequently became the pattern for American sanitary ordinances.

Health Care System Development in the United States

A relatively organized health care system as we know it today was long in developing. Most health-related services were initially reactive, responding to pressure of immediate needs, and uncoordinated from one locality to another. Over time, events and insights contributed to a gradually improving system of programs and services along with recognition that the health of individuals was affected by the health of the wider community.

PRECURSORS TO A HEALTH CARE SYSTEM

Early health care in the American colonies consisted of private practice with occasional (but infrequent) governmental action for the public good. Action was usually in the form of isolated local responses to specific dangers or nuisances such as the 1647 regulation to prevent pollution of Boston Harbor or the 1701 Massachusetts law requiring ship quarantine and isolation of smallpox patients. New York City in the late 1700s formed a public health committee to monitor, among other public concerns, water quality, sewer construction, marsh drainage, and burial of the dead.

The U.S. Constitution, adopted in 1789, made no direct reference to public health, nor was the federal government active in health matters. It was the responsibility of each sovereign state to manage its own health affairs. The first federal intervention for health problems was the Marine Hospital Service Act of 1798. It subsidized medical and hospital care for disabled seamen. During the early years a scourge of epidemics, especially yellow fever, smallpox, cholera, typhoid, and typhus, caused many deaths throughout the colonies. These "foreign" diseases were said to have decimated the early Native American population (Woodward, 1932). Slave trade further threatened the lives of colonists by introducing diseases such as yaws, yellow fever, and malaria (Marr, 1982). Quarantine efforts under local control proved ineffective. Congress, in 1873, finally instituted the national port quarantine system, which was regulated and enforced by the Marine Hospital Service. Epidemics were quickly brought under control, causing society to recognize the benefits of uniform central government policy. Improvements in public health and sanitation generally throughout the states, however, were held back by delayed progress in coping with other competing needs such as police and fire protection.

THE SHATTUCK REPORT

The **Shattuck Report**, a landmark document, made a tremendous impact on sanitary progress. Lemuel Shattuck, a layman and legislator, chaired a legislative committee that studied health and sanitary problems in the commonwealth of Massachusetts. In 1850, he produced the "Report of the Sanitary Commission of Massachusetts" (Shattuck, et al, 1850). It described public health concepts and methods upon which much of today's public health practice is based. Among his many recommendations, Shattuck advocated the establishment of state and local boards of health, environmental sanitation, collection, use of vital statistics, systematic study of diseases, control of food and drugs, urban planning, establishment of nurses' training schools (there were none before this time), and preventive medicine. Unfortunately, it was almost 25 years before the recommendations were appreciated and truly implemented. A similar report by John C. Griscom conducted about the same time concluded that illness, premature death, and poverty were directly related. He also recommended sanitary reform (Figure 2.1).

OFFICIAL HEALTH AGENCIES

The beginnings of an organized health care system in the United States came in the form of **official health agencies**, later called public health agencies. These were publicly funded and operated by state or local government with a goal of providing population-based health services. Development occurred initially at the local level. Many cities established local boards of health in the late 1700s and early to mid-1800s. Among the earliest were Baltimore, Maryland (1798), Charleston, South Carolina (1815), and Philadelphia (1818). As their efforts expanded from handling public "nuisances" to dealing with epidemics and complex public health problems, local health boards recognized that employment of full-time staff was needed and thus health departments were formed. The first full-time county health departments were established in 1911 in North Carolina and Washington states. Massachusetts formed the nation's first state board of health in 1869 and a few years later the first state department of health. At the national level, the Marine Hospital Service, now broadened in function, became the Public Health and Marine Hospital Service in 1902. Congress gave it a more clearly defined organizational structure and specific functions for its director, the surgeon general. In 1912 it was renamed the United States Public Health Service (USPHS).

Rapidly expanding through the years of World War I and the Great Depression, the Public Health Service

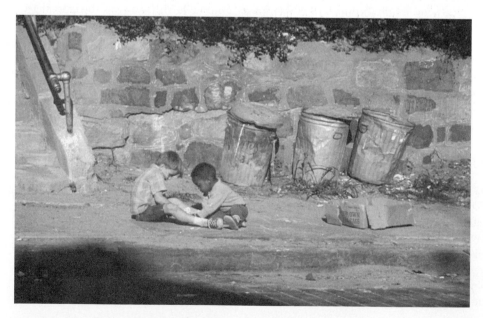

FIGURE 2.1. Poverty and environmental conditions have a direct influence on people's health.

strengthened its research activity based in the National Institutes of Health (NIH, founded in 1912), added demonstration projects, and initiated greater cooperation with the states. Responding to increasingly complex needs, the NIH added such programs significant to public health as the Children's Bureau (1912), the National Leprosarium at Carville, Louisiana (1917), examination of arriving aliens (1917), the Division of Venereal Diseases (1918), the Food and Drug Administration (1927), and the Narcotics Division (1929), which later became the Division of Mental Hygiene. Title VI of the 1935 Social Security Act promoted stronger federal support of state and local public health services including health manpower training.

As the number of health, welfare, and educational services proliferated, the need for consolidation prompted the creation of the Federal Security Agency in 1939. In 1953 it was enlarged and renamed the Department of Health, Education and Welfare (DHEW), established under President Eisenhower. In 1979, Education was made a separate cabinet-level department, and the DHEW was renamed the Department of Health and Human Services (DHHS). Other significant events included the establishment, during World War II, of the Communicable Disease Center in Atlanta, currently the National Centers for Disease Control and Prevention, and the development, after World War II, of the National Office of Vital Statistics, now called the National Center for Health Statistics.

VOLUNTARY HEALTH AGENCIES

The private sector actually responded first to America's health problems and to this day continues to complement and supplement the government's role in provision of health services. By the late 1800s **voluntary health agencies** (later called private agencies) began to emerge. They were privately funded and operated to address specific health needs. The first of these was the Anti-Tuberculosis Society of Philadelphia formed in 1892 to educate the public and the government about tuberculosis, then causing 10 percent of all deaths. Other agencies followed. The National Society to Prevent Blindness was formed in 1908, the Mental Health Association in 1909, the American Cancer Society in 1913, and several others, including the National Easter Seal Society for Crippled Children and Adults and the Planned Parenthood Federation of America in 1921. Also in the late 1800s, organized charities such as the Red Cross, previously denounced for promoting de-

pendent poverty, began to be recognized for their contributions to health and welfare. Philanthropy, too, became respected with the establishment of the Rockefeller Foundation (1913) followed by the Carnegie-Mellon, Kellogg, Robert Wood Johnston, and other foundations.

HEALTH-RELATED PROFESSIONAL ASSOCIATIONS

Many health-related professional associations over the years have influenced the quality and type of community health services delivery. Among these, the National Organization for Public Health Nursing (NOPHN), from 1912 to 1952, significantly influenced early preparation for and quality of public health nursing services (Fitzpatrick, 1975). The American Public Health Association, founded in 1872, to this day maintains a prominent role in the dissemination of public health information, influence on health policy, and advocacy for the nation's health. Other nursing and community health organizations that have promoted quality efforts in community health include the Association of State and Territorial Directors of Nursing (ASTDN), the Association of State and Territorial Health Officers (ASTHO), The National League for Nursing (NLN), the American Nurses Association (ANA), and the Association for Community Health Nursing Educators (ACHNE).

Health Organizations in the United States

The historical record demonstrates that for many centuries people attempted to address community health needs. Responsibility for these shifted between private groups and governing institutions. Each arm, public and private, offered a unique perspective, different skills, and different resources. Lack of coordination between them, however, and no method for comprehensive planning and delivery of health services left huge gaps in some areas, duplication in others. It has only been within the past century that the two arms have gradually begun to work together to create a loosely structured "system" of health care. Pickett and Hanlon speak of "the growing interdependence of the public and private sectors" (1990, p.185). How does that system work today? What are its strengths and weaknesses? To answer these questions, one must first examine its structure. Why look at structure? Because it becomes the operational base for assessment, diagnosis, planning, implementation, and evaluation of services, and because it provides a framework for intersystem and intrasystem communication and coordination.

Health services occur at four levels: local, state, national, and international. Like ever-widening concentric circles, these levels encompass broader and broader populations. The organization of health services at each level can be classified under one of two types, public or private.

PUBLIC SECTOR HEALTH SERVICES

Government health agencies, the tax-supported arm of the public health effort, perform a vital function in community health practice. They are the official public health agencies whose areas of jurisdiction and types of service are dictated by law. They coordinate and administer activities that often can be carried out only by group or community-wide action: for example, proper sewage disposal, the provision of sanitary water systems, or regulation of toxic wastes. Many community health activities require an authoritative legal backing to ensure enforcement (another useful function of public health agencies) of control in such areas as environmental pollution, highway safety practices, and proper food handling. Official or public health agencies provide important record-keeping services including the collection of and monitoring of vital statistics. They also conduct research, provide consultation, and sometimes financially support other community health efforts.

Core Public Health Functions

Public health services encompass a wide variety of activities but all can be grouped under one of three core public health functions. They are assessment, policy development, and assurance (Institute of Medicine, 1988; National Association of County Health Officials, 1993).

Assessment refers to measuring and monitoring the health status and needs of a designated community or population. As a core function it is a continuous process of collecting data and disseminating information about health, diseases, injuries, air and water quality, food safety, other health-related conditions, and available re-

sources. "The assessment function identifies trends in morbidity, mortality and causative factors; available health resources and their application; unmet needs; and community perceptions about health issues" (Plumb, 1994, p.14).

Policy development is the formation of a guide for action that determines present and future decisions affecting the public's health. As a core public health function, good public policy development builds on data from the assessment function and incorporates community values and citizen input. It provides leadership and administration for the development of sound health policy and planning.

Assurance is the process of translating established policies into services. This function ensures that population-based services are provided, whether by public health agencies or private sources. It also monitors the quality of and access to those services. The specific functions under assurance are listed in Table 2.1.

The roles of public health agencies vary by level, each level carrying out the core functions in different ways to form a partnership in protecting the public's health (Pickett and Hanlon, 1990). International health agencies focus on issues of global concern, setting policy, developing standards, and monitoring health conditions and programs. At the national level, government health agencies engage in similar functions aimed at regional or nationwide concerns. The federal level provides funds, such as through the Medicaid program, and develops policy, for instance air pollution policy, but depends on the states to implement them. Agencies at the federal level also develop facilities and programs for special groups, such as Native Americans, migrant workers, inmates of federal prisons, and military personnel and veterans, whose health care is not the direct responsibility of any one state or locality. State government health agencies function fairly autonomously while working within federal guidelines. They assess, develop, and monitor statewide health needs and services. At the local level, one may find a city government health agency, a county agency, or a combination of both to assess, plan for, and serve the health needs of that locality.

Unlike private organizations that tend to have a specific focus, government health agencies exist to accomplish a broad goal of protecting and promoting the health of the total population under their jurisdiction. Such a task requires a wide range of services and the combined talents of many types of professional disciplines. Among them are nurses, physicians, health

TABLE 2.1. *Core Public Health Functions*

Core Public Health Functions: Population-Wide Services	
Assessment	Health status monitoring and disease surveillance
Policy development	Leadership, policy, planning, and administration
Assurance	Investigation and control of diseases and injuries
	Protection of environment, workplaces, housing, food, and water
	Laboratory services to support disease control and environmental protection
	Health education and information
	Community mobilization for health-related issues
	Targeted outreach and linkage to personal services
	Health services quality assurance and accountability
	Training and education of public health professionals

Core Public Health Functions: Personal Services
Home visits for people at risk
Primary care for unserved and underserved people
Treatment services for targeted conditions—e.g., AIDS, alcohol and other drug abuse, mental illness
Clinical preventive services—e.g., immunization, STDs, family planning, WIC
Payments for personal services delivered by others

Source: The Core Functions Project, 1993.

educators, sanitarians, epidemiologists, statisticians, engineers, administrators, accountants, computer programmers, planners, sociologists, nutritionists, laboratory technicians, chemists, physicists, veterinarians, dentists, demographers, and even meteorologists. Furthermore, public health agencies must function not only on an interdisciplinary basis but on an interorganizational one as well. Other government services, education for example, can meet their goals fairly autonomously. Public health, on the other hand, "cannot accomplish its most important objectives without the cooperation of other agencies and organizations, both public and private" (Pickett and Hanlon, 1990, p.123). A case in point is the many organizations working together with public health to cope with the AIDS epidemic, including educational institutions, welfare agencies, mental health programs, home care services, Medicaid, and a variety of private groups.

Thus many different government agencies contribute to the health of a community. Most obvious are the local and state health departments, that provide a variety of direct and indirect health services, including community health nursing. Other tax-supported agencies that sponsor health care or health-related services include welfare departments, departments of public

works, public schools and hospitals, police departments, county agricultural services, and local housing authorities.

Local Public Health Agencies

At the grass-roots level, government health agencies vary considerably in structure and function from one locality to the next. This is due in part to variations in local needs and size of the community. For example, a rural community served by a county or state health department may have widely differing needs and services than a densely populated urban community. Differing health care standards and regulations as well as the type and stipulations of funding sources also contribute to variations in the structure and function of health agencies. Nonetheless, each local governmental health agency shares some commonly held responsibilities, functions, and structural features.

The primary responsibilities of the local health department are (1) to assess its population's health status and needs, (2) to determine how well those needs are being met, and (3) to take action toward satisfying unmet needs (Pickett and Hanlon, 1990). More specifically, local government health agencies should fulfill the core functions as follows (Institute of Medicine, 1988; National Association of County Health Officials, 1993):

■ Assess and monitor local health needs and the resources for addressing them.
■ Develop policy and provide leadership in advocating equitable distribution of resources and services, both public and private.
■ Assure availability, accessibility, and quality of health services for all members of the community.
■ Keep the community informed on how to access public health services.

The local health agency is a critical level of health services' provision because of its closeness to the ultimate recipients—health care consumers.

The structure of the local health department varies in complexity with the setting. Rural and small urban agencies need only a simple organization while large metropolitan agencies require more complex organizational structures to support the greater diversity and quantity of work. A local board of health generally holds the legal responsibility for the health of its citizens. Health board members may be appointed by the mayor if the board of health serves a city or by a board of supervisors if the board of health serves a county or they may be publicly elected. In turn, the board of health appoints a health officer, usually a physician with public health training, who employs the remaining staff of the health department, including public health nurses, environmental health workers, health educators, and office personnel. Others, like nutritionists, statisticians, epidemiologists, social workers, physical therapists, veterinarians, or public health dentists, may be added as needs and resources dictate.

Revenue to support local health department expenditures comes from a variety of sources. State and county general appropriations make up the largest share of the local health department's budget with additional funds provided through special levies and programs such as school health, Headstart, air pollution, toxic substance control, primary care, immunizations, fees, and private foundation grants. Federal funds provide another source of revenue targeted at specific efforts like AIDS research and services, family planning, child health, environmental protection, hypertension and nutrition programs. Fees and reimbursements and additional miscellaneous sources, such as state lab revenues and food supply supplements, make up the remaining portion of the budget. Figure 2.2 depicts the organization of one local health department serving a population of approximately 300,000.

State Public Health Agencies

State-level government health agencies, too, vary in structure and carrying out the core functions. Each state, as a sovereign government, establishes its own state health department that, in turn, determines its goals, actions, and administrative structure. The state health department is responsible for providing leadership in and monitoring of comprehensive public health needs and services in the state. It establishes statewide health policy standards, assists local communities, allocates funds, promotes state-level health planning, conducts and evaluates state-level health programs, promotes cooperation with voluntary (private) health agencies, and collaborates with the federal government for health planning and policy development (Pickett and Hanlon, 1990). Of the various levels of government health agencies, the states have recently played the most pivotal role in health policy formation (Institute of Medicine, 1988).

State health department functions can be listed generally to include (Pickett and Hanlon, 1990):

1. Statewide health planning
2. Intergovernmental and other agency relations
3. Intrastate agency relations
4. Certain statewide policy determination
5. Standard setting
6. Health regulatory functions

More specifically, the Institute of Medicine (1988) describes the role of state government related to health. Summarized, it includes the following.

■ Collect data statewide to assess health needs.
■ Assure an adequate statutory base for state health activities.
■ Establish statewide health objectives (holding localities accountable where power for implementation has been delegated).
■ Assure statewide development and maintenance of essential personal, educational, and environmental health services.
■ Solve problems that threaten the health of the state.
■ Support local health services (when needed to achieve adequate service levels) through subsidies, technical and administrative assistance, or direct action.

State public health agencies face a challenge in addressing the many health-related issues confronting them. Health insurance, long term care, organ trans-

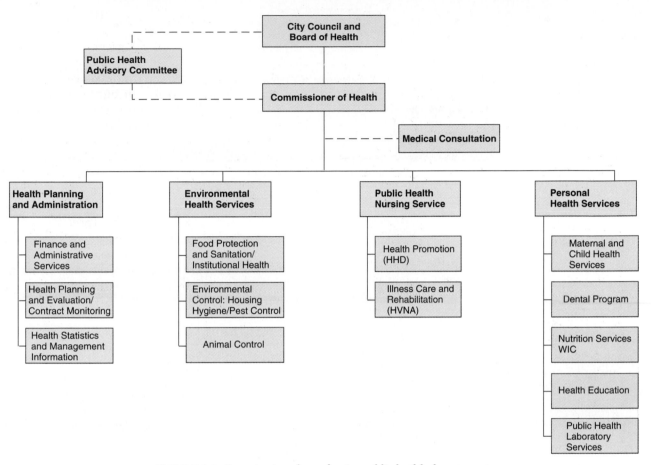

FIGURE 2.2. Organization chart of a city public health department.

plants and donations, AIDS, care of the **medically indigent** (those unable to pay for and totally lacking in medical services), malpractice, and certificates of need for new health services, are among the list of problems faced by most states. Clearly state health departments must collaborate closely with many other agencies, such as social services, education, public works, the legislature, housing bureau, and many others, to effectively solve such problems. Thus the solution of state health problems and delivery of health services requires the functioning of an interdependent network of organizations, many of which are not health agencies, per se.

Budgetary sources for operating a state health department include state generated funds, federal grants and contracts, and fees and reimbursements. A large source of federal monies to the states has come through the Department of Agriculture which has supported the supplemental nutrition program for women, infants, and children (WIC).

Each of the 50 state health departments in the United States has developed its own unique structure. Some are strongly centralized organizations and others are decentralized. All are overseen by a director of public health, but titles vary. Under the director are a number of divisions or bureaus. Those most commonly found in state health department organizational structures are environmental health, disease prevention and control, community health services, maternal and child health, health systems and technical services, laboratory services, and state center for health statistics. Figure 2.3 shows a state health department organizational chart.

National Public Health Agencies

The national level of public health organization consists of many government agencies. They can be clustered into four groups. First and most directly focused on health is the **Public Health Service** (PHS). It serves

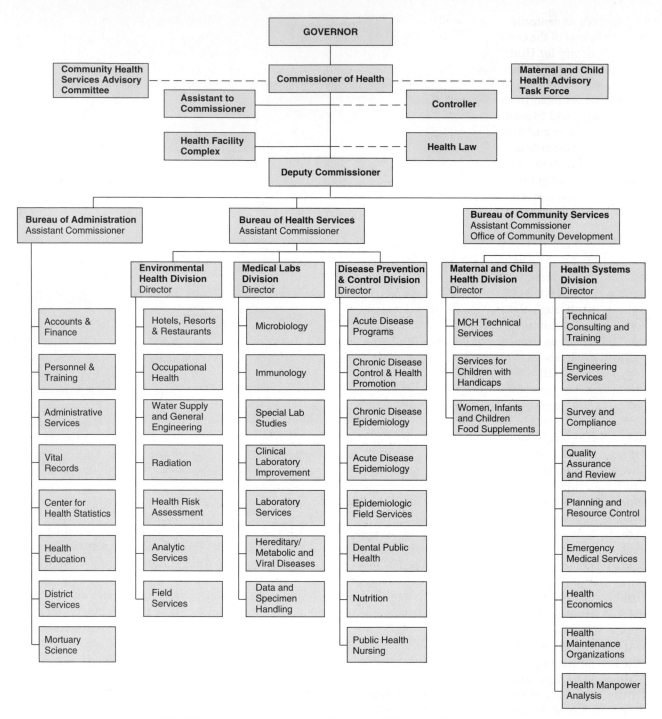

FIGURE 2.3. Organization chart of a state public health department.

an umbrella organization concerned with the broad health interests of the country and is directed by the Assistant Secretary for Health. The PHS is made up of six functional branches. They are the Centers for Disease Control and Prevention; the Food and Drug Administration; the National Institutes of Health; the Alcohol, Drug Abuse, and Mental Health Administration; the Health Resources and Services Administration; and the Agency for Toxic Substances and Disease Registry. One of its major functions through these six branches is the administration of grants and contracts with other government agencies, private organizations, and individuals. In some instances, as with the Indian Health Service, the PHS provides hospital, clinical, and other types of health services for Native Americans on reservations and for Eskimos. Through the Centers for Disease Control and the National Institutes of Health, it provides epidemiologic surveillance and numerous research programs. And through the Food and Drug Administration, the PHS monitors the safety and usefulness of various food and drug products as well as cosmetics, toys, and flammable fabrics.

Through its staff offices, the PHS offers other services. It has responsibility for health policy, planning and evaluation, health promotion, health services management, health research and statistics, intergovernmental affairs, legislation, population affairs, international health, and other matters of health concern to the nation. It provides financial assistance to the states through grants-in-aid—monies raised by Congress through taxes for specific purposes. It also offers consultation by means of a National Advisory Health Council and special advisory committees made up of lay experts. The PHS maintains ten regional offices to make its services more readily available to the states. These offices are located in New York, Boston, Philadelphia, Atlanta, Chicago, Kansas City, Dallas, Denver, Seattle, and San Francisco. Figure 2.4 portrays the PHS organizational structure.

At the federal level the primary agencies concerned with health are organized under the **Department of Health and Human Services** (DHHS). The PHS is one of five major units in this department. The other four are the Office of Human Development Services, the Health Care Financing Administration, the Social Security Administration, and the Family Support Administration. Figure 2.5 depicts this department's organization. In addition to the DHHS, a second cluster of federal agencies deals with the needs of special population groups such as the elderly (Administration on

Aging), farmers (Agricultural Extension Service), Native Americans (Bureau of Indian Affairs), and the military (Veterans Administration). A third cluster addresses special programs or problems. Examples are the Bureau of Labor Standards, the Office of Education, the Bureau of Mines, the Department of Agriculture, the Bureau of Labor Statistics, and the Social Security Administration. A final cluster of federal agencies focuses on international health concerns of interest to the nation. Two important ones are the Office of International Health, part of the PHS, and the Agency for International Development, under the Department of State.

PRIVATE SECTOR HEALTH SERVICES

The nongovernmental and voluntary arm of the health care delivery system includes many types of services. Private nonprofit health, which includes most hospitals, and welfare agencies make up one large group. Privately owned (proprietary) for-profit agencies are another. Private professional health care practice, composed largely of physicians in solo practice (about two fifths) and group practice (three fifths), forms a third group (DeLew, Greenberg, & Kinchen, 1992). These are the nontax-supported, nongovernmental dimension of community health care.

Private health services are complementary and supplementary to government health agencies. They often meet the needs of special groups, such as those with cancer or heart disease; they offer an avenue for private enterprise or philanthropy; they are freer than government agencies to develop innovations in health care; and they have been spurred to development, in part, by impatience or dissatisfaction with government programs. Their financial support comes from voluntary contributions, bequests, or fees.

For-Profit and Not-For-Profit Health Agencies

Proprietary health services are privately owned and managed. They may be nonprofit or for-profit. According to the Institute of Medicine study, 81% of nursing homes, 52% of psychiatric hospitals, 13% of acute care hospitals, and 35% of HMOs are for-profit (Institute of Medicine, 1988). Many hospitals and nursing homes offer nonprofit services but must generate sufficient revenues to keep ahead of operating costs. Often one or more special services offered by a hospital will generate enough income to cover the drain from more expensive

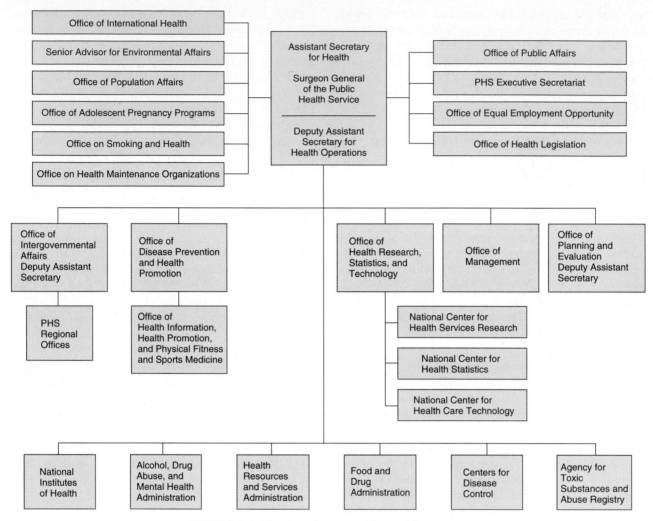

FIGURE 2.4. The United States Public Health Service.

programs or uncompensated care. As more hospitals have merged or been integrated into larger health conglomerates, the practice has often been to establish a separate for-profit corporation that generates revenues so that the basic organization can retain its nonprofit, tax-exempt status.

Examples of for-profit health services include a wide range of private practices by physicians, nurses, social workers, psychologists, laboratory and X-ray technologists, and many more. With the greater demand for home care services in the 1980s and 1990s we have also seen a major increase in new for-profit services, such as home care agencies, nursing personnel pools, and durable medical equipment supply companies.

Not-for-profit private health agencies are organizations established and administered by private citizens for some specific health-related purpose. Often this purpose is seen as a special need either not addressed or served inadequately by government. An example is visiting nurse associations that were formed to provide care for the sick in their homes. The contribution of the private, not-for-profit health agency then becomes complemental to public health services.

Several types of private, not-for-profit health agencies exist. Three have very specialized interests. First, there are some, such as the American Cancer Society and the American Diabetes Association, that are concerned with specific diseases. Second, there are others, such as the

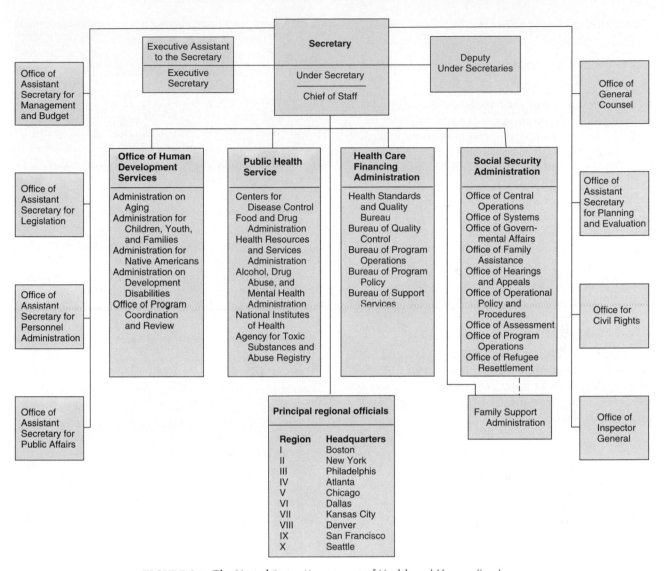

FIGURE 2.5. The United States Department of Health and Human Services.

National Society for Autistic Children, Planned Parenthood Federation of America, and the National Council on Aging, that focus on the needs of special populations. A third group, including agencies such as the American Heart Association and the National Kidney Foundation, is concerned with diseases of specific organs. All of these agencies are funded through private contributions.

Another group of private, not-for-profit agencies affecting health and health care includes the many foundations that support health programs, research, and professional education. Examples include the W. K. Kel-

logg Foundation, the Pew Charitable Trust, the Robert Wood Johnson Foundation, and the Bush Foundation. Some agencies, like the United Way, exist to fund other voluntary efforts. Still another group includes professional associations that work to improve the public's health through the promotion of standards, research, information, and programs. Examples are the American Public Health Association, the National League for Nursing, the American Nurses Association, and the American Medical Association. These organizations are funded primarily through membership dues, bequests, and contributions.

Functions of Private Sector Health Agencies

The general functions of private sector health agencies are as follows:

1. Detecting unserved needs or exploring better methods for meeting needs already addressed,
2. Piloting or subsidizing demonstration projects,
3. Promoting public knowledge,
4. Assisting official agencies with innovative programs not otherwise possible,
5. Evaluating official programs and assuming a public advocacy role,
6. Promoting health legislation,
7. Planning and coordinating to promote collaboration among voluntary services and between voluntary and official agencies, and
8. Developing well-balanced community health programs that seek to make services relevant and comprehensive.

In the future the functions of both private and public sectors will most likely remain much the same. However, the structure of the organizations within both sectors is changing dramatically. See the Issues in Community Health Nursing display.

International Health Organizations

The health of countries around the world cannot be ignored. Besides important humanitarian and moral concerns, there are pragmatic reasons for addressing health issues at the international level. We now live in an age when health, along with politics and economics, has become a global issue. The nations of the world are dependent on one another for goods and services, and as in any set of interdependent systems, a problem in one nation has repercussions on the others. Furthermore, as the constitution of the World Health Organization states: "The health of all peoples is fundamental to the attainment of peace and security." (World Health Organization [WHO], 1986)

International cooperation in health dates back to early concerns for epidemics. In 1851, representatives from 12 countries met in Paris for the First Interna-

Issues in Community Health Nursing
CHANGING HEALTH SYSTEM STRUCTURE

In recent years the lines have become increasingly blurred between hospitals and community-based services, for-profit and not-for-profit health organizations, and public and private sectors. The needs to reduce costs, increase efficiency and effectivness, and promote access have forced new structures and models of service delivery. Hospitals have merged together, some adding for-profit components and community-based services. Large umbrella organizations, such as Humana and Life Span, have purchased hospitals, clinics, and managed care organizations.

Public health agencies find it helpful to collaborate with private health organizations. A case in point is the partnerships formed between local health departments and private AIDS organizations in the community to provide more effective education, outreach, and casefinding. Another example is public health nursing agencies contracting for home health aides, physical and respiratory therapy, and other services from the private sector. Conversely, private companies, such as industries seeking worksite health programs, may contract for community health nursing services through the local health department.

Such partnerships and collaboration testify to a continuously changing system structure—one that community health nurses would do well to monitor carefully and seek to help shape.

tional Sanitary Conference. They later established a more permanent organization, the Office Internationale d'Hygiene Publique in 1907. Epidemics on the American continent also prompted representatives from 21 American republics to meet for the First International Sanitary Conference in Mexico City in 1902. In that same year they formed the International Sanitary Bureau, later renamed the Pan American Health Organization. After World War I, the League of Nations in 1921 formed a health organization with which the Office Internationale d'Hygiene Publique merged.

WORLD HEALTH ORGANIZATION

The **World Health Organization** (WHO), an agency of the United Nations, was developed to direct and coordinate the promotion of health worldwide. It was formed in 1948 and assumed the functions of the League of Nation's Health Organization. The Pan American Health Organization remained separate but became WHO's regional office for the Americas. WHO began its existence with 61 member nations, one of which was the United States and by 1988 had expanded its membership to 168 nations (WHO, 1988).

The responsibility or mission of WHO is to serve as "the one directing and coordinating authority on international health work" (Pickett & Hanlon, 1990, p. 74). From its inception, WHO has influenced international thinking with its classic definition of health as "a state of complete physical, mental, and social well-being and not merely the absence of disease or infirmity" (WHO, 1986). WHO's primary function is to help countries improve their health status and services by assisting them to help themselves and each other. To accomplish this, it provides member countries with technical services, information from epidemiology and statistics, advisory and consulting services, and demonstration teams.

The current goal for the World Health Organization is to achieve "Health for All by 2000." To accomplish this goal, WHO is emphasizing "the application of primary care, environmental health, control of infectious and diarrheal diseases, maternal and child health care, nutrition, injury prevention, and occupational health" (Pickett & Hanlon, 1990, p.75). These emphases point to a change in focus from primarily reactive programs, like stopping epidemics and instituting quarantines, to adding a more positive stance of promoting the health status of the global community.

In addition to its headquarters in Geneva, Switzerland, the World Health Organization has six regional offices. The office for the Americas, the Pan American Health Organization, is located in Washington, DC. The other regional offices are in Copenhagen for Europe, Alexandria for the eastern Mediterranean, Brazzaville for Africa, New Delhi for southeast Asia, and Manila for the western Pacific (Pickett & Hanlon, 1990). Its funding comes from member countries and from the United Nations. It holds an annual World Health Assembly (Figure 2.6) to discuss international health policies and programs (Pickett and Hanlon, 1990).

PAN AMERICAN HEALTH ORGANIZATION

The **Pan American Health Organization** (PAHO) serves as the central coordinating organization for public health in the Western Hemisphere. Founded in

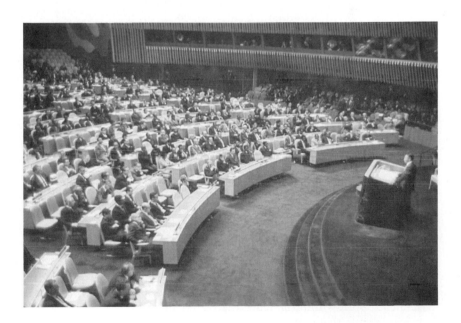

FIGURE 2.6. Delegates to the World Health Organization (WHO) have adopted a primary prevention approach to global health promotion.

1902, it is the oldest continuously functioning international health organization in the world. Its budget comes from assessments contributed by the American Republics member countries, augmented by funds from WHO, the United Nations, and a variety of other sources including private donations.

As WHO's regional office for the Americas, PAHO disseminates epidemiologic information, provides technical assistance, finances fellowships, and promotes cooperative research and professional education. An annual conference convened by PAHO provides an opportunity for delegates from all the member nations to discuss issues of concern and plan strategies for addressing health needs.

UNITED NATIONS INTERNATIONAL CHILDREN'S EMERGENCY FUND

Organized in 1946, the United Nations Children's Fund, now the *United Nations International Children's Emergency Fund* (UNICEF), was initially established as a temporary emergency program to assist children of war-torn countries. That focus has broadened and it has become a permanent agency. Now it promotes child and maternal health and welfare globally through a variety of programs and activities. Some include provision of food and supplies to underdeveloped countries, immunization programs in cooperation with WHO, disease control, prevention demonstrations, and, in particular, promotion of family planning in developing countries. Its International Children's Center, opened in the 1940s, has made a significant international impact with its teaching, research, publications, and cooperation on projects related to the health and welfare of children.

Many other organizations deal with health concerns at the international level (see World Watch display). The United Nations Educational, Scientific, and Cultural Organization (UNESCO) offers assistance on international health matters. The Southeast Asia Treaty Organization (SEATO) and the North Atlantic Treaty Organization (NATO) both have health components. The World Bank addresses health problems through funding and technical assistance. The Food and Agricultural Organization works to improve world food supplies. In addition to these international organizations, most developed countries have agencies that provide assistance, some in major proportions, to underdeveloped countries. The United States has many agencies, both within the federal government and the private sector, that provide other countries with health-

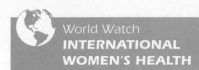

World Watch
INTERNATIONAL WOMEN'S HEALTH

A victory for international women's health was won at a conference held in Cairo, Egypt in September of 1994. Participants at the International Conference on Population and Development (ICPD) included 170 nations and thousands representing nongovernmental organizations (NGOs). A primary focus and hotly debated topic of the conference was abortion and reproductive health. Each year world-wide 500,000 women die from pregnancy-related complications. Of these complications, 15 to 20 percent are due to unsafe abortion. Unsafe abortion was defined as "a procedure for terminating unwanted pregnancy either by persons lacking the necessary skills or in an environment lacking the minimal medical standards or both" (The Nation's Health, 1994, p. 23). The ICPD's final report and Plan of Action emphasized the prevention of unwanted pregnancies and stated that abortion should not be promoted as a family planning method. At the same time the Plan urged all nations "to strengthen their commitment to women's health, to deal with the health impact of unsafe abortions as a major public health concern and to reduce the recourse to abortion through expanded and improved family planning services" (The Nation's Health: October, 1994, p. 23). It also promoted women's rights to decide the timing and number of pregnancies with access to safe means for accomplishing these goals. Overall, the conference made significant strides toward improving the health and well-being of women, particularly their reproductive health and empowerment.

related assistance. Government examples include the Office of International Health in DHHS, the Centers for Disease Control, the Fogarty International Center in the National Institutes of Health, and the Peace Corps housed in ACTION. Examples of private agencies include Project HOPE, International Planned Parenthood Federation, CARE, International Women's Health Coalition, as well as private foundations and missionary groups.

Significant Legislation

During the twentieth century in the United States, an ever-widening sense of responsibility for health in the public sector led to passage of an increasing amount of health-related legislation. Some acts are of particular significance to the financing and delivery of community health services.

The Shepard-Towner Act of 1921. The Shepard-Towner Act of 1921 provided federal grant-in-aid funds to the states for administration of programs to promote the health and welfare of mothers and infants. The act expired in 1929, but it set a pattern for maternal and child health programs that was later revived and strengthened through the successful and far-reaching efforts of the Children's Bureau, housed in the Department of Labor. Through the leadership of this Bureau many programs were instituted that enhanced children's health. Among them were services targeting prematurity, perinatal mortality, nutrition, mental retardation, audiology, rheumatic fever, cerebral palsy, epilepsy, dentistry, juvenile delinquency, and the problems of migrant workers' children (Eliot, 1962). The Children's Bureau maintained its impact through several administrative changes (moved to the Federal Security Agency in 1946 and to the Department of Health, Education and Welfare in 1953, becoming the Office of Child Development) but was phased out in 1972. For a number of years, federal advocacy for maternal and child health per se was considerably weakened.

The Social Security Act of 1935. The Social Security Act of 1935 had tremendous consequences for public health. In addition to its revolutionary welfare insurance and assistance programs, which particularly benefited high-risk mothers and children, Title VI of the act financially assisted states and localities in providing public health services. These funds were and still are allocated on the basis of population, public health problems, economic need, and need for training public health personnel. Many of the grants had to be matched by the states or localities serving to increase their knowledge of and commitment to health programs. The act strengthened local health departments and health programs in nearly all the states (Pickett and Hanlon, 1990).

The Hill-Burton Act (Hospital Survey and Construction Act) of 1946. The Hill-Burton Act of 1946 was an important breakthrough in nationwide health facilities planning. It marked the first real effort to link health planning with population need on a comprehensive basis. The act provided federal funds to states for hospital construction. Allocation of funds, however, was contingent upon the states forming planning councils to survey and document needs for new facilities and other capital expansion. The Hill-Harris Amendments in 1954 shifted the emphasis from purely construction to broader health planning based on needs assessment (Hyman, 1982).

The Maternal and Child Health and Mental Retardation Planning Amendments of 1963. The Maternal and Child Health and Mental Retardation Planning Amendments of 1963 opened the door for improved services to selected mothers and children. Recognizing the nation's high perinatal mortality rate as well as accompanying problems of premature births, handicapping conditions and mental retardation, Congress, by means of this law, authorized project grants to fund projects offering comprehensive care to high-risk, low income mothers and children. It also provided grants to states to design comprehensive programs addressing mental retardation.

The Heart Disease, Cancer, and Stroke Amendments of 1965 (PL. 89-239). The Heart Disease, Cancer, and Stroke Amendments of 1965 are noteworthy for their establishment of regional medical programs, one of the first real efforts at comprehensive health planning. Fifty-six regions in the United States were designated, each charged with the responsibility to evaluate the overall health needs of its region and cooperate with other regions for program development. Although the amendments were initially categorical in nature (limited to heart disease, cancer, and stroke), amendments in 1970 expanded the focus. The act was important for two additional reasons. It encouraged local participation in health planning, previously done at federal and state levels, and it funded program operations as well as planning.

The Social Security Act Amendments of 1965 (PL. 89-97). The Social Security Act Amendments of 1965 attempted to address a concern for some type of national health insurance. Title XVIII, *Medicare*, provides federally-funded health insurance for the elderly (65 and over) and disabled. Title XIX, *Medicaid*, is a joint federal-state welfare assistance program serving the blind, certain families with dependent children, the disabled, and eligible elderly. These two pieces of legislation (Medicare and Medicaid) have enabled many of the poor, disabled, and elderly to receive quality health care which they would otherwise not have had available to them (Davis, 1983, Pickett & Hanlon, 1990).

The Comprehensive Health Planning and Public Health Service Amendments Act (Partnership for Health Act) of 1966 (PL. 89-749). The Comprehensive Health Planning and Public Health Service Amendments Act (Partnership for Health Act) of 1966 promoted further advances in comprehensive health planning. It established comprehensive health planning agencies and attempted to coordinate the many categorical health and research efforts into an integrated system. It emphasized comprehensive health planning and cost containment at local, state, and regional levels. Its goals were improved efficiency and effectiveness of health care. Many problems, including unclear expectations, uncertain funding, and limited authority, prevented full accomplishment of these goals.

The Health Manpower Act of 1968 (PL. 90-490). The Health Manpower Act of 1968 sought to increase the supply of health personnel by providing federal money to educational institutions for construction, training, special projects, student loans, and scholarships. The act replaced several previous acts with similar goals but whose efforts were fragmentary in addressing the problem. Among them were the Nurse Training Act (1966) and the Allied Health Professions Personnel Training Act (1966). In 1976, Congress passed the Health Professions Education Assistance Act (PL. 94-484) to effect a better balance between the country's health needs and the supply of available health professionals. One of its major emphases was to address the problem of physician maldistribution between underserved (rural) and overserved (urban) areas through educational incentive programs.

The Occupational Safety and Health Act of 1970 (PL. 91-956). The Occupational Safety and Health Act of 1970 provides protection to workers against personal injury or illness resulting from hazardous working conditions. This and other acts affecting the working population, such as workers' compensation, toxic substance control, access to employee exposure and medical records, and "right-to-know" legislation, are discussed in Chapter 20.

The Professional Standards Review Organization Amendment to the Social Security Act of 1972 (PL. 92-603). The Professional Standards Review Organization Amendment to the Social Security Act of 1972 had two goals: cost containment and improved quality of care. Professional Standards Review Organization (PSRO) legislation created autonomous organizations, external to hospitals and ambulatory care agencies, to monitor and review objectively the quality of care delivered to Medicare and Medicaid patients. The PSRO review boards, composed mostly of physicians, examined such things as need for care, length of stay, and quality of care against predetermined standards developed locally. Failure to meet standards could mean denial of federal funding. The PSRO concept has created considerable controversy, partly because the two mandated goals, cost containment and quality of care, are potentially incompatible. The federal government's primary emphasis on costs frequently clashed with local concerns for quality. Also, the lack of criteria or standards for review as well as the primary governance by physicians has made it hard to evaluate the program's success. Some studies, however, indicated a substantial cost saving in Medicare expenditures (Hyman, 1982).

The Health Maintenance Organization Act of 1973 (PL. 93-222). The Health Maintenance Organization Act of 1973 added federal support to the concept of prepayment for medical care. Congress authorized funding for feasibility studies, planning, grants, and loans to stimulate growth among qualifying health maintenance organizations (HMOs). In addition, this act required a business employing 25 or more people to offer an HMO health insurance option, if such an option was available locally.

The National Health Planning and Resource Development Act of 1974 (PL. 93-641). The National Health Planning and Resource Development Act of 1974 was a major breakthrough in comprehensive health planning. Replacing the Partnership for Health Act, it combined Hill-Burton, comprehensive health planning agencies, and regional medical programs into a single new program. It fostered not only comprehensive health planning, but regulation and evaluation, and promoted collaborative efforts among regional, state, and federal governments. An important contribution of this act was its emphasis on consumer involvement in health planning. The act was divided into two titles. Title XV, National Health Planning and Development, established national health priorities and assisted the development of area-wide and state planning through health systems agencies and state health planning and development agencies. Title XVI, Health Resources Development, coordinated health facilities planning with health planning, replacing Hill-Burton (Hyman, 1982).

The National Center for Health Statistics (PL 93-353). The National Center for Health Statistics

(NCHS), established in 1974, arose from the earlier National Office of Vital Statistics and became part of the Centers for Disease Control under the Public Health Service in 1987. The NCHS operates eleven data collection systems that provide vital information for public health planning and service delivery. Table 2.2 lists these data collection systems.

The Omnibus Budget Reconciliation Act (OBRA) of 1981 (PL 97-35). The Omnibus Budget Reconciliation Act (OBRA) of 1981 had a profound effect on public health. In this act Congress halted the progress made in most of the public health laws of the previous 45 years; substantially reducing their funding authorization. The Reagan administration, in an attempt to shift more power to the states and to cut the budget, consolidated categorical grants into four block grants. The first block grant targeted general preventive health services; the second addressed alcohol, drug abuse, and mental health; the third focused on maternal and child health; and the fourth addressed primary care which covered federal support for community health centers. While block grants provide some advantages, these came with limiting restrictions on the amount and use

of the funds. The result was a significant reduction in funding for state and local health programs. Under OBRA, new legislation was introduced in 1987 to increase quality control in nursing homes and home care.

The Social Security Amendments of 1983 (PL. 98-21). The Social Security Amendments of 1983 became law in response to accelerating health care costs. The act represented a major reform in health care financing from retrospective to prospective payment. It introduced a billing classification system of 467 diagnosis related groups (DRGs) that provided Medicare payment to hospitals based on a fixed rate set in advance (Joel, 1983; Shaffer, 1988). The fixed payment could not be increased if hospital costs for care exceeded that amount. Conversely, if costs were less than the paid amount, the hospital could keep the difference (Davis, 1983). Thus, a positive incentive was introduced to reduce hospital costs at the same time offering a negative incentive for early patient discharge.

The Consolidated Omnibus Budget Reconciliation Act of 1985. The Consolidated Omnibus Budget Reconciliation Act of 1985 (COBRA) required employers to provide extended (up to 36 months) group

---

TABLE 2.2. *The National Center for Health Statistics Data Collection Systems*

1. *Basic vital statistics* are collected by each state on such things as births, deaths, pregnancy terminations, marriages, and divorces. The Center publishes monthly and annual reports on this data.

2. *Vital statistics follow-back surveys* are conducted periodically to obtain further information on previously gathered data.

3. *National Survey of Family Growth* studies such things as fertility, family planning practices, family formation and dissolution, and matters affecting maternal and child health.

4. *National Health Interview Survey* is a continuous nationwide survey of illness and disability— their amount, distribution, and affects–in the U.S. The results are published in Series 10 of *Vital Health Statistics*.

5. *National Medical Care Utilization and Expenditure Survey* was conducted once in 1980 to describe medical services' use and expenditures.

6. *National Ambulatory Medical Survey* occasionally gathers data from physicians on ambulatory services by specialty and target population.

7. *National Health and Nutrition Examination Survey* provides physical, physiological, and biochemical data related to nutrition of national population samples.

8. *National Hospital Discharge Survey* provides annual data on such things as length of stay, diagnosis, procedures performed, and patient use patterns

9. *National Nursing Home Survey* collects data from nursing home residents and staffs regarding need, level of care, costs, and use patterns.

10. *National Master of Facility Inventory* identifies and classifies by type of beds all facilities that offer 24-hour care including hospitals, nursing homes, and residential care facilities.

11. *National Health Professions Inventories and Surveys* draw from state data systems to describe the distribution and education of health personnel.

Statistics on mental health are collected through the National Institute of Mental Health.
Source: National Center for Health Statistics: Data systems of the National Center for Health Statistics, Series 1(16), DHHS Pub No (PHS) 82-1318, Hyattsville, MD, 1981, U.S. Department of Health and Human Services.

rate insurance coverage for laid-off workers and their dependents. The result was crippling costs to businesses with claims exceeding premiums by 83 percent in 1988 and 90 percent in 1990 (Medicine & Health, 1991).

The Gramm-Rudman-Hollings Balanced Budget & Emergency Deficit Control Act of 1985. The Gramm-Rudman-Hollings Balanced Budget & Emergency Deficit Control Act of 1985 caused reduced funding of Medicare and Medicaid programs.

Omnibus Budget Reconciliation Act Expansion of 1986. Omnibus Budget Reconciliation Act Expansion of 1986 promoted a prospective payment system for hospital outpatient service. In 1989, a further OBRA expansion regulated fee schedules for physicians encouraging less "high-tech" use. Under OBRA, the Agency for Health Care Policy and Research was also established in 1989 to study the effectiveness of health care services.

The Medicare Catastrophic Coverage Act of 1988 (PL. 100-360). The Medicare Catastrophic Coverage Act of 1988 (MCCA) expanded Medicare benefits significantly. Coverage was extended to include a portion of outpatient prescription drug costs and greater post-hospital extended care facility and home health benefits. MCCA also set limits on beneficiary liability, and provided increased inpatient hospital benefits.

The Family Support Act of 1988. The Family Support Act of 1988 assisted poor women and children by expanding their coverage and requiring states to extend Medicaid coverage

The Health Objectives Planning Act of 1990 (PL. 101-582). The Health Objectives Planning Act of 1990 was significant for its support of the Institute of Medicine's Report, *Healthy People 2000*, with funding to improve the health status of the nation. Funding for health promotion and disease prevention was added in the 1991 legislative session.

Implications for Community Health Nursing

The structure and functions of the health services delivery system as well as particular legislation have had a significant impact on community health nursing. Community health nurses have had to learn to adapt to a constantly changing system. They have developed innovative modes of service delivery, such as community-based nursing centers for health education, counseling, and screening of low income populations. They have learned to practice in a variety of settings extending beyond homes, worksites, schools, churches, clinics, and voluntary agencies. They have acquired skills in team work, leadership, and political activism. They have recognized the importance of outcomes research to document the value of nursing interventions with at-risk populations.

At the national, state, and local level, community health nursing has important ties with both private and public health agencies. Community health nurses may be employed by either type of organization. When serving in the public sector, they often provide consultation, serve on boards, volunteer their services, or collaborate with private sector health organizations to ensure quality and access of care to the broader community. Examples include joint efforts to promote certain types of health legislation or collaboration to produce and disseminate health education materials targeting specific populations. Sometimes community health nursing services operate within one organization that combines public and private sector organization and funding. An example is the Metropolitan Visiting Nurse Association of Minneapolis, Minnesota which has been a combined public-private agency supported by taxes as well as by voluntary funds.

Community health nurses also have many opportunities to serve in international health. Some work with WHO, PAHO, or other agencies to assist in direct care projects, such as famine relief, third world immunization efforts, or nutritional screening and education programs. Other nurses serve as health planners, assist with policy development, collaboratively conduct needs assessment projects and research efforts, or engage in program development.

Summary

Many factors and events have influenced the current structure, function, and financing of community health services. Understanding these gives the community health nurse a stronger base for planning for the health of community populations.

Historically health care has progressed unevenly, marked by numerous influences. Primitive practices of early centuries were replaced with more advanced sanitary measures by the Greeks and Romans. The Middle

Ages saw a serious health decline, with raging epidemics, leading to extensive nineteenth-century reform efforts in England and later in the United States.

Organized health care in the United States developed slowly. Public health problems, such as need for isolation of communicable disease and control of environmental pollution, prompted the gradual development of official interventions. For example, quarantines to control the spread of communicable disease were imposed in the late 1700s. Sanitary reform was pursued more vigorously during the 1800s. Local, then state, health departments were formed starting in the late 1700s. By the early 1900s the federal government had assumed a more active role in public health with a proliferation of health, education, and welfare services.

For many years efforts to address community health needs have been made by private individuals and public agencies. These two arms of service have not been coordinated in the past and only gradually during this century have begun to work together to form an emerging health care system.

The public arm of health services includes all government, tax-supported health agencies and occurs at four levels: local, state, national, and international. Each level deals with the health needs of the population that its boundaries encompass. Each level has a different structure and set of functions.

Private health services are the unofficial arm of the community health system. They include voluntary non-profit agencies as well as privately owned (proprietary) and for-profit agencies. Their financial support comes from voluntary contributions, bequests, or fees. Private health organizations often supplement and complement the work of official agencies.

The delivery and financing of community health services has been significantly affected by various legislative acts. These acts have prompted such innovations as health insurance and assistance for the poor, the elderly and the disabled; money to train health personnel and conduct health research; standards for health planning and delivery; health protection for workers on the job; and the financing of health services.

Activities to Promote Critical Thinking

1. Interview someone at your local health department. How do the services offered compare to those listed in this chapter? What is community health nursing's role?

2. Make an on-site visit to your state health department. Compare its functions to the core public health functions described in this chapter. Identify areas where improvement may be needed.

3. Conduct an interview on-site with someone at a private health agency. Compare their functions with those listed in this chapter for private health agencies. Describe how this agency works collaboratively with public health agencies.

4. Form two teams with your classmates and debate the pros and cons of a strong federal role in health care provision as opposed to decentralized (state and local) control.

REFERENCES

Davis, C.K. (1983) The federal role in changing health care financing. *Nursing Economics, 1*(1), 10–17.

DeLew, N., Greenberg, G., & Kinchen, K. (1992). A layman's guide to the U.S. health care system. *Health Care Financing Review, 14*(1), 151–169.

Elliot, M. (1962). The Children's Bureau: Fifty years of public responsibility for action in behalf of children. *American Journal of Public Health, 52,* 576.

Fitzpatrick, M.L. (1975). *The national organization for public health nursing 1912–1952: Development of a practice field.* New York: National League for Nursing.

Hecker, J.F.C. (1839). *The epidemics of the Middle Ages.* London: Trubner and Company.

Institute of Medicine. (1988). *The future of public health.* Washington, DC: National Academy Press.

Hyman, H. (1982). *Health planning: A systematic approach* (2nd ed.). Rockville, MD: Aspen Systems.

Joel, L.A. (1983). DRGs: The state of the art of reimbursement for nursing services. *Nursing and Health Care, 4,* 560–63.

Lewis, R.A. (1952). *Edwin Chadwick and the public health movement, 1832–1854.* New York: Longman's.

Marr, J. (1982). Merchants of death: The role of the slave trade in the transmission of disease from Africa to the Americas. *Pharos,* Winter, 31.

Medicine and Health (1991).

Pickett, G. & Hanlon, J. (1990). *Public health: Administration and practice* (9th ed.). St. Louis: Times Mirror/Mosby.

Plumb, D. (1994). The roles and responsibilities of state and local public health agencies. [position paper] *The Nation's Health.* American Public Health Association, September, 13–15.

Shaffer, F. (1988). DRGs: A new era for health care. *Nursing Clinics of North America, 23*(3), 453–463.

Shattuck, L., et al. (1850). *Report of the Sanitary Commission of Massachusetts.* Cambridge, MA: Harvard University Press (originally published by Dutton & Wentworth in 1850).

The Core Functions Project. (1993). *Health care reform and public health: A paper on population-based core functions.* Washington, DC: Office of Disease Prevention and Health Promotion, U.S. Public Health Service.

The Nation's Health. (1994). Cairo summit spells hope for women's health. *American Public Health Association*, October, 1, 23.

U.S. Department of Health and Human Services. (1991). *Healthy people 2000: National health promotion and disease prevention objectives.* DHHS publication PHS 91-50213. Washington, DC:Author.

Woodward, S.B. (1932). The story of smallpox in Massachusetts. *The New England Journal of Medicine, 206* (June 9), 1181.

World Health Organization. (1986). *Basic Documents.* (36th ed.). Geneva: Author.

World Health Organization. (1988). *World Health Statistics Annual.* Geneva: Author.

World Health Organization Study Group. (1991). *Community involvement in health development: Challenging health services.* WHO Technical Report no. 809. Geneva: Author.

SELECTED READINGS

Balinsky, W., & Starkman, J.L. (1987). The impact of DRGs on the health care industry. *Health Care Management Review, 12*(3), 61–74.

Barnhill, W. (1992). Canadian health care: Would it work here? *Arthritis Today,* Nov–Dec, 35–44.

Bergman, G. (1988). Standing alone: Why the U.S. has no national health system. *Grey Panther Network, 17*(1), 13, 18.

Brown, L.D. (1992). Political evolution of Federal health care regulation. *Health Affairs,* Winter, 17–37.

Chassin, M.R., Kosecoff, J., & Park, R.E. (1987). Does inappropriate use explain geographic variation in the use of health care services? *Journal of the American Medical Association, 258*(18), 2533–2537.

Edwardson, S.R., et al. (1988). Impact of DRGs on nursing: Report of the Midwest Alliance in Nursing. The impact of prospective payment systems on nursing care in community settings. U.S. Dept. of Health & Human Services Publication. Division of Nursing, Jul #HRP-0907178, 61–78.

Greenberg, G., & Kinchen, K. (1992). A layman's guide to the U.S. health care system. *Health Care Financing Review, 14*(1), 151–169.

Hash, M. (1988). Nursing practice in the 21st century. Structuring and financing of community health services. Community nursing organizations (CNOs). ANA Publication: American Nursing Foundation, No. CH-18, 36–40.

Jain, S.C. (1981). Introduction and summary: Role of state and local governments in relation to personal health services. *American Journal of Public Health, 71*(Supp.), 5–8.

Jonas, S. (1992). *An Introduction to the U.S. Health Care System* (3rd ed.). New York: Springer Publishing Company.

Kovner, A. (1990). *Health care delivery in the United States.* (4th ed.). New York: Springer Publishing Company.

Navarro, V. (1985). The public/private mix in funding and delivery of health services: An international survey. *American Journal of Public Health, 75*(11), 1318–20.

Phillips, E.K., et al. (1987). DRG ripple effects on community health nursing. *Public Health Nursing, 4*(2), 84–88.

Rosen, G. (1958). *A History of Public Health.* New York: MD Publications.

Shalala, D.E. (1993). Nursing and society: the unfinished agenda for the 21st century. *Nursing and Health Care, 14*(6), 289–291.

Shaffer, F. (1988). DRGs: A new era for health care. *Nursing Clinics of North America, 23*(3), 453–463.

Smith, J. P. (1990). The politics of American health care. *Journal of Advanced Nursing, 15*(4), 487–497.

Somers, A. R. (1986). The changing demand for health services: A historical perspective and some thoughts for the future. *Inquiry, 23*(4), 395–402.

Swinson, A. (1965). *The History of Public Health.* Exeter, England: A. Wheaton & Co.

U.S. Department of Health and Human Services. (1985). *Health: United States.* (1985). DHEW Pub. No. (PHS) 86-1232, December. Washington, DC: Author.

A Washington Seminar Report. (1987). *For profit and nonprofit health care: Are the distinctions blurring?* Washington, DC: National Health Council, Inc.

CHAPTER

3

Health Care Economics

LEARNING OBJECTIVES

Upon completion of this chapter, readers should be able to:

- Define the concept of health economics.
- Describe three sources of health care financing.
- Analyze the issues and trends influencing health care economics and community health services delivery.
- Explain the causes and effects of health care rationing.
- List the pros and cons of managed competition as opposed to a single payer system.
- Explain the philosophical implications of health care financing patterns on public health's mission and values.

KEY TERMS

- Competition
- Cost sharing
- Diagnosis-related groups
- Gross National Product
- Health economics
- Health Maintenance Organization
- Managed care
- Managed compction
- Medicaid
- Medicare

- National health insurance
- Preferred Provider Organization
- Prospective payment
- Rationing
- Regulation
- Retrospective payment
- Single payer system
- Third-party payments
- Universal coverage

Barbara Walton Spradley and Judith Ann Allender
COMMUNITY HEALTH NURSING: CONCEPTS AND PRACTICE, 4th ed.
© 1996 Barbara Walton Spradley and Judith Ann Allender

Nurses concerned with the delivery of needed community health services must also understand how those services are financed. In an era when health care resources are limited and provider organizations are competing for scarce dollars, it becomes essential for nurses to be knowlegeable about the issues related to health care financing as well as how to obtain funding to address identified health needs in the community.

Behind the financing of health care lies the science of health economics. The field of economics, as a whole, is a science that describes and analyzes the production, distribution, and consumption of goods and services. It is also concerned with a variety of related problems, such as finance, labor, and taxation. It studies and seeks to promote the best use of scarce resources for the greatest good of society. The science of **health economics** describes and analyzes the production, distribution, and consumption of health care goods and services in order to maximize the administration of scarce resources to benefit the most people. The goal of health economics, in some ways similar to that of public health, is to promote the greatest good for the greatest number using available resources and knowledge.

This chapter summarizes the changing picture of health care economics and its financial incentives and disincentives for enhancing the public's health. More extensive treatment of these important subjects can be found in the selected readings listed at the close of the chapter.

Economic Theories

One can better understand health economics by examining the two basic theories underlying the science of economics. The first is microeconomics and the second is macroeconomics.

MICROECONOMICS

Microeconomic theory is concerned with supply and demand. Economists using microeconomic theory study the supply of goods and services as these relate to consumer income allocation and distribution. They further study how this allocation and distribution affects consumer demand for these goods and services. Supply and demand influence each other and, in turn, affect prices. Increase in or over supply of certain products leads to less overall consumption (decreased demand)

and lowered prices. The opposite is also true. Limited availability of desired products means supply does not meet demand and prices increase. Microeconomic theory is useful for understanding price determination, resource allocation, and consumer income and spending distribution at the level of individuals and organizations.

MACROECONOMICS

Macroeconomic theory is concerned with the broad variables that affect the status of the total economy. Economists using macroeconimics study factors influencing employment, income, prices, and economic growth rates. Their focus is on the larger view of economic stability and growth. Macroeconomic theory is useful for providing a global or aggregate perspective of the variables affecting the total economic picture.

The economics of health care encompasses both micro- and macroeconomics by examining an intricate and complex set of interacting variables. It is concerned with supply and demand: Is the supply of available resources sufficient to meet the demand for use by consumers? It examines costs and benefits, cost effectiveness, and cost efficiency: Are the resources expended achieving the desired outcomes? It studies the allocation of scarce resources for health care: Where should resources, such as funding for health programs and services for at-risk populations, be applied when there are insufficient resources to address all the needs?

Health economics is a major field of study in and of itself. Health economists draw on economic theory to study and develop an understanding of the factors influencing the financing and delivery of health services. Macroeconomic theory has been useful in providing a large scale perspective on health care financing that has resulted in various proposals for national health plans, health care rationing, competition, managed care, and others. These concepts are described later in the chapter. Microeconomic theory may prove more useful if health care competition increases since the success of the supply and demand concept depends on a competitive market. The pros and cons of competition are also examined later in this chapter. Issues such as cost containment, competition between providers, accessibility of services, quality, and need for accountability have become targets of major concern for the 1990s. Further understanding of health economics and its impact on community health and community health nursing can come through examination of methods of health care financing, issues and trends influencing health care economics, and the effects of financing patterns on community health practice.

Sources of Health Care Financing: Public and Private

Financing of health care significantly affects community health and community health nursing practice. It influences the type and quality of services offered as well as the way those services are used. Sources of payment may be clustered into three categories: third-party payments, direct consumer payment, and private or philanthropic support.

THIRD-PARTY PAYMENTS

Third-party payments are monetary reimbursements made to providers of health care by someone other than the consumer who received the care. The organizations that administer these funds are called third-party payers because they are a third party, or external, to the consumer-provider relationship. Included in this category are four types of payment sources: private insurance companies, independent health plans, government health programs, and claims payment agents (Rapoport, Robertson, and Steward, 1982).

Private Insurance Companies

Private insurance companies market and underwrite policies aimed at decreasing consumer risk of economic loss because of a need to use health services. None directly delivers health services although some, such as John Hancock, do have subsidiary proprietary home health agencies. They are composed of three types. First are commercial stock companies that sell health insurance, generally as a sideline. They are private stockholder-owned corporations, such as Aetna, Travelers, and Connecticut General, that sell insurance nationally. Mutual companies, a second type that operates in the national marketplace, are owned by their policyholders. Examples are Mutual of Omaha, Prudential, and Metropolitan Life. The third type, nonprofit insurance plans, include companies such as Blue Cross, Blue Shield, and Delta Dental. These operate under special state enabling laws that give them an exclusive franchise to the whole

state (or some part of it) and to a specific type of insurance. Blue Cross, for example, in most instances sells only hospital coverage, Blue Shield only medical insurance, and Delta Dental only dental insurance. Because they are nonprofit, they are tax-exempt and at the same time subject to tighter state regulation than the commercial health insurance companies. Combined, the nonprofit and commercial carriers have sold the great majority of the private health insurance in the United States in recent years (DeLew, et al, 1992).

Independent Health Plans

Independent or self-insured health plans underwrite the remaining private health insurance in the nation. These plans have been offered through several hundred smaller organizations such as businesses, unions, consumer cooperatives, and medical groups. Health maintenance organizations (HMOs) and various company self-insured plans are also included in this category. They may sell only health insurance or, in some cases, may also provide health services; they focus on a very localized population. As a group, they generate a large amount of premium revenues but only a small percentage of the amount generated by the nonprofit and commercial health insurance companies.

All private health insurance companies combined (there were well over 1,000 in 1992) have provided coverage for the great majority, 74%, of the U.S. population. Of this group 61% obtained health insurance through their employers and 13% by direct purchase of nongroup coverage. A small portion of the total population, 13%, purchased both private and public health insurance, and 14% were uninsured (DeLew, et al, 1992). See Figure 3.1.

Government Health Programs

Government health programs make up the largest source of third-party reimbursement in the country. The government's four major health insurance programs have been Medicare, Medicaid, the Federal Employees Health Benefits Plan, and the Civilian Health and Medical Program of the Uniformed Services. Combined, they "account for more than 50 percent of the nation's hospital revenues and nearly a quarter of physician incomes" (Rapoport et al., 1982, p. 294). A third of the government's total third-party expenditures have gone for direct public medical services by the military, state hospitals, the Veterans Administration, public health

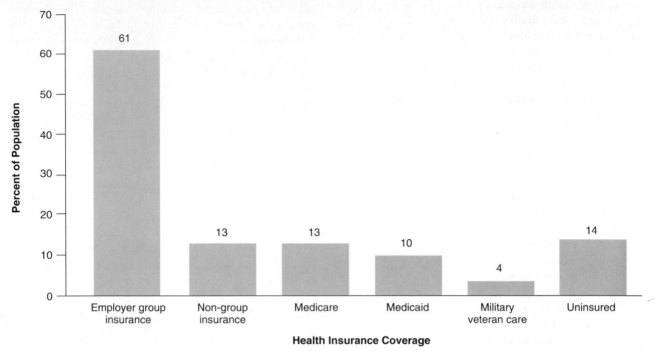

FIGURE 3.1. U.S. Health insurance coverage in 1990. Source: U.S. Department of the Census, 1991. Notes: Persons with more than one coverage are included more than once. Non-group is insurance purchased by individuals. Military includes dependents.

activities, and other "socialized" health services. Their primary target was what former Health and Human Services Secretary, Margaret Heckler, called "the most fragile Americans" ("Known Welfare Fraud," 1983, p. 42)—the elderly, the disabled, the poor, the very young, and the unemployed. Of the government's health insurance programs, Medicare and Medicaid constitute the largest.

Medicare, known as Title 18 of the Social Security Act Ammendments of 1965, provides mandatory federal health insurance for the elderly (65 and over) and certain disabled persons. "It is the single largest health insurer in the country, covering about 13 percent of the population, including virtually all the elderly 65 years of age or over (31 million people) and certain persons with disabilities or kidney failure (3 million people)" (DeLew, Greenberg & Kinchen, 1992, p. 152). It is administered by the Health Care Financing Administration of the U.S. Department of Health and Human Services. Part A of Medicare pays for hospitalization and limited nursing home and home care coverage to Social Security eligible participants. It is financed through trust funds derived from employment payroll taxes. Part

B, which is supplementary and voluntary, provides physician care and certain other health services to Medicare eligible enrollees. It is funded through enrollee monthly premiums (about 25%) and a tax-supported Federal subsidy (about 75%).

Medicare covers less than half of elderly persons' total medical expenses. It does not cover long-term nursing home care, outpatient prescription drugs, or routine eye care. Furthermore, participants must also pay coinsurance and deductibles. Consequently, "about 68 percent of Medicare beneficiaries have private supplemental health plans . . . and an additional 9 percent have Medicaid" (DeLew, et al, 1992, p.153).

Medicare funding, drawn primarily from working people's taxes to benefit the elderly, will need to find new revenue sources in the future. As the population of elderly increases, fewer workers will be available to support the program. In 1960 there were 5 workers for each Medicare beneficiary. Projections for the year 2000 say there will be 3 workers for each beneficiary and 1.9 by 2040 (DeLew, et al, 1992).

Medicaid, known as Title 19 of the Social Security Act Amendments of 1965, provides joint federal-state payment of health services for the blind, those permanently and totally disabled, the elderly who cannot afford to pay Part B of Medicare, and certain families with dependent children. Coverage includes preventive, acute, and long-term care services. Medicaid is funded jointly through taxes by federal and state governments but administered differently by each state under federal guidelines.

Potential Medicaid recipients must apply for coverage and prove their eligibility in terms of category and limited income. To be eligibile for Medicaid one must be poor as well as elderly, blind, disabled, pregnant, or the parent of a dependent child. "Mothers and dependent children comprise about 68 percent of Medicaid recipients, the elderly 13 percent, the blind and disabled 15 percent, and others 4 percent" (DeLew, et al, 1992, p.153). Eligibility is further defined by such things as maximum income and assets; thus more than half of the poor below Federal poverty levels are excluded from Medicaid. In some states the medically indigent, people with income below the poverty level who are unable to pay excessive medical expenses, are also eligible. Yet, since Medicaid has been the only public program financing long-term nursing home care, many middle-class elderly have qualified for nursing home care covered by Medicaid by intentionally shifting assets to their children and not using up their income on nursing home expenses (Burwell, 1991).

A federal health insurance program known as the Consolidated Omnibus Budget Reconciliation Act (COBRA) developed in 1985—this one designated to be self-financing—protects the unemployed who have lost their benefits. Another, workers' compensation, is a state-administered program that requires employers to pay health care costs of workers who sustain illness or injury associated with their jobs. In addition to third-party reimbursement, the government offers some direct health services to selected populations. They include Native Americans, military personnel, veterans, merchant marines, and federal employees.

Claims Payment Agents

Claims payment agents administer the claims payment process of government third-party payments. That is, the government contracts with private agents to handle the claims payment process. More than 80% of the government's third-party payments have been handled by these private contractors who are sometimes known as fiscal intermediaries (when processing Medicare hospital claims), carriers (when dealing with insurance under Medicare), or fiscal agents (as applied to Medicaid programs). As an example, Blue Cross plans, in addition to being private insurance companies, are also claims payment agents for Medicare.

DIRECT CONSUMER REIMBURSEMENT

A second major source of health care financing comes from direct fees paid by consumers. This refers to individual out-of-pocket payments made for several different reasons. One is payments made by individuals who have no insurance coverage so that fees must be paid directly for health and medical services. Another is for limited coverage and exclusions (services for which the consumer must bear the entire expense). For example, many individuals carry only major medical insurance and must pay directly for physician office visits, prescriptions, eye glasses, and dental care. In other instances, the insurance contract may include a deductible amount that must be paid by the insuree before reimbursement begins. The contract may be established on a copayment basis that determines a percentage to be paid by the insurer and the rest by the individual. Or the individual may pay the remainder of a health service bill after the insurer has paid a previously agreed-upon fixed amount such as a fixed coverage for labor and delivery. Direct consumer payment has accounted in recent years for approximately one-third of total personal health care expenditures in the United States. The amount of out-of-pocket payment in actual dollars is projected to continue rising (Congressional Budget Office, 1993). See Table 3.1.

PRIVATE SUPPORT

Private or philanthropic support, a third source, contributes both directly and indirectly to health care financing. Many private agencies, as discussed earlier in this chapter, fund programs, underwrite research, and provide benefits for people who would otherwise go without services. In addition, volunteerism, the efforts of numerous individuals and organizations who donate their time and services, provides tremendous cost savings to health care institutions. It also enables many individuals to receive services, such as home-delivered meals or transportation to health care facilities, at no charge. Philanthropic financing of health care has significantly decreased in the past two decades. However, continued private support is essential, particularly

TABLE 3.1. *Actual and Projected National Health Expenditures, by Source of Funds, Calendar Years 1990 to 2000*

Source of Funds	Actual		Projected								
	1990	1991	1992	1993	1994	1995	1996	1997	1998	1999	2000
BILLIONS OF DOLLARS											
Private											
Out-of-pocket	136	144	153	163	172	183	194	206	218	229	240
Private health insurance	222	244	266	288	313	339	368	400	432	465	499
Other	31	33	36	38	41	44	47	51	54	58	61
Total Private	390	422	455	490	526	566	610	656	704	752	800
Federal											
Medicare	111	123	138	156	178	200	223	246	272	301	332
Medicaid	43	56	70	82	94	106	119	133	148	165	184
Other	41	44	46	48	51	53	56	59	61	64	67
Total Federal	195	223	255	286	323	360	397	438	481	529	583
State and Local											
Medicaid	33	45	56	66	75	85	95	106	118	132	147
Other	58	62	66	70	74	78	83	87	92	97	102
Total State and Local	91	107	123	136	149	163	178	194	210	229	249
Total National Health Expenditures	675	752	832	912	998	1,089	1,185	1,288	1,395	1,510	1,631
ANNUAL PERCENTAGE CHANGE FROM PREVIOUS YEAR SHOWN											
Private											
Out of pocket	n.a.	5.7	6.2	6.5	5.2	6.3	6.4	6.2	5.6	5.2	4.8
Private health insurance	n.a.	10.0	8.8	8.4	8.6	8.4	8.6	8.4	8.1	7.7	7.1
Other	n.a.	6.0	7.8	7.6	7.2	7.1	7.0	7.2	6.8	6.5	6.3
Total Private	n.a.	8.2	7.8	7.7	7.4	7.6	7.7	7.6	7.2	6.8	6.4
Federal											
Medicare	n.a.	10.9	12.7	12.7	14.4	12.1	11.3	10.7	10.4	10.4	10.5
Medicaid	n.a.	30.6	25.8	16.8	14.4	13.2	11.7	11.7	11.4	11.5	11.5
Other	n.a.	7.8	4.3	5.1	4.9	4.9	4.8	4.7	4.6	4.5	4.4
Total Federal	n.a.	14.6	14.3	12.5	12.8	11.3	10.5	10.1	9.9	10.0	10.1
State and Local											
Medicaid	n.a.	36.6	26.0	16.8	14.4	13.2	11.7	11.7	11.4	11.4	11.4
Other	n.a.	7.9	6.1	5.8	5.6	5.8	5.7	5.6	5.3	5.2	5.0
Total State and Local	n.a.	18.3	14.4	10.9	9.9	9.5	8.8	8.8	8.7	8.7	8.7
Total National Health Expenditures	n.a.	11.4	10.7	9.6	9.6	9.1	8.8	8.6	8.4	8.2	8.0

Source: Congressional Budget Office.
Note: n.a. = not available.

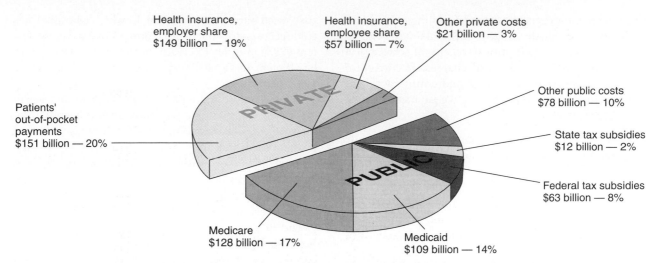

Health insurance, employer share $149 billion — 19%

Health insurance, employee share $57 billion — 7%

Other private costs $21 billion — 3%

Other public costs $78 billion — 10%

Patients' out-of-pocket payments $151 billion — 20%

State tax subsidies $12 billion — 2%

Federal tax subsidies $63 billion — 8%

Medicare $128 billion — 17%

Medicaid $109 billion — 14%

FIGURE 3.2. Public and private sources for payment of health care with estimated share of the $768 billion in health care expenditures in the fiscal year 1992. Based on data from the Department of Health and Human Services, Office of Management and Budget, and Joint Committee on Taxation.

when federal and state monies for health and social programs have been severely restricted in the recent past (Pickett & Hanlon, 1990). Figure 3.2 portrays differences in private and public payment sources.

Payment Concepts in Health Care

Reimbursement for health care services has generally been accomplished through one of two approaches, retrospective or prospective payment. Conceptually these approaches are opposite one another. It is helpful to understand their differences and their meaning for the financing and delivery of health services.

RETROSPECTIVE PAYMENT

A traditional form of reimbursement for any kind of service, including health care, is **retrospective payment** which means to reimburse for a service after it has been rendered. A fee may be established in advance. However, actual payment of that fee occurs after the fact, or retrospectively. We know this as the fee-for-service (FFS) approach.

In health care, limited accountability in the use of retrospective payment has created a number of problems. With third-party payers serving as intermediaries, nei-

ther consumers nor providers of health services were accountable for containing costs. Patients and providers alike often insisted on expensive and/or unnecessary tests and treatments. Since reimbursement was made retrospectively by the insuring agency, there was no incentive to keep a lid on this spending. Third-party reimbursement increased along with rising physician fees to create an inflationary spiral of escalating costs. Abuse of the FFS system made it more difficult to develop retrospective payment for other health care providers, including nurses.

A further problem associated with the FFS concept was its tendency to encourage sickness care, rather than wellness services. Physicians and other providers were rewarded financially for treating illness. There were few, if any, incentives for prevention or health promotion in an industry that reaped its revenues from keeping hospital beds full and caring for the sick and injured. While retrospective payment has worked well in other industries, from a cost containment as well as a public health perspective it has been problematic in health care.

PROSPECTIVE PAYMENT

Prospective reimbursement, while not a new concept, became central in the 1980s in response to the health care system's desperate need for cost containment. **Prospective payment** is a payment method based on rates derived from predictions of annual service costs that are set in advance of service delivery. Providers receive payment for services according to these fixed rates set in advance (Shaffer, 1988). Payments may be in the form of premiums paid prior to receipt of service or in response to fixed rate (not cost) charges. To correct unlimited reimbursement patterns and counteract disincentives to contain costs, prospective payment involves four steps (Dowling, 1979):

1. An external authority is empowered (by statute, market power, or voluntary compliance by providers) to set provider charges, third-party payment rates, or both.
2. Rates are set in advance of the prospective year during which they will apply and are considered fixed for the year (except for major, uncontrollable occurrences).
3. Patients, third-party payers, or both pay the prospective rates rather than the costs actually incurred by providers during the year (or charges adjusted to cover these costs).
4. Providers are at risk for losses or surpluses.

The concept of prepayment, or consumers paying in advance of health care, has existed for many years. As far back as 1933, prepaid medical groups were advocated to reduce costs and make services more accessible (Hyman, 1982). This pattern of prepayment for comprehensive services has continued ever since in a variety of forms. Examples of early plans were the Health Insurance Program of greater New York City and the Kaiser Plan. The success of these two plans, in particular, helped influence the growth of health maintenance organizations (HMOs), a type of managed care discussed later in this chapter.

Prospective payment, then, imposes constraints on spending and gives incentives for cutting costs. For these reasons the Federal government enacted into law a prospective payment plan (Social Security Amendments Act) in 1983. The plan, called **diagnosis-related groups**, is a billing classification system based on 23 major diagnostic categories and 467 diagnosis-related groups (DRGs) that provides fixed Medicare reimbursement to hospitals. Most Medicare-participating hospitals receive payment from Medicare on the basis of a fixed rate set in advance for each patient by diagnosis and based on hospital case mix (Joel, 1983; Shaffer, 1988). This system was enacted in an effort to curb Medicare spending in hospitals and to extend the program's solvency period. This regulatory approach changed Medicare hospital reimbursement "from a cost-based retrospective system, in which a hospital was paid its costs, to a fixed-price prospective payment system (PPS) in order to create incentives for hospitals to be efficient in the delivery of services" (DeLew, et al, 1992, p.162).

PPS has indeed reduced Medicare's rate of increase in inpatient hospital spending and increased hospital productivity (Coulam & Gaumer, 1992). It also reduced hospital stays and unnecessary admissions and created a boom in home health care (Fackelmann, 1987). A spinoff, however, was fierce competition among providers and mounting concern over quality of care—in hospitals, in ambulatory settings, and in home care.

The PPS concept has proven useful from a public health perspective as well. Prepaid services create incentives for providers to keep their enrollees healthy, thus reducing provider costs. An indirect benefit from fixed rates and reduced costs will be more of the health care dollar available for spending on prevention programs—a theme running through much of the Clinton administration health care reform debates.

Trends and Issues Influencing Health Economics and Financing of Health Services

COST CONTROL

Control of rapidly rising costs has been one of the largest driving forces behind health care reform in the 1980s and 1990s. Despite a variety of cost control strategies tried by public and private sector payors, health care costs have continued to rise. Health expenditures in 1980 accounted for 9.1% of the **Gross National Product** (GNP) which is the total value of all goods and services produced in the United States economy in one year. In 1990, health expenditures rose to about 12.2% of the GNP and by the year 2000 are projected to rise to 16% (Sonnefeld et al, 1991). "the United States spends more on health care services than does any other nation—on average, more than twice as much per person as the other OECD countries [Organization for Economic Cooperation and Development made up of 15 nations including the U.S.]" (DeLaw, et al 1992, p. 151). Of the United State's total health spending in 1990, about 39% was for hospital care, physician services were 19%, nursing home care was 8%, personal health spending was 22%, and non-personal health care, such as research and construction, made up 12% (Levit, et al, 1991). Table 3.2 depicts health expenditures by type of spending. Why are U.S. health care costs so high and what is being done to curb their growth?

Escalation of health care costs in the United States is due to multiple factors. Inflation has played a major role in driving up the price of goods and services associated with health care. Costs of tests, drugs, expensive technology and equipment, wages, and high-priced specialists are a few examples. Another factor in the escalation of health care costs has been the continuing dominant FFS payment system which encourages use of expen-

sive, unnecessary, and sometimes even dangerous procedures. Coronary artery bypass surgery was one of several procedures found in recent studies to be inappropriately used (Chassin, et al, 1987). Instances where medical interventions were shown in RAND Corporation studies to be inappropriate and/or unnecessary accounted for 15%–30% of medical procedures (Brook, et al, 1989, Merrick, et al, 1986). It has been estimated that the cost of clearly inappropriate medical procedures amounted to somewhere between $99 billion and $198 billion for the year 1990 (DeLew, et al, 1992).

Some argue that the high cost of medical malpractice premiums, another source of rising health care costs, has been responsible for inappropriate medical practice.

TABLE 3.2. *Actual and Projected National Health Expenditures, by Type of Spending, Selected Calendar Years, 1965 and 2000*

	Actual					Projected			
Type of Spending	1965	1980	1985	1990	1991	1992	1993	1995	2000
BILLIONS OF DOLLARS									
Hospital	14	102	168	258	289	321	351	421	644
Physician	8	42	74	129	142	156	171	205	309
Drugs, Other Nondurables	6	22	36	56	61	66	71	83	117
Nursing Home	2	20	34	53	60	67	75	91	137
All Other	12	64	110	179	201	222	244	290	425
National Health Expenditures	42	250	423	675	752	832	912	1,089	1,631
AVERAGE ANNUAL GROWTH RATE FROM PREVIOUS YEAR SHOWN (PERCENT)									
Hospital	n.a.	14.2	10.4	8.9	11.8	11.4	9.3	9.4	8.9
Physician	n.a.	11.5	12.1	11.7	10.2	9.6	9.9	9.5	8.5
Drugs, Other Nondurables	n.a.	9.1	10.8	9.0	9.0	8.2	8.1	7.9	7.2
Nursing Home	n.a.	17.9	11.3	9.3	12.4	12.1	11.4	10.2	8.5
All Other	n.a.	12.0	11.4	10.2	12.0	10.8	9.9	9.0	7.9
National Health Expenditures	n.a.	12.7	11.1	9.8	11.4	10.7	9.6	9.3	8.4
Memoranda:									
Gross Domestic Product (Billions of dollars)[a]	703	2,708	4,039	5,522	5,677	5,943	6,255	6,942	8,627
Average Annual Growth of Gross Domestic Product from Previous Year Shown (Percent)	n.a.	9.4	8.3	6.5	2.8	4.7	5.2	5.3	4.4
Ratio of National Health Expenditures to Gross Domestic Product	5.9	9.2	10.5	12.2	13.2	14.0	14.6	15.7	18.9

Source: Congressional Budget Office.
n.a. = not applicable.
[a] Economic assumptions reflect the Congressional Budget Office baseline of January 1993.

Defensive medicine, they say, is practiced by many physicians who order unnecessary procedures out of fear of malpractice suits. Defensive medicine has been estimated at 3% of health spending (American Medical Association, 1990). However, one study found that physicians' perceived probability of suit was significantly higher than actual experience warranted (Harvard Medical Practice Study, 1990). Others have argued that defensive medicine is also an opportunity to maximize FFS physician income.

Another source of rising costs has come through the extensive system of third-party insurance coverage. Third-party payment has shielded consumers from the real costs of health care, encouraging consumer demand. More important, the third-party concept created a mood of unlimited spending because someone else was paying the bill. Hospitals, physicians, and other providers could rely on payment regardless of what they spent, adding to the incentive to spend even more. Besides this are other cost-escalating features. The structure of U.S. health care is made up of a fragmented multipayer system. "The fragmented U.S. structure gives providers incentives to provide additional services and to bill for higher levels of service to increase revenues" (DeLew, et al, 1992, p.159). Associated with the complexity of the third-party payer system are high administrative costs, an added source of unnecessary health care expenditures. Also, large scale efforts in biomedical research and proliferation of new, expensive technologies further boost health care spending.

Numerous efforts to curb rising health care costs have met with mixed success. In the 1970s, strategies to control costs emphasized regulation and planning. State and local planning agencies, supported by Federal funds, designed measures to limit spending, particularly in hospitals and nursing homes. This approach was reversed in the 1980s with the introduction of competition as a cost containment strategy. Its aim was to create incentives so that both providers and insurers would become cost conscious. Because of the complexities and loopholes in the system, it has met with limited success. Nurses and other providers are encouraged to study their practice and find ways to cut costs while preserving quality. See the accompanying Research in Community Health Nursing display.

Cost sharing is a cost containment strategy in which consumers pay a portion of health care costs. Insurance deductibles of $100 to $500 per person per year are typical as are coinsurance rates of 20% per service (Employee Benefit Research Institute, 1990). Cost sharing has successfully reduced utilization of health services

Research in Community Health Nursing
CONSISTENCY AND COST OF HOME WOUND MANAGEMENT BY CONTRACT NURSES

Turner, J., et al (1994). Consistency and Cost of Home Wound Mangement by Contract Nurses. *Public Health Nursing*, 11(5):337–42.

The quality of nursing service delivered to clients in the community affects not only clients' health but also the costs associated with care. The numbers of community clients needing wound care in the home have increased as hospital stays have shortened and outpatient surgery has expanded. Yet inconsistency in wound management can slow healing and increase costs of care. Nursing research was conducted in a Visiting Nurse Association on the east coast to study consistency of wound care provided by contract registered nurses with physician orders and the agency wound care protocol. Data were collected by chart audit and observation over a five-month period. Two data collection instruments were designed and used to describe 117 home visits to 31 patients by 11 nurses. Study findings showed statistically significant differences between actual care observed and care documented in patients' records. Care consistency with a single client was high when given by one nurse but dropped when more nurses were involved. The researchers recommended several ways to improve wound care in the home that, based on their research, could potentially facilitate healing, improve efficiency of service, and reduce associated costs.

without having negative health effects. Utilization review techniques have further enhanced utilization, and cost control. However, cost sharing's usefulness when considering coverage for low-income and elderly persons appears to have limited value (DeLew, et al, 1992).

Coordinated, or managed, care is a cost control strategy used in both public and private sectors of health care. This approach includes the use of HMOs and PPOs and other alternative health care delivery models. In contrast to FFS, these models operate on a prospective payment basis and control costs by managing utilization and provider payments. The managed care model encourages the provision of services within fixed budgets, thus avoiding cost escalation. Nonetheless, as long as the system continues to reward increased FFS billings, managed care provides only a partial solution to controlling utilization.

An additional cost-control strategy used by many large employers is to self-insure. That is, the company pays for employees' health expenses instead of purchasing coverage through an insurance company. Under the Employee Retirement Income and Security Act (ERISA) of 1974, employers who self-insure their employees are exempted from certain state regulations, including mandated benefits and taxes on premiums. In addition to these savings, self-insured companies also save on the profit margins, marketing, and sales' costs that would have otherwise been passed on to them by the insurance companies. They further benefit financially by being able to invest the premiums and reserves normally secured by the other insurers. As of 1991, self-insurance provided more than one-half of all company group insurance coverage (Health Insurance Association of America, 1991).

Individual states have tried a variety of strategies to contain costs. One that has proven successful in Maryland, New Jersey, New York, and Massachusettes, is called all-payer rate setting for hospital services. This is a regulatory approach in which a system is established to set payment rates for treating each hospitalized patient (as in PPS) regardless of who pays (thus the term all-payer), or by directly setting annual budgets for hospitals. All-payer rate setting is designed to give hospitals enough revenue to cover all patients, even those without insurance; it prevents cost-shifting between payers, and it offers cost-containment incentives. Evaluations of this strategy have shown a per capita reduction in hospital cost growth rate greater than the national average (Anderson, 1992).

FINANCIAL ACCESS TO HEALTH SERVICES: THE UNINSURED AND UNDERINSURED

Associated with the rapid rise in inflation and health care costs, a growing segment of the U.S. population has had limited or no access to health care because they are without coverage for health services. Some of the poor, nearly poor, unemployed, and others who comprise the uninsured and underinsured make up between 15% and 20% of the United States' population (Relman, 1987). Fourteen percent have no insurance at all (U.S. Bureau of the Census, 1991).

The poor and the elderly are among the most vulnerable to access problems. Although PPS has had cost-saving benefits, it has also had negative effects. PPS has shortened hospital length of stays, on average by 24%. But RAND-UCLA researchers found "that under PPS elderly patients were 43 percent more likely to be discharged in an unstable condition than before" and that these patients' risk of dying was much higher than before (Warden, 1993). Medicare reimbursement cuts for doctors' office visits have resulted in more physicians restricting the number of Medicare patients that they see. These restrictions increased from 8% in 1990 to 12% in 1993 (Warden, 1993). Proposed cuts in Medicare spending, while aiming at cost control, could jeopardize access to health services for the 32 million Medicaid beneficiaries by widening the gap between public and private health insurance (Wagner, 1993). The Medicaid program, too, has recently lowered its reimbursement rates for the poor with further restriction of their access to health care. With growing numbers of homeless persons, a larger segment of the poor who might be eligible for services under Medicaid, also do not have access to health care. Furthermore, the system has yet to adequately protect the elderly from financial disaster associated with the costs of long-term care and catastrophic illness and to provide better access to these services.

In the private sector, a large number of firms do not offer health insurance to their employees. In fact, of all the uninsured, 75% are employees or their dependents of such firms (Short, Monheit, & Beauregard, 1989). Self-employed individuals also find it difficult to pay the higher costs of insurance premiums without the benefit of group rates. Consequently many of the self-employed have no access to health services except for expensive out-of-pocket payments. The current system does not provide even minimum basic coverage for these groups (Figure 3.2).

Advocates for the medically indigent, the disadvantaged, and the elderly are speaking out (Bergman, 1988); new groups have formed in recent years to study the issues and make policy recommendations (DeLew, et al, 1992; Relman, 1987). Among the issues being debated are controversial questions about such things as organ transplants: Who should receive them, and who will pay for them? Some form of universal coverage that will ensure access to health care for all citizens is a major concern for the 1990s and beyond. Meanwhile, many more individual states are considering passage of statewide health insurance policies to address some of these difficult access problems.

MANAGED CARE

The term **managed care** became popular in the late 1980s and 1990s and refers to systems that coordinate medical care for specific groups in order to promote provider efficiency and control costs. Care is "managed" by regulating the use of services and levels of provider payment. While the term may be relatively new, the concept has been practiced for many years through a variety of alternative health care delivery models.

Health Maintenance Organizations

Health maintenance organizations (HMOs) are systems in which participants prepay a fixed monthly premium to receive comprehensive health services delivered by a defined network of providers to plan participants. HMOs are perhaps the oldest model of coordinated or managed care. A number of HMOs have existed for decades but many more have developed in recent years. Enrollees benefit from lower costs, less cost-sharing, and minimal billing paperwork.

From 1930 to 1965, the HMO movement, supported initially by the private sector, gradually gained federal backing. Group plans were a part of Medicare and Medicaid bills and the Partnership for Health Act. The HMO Act of 1973 demonstrated stronger federal support. Amendments to this act in 1976 lifted restrictions and further encouraged HMOs.

The chief characteristics of an HMO are the following (Rapoport et al., 1982, p. 257):

1. There is a contract between the HMO and the consumers (or their representative), the so-called "enrolled population."
2. A regular (usually monthly) premium to cover specified (and typically broad) services is paid for or by each enrollee to the HMO; few additional charges are levied because the payment mechanism is not basically fee-for-service.
3. The HMO contracts with professional providers to deliver the services due the enrollees; the basis for reimbursing those providers varies among HMOs.

Official encouragement, government subsidies, and the pressures for cost control spurred the growth of HMOs. Some HMOs follow the traditional model that employs physicians, nurses and other professionals, builds their own hospital and clinic facilities, and serves only their own enrollees. Other HMOs provide some services while contracting for the rest. See Figure 3.3. HMO model variations include solo practice physicians

(some also continuing FFS medicine) who affiliate with hospitals. Americans enrolled in HMOs, whether through government programs like Medicare or employer-based or private insurers, constitute 15% of the population, numbering nearly 37 million (Porter, Ball, and Kraus, 1992).

HMOs have been viewed as a positive alternative delivery system because of their potential for conserving costs owing to their emphasis on prevention, health promotion, and ambulatory care, with a concomitant reduction in hospital and medical care utilization (DeLew, et al, 1992). However, some have questioned whether the cost-savings might be due in part to favorable selection of enrollees. Quality concerns have also been raised about the danger of underserving enrollees in order to stay within payment limits (DeLew, et al, 1992).

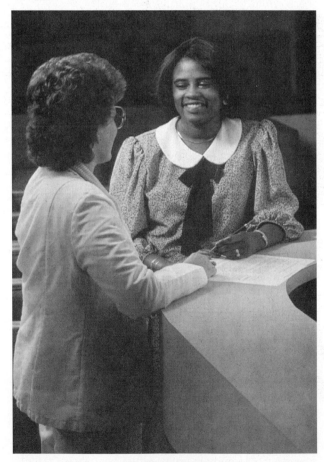

FIGURE 3.3. A community health nurse works collaboratively with another health team member to promote client health in a health maintenance organization.

Preferred Provider Organizations

Preferred provider organizations (PPOs) are another model of managed or coordinated care that developed more recently (Ellwood, 1985). A PPO is a network of physicians, hospitals and other health-related services that contracts with a third-party payor organization to provide comprehensive health services to subscribers on a fixed fee-for-service basis. Because of contractual fixed costs, employing organizations who subscribe can offer medical services to their employees at discounted rates. PPOs practice utilization review and use formal standards for selecting providers (DeLew, et al, 1992). Enrollment in PPOs has been growing. Among participants of medium and large employer health plans, 1% were enrolled in 1986 and 10% in 1989 (U.S. Department of Labor, 1990). Early use of PPOs appears to promote cost savings, but the long-range cost-effectiveness of this model has yet to be determined.

Other variations on managed care models continue to appear. One is the point-of-service (POS) network which combines HMO cost-containment with PPO freedom to choose providers. Enrollees may use their HMO's physicians or may select outside physicians by paying a higher coinsurance charge (DeLew, et al, 1992). Issues of cost, quality, extent of coverage, and freedom to choose providers remain dominant in discussions of the managed care concept.

HEALTH CARE RATIONING

The concept of **rationing** in health care refers to limiting the provision of adequate health services in order to save costs but in so doing jeopardizing the well-being of some groups of people (Wagner, 1993). Rationing implies that resources are limited and must therefore be used sparingly. Its effect is to restrict people's choices and deny access to beneficial services. While some consumer choice is involved, for the most part it is the providers and insurers of health services who are currently and unilaterally making rationing decisions in order to contain costs. When rationing occurs, there is always the danger of compromising what is acceptable to consumers and the quality of services they receive.

The practice of rationing in health care has been present for many years. With limited resources for health services delivery, government programs have had to establish strict eligiblity levels and monitor the use of these resources sparingly in order to ensure their most equitable distribution. In the past, private insurers, to maintain organizational viability and some kind of profit mar-

gin, have engaged in rationing to exclude enrollees at greatest risk of health problems (Warden, 1993). Advances in knowledge and technical capabilities through research and technology compounds rationing decisions. When several individuals need an organ transplant and only one organ is available, what criteria should be used to select the recipient? Now that we know certain lifestyle behaviors, such as smoking or driving without restraints, create health risks, should people who engage in these activities pay a higher price for health care or should they be excluded from certain services? Should a younger person needing specialized surgery take priority over an elderly person needing similar care? There are no easy answers. Providers and insurers have struggled with these difficult policy issues for many years. In today's health economics, the problems are even more complex. See the following Issues in Community Health Nursing display for more informtion.

COMPETITION AND REGULATION

Competition and regulation in health economics have often been viewed as antagonistic and incompatible concepts. **Competition** means a contest between rival health care organizations for resources and clients. **Regulation** refers to mandated procedures and practices affecting health services delivery that are enforced by law. In a society where freedom of choice and individualism have long been valued, competition provides opportunities for entrepreneurism, free enterprise, and scientific advancement. Yet, to promote the public good, oversee equitable distribution of health services, and foster community-wide participation, regulation also serves an important role.

From the 1950s through the 1970s the federal government assumed a strong role in the financing and regulation of health services. First, federal subsidy of health care costs increased and there was greater federal control of state programs. Health services became regionalized and more comprehensive. Federal appropriations supported operational as well as capital and planning costs. There was greater federal support for health research and the training of health professionals. Group medical practice multiplied as a cost-saving measure. Over 60% of the population was covered by some form of prepaid health insurance, largely because of the effects of Medicare and Medicaid. There was an increase in interagency health planning cooperation and improved health program evaluation. Neighborhood health centers, community mental health centers, and other programs developed to improve health care access

Issues in Community Health Nursing
HEALTH CARE RATIONING

Rationing has revived as a major issue in health economics. Health care providers and third-party insurers increasingly are making cost containment decisions that, intentionally or unintentionally, lead to limited access and negative outcomes for certain groups (Wagner, 1993). Decisions to raise premium prices, increase cost-sharing levels, or insist on exclusions for some types of services all have the effect of rationing health care. Insurees without the financial means to absorb these additional costs face limitations in and denial of needed health services. Further rationing occurs when beneficiaries are limited in choice of the physician, nurse, or other professional they are permitted to see.

A fundamental question of rationing is who gets to decide? Many argue that consumers have a right to informed choices (Grace, 1990) and to decide if or how they will ration their health spending. At the same time, public and private providers and insurers must contain costs (Warden, 1993). If some form of rationing is necessary, and current financial pressures would make that appear true, then an equitable solution must be found. Other countries employ selected rationing, such as in England where dialysis is not generally done for persons over age 55 or in Scandinavia where babies below a certain birth weight are not resuscitated. Health care reform debates in the U.S. have generated a variety of approaches with states such as Oregon and Vermont implementing deliberate forms of rationing.

ify and guide implementation" (Brown, 1992, p. 20); they are issued under the authority of law, and are part of most federal health care progams. Examples include regulations governing project grants such as HMO development, formula grants such as Hill-Burton, and entitlements such as Medicare and Medicaid. Regulatory *programs* are created from freestanding legislative enactments and are designed to accomplish specific goals such as accreditation and licensing rules for hospitals, public health agencies, and other health services providers. Regulatory *policies* are more broad in focus and involve "decisions that shape the health care system by constraining the flow of resources into it and setting limits on key players' freedom of action" (Brown, 1992, p. 21). Examples of regulatory policies can be found by reviewing state or federal budget proposals for funding programs such as health manpower training, research, and technology development.

In the early 1980s the passage of the Omnibus Budget Reconciliation Act caused dramatic changes affecting health care. The federal government, having failed to contain rising health care costs, shifted responsibility for the public's health and welfare back to state and local governments. Large amounts of federal funding for health research, health manpower training, and public health programs were withdrawn. Continued escalation of health care costs prompted a concentrated effort among public and private providers alike to find cost-containment measures. Out of all this grew the competition versus regulation debate.

Competition, its proponents say, offers wider consumer choice and positive incentives for cost containment and enhanced efficiency (DeLew, et al, 1992). That is, consumers are free to select among various health plans on the basis of cost, quality, and range of services. Competing providers must develop efficient production and distribution methods to stay in business, and consumers, because of the required cost sharing that is part of the competition model, are more likely to use only necessary services. Examples of competition are increasingly evident as a growing number of health plans, including HMOs and PPOs, vie with insurance companies for subscribers. Many hospitals, too, compete aggressively for patients. For example some hospitals now promote their services with advertisements depicting the new mother and father having a candlelight dinner in the hospital with their newborn infant in the bassinette beside them.

Although it appears that competition offers the best service for the least cost, regulation advocates argue

for everyone. Although costs were rising, it was a period of relative economic stability that emphasized quality of care. During this period the federal government assumed a major role regulating the planning, use, and reimbursement of health care services.

Health care incorporates four major kinds of regulation: (1) laws, (2) regulations, (3) programs, and (4) policies (Brown, 1992). *Laws* that regulate health care include any legislation that governs financing or delivery of health services such as legislation that regulates Medicare reimbursement to hospitals. *Regulations* "clar-

there are at least four problems associated with the competition model. (1) Consumers often don't make proper health care choices because of limited knowledge of health services. (2) Competition may discriminate against enrolling certain consumers, especially high-risk, high-cost patients, thus excluding those who may need services the most. (3) The competition model may not encourage enough teaching and research, expensive elements of our present system. (4) Quality may be sacrificed to keep down costs. (Weiss, 1982) Regulation advocates conclude that standardization and controls are needed to guarantee quality and equal access. Leaders in the field have concluded that both competition and regulation are needed (Ehlinger, 1982; Somers, 1986; Enthoven & Kronick, 1989; Reinhardt, 1993). With foresight McNerney said, "It is rapidly becoming apparent that what we need is a proper balance between competition and regulation with more effective links. . . . regulation [should be] used as a force to keep the market honest"(1980, p.1091).

Managed Competition

The idea of managed competition was born from the controversy over competition versus regulation and driven by the need for health care reform. **Managed competition**, the hope for the 1990s, would combine market competition to achieve cost savings with government regulation to achieve expanded coverage (Merline, 1993). This idea, whose origin is credited to economist Alain C. Enthoven of Stanford University, has played a major part in health care reform debates. It seeks to address the two fundamental issues driving reform—cost containment and universal access to health care.

Managed competition was seen as a market-based solution that placed accountability for resolving the health care crisis with the insurance industry. Under this concept, sponsors in the form of collective purchasing agents, represent consumers clustered into large groups. The sponsors negotiate with insurers or health plans to offer subscribers an array of choices based on costs and quality among various health plans. Insurers must accept all applicants without excluding those at poorer risk and at the same time must control costs (Mucklo, 1993).

Under managed competition consumers would choose between competing health insurance plans in the form of 'super-HMOs' that are privately owned and for-profit. These plans must "compete for managed care

contracts from large employers and group purchasers known as "health insurance purchasing cooperatives" (HIPCs) (Young, 1993, p.945). The proposed HIPCs would be mostly geographically-based (region or state), quasi-governmental organizations that would consolidate purchasing power in the health care market. HIPCs would contract only with insurers whose plans both meet federal guidelines and include a mandated package of basic benefits (Merline, 1993), hence the "managed" or regulated segment. Insurance companies would also have to prepare regular reports on the quality of their services to give consumers a basis for making an informed comparison among plans. Other common features of managed competition proposals include regulation that prevents screening out high-risk enrollees, penalties for companies that try to achieve better risk pools, community rating to prevent companies from setting rates by risk pool, and guaranteed coverage for all who apply (Congressional Budget Office, 1993).

Proponents of managed competition cite many advantages. Managed competition would encourage insurance companies to compete on price and quality of services to attract enrollees. It also would offer consumers tax incentive to purchase the lowest-cost plans that meet minimum benefits requirements. Managed competition, while market-driven, would be highly regulated to ensure quality and access. Besides HIPCs, some managed care proposals include the formation of two additional government bodies; "a National Health Board to set the minimum benefits package, and an Outcomes Management Standards Board to set standards for the health plans' reporting on the quality of their care" (Merline, 1993, p. 2). Thus managed competition, as a reform concept, could have the potential for reducing expenditures and improving access to health care coverage.

There are problems, however, with managed competition. It remains untested anywhere in the world and many believe that it will fail to achieve the needed cuts in health care spending growth. Similar models, such as HMOs and the Federal Employee Health Benefits Program, have failed to slow health care inflation (Kronick, et al, 1993). Nearly 25% of U.S. health care spending has gone to billing and bureaucracy because of the heavy administrative burden imposed by multiple private insurers; this is compared with only 11% of Canadian health care spending. Private insurance overhead in the U.S. averages 13% of premiums while for Medicare and Medicaid administration it is less than 3%

and for Canada's single-payer system it is less than 1%. Some critics believe managed competition's regulations will result in additional administrative layers increasing overhead and driving health care costs even higher (Young, 1993).

Some argue that managed care networks which enhance managed competition and enable health insurance plans to control cost and quality, would also limit consumers' choices in selecting their own providers and hospitals. Consumers would have to pay out-of-pocket if they choose services outside the network. Many people have not chosen managed care. A Harris poll conducted in 1990 showed that only 7% of those surveyed were "very interested" in joining an HMO and 63% were "hardly interested" or "not at all interested" (Merline, 1993). As of 1993, less than 20% of the U.S. population was enrolled in an HMO. Cost-saving incentives built into managed competition networks would further enhance the potential for reduced quality of services and denial of care to enrollees.

A major criticism of managed competition is its potential failure to provide equitable and universal coverage. Proposals differ about whether employers are required to provide health insurance coverage for their employees. One study done by the Employee Benefits Research Institute in 1993 showed that large employers would benefit financially under managed competition while small businesses would find the cost burden heavy and many individuals, such as the self-employed, would remain uninsured(Mucklo, 1993). Questions remain concerning the tax treatment of health insurance premiums, how sponsors should be organized, and what standard benefits should be offered. A basic benefits package, critics argue, must address special concerns affecting such groups as women and the elderly, including coverage for long term care, home care, mental health, abortions, and prescriptions. Competition among providers would be inefficient in rural areas with fewer providers, such as county nursing agencies and isolated small-town hospitals, scattered over great distances.

While the private insurance industry, many physicians, and others endorse the managed competition concept, a growing number of groups in the country strongly oppose it. Among the organizations against managed competition and supporting some kind of single-payer plan are the American Nurses' Association, the National League for Nursing, the National Women's Health Network, the American Public Health Association, Physicians for a National Health Program, the American Association for Retired Persons, and the Older Women's League. Dissatisfaction with managed competition as a reform solution has spurred a host of different proposals, all attempting to address cost savings and access issues.

Universal Coverage and a Single Payer System

A different approach to health care reform emphasizes universal health insurance coverage through a stronger role played by government. This so-called **single payer system** would replace the nearly 1500 health insurance companies in the U.S. with a single, public-sector insurer that would entitle all citizens to **universal coverage**. Efforts to accomplish this approach have been evident for many years.

Growing concern over the cost and accessibility of health services in the 1960s and again in the mid-1970s led to a renewed focus on **national health insurance (NHI)** as a solution whereby health insurance coverage would be provided for all citizens through a single payer system. NHI has been debated since 1912 as its proponents have sought comprehensive health care protection for the aged and needy in particular (Figure 3.4).Numerous attempts to pass some form of NHI have resulted in piecemeal legislation that added various benefits for Social Security recipients. The Kerr-Mills Bill (1960) set a precedent of public financing for elderly persons who were "medically needy" but not on public assistance. Medicare (1965) was the first compulsory NHI program in the United States. However, it reached only 10% of the population (Somers and Somers, 1977).

In the 1970s the debate over NHI revived in full force. Many proposed NHI bills were considered by Congress. The seeming consensus over the need for government to assure access to needed health services for the total population was misleading. Divergent interests and conflicting philosophies led to heated debate with four issues emerging as core areas of controversy. First was the public-private mix. What should be the amount and nature of private health insurance involvement in the public program? Second was the cost-sharing issue. To what extent, if any, should consumers share in the cost of the coverage? Third, what should be the amount and nature of cost and quality controls built into the program? And fourth, should an NHI program be used as a vehicle for reform of the health care provision system (Somers and Somers, 1977)? Resolution de-

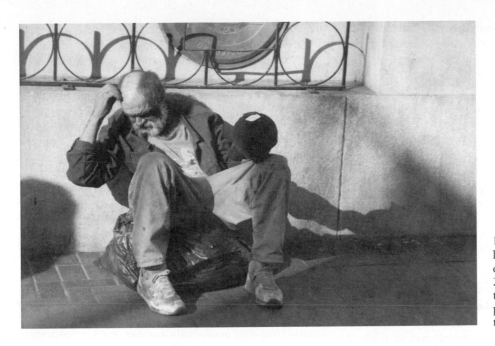

FIGURE 3.4. People who have little or no health insurance coverage make up between 15% and 20% of the U.S. population. National health insurance has been proposed as a way to alleviate the problem.

pended, in part, on reconciling the major roles of large private health insurers, hospitals, and the medical profession along with the nation's inherent aversion to direct government intervention.

In the decade of the 1980s, study of NHI as an important concept continued. Somers and Somers (1977) recommended that NHI in its ideal form should include the following:

1. Universal coverage regardless of income;
2. Equitable financing using multiple sources but channeled through one mechanism;
3. Comprehensive and balanced benefit structure;
4. Incentives for efficient and effective use of resources and discouragement of health care price inflation;
5. Controlled competition in the underwriting and administration of the program;
6. Appropriate and feasible consumer options;
7. Administrative simplicity;
8. Flexibility; and
9. Acceptability to providers and consumers.

These recommendations continue to be viable and have permeated health care reform discussions in the 1990s.

Some proponents of universal coverage point to Canada's health care system as a model to emulate. Under the Canada Health Act each provincial govern-

ment is responsible for providing health care to all citizens. Each province must develop a plan that meets the following criteria (Young, 1993):

1. Provides universal coverage that does not interfere with reasonable access;
2. Makes benefits transferable between provinces;
3. Provides insurance for all medically necessary services; and
4. Is publicly administered and nonprofit.

Canadian health services are primarily tax supported through provincial financing and national government subsidies. The system has been successful in the past but Canada now faces threats to that success in the form of a high national debt, a soaring budget deficit, rising health care costs, and an aging population which "account(s) for about 50 percent of all health care dollars spent" (Barnhill, 1992, p. 44). Still, the principle of spreading the financial risk for health care over the entire population has worked in many countries, including Canada. Furthermore, polls indicate that a majority of Americans "would prefer government-financed national health insurance" (Young, 1993, p. 946).

As a strategy for health care reform, proponents say a major advantage of the single payer approach is that accountability for cost saving, quality, and access lie with a single payer, most likely the government. This contrasts with accountability resting in multiple, competing insurers under managed competition. Other advantages include its more comprehensive approach to reform, its limiting the role of private insurance, and eliminating the tie between health insurance and employment. Furthermore, a single payer approach would significantly reduce administrative expenditures by eliminating the overhead costs of multiple private insurers. Supporters of a single payer system, including the nursing and public health professions, who are concerned for at-risk populations, believe it offers the best approach for getting rid of inequities in the system, providing universal access, and reducing soaring costs.

Those supporting universal health care and a single payer system stress certain guidelines to be incorporated into reform proposals. The Older Women's League summarizes them as follows:

- "universal access not tied to employment;
- comprehensive benefits including preventive, diagnostic, mental health and treatment services;
- long-term care avaliable at home and in institutions;
- choice of providers;
- cost controls;
- and public funding through a progressively financed plan and public administration"(1993, p.1).

HEALTH CARE REFORM

Consumers and professionals both agree that health care reform is needed in the U.S. The disagreement lies in what form it should take. At issue is a fundamental conflict in values between advocates of the managed competition model and advocates of the universal coverage, or single-payer plan. On the one hand are those who strongly value the competition model which insures a free market, individualism, and the right to choose the type of health care one desires.

On the other hand, proponents of universal coverage argue that more comprehensive benefits are needed to include the unemployed or physically or economically disadvantaged who cannot afford health care. Futhermore, they argue that universal coverage will emphasize prevention and primary health care as key factors in reducing long-range health care costs and, even more important, assuring improved levels of health for the public. *Nursing's Agenda for Health Care Reform* supported this emphasis by promoting nurses as primary providers of *health* care, a role enthusiastically endorsed

by Donna Shalala, who became U.S. Secretary of Health and Human Services in 1993, in a keynote address to the National League for Nursing's 20th Biennial Convention in 1991 (Shalala, 1993).

Designers of health reform have faced a difficult challenge in reconciling these conflicting views. As a result, elements of both models were used in an attempt to shape an improved system. Reform proposals included an incremental plan that allowed for a flexible transition and opportunities for states to experiment with both approaches.

Reinhardt (1993) points out the importance of separating the task of financing (how insurance funds are collected) from disbursement (how providers receive payment). Financing might be tried through an income-based premium that would go into a publicly-administered health insurance fund. Method of collection and administration are, of course, not yet decided. Japan and Germany have used a payroll-collection method for many years to successfully finance their health care. Supplemental financing (to adjust for low-income or no-income households) might come from an extra tax on the affluent or a tax on products that are known to contribute directly to health care costs, such as alcohol and tobacco. Disbursement of health insurance funds could occur in at least two ways. A strictly federal program could enroll all Americans who are not privately insured and disburse funds through a program like Medicare. A second option could be to disburse capitated funds from the federal government to states for payment to providers. In some cases state funds could supplement federal disbursement. Forms of either the single payer or managed competition models could be tried to accomplish disbursement, allowing states to adjust for local preferences and existing delivery systems (Reinhardt, 1993).

Another aspect of health care reform that has been considered is a global budget. This simply means that a single, nation-wide health budget, whose funding might come from the income-based premiums mentioned earlier plus supplemental sources, would help control certain aspects of national health spending. The amount of money in this budget would help determine the size of disbursements to federal programs, like Medicare, and to the states. States could still spend more on health care out of their own resources, if they chose.

A standard set of benefits, set by law, and enjoyed by the entire population, regardless of age, health, income and employment status, is an important health care reform element. Many countries have successfully implemented such a package under a plan called a "statutory" model. Various versions of this model have worked well in Austria, France, Belgium, Japan, Germany, the Netherlands, and Switzerland. In this model, health insurance falls under the rubric of social security and is funded through government mandated payroll premiums or taxes. Payment is made to private sector health insurers—called "sickness funds" in some countries. Individuals select among nationwide plans and choose their doctor and hospital. Reimbursement for services is made directly to providers by insurers. This model eliminates the need for separate programs such as Medicaid and Medicare. It also provides uniform and comprehensive benefits (Randal, 1993).

Other issues to be addressed in health reform include making the fee-for-service system more accountable, eliminating adverse risk selection, and providing informed choices to consumers. While reform is under way, there continues to be a need for advocates of universal access and cost containment to influence the process. Furthermore, health reform proposals must be encouraged to focus on the central question: do they fund the promotion of health and prevention of illness or simply pay for the diagnosis and treatment of those who are already ill? World Bank evaluations show that public health interventions have repeatedly been found to be more cost effective than medical services, yet health reform proposals have paid minimal attention to this critical issue (Freeman and Robbins, 1994). Community health nurses can play an influential role in emphasizing the importance of incorporating health promotion services into future health reform efforts through political involvement and policy development. An example of one such policy development is the international effort to control population expansion (see World Watch display).

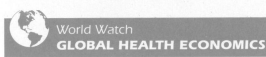

World Watch
GLOBAL HEALTH ECONOMICS

Health economics on a global scale is directly tied to an alarming rate of world population expansion. World population growth was relatively slow in earlier centuries taking hundreds of thousands of years to reach 10 million by about 8000 B.C. and 100 million about the time of Christ. By 1950 it was 2500 million and more than doubled to 5500 million by 1993. The urgency of the situation prompted representatives of the national academies of science throughout the world to convene a "science summit" on World Population in New Delhi, India in October of 1993. Participants developed a joint statement calling for the governments of all countries "to adopt an integrated policy on population and sustainable development on a global scale" (Mehra, 1994, p. 7). The Statement reflected "continued concern about the intertwined problems of rapid population growth, wasteful resource consumption, environmental degradation and poverty" (Mehra, 1994, p. 7). The scientists argued that worldwide social, economic, and environmental problems could not be successfully addressed without a stable world population and urged a goal of zero population growth by the end of the next generation. They recommended equality for women, free choice on family size, access to family planning and contraceptive options, and elimination of unsafe practices. They concluded that the responsibility lay with both the public and private sectors of the international community (Mehra, 1994).

Effects of Health Economics on Community Health Practice

Health economics has significantly affected community health and community health practice by advancing (1) disincentives for efficient use of resources, (2) incentives for illness care, and (3) conflict with public health values.

DISINCENTIVES FOR EFFICIENT USE OF RESOURCES

All the system structures that directly or indirectly promote cost escalation and prevent cost containment contribute to disincentives for efficient use of resources. For example, retrospective financial reimbursement, with its lack of limit setting, encourages spending on non-essential tests and treatments and drives up costs. Tax-deductible employer contributions for health care coverage and nontaxable employee health benefits encourage unnecessary use of services and drive up costs. Lack of cost sharing by consumers and no financial risk for decisions made by providers create further disincentives to keep costs down.

Community health has been affected in several ways. Abuse of resources in some parts of the system means a depletion in other areas. Community and public health programs have suffered greatly in recent years from diminished federal and state allocations and severe budget cuts affecting even basic community health services. Competition from the private sector in home care and other community services, such as health education programs, has forced traditional public health agencies to reexamine their programs and seek new avenues for service and new revenue sources. Costs indirectly affect even appropriate use of nursing personnel in community health. Failing to recognize the differences in skills of community health nurses and less prepared personnel, proliferating agencies in community health have often hired persons underqualified to give the kind of high-caliber and comprehensive care that is needed in many instances. Finally, the advent of prospective payment and limits on the length of stay have encouraged early hospital discharge with the result that an increasing number of more acutely ill people need home care services. The immediate effect has been an increase in the demand for highly skilled and more expensive home care services which requires changes in community health care provision patterns. The long-range effects of this phenomenon on family stress and caregiver health, on community health care reimbursement, and on the nature and structure of community health services, including the role of the community health nurse, have yet to be determined.

INCENTIVES FOR ILLNESS CARE

The traditional American health care system inadvertently tends to promote illness because health care providers have primarily been rewarded for treating problems, not for preventing them. Hospitals have had more income when their beds stayed full of sick or injured people. The bulk of most reimbursable health services has centered around treating illness or disability by hospitals, physicians, nursing homes, ambulatory care, and skilled nursing care in the home—settings in which the individual must play the role of patient. Health promotional nursing activities such as comprehensive prenatal, maternal, and infant care; health education; childhood immunizations; and home services to

enable the elderly to live independently have not been covered by most insurers.

A system that financially supports illness care affects community health practice in several ways. The number and severity of health problems in a community increase when individuals postpone care because they cannot afford visits to the doctor or clinic. It has been more difficult to encourage community clients to assume responsibility for their own health and to engage in self-care and prevention. Furthermore, such illness-oriented incentives create a basic societal valuing of illness care that, conversely, devalues wellness care. Health promotion and disease prevention efforts become second-ranked priorities in competition for scarce resources. In communities where a greater proportion of community health practice is spent on treatment of disorders and rehabilitation, resources are limited for prevention and health promotion. Prepayment methods and the growth of managed care have been positive moves in the direction of a more wellness-oriented financial incentive structure. An HMO has the incentive to offer preventive and health-promoting services such as early detection and treatment of symptoms, regular physical examinations, and health teaching. Health care reform proposals show promise of greater recognition of the cost-saving value of prevention efforts.

CONFLICT WITH PUBLIC HEALTH VALUES

Competition in health care is a reality with which community health practice must cope. Although competition offers a number of benefits, it poses some dilemmas for community health that are not easily resolved. Values underlying the competition model are in direct conflict with several basic public health values (Ehlinger, 1982). Competition, for example, encourages service providers to be adversarial—to win. Public health operates on the basis of collaboration and cooperation (Ray and Flynn, 1980). Competition serves a selected market determined, in part, by those able to purchase products or services. Public health is committed to serving all persons in need, regardless of ability to pay (Young, 1993, Beauchamp, 1975). The competition model focuses on individuals and is present-oriented; public health is concerned with aggregates and is future-oriented, emphasizing prevention. Competition establishes relatively fixed limits for service, while public health must remain flexible if it is to respond to the total population's health needs.

The effect of those philosophical differences plus the constraints, such as civil service restrictions and political influences, under which most public health agencies must operate, makes it very difficult for them to compete. They must remain committed to providing the health promotion and disease prevention services that are their public trust. Yet some aspects of competition seem necessary if they are to stay in business. Exclusion from health care competition, freedom from unreasonable constraints, and dependable financial support are needed to maintain the organizational viability of many public health agencies. Competition may also serve as a stimulus for new and innovative community health services and the possible introduction of new roles and revenue sources for traditional public health agencies. Health care reform implementation will need to address issues affecting delivery of public health services.

Summary

Health economics studies the production, distribution, and consumption of health care goods and services in order to maximize the use of scarce resources to benefit the most people. This science underlies the financing of the health care system. It is influenced by micro as well as macroeconomics.

Health care is funded through both public and private sources that fall into three categories: third-party payers, direct consumer payment, and private support.

Health care services have been reimbursed either retrospectively, typical of fee-for-service plans, or prospectively, typical of most HMOs.

Several issues and trends have influenced community health care financing and delivery and are important to understanding health economics and helping to improve community health. They include cost control, financial access, managed care, health care rationing, competition and regulation, managed competition, universal coverage and a single payer system, and health care reform.

The changing nature of health care financing in the past has adversely affected community health and its practice in three important ways. (1) Retrospective payment without limiting costs, tax-deductible employer contributions for health care coverage and nontaxable employee health benefits, plus a lack of consumer involvment in cost-sharing have all created disincentives for efficient use of resources. (2) Because the health care system has traditionally reimbursed only for treatment of the ill or disabled with no reward for health promotion and prevention efforts, it has promoted incentives to focus only on illness care. (3) The competition model that has for so long driven health care costs up and eliminated many groups of people from being able to afford health care services has generated a conflict with the basic public health values of health promotion and disease prevention for all persons. Health care reform efforts in the 1990s have focused on reversing these patterns by combining positive elements of competition, free-enterprise, and regulation to allow all individuals access to adequate health care.

Activities to Promote Critical Thinking

1. Compare and contrast the goal of public health with the goal of health economics.
2. Interview a community nursing administrator to determine the impact that escalating health care costs have had on community health and the delivery of community health nursing services.
3. Discuss the pros and cons of prospective payment versus retrospective reimbursement. How has each influenced community health and health care?
4. Form two teams with your classmates and debate the advantages and disadvantages of managed competition as opposed to universal coverage and a single payer system.
5. Read Freeman and Robbins (1993) from the reference list or a similar article on health reform and describe the risks of failure to include public health in reform proposals. What are some possible solutions that would incorporate public health?

REFERENCES

American Medical Association, (1990). *The Cost of Medical Professional Liability in the 1980s.* Chicago: AMA.

Anderson, G.F. (1992). All-payer rate setting: Down but not out. *Health Care Financing Review 1991 Annual Supplement.* HCFA Pub. No. 03322. Office of Research and Demonstrations. Washington DC: US Government Printing Office, March, 42–44.

Barnhill, W. (1992). Canadian Health Care: Would it work here? *Arthritis Today,* Nov–Dec, 35–44.

Beauchamp, D.E. (1975). Public health: Alien ethic in a strange land? *American Journal of Public Health, 65,* 1338–39.

Bergman, G. (1988). Standing alone: Why the U.S. has no national health system. *Grey Panther Network, 17*(1), 13, 18.

Brook, R., Kamberg, C., Mayer-Oakes, A., et al. (1989). *Appropriateness of Acute Medical Care for the Elderly: An Analysis of the Literature.* Santa Monica, CA: RAND.

Brown, L.D. (1992). Political evolution of Federal health care regulation. *Health Affairs,* Winter, 17–37.

Burwell, B. (1991). *Middle-class welfare: Medicaid estate planning for long-term care coverage.* Lexington, MA: SysteMetrics/McGraw-Hill.

Chassin, M.R., Kosecoff, J., & Park, R.E. (1987). Does inappropriate use explain geographic variation in the use of health care services? *Journal of the American Medical Association, 258*(18), 2533–2537.

Congressional Budget Office (1993). *Managed competition and its potential to reduce health spending,* May. Washington, DC: The Congress of the United States.

Coulam, R. & Gaumer, G.L. (1992). Medicare's prospective payment system: A critical appraisal. *Health Care Financing Review 1991 Annual Supplement,* HCFA Pub.No.03322. Office of Research and Demonstration. Washington, DC: US Government Printing Office.

DeLew, N., Greenberg, G., & Kinchen, K. (1992). A layman's guide to the U.S. health care system. *Health Care Financing Review, 14*(1), 151–169.

Dowling, W. L. (1979). Prospective rate setting: Concept and practice. *Topics in Health Care Financing, 3*(2), 35–42.

Ehlinger, E. (1982). Implications of the competition model. *Nursing Outlook, 30,* 518–21.

Ellwood, P. (1985). Alternative delivery systems: Health care on the move. *Journal of Ambulatory Care Management, 8*(4), 1–2.

Employee Benefit Research Institute (1990). *Fundamentals of Employee Benefit Programs.* Washington, DC: Author.

Enthoven, A. & Kronick, R. (1989). A consumer-choice health plan for the 1990s. *The New England Journal of Medicine,* Jan.5, 29–37, Jan.12, 94–101.

Fackelmann, K., & Sorian, R. (1987). Perspectives: Florida uproar shakes HMO movement. *McGraw-Hill's Medicine and Health,* May 4, *41*(18), Suppl. 4.

Freeman, P. & Robbins, A. (1994). National health care reform minus public health: A formula for failure. *Journal of Public Health Policy, 15*(3), 261–282.

Grace, H. (1990). Can health care costs be contained? *Nursing and Health Care, 11*(3), 125.

Harvard Medical Practice Study. (1990). *Patients, Doctors, and Lawyers: Medical Injury, Malpractice Litigation and Patient Compensation in New York.* Cambridge, MA: President and Fellows of Harvard College.

Health Insurance Association of America. (1991). *Source Book of Health Insurance Data.* Washington, DC: HIAA.

Hyman, H. (1982). *Health planning: A systematic approach.* (2nd ed.). Rockville, MD: Aspen.

Joel, L.A. (1983). DRGs: The state of the art of reimbursement for nursing services. *Nursing and Health Care, 4,* 560–63.

"Known welfare fraud is only the tip of the iceberg." (1983, November). *U.S. News & World Report,* 42–43.

Kronick, R., Goodman, D., Wennberg, J., & Wagner, E. (1993). The marketplace in health care reform: The demographic limitations of managed competition. *The New England Journal of Medicine, 328*(2), 148–52.

Levit, K., Lazenby, H., Cowan, C., et al. (1991). National health expenditures, 1990. *Health Care Financing Review, 13*(1), 29–54. HCFA Pub.No. 03341, Office of Research and Demonstration, Washington, DC: U.S. Government Printing Office.

McNerney, W.J. (1980). Control of health care costs in the 1980s. *The New England Journal of Medicine, 303,* 1088–95.

Mehra, L. (1994). Science academies call for action on population. *World Health, 47*(3), 7.

Merline, J. (1993). What is 'managed competition'? *Investor's Business Daily,* April 5, 1–3.

Merrick, N.J., Brook, R.H., Fink, A., et al. (1986). Use of carotid endarterectomy in five California Veteran's Administration Medical Centers. *Journal of the American Medical Association, 256*(18), 2531–2535.

Mucklo, M. (1993). Health care reform: managed competition and beyond. *Medical Benefits, 10*(7), 1–2, April 15.

Older Women's League (1993). Speak up on universal health care. *The Owl Observer, 13*(1), 1, Jan–Feb.

Pickett, G. & Hanlon, J. (1990). *Public health: Administration and practice.* (9th ed.). St. Louis: Times Mirror/Mosby.

Porter, M., Ball, P., & Kraus, N. (1992). *The Interstudy Competitive Edge.* Excelsior, MN: Interstudy.

Randal, J. (1993). Wrong prescription: why managed competition is no cure. *The Progressive,* May:22–25.

Rapoport, J., Robertson, R.L., & Stewart, B. (1982). *Understanding Health Economics.* Rockville, MD: Aspen.

Ray, D., & Flynn, B. (1980). Competition vs. cooperation in community health nursing. *Nursing Outlook, 28*(10), 626–30.

Reinhardt, U.E. (1993). An "all-American" health reform proposal. *Journal of American Health Policy,* May–June, 11–17.

Relman, A. S. (1987). The National Leadership Commission on Health Care. *The New England Journal of Medicine, 317*(11), 706–7.

Shalala, D.E. (1993). Nursing and society: the unfinished agenda for the 21st century. *Nursing and Health Care, 14*(6), 289–291.

Shaffer, F. (1988). DRGs: A new era for health care. *Nursing Clinics of North America, 23*(3), 453–463.

Short, P., Monheit, A., & Beauregard, K. (1989). *National medical expenditure survey: A profile of uninsured Americans.* Research findings. Rockville, MD: National Center for Health Services Research and Health Care Technology Assessment.

Somers, A.R., & Somers, H. (1977). *Health and health care: Policies in perspective.* Germantown, MD: Aspen.

Somers, A.R. (1986). The changing demand for health services: A historical perspective and some thoughts for the future. *Inquiry, 23*(4), 395–402.

Sonnenfeld, S., Waldo, D., Lemieux, J., et al. (1991). Projections of national health expenditures through the year 2000. *Health Care Financing Review, 13*(1), 1–27. HCFA Pub. No. 03321. Office of Research and Demonstrations, Health Care Financing Administration, Fall.

Turner, J., Larson, E., Korniewicz, D., Wible, J., Baigis-Smith, J., Butz, A., & Sennett, L. (1994). Consistency and cost of home wound management by contract nurses. *Public Health Nursing, 11*(5), 337–42.

U.S. Bureau of the Census. (1991). *Poverty in the United States: 1990.* Current Population Reports. Series P-60. No.175. Washington, DC: U.S. Government Printing Office.

U.S. Department of Labor. (1990). *Employee Benefits in Medium and Large Firms, 1989.* Bulletin Number 2363. Bureau of Labor Statistics. Washington, DC: U.S. Government Printing Office, June.

Wagner, L. (1993). HCFA's boss says drastic new cuts could undermine reform. *Modern HealthCare,* June 14, 14–15.

Warden, C. (1993). Is health-care rationing next? It might control costs but patients will suffer. *Investor's Business Daily,* July 2, 1–3.

Weiss, R.J. (1982). Competition in health care. *American Journal of Public Health,* I, 655.

Young, Q. (1993). Health care reform: a new public health movement. *American Journal of Public Health, 83*(7), 945–947.

SELECTED READINGS

Booth, R. (1985). Financing mechanisms for health care: Impact on nursing services. *Journal of Professional Nursing, 1*(1), 34–40.

Braunstein, J. (1991). National health care: necessary but not sufficient. *Nursing Outlook, 39*(2), 54–55.

Buerhaus, P. (1994). Managed competition and critical issues facing nurses. *Nursing and Health Care, 15*(1), 22–26.

Edwardson, S.R., et al. (1988). *Impact of DRGs on nursing: report of the Midwest Alliance in Nursing. The impact of prospective payment systems on nursing care in community settings.* Washington, DC: U.S. Dept. of Health & Human Services Publication. Division of Nursing, Jul #HRP-0907178, 61–78.

Frank, K.M. (1989). Rationally rationing health care: Effectiveness research by another name? *Nursing Economics, 7*(6), 289, 296.

Graham, K.Y. (1992). Health care reform and public health nursing. *Public Health Nursing, 9*(2), 73.

Harrington, C. (1990). Policy options for a national health care plan. *Nursing Outlook, 38*(5), 223–228.

Hash, M. (1988). *Nursing practice in the 21st century. Structuring and financing of community health services . . . community nursing organizations (CNOs).* ANA Publication: American Nursing Foundation No. CH-18, 36–40.

Johnson, P.A. (1990). A national health insurance program: A nursing perspective. *Nursing and Health Care, 1*(8), 416–429.

La Rochelle, D.R. (1989). The moral dilemma of rationing nursing resources. *Journal of Professional Nursing, 5*(4), 173, 236.

McGivern, D.O. (1988). Teaching nurses the language of the marketplace . . . economics. *Nursing & Health Care, 9*(3), 126–130.

Mundinger, M.O. (1994). Health care reform: Will nursing respond? *Nursing and Health Care, 15*(1), 28–33.

Navarro, V. (1985). The public/private mix in funding and delivery of health services: An international survey. *American Journal of Public Health, 75*(11), 1318–20.

Oda, D.S., et al. (1987). Documenting the effect and cost of public health nursing field services. *Public Health Nursing, 4*(3), 180–182.

Phillips, E.K., et al. (1987). DRG ripple effects on community health nursing. *Public Health Nursing, 4*(2), 84–88.

Porter-O'Grady, T. (1994). Building partnerships in health care: Creating whole systems change. *Nursing and Health Care, 15*(1), 34–38.

Primas, P., Mileham, T., Toronto, C., & McCoy, B. (1994). Breaking the cycle of disadvantage: A nursing system of health care. *Nursing and Health Care, 15*(1), 10–17.

Pruitt, R.H. (1987). Economics of health promotion. *Nursing Economics, 5*(3), 118–120, 122–123, 141.

Reis, J., et al. (1990). Care for the underinsured: who should pay? *Journal of Nursing Administration, 20*(3), 16–20.

Sofian, N.S. (1991). Health promotion can be a valuable strategy to assist in cost containment. *Occupational Health & Safety,* Dec., 24.

Starr, P. (1992). *The Logic of Health Care Reform.* Knoxville, TN: Grand Rounds Press.

A Washington Seminar Report. (1987). *For profit and nonprofit health care: Are the distinctions blurring?* Washington, DC: National Health Council, Inc.

Weiss, L.D. (1992). *No Benefit—Crisis in America's Health Insurance.* Boulder, CO: Westview Press.

Wood, C. (1991). Health care rationing: the Oregon experiment. *Nursing Economics, 9*(4), 239–243, 262.

Zwerdling, M. (1994). The health care delivery system in the year 2000: Nursing care for the societal client. *Nursing and Health Care, 15*(8), 422–24.

CHAPTER

Community Health Nursing: Past and Present

LEARNING OBJECTIVES

Upon completion of this chapter, readers should be able to:

- Describe the four stages of community health nursing's development.
- Analyze the impact of societal influences on community health nursing.
- Describe the primary characteristics of systems and adaptation theories as they relate to community health nursing practice.
- Explain the purpose and describe the variables that make up the conceptual framework for community health nursing presented in this chapter.
- Summarize the focus and nursing goals associated with the nursing models of Neuman, Orem, Pender, Roy, and Rogers.
- Explain six characteristics of community health nursing.

KEY TERMS

- Adaptation theory
- Collaboration
- Community health nursing
- Community health nursing dynamics
- Conceptual framework
- Coping mechanisms
- Health determinants
- Homeostasis
- Model
- Population-focused

- Practice interventions
- Practice priorities
- Public health nursing
- Scope of practice
- Self-care
- Stress
- Stressor
- System
- Systems theory
- Wellness

Barbara Walton Spradley and Judith Ann Allender
COMMUNITY HEALTH NURSING: CONCEPTS AND PRACTICE, 4th ed.
© 1996 Barbara Walton Spradley and Judith Ann Allender

As a specialty in nursing practice, community health nursing offers unique challenges and opportunities. For the nurse entering this field there is the challenge of understanding and the opportunity for enriching the heritage of early public health nursing efforts. There is the challenge of expanding one's nursing focus from the individual to encompass communities and the opportunity to impact the health status of those populations. There is the challenge of determining the needs of populations at risk and the opportunity for designing interventions to address their needs. There is the challenge of learning the complexities of the health care system and the opportunity to shape it's service delivery. Community health nursing is community-based and, most importantly, it is population-focused. Operating within an environment of rapid change and increasingly complex challenges, this field of nursing holds the potential for positively shaping the quality of community health services and improving the health of the general public.

This chapter examines the historical and philosophical foundations of community health nursing that undergird the dynamic nature of its practice. First, the chapter traces community health nursing's historical development and defines it as a specialty practice. The chapter also describes the societal influences that shaped early and evolving community health nursing practice and examines its theoretical and conceptual foundations. Then the chapter describes a conceptual framework for community health nursing and explores selected nursing models for their usefulness to this specialty's practice. Finally, the chapter discusses the salient characteristics of contemporary community health nursing.

Historical Development of Community Health Nursing

Before one can fully grasp the nature of community health nursing or define its practice, it is helpful to understand the roots and influencing factors that shaped its growth over time. Community health nursing is the product of centuries of responsiveness and growth. Its practice has adapted to accommodate the needs of a changing society, yet it has always maintained its initial goal of improved community health. Community health nursing's development, which has been influenced by changes in nursing, public health, and society,

can be traced through several stages. This section examines these stages.

The history of public health nursing since its inception in Europe and more recently in America encompasses continuing change and adaptation (Frachel, 1988). The historical record reveals a professional nursing specialty that has been on the cutting edge of innovations in public health practice and has provided leadership to public health efforts. A summary of public health nursing made in the early 1900s is still true today:

> "It is precisely in the field of the application of knowledge that the public health nurse has found her great opportunity and her greatest usefulness. In the nationwide campaigns for the early detection of cancer and mental disorders, for the elimination of venereal disease, for the training of new mothers and the teaching of the principles of hygiene to young and old; in short, in all measures for the prevention of disease and the raising of health standards, no agency is more valuable than the public health nurse" (Department of Philanthropic Information, 1938, p. 8).

In tracing the development of public health nursing and later community health nursing, it is clear how that leadership role has been evident throughout its history. Nurses in this specialty have provided leadership in planning and developing programs, in shaping policy, in administration, and in the application of research to community health.

Four general stages mark the development of public health/community health nursing: (1) the early home care stage, (2) the district nursing stage, (3) the public health nursing stage, and (4) the community health nursing stage.

EARLY HOME CARE STAGE (before mid 1800s)

Within the context of public health's historical development, described in Chapter Two, one can see early prototypes of home care nursing. For many centuries, the sick were tended at home by female family members and friends. The focus of this care was to reduce suffering and promote healing (Kalisch & Kalisch, 1986). The Bible cites numerous instances of visiting the sick and extols a woman of noble character as one who "opens her arms to the poor and extends her hands to the needy" (Proverbs 31:20) and who is "a helper of many" as Phoebe was described in the New Testament (Romans 16:2).

The early roots of home care nursing began with religious and charitable groups. Medieval times saw the development of various institutions devoted to the sick, including hospitals and nursing orders. In England, the Elizabethan Poor Law, written in 1601, provided medical and nursing care to the poor and disabled. Another example was the friendly visitor volunteers organized by St. Frances de Sales in the early 1600s in France. This association was directed by Madame de Chantel and assisted by wealthy women who cared for the sick poor at home (Dolan, 1978). In Paris, St. Vincent de Paul started the Sisters of Charity in 1617, an organization composed of nuns and lay women dedicated to serving the poor and needy. The ladies and sisters, under the supervision of Mademoiselle Le Gras in 1634, promoted the goal of teaching people to help themselves as they visited the sick in their homes. In its emphasis on preparing nurses and supervising nursing care as well as determining causes and solutions for clients' problems, their work laid a foundation for modern community health nursing. (Bullough & Bullough, 1978).

Unfortunately, the years that followed these accomplishments marked a serious setback in the status of nursing and care of the sick. From the late 1600s to the mid 1800s, the social upheaval following the Reformation caused a decline in the number of religious orders with subsequent curtailing of nursing care for the sick poor. Babies continued to be delivered at home by midwives, most of whom had little or no training. Concern over high maternal mortality rates prompted efforts to better prepare midwives and medical students. One midwifery program was begun in Paris in 1720 and another in London by Dr. William Smellie in 1741.

The Industrial Revolution created additional problems; among them were epidemics, high infant mortality, occupational diseases and injuries, and increasing mental illness both in Europe and America. Hospitals were built in larger cities and dispensaries developed to provide greater access to physicians. However, disease was rampant, mortality rates were incredibly high, and institutional conditions, especially prisons, hospitals, and "asylums" for the insane, were deplorable. The sick and afflicted were kept in filthy rooms without adequate food, water, cover, or care for their physical and emotional needs (Bullough & Bullough, 1978). Reformers like the Englishman, John Howard, who investigated the spread of disease in prisons and hospitals in 1779, revealed serious needs that would not be addressed until much later.

Both Catholic and Anglican religious nursing orders, although limited in number, continued their work of caring for the sick poor in their homes. For example, in 1812 the Sisters of Mercy organized in Dublin to provide care for the sick at home. But generally, with the status of women at an all time low, often only the least respectable women pursued nursing. In 1844 Charles Dickens, in *Martin Chuzzlewit,* portrayed the nurse, Sairy Gamp, as an unschooled and slovenly drunkard reflecting society's view of nursing at the time. It was in the midst of these deplorable conditions and in response to them that Florence Nightingale began her work.

Much of the foundation for modern community health nursing practice was laid through Florence Nightingale's remarkable accomplishments (see Figure 4.1).

Born in 1820 into a wealthy English family, her excellent education, including training at the first school for nurses in Kaiserwerth, Germany, and determination to serve the needy resulted in major reforms and improved status for nursing. During the Crimean War (1854–1856) her work with the wounded in Scutari is well documented (Woodham-Smith, 1951). Conditions in the military hospitals during the war were unspeak-

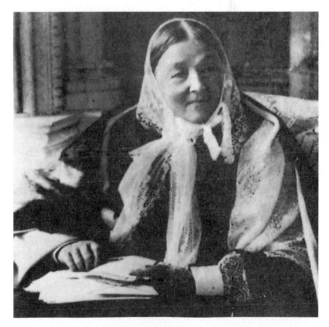

FIGURE 4.1. Florence Nightingale's concern for populations-at-risk as well as her vision and successful efforts at health reform provided a model for community health nursing today.

able. Thousands of sick and wounded men lay in filth without beds, clean coverings, food, water, or laundry facilities. Florence Nightingale organized competent nursing care and established kitchens and laundries that resulted in saving hundreds of lives. Her work further demonstrated that capable nursing intervention could prevent illness and improve the health of a population-at-risk—precursors to modern community health nursing practice. Her subsequent work for health reform in the military was supported by implementing another public health strategy, the use of biostatistics. Through meticulously gathered data and statistical comparisons, Miss Nightingale demonstrated that military mortality rates, even in peacetime, were double those of the civilian population due to the terrible living conditions in the barracks. This work led to important military reforms.

Miss Nightingale's concern for populations-at-risk included a continuing interest in the population of the sick at home. Her book, *Notes on Nursing,* published in England in 1858 (See Nightingale, 1992) was written to improve nursing care in the home (Bullough & Bullough, 1978).

Florence Nightingale made other contributions to community health nursing. Her exemplary influence on English politics and policy improved the quality of existing health care and set standards for future practice. Furthermore, in doing so, she demonstrated how population-focused nursing works. In her work to help establish the first school for nurses in 1860 at St. Thomas Hospital in London, she promoted a standard for proper education and supervision of nurses in practice.

DISTRICT NURSING
(mid 1800s to 1900)

The next stage in the development of community health nursing was the formal organization of visiting nursing, or district nursing. In 1859, William Rathbone, an English philanthropist, became convinced of the value of home nursing as a result of private care given to his wife (Kalisch and Kalisch, 1986). He employed Mary Robinson, the nurse who had cared for his wife, to visit the sick poor in their homes and teach them proper hygiene to prevent illness. But the need was so great it soon became evident that more nurses were needed. With Florence Nightingale's help and advice, Rathbone opened a training school for nurses connected with the Royal Liverpool Infirmary and established a visiting nurse service for the sick poor in Liverpool. As the ser-

vice grew, visiting nurses were assigned to districts in the city, hence the name district nursing. Subsequently, other British cities developed district nursing training and services as well. An example is the Nurse Training Institution for district nurses, founded in Manchester in 1864. Privately financed, the nurses were trained and then "dispensed food and medicine" . . . to the sick poor in their homes . . . "and were closely supervised by various middle- and upper-class women who collected the necessary supplies"(Bullough & Bullough, 1978, p.143).

In the United States, the first community health nurse, Frances Root, hired by the Women's Board of the New York Mission in 1877, pioneered home visits to the poor in New York City. In 1885, district nursing associations were founded in Buffalo and, in 1886, in Boston and Philadelphia. These district associations served the sick poor exclusively, because patients with enough money had private home nursing care. The English model, however, with standards for visiting nurses' education as well as practice, established in 1889 under Queen Victoria, was not followed in the United States. Instead, visiting nursing organizations sprang up in many cities without common standards or administration. Twenty-one such services existed in the United States in 1890.

Although district nurses primarily cared for the sick, they also taught cleanliness and wholesome living to their patients, even in that early period. Florence Nightingale referred to them as "health nurses". An example was the Boston program, founded by the Women's Educational Association, which "emphasized the teaching of hygiene and cleanliness, giving impetus to what was called instructive district nursing."(Bullough & Bullough, 1978, p.144) This early emphasis on prevention and "health" nursing became one of the distinguishing features of district nursing, and later of public health nursing, as a specialty.

The work of district nurses focused almost exclusively on the care of individuals. District nurses recorded temperatures and pulse rates and gave simple treatments to the sick poor under the immediate direction of a physician. (Figure 4.2) They also instructed family members in personal hygiene, diet and healthful living habits, and the care of the sick. The problems of early home care patients in the United States were numerous and complex. Increasing numbers of immigrants, crowded city slums, inadequate sanitation, unsafe and unhealthy working conditions all contributed to poverty and disease. Nursing educational programs

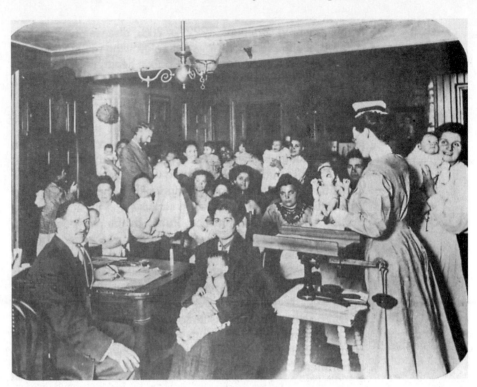

FIGURE 4.2. Examination of infants was part of early health department programs in which district nurses played a major role.

at that time did not truly prepare district nurses to cope with their patients' multiple health and social problems.

The sponsorship of district nursing changed over time. Early district nursing services in both England and the United States were founded by religious organizations. Later, sponsorship shifted to private philanthropy. Funding came from contributions and, in a few instances, from fees charged to patients on an ability-to-pay basis. Finally, visiting nursing began to be supported by public money. An early example occurred in Los Angeles where, in 1897, a nurse was hired as a city employee. Although one form of funding dominated, all three types of financing continued to exist as they still do today. While the government was beginning to assume more responsibility for the public's health, most district nursing services during this time remained private.

PUBLIC HEALTH NURSING (1900–1970)

By the turn of the century, district nursing had broadened its focus to include the health and welfare of the general public, not just the poor. This new emphasis was part of a broader consciousness about public health. Robert Koch's demonstration that tuberculosis was communicable led to Johns Hopkins Hospital hiring a nurse, Reba Thelin, in 1903 to visit the homes of tuberculosis patients. Her job was to ensure that patients followed prescribed regimens of rest, fresh air, proper diets, and to prevent possible infections (Sachs, 1908). A growing sense of urgency about the interrelatedness of health conditions and the need to improve the health of all people led to an increase in the number of private health agencies. These agencies supplemented the often limited work of government health departments. By 1910, new federal laws made states and communities accountable for the health of their citizens.

Specialized programs such as infant welfare, tuberculosis clinics, and venereal disease control were developed, causing a demand for nurses to work in these areas. Bullough and Bullough comment, "Although the hospital nursing school movement emphasized the care of the sick, a small but growing number of nurses were finding employment in preventive health care" (1978, p.143). In 1900 there were an estimated 200 public health nurses. By 1912 that number had grown to 3000 (Gardner, 1936). "This development was important: it brought health care and health teaching to the public, gave nurses an opportunity for more independent work, and helped to improve nursing education" (Bullough & Bullough, 1978, p.143).

The role of the district nurse expanded during this stage. Lillian Wald, a leading figure in this expansion, first used the term "public health nursing" to describe this specialty (Bullough and Bullough, 1978). District nurses, while caring for the sick, had pioneered in health teaching, disease prevention, and promotion of good health practices. Now, with a growing recognition of familial and environmental influences on health, public health nurses broadened their practice even more. Nurses working outside the hospital increased their knowledge and skills in specialized areas such as tuberculosis, maternal and child health, school health, and mental disorders.

Lillian D. Wald's (1867–1940) contributions to public health nursing were enormous. A graduate of the New York Hospital Training School, she started teaching home nursing but quickly changed to a career of social reform and nursing activism. Appalled by the conditions of an immigrant neighborhood in New York's Lower East Side, she and a nurse-friend Mary Brewster started the Henry Street Settlement in 1893 to provide nursing and welfare services. Her book, *The House on Henry Street,* portrays her work and views on public health nursing. Nursing visits conducted through her organization were supervised by nurses in contrast to earlier models in which nursing services were administered by lay boards and actual care supervised by lay persons. Demonstrating that nursing could reduce illness-caused absenteeism, Wald convinced the New York City Board of Education to hire the first school nurse in the United States in 1902. Her suggestion that nurse intervention could reduce death rates resulted in the Metropolitan Life Insurance Company starting a visiting nurse service in 1909 for policy holders (Kalisch & Kalisch, 1986).

The legendary accomplishments of Lillian Wald reflect her driving commitment to serve needy populations. Through her efforts the New York City Bureau of Child Hygiene was formed in 1908 and later the Children's Bureau at the federal level in 1912. Wald's emphasis on illness prevention and health promotion through health teaching and nursing intervention as well as her use of epidemiologic methodology established these actions as hallmarks of public health nursing practice. She promoted rural nursing and family-focused nursing and encouraged improved coursework at Teachers College of Columbia University to prepare public health nurses for practice. Through her influence improvements were made in child labor and pure food laws, tenement housing, parks, city recreation centers, immigrant handling, and teaching of mentally handicapped children. In 1912 she also helped to found and was first president of the National Organization for Public Health Nursing (NOPHN), an organization that set standards and guided public health nursing's further development and impact on public health (Kalisch & Kalisch, 1986). Her exemplary accomplishments truly reflect a concern for populations-at-risk. They further demonstrate how nursing leadership, involvement in policy formation, and use of epidemiology, can lead to improved health for the public.

By the 1920's public health nursing was acquiring more professional stature, in contrast to its earlier association with charity. Nursing as a whole was gaining professional status as a science in addition to being an art. National nursing organizations began to form during this stage and contributed to nursing's professional growth. The first of these emphasized establishing education standards for nursing. Called the Society of Superintendents of Training Schools of Nurses in the United States and Canada, it was started by Isabel Hampton Robb in 1893, and later became known as the National League for Nursing (NLN). In 1895 the Nurses' Associated Alumnae of the United States and Canada, later to be named the American Nurses Association (ANA), was formed to promote nursing education and practice standards. The previously mentioned NOPHN, founded by Lillian Wald and Mary Gardner merged with the NLN (1952). These three organizations, in particular, strengthened ties between nursing groups and improved nursing education and practice.

As nursing education became increasingly rigorous, collegiate programs began to include public health as essential content in basic nursing curricula. The first collegiate program with public health content to be accredited by the NLN began in 1944 (NOPHN, 1944). Previously, only postgraduate courses in public health nursing had been offered for nurses choosing this specialty. The first of such courses had been developed by Adelaide Nutting in 1912 at Teachers College in New York in affiliation with the Henry Street Settlement. A group of agencies met in 1946 to establish guidelines for public health nursing and by 1963 public health content was required for NLN accreditation in all baccalaureate nursing programs. The nurse practitioner movement, starting in 1965 at the University of Colorado, was initially a part of public health nursing and emphasized primary health care to rural and underserved populations. Educational programs to prepare nurse practitioners (NPs) increased in number with some NPs continuing in public health and others moving into different clinical areas.

During this period, as a result of Lillian Wald's and other nursing leaders' influence, the family began to emerge as a unit of service. The multiple problems faced by many families impelled a trend toward nursing care generalized enough to meet diverse needs and provide holistic services. Public health nurses gradually gained more autonomy in such areas as home care and instruction of good health practices to families and community groups. Their collaborative relationships with other community health providers grew as the need to avoid gaps and duplication of services became apparent. Public health nurses also began keeping better records of their services.

Industrial nursing, another form of public health nursing, also expanded during this period The first known industrial nurse, Philippa Flowerday (later married to William Reid), was hired in Norwich, England by J. and J. Colman in 1878. Her job was to assist the company physician and visit sick employees and their families in their homes. In the United States the Vermont Marble Company was first to begin a nursing service in 1895; other companies followed soon after. By 1910, 66 firms in the United States employed nurses. During World War I the number of industrial nurses greatly increased with recognition that nursing service reduced worker absenteeism (Bullough & Bullough, 1978).

During this stage, the institutional base for much of public health nursing shifted to the government. By 1955, 72% of the counties in the continental United States had local health departments. Public health nursing constituted the major portion of these local health services and emphasized health promotion as well as care for the ill at home (Pickett and Hanlon, 1990). Some of the district nursing services, now known as visiting nurse associations (VNAs), remained privately funded and administered, offering their own home nursing care. In some places, city or county health departments joined administratively and financially with VNAs to provide a combination of services, such as home care of the sick and health promotion, to families.

Rural public health nursing, which had already been organized around 1900 in Great Britain, Germany, and Canada, also expanded in the United States. Initially, starting in 1912, rural nursing was privately financed and largely administered through the Red Cross and the Metropolitan Life Insurance Company but responsibil-

ity had shifted to the government by the 1940s (Bullough & Bullough, 1978). An innovative example of rural nursing was the Frontier Nursing Service (FNS), started by Mary Breckenridge in 1925 to serve mountain families in Kentucky. From six outposts, nurses on horseback visited remote families to deliver babies and provide food and nursing services. Over the years the service has expanded to provide medical and dental as well as nursing care (Tirpak, 1975). The FNS continues to the present in its remarkable accomplishments of reducing mortality rates and promoting health among this disadvantaged population (see Fig. 4.3).

The public health nursing stage was characterized by service to the public, with the family targeted as a primary unit of care. Official health agencies, which placed greater emphasis on disease prevention and health promotion, provided the chief institutional base.

COMMUNITY HEALTH NURSING (1970 to present)

The emergence of the term community health nursing heralded a new era. While public health nurses continued their work in public health, by the late 1960s and early 1970s many other nurses, not necessarily practicing public health, were based in the community. Their practice settings included community-based clinics, doctors' offices, work sites, schools, and more. To provide a label that encompassed all nurses in the community, the American Nurses Association and others called them community health nurses. This and other events led to confusion about the nature of community health nursing as a specialty practice.

Nursing education, recognizing the importance of public health content, now required course work in public health for all baccalaureate students. This change meant that graduates were expected to incorporate public health principles such as health promotion and disease prevention into nursing practice, regardless of their sphere of service. Consequently, some people questioned whether public health nursing retained any unique content. Although leaders like Carolyn Williams had clearly stated that community health nursing's specialized contribution lay in its focus on populations (Williams, 1977), this concept did not appear to be widely understood or practiced.

Another source of confusion arose around the issues of community health nursing being a generalized versus a specialized practice. Graduates from baccalaureate nursing programs were inadequately prepared to prac-

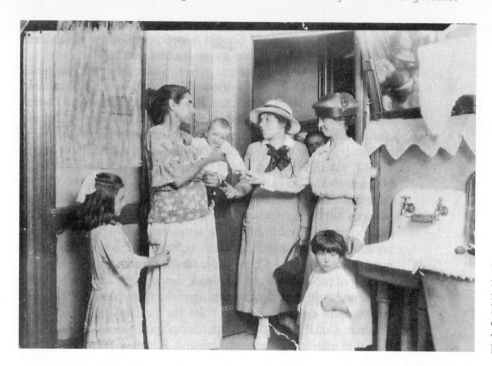

FIGURE 4.3. The public health nurse, carrying her bag of equipment and supplies, makes regular home visits to provide physical and psychological care as well as health lessons to families.

tice in public health; their education had emphasized individualized and direct clinical care and provided little or no understanding of applications to populations and communities. By the mid-1970s various community health nursing leaders had identified knowledge and skills needed for more effective community health nursing practice (Roberts & Freeman, 1973). These leaders valued promoting the health of the community, but both education and practice continued to emphasize direct clinical care to individuals, families, and groups in the community (de Tornyay, 1980). Reflecting this view, the ANA's Division of Community Health Nursing developed *A Conceptual Model of Community Health Nursing* in 1980. This document distinguished generalized community health nursing preparation at the baccalaureate level and specialized community health nursing preparation at the masters or post-graduate level. The generalist was described as one who provided nursing service to individuals and groups of clients while keeping "the community perspective in mind" (ANA, 1980, p. 9).

Yet another area of confusion lay in distinguishing between public health nursing and community health nursing. The terms were being used interchangeably and yet held different meanings for many in the field. In 1984 the Division of Nursing convened a Consensus Conference on the Essentials of Public Health Nursing

Practice and Education in Washington, DC. (1985). This group concluded that community health nursing was the broader term referring to all nurses practicing in the community regardless of their educational preparation. Public health nursing, viewed as a part of community health nursing, was described as a generalist practice for nurses prepared with basic public health content at the baccalaureate level and a specialized practice for nurses prepared in public health at the masters level or beyond.

Finally, confusion arose over the changing roles and functions of community health nurses. Accelerated changes in health care organization and financing, technology, and social issues made increasing demands on community health nurses to adapt to new patterns of practice. Many new kinds of community health services appeared. Hospital-based programs reached into the community. Private agencies proliferated offering home care and other community-based services. Other community health professionals assumed responsibilities that had traditionally been the domain of public health nursing. Some school counselors in Oregon, for example, began coordinating home visits previously done by school nurses, and health educators, who were part of a more recently developed discipline, took over large segments of client education (Chavigny and Kroske, 1983). Social workers, too, provided services that appeared to overlap with community health nursing roles. Health educators, counselors, social workers, epidemiologists, nutritionists, and others working in community health came prepared with different backgrounds and emphases in their practice. Their contributions were and still are important. Their presence, however, forced community health nurses to reexamine their own contribution to the public's health and incorporate stronger interdisciplinary and collaborative approaches into their practice.

The debate over these areas of confusion continued through the 1980s with some issues yet unresolved today. Still, the direction in which public health and community health nursing must move remains clear—to care for, not simply in, the community. **Public health nursing** continues to mean the synthesis of nursing and the public health sciences applied to promoting and protecting the health of populations. Community health nursing, for some, refers more broadly to nursing in the community. In this text the term **community health nursing** is used synonymously with public health nursing and refers to specialized population-focused nursing practice which applies public health sciences as well as nursing sciences. A possible distinction between the two terms might be to view community health nursing as a beginning level of specialization and public health nursing as an advanced level. Clarification and consensus on the meaning of these terms will help to avoid misconceptions and misuse. Whichever term is used to describe this specialty the fundamental issues and defining criteria remain: (1) are populations and communities the target of practice? and (2) are the nurses prepared in public health and engaging in public health practice?

As community health nursing continues to evolve, many signs of positive growth are evident. Community health nurses are carving out new roles for themselves in primary health care. Collaboration and interdisciplinary teamwork are recognized as crucial to effective community nursing. Practitioners work through many kinds of agencies and institutions, such as senior citizen centers, ambulatory services, mental health clinics, and family planning programs. Community needs assessment, documentation of nursing outcomes, program evaluation, quality improvement, public policy formulation, and community nursing research are high priorities. This field of nursing is assuming responsibility as a full professional partner in community health.

Table 4.1 summarizes the most important changes that have occurred during community health nursing's four stages of development. It shows these changes in terms of focus, nursing orientation, service emphasis, and institutional base.

The Specialty of Community Health Nursing

The two characteristics of any specialized nursing practice are (1) specialized knowledge and skills, and (2) focus on a particular set of people receiving the service. These two characteristics are true for community health nursing. As a specialty, community health nursing adds public health knowledge and skills that address the needs and problems of communities and aggregates, and focuses care on communities and vul-

*TABLE 4.1. **Development of Community Health Nursing***

Stages	Focus	Nursing Orientation	Service Emphasis	Institutional Base (Agencies)
Early home care (Before mid 1800s)	Sick poor	Individuals	Curative	Lay and religious orders.
District nursing (1860–1900)	Sick poor	Individuals	Curative; beginning of preventive	Voluntary; some government
Public health nursing (1900–1970)	Needy public	Families	Curative; preventive	Government; some voluntary
Emergence of community health nursing (1970–present)	Total community	Populations	Health promotion; illness prevention	Many kinds; some independent practice

nerable populations. Confusion over the meaning of "community health nursing" arises when the practice is defined only in terms of *where* it is practiced. As health care services have shifted from the hospital to the community, many nurses practicing other specialties now practice *in* the community. Examples of these practices include home care, mental health, geriatric nursing, long term care, or occupational health. Although community health nurses today practice in the same or similar settings as other specialties, the real difference lies in applying the public health sciences to large groups and communities of people. Most basic nursing specialties focus on individuals or perhaps families and small groups whereas community health nursing's unique contribution comes from serving the needs of the larger community. For nurses moving into this specialty it requires a shift in focus—from individuals to aggregates.

Community health nursing, then, as a specialty combines nursing science with public health science to formulate a practice that is community-based and population-focused (Williams, 1992). It "synthesizes the body of knowledge from the public health sciences and professional nursing theories" to improve the health of communities and vulnerable populations (American Public Health Association, 1982).

Community health nursing is grounded in both public health science and nursing science, which makes its philosophical orientation and the nature of its practice unique. It has been recognized as a subspecialty of both fields. Recognition of this specialty continues today with an even greater awareness of the important contributions community health nursing can make to the health of the public (Anderson, 1991, Zerwekh, 1992).

Societal Influences on Community Health Nursing Development

Many factors influenced the growth of community health nursing. To understand better the nature of this field, one must recognize the forces that began and continue to shape its development. Six are particularly significant: advanced technology, progress in causal thinking, changes in education, the changing role of women, the consumer movement, and economic factors.

ADVANCED TECHNOLOGY

Advanced technology has contributed in many ways to shaping the practice of community health nursing. For example, technological innovation has greatly improved health care, nutrition, and life-style and caused a concomitant increase in life expectancy. Consequently, community health nurses direct an increasing share of their effort toward meeting the needs of the elderly population and addressing chronic conditions. Advanced technology has also been a strong force behind industrialization, large-scale employment, and urbanization. We are now primarily an urban society; health planners project that 75% of the world's population will live in urban areas by the year 2000 (United Nations, 1987). Population density leads to many health-related problems, particularly the spread of disease and increased stress. Community health nurses are learning how to combat these urban health problems. In addition, changes in transportation and high job mobility have affected the health scene. As people travel and relocate, they are separated from families and traditional support systems; community health nurses design programs to help urban populations cope with the accompanying stress. New products, equipment, methods, and energy sources in industry have also increased environmental pollution and industrial hazards. Community health nurses have become involved in related research, occupational health, and preventive education. Technological innovation has helped promote medicine's complex diagnostic and treatment procedures, thus making illness-oriented care more dramatic and desirable, as well as more costly. Community health nurses face a challenge to demonstrate the physical and economic value of wellness-oriented care.

Finally, innovations in communications and computer technology have shifted America from an industrial society to an "information society" (Naisbitt & Aburdene, 1990). Our economy is now built on information—the production and marketing of knowledge. Community health nurses, now more than ever, are in the business of information distribution and use new computer technologies to enhance the efficiency and effectiveness of their services. Associated with high use of technology are societal needs for "high touch" (Powell, 1984; Naisbitt & Aburdene, 1990). Interacting with machines creates a greater need for human contact; technologic complexity, speed, and impersonality can all induce stress. Stress management, and interventions for other technology-induced health problems will continue to shape the role of community health nursing in the future.

PROGRESS IN CAUSAL THINKING

Relating disease or illness to its cause is known as causal thinking in the health sciences. Progress in the study of causality, particularly in epidemiology, has significantly affected the nature of community health nursing, (Turner and Chavigny, 1988). The germ theory of disease causation, established in the late 1800s, was the first real breakthrough in control of communicable disease. At that time it was established that disease could be spread or transmitted from patient-to-patient or nurse-to-patient by contaminated hands or equipment. Nurses incorporated the teaching of cleanliness and personal hygiene into basic nursing care. A second advance in causal thinking was initiated by the tripartite view that called attention to the interactions between a causative agent, a susceptible host, and the environment. This information offered community health nursing new ways to control and prevent health disorders. For example, nurses could decrease the vulnerability of individuals (host) by teaching them healthier life-styles. They could instigate measles vaccination programs as a means of preventing the organism (agent) from infecting children. They could promote proper disinfection of a school's swimming pool (environment) to prevent disease. Further progress in causal thinking led to the recognition that not just one single agent but many factors—a multiple causation approach—contribute to a disease or health disorder. A food poisoning outbreak that is associated with a restaurant might be caused not only by the salmonella organism but also by improper food handling and storage, lack of adherence to minimum food preparation standards, and lack of adequate health department supervision and enforcement.

Community health nurses can control health problems by examining all possible causes and then attacking strategic causal points. AIDS prevention efforts provide a dramatic case in point. Contact reporting, condom use, protection of health workers serving HIV infected patients, HIV screening and public education about AIDS are examples of a multi-faceted approach. Current causal thinking has led to a broader awareness of unhealthy conditions; in addition to disease, problems such as accidents and environmental pollution are major targets of concern. As a result, work-related stress, environmental hazards, chemical food additives, and alcohol and nicotine consumption during pregnancy are all examples of concerns in community health nursing practice.

Nursing's contribution to public health adds a further application of causal thinking. That is, nursing seeks to identify and implement the causes, or contributing factors, of wellness. Community health nurses do more than prevent illness; they seek to promote health. By conducting research and applying research findings, community health nurses promote health-enhancing behaviors. These include promoting healthier life-style practices such as eating low-fat diets, exercising, and maintaining social support systems, promoting healthy conditions in schools and work sites, and designing meaningful activities for adolescents and the elderly.

CHANGES IN EDUCATION

Changes in education, especially those in nursing education, have had an important influence on community health nursing practice. Education, once an opportunity for a privileged few, has become widely available; it is now considered a basic right and a necessity for a vital society. When people's understanding of their environment grows, an increased understanding of health is usually involved. For the community health nurse, health teaching has steadily assumed greater importance in practice. For the learner, education has led to much more responsibility. As a result, people feel that they have a right to know and question the reasons behind the care they receive. Community health nurses have shifted from planning for clients to collaborating with clients.

Education has had other effects. Scientific inquiry, considered basic to progress, has created a dramatic increase in knowledge. The wealth of information relevant to community health nursing practice means that nursing students have more content to assimilate, and practicing community health nurses have to make greater efforts to keep abreast. In contrast to earlier times when nurses were trained to work as apprentices in hospitals or health agencies and perfunctorily follow orders, today's educational programs, including continuing education, prepare nurses to think for themselves in the application of theory to practice. Community health nursing has always required a fair measure of independent thinking and self-reliance; now community health nurses need skills in such areas as population assessment, policy making, political advocacy, research, management, and collaborative functioning. As the result of expanding education, community health nurses have had to reexamine their practice and clarify their roles.

CHANGING ROLE OF WOMEN

The changing role of women has profoundly affected community health nursing. In the past century, the women's rights movement made considerable progress; women achieved the right to vote and gained greater economic independence by moving into the labor force. Today 67% of women with children work and 79% of women without children under 18 work, compared to 74% of men who work (Naisbitt & Aburdene, 1990). Women today have more education and consequently more influence than did women of the past. The percentage of women entering professions such as medicine (40% of medical students in the United States are women) and law (42.7% of law students in 1991–92 were women) is increasing (Griffin, 1993). Naisbitt and Aburdene describe the 1990s as the "decade of women in leadership." They write, "In business and many professions women have increased from a minority as low as 10 percent in 1970 to a critical mass ranging from 30 to 50 percent in much of the business world, including banking, accounting, and computer science"(1990, p.217). Yet women continue to be paid less than men. For example, Department of Labor Statistics figures show that women attorneys earn 75 cents for every dollar earned by male attorneys. Women physicians in private practice earned 34% less median income than their male counterparts in 1991 (Griffin, 1993). All of these changes mean that many more women must manage dual roles of career and family, often under disadvantaged economic conditions.

While the diversity of career options and employment opportunities for women has been a positive factor, these gains have decreased the number of women entering nursing. As a profession, nursing's contributions and status have improved but it's ability to compete with higher-paying and higher-status careers remains a problem. Changes resulting from the women's movement continue to occur. Nurses still struggle for equality—equality of recognition, respect, and autonomy as well as job selection, equal pay for equal work, and equal opportunity for advancement in the health field. If community health nurses are to influence the field of community health, they need status and au-

thority equal to that of their colleagues. This step will require nurses to demonstrate their competence and learn to be assertive in assuming roles as full professional partners (see Research in Community Health Nursing display). In community health, as in society generally, women hold fewer administrative (39%) or policy-making positions than men do (Bureau of Labor Statistics, 1989). Although only 4% of registered nurses are male, they hold 33% of nursing administrative positions. This may be influenced by a larger proportion of women in nursing having less than full-time careers (Christman, 1988). The women's movement has contributed to community health nursing's gains in assuming leadership roles, but a need for much greater influence and involvement remains.

CONSUMER MOVEMENT AND CHANGING DEMOGRAPHICS

The consumer movement has also affected the nature of community health nursing. Consumers have become more aggressive in demanding quality services and goods; they assert their right to be informed about goods and services and to participate in decisions that affect them regardless of sex, race, color, or socioeconomic level. This movement has stimulated some basic changes in the philosophy of community health nursing. Health care consumers are viewed as active members of the health team, rather than as passive recipients of care. They may contract with the community health nurse for family care or group services, represent the community on the local health board, or act as ombudsmen by serving as representatives or advocates for their community constituents: for example, to investigate complaints and report findings in order to protect the quality of care in a local nursing home. This assumption of consumers' responsibility for their own health means that the community health nurse supplements, in contrast to primarily supervising, clients' services.

Changing demographics, such as shifting patterns in immigration, numbers of births and deaths, and a rapidly increasing population of elderly persons, affect community health nursing planning and programming efforts. Monitoring these changes is essential for relevant and effective nursing services.

The consumer movement and changing demographics have also contributed to increased concern for the quality of health services including a demand for more humane, personalized health care. Dissatisfied with

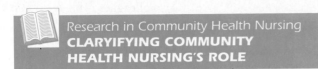

Research in Community Health Nursing
CLARYIFYING COMMUNITY HEALTH NURSING'S ROLE

Beddome, G., H. Clarke, and N. Whyte (1993). Vision for the future of public health nursing: A case for primary health care. *Public Health Nursing*, 10(1): 13–18.

Primary health care is seen as the means to achieve health for all—a goal proposed by the World Health Organization and supported by most other publicly concerned organizations. Primary health care refers to essential health care services (promotive, curative, rehabilitative, and supportive) made universally accessible and affordable. It requires a shift from direct care to a greater emphasis on health promotion and community development. Since public health nursing's role in this effort has not been clear, the authors surveyed over 100 public health nurses (only those engaged in population-based and health promoting practice) in British Columbia using a two-wave Delphi approach. The responses were coded, statistically analyzed, compared to the literature, and ranked in order of their importance for the future of public health nursing. The top 10 were: (1) more preventive funding, (2) more public health nurse involvement in planning, (3) more client self-responsibility, (4) better integration of community health services, (5) clearer role definition for public health nurses, (6) greater public health nurse enabling/empowerment of clients, (7) increased public education, (8) improved public health nurse research, (9) increased teamwork, and (10) more supportive public health nurse work environment.

The respondents' vision for public health nursing was consistent with concepts of primary health care and community development. The study findings have important implications for community health nursing practice and education.

workers, nutritionists, recreational therapists, nurses, and other callers ascertaining a variety of specific needs and starting a variety of separate programs. Community health nurses seek to provide holistic care by collaborating with others to offer more coordinated, comprehensive, and personalized services—a case management approach.

ECONOMIC FORCES

Myriad economic forces have affected community health nursing practice. Unemployment and rising costs of living combined with mounting health care costs have spawned great numbers of people who are underinsured or not insured at all. With limited or no access to needed health services, these populations are especially vulnerable to health problems and further economic stress. Other economic forces affecting community health nursing are changing health care financing patterns (including prospective payment and DRGs); decreased federal, state, and local subsidy of public health programs; pressures for cost containment in health care; and increased competition among providers of health services. (See Chapter 3 for further explanation of health economics).

Global economic forces also influence community health nursing practice. As the United States experiences increasing interdependence with foreign countries for trade, investments, and production of goods, there is also growing population mobility and increased immigration, particularly among Hispanic and Asian populations. Under these conditions, the spread of communicable disease poses a serious threat, as do problems associated with unemployment and poverty. Furthermore, the fastest growing sector of the job market is in technical areas that require new or retrained workers, and these jobs are frequently accompanied by high-tech and stress-related health problems.

Community health nursing has responded to these economic forces in several ways. One is by assuming new roles, such as health educators in industry or case managers for Alternative Care or other government-sponsored programs for the elderly. Another is by directly competing with other community health service providers, particularly in such areas as ambulatory care or home care. Still another is by developing new programs and service emphases. Elder day care, respite care, teen pregnancy and drug prevention projects, and homeless programs are a few examples of community

fragmented services offered by an array of health workers, consumers now seek more comprehensive, coordinated care. For example, senior citizens in a high-rise apartment building need more than a series of social

health nursing's response to changing community needs created by economic forces. Yet another community health nursing response has been to develop new revenue-generating services, such as workplace wellness or health screening programs, to augment depleted budgets.

Economic factors continue to play a significant role in shaping community health nursing practice. Limited dollars for health promotion services and increased demands for home care have drawn some public health agencies into more illness-oriented than wellness-oriented services. Yet community health nurses continue to be resourceful in finding ways to foster the community's optimal health while adapting to changing economic conditions.

Theoretical Bases for Community Health Nursing

What is a theory and why is it important for nursing practice? A theory is a set of systematically interrelated concepts or hypotheses that seek to explain and predict phenomena. A concept is a generalized idea about an abstract or concrete set of objects. Combining concepts and theories into relevant wholes provides community health nursing with greater understanding of human-environment interactions and guides practice decisions. A clustering of concepts with a set of explanations that describe their relationships is called a **conceptual framework**. The same is true for a theoretical framework. Stevens and Hall argue, "We need theoretical frameworks that can guide our practice with communities in the face of . . . serious public health challenges" (1992, p.2). For community health nursing, the issues we must address, such as inequitable health care access, the effects of poverty, or the destruction of the environment, require a broader, more comprehensive view of health. Stevens and Hall go on to say:

> "We can no longer be satisfied with the exclusive focus on individuals and their immediate milieus that characterizes traditional nursing theories. The future of community health nursing depends on two things: (1) our ability to recognize social, economic, and political aspects of the environment as they affect health and (2) our willingness to intervene at the community level for structural change" (1992, p.3).

Critical theories that draw from both reflection and action; that are grounded in real life circumstances will empower community health nurses and the communities they serve to effect health-enhancing changes (Stevens and Hall, 1992). Some of these theories are described in context in later chapters.

SYSTEMS THEORY AND COMMUNITY HEALTH NURSING

Of the many theories underlying community health nursing practice, systems theory proves to be one of the most pivotal. **Systems theory**, which states that every living system is a whole and its wholeness is made up of interdependent parts in interaction, (von Bertanlanffy, 1968), provides the foundation for understanding how communities function as living systems.

Systems theory as it applies to community health nursing includes the following attributes. A **system** is a regularly interacting and interdependent group of parts forming a unified whole (Buckley, 1968; Helvie, 1994). Community health nursing practice must address many sizes of systems, ranging from an individual and family to populations and larger aggregates. Each is a whole that functions as such by virtue of the relationships between its parts. Living systems, such as humans, animals, plants, or groups of people, are known as open systems because they exchange matter, energy, and information with their environment. A closed system, such as a rock, does not have such an exchange and remains self-contained, isolated, and relatively unaffected by its environment. Community health nursing deals with systems that are open.

Open systems experience hierarchical ordering with other systems from simple to complex and from small to large. Such order is interlocking and interacting (Putt, 1978). For example, various human cells together make up larger systems such as the musculoskeletal or circulatory systems that, in turn, make up the body as a system. Similarly, people organize themselves into groups, such as the health system or the legal system, which are subunits of a larger community. Communities themselves are parts of larger systems in the same way that a school of fish is part of undersea life systems.

Living systems form boundaries, or lines of demarcation, that distinguish them from other systems and from their environment. Boundaries may be visible, such as human skin or a county line, or they may be understood, such as the composition of a group or community. A system's boundary serves as a means of identifying the system and acts as a filter for exchanging energies, in the form of materials or information, with its environment.

Energy exchange is a critical attribute of living systems, since the input-output phenomenon enables the system to function toward the purpose for which it exists. Energy exchange occurs at varying rates depending on the ability of the system to absorb energy from and release energy into its environment. Through energy absorption all living systems may potentially increase their order or complexity. The reverse is also true. A boundary may contract or expand depending on the system's goals and needs, thus establishing one of a system's functions, that of boundary maintenance. Systems need to monitor the input-output exchange with the environment to assure adequate functioning. A community, for example, may increase its health and social services as its population grows but may decrease these at a later date if emigration occurs. Community health nurses assess and seek to facilitate their client systems' ability to maintain their boundaries and engage in healthy exchanges with their environment.

All systems have structure, which is the way their component parts are arranged. The structure of a group, for instance, may consist of its leadership and a described set of followers. A community's structure is generally much more complex and consists of some kind of overall governance by an authority such as a president, governor, or mayor. The community's structure will also coexist with many subsystems, such as education or social services, that have their own internal structures. The parts of a system, sometimes called subparts or subsystems, are interrelated and interdependent and function together to maintain the whole (Helvie, 1994). Thus, a change in one part can affect the operation of other parts or the total system. A change in one family member's life-style, such as unemployment, will likely affect the entire family system. Nurses, as change agents, seek to introduce many positive changes in community systems and need to understand the effects of these changes on system functioning. They also need to understand how to manage these changes most effectively. Chapter 25 describes the community health nurse's role as an agent of change.

Systems may be stable or adaptive. As a system grows and learns, its ability to adapt increases. Too much flexibility, however, can lead to instability and disruption of functioning. A living system seeks **homeostasis**, a relatively stable state of equilibrium between its interdependent parts, to which it returns after adaptation. An example is the human body's return to normal temper-

ature after a fever or a community's rebuilding after a devastating flood. To accomplish this, systems often employ a feedback loop for self-correction. That is, they retain some portion of energy in the exchange to enable them to adjust.

Although living systems may be very different from one another, they often share similar components. This attribute, known as isomorphism (Putt, 1978), enables nurses to use knowledge of one system as a basis for understanding another system. Community health nurses can generalize from their knowledge of the "universal traits" of individuals, families, and groups as systems to increase their effectiveness in working with larger community systems. See the Issues in Community Health Nursing display.

ADAPTATION THEORY AND COMMUNITY HEALTH NURSING

Life involves response to constant change and this response is called adaptation. **Adaptation theory** draws in large measure from systems theory and states that human beings, whether individuals or groups, are adaptive systems (Roy, 1984). Every living system—whether an individual, a family, a community, or a nation—must cope with internally and externally imposed conditions; these are called inputs or stimuli. For example, an individual might experience being laid off from work or a community might face the aftermath of a devastating tornado. The control processes by which people deal with various stimuli are called **coping mechanisms**. The unemployed person, for instance may become depressed and escape into alcohol use while the community hit by the tornado may mobilize cleanup and rebuilding efforts. When people cope or respond to stimuli in a healthy manner, that is, in a way that promotes growth and new levels of mastery, it is called adaptive. If not, the response is maladaptive. These effective or ineffective responses become the output in the adaptation process. The ability of people to cope at any given point in time is called their adaptation level, a level that is constantly fluctuating (Helson, 1964). This level influences the feedback loop giving information back to the point of input and directing overall functioning.

An early influence on the development of adaptation theory was Hans Selye's work on stress (1956). He stated that people's survival depends on their capacity to adapt to environmental demands. **Stress**, he said, is a physical and emotional state always present in people which increases in the presence of internal or external

There were once two sisters who inherited a large tract of heavily forested land from their grandmother. In her will, the grandmother stipulated that they must preserve the health of the trees. One sister studied tree surgery and became an expert in recognizing and treating diseased trees. She was also able to spot conditions that might lead to problems and prevent them. Her work was invaluable in keeping single or small clusters of trees healthy. The other sister became a forest ranger. In addition to learning how to care for individual trees, she studied the environmental conditions that affected the well-being of the forest. She learned the importance of proper ecological balance between flora and fauna and the impact of climate, geography, soil conditions, and weather. Her work was to oversee the health and growth of the whole forest. While she spent time walking through the forest assessing conditions, her aerial view from their small plane was equally important for spotting fires, signs of disease or other potential problems. Together, the sisters preserved a healthy forest.

Nursing also has tree surgeons and forest rangers. Various nursing specialties, like the tree surgeons, serve the health needs of individuals and families. Community health nurses, like the forest rangers, study and address the needs of populations. Both are needed and must work together to ensure healthy communities.

environmental changes or threats that require additional response. Human beings have built-in or acquired self-regulatory mechanisms that assist them in this response and adaptation process. Examples might be the body's inflammatory response to an infectious organism or a city's laws protecting its citizens against crime. When adequate regulatory mechanisms are present, certain amounts of stress are manageable and can be constructive. Excessive stress (as defined by the persons affected), on the other hand, can tax people beyond their ability to cope (Veninga and Spradley, 1981).

Selye described two types of responses to stress, local and general. When a **stressor**, the tension-producing stimulus causing stress, could be handled locally, like the body walling off a local infection, or local police apprehending a drug dealer, each system was responding positively. He called this the Local Adaptation Syndrome. When stressors could not be handled locally then a larger system had to respond to ensure survival. Using our previous examples, it would be like the whole body needing to fight the infection systemically or the entire city's police force attacking a ring of drug dealers. This larger response Selye called the General Adaptation Syndrome.

Adaptation theory has many useful applications for community health nursing. It forms a basis for understanding how human systems function. It provides a means for assessing clients' coping abilities and designing nursing actions to facilitate positive adaptation. Roy has pioneered in the use of adaptation theory to nursing and has developed a model described later in this chapter (Roy, 1970, 1991).

Conceptual Framework for Community Health Nursing

Community health nursing combines theories, concepts, and principles from nursing, public health, and other sciences to form the basis for its practice. A set of concepts integrated into a meaningful configuration called a conceptual framework helps one interpret behaviors or situations. This section summarizes the concepts underlying community health nursing to evince a conceptual framework for understanding its nature and practice. Developed by White (1982), they are grouped into five sets of variables: (1) practice priorities, (2) practice interventions, (3) scope of practice, (4) health determinants, and (5) community health nursing dynamics.

PRACTICE PRIORITIES

Three fundamental concepts underlie public health practice and form its **practice priorities**: prevention, protection, and promotion (Ibid.). *Prevention* includes three levels of activities. Primary prevention seeks to avoid the occurrence of illness or injury, such as enforcement of seat belt use to prevent injuries. Secondary prevention aims to find and treat existing health problems at the earliest stage possible. Use of mammograms and Pap smears are examples. Tertiary prevention seeks to reduce or minimize the effects of illness as much as possible, as with stroke rehabilitation programs. The concept of prevention and its three levels were discussed in Chapter 1. *Health protection*, the second fundamental concept, involves efforts to shield the public from harmful health effects of elements in the environment. These elements can range from obviously harmful physical agents, such as cigarette smoke or lead in furniture paint that may be ingested by teething toddlers, to less obvious agents, such as work stress and bereavement. *Health promotion*, the third concept, refers to activities that maintain and enhance the community's level of wellness. These, too, cover a wide range, from such efforts as a community-wide parks improvement program to family planning. These practice priorities make up one aspect of community health nursing's distinctive emphasis, the long-range goal and priority of moving the community or some population-at-risk ever nearer wellness on the wellness-illness continuum.

PRACTICE INTERVENTIONS

To accomplish the practice priorities, community health nurses use three categories of **practice interventions**: education, engineering, and enforcement (Ibid.). They provide varying degrees of "persuasion" for enhancing the accomplishment of public health goals. *Education* means the nursing actions of providing information to encourage people to voluntarily modify their behavior in health-promoting ways; typical is encouraging proper diet and exercise. *Engineering* is a stronger form of persuasion. Nursing actions directly or indirectly manage the variables in the environment to reduce health risks. That is, specific actions are taken, such as immunization against disease, to prevent health problems. *Enforcement* uses more coercive measures, such as laws prohibiting child abuse or intake of harmful chemicals. Community health nursing employs all three interventions (singly or in combination) to protect the public, prevent illness or disability, and promote health. These varying levels of persuasion are discussed in Chapter 25 as three types of change strategies in community health nursing practice.

SCOPE OF PRACTICE

Community health nursing's **scope of practice** refers to the extent or range of nursing activity and influence. What does it encompass? One can understand the scope of practice by answering the questions, "what is practiced?" and "for whom?" Answering "what is practiced?" focuses on protection from health-endangering agents, prevention of illness and disability, and promotion of wellness. These practice priorities represent a trend, as was evident in the historical review of community health nursing, away from a curative emphasis to a strong emphasis on the preventive and health promotive end of the scale. The answer to "for whom?" in community health nursing practice involves a broad range from individuals to worldwide aggregates but always maintains a conscious aggregate commitment. The nurse always asks, "what populations are affected or at risk? What are their needs? How can those needs best be served?" For example, a community health nurse working with a day care center, when truly population focused, does not limit practice to his/her charges in that center. Instead, the nurse considers the day care staff, its children, and their parents as three related population groups for assessment and intervention. Furthermore, the nurse with an aggregate orientation looks beyond the single day care center to clusters of day care centers in the community as potential populations for service. It is the goal of public health to reduce premature death, disease, disability, and discomfort and to protect, restore, and promote people's health for the good of the entire community (Institute of Medicine Committee, 1988). Figure 4.4 illustrates the scope of community health nursing practice in the context of other health disciplines.

HEALTH DETERMINANTS

A further set of variables in the conceptual framework must be considered—they are **health determinants** or factors that influence health positively or negatively. The following four influencing elements were identified by the Canadian government in 1974 and studied in the United States (Public Health Service, 1979); they form the basis for the health determinants in this conceptual framework (White, 1982):

1. *Human biological determinants,* those physiological defenses and vulnerabilities that influence who is at risk. An example is genetic predisposition to certain diseases.
2. *Environmental determinants* which are any external agents or conditions, such as persons living in an earthquake zone or in poverty, capable of enhancing or inhibiting health.
3. The adequacies and inadequacies of the health care system, the *medical-technological-organizational determinants.* Examples include inadequate

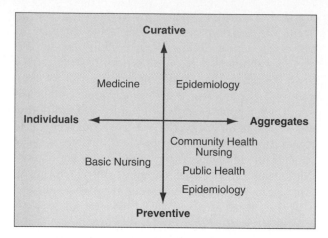

FIGURE 4.4. The scope of community health nursing practice. Basic nursing and medicine emphasize interventions with individuals. Medicine is mostly curative; nursing emphasizes restorative and preventive services. Epidemiology shifted its focus from acute disease to include chronic and disabling conditions, injuries, and prevention. Its concern is always with aggregates. Public health and community health nursing emphasize aggregates and the promotion of high-level wellness.

access to services in rural areas and the expense of high tech equipment in hospitals.

4. *Psycho-socio-cultural determinants,* such as lifestyles and racially-determined practices, that influence health.

Study of the above four variables suggests that the largest contributor to death in the United States (based on the ten leading causes) is unhealthy behaviors or life-style (accounting for about 50% of deaths). Environmental determinants account for 20% of deaths, human biologic determinants for about 20%, and inadequacies in the health care system for about 10% (Public Health Service, 1979; U.S. Department of Health and Human Services, 1991).

COMMUNITY HEALTH NURSING DYNAMICS

Two **community health nursing dynamics**, the nursing process and the valuing process, are the driving forces that energize nursing practice (White, 1982).

The *nursing process,* which includes assessment, diagnosis, planning, implementation, and evaluation, provides the means for analyzing health needs and solving health problems of communities and populations-at-risk. Chapter 11 explores the nursing process in

greater depth as a tool for enhancing community health. Its application to community health problem solving and community health nursing practice can be seen throughout the book.

The *valuing process,* a second dynamic, guides community health nursing actions. To value something is to judge it worthy. What one values determines one's priorities, commitments, and behavior. Public health holds to several significant values, some of which are discussed in Chapters 3 and 8. For example, public health subscribes to the greatest good for the greatest number, a concept that conflicts with our society's emphasis on individualism (Beauchamp, 1976). Public health bases its practice on collaboration and cooperation and believes in advocacy for the underserved and disadvantaged (Pickett & Hanlon, 1990). Values also influence consumers' attitudes and behaviors and dictate their responses to health care interventions. Chapter 8 examines values and health.

These are the variables needed to describe the nature of community health nursing practice. Figure 4.5 exhibits them in a conceptual model that incorporates the practice priorities, interventions, scope, and health determinants with the nursing process and valuing dynamics.

Nursing Models for Community Health Nursing Practice

To enhance one's understanding and use of the conceptual framework just described, this section turns to an examination of selected nursing models that have special relevance to community health nursing. A **model** is a description or analogy used as a pattern to enhance understanding of some reality. Each of the five models selected emphasizes a particular conceptual focus; (1) Neuman's model enhances an understanding of systems' functioning, (2) Rogers' emphasizes the Science of Unitary Man, (3) Pender's model reinforces health promotion, (4) Roy's model focuses on adaptation, and (5) Orem's model promotes self-care.

NEUMAN'S HEALTH CARE SYSTEMS MODEL

Drawing on systems theory, Betty Neuman has proposed a model for understanding and assisting clients (Neuman, 1980) that can enhance one's use of the community health nursing conceptual framework just

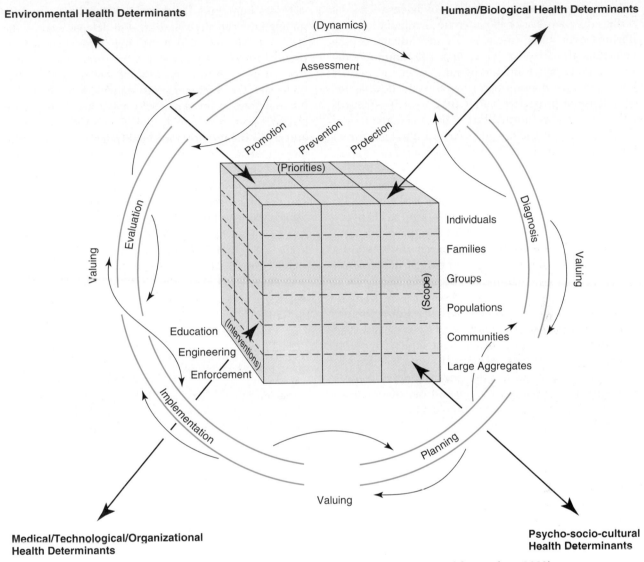

FIGURE 4.5. A conceptual model of community health nursing (adapted from White, 1982).

presented. (The discussion of Neuman's model here is adapted to viewing clients as aggregates or population groups.) Neuman provides a holistic, or total system, view of clients receiving nursing care.

With the Neuman model, each client is seen as a whole system that is greater than the sum of its parts. Four sets of variables, or influences, make up each client's "whole." These are physiological, psychological, sociocultural, and developmental variables, similar to the health determinants presented in the community health nursing conceptual framework. Given these variables, each client has a unique response to stressors,

those tension-producing stimuli that may potentially cause disequilibrium or illness.

A client's response to stressors is depicted as a series of concentric circles. In the center is a core of basic survival abilities, such as an individual's genetic responses and normal system functioning or a community's ability to make the best use of its natural resources. Surrounding the core are three boundaries. The first, or innermost, boundary is a set of flexible lines of resistance. These are the client's internal defense mechanisms against stress, such as an individual's immune response or a community's collective sense of responsibility. The second boundary is the normal line of defense. This describes the client's learned pattern for maintaining equilibrium over time, such as an individual's coping behaviors and adaptive life-style or a community's development of police and fire-fighting systems. The third boundary is a dynamic outer ring called the flexible line of defense, a protective buffer that prevents stressors from invading the normal line of defense. Examples of this boundary are adequate sleep and nutrition for an individual or regular maintenance of roads and support of schools within a community.

Neuman's model describes stressors as originating from a two-part environment. One part is the client's internal environment, where factors within the client become stressors. Examples of these intrapersonal stressors might be age level, maladaptive responses, or poor system maintenance. The second part of the environment, or external environment, produces two types of stressors. One is interpersonal stressors arising from interaction with other people or systems. For a population group, these might include such factors as stressful intergroup relationships, inadequate support systems, or maladaptive cultural patterns. The second type of stressor originating within the external environment is extrapersonal stressors which arise from the environment itself, such as economic problems, tornado damage, or a nuclear spill.

Neuman describes people as open systems which constantly interact with their environment, both influencing and being influenced by it. People respond to environmental stressors by either adapting themselves to the environment or changing the environment to meet their needs. People are healthy, according to Neuman (1982), when they have achieved a state of harmony between themselves and their environment—when they have successfully adapted to or changed their environment to meet their needs.

Nursing interventions in this model focus on assisting clients to remain stable within their environment (Neuman, 1983). Corresponding to our conceptual framework, nursing's goals include (1) prevention: helping clients to remove or minimize environmental stressors; (2) health promotion: strengthening clients' defenses; and (3) protection: promoting recovery (stability) when clients have responded to a stressor.

An adaptation of Neuman's model (Ross and Helmer, 1988) provides a useful means for applying the nursing process to population-focused practice. The community health nurse assesses and collects data on the population's perception of its situation. What are the perceived stressors impinging on their health and what are the population's reactions and lines of defense against the stressors? The nurse identifies her or his own perceptions of the stressors and then interprets and summarizes all the data in terms of their interpersonal, intrapersonal, and extrapersonal dimensions. Next, the nurse organizes the data into categories of influence: physiological, psychological, sociocultural, and developmental. Using our conceptual framework, we would incorporate all four health determinants (biological, psycho-socio-cultural, medical/technological/organizational, and environmental) into this data categorization. The nursing diagnosis clarifies the differences in perception between the client population and the nurse and, based on the diagnosis, the nurse works collaboratively with other health professionals to design a care plan. Throughout the design, implementation, and evaluation of the plan, the nurse seeks to reduce the effect of stressors through primary, secondary, and tertiary prevention.

ROGERS'S MODEL OF THE SCIENCE OF UNITARY MAN

Martha Rogers developed a conceptual model in 1970 based on systems theory and emphasized that the whole is greater than the sum of its parts. To focus on parts of a person, their gastrointestinal and respiratory systems for instance, or parts of a community, such as its health care and political systems, does not provide an adequate picture of their totality. Rogers developed her model around four components which she called (1) universe of open systems, (2) energy fields, (3) pattern and organization, and (4) four dimensionality (Rogers, 1980). Universe of open systems refers to the constant interaction between people and their environment. Energy fields refer to the wave patterns of energy given off by people and their environment. Pattern and organization refers to the way these energy fields take shape. Four dimensionality refers to the energy fields transcending time and space.

Rogers also incorporated developmental theory into her model by describing the development of unitary persons. From homeodynamics she drew the principles of helicy (life proceeds one-directionally along a rhythmic spiral), resonancy (energy fields follow a certain wave pattern and organization) and complementarity (human and environmental energy fields interact simultaneously and mutually, leading to completeness and unity). While the terms in Rogers's model may be difficult to understand, the concepts are useful for community health nursing. Using this model one can focus on client-environment interaction and see the client (whether group or community) as functioning interdependently with others and the environment. Community health nursing's goal is to promote holistic health and client-environment interaction in order to maximize client health potential.

PENDER'S HEALTH PROMOTION MODEL

The meaning and application of health promotion, a practice priority in the conceptual model, is especially important for community health nursing. Pender defines health promotion as action "directed toward increasing the level of well-being and self-actualization of a given individual or group" (Pender, 1987, p.57). This is in contrast to health protection, another important variable in our conceptual framework, which Pender describes as actions "directed toward decreasing the probability of experiencing illness by active protection of the (system) against pathological stressors or detection of illness in the asymptomatic stage" (p.57).

Pender describes health promotion as a proactive set of behaviors in which people *act* on their environment rather than *react* to stressors arising from the environment (see Figure 4.6). Pender's Health Promotion Model seeks to explain this behavior. The model is based on social learning theory that stresses cognitive mediating processes which help to regulate behavior. Health-promoting behaviors are determined by two sets of variables. First are cognitive-perceptual factors or the individual perceptions people have that directly influence their motivation to start and continue health-promoting behaviors. The model addresses seven perceptions: (1) the way people view the importance of health, (2) their perceived control of their health, (3) their perceived self-efficacy (how strongly they believe they can successfully engage in the behavior and achieve the desired outcomes), (4) their definition of health (ranging from "absence of illness" to self-actualization), (5) their perceived health status (perceptions of being in "good health" appear to increase the likelihood of engaging in health-promoting behavior), (6) their perceived benefits of health-promoting behavior, and (7) their perceived barriers to health-promoting behavior. Each of these perceptions directly affects people's likelihood of engaging in health-promoting behaviors.

The second set of variables in Pender's model is called modifying factors. These include demographic factors (e.g.: age, sex, ethnicity), biological characteristics (e.g.: body fat and weight), interpersonal influences (e.g.: expectations of others, family patterns), situational factors (e.g.: availability of healthy foods, opportunity to exer-

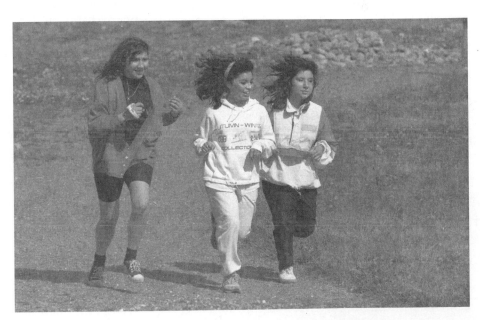

FIGURE 4.6. Health promotion and disease prevention can be enhanced through regular exercise.

cise), and behavioral factors (e.g.: stress-coping patterns). These modifying factors work indirectly to influence the first set of variables that, in turn, directly affect people's likelihood of engaging in health-promoting behaviors.

While Pender's testing of this model is with individuals, one can make applications to families and communities. Community health nurses can encourage health promoting behaviors among their clients by careful assessment of the model's variables to determine perceptions and the modifying factors that might influence the likelihood of clients engaging in health-promoting behaviors. Group interview, or surveys are two possible data collection methods. Clients should be involved in the entire process of assessing, planning, implementing, and evaluating health promotion efforts. Furthermore, promoting levels of wellness among groups and communities can be achieved through all three practice interventions, education, engineering and enforcement, described in the conceptual framework.

A final note. Research has shown that people who already engage in health-promoting behaviors tend to continue these activities as a part of their life style (Pender, 1987). This suggests that as one moves people toward healthier living it may increase the chances of these behaviors continuing and perhaps becoming more self-reinforcing—a worthy goal for community health nursing and an idea worth testing for improving community health.

ROY'S ADAPTATION MODEL

Sr. Callista Roy's model builds on adaptation, systems, and interactionist theories. People, as open and adaptive systems, she says, experience stimuli (inputs), develop coping mechanisms (control processes), and produce responses (outputs). These responses may be adaptive or maladaptive. In turn, the responses determine people's adaptation level providing information (feedback) and standards that determine the amount and type of stimuli they can handle next time (Roy, 1991).

In discussing coping mechanisms, Roy describes two processes that influence people's responses to stimuli. She calls them the regulator and the cognator processes. The *regulator* receives stimuli from the external environment and from within the system and then processes this combination of information to produce a response. For an individual, Roy describes the regulator process-

ing as going through neural-chemical-endocrine channels and goes on to say, "by some unknown process, the neural inputs are transformed into conscious perceptions in the brain. Eventually this perception leads to psycho-motor choices of response which activate a body response" (1984, p.33). A simple example of a regulator is the hunger sensation (stimulus) that promotes appetite (regulator) leading to nutritional intake (response). But Roy is quick to warn that "regulator mechanisms seldom act alone, but are most often interactive with other human control processes" (1984, p.33). Appetite, for instance, is also influenced by culture, emotional state, whether one is dieting, how appetizing the food looks, and so on. On a community level, an example of a regulator process might be the desire to keep adolescents from smoking (stimulus) that promotes a city's ordinance against minors purchasing cigarettes (regulator) that leads to lowered level of smoking (response) among this population.

The other coping process Roy calls the *cognator*. Using the cognator mechanism, people apply perception, learning, judgment, and emotion to process internal and external stimuli and arrive at a response. An example of the cognator process with an individual might be when a woman learns that she is unexpectedly pregnant. She applies her perception about this information and her previous learning about what being pregnant will mean to her physically, emotionally, economically, etc. She also applies judgment (her ability to solve problems and make decisions) and emotion (her affective assessments) to arrive at a response which may be adaptive or maladaptive. A community similarly may apply the cognator process to the stimulus of a potential flood using these four channels (perception, learning, judgment, and emotion). Community members will develop perceptions about the continuing rainfall and rising river levels. They will draw on their memory of previous floods. They will apply learning and their previous insights about dealing with floods. Community leaders will draw on collective judgment to solve the problem and decide to evacuate people living near the river and build sandbag reinforcements to protect homes and businesses. Finally, they will use emotion, their affective appraisal of the situation, to respond to the crisis by encouraging preventive action and avoiding fear and panic. This would be an adaptive community response.

Roy explains that cognator and regulator processes act in relation to four effector modes: physiological function, self-concept, role function, and interdependence. These variables further shape the nature of people's coping and help determine whether their response will be adaptive or ineffective.

When one applies Roy's model to community health nursing, it is important to remember that people, as systems, are wholes made up of many parts and influenced by many variables. Roy also points out that people's adaptation levels are constantly changing, influenced by all these factors. Whether the client is an individual, a group, or a community, the community health nurse must assess clients' coping mechanisms and help people to more effectively use their abilities to promote adaptation. If a person is dealing with stress by smoking or a community is responding to increased numbers of teen pregnancies by doing nothing, nursing actions can be designed to encourage healthier coping patterns and adaptive responses.

OREM'S SELF-CARE MODEL

This model for nursing practice focuses on the concept of self-care. It draws from developmental and systems theory. Orem first described people who needed nursing care as those who lacked ability in self-care (1959). She developed her model to include other related concepts. **Self-care** she defined as the actions people take to preserve and promote their health, life, and state of well-being. The ability of people to engage in these actions, or to care for themselves, she called *self-care agency*. The total set of self-care actions that a person might need at a given point in time she called that person's *therapeutic self-care demand*. When the therapeutic self-care demand exceeded the person's self-care agency, then they experienced a *self-care deficit*. At this point nursing intervention was appropriate and the goal of nursing action was to address people's self-care demand until they were able to take over that function for themselves (Orem, 1991).

Orem further describes self-care in terms of three types of requirements that influence people's self-care ability:

1. Universal requirements—self-care activities required to meet physiological and psychosocial needs.
2. Developmental requirements—self-care activities necessary to help people progress developmentally.
3. Health deviation requirements—self-care activities needed to help people deal with a diminished level of wellness.

While Orem applied her model primarily to individuals as systems, one can again draw applications for community health nursing. Families, groups, populations, and communities all have similar characteristics as those portrayed in Orem's model. Each aggregate also has a collective set of actions (self-care) and requirements that promote its well-being as a total group. That group's ability to engage in these actions could be called its self-care agency and the self-care actions needed to maintain its level of health in response to its requirements would be the group's self-care demand. When the group's need is greater than the demand, community health nursing intervention would be indicated.

Using this model one can define community health nursing's goal as assisting people until they can take care of themselves. One might, for example, work with a school population of teens using drugs and seek, through education and engineering, collaborative approaches to helping them get off drugs and into healthy and meaningful activities. The goal is to promote people's collective independence and self-care ability. Table 4.2 compares the five nursing models in terms of their main concepts, theoretical base, and nursing goals and interventions.

Characteristics of Community Health Nursing

Six characteristics of community health nursing are particularly salient to the practice of this specialty: (1) it is a field of nursing; (2) it combines public health with nursing; (3) it is population-focused (4) it emphasizes wellness; (5) it involves interdisciplinary collaboration; and (6) it promotes clients' responsibility and self-care.

FIELD OF NURSING

Community health nursing is a field of nursing; its basic knowledge and skills are those of professional nursing practice. It seeks to give humanistic, accessible, and holistic care. For instance, community health nurses are nursing when their concern for homeless individuals sleeping in a park leads to development of a program providing food, shelter and other services for this population. Community health nurses are nursing when they collaborate to institute an AIDS education

TABLE 4.2. *Components of Selected Nursing Models*

	Concepts for Community Health Nursing	Theory Base	Nursing Goal and Action
Neuman	Holism Prevention	Systems theory	To reduce effect of stressors through 3 prevention levels
Orem	Self-care	Systems and Developmental theories	To achieve clients' self-care agency by facilitating recovery from self-care deficit and promoting self-care ability
Pender	Health promotion	Social Learning theory	To enhance likelihood of people engaging in health promoting behaviors by assessing and influencing perceptual and modifying factors
Rogers	Holism Client-environment interaction	Systems theory	To maximize integrity and health potential by facilitating complementary client-environment interaction
Roy	Adaptation coping mechanisms	Adaptation, systems, and interactionist theories	To promote healthy coping patterns and adaptive responses

curriculum in the local school system. When they assess the needs of elderly people in retirement homes to ensure necessary services and provide health instruction and support, they are again nursing.

Community health nursing is a nursing specialty; nursing theories undergird its practice and the nursing process is one of its basic tools, but community health nursing synthesizes concepts, knowledge, and skills from public health to become a distinctive practice (see Levels of Prevention display) (Hanchett and Clarke, 1988).

COMBINES PUBLIC HEALTH WITH NURSING

Knowledge of the following elements of public health is essential to community health nursing (Pickett & Hanlon, 1990; White, 1982; Williams, 1977, 1983, 1992):

1. The history and philosophy of public health, including emphasis on the greatest good for the greatest number;
2. The concept of aggregates—assessing needs, planning and providing services, and evaluating services' impact on population groups—including aggregate-level decision making;
3. Priority of preventive, protective, and health-promoting strategies over curative strategies;

4. The means for measurement and analysis of community health problems, including epidemiologic concepts and biostatistics;
5. Influence of environmental factors on aggregate health;
6. Principles underlying management and organization for community health, since the goal of public health is accomplished through organized community efforts;
7. Public policy analysis and development;
8. Health advocacy and the political process.

There are many ways in which community health nursing incorporates public health knowledge into its practice. For example, prior to immunization laws, some school nurses who were working with the city of Cincinnati health authorities were concerned with the failure of many children to receive adequate immunization. They used health statistics, specifically a review of school immunization records, to determine immunization needs of school-aged children. Next, they set up an immunization program that successfully met the needs of the community (Anthony, Reed, Leff, Huffer, and Stephens, 1977). They effectively combined biostatistics with a community focus to carry out their goals. Another group of community health nurses designed an experimental study to test the effectiveness of breast self-examination (BSE) instruction given to healthy women in their community (Shamian and Edgar, 1987). They tested the women's knowledge of the signs and

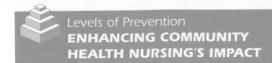

Levels of Prevention
ENHANCING COMMUNITY HEALTH NURSING'S IMPACT

GOAL

To avoid misunderstanding and misuse of community health nursing by clarifying and enhancing its role in the delivery of health services.

PRIMARY PREVENTION

To prevent misunderstanding and misuse from occurring. Proactively develop knowledge and skills and participate in policy formation, political activism, collaborative program development, and defining community health nursing's role. Conduct research on health and nursing outcomes to ensure theory-based practice, to establish credibility in the community, and to acquire funding for programs.

SECONDARY PREVENTION

To detect early signs of misunderstanding and misuse and correct them. Identify agencies where community health nurses could more fully practice population-based nursing and have a greater impact on promoting the community's health. Develop measures to enlarge the nurses' vision and to promote aggregate-level interventions. Foster nurse involvement on community boards, in politics and policy formation, in program development, and in research and collaboration with community colleagues.

TERTIARY PREVENTION

To identify misunderstanding and misuse, minimize their impact, and improve nursing function. Identify community health nurses who lack vision or clarity of their role. Through education, staff development, or reassignment provide opportunities for developing vision, knowledge and skills to enlarge their role and impact on the health of populations.

symptoms of breast cancer and how to do BSE. They also examined how frequently these women did BSE. After they obtained this information the women were provided a BSE education session. Findings obtained after the educational program provided by the nurses indicated that it positively influenced the women's knowledge base and frequency of BSE practice. This epidemiologic study combined public health and nursing practice to show that nurses can be agents for change in community health.

As community health nurses carefully assess group and community needs, establish priorities, and plan, implement, and evaluate services, they are using public health management and organizational principles. For example, one community health nurse discovered a concern about the high incidence of dental decay among the school children in the community whose needs she was assessing. Because of the relationships she had already established within the community, she was able to help form a committee that studied the problem. The committee initiated a pilot dental health program in one school that was to be evaluated a year later. She then continued to assist this committee in its efforts (Flynn, Gottschalk, Ray, and Selmanoff, 1978).

Each of the nurses mentioned here has demonstrated an important characteristic of community health nursing—the combination of fundamental public health concepts and nursing.

POPULATION-FOCUSED

The central mission of public health practice is to improve the health of population groups (Last, 1987). Community health nursing shares this essential feature: it is **population-focused** meaning that it is concerned for the health status of population groups and their environment. A population may consist of the elderly living throughout the community or Southeast Asian refugees clustered in one section of a city. It may be a scattered group with common characteristics, such as people at high risk of developing coronary heart disease, or battered women living throughout a county. It may include all the people living in a neighborhood, district, city, state, or province. Community health nursing's specialty practice serves populations and aggregates of people.

Working with individuals and families as parts of aggregates has been common in the past for community health nursing; however, such work must expand to incorporate a population-oriented focus, a feature that distinguishes it from other nursing specialties. The difference lies in two areas: The first is it's specialized knowledge and skill in public health, as discussed above. Secondly is its focus. Basic nursing focuses on individuals, and community health nursing focuses on aggregates (Williams, 1992; Hanchett and Clarke,

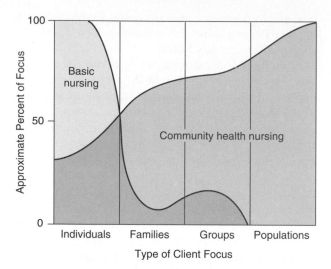

FIGURE 4.7. Difference in client focus between basic nursing and community health nursing.

1988), but the many variations in community needs and nursing roles inevitably cause some overlap. Figure 4.7 shows the distinctions between basic and community health nursing.

A population-oriented focus requires the assessment of relationships. When working with groups and communities, the nurse does not consider them separately but rather in context, that is, in relationship to the rest of the community. When an outbreak of hepatitis occurs, for example, the community health nurse does more than simply work with others to treat it. The nurse tries to stop spread of the infection, locate possible sources, and prevent its recurrence in the community. As a result of their population-oriented focus, community health nurses seek to discover possible groups with a common health need, such as expectant mothers, or groups at high risk of developing a common health problem, such as potential diabetics or child abuse victims. Community health nurses continually look for problems in the environment that influence community health and seek ways to increase environmental quality. They work to prevent health problems, such as promoting education about safe sex in schools or nutrition counseling for groups of seniors.

A population-oriented focus involves a whole new outlook and set of attitudes. Individualized care is important, but prevention of aggregate problems in community health nursing practice reflects more accurately its philosophy and benefits a larger number of people. The community or population-at-risk is the client. Fur-

thermore, since community health nurses will be concerned about a number of aggregates at the same time, service will, of necessity, be provided to multiple and overlapping groups.

EMPHASIZES WELLNESS

Another distinguishing characteristic of community health nursing is its emphasis on positive health, or **wellness** (Hanchett and Clarke, 1988). Chapter 1 described the wellness-illness continuum. Medicine and acute care nursing deal primarily with the illness end of that continuum. In contrast, community health nursing has a primary charge to prevent health problems from occurring and to promote a higher level of health. For example, although a community health nurse may assist a population of new mothers in the community with postpartum fatigue and depression, the nurse also works to prevent such problems among women of child-bearing age by developing health education programs, establishing prenatal classes, and encouraging proper rest, nutrition, adequate help, and stress reduction.

Community health nurses concentrate on the wellness end of the wellness-illness continuum in a variety of ways. They teach proper nutrition or family planning, promote immunizations among preschool children, encourage regular physical and dental checkups, assist with starting exercise classes or physical fitness programs, and promote healthy interpersonal relationships. Their goal is to help the community reach its optimal level of wellness.

This emphasis on wellness changes the community health nursing role from a reactive to a proactive stance. It places a greater responsibility on community health nurses to find opportunities for intervention. In clinical nursing and medicine, the patients seek out professional assistance because they have health problems. As Williams puts it, "Patients select themselves into the care system, and the providers' role is to deal with what the patients bring to them"(1977, p. 251). Community health nurses, in contrast, seek out potential health problems. They identify high-risk groups and institute preventive programs. They watch for early signs of child neglect or abuse and intervene when any occur, often long before a request for help is made. They look for possible environmental hazards in the community, such as smoking in public places, and work with appropriate authorities to correct them. A wellness emphasis requires taking initiative and making sound judgments, which are characteristics of effective community health nursing.

INVOLVES INTERDISCIPLINARY COLLABORATION

Community health nurses must work in cooperation with other members of the health team, coordinating services and addressing the needs of population groups. This interdisciplinary **collaboration** among health care workers and professionals is essential to establishing effective programs. Individualized efforts and specialized programs, when planned in isolation, can lead to fragmentation and gaps in health services. For example, without collaboration, a well-child clinic may be started in a community that already has a strong early and periodic developmental screening and testing program; yet, at the same time, community prenatal services may be nonexistent. Interdisciplinary collaboration is important in individualized practice, since nurses need to plan with the physician, social worker, physical therapist, or other involved health professional and keep them informed of clients' health status; however, it is an even greater necessity in working with population groups.

Effective collaboration requires team members who are strong individuals with various areas of expertise and who can make a commitment to team goals. Community health nurses who think and act interdependently make a great contribution to the team effort. In appropriate situations, community health nurses also function autonomously, making independent judgments. Collaboration involves working with members of other disciplines on community advisory boards, health planning committees, needs assessment surveys, policy development efforts, and many more.

Interdisciplinary collaboration requires clarification of each team member's role, a primary reason for community health nurses to understand the nature of their practice. When planning a city-wide immunization program with a community group, for example, community health nurses need to explain the ways they might contribute to the program's objectives. They can offer to contact key community leaders, with whom they have established relationships, in order to build community acceptance of the program. They can share their knowledge of the public's preference about times and locations for the program. They can help organize and give the immunizations, and they can influence planning for follow-up programs. Collaboration is discussed further in Chapter 13.

PROMOTES CLIENTS' RESPONSIBILITY AND SELF-CARE

The goal of public health, "to protect, promote, and restore people's health" (U.S. Department of Health and Human Services, 1991), requires a partnership effort. Just as learning cannot take place in schools without student participation, the goals of public health cannot be realized without consumer participation. Community health nursing's efforts toward health improvement can go only so far. Clients' health status and health behavior will not change unless people accept and apply the proposals of the community health nurse.

Community health nurses can encourage individual's participation by promoting their autonomy, rather than allowing dependency to occur. For example, elderly persons attending a series of nutrition or fitness classes can be encouraged to take the initiative and develop health or social programs on their own. Independence and feelings of self-worth are closely related. By treating people as independent adults, with trust and respect, community health nurses help promote self-reliance and the ability to function independently.

A characteristic of community health nursing that is sometimes overlooked is encouraging clients to take responsibility for their own health. The earlier discussion of the consumer movement emphasized consumers' rights to health care and to involvement in decision making about health care. However, consumers are frequently intimidated by health professionals and uninformed about health and health care. They do not know what information to ask for and are hesitant to act assertively. For example, a woman brought her two-year-old son, who had symptoms resembling those of scurvy, to a clinic. Recognizing a vitamin C deficiency, the physician told her to feed the boy large quantities of orange juice but gave no explanation. Several weeks later, she returned; the child was much worse. After questioning her, the nurse discovered that the mother had been feeding the child large amounts of an orange soft drink, not knowing the difference between that and orange juice. Obviously, the quality of care is affected when the consumer does not understand and cannot participate in the health care process.

When people believe their health and that of the community are their own responsibility, not just of health professionals, they will take a much more active interest in promoting it. The process of taking responsibility for developing one's own health potential is called self-care (Levin, 1978; Norris, 1979; Goeppinger, 1982,

Orem, 1991), a concept discussed earlier. As people maintain their own life, health, and well-being they are engaging in self-care. Some examples of self-care activities at the aggregate level include a community building safe playgrounds, developing teen employment opportunities, and providing senior exercise programs. When people's ability to continue self-care activities drops below their need, they experience a self-care deficit. At this point nursing may appropriately intervene. However, nursing's goal is to assist clients to return to or reach a level of functioning where they can attain optimal health and assume responsibility for maintaining it (Orem, 1991). To this end, community health nurses foster their clients' sense of responsibility by treating them as adults capable of managing their own affairs. Nurses can encourage people to negotiate health care goals and practices, develop their own programs, contact their own resources (such as support groups or transportation services), identify and implement life-style changes that promote wellness, and learn ways to monitor their own health.

Client participation is promoted when people serve as partners on the health care team. An aim of community health nursing is to collaborate with people rather than do things for them. As consumers of health services are treated with respect and trust and, as a result, gain confidence and skill in self-care—promoting their own health and that of their community—their contribution to health programs will become increasingly valuable. The consumer perspective in planning and delivering health services makes those services relevant to consumer needs. Community health nurses encourage the involvement of health care consumers by soliciting their ideas and opinions, by inviting them to participate on health boards and committees, and by finding ways to promote their participation in decisions affecting their collective health.

Summary

The specialty of community health nursing developed historically through four stages. The early home care stage (prior to the mid 1800s) emphasized care to the sick poor in their homes by various lay and religious orders. The district nursing stage (mid 1800s) included voluntary home nursing care for the poor by specialists or "health nurses" who treated the sick, and taught wholesome living to patients. The public health nurs-

ing stage (1900–1970) was characterized by an increased concern for the health of the general public. The community health nursing stage (1970 to present) included increased recognition of community health nursing as a specialty field with focus on communities and populations.

Community health nursing combines knowledge and skills from nursing science and public health science to form a specialty nursing practice. Its goal is to prevent illness and to protect and promote the health of communities and populations-at-risk.

Six major societal influences have shaped the development of community health nursing. They are advanced technology, progress in causal thinking, changes in education, the changing role of women, the consumer movement, and economic factors, such as health care costs, access, limited funds for public health, and increased competition among health service providers.

The theoretical base of community health nursing practice draws from many theories and disciplines. Two that are especially relevant are systems theory and adaptation theory. Systems theory provides understanding of the interdependent interactions of human communities as systems. Adaptation theory describes and explains human beings' adaptive or maladaptive responses to changes in their environment.

A conceptual framework for community health nursing encompasses five sets of variables: (1) practice priorities include prevention, protection, and promotion, (2) practice interventions are education, engineering, and enforcement, (3) scope of practice encompasses the range from individuals to aggregates, emphasizing the aggregate end of the individual-to-aggregate scale and the preventive end of the curative-preventive scale, (4) four health determinants are human biological, environmental, medical-technological-organizational, and social-behavioral determinants, (5), two essential dynamics, the nursing process and the valuing process, guide community health nursing practice.

Five nursing models have particular relevance for community health nursing. Neuman's health care system model draws on systems theory and focuses on environmental stressors and people's reaction to them. Nursing's goal is to help clients remain stable in their environment and to reduce the effect of stressors through primary, secondary, and tertiary prevention. Rogers's science of unitary man model, also based on systems theory, focuses on client-environment interaction and holistic health. Nursing's goal is to maximize people's integrity and health potential by facilitating complementary client-environment interaction. Pender's health promotion model draws from social learning theory and focuses on the development of health promoting behaviors in people. Nursing's goal is to enhance the likelihood of people engaging in health promoting behaviors by assessing and influencing perceptual and modifying factors. Roy's adaptation model is based on adaptation theory as well as systems and interactionist theories. Nursing's goal is to promote healthy coping mechanisms and adaptive responses. Orem's self-care model draws from developmental and systems theories. It emphasizes people's need to care for themselves. Nursing's goal is to promote client self-care ability.

Six important characteristics of community health nursing are:

1. It is a specialty field within nursing.
2. Its practice combines public health and nursing sciences.
3. It has a population-oriented focus.
4. It emphasizes wellness rather than disease or illness.
5. It involves interdisciplinary collaboration.
6. It promotes client self-care.

Activities to Promote Critical Thinking

1. Select one societal influence on the development of community health nursing and explore its continuing impact. What other events are occurring today that shape community health nursing practice? Support your arguments with documentation.

2. Describe a situation in community health nursing practice in which use of the practice intervention of education would be most appropriate. Do the same with engineering and enforcement. Discuss what made you match each situation with that intervention.

3. Assume you have been asked to make a home visit to a 75-year-old man living alone whose wife recently died. Besides assessing his individual needs, what additional factors should you consider for assessment and intervention that would indicate an aggregate or population-focused approach?

4. Interview a community health nursing director to determine what population-based programs are currently offered in your locality. Explore nursing's role in the assessment, development, implementation, and evaluation of these programs. Discuss with the director how community health nurses might expand their population-focused interventions.

REFERENCES

American Nurses Association, Community Health Nursing Division. (1980). *A conceptual model of community health nursing,* (Pub. No. CH-10 2M 5/80). Kansas City, MO: Author.

American Nurses Association. (1981). *Standards: Community health nursing practice,* Kansas City, MO: Author.

American Public Health Association. (1982). Definition and role of public health nursing in the delivery of health care (Policy Statement No. 8132). *American Journal of Public Health,* 72, 210–12.

Anderson, E.T. (1991). A call for transformation. *Public Health Nursing, 8*(1), 1

Anthony, N., Reed, M., Leff, A., Hoffer, J., & Stephens, B (1977). Immunization: Public health programming through law enforcement. *American Journal of Public Health, 67,* 763–64.

Beauchamp, D.E. (1976). Public health as social justice. *Inquiry, 13,* 3–14.

Beddome, G., Clarke, H., & Whyte, N. (1993). Vision for the future of public health nursing: A case for primary health care. *Public Health Nursing, 10*(1), 13–18.

Buckley, W. (Ed.). (1968). *Modern systems research for the behavioral scientist.* Chicago: Aldine.

Bullough, V. & Bullough, B. (1978). *The care of the sick: The emergence of modern nursing.* New York: Neale, Watson.

Bureau of Labor Statistics. (1989). Employed civilians by occupation, sex, and age. *Employment and Earnings, 36*(2), 31. U.S. Department of Labor.

Chavigny, K. H. & Kroske, M. (1983). Public health nursing in crisis. *Nursing Outlook, 31*(5), 312–16.

Christman, L. (1988). Men in nursing. *Imprint, 35*(3), 75.

Concensus Conference on the Essentials of Public Health Nursing Practice and Education, (1985). Rockville, MD: U.S. Department of Health and Human Services, Bureau of Health Professions, Division of Nursing.

Department of Philanthropic Information, Central Hanover Bank and Trust Company, (1938). *The Public Health Nurse,* New York: reprinted by the National Organization for Public Health Nursing.

de Tornyay, R. (1980). Public health nursing: the nurse's role in community-based practice. *Annual Review of Public Health, 1,* 83.

Dickens, C. (1910). *Martin Chuzzlewit,* New York: Macmillan.

Dolan, J.A. (1978). *Nursing in Society: A historical perspective.* Philadelphia: W.B. Saunders.

Flynn, B., Gottschalk, J., Ray, D., & Selmanoff, E. (1978). One masters curriculum in community health nursing. *Nursing Outlook, 26*(6), 633–37.

Frachel, R. R. (1988). A new profession: The evolution of public health nursing. *Public Health Nursing, 5*(2), 86–90.

Gardner, M.S. (1936). *Public health nursing* (3rd ed.). New York: Macmillan.

Goeppinger, J. (1982). Changing health behaviors and outcomes through self-care. In J. Lancaster & W. Lancaster, (Eds.), *Concepts for advanced nursing practice: The nurse as a change agent.* St. Louis: C. V. Mosby.

Griffin, G. (1993). Women and doctors and lawyers. *Capitol Bulletin of the Minnesota Women's Consortium,* #583, Mar 10.

Hanchett, E.S., & Clarke, P.N. (1988). Nursing theory and public health science: Is synthesis possible? *Public Health Nursing, 5*(1), 2–6.

Helson, H. (1964). *Adaptation level theory.* New York: Harper & Row.

Helvie, C.O. (1994). *Community health nursing: Theory and process.* Philadelphia: Harper & Row.

Kalisch, P. & Kalisch, B. (1986). *The advance of American nursing.* (2nd ed.). Boston: Little, Brown.

Institute of Medicine Committee for the Study of the Future of Public Health. (1988). *The future of public health.* Washington, DC: National Academy Press.

Last, J.M. (1987). *Public health and human ecology.* East Norwalk, CT: Appleton & Lange.

Levin, L. (1978). Self-care: An emerging component of the health care system. *Hospital & Health Services Administration, 23,* 17.

Naisbitt, J. & Aburdene, P. (1990). *Megatrends 2000.* New York: William Morrow.

National Organization for Public Health Nursing (1944). Approval of Skidmore College of Nursing as preparing students for public health nursing. *Public Health Nursing, 36,* 371, July.

Neuman, B. (1980). The Betty Neuman health care systems model: A total person approach to patient problems. In J. Riehl & S. Roy (Eds.), *Conceptual models for nursing practice.* (2nd ed.). New York: Appleton-Century-Crofts.

Neuman, B. (1982). *The Neuman systems model: Application to nursing education and practice.* Norwalk, CT: Appleton-Century-Crofts.

Neuman, B. (1983). Family intervention using the Betty Neuman health care systems model. In I. W. Clements & F. Roberts, *Family health: A theoretical approach to nursing care.* New York: Wiley.

Nightingale, F. (1992). *Notes on Nursing* (Commemorative Edition). Philadelphia: Lippincott.

Norris, C. M. (1979). Self-care. *American Journal of Nursing,* 79: 486–89.

Orem, D. (1959). *Guides for developing curriculum for the education of practicing nurses.* Washington, DC: U.S. Government Printing Office.

Orem, D. (1991). *Nursing: Concepts of practice* (4th ed.). New York: McGraw-Hill.

Pender, N.J. (1987). *Health Promotion in Nursing Practice* (2nd ed.). Norwalk, CT: Appleton & Lange.

Pickett, G. & Hanlon, J. (1990). *Public Health: Administration and Practice* (9th ed.). St. Louis: Times Mirror/Mosby.

Powell, D.J. (1984). Nurses—"High touch" entrepreneurs. *Nursing Economics, 2*(1), 33–36.

Public Health Service. (1979). *Healthy people: The surgeon general's report on health promotion and disease prevention.* (DHEW Publication No. PHS 79-55071).Washington, DC: U.S. Government Printing Office.

Putt, A.M. (1978). *General systems theory applied to nursing.* Boston: Little, Brown.

Roberts, D. & Freeman, R. (Eds.). (1973). *Redesigning nursing education for public health: Report of the conference.* (Pub. No. [HRA] 75-75). Bethesda: U.S. Department of Health, Education and Welfare.

Rogers, M. (1980). Nursing: A science of unitary man. In Riehl, J. & C. Roy (Eds.), *Conceptual models for nursing practice.* New York: Appleton-Century-Crofts.

Ross, M. M., & Helmer, H. (1988). A comparative analysis of Neuman's model using the individual and family as the units of care. *Public Health Nursing, 5*(1), 30–36.

Roy, Sr. C (1970). Adaptation: A conceptual framework for nursing. *Nursing Outlook, 18*(3), 43–45.

Roy, C. (1984). *Introduction to nursing: An adaptation model* (2nd ed.). Englewood Cliffs, NJ: Prentice-Hall.

Roy, C. & Andrews, H. (1991). *The Roy Adaptation Model: The definitive statement.* Norwalk, CT: Appleton and Lange.

Sachs, T.B. (1908). The tuberculosis nurse. *American Journal of Nursing,* 8, 597.

Selye, H. (1956). *The stress of life.* New York: McGraw-Hill.

Shamian, J., & Edgar, L. (1987). Nurses as agents for change in teaching breast self-examination. *Public Health Nursing,* 4(1), 29–34.

Stevens, P. & Hall, J. (1992). Applying critical theories to nursing in communities. *Public Health Nursing,* 9(1), 2–9.

Tirpak, H. (1975). The Frontier Nursing Service—Fifty years in the mountains. *Nursing Outlook,* 33(3), 308–310.

Turner, J.G., & Chavigny, K.H. (1988). *Community health nursing: An epidemiologic perspective through the nursing process.* Philadelphia: Lippincott.

United Nations. (1987). *The prospects of world urbanization.* New York: United Nations Publication #ST/ESA/SER.A/101, Department of International Economic and Social Affairs.

U.S. Department of Health and Human Services. (1991). *Healthy People 2000: National Health Promotion and Disease*

Prevention Objectives. (DHHS publication PHS 91-50213). Washington, DC: Author.

Veninga, R. & Spradley, J. (1981). *The Work Stress Connection: How to cope with job burnout*. Boston: Little, Brown.

von Bertalanffy, L. (1968). General systems theory: A critical review. In W. Buckley (Ed.), *Modern systems research for the behavioral scientist*. Chicago: Aldine.

White, M. S. (1982). Construct for public health nursing. *Nursing Outlook, 30*, 527–30.

Williams, C. A. (1977). Community health nursing—What is it? *Nursing Outlook, 25*, 250–54.

Williams, C. A. (1983). Making things happen: Community health nursing and the policy arena. *Nursing Outlook, 31*, 225–28.

Williams, C.A. (1992). Community-based, population-focused practice: The foundation of specialization in public health nursing. In Stanhope, M. & J. Lancaster. *Community Health Nursing: Process and Practice for Promoting Health*. St. Louis: Mosby Year Book.

Woodham-Smith, C. (1951). *Florence Nightingale*. New York: McGraw-Hill.

Zerwekh, J.V. (1992). Community health nurses—A population at risk. *Public Health Nursing, 9*(1), 1.

SELECTED READINGS

Baumann, L.C. & Schmelzer, M. (1994). Writing to learn in community health nursing: The aggregate. *Public Health Nursing, 11*(4), 255–58.

Bracht, N. (Ed.). (1990). *Health Promotion at the Community Level*. Newbury Park, CA: Sage.

Buhler-Wilkerson, K. (1988). Public health nursing: A photographic study. Turn-of-the-century visiting nurses. *Nursing Outlook, 36*(5), 241–43.

Hamilton, P. & Keyser, P. (1992). The relationship of ideology to developing community health nursing theory. *Public Health Nursing, 9*(3), 142–48.

Henry, V., Schmitz, K., Reif, L., & Rudie, P. (1992). Collaboration: Integrating practice and research in public health nursing. *Public Health Nursing, 9*(4), 218–222.

Matuk, L. & Horsburgh, M. (1992). Toward redefining public health nursing in Canada: Challenges for education. *Public Health Nursing, 9*(3), 149–154.

McKnight, J. & Van Dover, L. (1994). Community as client: A challenge for nursing education. *Public Health Nursing, 11*(1), 12–16.

Rothman, N. (1990). Toward description: Public health nursing and community health nursing are different. *Nursing & Health Care, 11*(9), 481–83.

Salmon, M. (1989). Public health nursing: the neglected specialty. *Nursing Outlook, 37*(5), 226–29.

Salmon, M. (1993). An open letter to public health nurses. *Public Health Nursing, 10*(4), 211–12.

Spradley, B. (1991). *Readings in community health nursing*, (4th ed.). Philadelphia: Lippincott.

Wald, L. (1971). *The House on Henry Street*. New York: Dover Publications, Inc. (reprinted from 1915 edition published by Henry Holt and Co., New York).

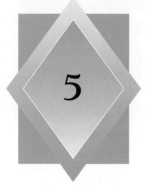

5

Roles and Settings for Community Health Nursing Practice

LEARNING OBJECTIVES

Upon completion of this chapter, readers should be able to:

- Describe and differentiate between seven different roles enacted by community health nurses.
- Explain the importance of each role for influencing people's health.
- Identify and discuss factors that affect nurses' selection and practice of roles.
- Describe six settings in which community health nurses practice.
- Discuss the nature of community health nursing, the common threads basic to its practice, woven throughout all roles and settings.

KEY TERMS

- Advocate
- Case management
- Clinician
- Collaborator
- Conceptual skills
- Controller
- Educator
- Evaluator

- Human skills
- Leader
- Manager
- Organizer
- Planner
- Researcher
- Technical skills

Barbara Walton Spradley and Judith Ann Allender
COMMUNITY HEALTH NURSING: CONCEPTS AND PRACTICE, 4th ed.
© 1996 Barbara Walton Spradley and Judith Ann Allender

Historically, community health nurses engaged in many roles. From the beginning, nurses in this profession provided care to the sick, taught positive health habits and self-care, advocated on behalf of needy populations, developed and managed health programs, provided leadership, and collaborated with other professionals to implement change in health services. The settings, too, in which these nurses practiced varied. The home was certainly one site for practice but so too were clinics, schools, factories, and other community-based locations. Today professional community health nurses practice in an even wider variety of settings and their roles have also expanded.

This chapter examines how the conceptual foundations of community health nursing are integrated into the various roles and the settings in which community health nurses practice. It is an opportunity for the reader to gain greater understanding about how and where community health nursing is practiced. Furthermore, it promotes an expanded awareness of the many existing and future possibilities for community health nurses to positively improve the public's health (see accompanying display).

Roles of Community Health Nurses

One could say that community health nurses wear many hats while conducting day-to-day practice. In other words, community health nursing incorporates a variety of roles. At times, one role is primary. For example, the nurse may assume a set of responsibilities in a specialized role such as that of full-time manager. More often, however, a number of roles are assumed simultaneously. Furthermore, several factors influence what and how roles are performed. This chapter examines seven major roles: (1) clinician, (2) educator, (3) advocate, (4) manager, (5) collaborator, (6) leader, and (7) researcher. Then it examines the factors that influence the selection and performance of those roles.

CLINICIAN ROLE

The most familiar community health nurse role is that of clinician or provider of care; however, giving nursing care takes on new meaning in the context of community health. The **clinician** role in community health means that the nurse ensures health services are

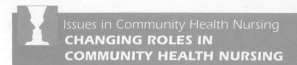

Issues in Community Health Nursing
CHANGING ROLES IN COMMUNITY HEALTH NURSING

With the advent of health care reform, community health nursing's roles are being positively challenged. The need for change in health care delivery systems, universal access to care, and assurance of quality services all call for community health nursing involvement. Herein lie opportunities for nurses to shape health care reform and public policy through enhanced advocacy and leader roles. Designing a system that is responsive to public health needs will call for formation of coalitions and community partnerships; exercising the collaborator role in new ways. Salmon (1993) challenges public health nurses with a vision of what they can do and be in the twenty first century. Reverby (1993), too, describes nursing's roles and contributions to community health in the past and it's potentially expanded influence for the future. The needs are great and community health nurses' roles and expertise position them for positive change affecting the future of the public's health.

provided, not just to individuals and families but also to groups and populations. Nursing service is still designed for the special needs of clients; however, when those clients comprise a group or population, clinical practice takes different forms. It requires different skills to assess collective needs and tailor service accordingly. For instance, a community health nurse might visit elderly persons in a seniors' high rise apartment building. This is an opportunity for the nurse to assess the needs of that entire aggregate and design appropriate services.

For community health nurses the clinician role involves certain emphases different from basic nursing. Three, in particular, are useful to consider here. They are the clinician's emphasis on holism, health promotion, and skill expansion.

Holistic Practice

Most clinical nursing seeks to be holistic. In community health, however, a holistic approach means considering the broad range of interacting needs that affect the collective health of the "client" as a larger system. The client is a composite of people whose relationships and interactions with each other must be considered in totality. Holistic practice must emerge from this systems perspective (Anderson and McFarlane, 1988). For example, a community health nurse may be working with a group of pregnant teenagers living in a juvenile detention center. The nurse would consider the girls' relationships with each other, their parents, the fathers of their unborn children, and the detention center staff. The nurse would evaluate their age levels, developmental needs, and peer influences, as well as their knowledge of pregnancy, delivery, and issues related to the choice of keeping or giving up their babies. The girls' reentry into the community and their future plans for school or employment would also be considered. Holistic service would go far beyond the physical condition of pregnancy and childbirth. It would incorporate consideration of pregnant adolescents in this community as a population-at-risk. What factors contributed to these girls' situations and what preventive efforts could be instituted to protect other teenagers? The community health nurse's clinician role involves holistic practice from an aggregate perspective.

Focus on Wellness

The clinician role in community health is also characterized by its focus on wellness (Birmingham, 1987). As discussed in Chapter 1, the community health nurse provides service along the entire range of the wellness-illness continuum but especially emphasizes promotion of health and prevention of illness. Nursing service includes seeking out clients with potential risk of poor health in order to offer preventive and health promoting services, rather than waiting for them to come for help after problems arise (Mullen, 1986; Wickizer, et al, 1993). Community health nurses identify people who are interested in achieving a higher level of health and work with them to accomplish that goal. They may help employees of a business learn how to live healthier lives, or they may work with a group that wants to quit smoking. They may hold seminars with a men's group on enhancing fathering. They may assist several families with terminally ill members to develop positive acceptance of dying and death. Community health nurses also identify groups and populations that may be vulnerable to certain health threats and design preventive and health-promoting programs. Examples include immunizing preschoolers, family planning programs, cho-

lesterol screening, drug education, and prevention of adolescent problem behaviors (Hurrelmann, 1990). Protecting and promoting the health of vulnerable populations is an important component of the community health nurse's clinician role and is addressed extensively in Chapter 24.

Expanded Skills

The nurse uses many different skills in the community health clinician role. In the early years of community health nursing, great emphasis was placed on physical care skills. As time went on, skills in observation, listening, communication, and counseling became integral to the clinician role as it grew to encompass an increased emphasis on psychological and sociocultural factors. Recently, environmental and community wide considerations, such as problems caused by pollution, violence and crime, drug abuse, unemployment, and limited funding for health programs, have created a need for stronger skills in assessing the needs of groups and populations and intervening at the community level (Rivera & Palmer-Willis, 1991). The clinician role in population-based nursing also requires skills in collaboration with consumers and other professionals, use of epidemiology and biostatistics, community organization and development, research, program evaluation, administration, leadership, and effecting change. These skills are addressed in greater detail in later chapters.

EDUCATOR ROLE

A second important role of the community health nurse is that of **educator** or health teacher. It is widely recognized that health teaching is part of good nursing practice and one of the major functions of the community health nurse (Brown, 1988). The educator role is especially useful in promoting the public's health for at least two reasons. First, community clients tend not to be in the most acute state of illness and are potentially better able to absorb and act on health information. For example, a class of expectant parents, unhampered by significant health problems, can grasp the relationship of diet to fetal development. They will understand the value of specific exercises to the childbirth process and then more likely perform those exercises. Thus the educator role has the potential for finding greater receptivity and providing higher yield results. Second, the educator role in community health nursing is significant because a wider audience can be reached. With an emphasis on populations and aggregates, community health nursing's educational efforts are appropriately targeted to reach many people. Instead of limiting teaching to one-on-one or small groups, the nurse has the opportunity and mandate to develop educational programs based on community needs and that seek a community-wide impact. Community-wide AIDS education, anti-smoking campaigns, and breast self-examination efforts (Coleman, et al, 1991) provide useful models for implementing the educator role at the population level and demonstrate its effectiveness in reaching a wide audience (See Figure 5.1).

One factor that enhances the nurse's educator role is the higher level of health consciousness many citizens have acquired. Through plans ranging from the President's Physical Fitness Program to local antismoking campaigns, people are recognizing the value of health and are increasingly motivated to achieve higher levels of wellness. When a middle-aged man, for example, is discharged from the hospital following a heart attack, he is likely to be more interested than he was before the attack in learning how to prevent occurrence of an attack. He can learn how to reduce stress, develop an appropriate and gradual exercise program, and alter his eating habits. Families with young children are often interested in learning about children's growth and development; many young parents want to raise happier,

healthier children. Health education can affect the health status of people of all ages (Coleman, et al, 1991; Ostwald, 1990). In an increasing number of businesses and industries nurses promote the health of employees through active wellness education programs (Kirkpatrick, 1985; Chen, 1988). The companies recognize that improved health of their workers means less absenteeism and higher production levels in addition to other benefits (White, 1986). Some companies even provide exercise areas and equipment for employee use.

Nurses in acute care teach patients about such things as personal care, diet, and medications. Community health nurses, however, go beyond these topics to educate people in many areas. Community clients need and want to know about a wide variety of issues such as family planning, weight control, smoking cessation, and stress reduction. Aggregate level concerns also include such topics as environmental safety, sexual discrimination and harassment at school or work, violence, and drugs. What foods and additives are safe to eat? How can people organize the community to work for reduction of violence on television? What are health consumers' rights? Topics taught by community health nurses extend from personal and family health to environmental health and community organization.

As educators, community health nurses seek to facilitate client learning. They share information with

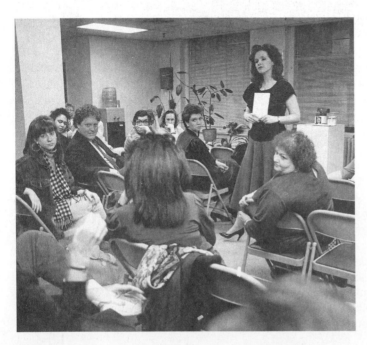

FIGURE 5.1. A community health nurse conducts smoking cessation classes.

clients both formally and informally. They act as consultants to individuals or groups. They may hold formal classes to increase people's understanding of health and health care. Community health nurses may use established community groups in their teaching. For example, they may teach parents and teachers at a Parent and Teachers' Association (PTA) meeting about signs of drug abuse, discuss safety practices with a group of industrial workers, or give a presentation on the importance of early detection of child abuse to a health planning committee considering the funding of a new program. At times, the community health nurse facilitates client learning through referral to more knowledgeable sources or through use of experts on special topics. The community health nurse also facilitates clients' self-education; in keeping with the concept of self-care, clients are encouraged and helped to use appropriate health resources and to seek out health information for themselves. The emphasis throughout the health teaching process continues to be placed on illness prevention and health promotion. Health teaching as a tool for community health nursing practice is discussed in Chapter 14.

ADVOCATE ROLE

The issue of clients' rights is important in health care today. Every patient or client has the right to receive just, equal, and humane treatment. Our present health care system is often characterized by fragmented and depersonalized services and many clients are frequently unable to achieve their rights, especially the poor and disadvantaged. They become frustrated, confused, degraded, and unable to cope with the system on their own. The community health nurse often must act as **advocate** for clients, pleading the cause or acting on behalf of the client group. There are times when health care clients need someone to explain what services to expect and which services they ought to receive. They need someone to guide them through the complexities of the system and someone to assure the satisfaction of their needs. This is particularly true for minorities and disadvantaged groups (Lythcott, 1985).

Advocacy Goals

Kosik (1972) a number of years ago described two underlying goals in client advocacy that remain true today. One is to help clients gain greater independence or self-determination. Until they can discover this information and access these services for themselves, the community health nurse acts as an advocate for the clients by showing them what services are available, which ones they are entitled to, and how to obtain them. A second goal is to make the system more responsive and relevant to the needs of clients. By calling attention to inadequate, inaccessible, or unjust care, the community health nurse can influence change.

Consider the experience of the Martin family. Gloria Martin and her three small children had gone to the Westside Clinic on Wednesday. On Tuesday morning, the baby, Tony, had suddenly started to cry. Nothing would comfort him. Gloria called the clinic and was told to come in the next day. The clinic did not take appointments and was too busy to see any more patients that day. The rest of that day and night Tony cried almost incessantly. On Wednesday there was a 45-minute bus ride and a wait of three-and-a-half hours in the crowded reception room, a wait punctuated by intake workers' interrogations. The children were restless, and the baby was crying. Finally they saw the physician. Tony had an inguinal hernia that could be gangrenous. The doctor admonished the mother that the baby should have been brought in sooner. Now immediate surgery was necessary. Someone at the clinic told Gloria that Medicaid would pay for it. Someone else told her that she was ineligible because she was not a registered clinic patient. By now all the children were crying. Gloria had been up most of the night. She was frantic, confused, and felt that no one cared. This family needed an advocate.

Advocacy Actions

The advocate role incorporates four characteristic actions: (1) being assertive, (2) taking risks, (3) communicating and negotiating well, and (4) identifying resources and obtaining results. First, advocates must be *assertive*. In the Martins' dilemma, a community health nurse took the initiative to identify their needs and find appropriate solutions. She contacted the right people and helped them establish eligibility for coverage of surgery and hospitalization costs. She helped Gloria make arrangements for the baby's hospitalization and the other children's care. Second, advocates must *take risks*, go out on a limb if need be, for the client. The community health nurse was outraged at the kind of treatment that the Martins had received—the delays in service, the impersonal care, and the surgery that might have been prevented. She wrote a letter describing the details of the Martins' experience to the clinic director, the chairman of the clinic board, and the nursing director. It resulted in better care for the Martins and a series of meetings aimed at changing clinic procedures and providing better initial screening. Third, advocates must *communicate and negotiate well* by bargaining thoroughly and convincingly. The community health nurse helping the Martins was able to state the problem clearly and argue for its solution. Finally, advocates must *identify and obtain resources* for the client's benefit. By contacting the most influential people in the clinic and appealing to their desire for quality service, the nurse concerned with the Martins was able to facilitate change.

Advocacy at the population level incorporates the same goals and actions. Whether the population is homeless people, battered women, migrant workers, or some other group, the community health nurse in the advocate role speaks and acts on their behalf (see Figure 5.2). The goals remain the same—to promote clients' self-determination and to shape a more responsive system. Advocacy may take the form of presenting public health nursing data to encourage program funding (Ekstrand, et al, 1992). It may mean conducting a needs assessment to demonstrate the necessity for a shelter and multi-service program for the homeless. It may mean that the nurse testifies before the legislature to create awareness of the problems of battered women and the need for more protective laws. It may mean organizing a lobbying effort to require migrant workers' employers to provide proper housing and working conditions. In each case, the nurse works with representatives of the population to gain their understanding of the situation and to ensure their input.

MANAGER ROLE

Community health nurses, like all nurses, engage in the role of managing health services. As a **manager** the nurse exercises administrative direction toward the accomplishment of specified goals by assessing clients' needs, planning and organizing to meet those needs, directing and leading to achieve results, and controlling and evaluating the progress to assure that goals are met. Nurses serve as managers when they oversee client care, supervise ancillary staff, do case management, manage caseloads, run clinics, or conduct community health needs assessment projects. In each instance, the nurse engages in four basic functions that make up the man-

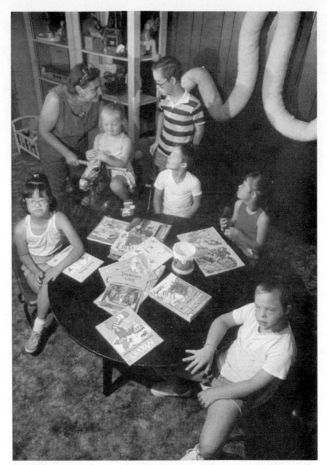

FIGURE 5.2. A community health nurse evaluates a day care facility for mentally challenged children.

agement process. The management process, like the nursing process, incorporates a series of problem-solving activities or functions: planning, organizing, leading, and controlling/evaluation. These activities are sequential and yet also occur simultaneously for managing service objectives (Robbins, 1993; Rowland & Rowland, 1985). While performing these functions, community health nurses most often are participative managers; that is, they participate with clients, other professionals, or both, to plan and implement services.

Nurse as Planner

The first function in the management process is planning. As **planner** the nurse sets the goals and direction for the organization or project and determines the means for achieving them. More specifically, planning includes defining goals and objectives, determining the strategy for reaching them, and designing a coordinated set of activities for implementing and evaluating them. Planning may be *strategic*, which tends to include broader and more long range goals (McKnight, et al, 1991). An example of strategic planning would be setting two-year agency goals to reduce teen pregnancies in the county by 50%. Or planning may be *operational*, which focuses more on short term planning needs. An example of operational planning would be setting six month objectives to implement a new computer system for client record keeping.

The community health nurse engages in planning as a part of the manager role when supervising a group of home health aides working with home care clients. Plans of care must be designed that include setting short term and long term objectives, describing actions to carry out the objectives, and designing a plan for evalating the care given. With larger groups, such as a program for a homeless mentally ill population, the nurse uses the planning function in collaboration with other professionals in the community to determine appropriate goals for shelter and treatment and to develop an action plan to carry out and evaluate the program (Ervin & Kuehnert, 1993; Pearson, et al, 1991). The concept of planning is discussed further in Chapter 11.

Nurse as Organizer

The second function of the community health nurse's manager role is as **organizer** which involves providing a structure within which people and tasks can function to reach the desired objectives. A manager must arrange matters so that the job can be done. People, activities, and relationships have to be assembled in order to put the plan into effect (Rowland and Rowland, 1985). Organizing includes deciding the tasks to be done, who will do them, how to group the tasks, who reports to whom, and where decisions will be made (Robbins, 1993). In the process of organizing, the nurse provides a framework for the various aspects of service so that each will run smoothly and accomplish its purpose. The framework is a part of service preparation. When a community health nurse manages a well-child conference (WCC), for instance, the organizing function involves making certain that all equipment and supplies are present, required staff are hired and on duty, and staff responsibilities are clearly designated.

Nurse as Leader

In the manager role, the community health nurse must also act as a leader to work with people who need direction and coordination to achieve positive health outcomes. In this context leading means moving individuals as a group toward a goal. The leading function includes motivating people, directing activities, ensuring effective two-way communication, resolving conflicts, and coordinating the plan. Coordination means bringing people and activities together so that they function in harmony while pursuing desired objectives.

The nurse acts as leader when she or he directs and coordinates the functioning of a hypertension screening clinic, a weight control group, or a three-county mobile health assessment unit. At the community-wide level, the nurse's leading function may involve working with a team of professionals to direct and coordinate such projects as a campaign to eliminate smoking in public areas or to lobby legislators for improved handicapped facilities. In each case the leading function requires motivating the people involved, keeping clear channels of communication, negotiating conflicts, and directing and coordinating the activities established during planning so that the desired objectives can be accomplished.

Nurse as Controller and Evaluator

The fourth management function in the manager role is to control and evaluate projects or programs. As **controller** the nurse monitors the plan and ensures that it stays on course. The nurse engaged in this function must realize that plans don't always proceed as intended and may need adjustments or corrections to reach the desired results or goals. Monitoring, comparing, and adjusting make up the controlling part of this function. At the same time the nurse must compare and judge performance and outcomes against previously set goals and standards—a process that forms the **evaluator** aspect of this management function.

An example of the controlling and evaluation function was evident in a program started in several preschool day care centers in a city in the Midwest. The goal of the project was to reduce the number of illnesses among the children through intensive physical and emotional preventive health education with staff, parents, and children. The two community health nurses managing the project were pleased with the progress of the classes and monitored the application of the prevention principles in day-to-day care. However, after several weeks, staff became busy and some plans were not being followed carefully. Preventive activities were not being closely monitored, such as ensuring that the children covered their mouths if they coughed or washed their hands after using the bathroom and before eating. Several children who were clearly sick had not been kept at home. Touching and inclusion of lonely children was sometimes overlooked. The nurses worked with staff and parents to motivate them and get the project back on course. One activity was to establish competition between the centers for the best health record with promise of a photograph of the winning center's children and a covering article in the local newspaper. Their efforts were successful.

Management Behaviors

As managers, community health nurses engage in many different types of behaviors. These behaviors or parts of the manager role were first described by Mintzberg (1973). He grouped them into three sets of behaviors: (1) decision making, (2) transferring of information, and (3) engaging in interpersonal relationships.

Decision-making behaviors. Mintzburg identified four types of decisional roles or behaviors—entrepreneur, disturbance handler, resource allocator, and negotiator. Community health nurses as managers serve in the *entrepreneur* role when they initiate new projects. Starting a nursing center to serve a homeless population is an example. They play the *disturbance-handler* role when they manage disturbances and crises, particularly interpersonal conflicts among staff or between staff and clients. By determining the distribution and use of human, physical and financial resources, they play the *resource-allocator* role. And they play the *negotiator* role when negotiating, perhaps with higher levels of administration or a funding agency, for new health policy or budget increases to support expanded services for clients.

Transfer of information behaviors. Mintzburg described three informational roles or behaviors—monitor, information disseminator, and spokesperson. In the *monitor* role community health nurses collect and process information such as gathering on-going evaluation data to determine whether a program is meeting its goals. In the *disseminator* role they transmit the collected information to people involved in the project or organi-

zation. And in the *spokesperson* role they share information on behalf of the project or agency with outsiders.

Interpersonal behaviors. While engaging in various interpersonal roles, the community health nurse may function as figurehead, leader, and liaison (Ibid.). In the *figurehead* role they act in a ceremonial or symbolic capacity, such as participating in a ribbon-cutting marking the opening of a new clinic, or representing the project or agency for news media coverage. In the *leader* role they motivate and direct people involved in the project. And in the *liaison* role they maintain a network with people outside of the organization or project for information exchange and project enhancement.

Management Skills

What types of skills and competencies does the community health nurse need in the manager role? Three basic management skills are needed for successful achievement of goals; they are human, conceptual, and technical (Robbins, 1993). **Human skills** refer to the ability to understand, communicate, motivate, delegate, and work well with people. An example is a nursing supervisor or team leader's ability to gain the trust and respect of staff and promote a productive and satisfying work environment. Community health nurses as managers only accomplish goals *through* other people. Thus human skills are essential to successful performance of the manager role. **Conceptual skills** refer to the community health nurse's mental ability to analyze and interpret abstract ideas for the purpose of understanding and diagnosing situations and formulating solutions. Examples are analyzing demographic data for program planning purposes or developing a conceptual model to describe and improve organizational function. Finally, **technical skills** refer to the nurse's ability to apply special management-related knowledge and expertise to a particular situation or problem. Such skills might include implementing a staff development program or developing a computerized management information system.

Case Management

Case management has become increasingly important in community health nursing (Sager, 1990). **Case management** refers to a systematic process by which the nurse assesses clients' needs, plans for and coordinates services, refers to other appropriate providers, and monitors and evaluates progress to ensure that clients' multiple service needs are met (Knollmueller, 1989). As clients leave hospitals earlier, as families struggle with multiple and complex health problems, as increasing numbers of elderly persons need alternatives to nursing home care, and as competition and scarce resources contribute to fragmentation of services, there is a growing need for someone to oversee and coordinate all facets of needed service. Community health nurses, through case management, address this need (Pickett & Hanlon, 1990; Knollmueller, 1989).

The activity of case management often follows discharge planning as a part of continuity of care. When applied to individual clients it means overseeing their transition from the hospital back into the community and following them to ensure that all their service needs are met. Case management also applies to aggregates. This involves overseeing and assuring that a group's or population's health-related needs are met, particularly those at high-risk of illness or injury. For example, a community health nurse may work with battered women who come to a shelter. First the nurse must assure that their immediate needs for safety, security, food, finances, and care for their children are met. Then the nurse must work with other professionals to provide more permanent housing, employment, on-going counseling, and financial and legal resources for this group of women. Whether applied to families or aggregates, case management like other applications of the manager role, uses the three sets of management behaviors and engages the nurse as planner, organizer, leader, controller and evaluator.

COLLABORATOR ROLE

Community health nurses seldom practice in isolation. They must work with many people, including clients, other nurses, physicians, social workers, physical therapists, nutritionists, occupational therapists, psychologists, epidemiologists, biostaticians, attorneys, secretaries, environmentalists, city planners, legislators, and many more. As a member of the health team (Farley 1993; Williams, 1986), the community health nurse assumes the role of **collaborator** which means to work jointly with others in a common endeavor, to cooperate as partners (See Figure 5.3). Successful community health practice depends on this multidisciplinary collegiality (Turner and Chavigny, 1988). Everyone on the team, including the community health nurse, has an important and unique contribution to make to the health care effort. As on a championship ball team, the better all members play their individual positions and cooperate with other members, the more likely the health team is to win.

The community health nurse's collaborator role requires skills in communicating, in interpreting the nurse's unique contribution to the team, and in acting

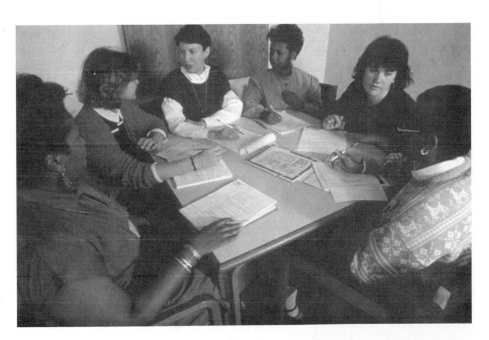

FIGURE 5.3. Community health nurses frequently collaborate with other health professionals.

assertively as an equal partner. The collaborator role may also involve functioning as a consultant.

The following examples show a community health nurse functioning as collaborator. Three families needed to find good nursing homes for their elderly grandparents. The community health nurse met with the families, including the elderly members, made a list of desired features, such as as shower and access to walking trails, and then worked with a social worker to locate and visit several homes. The grandparent's respective physicians were contacted for medical consultation, and in each case the elderly member made the final selection. In another situation, the community health nurse collaborated with the city council, police department, neighborhood residents, and manager of a senior citizens' high-rise apartment building to help a group of elderly people organize and lobby for safer streets. In a third example, a school nurse noticed a rise in the incidence of drug use in her schools. She initiated a counseling program after joint planning with parents, teachers, school psychologist, and local drug rehabilitation center.

LEADER ROLE

Community health nurses are becoming increasingly active in the leader role. As a **leader**, the nurse directs, influences, or persuades others to effect change that will positively affect people's health. The leadership role's primary function is to effect change; thus, the community health nurse becomes an agent of change. (Chapter 25 elaborates on this role.) As leaders, nurses seek to initiate change that will positively affect people's health. They also seek to influence people to think and behave differently about their health and the factors contributing to it. When they guide community health decision making, stimulate an industry's interest in health promotion, initiate group therapy, direct a preventive program, and influence health policy, they assume the leader role. For example, a community health nurse started a rehabilitation program that included self-esteem building, career counseling and job placement to help women in a half-way house who were recently released from prison.

The role of leader assumes a different form in another situation. One community health nurse determined that there was a need for a mental health program in her district. She planned to implement it through the agency for which she worked. But certain individuals on the health board were opposed to adding any new programs because of cost. Her approach was to gather considerable data to demonstrate the program's need and cost-effectiveness. She lunched individually with key board members in order to convince them of the need. She prepared written summaries, graphs and charts and, at a strategic time, presented her case at a board meeting. The mental health program was approved and implemented.

As leaders, community health nurses also exert influence through health planning (Ervin & Kuehnert, 1993; McLemore, 1980) . The need for coordinated, accessible, cost-effective health care services creates a challenge and an opportunity for community health nurses to become more involved in health planning at all levels—organizational, local, state, national, and even international. Nurses need to exercise their leadership responsibility and assert their right to share in health decisions (Farley, 1993).

RESEARCHER ROLE

In the **researcher** role community health nurses engage in systematic investigation, collection, and analysis of data for the purpose of solving problems and enhancing community health practice. But, it may be asked, how can research be combined with practice? Although technically research involves a complex set of activities conducted by persons with highly developed and specialized skills, research also means applying that technical study to real-practice situations. It is an investigative process in which all community nurses can become involved in asking questions and looking for solutions. Collaborative practice models between academics and practitioners combine research methodology expertise with practitioners' knowledge of problems to make community health nursing research both valid and relevant (Misener, Watkins & Ossege, 1994).

Research literally means to search—to investigate, discover, and interpret facts. All research in community health, from the simplest inquiry to the most complex epidemiologic study, uses the same fundamental process. Most simply put, the research process involves the following steps: (1) identify an area of interest, (2) specify the research question or statement, (3) review the literature, (4) identify a conceptual framework, (5) select a research design, (6) collect and analyze data, (7) interpret the results, and (8) communicate the findings (see Chapter 26).

Investigation builds on the nursing process, that essential dynamic of community health nursing practice, using it as a problem-solving process (Polit and Hungler, 1991). That is, the nurse identifies a problem or question, investigates by collecting and analyzing data, suggests and evaluates possible solutions, and selects a solution or rejects them all and starts the investigative process over again. In one sense the nurse is gathering data for health planning—investigating health problems in order to design wellness-promoting and disease-preventing interventions for community populations.

Community health nurses practice the researcher role at several levels. In addition to everyday inquiries, community health nurses often participate in agency and organizational studies to determine such matters as the effectiveness of a screening program or the needs of homeless minority women (Nyamanthi et al, 1992). Some community health nurses initiate more complex research on their own or in collaboration with other health professionals (Selby et al, 1990). The researcher role, at all levels, helps to determine needs, evaluate effectiveness of care, and develop theoretical bases for community health nursing practice. Chapters 12 and 26 explain community health research in greater detail.

Attributes of the Researcher Role

A *questioning attitude* is a basic prerequisite to good nursing practice. There have probably been many times when a nurse revisited a patient and noticed some change in his condition such as restlessness or pallor. Consequently, the nurse wondered what was causing this change and what could be done about it. In everyday practice, community health nurses encounter numerous situations that challenge them to ask questions. Consider the following examples:

"Today's paper reports another group of kids arrested for doing drugs. Is there an increase in the incidence of drug abuse in the community?"

"Several day care children appear to have excessive bruises on their arms and legs. What is the incidence of reported child abuse in this community? What could be done to promote earlier detection and improved reporting?"

"There are several elderly persons living alone and without assistance in this neighborhood. How prevalent is this situation and what are this population's needs?"

"While driving through this part of the city, I haven't seen a single playground for miles. I wonder where the kids play?"

Each of these questions places the community health nurse in the role of investigator. They express the fundamental attitude of every researcher: a spirit of inquiry.

A second attribute, *careful observation*, is also evident in the examples just given. The community health nurse develops a sharpened ability to notice things as they are, including deviations from the norm and even subtle changes that suggest the need for some nursing action. Coupled with observation is open-mindedness, another attribute of the researcher role. In the case of the daycare childrens' bruises, the community health nurse's observations suggest child abuse as a possible cause. But open-mindedness requires consideration of other alternatives, and as a good investigator, the nurse explores these as well.

The community health nurse also uses *analytic skills* in this role. In the drug abuse example, the nurse has already started to analyze the situation by trying to determine its cause-and-effect relationships. Successful analysis depends on how well the data have been collected. Insufficient information can lead to false interpretations, so the nurse is careful to seek out the needed data. Analysis, like a jigsaw puzzle, involves studying the pieces and fitting them together until the meaning of the whole picture can be described.

Finally, the researcher role involves *tenacity*. The community health nurse persists in an investigation until facts are uncovered and a satisfactory answer is found. Noticing an absence of playgrounds and wondering where the children play is only a beginning. The nurse, concerned about the children's safety and need for recreational outlets, gathers data about location and accessibility of play areas as well as felt needs of community residents. A fully documented research report may result. If the data support a need for additional play space, the report can be brought before the proper authorities.

Settings for Community Health Nursing Practice

The previous section examined community health nursing from the perspective of its major roles. Now the roles can be placed in context by viewing the settings in which they are practiced. The types of places in which community health nurses practice are increasingly varied including a growing number of non-traditional settings and partnerships with non-health groups. Employers of community health nurses range from state and local health departments and home health agencies to managed care organizations, businesses and industry. For purposes of discussion, however, these various settings can be grouped into six categories: (1) homes, (2) ambulatory service settings, (3) schools, (4) occupational health settings, (5) residential institutions, and (6) the community at large.

HOMES

For a long time the most frequently used setting for community health nursing practice was the home. In the home all of the community health nursing roles, to varying degrees, are performed. Clients discharged from acute care institutions, such as hospitals or mental health facilities, are regularly referred to community health nursing for continued care and follow-up. Here the nurse can see clients in a family and environmental context, and service can be tailored to clients' unique needs. For example, Mr. White, 67 years of age, was discharged from the hospital with a colostomy. Doreen, the community health nurse from the county public health nursing agency, immediately started home visits. She met with Mr. White and his wife to discuss their needs as a family and to plan for Mr. White's care and adjustment to living with a colostomy. Practicing the clinician and educator roles, she reinforced and expanded on the teaching started in the hospital for colostomy care, including bowel training, diet, exercise, and proper use of equipment. As part of a total family care plan, Doreen provided some forms of physical care for Mr. White as well as counseling, teaching, and emotional support for both the Whites. In addition to consulting with the physician and social services, she arranged and supervised home health aide visits that gave personal care and homemaker services. She thus performed the manager, leader, and collaborator roles.

The home is a setting for health promotion as well. Many community health nursing visits focus on assisting families to understand and practice healthier living. They may, for example, include instruction in parenting, infant care, child discipline, diet, exercise, coping with stress, or managing grief and loss.

The character of the home setting is as varied as the clients whom the community health nurse serves. In one day the nurse may visit an elderly, well-to-do widow in her luxurious home, a middle-income family in their modest bungalow, and a transient in his one-room fifth-story walk-up. In each situation, community

health nurses can view their clients in perspective and, therefore, better understand their limitations, capitalize on their resources, and tailor health services to meet their needs. In the home, unlike most other health care settings, clients are on their own turf. They feel comfortable and secure in familiar surroundings and are often better able to understand and apply health information. Client self-respect can be promoted, since the client is host while the nurse is a guest.

Health care reform along with shifting health economics and service delivery, discussed in Chapter 3, is changing community health nursing's use of the home as a setting for practice. The increased demand for high tech acute care in the home requires specialized skills best delivered by nurses with this expertise. Community health nurses with skills in population-based practice serve the public's health best by focusing on sites where they can have the greatest impact. At the same time, they can collaborate with various types of home care providers, including hospitals, other nurses, physicians, rehabilitation therapists, and durable medical equipment (DME) companies to ensure continuous and holistic service. They continue to supervise home care services and engage in case management. An innovative example is the Block Nurse Program described below. Chapter 22 further examines the nurse's role in the home setting.

AMBULATORY SERVICE SETTINGS

Ambulatory service settings include a variety of places for community health nurses' practice in which clients come for day or evening services, but that do not include overnight stays. Community health centers are an example of an ambulatory setting. Sometimes multiple clinics, offering comprehensive services, are community-based or located in outpatient departments of hospitals and medical centers. They may also be based in comprehensive neighborhood health centers (See Figure 5.4). A single clinic, such as a family planning clinic or well-child conference, may be found in a location more convenient for clients, perhaps a church basement or empty storefront. Some kinds of day care centers, such as those for physically handicapped or emotionally disturbed adults, utilize community health nursing services. Additional ambulatory care settings include health departments and community health nursing agencies where clients may come for assessment and referral or counseling.

Offices are another type of ambulatory care setting. Some community health nurses provide service in con-

Research in Community Health Nursing
EVALUATION OF THE BLOCK NURSE PROGRAM

Jamieson, M.K. (1990). Block Nursing: Practicing autonomous professional nursing in the community. *Nursing & Health Care*, 11(5): 250–253.

This evaluation study describes an example of innovative community health nursing in the home setting. It is the Block Nurse Program in St. Paul, Minnesota. Begun in 1982, this community-based service to elderly clients was conceived, implemented, and is primarily managed by nurses. Staffing for the program comes through trained Block Volunteers, Block Companions, and Block Nurses, all of whom are residents of the neighborhood in which the program is located. Elderly clients receive a range of services in their homes from such things as a bladder control program or respite care to grocery delivery and transportation to doctor's appointments or concerts. The program has proven highly successful in maintaining the elderly population in their homes, 85% of whom would otherwise have been forced to enter nursing homes. Costs of the program are at least 24% lower than minimum nursing home costs without nursing services. The Block Nurse Program has been replicated in three other sites and all have drawn their funding from several sources including Medicaid, Medicare, client fees, grants, and the Veterans Administration. Block Nurses practice all of the seven community health nursing roles, particularly the clinician, advocate, collaborator, and manager roles. They plan and oversee clients' services and work with neighborhood businesses and personnel to provide comprehensive and caring support.

junction with a medical practice; for example, a community health nurse associated with an HMO sees clients in the office and undertakes screening, referrals, counseling, health education, and group work. Others establish independent practices by seeing clients in nursing centers as well as making home visits (Anderson, 1989; Buchanan et al, 1989; Gloss and Fielo, 1987; Thibodeau, 1987).

Another type of ambulatory service setting includes places where services are offered to selected groups. For example, community health nurses practice in migrant camps, Native American reservations, correctional facilities, children's day care centers, through churches as parish nurses (Denny, 1990; Miller, 1987), and in remote mountain and coal-mining communities. Again, in each ambulatory setting all the community health nursing roles are used to varying degrees.

SCHOOLS

Schools of all levels make up a major group of settings for community health nursing practice. Nurses from community health nursing agencies frequently serve private schools of elementary and intermediate levels. Public schools are served by the same agencies or by community health nurses hired through the public school system. Community health nurses may work with groups of children in preschool settings, such as Montessori schools, as well as in vocational or technical schools, junior colleges, and college and university settings. Specialized schools, such as those for the handicapped, are another setting for community health nursing practice.

Community health nurses' roles in school settings are changing. School nurses, whose primary role was initially that of clinician, are widening their practice to include more health education, collaboration, and client advocacy. For example, one school had been accustomed to using the nurse as a first-aid giver and record keeper. Her duties were handling minor problems, such as headaches and cuts, and keeping track of such events as immunizations. This nurse sought to expand her practice and, after consultation and preparation, collaborated with a health educator and some of the teachers to offer a series of classes on personal hygiene, diet, and sexuality. She started a drop-in health counseling center in the school and established a network of professional contacts for consultation and referral. Community health nurses in school settings are also beginning to assume managerial and leadership roles and to recognize that the researcher role should be an integral part of their practice. The nurse's role with preschool and school-age populations is discussed in greater detail in Chapter 19.

OCCUPATIONAL HEALTH SETTINGS

Business and industry provide another group of settings for community health nursing practice. Employee health has long been recognized as making a vital contribution to individual lives, productivity of business,

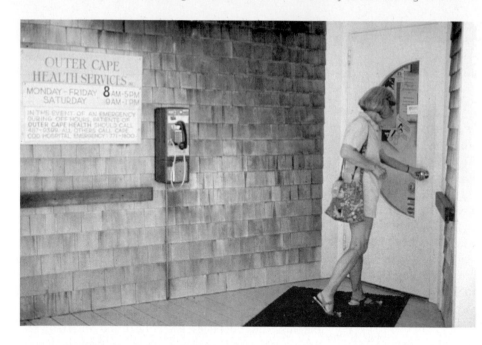

FIGURE 5.4. This neighborhood health center serves an island community.

and the well-being of the entire nation. Organizations now are expected to provide a safe and healthy work environment in addition to offering insurance for health care. An increasing number of companies, recognizing the value of healthy employees, go beyond offering traditional health benefits to supporting health promotional efforts. Some businesses, for example, offer healthy snacks such as fruit at breaks and promote jogging during the noon hour. A few larger corporations have built exercise facilities for their employees, provide health education programs, and offer financial incentives for losing weight or staying well.

Community health nurses in occupational health settings practice a variety of roles. Early industrial nursing, which started in 1895 when the first nurse, Ida M. Stewart, was hired by the Vermont Marble Company, mostly involved visiting mothers and infants as well as sick workers in their homes (Pickett & Hanlon, 1990). The clinician role was primary for many years as nurses continued to care for sick or injured employees at work. However, recognition of the need to protect employees' safety, and later, to prevent their illness led to the inclusion of health education in the occupational health nurse role. Now occupational health nurses also act as employee advocates, assuring appropriate job assignments for workers and adequate treatment for job-related illness or injury. They collaborate with other health care providers and company management to offer better services to their clients. They act as leaders and managers in developing new health services in the work setting endorsing programs such as hypertension screening or weight control. Occupational health settings range from industries and factories, such as an automobile assembly plant, to business corporations and even large department stores. The field of occupational health offers a challenging opportunity, particularly in smaller businesses where nursing coverage usually is not provided. Chapter 20 more fully describes the role of the nurse serving the working population.

RESIDENTIAL INSTITUTIONS

Any facility where clients reside can be a setting in which community health nursing is practiced. Residential institutions can include a half-way house in which clients live temporarily while recovering from drug addiction, or an inpatient hospice program in which terminally ill clients live. Some residential settings, such as hospitals, exist solely to provide health care, others provide other services and support. Community health nurses based in a community agency maintain continuity of care for their clients by collaborating with hospital personnel, visiting clients in the hospital, and helping plan care during and following hospitalization. Some community health nurses may serve one or more hospitals on a regular basis by providing a liaison with the community, consultation for discharge planning, and periodic in-service programs to keep hospital staff updated on community services for their clients. Other community health nurses with similar functions are based in the hospital and serve the hospital community.

A long term care facility is another example of a residential site providing health care that may use community health nursing services. In this kind of setting, where residents are usually elderly with many chronic health problems, community health nurses function particularly as advocates and collaborators to improve services. They will coordinate available resources to meet the needs of residents and their families and help safeguard the maintenance of quality operating standards. Sheltered workshops and group homes for mentally ill or retarded adults are other examples of residential institutions that serve clients who share specific needs.

Community health nurses also practice in settings where residents are gathered for purposes other than receiving care. Health care is offered as an adjunct to the primary goals of the institution. For example, many nurses work with camping programs for children and adults offered by churches and other community agencies, such as the Boy Scouts, Girl Scouts, or the YMCA. As camp nurses, community health nurses practice all available roles, often under interesting and challenging conditions.

Residential institutions provide unique settings for community health nurses to practice health promotion. Their clients are a "captive" audience whose needs can be readily assessed and whose interests can be stimulated. These settings offer community health nurses the opportunity to generate an environment of caring and optimal-quality services.

COMMUNITY AT LARGE

Unlike the five settings already discussed, the sixth setting for community health nursing practice is not confined to a specific location or building. When nurses work with groups, populations, or the total community, they may practice in many different places. For example, a community health nurse, as clinician and health educator, may work with a parenting group in a church or town hall. Another nurse, as client advocate, leader, and researcher, may study the health needs of a neighborhood's elderly population by collecting data throughout the area and meeting with resource people in many places. Again, the community at large becomes

the setting for practice of a nurse who serves on health care planning committees, lobbies for health legislation at the state capitol, runs for a school board position, or assists with flood relief in Pakistan (see World Watch display below).

Although the term 'setting' implies place, it is important to remember that community health nursing practice is not limited to a specific site. Community health nursing is a specialty of nursing defined by the nature of its practice, not it's location (Anderson and Meyer, 1985; Williams, 1992); it can be practiced anywhere.

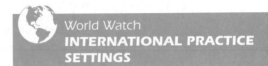

World Watch
INTERNATIONAL PRACTICE SETTINGS

For many decades community health nurses have practiced in other countries as well as their country of origin. Organizations such as the World Health Organization, Pan American Health Organization, Project Hope, American Refugee Committee, the Peace Corps, hunger relief groups, missionary organizations, and many others have engaged public health nurses in work overseas. Some have gone primarily as clinicians to develop and provide direct services; many third world countries have had desperate need for screening and treatment clinics, nutrition counseling, and family planning assistance. Most community health nurses practicing in international settings combine the clinician role with that of manager, educator, advocate, collaborator, and researcher. The variety and complexity of health-related needs in countries experiencing famine, floods, AIDs and other communicable disease epidemics, war and poverty challenge nurses to practice multiple roles simultaneously.

International community health nursing continues to offer a challenging and rewarding arena for practice. Today nurses serve in almost every country of the world, many under difficult and even dangerous conditions. The needs are great and nursing's impact on the health of disadvantaged populations in developing countries, in particular, can be tremendous.

Summary

Community health nurses play many roles including that of clinician, educator, advocate, manager, collaborator, leader, and researcher. Each role entails special types of skills and expertise. The type and number of roles that are practiced vary with each set of clients and each specific situation, but the community health nurse should be able to successfully function in each of these roles as the particular situation demands. The role of manager is one that the community health nurse must play in every situation because it involves assessing clients' needs, planning and organizing to meet those needs, directing and leading cients to achieve results, and controlling and evaluating the progress to assure that the goals and clients's needs are met. A type of comprehensive management of clients has become known as case management and is now an integral part of community health nursing practice today.

As a part of the manager role, the community health nurse must engage in three crucial management behaviors: decision making, transferring information, and relationship building. The nurse must also use a comprehensive set of management skills: human skills that allow the nurse to understand, communicate, motivate, and work with people; conceptual skills that allow the nurse to interpret abstract ideas and apply them to real situations to help formulate solutions; and technical skills which allow the nurse to apply special management-related knowledge and expertise to a particular situation or problem.

There are also many types of settings in which the community health nurse must practice and in which the above roles are enacted. Setting does not necessarily mean a specific location or site but rather a particular situation. These situations can be grouped into six major categories: homes, ambulatory service settings where clients come for care but do not stay overnight, schools, occupational health settings which serve business and industry employees, residential institutions such as hospitals, longterm care facilities, half-way houses, or any other institutions in which people live and sleep, and the community-at-large which can be found in a variety of locations.

Activities to Promote Critical Thinking

1. Discuss some ways that a community health nurse can make service holistic and focused on wellness with a group of chemically-dependent adolescents.

2. Select one community health nursing role and describe its application in meeting your next-door-neighbor's needs.

3. Describe a hypothetical or real situation in which you, as a community health nurse, would combine the roles of leader, collaborator, and researcher (investigator). Discuss how each of these roles might be played.

4. If your community health nursing practice setting is the community-at-large, will your practice roles be any different from those of the nurse whose practice setting is the home? Why? What determines the roles played by the community health nurse?

5. Interview a practicing community health nurse and determine which roles she or he plays over a period of a month of practice. Describe the ways in which each role is enacted. How many instances of this nurse's practice were aggregate-focused? If you were a public health consultant what suggestions might you make to expand this nurse's roles into aggregate level practice?

REFERENCES

Anderson, E. & McFarlane, J. (1988). *Community as client.* Philadelphia: Lippincott.

Anderson, E. & Meyer, A.T. (1985). Report of the Conference. *Consensus conference on the essentials of public health nursing practice and education.* Rockville, MD: U.S. Department of Health and Human Services.

Anderson, S.J. (1989). *Nursing centers: meeting the demand for quality health care. Geriatric education and health management clinic: synergy in a nursing center.* National League for Nursing Publication, #21-2311, 129–34.

Birmingham, J.J. (1987). The wellness frontier: The community. *Nursing Administration Quarterly, 11*(3), 14–18.

Brown, M.A. (1988). Health promotion, education, counseling and coordination in primary health care nursing. *Public Health Nursing, 5*(1), 16–23.

Buchanan, M., et al. (1989). *Nursing centers: meeting the demand for quality health care. Community wellness outreach: family health through empowerment.* National League for Nursing Publication, #21-2311, 111–6.

Chen, M.S., Jr. (1988). Wellness in the workplace: Beyond the point of no return. *Health Values, 12*(1), 16–22.

Coleman, E.A., et al. (1991). Efficacy of breast self-examination teaching methods among older women. *Oncology Nursing Forum, 18*(3), 561–6.

Denny, M. (1990). Church-based geriatric care. *Nursing Administration Quarterly,* Winter, *14*(2), 64–7.

Ekstrand, C., et al. (1992). Using public health nursing data for program advocacy. *Journal of Nursing Administration, 22*(4), 32–6.

Ervin, N. & Kuehnert, P. (1993). Application of a model for public health nursing program planning. *Public Health Nursing, 10*(1), 25–30.

Farley, S. (1993). The community as partner in primary health care. *Nursing and Health Care, 14*(5), 244–9.

Gloss, E.F., & Fielo, S.B. (1987). The nursing center: An alternative for health care delivery. *Family and Community Health, 10*(2), 49–58.

Hurrelmann, K. (1990). Health promotion for adolescents: preventive and corrective strategies against problem behavior. *Journal of Adolescence, 13,* 321–50.

Jamieson, M.K. (1990). Block nursing: practicing autonomous professional nursing in the community. *Nursing and Health Care, 11*(5), 250–3.

Kirkpatrick, S.L. (1985). Nurses: Leaders in wellness health promotion at the worksite. *Occupational Health Nursing, 33*(9), 450–52.

Knollmueller, R.N. (1989). Case management: What's in a name? *Nursing Mangement, 20*(10), 38–42.

Kosik, S.H. (1972). Patient advocacy or fighting the system. *American Journal of Nursing, 72,* 694–96.

Lythcott, G. (1985). Health advocacy among minority groups. In J. H. Marks (Ed.). *Advocacy in Health Care.* Clifton, NJ: Humana Press.

McKnight, J., et al. (1991). The delphi approach to strategic planning. *Nursing Management, 22*(4), 55–7.

McLemore, M. (1980). Nurses as health planners. *Journal of Nursing Administration, 1,* 13–17.

Miller, J.T. (1987). Wellness programs through the church: Available alternative for health education. *Health Values, 11*(5), 3–6.

Mintzberg, H. (1973). *The Nature of Managerial Work.* New York: Harper and Row.

Misener, T., Watkins, J., & Ossege, J. (1994). Public health nursing research priorities: A collaborative delphi study. *Public Health Nursing, 11*(2), 66–74.

Mullen, K.D. (1986). Wellness: The missing concept in health promoting programming for adults. *Health Values, 10*(3), 34–37.

Nayamathi, A.M., et al. (1992). A community-based inventory of current concerns of impoverished homeless and drug addicted minority women. *Research in Nursing and Health, 15*(2), 121–9.

Ostwald, S.K., et al. (1990). The impact of health education on health status: an experimental program for elderly women in the community. *Journal of Community Health Nursing, 7*(4), 199–213.

Pearson, M., et al. (1991). Program evaluation application of a comprehensive model for a community-based respite program. *Journal of Community Health Nursing, 8*(1), 25–31.

Pickett, G. E. & Hanlon, J.J. (1990). *Public health: Administration and practice* (9th ed.). St. Louis: Times Mirror/Mosby.

Polit, D., & Hungler, B. (1991). *Nursing research: Principles and methods* (3rd ed.). Philadelphia: Lippincott.

Reverby, S.M. (1993). From Lillian Wald to Hillary Rodham Clinton: what will happen to public health nursing? (editorial) *American Journal of Public Health, 83*(12), 1662–3.

Rivera, S.J. & Palmer-Willis, H. (1991). County nursing service assessment tool: An overview. *Public Health Nursing, 8*(4), 264–6.

Robbins, S.P. (1993). *Organizational behavior* (6th ed.). Englewood Cliffs, NJ: Prentice-Hall.

Rowland, H.S., & Rowland, B.L. (1985). *Nursing administration handbook* (2nd ed.). Rockville, MD: Aspen Systems.

Sager, D. (1990). The business of case management. *The Case Manager, 1*(1), 36–40.

Salmon, M. (1993). An open letter to public health nurses (editorial). *Public Health Nursing, 10*(4), 211–12.

Selby, M., et al. (1990). Public health nursing interventions to improve the use of a health service: Using a plot study to guide research. *Public Health Nursing, 7*(1), 3–12.

Thibodeau, J.A., et al. (1987). Evolution of a nursing center. *Journal of Ambulatory Care Management, 10*(3), 30–39.

Turner, J., & Chavigny, K. (1988). *Community health nursing: An epidemiologic perspective through the nursing process.* Philadelphia: Lippincott.

White, D.M. (1986). Health promotion pays: 3 to 1 return seen in stress management programs. *Occupational Health and Safety, 55*(8), 18–19, 55.

Wickizer, T., Von Korff, M., Cheadle, A., Maeser, J., Wagner, E., Pearson, D., Beery, W., & Psaty, B. (1993). Activating communities for health promotion: a process evaluation method. *American Journal of Public Health, 83*(4), 561–7.

Williams, E. (1986). Teamwork: Reinventing the wheel. *Community Outlook,* September: 36, 38.

Williams, C. (1992). Community-based population-focused practice: The foundation of specialization in public health nursing. In M. Stanhope & J. Lancaster (Eds.). *Community health nursing: process and practice for promoting health* (3rd ed.). St. Louis: Mosby Year Book.

SELECTED READINGS

American Nurses Association. (1986). *Standards: Community health nursing practice.* Kansas City, Mo.: Author.

Association of Community Health Nursing Educators Committee on Practice. (1993). *Differentiated nursing practice in community health.* Lexington, KY: Association of Community Health Nursing Educators.

Beddome, G., Clarke, H., & Whyte, N. (1993). Vision for the future of public health nursing: a case for primary health care. *Public Health Nursing, 10*(1):13–18.

Cairns, A., et al. (1990). Unique and changing roles for the CHN today. *Journal of Community Health Nursing, 7*(3), 121–2.

Coss, C. (1993). Lillian D. Wald: Progressive Activist. *Public Health Nursing, 10*(2), 134–7.

Crosby, J.M. (1990). Helping older learners learn. *Home Healthcare Nurse, 8*(3), 42–5.

Ethridge, P. (1991). A nursing HMO: Carondelet St. Mary's experience. *Nursing Mangement, 22*(7), 22–7.

Faherty, B. (1993). Now is the time to advocate. *Nursing Outlook, 41*(6), 248–9.

Farley, S. (1993). The community as partner in primary health care. *Nursing & Health Care, 14*(5), 244–9.

Gaines, S., Rice, M., & Carmon, M. (1993). A model of health care delivery in a child day-care setting. *Public Health Nursing, 10*(3), 166–9.

Gleavey, D. (1990). The nursing role in epidemiology, risk management, and patient-public education. *Journal of Opthalmic Nursing Technology, 9*(5), 215–19.

Lyons, N.B. et al. (1990). Too busy for research? Collaboration: An answer. *Maternal Child Nursing, 15*(2), 67–8, 70, 72.

Lunin, L.F. (1987). Where does the public get its health information? *Bulletin of New York Academy of Medicine, 63*(10), 923–38.

Maglacas, A. M. (1988). Health for all: Nursing's role. *Nursing Outlook, 36*(2), 66–71.

Mahon, J., McFarlane, J., & Golden, K. (1991). De Madres a Madres: A community partnershp for health. *Public Health Nursing, 8*(1), 15–19.

Michielutte, R. & Beal, P. (1990). Identification of community leadership in the development of public health education programs. *Journal of Community Health, 15*, 59–68.

Nelson, M.L. (1988). Advocacy in nursing. *Nursing Outlook, 36*(3), 136–141.

Novak, J.C. (1988). The social mandate and historical basis for nursing's role in health promotion. *Journal of Professional Nursing, 4*(2), 80–87.

Riner, M.B. (1989). Expanding services: the role of the community health nurse and the advanced nurse practitioner. *Journal of Community Health Nursing, 6*(4), 223–30.

Riportella-Muller, R., Selby, M., Salmon, M., Quade, D., & Legault, C. (1991). Specialty Roles in Community Health Nursing: A national survey of educational needs. *Public Health Nursing, 8*(2), 81–89.

Solari-Twadell, A., et al. (1991). Body, mind, and soul: the parish nurse offers physical, emotional, and spiritual care. *Health Progress, 72*(7), 24–28.

Williams, C. A. (1977). Community health nursing—What is it? *Nursing Outlook, 25*, 250–54.

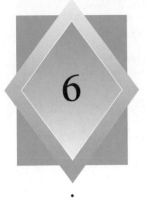

CHAPTER

6

Environmental Health and Safety

LEARNING OBJECTIVES

Upon completion of this chapter, readers should be able to:

- Discuss the significance of systems theory and the significance of an ecological perspective on understanding human-environment relationships.
- Explain the concepts of prevention and long-range environmental impact and their importance for environmental health.
- Identify at least six areas of environmental health concern to community health nursing and describe hazards associated with each area.
- Relate the effect of the above hazards on people's health.
- Discuss appropriate interventions for addressing the above environmental health problems including community health nursing's role.
- Identify at least six national health objectives for the year 2000 targeted at environmental health.
- Describe strategies for nursing collaboration and participation in efforts to promote and protect environmental health.

KEY TERMS

- Contaminant
- Ecological perspective
- Ecosystem
- Environment
- Environmental health
- Environmental impact
- Hazard
- Pollution
- Toxic agent
- Vectors

Barbara Walton Spradley and Judith Ann Allender
COMMUNITY HEALTH NURSING: CONCEPTS AND PRACTICE, 4th ed.
© 1996 Barbara Walton Spradley and Judith Ann Allender

The conditions within which people live and work (the **environment**) strongly influence people's health status, including the quality of the air, water, food, and even working conditions. Consequently the study of environmental health has tremendous meaning for community health nurses. Broadly defined, "**environmental health** is the subfield of public health concerned with assessing and controlling the impacts of people on their environment and the impacts of the environment on them"(Moeller, 1992, p.1). The field of environmental health is concerned with all those elements of the environment that influence people's health and well-being. The conditions of workplaces, homes, or communities, including the many forces—chemical, physical, and psychological—present in the environment that affect human health are important considerations.

Different environments pose different health problems and benefits. Consider the effects of acid rain, soil erosion, and insect invasions on a rural community or the effects of industrial toxic wastes, auto emissions, and airport noise on urban residents. The health effects of a hot, dry climate are different from those of an arctic area, and the environmental conditions of an industrialized nation are dramatically different from those of a developing country.

This chapter describes conceptual and theoretical approaches to environmental health, examines historical perspectives, and the primary environmental areas of concern to community health nurses. These areas include air pollution, water pollution, unhealthy and contaminated food, waste disposal, insect and rodent control, and safety in the home, worksite, and community.

Conceptual and Theoretical Approaches to Environmental Health

Assessing environmental health means more than looking for illness or disease-causing agents; it also means examining the quality of the environment. Do the conditions of both the person-made and the natural environment combine to provide a health-enhancing milieu? Are people's surroundings safe and life-sustaining? Are they clean and aesthetically enriching? Is the environment not only physically but also psychologically health enhancing? To answer these questions and gain greater understanding, the nurse needs to consider conceptual and theoretical approaches essential to assessing and controlling environmental health.

PREVENTIVE APPROACH

The study of environmental health has become increasingly complex as people's influence on the environment has increased. With the unprecedented advances in science and technology that have taken place in the past few decades, society's ability to affect the environment has expanded and the implications are not fully comprehended. New forms of energy and new synthetic chemical substances appear each year with such rapidity that it is nearly impossible to anticipate all the potential side effects on the environment and in turn on people's health. For each advance and "improvement" the toll to be paid is frequently unknown.

Thus, the concept of prevention is vital to environmental health. Scientists must use foresight as they design innovations; government, business, and citizens must play watchdog; and those concerned with human and environmental health must monitor new developments and intervene to prevent problems from occurring. Health practitioners need to determine causal links between people and their environment with an eye to improving the health and well-being of both. Nurses, in particular, must be aware of environmental factors that have the potential to either promote or adversely affect the health of communities. All three (primary, secondary, and tertiary) levels of prevention must be employed but most important is primary prevention. Primary prevention, that is, preventing a disease or **hazard** (a source of danger and risk particularly affecting human health) from occuring at all, has the greatest benefit to the community. See Figure 6.1.

While small scale preventive and health promoting measures, such as safety education in the home or workplace, are important, the larger environmental health picture must also be addressed. It is the larger environmental problems that ultimately place many if not all the members of a given community at risk. Community health nurses can develop an understanding of these environmental threats as well as the collaborative skills needed to work with other members of the public health team to prevent or alleviate them.

SYSTEMS/ECOLOGICAL PERSPECTIVE

When considering environmental health it is important to keep in mind the total relationship or patterns of relationships between people and their environment,

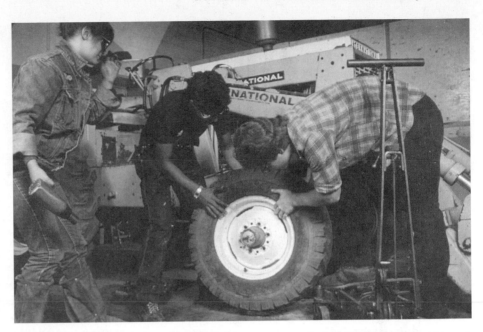

FIGURE 6.1. Safety goggles and appropriate clothing and footwear protects against workplace hazards.

also known as an **ecological perspective**. The application of systems theory and an ecological viewpoint are needed to provide this perspective (Benarde, 1989). Environmental health efforts may focus on a specific health hazard or environmental factor that poses a health threat; nonetheless, a broad view of human-environment relationships must be maintained. Environmental conditions and their effect on people must be considered holistically. One cannot isolate a single causal factor in most cases, since there may be many causal relationships. An outbreak of food poisoning, for example, may be attributed to the *salmonella* organism. However, it is most likely also associated with improper food handling and restaurant standards which, in turn, may be affected by inadequate inspections and monitoring. The multiple relationships present in any environmental situation have been referred to as a web (Benarde, 1989) and the multiple causes of a problem as a web of causation. This concept is discussed further in Chapter 12.

By taking a systems or ecological approach in studying environmental health, the community health nurse can examine the interrelatedness between humans and their environment. This ecological perspective recognizes that people can affect their environment and the environment can affect them. Further, the ecological perspective recognizes that preventive and health promotive measures may be applied to all aspects of the environment as well as to the people in it (Moeller, 1992). An ecological perspective takes into account the inter-connectedness of all living organisms and their physical environment. It recognizes that any manipulation of one element or organism may have hazardous effects on the rest of the environment, upsetting the balance of this aggregation of links known as the ecosystem. The **ecosystem** consists of a community of living organisms and their interrelated physical and chemical environment; no one factor, whether organism or substance, can be viewed in isolation from the rest of its environment. For example, several years ago an illegal application of pesticides on a watermelon crop on the west coast of the United States resulted in a serious outbreak of anticholinesterase intoxication. The food-borne pesticide caused 264 reported cases in Oregon, Washington, and California. After eating aldicarb-contaminated watermelons, people experienced nausea, vomiting, abdominal pain, diarrhea, blurred vision, dysarthria, and other neurological signs (Green et al., 1987). People must keep in mind that their actions affect other living organisms. Humans share this planet with millions of other living creatures, and must consider the ecological balance and anticipate the far-reaching consequences of their actions before introducing environmental change.

LONG-RANGE ENVIRONMENTAL IMPACT

When studying environmental health it is important to consider the effect of positive or negative changes on the environment and on the people, animals, and plants living in it; this is known as the **environmental impact**. This must be viewed not only in terms of its consequences for people living now but its long range impact on the human species. One must consider the health of future generations as well as present ones. Considerations should include food and fuel limitations of the natural environment, attendance to conservation by balancing present and future needs, and preventing the consequences of environmental abuse. This last point broadens the focus even more. Certainly one should determine how current practices and toxins are hurting humans, but it is also imperative to discover what threats they pose to the biosphere and thus to future generations—their long-range environmental impact. For example, carbon monoxide gas given off by factories and automobiles is toxic and can be lethal causing dizziness, headaches, and lung diseases in humans who inhale it at certain concentrations and has been found to reduce the atmosphere's ozone layer which protects us against ultraviolet irradiation. It poses a serious ecological threat for the future. See Figure 6.2.

Historical Perspectives

Environmental influences on people's health span all of human history. People's interactions with their environment and the conditions of that environment have shaped their mental, emotional, and physical health since the beginning of time. From ancient tribal practices of burial of excreta to modern-day sewage treatment, humans have been concerned with how the environment would provide for their needs and affect their well-being.

In an effort to promote human health, people have taken steps to control, alter, and adapt to their environment. Demonstrations of this concern go back to Biblical times, when the Israelites observed strict rules governing food preparation, practiced sanitation, and quarantined people with infectious diseases, such as leprosy.

As populations became more settled and urbanized, many different environmental health concerns developed. Community actions to deal with these developments have been recorded as far back as 2500 B.C. Archeologists have discovered remnants of sophisticated water and waste systems in ancient cities of northern India and in the Middle Kingdom of Egypt. Early

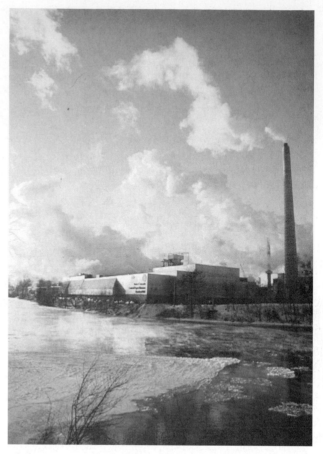

FIGURE 6.2. Industries are now regulated to prevent the environmental impact of carbon monoxide pollution.

Roman engineers built aqueducts for supplying fresh water, and they developed management operations for overseeing water and sewage systems (McGrew, 1985).

A major environmental issue in the medieval world was the spread of infectious diseases brought about by the growth of cities, increased trade, and wars. "Plague, spread by rodents, appears in the writings of Dionysius in the third century" (Blumenthal & Ruttenber, 1994). The most severe infectious diseases were outbreaks of leprosy and bubonic plague during the thirteenth and fourteenth centuries (McGrew, 1985). As leprosy spread and peaked in Europe in the early thirteenth century, people recognized a connection between the environment and the spread of the disease. They instituted epidemic control by isolating people with signs of the disease and checking newcomers to the community. Thus, long before science had discovered the true cause of these diseases, people were instinctively changing or avoiding harmful environmental circumstances in an effort to promote health (Purdom, 1980). Simple city ordinances restricted locals from washing their clothes or tanners from cleaning their skins in rivers that supplied drinkng water. A law passed in London in 1309 governed the disposal of wastes into the Thames river. Similarly, people passed rules governing the sale of old or spoiled meat to local residents, and "in Basel, leftover fish were displayed at a special inferior food stall and sold only to strangers" (McGrew, 1985, p. 139). This early concern for sanitary conditions became a major focus in public health, reaching its peak between 1840 and 1880.

The social hygiene movement called for societal transformation to create a truly healthful environment (Ibid.). During the mid- to late-1800s, Florence Nightingale in England and Dr. Ignace Semmelweiss in Vienna pioneered the promotion of clean hospital and surgical conditions to prevent illness. Oliver Wendell Holmes made the connection between exposure to sepsis and childbed fever in Boston in 1843. John Snow first documented environmental spread of disease in London in 1850 when he linked the spread of cholera with contaminated drinking water (Moeller, 1992). The work of Pasteur and Koch demonstrated the role of bacteria in disease. All of these, in addition to greater use of the microscope, shed further light on the relationship of the environment to health.

Awareness of environmental impact on health was first documented in a "Report on an Inquiry into the Sanitary Conditions of the Labouring Population of Great Britain" by Edwin Chadwick in 1842 (Pickett & Hanlon, 1990). This document addressed the necessity for a healthy environment. About the same time, a similar report in the United States called "Report of the Sanitary Commission of Massachussetts," by Lemuel Shattuck, provided original insights into environmental health issues including smoke prevention, pest control, sanitation programs, and food regulations (Ibid.). These documents marked the first organized concern for public health and environmental health controls. Since that time, the focus has gradually expanded from sanitation to the problems generated by advances in technology, chemical production, and pollution which are discussed in this chapter

In the United States, all levels of government have worked diligently to assess, prevent, and correct environmental health hazards. The major environmental health efforts of the federal government have come primarily since the early 1970s. Local governments assume responsibility for proper waste disposal, pure water supply, and efficient sanitary and safety conditions within the community. State governments, represented by different agencies, handle broader issues that deal with the creation of state regulations, policies, and supervision of local health efforts (Pickett & Hanlon, 1990). The federal government is charged with establishing and enforcing health standards and regulations. During the past twenty years the public concern for people's health in relation to the environment, as well as concern for the environment itself, has stimulated increased government actions. The Environmental Protection Agency (EPA) was established in 1971 and was given extensive authority over all environmental concerns and protection of public health. Other related agencies included incorporation of the Food and Drug Administration (FDA) within the Public Health Service in 1968, the Occupational Safety and Health Administration (OSHA) for regulation and the National Institute for Occupational Safety and Health (NIOSH) for research both established in 1970. The Public Health Service under the U.S. Department of Health and Human Services has helped to focus environmental control efforts through development of objectives published in 1979 and again in 1991. Its 1991 document, *Healthy People 2000: National Health Promotion and Disease Prevention Objectives*, lists objectives in major target areas. One related to environmental health can be found in the Levels of Prevention display.

An important international agency, the World Health Organization, was created in 1948 and has helped to identify and address world health problems, including issues of environmental concern. Since many modern technological discoveries cause far-reaching health hazards that affect the environment and the health of the entire global population, this organization and others like it will play increasingly important roles in the future (WHO, 1986).

Private business has become more conscious of health and safety issues as those isues have been enhanced by legislation such as the Products Liability Law and monitored by the Products Safety Commission. Private business and industry have often been accused of having total disregard for the health of the environment and its effect on human health but this image seems to be changing slowly. Many companies, confronted by concerned environmentalists or consumer protection groups that have formed in recent years, have been

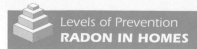

Levels of Prevention
RADON IN HOMES

GOAL

By the end of a year to increase the percent of homes in the city to 50 or more that have demonstrated safe levels of radon concentration.

PRIMARY PREVENTION

Conduct community education regarding the nature and dangers of inhaling the solid, radioactive decay products of radon gas. Require home testing for radon concentrations. Require sealed basement construction to avoid release of radon into buildings from underlying soil.

SECONDARY PREVENTION

Circulate air with electric fans in homes where radon concentrations are low. Use fan in combination with a positive-ion generator to more effectively reduce inhaled concentrations of airborne radon decay products. Periodic testing to ensure minimal levels of radon concentrations.

TERTIARY PREVENTION

Require building modifications where radon concentrations are high (ten or more times remedial action level). Seal cracks in basement floors and walls. Install subslab exhaust systems below basement floors.

---

forced to change their practices. Boycotts of products, listings of environmentally conscientious firms, and general public outrage have put a stop to many harmful practices. A number of companies have been concerned for some time with the environmental impact of their business operations; they have sought not only reduction of health hazards but also ways to promote environmental and public health. Timber companies, for example, have actively engaged in reforestation projects. Private business has been a major contributor to many nonprofit environmentally concerned projects and agencies, such as the Sierra Club.

Maintaining a healthy environment and balanced ecology, and promoting the health of those living in it, remains challenging. Past efforts to accomplish these goals have been only partially successful. However, increased public awareness and concern for future generations has exerted tremendous pressure to create new and more effective measures.

Environmental Health Areas of Concern

There are six major environmental health areas of concern with which community health nurses should be familiar: (1) air pollution, (2) water pollution, (3) unhealthy or contaminated food, (4) waste disposal, (5) insect and rodent control, and (6) safety in home, worksite, and community.

AIR POLLUTION

For many centuries people have known that air quality affects human health. In Europe and America in the 1800s and early to mid 1900s, documented episodes of concentrated air pollution due to thermal atmospheric inversion caused many reported deaths (Moeller, 1992). **Pollution** refers to the act of contaminating or defiling the environment so that it negatively affect people's health. Air pollution is now recognized as one of the most hazardous sources of chemical contamination. It is especially prevalent in highly industrialized and urbanized areas where concentrations of motor vehicles, and industry produce large volumes of gaseous pollutants. Decades of environmentally insensitive industrial development in eastern Europe and the Soviet Union as it was known then has caused serious life- and health-threatening air pollution in recent years (French, 1991). There is evidence that tens of thousands of people in these countries have developed respiratory and cardiovascular problems from airborne contaminants and 75% of the children in many industrial areas of these countries have respiratory disease (Munson, 1990). Even in the United States where controls have been more stringent, estimates indicate that "up to 8 percent of Americans suffer from chronic bronchitis, emphysema, or asthma either caused or aggravated by air pollution" (Moeller, 1992, p. 211). Airborne pollutants have adverse effects on many areas of human life; costs to property, productivity, quality of life, and especially human health are enormous.

Most air pollution results from industrial and automotive emissions. Pollutants include lead, ozone, carbon monoxide, sulfur dioxide, hydrocarbons, nitrogen oxides, and particulates such as dust and ash. The list of diseases and symptoms of ill health associated with specific air pollutants is lengthy, ranging from minor nose and throat irritations, respiratory infections, and bronchial asthma, to emphysema, cardiovascular disease, lung cancer, and genetic mutations. See Figure 6.3.

As with other toxic chemicals, it is often difficult to establish a cause-effect relationship between air pollution and illness. A relatively short, high level of exposure is normally easier to identify. There have been a number of poignant examples. One occurred in London in 1952, when an atmospheric inversion trapped coal-burning smoke and fog over the city for nearly a week. Four thousand people, mostly the elderly and those vulnerable from respiratory and cardiac diseases, died as a result (Moeller, 1992). Another incident occurred in Bhopal, India, in 1984 in which a chemical plant leaked methyl isocyanate into the atmosphere, taking approximately two thousand lives (Green & Anderson, 1986). Although these disasters and others like them are dramatic and frightening, the effects of long-term exposure to low levels of pollution are perhaps even more threatening. They are definitely more difficult to record, measure, understand, define, correlate, and control. It may be impossible to ever document their total effects.

Certain geographic areas are more susceptible to the ill effects of air pollution because of weather conditions or physical terrain. The episode in London occurred when a lack of wind combined with low temperatures to create a temperature inversion—a phenomenon in which air that normally rises is trapped under a layer of warm air, allowing air contaminants to build up to intolerable levels. Los Angeles, another city troubled by air pollution, is surrounded by mountains that prevent winds from clearing away smoke and fumes. A further condition occurs in urban areas where city buildings create a "heat island effect" in which warm air traps pollution in the atmosphere around the city (Blumenthal & Ruttenber, 1994). Thus, in examining the effects of air pollution, it is necessary to take into account the climate conditions and topography of an area.

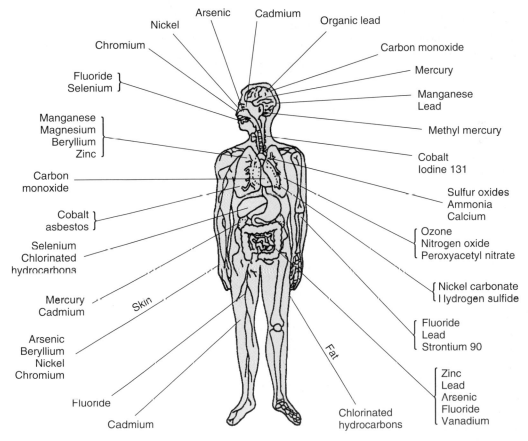

FIGURE 6.3. Body system targets of major air pollutants.

Air Pollutants Which Cause Illness

Dusts can contain numerous types of chemical irritants and poisons. Many hazardous dusts are associated with the workplace; for example, coal miners have developed black lung disease from inhaling coal dust, and a respiratory disease called silicosis is caused by exposure to silica dust (common in mining, sandblasting, and tunnel work). Asbestos fibers, which are found in insulation and fireproofing materials, textiles, and many other products, have been associated with lung cancer. Exposed individuals who smoke are at 30 times greater risk of developing lung cancer than those who do not smoke (Green & Anderson, 1986). Dusts are also associated with farming and grain elevator work, as well as highway construction.

Although much air pollution results from some type of human activity, naturally occurring dusts and ash can also pose problems. Elements in the environment, such as pollen from plants and flowers, ash from volcanic eruptions, or airborne microorganisms, can have ill effects on health.

A long list of gaseous pollutants, including sulfur oxides and nitrogen oxides produced by industrial emissions, pose additional problems for community health. Not only do such gases cause respiratory disease, asphyxiation, or are toxic in humans, but they can harm plant and animal life as well. Other gases, including chlorine, ozone, sulfur dioxide, and carbon monoxide, are all harmful to individual health as well as to the broader environment and the ecosystem.

Another gas that has been a topic of concern in recent years is radon. This colorless, odorless radioactive gas is formed by uranium breakdown in soil and rock. Radon enters buildings through cracks in basement walls or through sewer openings. Furnaces and exhaust fans can help pull radon into a house, although the highest levels tend to be found in basements where the gas enters. Home testing for radon was recommended by the EPA and the U.S. Public Health Service starting in 1988 (Weinstein et al., 1988). Sealing the cracks in basement walls and covering dirt floors can substantially reduce radon levels.

Air Pollutants Which Upset the Ecosystem

The emission of hazardous chemicals into the earth's atmosphere has a serious effect on the environment. Air pollutants, such as sulfur dioxide from power plant emissions or nitrogen oxides from motor vehicle exhaust, combine with water vapor to produce sulfuric and nitric acid, known as "acid rain," in many parts of the northern United States (Last, 1987). Although acid rain does not seem to pose any direct danger to humans, it kills small forms of life and endangers the forest and fresh water ecologies. An increased accumulation of carbon dioxide in the atmosphere from fuel combustion is altering the climate. Scientists believe that this carbon dioxide buildup traps infrared heat near the earth's surface and raises the earth's temperatures (Lemonick, 1987). Known as the "greenhouse effect," this too could have catastrophic consequences (Last, 1987) for the world's food supply and living conditions.

Government's Role

Government regulation of air pollution has been relatively slow. In 1963 the federal government passed a series of Clean Air Acts. These set standards for air quality and industrial emissions, and delegated funds to assist in pollution control programs. Although progress has been made, further public health efforts are needed to help identify pollution sources and related health hazards (Bingham & Meader, 1990; Rabe, 1990).

Nurse's Role

Community health nurses can influence air quality through detection, community education, and lobbying for appropriate legislation. People are exposed to numerous impurities in the air in their homes and workplaces. Nurses can promote health by helping to detect indoor pollutants and inform people of existing or potential dangers. Many household products and building materials emit vapors that can cause problems. Cigarette and cigar smoke are common indoor pollutants that can have ill effects on nonsmokers as well as smokers. Infants and other vulnerable persons are at risk to such exposure (Chilmonczyk et al., 1990). Carbon monoxide poisoning may result from stove and furnace emissions or car exhaust accumulating in a garage. Radon gas trapped in basements or tightly insulated homes is also a concern (Adelson, 1991; AMA, 1991). Nurses can assist with prevention or elimination of these health hazards by ensuring a well-ventilated (oxygenated) indoor environment, properly maintained heating equipment, and by looking for possible sources of pollution (see Issues in Community Health Nursing display).

1. Reduce asthma morbidity, measured by reduced asthma hospitalizations, to no greater than 160 per 100,000 population.
   Special target populations:
   Blacks and Nonwhites
   Children

2. Reduce prevalence of serious mental retardation among school-aged children to no more than 2 per 1,000 children.

3. Reduce outbreaks of waterborne disease from infectious agents and chemical poisoning to no more than 11 per year.
   Special target populations:
   People served by public or investor-owned water systems.

4. Reduce the prevalence of blood lead levels exceeding 15 ug/dL and 25 ug/dL among children aged 6 months through 5 years to no more than 500,000 and zero respectively.
   Special target population—Inner-city, low-income, black children

5. Reduce human exposure to criteria air pollutants, measured by an increase to 85% or more in the proportion of people who live in counties where any Environmental Protection Agency standard for air quality has not been exceeded in the past 12 months.
   Target air pollutants
   Ozone, carbon monoxide nitrogen dioxide, sulfur dioxide, particulates, lead.

6. Increase the proportion of homes to 40% or more where owner or occupant radon testing shows minimal risk or has been modified to reduce health risk.
   Target populations at 50%.
   Homes with smokers and former smokers
   Homes with children

7. Reduce human exposure to toxic agents by confining total pounds of toxic agents released into the air, water, and soil each year. Goal is no more than:
   0.24 billion pounds of toxic agents on DHHS carcinogens list
   2.6 billion pounds of toxic agents on Agency for Toxic Substances and Disease Registry list for most toxic chemicals

8. Reduce human exposure to solid waste-related water, air, and soil contamination. This will be measured by a reduction in average pounds of municipal solid waste produced per person per day to no more than 3.6 pounds.

9. Increase the proportion of people to at least 85% who receive safe drinking water supplies measured by EPA standards.

10. Reduce potential risks to human health from surface water. This will be measured by a decrease in the proportion of surface waters (lakes, streams, etc) to no more than 15% that do not support beneficial uses, such as fishing and swimming.

11. Provide testing for lead-based paint in at least 50% of homes built before 1950.

12. Expand the number of states to at least 35 where 75% of local jurisdictions have adopted construction standards and techniques to minimize elevated indoor radon levels.

13. Increase the number of States to at least 30 that require disclosure of lead-based paint and radon concentrations to prospective buyers of buildings for sale.

14. Eliminate significant health risks from hazardous waste sites on the Environmental Protection Agency's National Priority List. This will be measured by performing site clean-ups sufficient to eliminate specified health threats.

15. Establish programs for recyclable materials and household hazardous waste in at least 75% of counties.

16. Establish and monitor plans to define and track sentinel environmental diseases in at least 35 states. (These diseases include lead poisoning, other heavy metal poisoning, pesticide poisoning, carbon monoxide poisoning, heatstroke, hypothermia, acute chemical poisoning, methemoglobinemia, and respiratory diseases due to environmental factors.)

(Source: U.S. Department of Health and Human Services. (1991). Healthy People 2000: National health promotion and disease prevention objectives. Washington, DC: Government Printing Office.)

WATER POLLUTION

Water is such an essential element to human survival that the available quantity and quality of water within a community becomes a prime environmental health issue. In the Middle Ages disease epidemics spread as people drank water contaminated by human waste; this is still a problem in developing countries today. Water has many uses other than consumption by humans. It serves as a means of transportation. It cleans and cools the body or other objects. It is the basis for many forms of recreation and sports such as swimming and boating, and it provides a vehicle for disposing of human and industrial wastes and controlling fires. Apart from serving human needs, water also serves as a medium for sustaining other living organisms, a home to plant and animal life, and as a means of carrying and distributing necessary nutrients in the environment. Although nursing's environmental health concerns the safe consumption of water by humans, it is important, taking an ecological perspective, to keep in mind water's other uses and users.

Drinking water comes from two main sources: surface water, such as lakes and streams, and underground sources, called groundwater collected in areas known as aquifers; it comes to the surface through wells and springs. In general, underground sources are thought to be less subject to contamination than are surface sources, which are open to runoff from agricultural pesticides or industrial wastes. But groundwater, too, may be contaminated when seepage occurs. A **contaminant** is organic or inorganic matter that enters a medium, such as water or food, and renders it impure. Well water, for example, may contain fecal contaminants from improper septic tank drainage. A **toxic agent** is a poisonous substance in the environment that produces harmful effects on human health. Examples of toxic agents affecting groundwater include buried hazardous wastes or nitrate contamination of wells in rural areas (Johnson, 1990).

In most industrialized nations lack of sufficient water for drinking has not been a serious issue. Areas with limited water supplies have devised facilities to store water during high flow periods so that it would be available to satisfy the year-round needs of a given community. Adequate water supply to meet agricultural demands still has not been achieved, however.

The major concern with regard to water is its purity. Water can be contaminated and made unsafe for drinking in many different ways (Seymour, 1990). Three are discussed here.

1. Water may be infected with bacteria or parasites which cause disease. Giardia lamblia is a parasite shown to enter water supply by contamination from human or wild animal feces and which can cause giardiasis, a gastrointestinal disease that results in diarrhea and malabsorption of nutrients. One study showed an association between the risk of giardiasis and unfiltered surface water systems (Kent et al., 1988). Beavers in the north Cascade mountains often contaminate water (Blumenthal & Ruttenber, 1994) and make it essential for humans using the area for recreation to treat the water with iodine before drinking it. Water may also be contaminated with bacteria such as vibrio cholerae, resulting in cholera, or with viruses leading to hepatitis-A (Moeller, 1992).

2. Toxic substances introduced by humans into water systems are another source of water pollution and include farming pesticides as well as other chemicals which may contaminate streams, lakes, and wells (Johnson, 1990). Industrial pollutants may also enter drinking water through oil spills, careless dumping, or buried hazardous wastes that seep into underground water sources. Such wastes not only harm the quality of the water, they have been linked to causing disease such as leukemia (Fagliano et al., 1990) and can contaminate local fish and shellfish, making them unfit for consumption. Mercury poisoning from contaminated seafood on the Atlantic coast is a case in point. By 1988 one third of the nation's shellfish beds had been closed because of pollution.

3. Pollutants may upset the ecosystem affecting natural organisms which help purify water systems (Nadakavukaren, 1990). Power plants or other industries dissipate excess heat into lakes and streams which causes water temperatures to rise negatively affecting beneficial organisms in the water (thermal pollution).

In response to the various potential water pollutants, most cities and local communities with public or semipublic water systems in operation have set up water testing and treatment purification centers to ensure safe drinking water (Jones et al., 1991; Whyatt, 1990). Unfortunately, testing for bacteria and toxins often does not occur until after illness has been reported. Another major problem arises in rural areas where most water supplies are private and thus not assured of systematic testing and treatment. Testing water for coliforms as indicator organisms has proven useful. Water frequently is treated with chlorine to disinfect it but this, too, has led to risk of chloroform exposure from multiple uses of chlorinated tap water (Jo et al., 1990). Research also shows that carcinogens are produced from the reaction of chlorine to humic acids found in treated waters (Purdom, 1980).

Recreational uses of water, such as public swimming, have health implications. Lakes, oceans, rivers, and even hot tubs often carry infectious agents and result in a number of health problems including swimmers' itch and diarrheal diseases (Moeller, 1992; WHO, 1986). Many disease outbreaks have been caused by polluted water systems serving campgrounds, parks, and other public areas (DeWailly et al., 1986).

Government's Role

Most of the responsibility for maintaining water quality rests with state and local governments. The federal government took a needed step in 1974 by passing the Safe Drinking Water Act, which gave the Environmental Protection Agency (EPA) authority to establish water standards and to ensure that these standards were upheld. The federal government also provided funds to assist state and local governments in this effort. However, policies related to groundwater quality protection need continued monitoring (Huang & Uri, 1990).

On an international scale, because of enormous health problems in developing nations due to unclean water, the World Health Organization (WHO) declared the 1980s as the International Clean Water Decade and established a goal to have safe drinking water for all by the year 1990 (Blumenthal & Ruttenber, 1994; Last, 1987). Efforts to address water purity at the international level continue to assume high priority.

Nurse's Role

What role can community health nurses play in the effort to keep water safe? As nurses work in a community, they can help by examining household or city drinking water. Is there a strange odor or discoloration? Are particles or sediment visible in the water? Being aware of drinking water quality and possible contaminants in a given locality alerts the nurse to consider possible causal relationships if a problem exists. Asking clients to observe and report changes in water quality further assists the nurse in the monitoring process. When such changes occur, the proper authorities, such as health department officials, should be notified and

water samples tested. Community health nurses can also be alert to increased incidence of illnesses that might be water related. For example, if several children exhibit similar symptoms, the nurse might inquire as to whether all have been swimming in the same pool or drinking from the same water fountain. While water quality monitoring is ultimately the responsibility of environmental health authorities, it behooves the nurse, as a contributing member of the health team, to observe and report any information that would further the goal of safe and healthy water for communities.

UNHEALTHY OR CONTAMINATED FOOD

This section describes how the supply of food, particularly the quality of that food, is affected by the environment, and what health hazards are associated with food. The community health nurse needs to ask: "How does the environment influence the safety of food for human consumption?" Three types of hazardous foods must be considered when examining food as a possible health problem: inherently harmful foods, contaminated foods, and foods with toxic additives.

Inherently Harmful Foods

Poisonous foods such as certain types of mushrooms or inedible berries, do not pose a serious threat to most people. The general public can identify and avoid harmful plants and substances, so that cases of poisonings are rare (Green & Anderson, 1986).

Contaminated Food

Contaminated foods pose a more serious health problem. Food may contain harmful bacteria such as *Salmonella enteritidis*, *Staphylococcus aureus*, or *Clostridium botulinum*, causing outbreaks of salmonellosis or botulism. An estimated five million *Salmonella* infections alone occur annually in the United States (Benenson, 1990). Salmonellosis is characterized by sudden onset of headache, abdominal pain, diarrhea, nausea, vomiting, fever, and dehydration. The acute enterocolitis may develop into septicemia or a severe focal infection, such as endocarditis, meningitis, pneumonia, or pyelonephritis. Infants, elderly, and debilitated persons are at greatest risk for death. Blumenthal reported that nationally in one year 33% poultry, 15% pork, and close to 10% beef products were contaminated with *Salmonella* (1994) because of inadequate processing and shipping methods. Cooking destroys the organism, but problems may be caused by undercooking foods, such as rare roast beef, or handling raw meats. Viral food transmission is rare. Parasitic transmission generally takes the form of trichinosis, caused by ingesting *Trichinella spiralis* in undercooked pork. Various types of worm infestations have created serious health problems, particularly in developing countries. Different types of chemical food contamination result from improper food handling or processing. Examples include dirty machines used in food processing factories, pesticides and herbicides used by farmers to grow their crops, and mercury in fish that live in polluted water (WHO, 1986).

Food with Toxic Additives

A third health hazard from food comes from the intentional introduction of additives to food products. Because present-day consumers demand convenience foods and time-saving devices, and businesses want to produce food items with long shelf lives, enhanced flavor, and lasting, vibrant colors, many foreign chemicals and synthetic products have been added to foods. Animals that are raised for food, such as chickens, pigs, and beef cattle, are often fed or injected with substances to speed their growth. As consumers shift toward healthier eating, they do not know and are only starting to question the effects these additives may have over time. For example, red dye #2 once was added to improve the color of certain food products but has since been proven carcinogenic. Preservatives and chemical flavorings such as saccharin have also proven hazardous in large doses. It is still questionable what small doses may do with prolonged use. Recently, questions have been raised about potential long-range effects of NutraSweet, a sugar substitute. Furthermore, such natural flavor enhancers as salt and processed sugars appear in excessive quantities in some canned and packaged foods and are linked to unhealthy dietary consequences such as hypertension or obesity. In small doses these additives may not be harmful, but when additives are consumed in combination over prolonged periods of time, they may create serious health consequences.

Government's Role

It is the legal responsibility of food producers, processors, and manufacturers to guarantee the quality and safety of food products. However, conflicting motives, such as concern over loss of profit, often lead to careless or inadequate monitoring (Green & Kreuter, 1991). Governmental regulatory agencies exist on the local, state, and federal level to set standards and control the quality of food sold to the public. Such public health authorities as the Food and Drug Administration and the Departments of Agriculture and Health and Human Services are all necessary to help ensure the purity of commercial food products. Included in their jurisdiction is the supervision of the food service industry. Licensing requirements, sanitation standards, and inspections serve as control measures.

Governmental agencies cannot cover all the bases, however. Inadequate inspection of the quality of commercial fish sold for food, for example, has led to numerous outbreaks of hepatitis A and other illnesses. With the wide variety of possible contaminants and potential dangers, consumers' best protection is to supervise their own food quality.

Nurse's Role

Community health nurses can have a significant impact through health education. Most bacterial and viral food-borne diseases can be prevented if people know and practice proper cooking and storage of food as well as proper personal hygiene. See Table 6.1.

Nurses can teach the basics of keeping perishable products sufficiently refrigerated, discarding foods that may be old or spoiled, cooking foods thoroughly, and

---

TABLE 6.1. *Ten Golden Rules for Safe Food Preparation*

To prevent and control foodborne disease the World Health Organization has developed the following rules:

1. Choose food processed for safety.
2. Cook food thoroughly.
3. Eat cooked food immediately.
4. Store cooked food carefully.
5. Reheat cooked foods thoroughly.
6. Avoid contact between raw foods and cooked foods.
7. Wash hands repeatedly.
8. Keep all kitchen surfaces meticulously clean.
9. Protect foods from insects, rodents, and other animals.
10. Use pure water.

Source: Benenson, A., (ed) (1990). Control of Communicable Diseases in Man, (15 ed.) Washington, D.C.: American Public Health Association, p. 171.)

bringing water to a full boil when appropriate to be certain of eliminating microbes. Nurses can emphasize washing and cleaning produce and tools used in food processing, including the preparer's own hands. Finally, nurses can educate people to watch for signs of contamination. A dented can, for example, may signal the presence of living bacteria using the oxygen within the container and contaminating its contents. Nurses can raise public awareness regarding the conditions of supermarkets, restaurants, and other food handlers. They can also help promote community standards, enabling legislation, and policies for safer food supplies.

WASTE DISPOSAL

The United States generates more solid and hazardous waste per capita than any other industrialized nation (Moeller, 1992). On average "each person in the United States produces 1000–1500 pounds of municipal solid waste, including almost 100 pounds of plastics, per year" and "industry produces the equivalent of over one ton of hazardous waste per person each year." (Ibid., p.104) (See Figure 6.4) With the vast amounts of waste produced in the form of household garbage, human excreta, and agricultural and industrial by-products, including hazardous chemical and radioactive substances, it is no wonder that waste management and disposal has become an important and pressing topic in recent decades. New technology has effectively addressed some of the problems but there is still much need for improvement. Solid and hazardous wastes pose a wide range of public health concerns. Therefore, it is imperative that health officials, including nurses, become aware of the possible health hazards that these wastes present to individuals and to communities.

Disposal of Human Waste

One of the oldest environmental health hazards comes from improper disposal of human excreta. Although industrialized nations successfully address the problem, it continues to be a widespread problem in developing nations and in rural, poverty-stricken communities. Human wastes, particularly feces, provide a perfect environment in which bacteria and disease-causing parasites can live and reproduce. Therefore, contaminated drinking water, food grown in contaminated soil, and even direct contact with the soil can cause infections. For example, hookworm, a problem in the United States in the early part of the twentieth century, usually

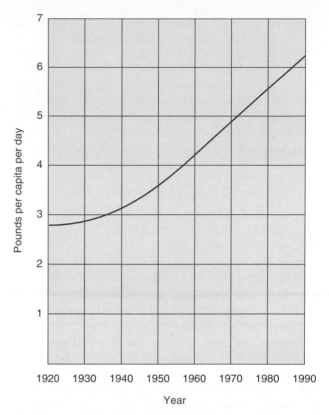

FIGURE 6.4. United States trend in per capita refuse production.

entered the body through the skin of bare feet (Blumenthal & Ruttenber, 1994).

In most modernized urban areas the public sewage system handles waste by treating raw sewage and disposing it into a body of water. In most instances in the United States, state health departments oversee proper waste treatment and disposal. In rural areas where individuals usually have private cesspools or septic tanks, the supervision of proper waste handling is difficult and not as consistent. Health workers in rural settings should be alert to the potential dangers posed by inconsistent monitoring.

Disposal of Garbage

Dumping and burning are the most common solid waste disposal methods. Dumping is problematic because garbage dumps provide perfect conditions for the breeding of rats, flies, and other disease-carrying organisms and may potentially be a source of water contamination from run-off. Dumps also are eyesores that take up valuable land resources. Burning, although it reduces the volume of garbage, produces noxious odors and pollutes the air. Sanitary landfills have generally replaced dumps as a more effective way to dispose of refuse by burying it. With proper handling, including covering and daily sealing (to prevent insect and rodent breeding), this method has proven satisfactory for handling of solid waste.

Hazardous Waste Disposal

Disposal of toxic chemical and radioactive wastes produced by industry is another grave concern. The threat is serious since one cannot be certain of all the effects of these wastes, or whether present methods of disposal are foolproof. Furthermore, many of these wastes escape containment or accidentally leak into water systems and into the soil to contaminate drinking water and food.

Primary methods of hazardous waste disposal include burial in double-lined cells in landfills, surface impoundments for special treatment and storage, waste-injected underground steel and concrete lined wells, solid waste piles, and land treatment facilities. Some hazardous wastes are incinerated before disposal. With the disposal of hazardous waste it is always a concern that storage containers may not be leakproof, and interference with dump sites or storage facilities may expose the environment to these toxic substances. Examples of chemical contamination have been discovered in communities such as Elizabeth, N.J., Times Beach, Mich., Love Canal, N.Y., and Minamata, Japan, where residents developed cancer and other health problems because of exposures to toxic chemicals (Blumenthal & Ruttenber, 1994). There is also the continuing problem of securing disposal sites for the increasing volume of hazardous wastes. Communities seek the advantages of new technology but do not wish to bury the resulting wastes in their backyards. In many instances legislators and public officials have faced serious conflict in their efforts to locate acceptable toxic waste dump sites.

With burgeoning industry and new technology in the world today, society has developed more sophisticated means of energy production, more labor-saving devices, and more practical and innovative products. This massive new product development has created a problem for the environment: how to handle the vast amount of waste created from discardable goods, by-products of production, and the "throw-away" mentality. For example, about 18 billion disposable diapers, which alone are estimated to be 2% of municipal wastes, are used each year in the United States. Made of durable plastics, these diapers are estimated to resist deterioration up to five centuries after burial in a landfill (Nadakavukaren, 1990). Not only does the development of such products take an enormous toll on natural resources, but the quantity and nature of the resulting wastes also pose serious health hazards and environmental problems. Improper disposal of domestic products, such as toxic insect sprays or some household cleaners, causes health dangers (Tuthill et al., 1987). Surveys show that 99% of disposable diaper users discard them directly into the trash instead of flushing fecal material down the toilet (Nadakavukaren, 1990). Consequently, a large amount of raw untreated sewage is ending up in landfills with the potential for serious problems in the future.

Government's Role

The government's role is to establish standards for safe waste disposal and to monitor and enforce compliance. More research is needed to determine the effects of various disposal methods and to improve disposal practices. It is imperative that people learn not only to dispose of wastes safely—to protect humans, the environment, and future generations—but that they also look seriously at other options. More emphasis must be placed on transforming waste into usable products, increasing the amount and kinds of recycling done, and reducing the amount of refuse produced in the first place.

Nurse's Role

Community health nurses can encourage the above actions by educating the public and lobbying for enabling legislation. Nurses can promote greater sensitivity among citizens to the problems of accumlating waste with its potential health hazards, encourage clients to buy products that can be recycled, and discourage use of aerosol spray containers, plastics, and other non-recycleable items.

INSECT AND RODENT CONTROL

All human communities are affected by the insects and rodents living in their environment. Not only are these creatures a nuisance in people's homes, but they may cause economic damage and create serious health hazards as well. On the least dangerous level they serve as annoying pests that may cause irritation, such as mosquito or fly bites, and discomfort, such as infestations of bedbugs or lice. They can also pose a direct threat to health through such things as attacks by diseased rats or squirrels. They can consume and, in turn, contaminate food. But by far the most serious health hazard that they impose is through their role as **vectors** which are nonhuman carriers of disease organisms that can transmit these organisms directly to humans (Blumenthal & Ruttenber, 1994). The most common vectors are mosquitos, flies, ticks, roaches, fleas, rats, mice, and ground squirrels. All of these agents can serve as reservoirs for germs that they then transmit through physical contact with humans or by contaminating human foodstuffs or water. Table 6.2 summarizes some of the diseases spread by vectors. Cases of vector-spread diseases range from the fourteenth-century bubonic plague epidemic spread by rat fleas, which killed a quarter of the European population, to the continuing problem of mosquito-spread malaria in nonindustrialized nations.

Government's Role

Vector surveys, research, and control are usually left to local and state health departments. These agencies have also implemented community awareness and pest control programs. Once vectors have been found, health workers can attempt to control them through many methods. Approaches used in the past include trapping rodents, poisoning, spraying with pesticides, and eliminating areas where vectors breed, by draining or filling marshes to control mosquito populations, for example. It is essential in planning any approach to consider the possible health hazards to humans or other living organisms and the effect the method will have on the ecosystem—how it may upset the ecological balance.

"The most fundamental and effective approach is to improve sanitary conditions and practices to the extent that conditions no longer exist that encourage the multiplication of insects and rodents" (WHO, 1986, p. 110).

TABLE 6.2. *Some Insect Vectors and Diseases Transmitted by Them*

Vector	Disease	Pathogen
Mosquitoes		
Anopheles sp.	Malaria	*Plasmodium sp.* (protozoa)
Culex sp.	Filariasis	*Wucheraria bancrofti* and *malayi* (nematodes)
Culex sp.	Encephalitis	arbovirus
Aedes aegypti	Yellow fever	arbovirus
Aedes aegypti	Dengue	arbovirus
Biting Flies		
Deerfly	Filariasis	*Loa loa* (nematode)
Black fly	River blindness	*Onchocerca volvulus* (nematode)
Tsetse fly	Sleeping sickness	*Trypanosoma gambiense* and *rhodesiense* (protozoa)
Sand fly	Kala-azar	*Leishmania donovani*
	Tropical ulcer	*Leishmania tropica*
	Cutaneous leishmaniasis	*Leishmania mexicana*
	Espundia	*Leishmania braziliense* (protozoa)
	Phlebotomus fever	arbovirus
Other Insects		
Gnats	Filariasis	*Mansonella ozzardi* (nematode)
Rat flea	Plague	*Yersinia pestis* (bacteria)
	Murine typhus	*Rickettsia mooseri*
Body louse	Epidemic typhus	*Rickettsia prowazekii*
	Trench fever	*Rickettsia quintana*
Tick	Rocky Mountain spotted fever	*Rickettsia rickettsia*
Tick	Colorado tick fever	arbovirus
Mite	Riskettsialpox	*Rickettsia akari*

Source: Blumenthal, D. and Ruttenber, J. (1994). *Introduction to Environmental Health,* (2nd ed.). New York: Springer.

Nurse's Role

The community health nurse can contribute through awareness of the presence and possible health threat of rodents and insects. By remaining alert to the presence of rodents and insects in homes, schools, and communities, nurses can take measures to educate affected persons and notify proper authorities when corrective action is needed. Nurses can assist this effort by surveying homes and neighborhoods for exposed rubbish or conditions that might attract insects and rodents. They can also promote preventive efforts through education and influencing policy makers.

SAFETY IN THE HOME, WORKSITE, AND COMMUNITY

The environment of the home, the workplace, and the community at large significantly affects people's health. Protection from impure air, water, food, dangerous wastes, and vectors have been discussed in previous sections. This section addresses four additional areas affecting people's safety: exposure to toxic chemicals, radiation exposure, injury control and safety, and psychological hazards.

Exposure to Toxic Chemicals

The list of chemicals, both natural and synthetic, in the environment and the threats they pose to human and environmental health are overwhelming.

"Approximately 55,000 chemicals are in use in the United States; of these, 1000 to 1500 constitute the greatest part of hazardous exposures, but only about 450 have established threshold limit values and adequate toxicity testing. Several hundred new chemicals come into use each year, basically untested" (Last, 1987, p. 146).

This section presents a general overview of the different categories of environmental chemicals, where they are found, the dangers they impose, and community health nurses' role in forestalling or detecting those dangers.

Toxic chemicals include those that do not contain carbon, are not derived from living matter, and are usually of mineral composition. Substances such as zinc, cadmium, lead, iron, calcium, sodium, potassium, magnesium, and copper often play an important and healthful role in human physiology, but they become toxic if a person is exposed to large quantities.

Lead is a toxic agent frequently found in occupational or industrial settings. Workers must be careful to avoid inhaling lead fumes and exposing their families to lead dust on their clothing. Lead was once widely used in paint, and can still be found in leaded gasoline, and batteries. Lead poisoning usually produces symptoms of cerebral or central nervous system disorders. It is especially dangerous in children, whose high metabolic activity makes them more susceptible (Barker, et al.,1990; Last, 1987). Even low level exposure to lead has a dangerous cumulative effect (Lee, et al., 1990) such as that acquired by children playing near roadways where dirt has absorbed lead from gasoline. In utero lead exposure is another concern (Brown, et al., 1990). Community health nurses need to check with clients for possible exposure, and examine client homes for lead-based paint, now restricted in residential use. In particular, nurses can warn parents to keep their young children from eating paint chips from windowsills, walls, or furniture painted with lead-based paint and to keep them away from lead-infused dirt near roads.

Mercury is also highly toxic. It is used in many scientific instruments, electronic equipment, crop fungicides, and the processing of dental fillings. Inorganic mercury can be changed through bacterial action in industrial processes to more toxic organic compounds, as in the bleach used for paper manufacturing. Toxic mercurials then escape into the environment and contaminate the food chain. In Minanata Bay, Japan, for example, many persons were crippled with nervous system disorders caused by eating mercury-contaminated seafood.

Other harmful metals include aluminum, which recently has been associated with certain mental disorders and has been found in high levels in the brain tissue of patients with Alzheimer's disease (Last, 1987). Chromium, nickel, and arsenic are included among other toxic compounds. (See Table 6.3).

Many toxic chemicals are by-products of the petroleum industry, including many alcohols, ethers, hydrocarbons such as benzene, medicines, and plastics which contain carbon. Ingestion or exposure may cause cancer, liver and kidney disease, birth defects, and many other health problems. Pesticides for household and crop use, particularly DDT (Dichlorodiphenyl Trichloroethane), have created major health hazards (Blumenthal & Ruttenber, 1994). DDT, a very dangerous chemical used for pest control, was banned in 1972 in the U.S. because of environmental and health concerns. However, it is still present in the environment and

TABLE 6.3. *Occupational Carcinogens*

Carcinogen	Cancer Site	Examples of Exposed Occupations
4-Aminodiphenyl Auramine B-napthylamine Magenta Benzidine	Bladder	Dye manufacturing; rubber manufacturing
Arsenic	Skin; lung; liver	Metal smelting; arsenic pesticide production; metal alloy workers
Asbestos	Lung; mesothelium; gastrointestinal tract	Asbestos miners; insulators; shipyard workers
Benzene	Leukemia (blood-forming organs)	Petrochemical workers; chemists
Bischloromethyl ether (BCME)	Lung	Organic chemical synthesizers
Cadmium	Prostate	Cadmium alloy workers; welders
Chromium/Chromates	Lung; nasal sinuses	Chromate producers; metal workers
Coke oven emissions	Lung; kidney	Coke oven workers
Foundry emissions	Lung	Foundry workers
Leather dust	Nasal cavity; nasal sinuses; bladder	Shoe manufacturing
Nickel	Lung; nasal passages	Nickel smelting; metal workers
Radiation (x-rays)	Leukemia (blood-forming organs); skin; breast; thyroid; bone	Radiologists; industrial radiographers; atomic energy workers
Radon gas	Lung	Uranium and feldspar miners
Soots, tars, and oil (aromatic hydrocarbons)	Skin; lung; bladder; scrotum	Roofers; chimney sweepers; petroleum workers; shale oil workers
Ultraviolet light	Skin	Outdoor workers
Vinyl chloride	Liver; brain; lung	Polyvinyl chloride synthesizers; rubber workers
Welding fumes	Lung	Welders
Wood dust	Nasal passages	Hardwood workers; furniture makers

Source: Blumenthal, D. and Rutenber, J. (1994). *Introduction to Environmental Health*, (2nd ed.). New York: Springer.

continues to be used illicitly, posing a danger to farmers and migrant farmworkers in particular. It has also been used legally in certain countries to control malaria.

Exposure to toxic chemicals can have far-reaching effects on humans. People may come in contact with them in their homes through building materials, cleaning products, or airborne dust. Another source is the workplace, where many different compounds are created and used each day. Toxic substances also may be transferred home from the workplace in motor vehicles and on clothing or shoes. In the greater community, pollutants in the air and food chain create further hazards. Toxic chemicals can cause illness when they are inhaled, come into contact with the skin (as in industrial accidents where chemicals are spilled), or ingested (as when a child drinks from a liquid cleaning solvent bottle).

Radiation Exposure

Radiation can be found in many areas of the environment. It occurs naturally as background radiation from the sun, soil, and minerals. The largest natural source of radiation exposure is airborne radon. Radiation in its personmade form has numerous beneficial uses in science and industry for lasers, radiographs which help in the diagnosis of disease (Boice, et al., 1991), and in the production of nuclear energy. It is found in many home electronic devices, such as television sets, smoke detectors, and microwave ovens.

Regardless of its source, radiation is a threat to human health in the workplace and in the general environment. The extent of danger depends on the dose and type of radiation. For example, casualties among miners can be attributed to their prolonged and intense exposure to radioactive minerals such as uranium. Prolonged exposure may cause skin ulcers, damage to cells, cancer, premature aging, kidney dysfunction, and genetic disorders in the children of those whose cells have been damaged. Naturally occurring radioactive materials are present in tobacco and further threaten the health of smokers. A two-pack per day cigarette smoker receives more than ten times the long-term dose-rate limit for radiation exposure (Moeller, 1992).

A major area of concern centers on the problems associated with nuclear energy and nuclear weapons. The production of radioactive wastes, the threat of accidental exposure from unsafe reactors, and possible fallout from weapons testing generate real fears. These fears have been confirmed by such incidents as Three Mile Island and Chernobyl nuclear reactor accidents which allowed radioactive ions to escape into the atmosphere.

> "Such accidents, however, are not very common. Further, the normal operation of nuclear power plants exposes the population to considerably less radiation than other manmade sources, such as medical radiation, or natural radiation." (WHO, 1986, p.18)

Research in Community Health Nursing
UNINTENTIONAL INFANT INJURIES

Harris, M.J., & Kotch, J.B. (1994). Unintentional infant injuries: sociodemographic and psychosocial factors. *Public Health Nursing,* 11(2): 90–97.

A prospective study examined risk factors for unintentional injuries occurring to infants in or around their homes. Subjects, 367 mothers, were interviewed six to eight weeks postpartum and again in a year. During that time, 132 infants (36%) were reported injured from burns, poisoning, serious falls, or airway problems. Family conflict proved to be the most significant predictor of unintentional infant injuries. The second risk factor was less than two siblings living at home and the third was maternal unemployment. Furthermore, for mothers experiencing high stress, fewer unintentional infant injuries resulted when social supports, such as relatives, friends, or spiritual sources, were used. This study supports the importance of modifying the social and psychological environment to prevent injuries.

Injury Control and Safety

An environmental characteristic that must be considered in assessing health risks is a community's level of physical safety. How likely is it that injuries will occur? This is a very important question when one considers that the fourth leading cause of death in the United States is unintentional injury. Also, "nonfatal injuries are responsible for one of every six hospital days and one of every 10 hospital discharges." (U.S.Department of Health and Human Services, 1990, p.64) Groups at highest risk are the young and the elderly, the poor, minorities, and rural residents (see accompanying display). Motor vehicle collisions cause nearly half the deaths from unintentional injuries. The second ranked cause of injury death is from falls. Deaths from poisoning, drowning, and residential fires follow in ranking, respectively. Alcohol plays a major role in many of these injuries and subsequent deaths, particularly with motor vehicle collisions and drownings (U.S. Department of Health and Human Services, 1990).

Another area of safety concern is injury and death from violence. Individuals, families, and communities are frequently at risk for violent acts stemming from domestic quarrels and abuse, dysfunctional behavior, and crime. Violence and the injuries and deaths it causes is becoming one of the most urgent health problems in the United States. Use of handguns and domestic abuse make women, children, and the elderly particularly at risk for injury and death. Community health nurses have a responsibility to assess situations for the threat of potential physical harm and work with other professionals to design preventive measures. The subject of violence is discussed further in Chapter 24.

Psychological Hazards

A discussion of environmental health and safety would not be complete if it overlooked the psychological hazards that people must face in their environments. Environment plays a significant role in the mental health of a community. The psychological variables that affect individuals often lead to physiological illnesses. Such elements as noise, overcrowding, traffic, lack of privacy, unavailability of work, lack of natural beauty, and boredom can be detrimental to peoples' well-being.

Noise has been cited as a major environmental health problem. Extremely loud noises, such as pneumatic drills or loud rock music, can cause temporary or permanent hearing loss (Moeller, 1992). Other noises, perhaps from machinery at the workplace or residential exposure to airport traffic, can lead to headaches, sleep disruption, lowered body resistance to disease, ulcers, and aggravation of existing physical disorders (Clark, 1984). The effects vary in severity depending on the intensity and duration of the noises and the disposition of the individuals concerned.

Another psychological hazard is urban crowding. Early studies on crowding done by J. B. Calhoun demonstrated serious effects on behavior. When healthy, naturally clean laboratory mice were forced to live in overcrowded conditions, they experienced dramatic behavior changes (Pickett & Hanlon, 1990). Gross insanitation led to aggressive behavior, strong mice attacking the weak, symptoms of regression and mental disturbance, mating decline, and neglect or cannibalization of weaker offspring. Although this is an extreme example, it perhaps provides some insight into the conditions of urban areas and the psychological stress that urban conditions may create.

The daily psychological stresses of the modern world are innumerable. Excessive stimulation comes from rapid societal changes created by new technology, an accelerated pace of living, increased work production demands, and other causes. All can create potential health hazards.

Government's Role

The government plays an active role in promoting public safety. Standards and regulations have been set at the federal level regarding toxic chemicals, radiation exposure, occupational safety practices, noise abatement, and other safety issues. State and local governments seek to enforce business, industry, and community compliance with these standards. Health departments and other government agencies assist with monitoring of chemical use and production as well as promotion of public education programs to alert people to the presence and potential dangers of toxic chemicals and exposure to radiation in the environment. Research is examining the biological effects of chemicals and radiation. The medical and dental fields have developed simple safety procedures, such as having patients wear lead aprons during X-rays and having technicians stand behind metal walls. The United States Public Health Service holds responsibility for monitoring nuclear plants and other possible sources of radiation to protect the public.

Because the government holds companies liable for the safety of their products, industry now invests considerable resources into researching and designing safe goods. Many products have been modified to make them more safe such as childproof caps on medication bottles, flame-retardant children's clothing, and seat belts and airbags in automobiles. Industry must also warn consumers if a product is inherently dangerous, as when toys have sharp edges or parts are small enough to be ingested by toddlers. Bright orange frowning faces on bottles that contain harmful substances have helped to warn consumers and reduce the number of poisonings. Children learn to avoid poisonous plants and other potential hazards through school and community education efforts.

Community safety organizations, government agencies, and public health officials all play their part in assessing community safety and taking measures to prevent accidents. Organizations such as the Consumer Protection Agency, and consumer advocates like Ralph Nader continue to watchdog environmental safety. Federal and state legislation to enforce speed limits has helped to reduce the number of automobile accidents, and supervision of recreational and occupational areas has led to discovery of health hazards and promoted the development of safety programs. State-established boating safety regulations, or the assigning of adequate lifeguards to monitor busy swimming beaches, are measures that help to reduce the number of recreational accidents. Community surveys of intersections where multiple traffic accidents have occurred have led to installation of traffic signals and a reduction of accidents.

The role of government in reduction or control of violence and psychological hazards has been less effective. Certain federal-level agencies, such as the National Institute for Mental Health, the National Institute for Occupational Safety and Health, the Departments of Labor, Commerce, and Transportation influence standards and regulations affecting psychological well-being. Legislation regarding firearm use and penalties associated with domestic abuse and physical violence have become more stringent. Nonetheless, both violence and psychological hazards continue to be serious public health problems that are preventable and deserve greater attention.

Nurse's Role

It is difficult to monitor all the possible contacts a person or community may be experiencing with toxic chemicals or radiation, but such monitoring is necessary in order to estimate health risks and establish correlations. Multiple exposures in small doses from many different sources may add up. Are clients' homes well ventilated? Is the burning of fossil fuels polluting the air with sulfur oxides? Does home, school, or work-site insulation contain asbestos? Are all household chemical agents stored in a childproof place? Monitoring difficulties arise from the many opportunities for exposure to toxic chemicals or radiation, cumulative exposure over time, and the fact that disease symptoms may not appear until years after exposure, when the agent may no longer be in the immediate environment. The best protection is to promote and monitor the safe use and disposal of chemical hazards and limit radiation exposure to prevent health problems from occurring.

Community health nurses can promote environmental safety and prevent injuries in many ways. Six target area settings in which to concentrate preventive measures are highways, homes, worksites, schools, farms, and recreational sites. Working with the police, fire personnel, social services, schools, drug rehabilitation counselors, and many other community groups, the nurse can help to develop programs targeted at preventing drunk driving, firearm misuse, failed smoke detectors, unsafe playground equipment, and much more. In homes, nurses can encourage safe storage of toxic materials. Railings can be installed on stairways and in bathrooms used by the elderly. Gates at the tops of stairways and window guards can prevent small children from falling. Non-skid decals can be used in bathtubs to prevent slipping.

Safety education offers one of the most vital preventive measures. When people are made aware of possible dangers and unsafe areas, they can avoid injuring themselves. Local community programs to educate people on the dangers of driving while intoxicated, to instruct them on the proper handling of home machinery such as chainsaws, or to encourage safe use of fireworks during holiday celebrations can also help to reduce injuries. In the event that an injury does occur, educating the public about appropriate actions to take can help to reduce its potential impact. Promoting first-aid and CPR classes can be beneficial.

Education as a preventive measure against injuries applies particularly in the case of natural disasters. Although a tornado or earthquake cannot be prevented, people can be prepared in the event that one does occur. By running fire drills in schools and workplaces, informing people of the location of safe and unsafe places to take shelter during an electrical storm or hurricane, and of what to do in an earthquake or flood, nurses can help to forestall or minimize tragic events.

It is necessary for community health nurses to be aware of psychological hazards in the environment, to recognize the potential they have for affecting both psychological and physiological health, and to encourage stress reduction wherever possible. Some specific ways that community health nurses can promote a psychologically healthy environment include active lobbying for control and prevention of domestic abuse and violence (see Figure 6.5), neighborhood crime prevention, reduction of workplace stressors, and development of educational and support programs to reduce life-style stressors.

Role of the Community Health Nurse in Environmental Health

Each of the preceding sections has discussed actions and given examples of ways that the community health nurse can be involved in environmental health. To summarize, the nurse has a two-part challenge: (1) to help protect the public's health from potential threats in the environment and (2) to help protect and promote the health of the environment itself so that it can be life and health enhancing for its human inhabitants. The following strategies for collaboration and participation provide a summary of the nurse's role and can assist the nurse in addressing this two-part goal.

STRATEGIES FOR NURSING COLLABORATION AND PARTICIPATION

1. Learn about possible environmental health threats. The nurse has a responsibility to keep abreast of current environmental issues and know the proper authorities to whom problems should be reported.

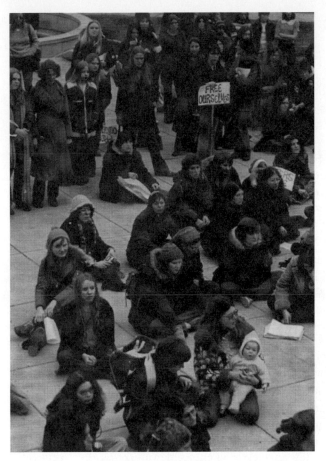

FIGURE 6.5. A group peacefully demonstrates to call attention to domestic violence.

2. Assess clients' environment and detect health hazards. Careful observation and an environmental checklist can assist in this assessment.

3. Plan collaboratively with citizens and other professionals to devise protective and preventive strategies. Remember that environmental health work is generally a team effort.

4. Assist with the implementation of programs to prevent health threats to clients and the environment.

5. Take action to correct situations in which health hazards exist. Nurses can use direct intervention, as with an unsafe home situation, notify proper authorities, or publicly protest when corrective measures are beyond their sphere.

6. Educate consumers and assist them to practice preventive measures. Examples of preventive measures include radon testing in homes or well water testing in rural communities.

7. Take action to promote development of policies and legislation that enhance consumer protection and a healthier environment.

8. Assist with and promote program evaluation to determine effectiveness of environmental health efforts.

9. Apply environmentally-related research findings and participate in nursing research.

Summary

Environmental health is a discipline encompassing all the elements of the environment that influence the health and well-being of its inhabitants. Public health workers, including community health nurses, need to monitor and determine causal links between people and their environment with a concern as to how they may promote the health and well-being of both.

A systems theory or ecological perspective of environmental health is important to understand the human-environment relationship and how the health of one impacts the health of the other. Prevention and strategic or long-range concerns are also important in considering environmental health because what is done today may impact the health of many generations in the future.

There are six primary areas of concern today in environmental health: air pollution, water pollution, unhealthy or contaminated food, waste disposal, insect and rodent control, and safety in the home, worksite and community. Each has its own set of problems, concerns, and solutions.

Both public and private sectors are involved in regulating, monitoring, and preventing environmental health problems and have accomplished much during the past twenty years. Much, however, is still left to be done and new problems continue to develop. The community health nurse is an important member of the team of health professionals promoting and protecting the reciprocal relationship between the environment and the public's health. The nurse can follow several important strategies to accomplish the two-part goal of (1) protecting the public's health from environmental threats and (2) promoting a healthy and health-enhancing environment.

Activities to Promote Critical Thinking

1. You are planning a visit to a young family who live in an older home. You know that older homes may have radon, lead pipes and lead-based paint, asbestos insulation, and other safety, fire, and health threats. Using the nursing process, design a plan for (a) determining whether any of these threats are present, (b) what actions should be taken if the dangers exist, (c) how to assist the family in taking corrective action, and (d) evaluating successful removal of existing threats.

2. Data from the local health department show that in the past year five people from the same rural portion of the county all died of cancer. What collaborative actions would be appropriate for you to take to determine whether there is an environmental relationship? What other members of the health team should be involved in the investigation? Write a letter to the Mayor and the County Commissioners to justify why nurses should be involved in this study.

3. Select an article from the mass media (newspaper, weekly news magazine, etc) that deals with an 'environmental health' problem. Analyze and critique the article by answering the following questions: What are the characteristics of the community involved? What appear to be the sources of the problem? What evidence is provided in the article to substantiate the cause? Does the news coverage describe health effects? What population is at risk? Does the coverage provide adequate information for consumers to understand the problem and seek any needed assistance? What suggestions do you have for improving the article?

4. Design a list of items to include in a checklist for assessing clients' home, school, or worksite environments. Consider each of the environmental areas of concern described in this chapter and what potential health threats might be present in each area. Review this list with an environmental health expert for accuracy and completeness. Use the list as a teaching tool with two different sets of clients and evaluate its effectiveness for assessment and diagnosis of environmentally-related health hazards.

5. Identify an environmental health problem in your community or state. Become informed about this problem by talking with experts in the area and reading recent literature and research reports on the problem. Meet with a senator or congressperson who has been involved in legislation related to the problem and learn what they plan to do about it. Summarize what you have learned and present it in writing as a letter to the editor of your city newspaper.

REFERENCES

Adelson, O. (1991). Occupational and environmental exposures to radon: Cancer risks. *Annual Review of Public Health, 12*, 235–55.

American Medical Association (1991). Health effects of radon exposure. Report of the AMA Council on Scientific Affairs. *Archives of Internal Medicine, 151*(4), 674–7.

Barker, P.O., et al. (1990). The management of lead exposure in pediatric populations. *Nurse Practitioner, 15*(12), 8–10, 12–13, 16.

Benarde, M.A. (1989). *Our precious habitat: Fifteen years later.* New York: Wiley.

Benenson, A.S. (Ed.). (1990). *Control of communicable diseases in man* (15th ed.). Washington, DC: American Public Health Association.

Bingham, E. & Meader, W. (1990). Governmental regulation of environmental hazards in the 1990s. *Annual Review of Public Health, 11*, 419–34.

Blumenthal, D. & Ruttenber, J. (1994). *Introduction to environmental health* (2nd ed.). New York: Springer

Boice, J.D., Morin, M.M., Glass, A.D. & Friedman, G.D. (1991). Diagnostic x-ray procedures and risk of leukemia, lymphoma, and multiple myeloma. *Journal of the American Medical Association, 265*, 1290–94.

Brown, M.J., et al. (1990). In utero lead exposure. *Maternal Child Nursing, 15*(2), 94–6.

Chilmonczyk, B.A., et al. (1990). Environmental tobacco smoke exposure during infancy. *American Journal of Public Health, 80*(10), 1205–8.

Clark, C.R. (1984). The effects of noise on health. In D.M. Jones & A.J.Chapman (Eds.). *Noise and Society*. New York: Wiley.

Dewailly, E., Poirier, C. & Meyer, F. (1986). Health hazards associated with windsurfing on polluted water. *American Journal of Public Health, 76*(6), 690–91.

Fagliano, J. et al. (1990). Drinking water contamination and the incidence of leukemia: an ecologic study. *American Journal of Public Health, 80,* 1209–12.

French, H. (1991). Eastern Europe's clean break with the past. *World-Watch, 4*(2), 21–7.

Green, L.W., & Anderson, C.L. (1986). *Community health.* St. Louis: Times Mirror/Mosby.

Green, L.W. & Krueter, M.W. (1991). *Health promotion planning: An educational and environmental approach,* (2nd ed.). Mountain View, CA: Mayfield Pub.

Green, M., et al. (1987). An outbreak of watermelon-borne pesticide toxicity. *American Journal of Public Health, 77,* 1431–34.

Huang, W.Y. & Uri, N.D. (1990). An analytical framework for assessing the benefits and costs of policies related to protecting groundwater quality. *Environmental Planning, 22,* 1469–86.

Jo, W.K., et al. (1990). Chloroform exposure and the health risk associated with multiple uses of chlorinated tap water. *Risk Analysis, 10*(4), 581–5.

Johnson, C.J., et al. (1990). Continuing importance of nitrate contamination of groundwater and wells in rural areas. *American Journal of Industrial Mededicine, 18*(4), 449–56.

Jones, T.D., et al. (1991). Protection of human health from mixtures of radionuclides and chemicals in drinking water. *Archives of Environmental Contamination Toxicology, 20*(1), 143–50.

Kent, G., Greenspan, J., Herndon, J., Mofenson, L., Harris, J., Eng, T., & Waskin, H. (1988). Epidemic giardiasis caused by a contaminated public water supply. *American Journal of Public Health, 78,* 139–43.

Last, J.M. (1987). *Public health and human ecology.* East Norwalk: Appleton and Lange.

Lee, W.R., et al. (1990). Low level exposure to lead: the evidence for harm accumulates. *British Medical Journal, 301*(6751), 504–5.

Lemonick, M. D. (1987). The heat is on: Chemical wastes spread into the air threaten the earth's climate. *Time,* (Oct 19), 53–67.

McGrew, R (1985) *Encyclopedia of medical history* New York: McGraw-Hill, pp. 137–141.

Moeller, D.W. (1992). *Environmental Health.* Cambridge,MA: Harvard University Press.

Munson, H. (1990). Pollution in the Soviet Union. *ECON: Environmental Contractor 5*(8), 24–29.

Nadakavukaren, A. (1990). *Man and environment: A health perspective* (2nd ed.). Prospect Heights, IL: Waveland Press.

Pickett, G., & Hanlon, J. (1990). *Public health: Administration and practice* (9th ed.). St.Louis: Times Mirror/Mosby.

Purdom, P. W. (1980). *Environmental health.* New York: Academic Press.

Rabe, B. (1990). Environmental health policy. In G. Pickett & J. Hanlon. *Public health administration and practice.* (9th ed.). St. Louis: Times Mirror/Mosby.

Seymour, J. (1990). Water, water everywhere . . . environmental hazards. *Nursing Times, 86*(44), 60–1.

Tuthill, R., Stanekill, E., Willis, C., & Moore, G., (1987). Degree of public support for household hazardous waste control alternatives. *American Journal of Public Health, 77,* 304–6.

U.S. Department of Health and Human Services (1991). *Healthy people 2000: National health promotion and disease prevention objectives.* Washington, DC: Government Printing Office.

Weinstein, N., Klotz, M., & Sandman, P. (1988). Optimistic biases in public perceptions of the risk from radon. *American Journal of Public Health, 78*(7), 796–800.

Whyatt, R.M. (1990). Setting human-health-based groundwater protection standards when toxicological data are inadequate. *American Journal of Indian Medicine, 18*(4), 505–10.

World Health Organization. (1986). *Health and the environment.* Vienna: WHO Regional Publications, European Series, No. 19, 12–16.

SELECTED READINGS

Briasco, M.E. (1990). Indoor air pollution: Are employees sick from their work? *American Association of Occupational Health Nursing Journal, 38,* 375–80.

Brown, R.S., & Garner, L.E. (1988). *Resource guide to state environmental management.* Lexington, KY: Council of State Governments.

Carnes, S., & Watson, A. (1989). Disposing of the U.S. chemical weapons stockpile. *Journal of the American Medical Association, 262,* 653–9.

Cohen, S. (1981). Sound effects on behavior. *Psychology Today, 15,* 38–46.

Elson, D. (1987). *Atmospheric air pollution: Causes, effects, and control policies.* New York: Basil Blackwell.

Farfel, M. & Chisholm, J., Jr. (1990). Health and environmental outcomes of traditional and modified practices for abatement of residential lead-based paint. *American Journal of Public Health, 80*(10), 1240–5.

Gibbons, W. (1991). Low level radiation: Higher long-term risk? *Science News, 139,* 181.

Godish, D. (1989). Asbestos exposure in schools. *Journal of School Health, 59*(8), 362–3.

Goldsmith, J. R. (Ed.). (1986). *Environmental epidemiology. Epidemiological investigation of community environmental health problems.* Boca Raton, FL. CRC Press.

Gordis, L. (1988). *Epidemiology and health risk assessment.* New York: Oxford University Press.

Gorey, F. (1990). Environmental advocacy. *Australian Nurses Journal, 19*(10), 15–6.

Greenberg, M.R. (1987). *Public health and the environment: The U.S. experience.* New York: The Guilford Press.

Hall, J.M. & Stevens, P.E. (1992). A nursing view of the U.S.-Iraq war: psychosocial health consequences. *Nursing Outlook, 40,* 113–120.

Labonte, R.N. (1989). Pesticides and healthy public policy. *Canadian Journal of Public Health, 80*(4), 238–42.

Loehr, R.C. (1989). Groundwater contamination—the problem and potential solutions. *National Forum, LXIX*(1), 26–8.

Macinick C.G., et al. (1987). Toxic new world: what nurses can do to cope with a polluted environment. *International Nursing Review, 34*(2/272), 40–2.

Mortality Morbidity Weekly Reports (1992). *Hazardous waste sites: Priority health conditions and research strategies—U.S. Department of Health and Human Services, Centers for Disease Control,* Feb. 7, *41*(5), 72.

Nelson, D. (1990). Mitigating disasters: power to the community. *International Nursing Review 37*(6), 371.

Neufer, L. (1994). The role of the community health nurse in environmental health. *Public Health Nursing 11*(3):155– 62.

Page, G.W., III. (1987). Water and health. In M.R. Greenberg (Ed.). *Public health and the environment.* New York: Guilford Press.

Pope, K. & Olson, K. (1990). Pesticides and their control. *American Association Occupational Health Nursing Journal, 38,* 353–9.

Probart, C.K. (1989). Issues related to radon in schools. *Journal of School Health, 59*(10), 441–3.

Proceedings of the Conference on Pesticides, Groundwater, and Health. (1987). Pesticides: Balancing risks and benefits. *Health and Environment Digest, 1*(1), 1–5.

Pucci, J. et al. (1990). Radon: A health problem. *Home Healthcare Nurse, 8*(1), 40–4.

Raloff, J. (1991). Air pollution: a respiratory hue and cry. *Science News, 139,* 203.

Roderick, P., et al. (1991). Is housing a public health issue? A survey of directors of public health. *British Medical Journal, 302*(6769), 157–60.

Schnorr, T., Grawjewski, P., Hornung, P., & Thun, M. (1991). Video display terminals and the risk of spontaneous abortion. *New England Journal of Medicine, 324,* 727–33.

Stevens, P.E. & Hall, J.M. (1992). Applying critical theories to nursing in communities. *Public Health Nursing, 9,* 2–9.

Vallely, B. (1991). Women, health, and the environment. *Health Visitor, 64*(2), 44–6.

Walker, B. (1990). Environmental health policies in the 1990s. *Journal of Public Health Policy, 11,* 438–47.

Walker, B. (1994). Impediments to the implementation of environmental policy. *Journal of Public Health Policy, 15*(2): 186–202.

CHAPTER

7

Influence of Culture on Community Health

LEARNING OBJECTIVES

Upon completion of this chapter readers should be able to:

- Define and explain the concept of culture.
- Identify five characteristics shared by all cultures.
- Discuss the meaning of cultural diversity and its significance for community health.
- Describe the meaning and effects of ethnocentrism on community health nursing practice.
- Contrast the health-related values, beliefs, and practices of culturally diverse populations with those of the dominant U.S. culture.
- Conduct a cultural assessment.
- Apply transcultural nursing principles in community health nursing practice.

KEY TERMS

- Cultural assessment
- Cultural diversity
- Cultural relativism
- Cultural self-awareness
- Cultural sensitivity
- Culture
- Culture shock
- Dominant values
- Enculturation
- Ethnic group
- Ethnicity
- Ethnocentrism
- Microculture
- Minority Group
- Race
- Subcultures
- Tacit
- Transcultural Nursing
- Value

Barbara Walton Spradley and Judith Ann Allender
COMMUNITY HEALTH NURSING: CONCEPTS AND PRACTICE, 4th ed.
© 1996 Barbara Walton Spradley and Judith Ann Allender

American society values individuality. People are delighted to see children grow and develop in unique ways. They applaud someone's creative achievement. Each has personalized preferences about food, dress, or the vehicle one drives. The right to be oneself and different from others is highly valued. Although individuality is part of the dominant culture, there are limits to the range of acceptable differences. People whose behavior falls outside that acceptable range are labelled as deviants or misfits. For example, United States' culture approves moderate social drinking but not alcoholism. These beliefs and sanctions are based on **dominant values** which are the values of the dominant or majority culture. In the United States the dominant culture is largely made up of Anglo Saxons whose values include the work ethic, thrift, success, independence, initiative, respect for others, privacy, cleanliness, youthfulness, attractive appearance, and a focus on the future.

Cultural values are important to consider in the practice of community health because cultural values shape people's thoughts and behaviors. In community health why are some client behaviors acceptable to health professionals and others not? Why do nurses have such difficulty persuading certain clients to accept new ways of thinking and acting? Explanations can be found by examining the concept of culture; its influence on community health and on nursing practice.

The Meaning of Culture

Culture refers to the beliefs, values, and behavior that are shared by members of a society and that provide a design or "map" for living. It is culture that tells people what is acceptable and unacceptable in a given situation. It is culture that dictates what to do, or say, or believe. Culture is learned. As children grow up they learn from their parents and others around them how to interpret the world. In turn, these assimilated beliefs and values prescribe desired behavior.

Anthropologists describe culture as "the acquired knowledge that people use to generate behavior and interpret experience." (Spradley & McCurdy, 1994, p.4) This knowledge is more than simply custom or ritual, it is a way of organizing and thinking about life. It gives people a sense of security about their behavior; without having to consciously think about it, they know how to act. Culture also provides the underlying values and beliefs upon which people's behavior is based. For example, culture determines the value one places on achievement, independence, work, and leisure. It forms the basis for one's definitions of male and female roles. It influences a person's response to authority figures, dictates religious beliefs and practices, and shapes child-rearing. Culture, as Benjamin Paul has described it, "is a blueprint for social living." (cited in Landy, 1977, p.233)

CULTURAL INFLUENCE ON BEHAVIOR

Every community, every social or ethnic group, has its own culture. Furthermore, all the individual members believe and act based on what they have learned within that specific culture. As anthropologist Edward Hall said, "Culture controls our lives." (1959, p.38) Even the smallest elements of everyday living are influenced by one's culture. For instance, culture determines the distance to stand from another person while talking (Meisenhelder, 1982). A comfortable talking distance for Americans is at least two and a half feet (Figure 7.1), while Latin Americans prefer a shorter distance, often only 18 inches, for dialogue. Culture also influences people's perception of time. In American culture when someone makes an appointment they expect the other person to be on time or not more than a few minutes late. To keep a person waiting (or to be kept waiting) for 45 minutes or an hour is insulting and intolerable. Yet there are other cultural groups, including Native Americans and Asians, whose response to time is much more flexible; their members think nothing of waiting or keeping someone else waiting for an hour or two. Clearly, culture is the knowledge people use to design their own actions and, in turn, to interpret others' behavior (Spradley & McCurdy, 1994).

Cultural Diversity

Cultural diversity not only occurs between countries or continents, it can and does occur within developed countries such as the United States (Bernal, 1993). **Cultural diversity** means that a variety of cultural patterns coexist within a designated geographic area. It is sometimes called cultural plurality. Cultural diversity exists when a variety of racial or ethnic groups join a common larger group. **Race** refers to a biologically designated group of people whose distinguishing features, such as

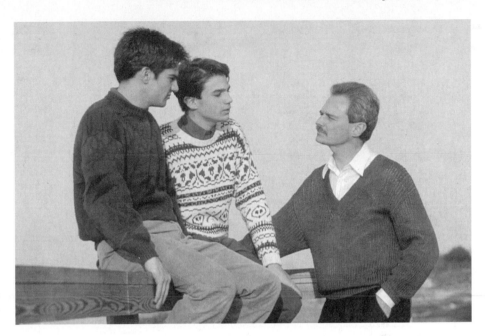

FIGURE 7.1. A comfortable distance between people in conversation is determined by culture.

skin color, are inherited. An **ethnic group** is a collection of people with common origins and with shared culture and identity. **Ethnicity** means possessing the qualities that mark one's association with an ethnic group.

Immigration patterns over the years have contributed to marked cultural diversity in the United States. Early settlers came primarily from British and European countries in the 1800s peaking in numbers just after the turn of the century (See Figure 7.2). Immigration decreased considerably during the years of World War I and II but increased again in the 1960s with the largest number from Mexico. During the 1970s, roughly half a million immigrants legally entered the United States. By the end of the 1980s over a million more had been admitted (Statistical Yearbook, 1993).

As shown in Figure 7.3, Asian and South American immigrants were by far the largest groups to enter the United States in the 1980s. *The Harvard Encyclopedia of American Ethnic Groups* (1980) listed one hundred different ethnic groups living in the United States, 50 of which were significant in size. According to the United States Census Bureau (1990), two of the largest minorities include Hispanic Americans, numbering over 22 million officially (with more entering illegally), representing approximately 9% of the population, and Asian-Americans, numbering slightly more than 7 million, or approximately 3% of the population. The largest ethnic group in the United States continues to be African American, numbering close to 30 million, or about 12% of the population (U.S. Census Bureau, 1990).

As immigration patterns and laws have changed, so too has the mix of cultural diversity in the United States. The Immigration Reform and Control Act of 1986 (Public Law 99-603) and the Immigration Act of 1990 (Public Law 101-649) have limited the total number of immigrants being admitted. Futhermore, the laws' greater stringency places annual numerical ceilings on certain immigrant groups while authorizing increases in such areas as highly skilled workers or family members of aliens who have been recently legalized. Population trends indicate that the fastest growing ethnic group is of Hispanic origin followed by African American and then Asian/Pacific Islander. By the year 2050 Hispanic Americans are expected to reach 21% of the United States population, African Americans will make up 15%, and Asian Americans 10% (Current Population Reports, 1992).

Although broad cultural values are shared by most large national societies, within those societies are smaller cultural groups called **subcultures**. Subcultures are relatively large aggregates of people within a society who share separate distinguishing characteristics such as ethnicity (African or Hispanic Americans), occupation (farmers or physicians), religion (Catholics or Muslims), geographic area (New Englanders or Southerners), age (the elderly or school children), sex or sex-

(text continues on page 148)

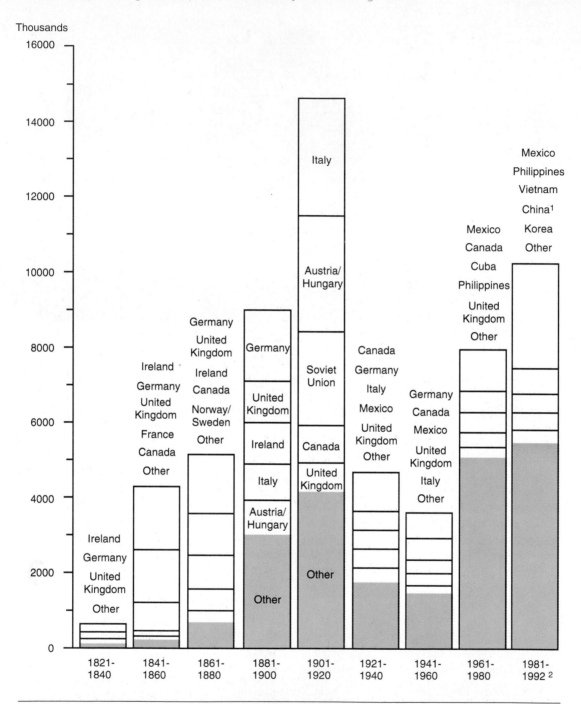

¹China includes mainland China and Taiwan.   ²Twelve-year period.

FIGURE 7.2. Immigrants admitted to the United States from the top five countries of last residence: 1821 to 1992. Source: 1986 Statistical Yearbook of the Immigration and Naturalization Service: United States Immigration and Naturalization Service, Washington, D.C.

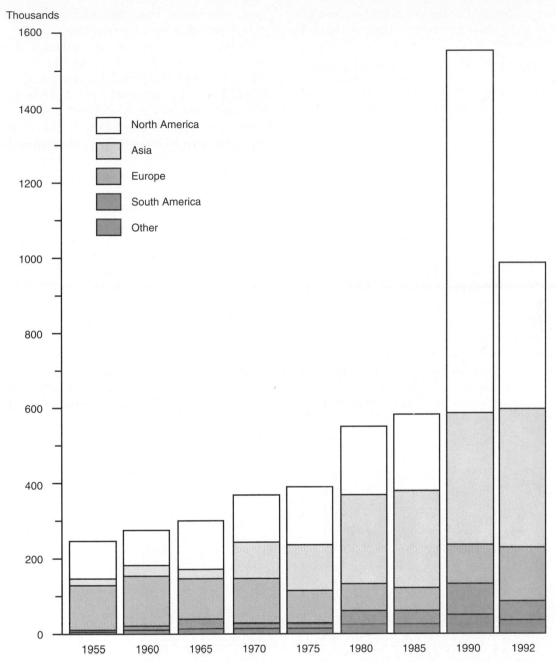

FIGURE 7.3. Immigrants admitted by region of birth: selected fiscal years 1955–1992. Source: 1986 Statistical Yearbook of the Immigration and Naturalization Service: United States Immigration and Naturalization Service, Washington, D.C.

ual preference (women or gay men). Within these sub-cultures are yet smaller groups called **microcultures** by anthropologists.

> "Microcultures are systems of cultural knowledge characteristic of subgroups within larger societies. Members of a microculture will usually share much of what they know with everyone in the greater society but will possess a special cultural knowledge that is unique to the subgroup" (Spradley and McCurdy, 1994, p.15).

Examples can range from a group of Hmong immigrants adopting selected aspects of United States culture to a third-generation Norwegian American community whose members share unique foods, dress, and values.

The members of each subculture and microculture retain some of the characteristics of the society from which they came or in which their ancestors lived (Mead, 1960). Some of their beliefs and practices, such as the food they eat, the language they speak at home, the way they celebrate holidays, or their ideas about sickness and healing, remain an important part of their everyday life. Native American groups have retained some aspects of their traditional cultures (Figure 7.4). Mexican Americans, Irish Americans, Swedish Americans, Italian Americans, African Americans, Puerto Rican Americans, Chinese Americans, Japanese Americans, Vietnamese Americans, and many other ethnic groups have their own microcultures.

Furthermore, certain customs, values, and ideas are unique to the poor, the rich, the middle class, women, men, youth, and the elderly. Many deviant groups, such as narcotic addicts, criminals, and skid row alcoholics, have developed their own microcultures. Regional microcultures, such as that of the Kentucky mountain people, also have distinctive ways of defining the world and coping with life. Other microcultures, such as those of rural migrant farm workers and urban homeless street people, acquire their own sets of beliefs and patterns for dealing with their environments. Many religious groups have their own microcultures. Even occupational and professional groups develop their own special languages, beliefs, and perspectives such as nurses or other health professionals.

Ethnocentrism

There is a difference between a healthy cultural or ethnic identification and **ethnocentrism**. Anthropologists explain that, "ethnocentrism is the belief and feel-

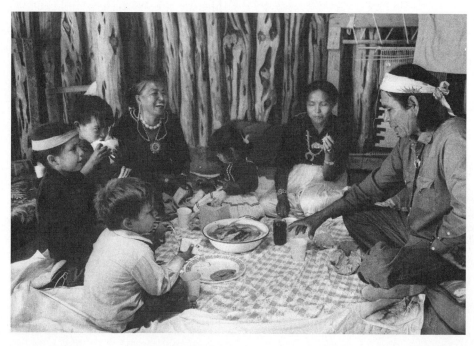

FIGURE 7.4. Native Americans celebrating a festive occasion.

ing that one's own culture is best. It reflects our tendency to judge other people's beliefs and behavior using values of our own native culture" (Spradley & McCurdy, 1994, p.16). It causes people to believe that their way of doing things is right and to judge others' methods as inferior, ignorant, or irrational. Ethnocentrism blocks effective communication by creating biases and misconceptions about human behavior. In turn, this can cause serious damage to interpersonal relationships and interfere with nurse effectiveness (Eliason, 1993; Leininger, 1991). See the Issues in Community Health Nursing display below.

Issues in Community Health Nursing
ETHNOCENTRISM

One of the most dangerous and subtle barriers to effective community health nursing service is ethnocentrism. This refers to the conscious or unconscious belief that one's own beliefs and ways of doing things are best. It also involves a lack of understanding or appreciation of other cultural beliefs and practices. The potential dangers of ethnocentrism can be seen in the following situations:

- The young community health nurse, wanting to be friendly, calls a group of newly immigrated elderly Southeast Asian refugee women by their first names. She has not learned that this is disrespectful in their culture and she fails to gain their trust.
- Conducting health education classes with Mexican American migrant workers, the community health nurse discourages use of herbal and folk remedies. She does not recognize their possible value or meaning for this cultural group who find this approach belittling of important traditions.
- In a community planning session with a Native American group the community health nurse breaks in during silences and assertively offers solutions. To the group this is offensive and a sign of immaturity.

These types of situations can be prevented by developing cultural self-awareness and learning and respecting the client culture.

Significance of Culture in Health Care

Culture, because it so profoundly influences thinking and behavior, has an enormous impact on the effectiveness of health care. Just as physical and psychological factors determine clients' needs and attitudes toward health and illness, so too does culture. Kark emphasized that "culture is perhaps the most relevant social determinant of community health" (1974, p.149). Culture influences diet and eating practices. In fact, partly because of culturally derived preferences, "one of the most difficult problems is changing eating habits" (Pickett & Hanlon, 1990, p.373). Culture determines how people rear their children, react to pain, cope with stress, deal with death, respond to health practitioners, and value the past, present, and future. Yet health care consumers' cultures are often misunderstood or ignored in the delivery of health care (Leininger, 1994a). Nurses must be careful to avoid ethnocentric attitudes and attempt to understand and bridge cultural differences when working with others. They must develop knowledge and skill in serving multicultural clients.

Overcoming ethnocentrism requires a concerted effort on the nurse's part to see the world through the eyes of clients. It means being willing "to examine one's own culture carefully and become aware that alternative viewpoints are possible" (Eliason, 1993, p.226). It means attempting to understand the meaning of other people's culture for them, and it means appreciating their culture as important and useful to them. Ignoring consideration of clients' different cultural origins can often have devastating results as illustrated by the case study of Maria Juarez.

Characteristics of Culture

In their study of culture, anthropologists and sociologists have made significant contributions to the field of community health. Their findings shed light on why and how culture influences behavior. Five characteristics shared by all cultures are especially pertinent to nursing's efforts to improve community health: culture is (1) learned, (2) integrated, (3) shared, (4) tacit, and (5) dynamic.

CASE STUDY

MARIA JUAREZ

Maria Juarez, a 53-year-old Mexican-American widow, was referred to a community health nursing agency by a clinic. Her married daughter reported that Mrs. Juarez was having severe and prolonged vaginal bleeding and needed medical attention. The daughter had made several appointments for her mother at the clinic, but Mrs. Juarez had refused at the last minute to keep any of them.

After two broken home visit appointments, the community health nurse made a drop-in call and found Mrs. Juarez at home. The nurse was greeted courteously and invited to have a seat. After introductions, the nurse explained that she and the others were only trying to help. Mrs. Juarez had caused a lot of unnecessary concern to everyone by not cooperating, she scolded in a friendly tone. Mrs. Juarez quickly apologized and explained that she had felt fine on the days of her broken appointments and saw no need "to bother" anyone. Questioned about her vaginal bleeding, Mrs. Juarez was evasive. "It's nothing," she said, "it comes and goes like always, only maybe a little more." She listened politely, nodding in agreement as the nurse explained the need for her to see a physician. Her promise to come to the clinic the next day, however, was not kept. The staff labeled Mrs. Juarez unreliable and uncooperative.

Mrs. Juarez had been brought up in traditional Mexican-American culture that taught her to be submissive and in-terested primarily in the welfare of her husband and children. She had learned long ago to ignore her own needs and, in fact, found it difficult to identify any personal wants. Her major concern was to avoid causing trouble for others. To have a medical problem, then, was a difficult adjustment. The pain and bleeding had caused her great apprehension. Many Mexican Americans have a particular dread of sickness and especially hospitalization. Furthermore, Mrs. Juarez's culture had taught her the value of modesty. "Female problems" were not discussed openly. This cultural orientation meant that the sickness threatened her modesty and created intense embarrassment. Conforming to Mexican-American cultural values, she had first turned to her family for support. Often it is only under dire circumstances that members of this cultural group seek help from others; to do so means sacrificing pride and dignity. Mrs. Juarez agreed to go to the clinic because refusal would have been disrespectful, but her fear of physicians as well as her extreme reluctance to discuss such a sensitive problem kept her from going. Mrs. Juarez was being asked to take action that violated a number of deeply felt cultural values. Her behavior was far from unreliable and uncooperative. With no opportunity to discuss and resolve the conflicts, she had no other choice.

CULTURE IS LEARNED

Patterns of cultural behavior are acquired, not inherited. Rather than being genetically determined, the way people dress, what they eat, how they talk—all are learned. Spradley and McCurdy offer the following explanation:

"At the moment of birth, we lack a culture. We don't yet have a system of beliefs, knowlege, and patterns of customary behavior. But from that moment until we die, each of us participates in a kind of universal schooling that teaches us our native culture. Laughing and smiling are genetic responses, but as infants we soon learn when to smile, when to laugh, and even how to laugh. We also inherit the potential to cry, but we must learn our cultural rules for when crying is appropriate" (1994, p.14).

Each person learns their culture through socialization with their family or significant group, a process called **enculturation**. As a child grows up in a given society, she or he acquires certain attitudes, beliefs, and values and learns how to behave in ways appropriate to that group's definition of the female or male role; they are learning their culture (See Fig. 7.5).

Although culture is learned, the process and results of that learning are different for each person. Each individual has a unique personality and experiences life in a singular way; these factors influence acquisition of culture. Families, social classes, and other groups within a society differ from one another, and this sociocultural variation has important implications for planned change. Since culture is learned, it is possible for parts of it to be relearned. People might change certain cultural elements or adopt new behaviors or values. Some individuals and groups will be more willing than others to try new ways and thus potentially influence change.

CULTURE IS INTEGRATED

Rather than an assortment of various customs and traits, a culture is a functional, integrated whole. As in any system, all the parts of a culture are interrelated and interdependent. The various components of a culture, such as its social mores or religious beliefs, perform separate functions, comingling in relative harmony with

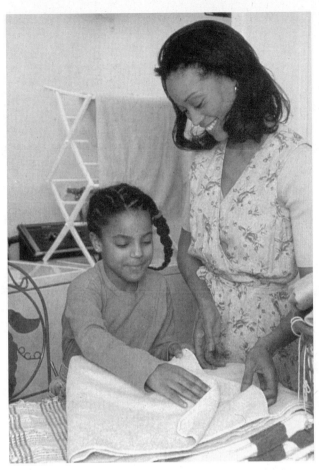

FIGURE 7.5. Children are socialized into the roles of their culture by imitating behavior of the same sex parent.

each other to form an operating and cohesive whole. In other words, to understand culture, one cannot simply describe single traits. Each part must be viewed in terms of its relationships to other parts and to the whole.

A person's culture is an integrated web of ideas and practices. For example, a nurse may promote the consumption of three balanced meals a day, a practice tied to her belief that nutrition leads to good health and that prevention is better than cure. These cultural traits, in turn, are related to her values about health. Health, the nurse believes, is essential for maximum energy output and productivity at work. Productivity is important because it enables people to reach goals. These values are linked to social or religious beliefs about hard work and taboos against laziness. Thus these ideas and beliefs about nutrition, health, economics, religion, and family are all interrelated and work to motivate one's behavior.

Parents who are Jehovah's Witnesses refusing a blood transfusion for their child is another example of culturally determined behavior. Their actions might seem irrational or ignorant to those who do not understand their religious beliefs. However, that choice represents behavior consistent with the couple's cultural values and standards. The single behavior of refusing blood transfusions, when viewed in context, is part of a larger religious belief system and a basic component of their culture.

In some cultural groups modesty for women may make it uncomfortable and perhaps traumatic to be examined by a person of the opposite sex, as was the situation with Mrs. Juarez whose case study was related earlier. Asking certain Native American groups to comply with rigid appointment scheduling means requiring them to reframe their concept of time. It also violates their values of patience and pride. Before nurses attempt a change in a person's or group's behavior, they need to ask how that change will affect the people involved through its influence on other parts of their culture. Extra time and patience or different strategies may be needed if change is still indicated. Nurses may often find that their own practice system can be modified to preserve clients' cultural values.

CULTURE IS SHARED

Culture is the product of aggregate behavior, not individual habit. Certainly, individuals practice a culture, but customs are phenomena shared by all members of the group (see Fig. 7.6). The anthropologist, Murdock, in his seminal work explains:

"Culture does not depend on individuals. An ordinary habit dies with its possessor, but a group habit lives on in the survivors, and is transmitted from generation to generation. Moreover, the individual is not a free agent with respect to culture. He is born and reared in a certain cultural environment, which impinges upon him at every moment of his life. From earliest childhood his behavior is conditioned by the habits of those around him. He has no choice but to conform to the folkways current in his group" (1972, p. 258).

A culture's values are among its most important elements. A **value** is a notion or idea designating relative worth or desireability. Each culture classifies phenomena "into good and bad, desirable and undesirable, right and wrong" (Foster, 1962, p.18). When people respond in favor of or against some practice, they are reflecting their culture's values about that practice. One person may eagerly anticipate eating a steak for dinner. An-

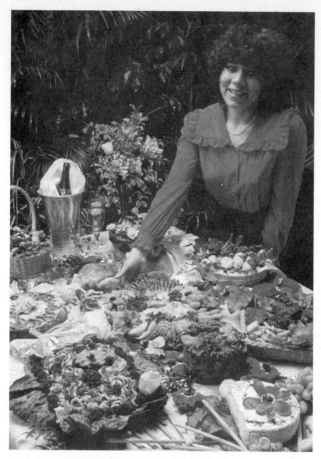

FIGURE 7.6. Serving special foods to guests connotes appreciation and respect.

other, who believes that eating meat is sacrilegious or unhealthy, will experience revulsion at the idea. Some American subcultures think that loud, vocal expressions are a necessary way to deal with pain. Others value silence and stoicism. Some have high regard for speed and efficiency while others prefer patience and thoughtfulness. Either way, values serve a purpose. Shared values give people in a specific culture stability and security; they provide a standard for behavior. From these values members know what to believe and how to act. The normative criteria by which people justify their decisions are based on values which are more deeply rooted than behaviors and consequently more difficult to change.

Knowing that culture is shared helps one to understand human behavior. For example, a community health nurse tried unsuccessfully to persuade a mother to stop heavily oiling her infant's skin (Taylor, 1973).

She discovered that the mother was acting in a tradition of her rural subculture that held that oil promoted good health. The fact that all the other mothers in that religious group also used oil on their babies proved a powerful deterrent to the change requested by the nurse. Individual health behavior is always influenced by other people of the same culture. Thus, it becomes very difficult for one person to eliminate some cultural practice when it will continue to be reinforced by other group members. In fact, group acceptance and a sense of membership almost always depend on conforming to shared cultural practices (Spradley & McCurdy, 1994).

Thus community health nursing may need to focus on an entire group's health behavior to affect individual practices. The pattern of oiling young infants, for instance, ceased when the nurse worked with the entire church group. She began with a well-recognized cultural strategy: to work through formal or informal leaders. She contacted the minister and discussed the cultural practice. He admitted that anointing with oil, a Biblical teaching, was one of their beliefs. When she explained her concerns, he agreed that a drop of oil on the head was all that was needed. He clarified this teaching in his next sermon, and as a result, additional health problems also cleared up when other members of the group stopped rubbing oil into wounds and infections (Taylor, 1973).

CULTURE IS MOSTLY TACIT

Culture provides a guide for human interaction that is mostly unexpressed and at the unconsious level, or **tacit**. Members of a cultural group, without the need for discussion, know how to act and what to expect from one another. Culture provides an implicit set of cues for behavior, not a written set of rules. Spradley and McCurdy explain that culture is often "so regular and routine that it lies below a conscious level" (1994, p.16). It is like a memory bank where one stores knowledge for recall when the situation requires it, but this recall process is most often unconscious. Culture teaches one the proper tone of voice to use for each occasion. It prescribes how close to stand when talking with someone. Individuals learn to make responses that are appropriate to their sex, role, and status. They know what is right and wrong. All of these attitudes and behaviors are so ingrained, so tacit, that people seldom, if ever, need to discuss them.

Because culture is mostly tacit, it is difficult to realize which of one's own behaviors may be offensive to people from other groups. It is also difficult to know the meaning and significance of other cultural practices. Silence in some groups, such as Native American women, is valued but may make others uncomfortable. Offering food to a guest in many cultures is not merely a social gesture but an important symbol of hospitality and acceptance (see Fig. 7.6) and to refuse, for any reason, may be an insult and a rejection. Touching or calling someone by their first name may be a demonstration of caring for some but be viewed as disrespectful and offensive by others. Consequently, community health nurses have a twofold task in developing cultural sensitivity; not only must they try to learn clients' culture, but they must also try to make their own culture less tacit and more explicit. Cross-cultural tension can be resolved through conscious efforts at developing awareness, patience, and acceptance of cultural differences. See the World Watch discussion of culture shock.

CULTURE IS DYNAMIC

Every culture undergoes change; none is entirely static. Within every cultural group are individuals who generate innovations. More important, there are members who see advantages in different ways of doing things and are willing to adopt new practices. Each culture, including our own, is an amalgamation of ideas, values, and practices from a variety of sources. This process depends, of course, on the extent of exposure to other groups. Nonetheless, every culture is in a dynamic state of adding or deleting components. Functional aspects are retained; less functional ones are eliminated.

When this adaptation does not occur the cultural group may face serious difficulty. For example, many Southeast Asian refugees in the United States have continued to prepare and eat food in their traditional fashion. Uncooked pork is a part of that diet. As a result, a study showed that "between 1975 and 1984, the incidence of trichinosis in the United States was 25 times greater for the Southeast Asian refugee population than for the general United States population" (Stehr-Green & Schantz, 1986, p.1238). Other outbreaks of trichinosis among this population in recent years reinforce the need for futher education and control measures (McAuley, et al, 1992).

The dynamic nature of culture is useful to community health nursing for several reasons. Cultures and subcultures do indeed change over time. Patience and persistence are probably key attributes to cultivate

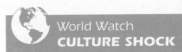

World Watch
CULTURE SHOCK

An increasing number of immigrants and refugees from many different countries have been assimilated into American culture in recent years. While they quickly adapt in many respects, learning the language, seeking housing and employment, they continue to operate within the framework of their own cultural beliefs and behaviors. The conflict between their culture and American culture often causes **culture shock**, "a state of anxiety that results from cross-cultural misunderstanding . . . and an inability to interact appropriately in the new context" (Spradley & McCurdy, 1994, p.16). Immigrants and refugees find themselves in a strange setting with people who act in unfamiliar ways. Speaking their own language in their homes, retaining values and familiar practices all help to promote some sense of security in the new environment. The same is true for nurses and others working overseas in unfamiliar countries. No longer are the small but important cues available that orient one to appropriate behavior. Instead a person may feel isolated and anxious and even become dysfunctional or ill. Immersion in the culture over time and making an effort to learn the new culture are the major remedies. As adjustment occurs, old beliefs and practices that are still functional in the new setting can be retained while others that are not functional must be replaced.

when working toward improvement of health behaviors. Another point to remember is that cultures change as their members see greater advantages in the "new ways." Discussing these advantages will have to be done in a language they understand and in the context of their own cultural value system. This is an important reason for nurses to develop an understanding of their clients' culture (Bernal, 1993; Eliason, 1993; Leininger, 1991b & 1994a). Furthermore, change within a culture is usually brought about by certain key individuals who are receptive to new ideas and able to influence their peers. These same key persons can adapt the change process so that "new" practices are culturally consistent and fit with group values. Tapping this resource becomes imperative for successful change. Finally, the health care culture can, and perhaps should, change, too. Consider its changes in the past. Nurses can learn a great deal from their clients and their cultures. And as nurses discover more effective ways of working with clients, they can and may choose to modify their own practices.

Cultural Communities

An examination of the meaning and nature of culture clearly underscores the need to recognize cultural differences and understand clients in the context of their cultural backgrounds. Practically speaking, however, how can knowledge of cultural diversity be integrated into everyday community health nursing practice? Who are the diverse cultural communities served by community health nurses? What are their differences? Do they share some features in common? This section describes select clusters of cultural communities to provide insights and answers to these questions. Descriptions are kept intentionally brief to remind the reader that each culture is complex and unique and deserves much more comprehensive study than is possible within the scope of this chapter. The reader is encouraged to pursue further information provided in the references and selected readings.

NATIVE AMERICANS

Native Americans, the first known settlers of this continent, form a large cluster of tribal groups whose members were born and live in the United States. They number close to two million and are scattered across the continental United States, Alaska, and the Aleutian Islands (U.S. Census Bureau, 1990). Native Americans have adopted many Anglo American values and practices, yet preserve large aspects of their own culture.

Population Characteristics and Culture

Native Americans, or American Indians, are a diverse group made up of 270 different tribes. They are scattered throughout 26 states in the United States with more than half living in Arizona, California, New Mexico, North Carolina, and Oklahoma (West, 1993). Each tribe or nation has its own distinct language, beliefs, customs, and rituals. Thus the community health nurse

TABLE 7.1. *Native American Cultural Similarities*

Value dignity of the individual
Value family and community
Respect for increasing age, elders are leaders
Live in harmony with nature, respect the environment
Value symbolic arts and crafts
Live in the present, little concern for the distant future
Value generosity and sharing, discourage competition
Integrate religion into everyday life
Treat body and soul as one unit
Use herbal medicines and traditional healing practices.
Value rituals and ceremonies
Practice periods of silence, value thoughtful speech
Value patience

(Sources: Bell, 1994; Orque, et al. 1983; West, 1993)

cannot assume that knowledge of one group can be generalized to others. Knowledge of certain similarities (see Table 7.1) among the various Native American cultures can assist the nurse in working with the members of a specific tribe (Bell, 1994; Primeaux & Henderson, 1981; West, 1993). For many Native American groups their large extended family networks serve to reinforce cultural standards and expectations as well as provide emotional support and practical assistance (Seideman, et al, 1994).

Health Problems

Health problems among Native Americans tend to be both chronic and socially related (West, 1993). The highest ranking health problems in children include dysentery, impetigo, intestinal infectious diseases, skin diseases, staphylococcal infections, respiratory disease, influenza, and pneumonia. For adults, trachomatous conjunctivitis poses a serious health threat not common in the rest of the U.S. population. Tuberculosis, diabetes, and obesity all rank higher among Native Americans than in the general population. Poor sanitation, crowded housing, and low immunization levels all contribute to a variety of communicable diseases. Heart disease is lower among Indians than whites. Alcoholism, however, is a major health problem with a related high incidence of fetal alcohol syndrome (FAS) and fetal alcohol effects (FAE) along with a high incidence of violence and injuries. Substance abuse, increasingly among children, is prevalent among those living on reservations.

Health Beliefs and Practices

Native Americans as a group tend to prefer traditional healing practices and folk medicine over Western medicine. As many as "90% of Indians today still seek out a medicine man before going to a health clinic" (West, 1993, p.231). Many of their beliefs about health and illness have supernatural explanations and their health and dietary practices are closely tied to cultural and religious beliefs. Herbal teas, charms and fetishes are used as preventive measures. Because of decades of racism and government paternalism, many Native Americans feel oppressed, dehumanized, and carry considerable resentment and lack of trust toward whites. As a result many maintain a degree of separateness from overall American culture. Nurses must overcome these barriers through patience, acceptance, and respect for their culture as illustrated in the case study of Mrs. Brown.

CASE STUDY

MRS. BROWN

Consider the following experience of a community health nurse with one Native American community.

As she drove up the dirt road and parked her car next to the community hall, Sandra felt apprehensive. She had been warned by the previous community health nurse that these Indian people were hard to work with: "This tribe is lazy and unappreciative. You can't get anywhere with them." It was only through the urging of an Indian community aide, Mrs. Brown, that a group of the women had reluctantly agreed to meet with the new nurse. They would see what she had to say.

Sandra's steps echoed hollowly as she walked across the wooden floor of the large room to the far corner where a group of women sat silently in a circle. Only their eyes turned; their faces remained impassive. Mrs. Brown rose slowly, greeted the nurse, and introduced her to the group. Swallowing her fear, Sandra smiled. She told them of her background and explained that she had not worked with Indian people before. There was a long silence. No one spoke. Sandra continued, "I'd like to help you if I can, maybe with problems about care of your children when they are sick or questions about how to keep them healthy, but I don't know what you need or want." Silence fell again. She would like to learn from them, she repeated. Would they help her? Again an uncomfortable silence ensued.

Then one woman began to speak. Quietly, but with deep feeling, she described several bad experiences with the previous nurse and the county social worker. Then others spoke up: "They tell us what we should do. They don't listen. They say our way is not good." Seeing Sandra's interest and concern, the women continued. One of their main concerns was their children's health. Another was the high incidence of accidents and injuries on the reservation. They wanted to learn how to give first aid. Other concerns were expressed. The group agreed that Sandra could help them by teaching a first-aid class.

In the weeks that followed, Sandra taught several classes on first aid and emergency care. She then began a series of sessions on child health. Each time she would ask the women to choose a topic or problem for discussion then elicit from them their accustomed ways of dealing with each problem, for example, how they handled toilet training or taught their children to eat solid foods. Her goal was to learn as much as she could about their culture and incorporate that information into her teaching, which preserved as many of their practices as possible. Sandra also visited informally with the women in their homes and at community gatherings. She learned about their way of life, their history, and their values. For example, patience was highly valued. It was important to be able to wait patiently, even if a scheduled meeting was delayed as much as two hours. It was also important for others to speak, which explained the Indian women's comfort with silences during a conversation. Other values influenced their way of life. Courage, pride, generosity, and honesty were all important determinants of behavior. These were also values by which they judged Sandra and other professionals. Sandra's honesty in keeping her promises enabled the women to trust her. Her generosity in giving her time, helping them occasionally with some household task, and arranging for child care during classes won their respect.

The women came to accept her, and Sandra was invited to eat with them and share in tribal get-togethers. The women criticized and advised her on acceptable ways to speak and act. Her openness and patience to learn and her respect for them as a people had paved the way to improving their health. At first, Sandra felt that her progress was very slow, but this slowness was actually an advantage. She had built a solid foundation of cross-cultural trust, and in the months that followed, she saw many changes in their health practices.

AFRICAN AMERICANS

A second cultural group includes black Americans, also called African Americans. Unlike Native Americans, this group originally came from other countries although most African Americans living today were born in the United States. Their ancestors first came to this continent in 1619 as free settlers (Bennett, 1962) but the great majority who followed came as slaves from West Africa. Today, black immigrants come from Caribbean as well as African and other countries.

Population Characteristics

In 1990 African Americans, numbering about 30 million, constituted 12% of the United States population with projections showing an increase to 15% by the year 2050 (*Current Population Reports,* 1992). One third of the African American population is under the age of 18 years with a predominance of that group being males (see Fig. 7.7). Slightly more than 8% are in the 65 and over age group with a majority being older women. Over half of black children live with their mothers only, compared to one in six white children who live with their mothers only.

Economic Conditions and Education

Despite improvements in the legal and social climate for African Americans, great disparities still exist. Aver-

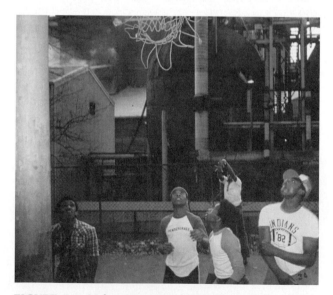

FIGURE 7.7. Males constitute the majority of the African American population less than 18 years old.

age family income for African Americans is 56% of the income earned by white families. More than 33% of African Americans live in poverty contrasted with 10% of whites. While they are 12% of the population, blacks make up 50% of prison inmates. Close to 44% of all African American children as well as most female-headed families live below the poverty level (*Current Population Reports,* 1993). Unemployment among African Americans is around 11% compared to about 4% for whites with rates for men being slightly higher than for women.

Educational disparities also exist. Two thirds of African Americans complete high school compared to 80% of whites. Far fewer African Americans enroll in and complete college than whites. African American women acquire more educational training than their male counterparts; however, their earnings are much lower than black men.

Culture

Like Native Americans and Asians, there is no single African American culture; rather, this group forms a heterogeneous community of people. Like other large ethnic and racial groups, many factors influence their culture and thus result in much diversity within the African American population. Among the variables determining specific microcultures within the African American community are economic level, religious background, education, occupation, social class identity, geographic origin, and residence in an integrated or segregated neighborhood (Porter & Villarruel, 1993). For community health nurses this means that specific groups of African Americans will have their own unique values, character, life style, and health needs.

The primary language of most African Americans is English. More recent black immigrants from Caribbean or other countries may retain the language of their country of origin but generally learn English as well. Many African Americans speak variations of soul talk, also called black English or black creole. It evolved from pidgin spoken during the era of slavery and has become a dynamic and meaningful language of its own. For some African Americans, soul talk symbolizes racial pride and identity.

Health Beliefs

While African Americans have absorbed most of the dominant culture in the United States, some still retain aspects of their ancestors' traditional values and practices. Some, for example, hold to traditional African beliefs about health being a sign of harmony with nature and illness being evidence of disharmony. Evil spirits, the punishment of God, or a hex placed on the person might account for this disharmony. Healers treat body, mind and spirit. Prayer, laying on of hands, home remedies, magic or other rituals, special diets, wearing of preventive charms or copper bracelets, ointments and other folk remedies are sometimes practiced. Each African American community has its own set of health beliefs and practices which must be determined before planning any community health nursing interventions.

Health Problems

African Americans have much higher mortality rates than whites and a life expectancy of 69.1 years contrasted with 75.6 years for whites. Their major health problems include cardiovascular disease and stroke, cancer, diabetes mellitus, cirrhosis, a high infant mortality rate (twice that of whites), homicide and accidents, and malnutrition. A number of factors contribute to these problems. Stress and discrimination, poverty, lack of education, high rates of teen pregnancies, inadequate housing, and inadequate insurance for health care are among the risk factors influencing the health of this population. In the last three decades, a dramatic increase in black female-headed households, out-of-wedlock births, and a limited presence of male role models further exacerbated family vulnerability (Friedman, 1990).

Mortality rates for communicable diseases, including AIDS, are also higher for blacks than whites. African Americans with AIDS make up nearly one third of reported cases and 80% of those are black men (National Center for Health Statistics, 1993). The incidence of tuberculosis among this population is also rising.

ASIAN AMERICANS

A third cultural cluster is composed of immigrants and refugees from various Pacific Rim countries. Coming from China, Korea, Japan, Thailand, Laos, the Philippines, Vietnam, Cambodia, and other Asian countries, some of these people have more recently been transplanted from their own cultures to an entirely different culture while others may have lived here many years or been born in America. In 1990 there were over 7 million Asians and Pacific Islanders living in the United States. By far the largest groups were Chinese, numbering well over a million and a half persons, and Filipinos, numbering just under a million and a half persons (U.S. Bureau of the Census, 1990). Each group represents a distinct culture with its own unique challenges for community health nurses as illustrated in the case study of Mrs. Kim.

Asian Culture

While each Asian culture is distinct in language, values, and customs, some general traits are shared in common by many Asians. Traditional Asian families tend to be patriarchal, the father is the head of the household, and patrilineal, the geneology is carried through the male line. Males are valued over females. Elders are respected. The male role is generally the provider while the female role is that of homemaker. Traditional Asians value achievement because it brings honor to the family name. Saving face or preserving dignity and family pride is very important. Cooperation is valued over competition.

Health Problems

Health problems for Asian Americans include malnutrition, tuberculosis, mental illness, cancer, respiratory infections, arthritis, and parasitic infestations as well as chronic diseases associated with aging. Suicide rates and stress-related illness are particularly high among Asian refugee groups who have had to flee their countries under extremely stressful conditions. However Asians view mental illness as shameful and the stigma attached to it prompts them to somaticize it or hide it as long as possible.

Health Beliefs and Practices

Asian health beliefs vary between cultures. Many Asians believe in the Chinese concepts of Yin (cold) and Yang (hot) which refer not to temperature but to the opposing forces of the universe regulating normal flow of energy. A balance of Yin and Yang results in Qi (pronounced chee) which is the desired state of harmony. Illness results when there is an imbalance in these forces. If the imbalance means an excess of Yin then "cold" foods, such as vegetables and fruits are avoided and "hot" foods, such as rice, chicken, eggs, and pork are offered. Some Asians view western medicines as "hot" and eastern folk medicines and herbal treatments as "cold"

CASE STUDY

MRS. KIM

The following experience illustrates some of the challenge of transcultural nursing with one Asian culture for the community health nurse.

Armed with enthusiasm and pamphlets on pregnancy and prenatal diet, the community health nurse began home visits to the Kim family. Her initial plan was to discuss pregnancy and fetal development, teach diet, and prepare the mother for delivery. Mr. Kim, a graduate student, was present to interpret since Mrs. Kim spoke very little English. Their two boys, three years and one and one half years of age, played happily on the kitchen floor. The family offered tea to the nurse and listened politely as she explained her reasons for coming and added, "How can I be most helpful to you? What would you like from my visits?"

The Kims were grateful for this approach. Hesitant at first, they hinted at Mrs. Kim's fears of American doctors and hospitals; her first two children had been born in Korea. None of the family had any experience with Western medicine. They shared some concerns about adjustment to living in the United States. It was difficult to shop in American food stores with their overwhelming variety of foods, many of which the Kims found unfamiliar. Mrs. Kim, who had come from a family whose servants prepared the food, was an in-experienced cook. Servants had also cared for the children, and her role had been that of an aristocrat in hand-tailored silk gowns.

Listening carefully, the nurse began to realize the striking differences between her own and her clients' culture. Her care plans changed. In subsequent visits she determined to learn about Korean culture and base her nursing intervention on that knowledge. She learned about their traditional ways of raising children, male and female roles, and practices related to pregnancy and lactation. She respected their value of "saving face" and attempted never to offend their pride or dignity (Sich, 1988). As time went on, her interest and respect for their way of life won their trust. She inquired about their cultural practices before attempting any intervention. As a result, the Kims were receptive to her suggestions. Whenever possible, she adapted her teaching and suggestions to comply with the Kim's culture. Appropriate changes were made in Mrs. Kim's diet, for example, that were still compatible with her food preferences and cultural eating patterns. Because she was not accustomed to drinking milk, she increased her calcium intake by learning to prepare custards (which disguised the milk flavor) and by eating more green, leafy vegetables. After five months, a strong, positive relationship had been established between this family and the nurse. Mrs. Kim delivered a healthy baby girl and looked forward to continued supportive visits from the community health nurse.

which may explain why some groups practice both for balance. The Vietnamese have a similar hot and cold belief but call it *Am* and *Dong*. Other Asian groups, such as the Filipinos, view illness as an act of God and pray for healing. The Khmer of Cambodia believe illness reflects one's deviation from moral standards and the Hmong consider illness a visitation by spirits. All have traditional healers which, depending on the culture, include acupuncturists, herbalists, herb pharmacists, spirit and magic experts, or a shaman. Most Asian cultures also exercise traditional self-care practices which include herbal medicines and poultices, types of acupuncture, and massage (Lin-Fu, 1991). Southeast Asians also practice dermabrasive techniques of cupping, pinching, rubbing, and burning. These are used to relieve headaches, sore throats, coughs, fever, diarrhea and other symptoms by bringing toxins to the skin surface or compensating for heat lost. They can be mistaken for physical abuse (Muecke, 1983). Each client requires careful cultural assessment before implementing nursing action.

HISPANIC AMERICANS

A fourth cultural cluster comprises groups who are of Hispanic origin and have immigrated to the United States. In 1990 this group numbered well over 22 million and amounted to 9% of the U. S. population. More than half came from Mexico with the next largest groups of immigrants coming from Puerto Rico and Cuba (U. S. Bureau of the Census, 1990). Those with Mexican and Central American backgrounds are generally referred to as Latinos (Friedman, 1990). Hispanics are the fastest growing ethnic group in the United States and are predicted to reach 21% of the population by 2050 (*Current Population Reports*, 1992).

Culture

Hispanics share Spanish as their common and primary language, nonetheless, their diverse cultural and linguistic backgrounds account for diversity in dialects

(Magar, 1990). Latinos value extended cohesive families. Families have been patriarchal with males perceived as superior and females seen as a family bonding life force. These traditional family structures are changing with migration, urbanization, women in the work force, and social movements. Spousal roles are becoming more egalitarian (Friedman, 1990). However, vestiges of the machismo male and the self-sacrificing female are still evident in Latino culture and continue to shape behavior.

Health Problems

Health problems among the Hispanic population are complicated by experiences in their countries of origin as well as socioeconomic and life style factors in this country. Tuberculosis is very high in this group, especially among those under 35 years of age. Hypertension, diabetes, and obesity are major concerns. Other problems include infectious diseases, particularly AIDS and pneumonia, parasitic infections, malnutrition, gastroenteritis, alcohol and drug abuse, accidents, and violence. Post-traumatic stress disorder is a major problem among refugees from Central and South America who have experienced war and physical and emotional torture (Magar, 1990).

Health Beliefs and Practices

Religion plays an important part in Latino culture. For most Latinos, Catholicism is the dominant religion (95% of Mexican-Americans are Catholic) but it is often "a blend of both Catholicism and Pre-Cortesian Indian beliefs and ideology" (Friedman, 1990, p.221). Latinos believe in submission to the will of God and that illness may be a form of "castigo" or punishment for sins. They cope with illness through prayers and faith that God will heal. Their religion also determines the rituals used in healing. For example, "solisto" which is a condition of depression in women (similar to midlife depression in American culture) is treated by having the patient lie on the floor while her body is stroked by the curandero (native healer) until the depression passes. Latino culture includes beliefs that witchcraft, or "brujeria", and evil eye, or "mal ojo", are supernatural causes of illness that cannot be treated by 'Anglo' medicine. "Empacho", a stomachache ailment in children that occurs after a traumatic event is treated by the curandero with herbal mixtures made into teas. After tender loving care and a bowel movement, the child is "healed." Like Asians, Latinos believe in "hot" and "cold" categories of foods that influence their diet during illness. Many Latinos tend to be present-oriented and not as concerned about keeping time schedules or preparing for the future.

DISADVANTAGED POPULATIONS

A final cultural community is made up of groups of people who are economically, physically, or emotionally disadvantaged. Each of these groups also can be said to have their own subcultures or microcultures. The poor, the homeless, and migrants who are economically disadvantaged, as well as the mentally retarded, the deaf, the blind, or persons physically challenged in other ways often form their own communities with certain distinct beliefs and practices that characterize their culture.

Economically Disadvantaged Populations

The microcultures of low-income populations can easily be misunderstood by health professionals. Although they may share the same values as the dominant culture, the poor are unable to act on these values and exist in separate microcultures that are diverse and unique. People who are economically disadvantaged come from many ethnic and racial backgrounds and bring the values, beliefs, and customs of their backgrounds with them. Because of this diversity, some have challenged the notion of a culture of poverty, warning of the dangers of stereotyping (Carney, 1992; Martin & Henry, 1989; Pesznecker, 1984). As in any culture, individual variations exist because people belong to overlapping groups even within a specified culture. The nurse needs to be careful to avoid stereotyping the poor, as this may lead to inaccurate assessments and interventions. What, then, characterizes the poor? Poverty is a state of being economically disadvantaged or, because of extremely limited resources, being unable to obtain adequate food, shelter, clothing, employment, or health care. But the microculture of those in poverty is more than economic. Culture, as was previously discussed, comprises the ideas, values, and behaviors that a group shares and that provides a design for living. When a person or group of persons is poor, regardless of the circumstances leading to that poverty, those individuals learn a set of behaviors and practices enabling them to cope with life. It is these behaviors and practices that make up the microculture of the poor.

Three attributes, in particular, tend to characterize the poor. One is that people experiencing poverty live mostly in the present (Strauss, 1967). Much of the health practitioner's emphasis tends to be preventive and thus future-oriented. Taking vitamins, eating well balanced meals, or getting a routine mammogram all involve a future-orientation, a view conflicting with the priorities of most people in poverty. Economically disadvantaged persons may have an orientation to the present because frequently they must meet immediate needs at the expense of long-term gains.

A second attribute is that the lives of many in poverty "are uncertain, dominated by recurring crises" (Strauss, 1967, p.10). Our larger society espouses a value of ordered, controlled, and well-planned lives. We advocate crisis prevention. For the poor, including migrant farm workers and urban homeless people (see Fig. 7.8), the demands of daily living with limited resources require adaptation on a day-to-day and even moment-by-moment basis. The poor experience a barrage of stressors, such as inability to find employment, housing, respectful treatment, or freedom from violence, that limit their ability to cope (Pesznecker, 1984). In many instances, positive health may be valued by this group but unattainable; thus they learn to live with illness and crisis.

A third attribute for many of the economically disadvantaged is the lack of a stable environment. Certain groups, the homeless, migrants, and vagrants in particular, have no permanent housing; their lives are characterized by a high rate of mobility. Migrant farm laborers work the southern states in the winter and then move northward in the summer months. Their mobility makes it difficult to provide continuous or comprehensive health services which, in turn, accounts for "a higher rate of respiratory, infectious, and digestive diseases than the general population" (Watkins, et al, 1990, p. 568). The migrant farmworker population in the United States, an estimated 3 million, includes whites, American blacks, Hispanics, Haitians and a small percentage of other minorities although most migrants are from Mexico (Watkins, et al, 1990). Migrant groups may retain some of their ethnic heritage but add their own cultural characteristics.

Many of the poor have learned to accept their life conditions and to make the most of them. Despite limited resources and often limited education, some have positive health practices although most have "compromised physical or pyschosocial health. . . . Lack of resources and options for coping lead to poor nutritional and other health habits that become extremely difficult to change" (Carney, 1992, p.74). Some religious groups choose poverty as a way of life and others, while poor economically, have learned to accept and live happily with limited material resources. Differences in life-style, dress, and behavior can easily lead the nurse to make

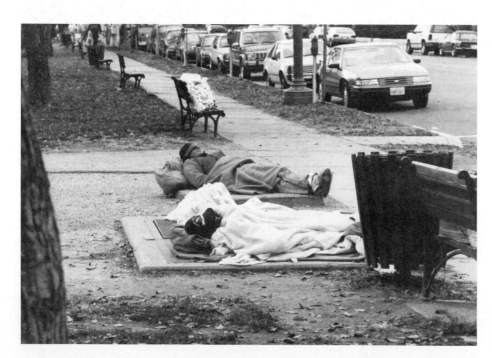

FIGURE 7.8. Homeless city dwellers try to keep warm in a public park.

assumptions about this group that are not necessarily correct. For instance, the poor have been characterized as having low self-esteem (Robertson, 1969). While this may be true in some instances, it is not fair or accurate to make such a generalization. Rather, these groups need caring professionals who understand and appreciate their values and needs and who offer health assistance within the context of their unique microcultures.

Physically or Mentally Challenged Populations

Persons with varying disabilites often form their own communities for employment, recreation, and mutual support. In turn, these communities develop their own microcultures. These include the deaf community (Holm, 1991), the handicapped community, the community of retarded persons, disabled veterans, the blind, and others. A problem created by well-meaning parents, teachers, and health professionals is to try to "fix" these people to be as "normal" as possible. While this might seem reasonable in some respects, the implication is that they are deficient or inferior. Physically challenged people find this approach deeply debilitating and oppressive. It is a form of ethnocentrism. For the deaf community the attempt to normalize, which is the integration model, is being challenged.

> "Many believe that a bi-lingual and bi-cultural model should be substituted for the integration model. This involves a profound shift in thinking. Deafness would be celebrated as a distinct, unique culture, rather than treated as a problem to be fixed. A bi-cultural model views Deafness as qualitatively different, but not worse and not broken" (Conflict and Change Center, 1992).

In 1994 Disabilities Services at the University of Minnesota proposed replacing the medical model with an interactional model, displayed in Table 7.2, that implicitly supports the bi-cultural view.

Transcultural Community Health Nursing Principles

The previous discussions have highlighted two important facts. One is that culture is a universal experience. Each person is part of some group and that group helps to shape the values, beliefs, and behaviors that make up their culture. The second is that every cultural group is different from all others. Even within fairly homogeneous cultural groups there are subcultures and microcultures that each have their own distinctive characteristics. Further differences, based on such factors as socioeconomic status, social class, age, or degree of acculturation, can be found within microcultures. These latter differences have been called intraethnic variations (Friedman, 1990), and only serve to underscore the range of culturally diverse clients that community health nurses serve.

Given such diversity, community health nurses face a considerable challenge in providing service to cross cultural groups. This kind of practice, known as **transcultural nursing**, means culturally sensitive nursing service to people of an ethnic or racial background different than the nurse's. Several principles can guide community health nurses in transcultural practice with client groups. They are (1) develop cultural self-aware-

TABLE 7.2. *Cultural Views of People With Disabilities*

Medical Model	Interaction Model
Disability is a deficiency or abnormality.	Disability is a difference.
Being disabled is negative.	Being disabled, in itself, is neutral
Disability resides in the individual.	Disability derives form interaction between the individual and .society
The remedy for disability-related problems is cure or normalization of the individual.	The remedy for disability-related problems is a change in the interaction between the individual and society.
The agent of remedy is the professional.	The agent of remedy can be the individual, an advocate, or anyone who affects the arrangements between the individual and society.

(Source: Workshop on meaningful access for people with disabilities. University of Minnesota Disabilities Services, Minneapolis, MN, May 18, 1994.)

ness, (2) cultivate cultural sensitivity, (3) assess client group's culture, (4) show respect and patience while learning about other cultures, (5) examine culturally-derived health practices.

DEVELOP CULTURAL SELF-AWARENESS

The first transcultural nursing principle focuses on the nurse's own culture. Self-awareness is crucial for the nurse working with people from other cultures (Leininger, 1994a). "A first step in developing cultural sensitivity is to examine one's own culture carefully and become aware that alternative viewpoints are possible" (Eliason, 1993, p.226). Nurses must remember that their culture is often sharply different from the culture of their clients. **Cultural self-awareness** means recognition of one's own values, beliefs, and practices that make up one's culture. It also means becoming sensitive to the impact of one's culturally-based responses on others. The nurse who assisted Mrs. Juarez probably thought she was being friendly, efficient, and helpful. In terms of her own culture, this nurse's behavior was intended to reassure clients and meet their needs. Unaware of the negative consequences of her behavior, the nurse caused damage rather than met needs.

Cultural Self-Assessment

To gain skill in understanding their own culturally-based behavior, nurses can benefit from conducting a cultural self-assessment by analyzing the following points.

- Influences from own ethnic/racial background
- Own typical verbal and non-verbal communication patterns
- Own cultural values and norms
- Own religious beliefs and practices
- Own health beliefs and practices

Start with a detailed list of values, beliefs, and practices relative to each point. Next enlist one or more close friends to call attention to selected behaviors to bring these to a more conscious level. Video taping practice interviews with colleagues and even actual interviews with selected clients can create further awareness of the nurse's culturally-based unconscious responses. Finally, ask selected clients to critique nursing actions in contrast with client culture. Feedback from clients' perspectives can bring many of the nurse's own cultural responses to light.

Since culture is mostly tacit, as discussed earlier in this chapter, it takes conscious effort and hard work to bring one's own culture to the surface. The rewards of this effort, however, are to first make the nurse far more effective in understanding herself or himself and, in turn, to providing culturally relevant service with clients.

CULTIVATE CULTURAL SENSITIVITY

The second transcultural nursing principle seeks to expand the nurse's awareness of the significance of culture on behavior. Nurses' beliefs and ways of doing things frequently conflict with those of their clients. A first step toward bridging cultural barriers is recognition of those differences and the development of cultural sensitivity. **Cultural sensitivity** requires recognizing that culturally-based values, beliefs, and practices influence people's health and life styles and need to be considered in plans for service (Spradley, 1988). Mrs. Juarez's values and health practices sharply contrasted with those of the clinic's staff. Failure to recognize these differences led to a breakdown in communication and ineffective care. Once differences in culture are recognized, it is important to accept and appreciate them. A nurse's ways are valid for the nurse; clients' ways work for them. The nurse visiting the Kims avoided the dangerous ethnocentric trap of assuming that her way was best, and she consequently developed a fruitful relationship with her clients.

As a part of developing cultural sensitivity, nurses need to try to understand clients' points of view. They need to stand in their shoes, to try to see the world through their eyes. As the nurse listens, observes, and gradually learns other cultures, she or he must add a further step of choosing to avoid ethnocentrism. Otherwise the nurse's view of a different culture will remain distorted and perhaps prejudiced. The ability to show interest, concern, and compassion enabled Sandra to win the trust and respect of the Native American women. It told the Kims that their nurse cared about them. These nurses attempted to understand the feelings and ideas of their clients thus establishing a trusting relationship and opening the door to the possibility of the clients adopting healthier behaviors.

ASSESS CLIENT GROUP'S CULTURE

A third transcultural nursing principle emphasizes the need to learn clients' cultures. All clients' actions, like our own, are based on underlying culturally learned beliefs and ideas. Mrs. Kim did not like milk because her culture had taught her that it was distasteful. The Native American women's response to waiting or keeping someone else waiting was influenced by their value of patience. There is usually some culturally based reason that causes clients to engage in (or avoid) certain actions. Instead of making assumptions or judging clients' behavior, the nurse must first learn about the culture that guides that behavior (Calhoun, 1986). Called **cultural assessment**, it means obtaining health-related information about a designated cultural group concerning their values, beliefs, and practices. See Research in Community Health Nursing display below. One study showed that client behavior was interpreted differently by professionals of a different culture than by professionals of the clients' culture (Tripp-Reimer, 1982). Learning clients' culture first is critical to effective nursing practice. When nurses interview members of a subcultural group, as in Robertson and Cousineau's (1986) study of the homeless, it can provide valuable data for enhanced understanding in order to plan interventions.

Research in Community Health Nursing
CROSS CULTURAL PARENTING

Seideman, R., Williams, R., Burns, P., Jacobson, S., Weatherby, F., & Primeauz, M. (1994). Culture sensitivity in assessing urban Native American parenting. *Public Health Nursing*, *11*(2), 98–103.

To assess the quality of parenting in a cross-cultural group poses a challenge to community health nurses. It is impractical to develop new assessment instruments for each cultural group so several nurses conducted a study to test the use of two existing instruments that are widely used in community health nursing. They were the home observation for measurement of the environment (HOME) and nursing child assessment teaching scale (NCATS). These instruments were used with 63 Native American families. Findings from the study showed that the instruments were useful with Native American parents "when accompanied by discussion of findings with them, and nurse awareness of common family structures and traditional values" (Ibid. p.98).

To fully understand a group's culture one should study it in depth, as Bernal maintains:

"Although a general knowledge base and skills are applicable transculturally, immersion in a given culture is necessary to understand fully the patterns that shape the behavior of individuals within that group. Experience with one group can be helpful in understanding the concept of diversity, but each group must be understood within its own ecologic niche and for its own historical and cultural reality" (1993, p.231).

Cultural Assessment

Practically speaking, however, it is not possible to study all the cultural groups the nurse encounters in depth. Instead, the nurse can conduct a cultural assessment of clients' cultures through questioning key informants, observation of the cultural group, and reading additional information in the literature. This data can be grouped into six categories:

1. Ethnic or racial background. Where did the client group originate and how does that influence their status and identity?
2. Language and communication patterns. What is the preferred language spoken and what are their culturally-based communication patterns?
3. Cultural values and norms. What are their values, beliefs, and standards regarding such things as roles, education, family functions, child-rearing, work and leisure, aging, death and dying, and rites of passage?
4. Biocultural factors. Are there physical or genetic traits unique to this cultural group that predispose them to certain conditions or illnesses?
5. Religious beliefs and practices. What are the group's religious beliefs and how do they influence life events, roles, health, and illness?
6. Health beliefs and practices. What are the group's beliefs and practices regarding prevention, causes, and treatment of illnesses?

The cultural assessment guide, presented in Table 7.3, gives suggestions for more detailed data collection.

Other cultural assessment guides are also available (Bloch, 1983; Brownlee, 1978; Gagnon, 1983; Leininger, 1994a; Orque, 1983; Tripp-Reimer, 1985). Tripp-Reimer et al. (1984) suggest that a thorough cultural assessment may be too time-consuming and costly. Instead, they propose the two-phase assessment process outlined in Table 7.4. Categories to explore in the assessment include values, beliefs, customs, and social structure components. Two methods that have proven highly effective for in-depth study of cultural groups are

TABLE 7.3. **Cultural Assessment Guide**

Category	Sample Data
Ethnic/racial background	Country(s) of origin Mostly native-born or U.S. born? Reasons for emigrating if applicable Racial/ethnic identity Experience with racism or racial discrimination?
Language and communication patterns	Language(s) of origin Language(s) spoken in the home Preferred language for communication How verbal communication patterns affected by age, sex, other? Preferences for use of interpreters Non-verbal communication patterns (eg: eye contact, touching, etc)
Cultural values and norms	Group beliefs and standards for male and female roles and functions Standards for modesty and sexuality Family/extended family structures and functions Values re work, leisure, success, time Values re education and occupation Norms for child-rearing and socialization Norms for social networks and supports Values re aging and treatment of elders Values re authority Norms for dress and appearance
Biocultural factors	Group genetic predisposition to health conditions (eg: hypertension, anemia) Socioculturally associated illnesses (eg: AIDS, alcoholism) Group attitudes toward body parts and functions Group vulnerability or resistance to health threats? Folk illnesses common to group? Group physical/genetic differences (eg: bone mass, height, weight, longevity)
Religious beliefs and practices	Religious beliefs affecting roles, childbearing and rearing, health and illness? Recognized religious healers? Religious beliefs and practices for promoting health, preventing illness, or treatment of illness Beliefs and rituals re conception and birth Beliefs and rituals re death, dying, grief
Health beliefs and practices	Beliefs re causes of illness Beliefs re treatment of illness Beliefs re use of healers (traditional and Western) Health promotion and illness prevention practices Folk medicine practices Beliefs re mental health and illness Dietary, herbal, and other folk cures Food beliefs, preparation, consumption Experience with Western medicine

ethnographic interviewing and participant observation (Spradley, 1979, 1980).

SHOW RESPECT AND PATIENCE WHILE LEARNING ABOUT OTHER CULTURES

The fourth transcultural nursing principle emphasizes key behaviors for the nurse to practice during the cultural learning process. Respect is the first behavior

and it is shown in many ways. When Sandra involved the Native American women in decisions and gave them choices, she was showing respect. When the nurse gave positive recognition to the importance of the Kims' culture, she was showing respect. Attentive listening is a way to show respect as well as a way to learn about their culture (Eliason, 1993). Within the United States, people of minority groups particularly need respect. A **minority group** is part of a population that differs from the

TABLE 7.4. Two-phased Cultural Assessment Process

Phase I—Data Collection

Stage 1	Assess values, beliefs, and customs (e.g., ethnic affiliations, religion, decision-making patterns)	
Stage 2	Collect problem-specific cultural data (e.g., cultural beliefs and practices related to diet and nutrition). Make nursing diagnosis.	
Stage 3	Determine cultural factors influencing nursing intervention (e.g., child-rearing beliefs and practices that might affect nurse teaching toilet training or child discipline).	

Phase II—Data Organization

Step 1	Compare cultural data with —standards of clients' own culture (e.g., clients' diet compared to cultural norms); —standards of the nurse's culture —standards of the health facility providing service.	
Step 2	Determine incongruities in above standards.	
Step 3	Seek to modify one or more systems (clients', nurse's, or the facility's) to achieve maximum congruity.	

majority and often receives differential and unequal treatment. Their ways are in contrast to the dominant culture. It is difficult for them to retain pride in their lifestyles, or in themselves, when the majority culture suggests they are inferior. The message may be only implied or even unintentional. Such was the case for Mrs. Juarez as described in the earlier case study. The clinic's routine and the manner of the staff were certainly not meant intentionally to show disrespect. They did, nevertheless, and Mrs. Juarez was intimidated and unable to receive the help she needed. Everyone needs respect to enhance pride, dignity, and self-esteem; it is an important contributor to good mental health. Showing respect is also an important means for breaking down barriers in cross-cultural communication. For community health nurses, culturally relevant care means practicing cultural relativism. **Cultural relativism** is recognizing and respecting alternative viewpoints and understanding values, beliefs, and pratices within their cultural context.

Besides respect, patience is essential. It takes time to build trust and effect cultural change. It can be difficult to establish the nurse-client relationship when it involves two different cultures. Trust must be won, and winning it may take weeks, months, or even years. Time must be allowed for both the nurse and clients to learn how to communicate with one another, to test each other's trustworthiness, and to learn about each other. Change in behavior (learned aspects of the culture) occurs gradually. Some aspects of both the nurse's and the client's cultures can, and probably will, change. The Kims' nurse, for example, modified some of her usual practices and adapted them to the Kims' culture and needs. They, in turn, began to assume some American practices and values. However, the process took several months. Time, respect, and patience help to break down cultural barriers.

EXAMINE CULTURALLY DERIVED HEALTH PRACTICES

The final transcultural nursing principle involves scrutiny of the client group's cultural practices as they affect the group's health status. Once the community health nurse has assessed the culture of the client group, further determinations must be made. Cultural practices affecting the health of the client group need to be examined. Are these behaviors preserving and enhancing the group's health or are they harmful to their health? Some traditional practices, such as customary diet, birth rituals, and certain folk remedies, may promote both physical and psychological health. These can be considered healthful. Other practices may be neither harmful nor particularly health promoting but serve a useful purpose in preserving the culture, security, and sense of identity of a particular ethnic group. Then some traditional practices may be directly harmful to health. An example might be the use of herbal poultices to treat an infected wound or "burning" the abdomen to compensate for heat lost with diarrhea.

It is important for the community health nurse to remember that cultural assessment and aggregate health assessment need to go hand in hand. If the group is experiencing a high incidence of low birth weight babies, pregnancy complications, skin infections, mental illness, or other evidence of health problems, these can be clues to prompt an examination of cultural health practices. Those that are clearly damaging to health can be discussed with group leaders and healers. It is here that knowing their cultural norms for authority and decision making can be helpful. Often a cultural practice can be continued or modified and combined with Western medicine so that respect for the culture is maintained while full treatment efficacy is accomplished.

Summary

Community health clients belong to a variety of cultural groups. A culture is a design for living and provides a set of norms and values that offer stability and security for members of a society and plays a major role in motivating behaviors. The increase in and great variety of cultural groups reinforce the need for community health nurses to understand and appreciate cultual diversity. Ethnocentrism is the bias that one's own culture is best and others are wrong or inferior. It can create serious barriers to effective nursing care. Understanding cultural diversity and being sensitive to the values and behaviors of cultural groups can often be the key to effective community health intervention.

Culture has five characteristics; it is learned from others; it is an integrated system of customs and traits; it is shared; it is tacit; and it is dynamic. Every culture preserves its integrity by deleting nonfunctional practices and acquiring new components that will better serve the group. Nurses must strive to introduce improved health practices that are presented in a manner consistent with clients' cultural values in order to gain acceptance.

Five transcultural nursing principles, drawn from an understanding of the concept of culture, can guide community health nursing practice:

1. Develop cultural self-awareness.
2. Cultivate cultural sensitivity.
3. Assess client group's culture.
4. Show respect and patience while learning other cultures.
5. Examine culturally-derived health practices.

Activities to Promote Critical Thinking

1. Based on your own cultural background, how would you feel and what behaviors would you exhibit if you were:
   a. A client sitting in a clinic waiting room in a foreign country whose language you didn't know?
   b. Part of a nutrition class being told to eat foods you had never heard of before?
   c. Visited in your home by a nurse who told you to discipline your child in a way that contradicted everything you had been reared to believe about parenting?

2. Describe three tacit cultural rules that govern your own behavior. How might these affect your interaction with clients from another culture?

3. What does the term ethnocentrism mean to you? Have you ever experienced someone else being ethnocentric in their attitude toward you? If so, describe that experience.

4. Imagine that you are assigned to work with a Mexican American migrant population. What are the steps you would take to gather the appropriate information to provide culturally relevant nursing service? What sources might provide that information?

5. A Hmong father, who severely beat his 12 year old son with a belt leaving cuts and bruises, is charged with child abuse. "If I can't discipline my son, how can he be a good kid?", said the father.(Bonner, 1994, p.1) What nursing responses would show respect for this cultural group's norms and values and yet be constructive in resolving the culture conflict?

REFERENCES

Bell, R. (1994). Prominence of women in Navajo healing beliefs and values. *Nursing and Health Care, 15*(5), 232–40.

Bennett, L. (1962). *Before the Mayflower: A history of the Black American, 1619–1962.* Chicago: Johnson.

Bernal, H. (1993). A model for delivering culture-relevant care in the community. *Public Health Nursing 10*(4), 228–32.

Bloch, B. (1983). Bloch's assessment guide for ethnic/culture variations. In M. Orque and B. Bloch (Eds.), *Ethnic nursing care.* St. Louis: C. V. Mosby.

Bonner, B. (1994). Hmong parents feeling pressure to spare the rod. *St. Paul Pioneer Press, 146*(54), 1A, 5A.

Brownlee, A. T. (1978). *Community, culture, and care.* St. Louis: C. V. Mosby.

Calhoun, M. S. (1986). Providing health care to Vietnamese in America: What practitioners need to know. *Home Healthcare Nurse, 4*(5), 14–22.

Carney, P. (1992). The concept of poverty. *Public Health Nursing, 9*(2), 74–80.

Conflict and Change Center, (1992). Conflict and change in the deaf and hearing cultures. *Conflict/Change Process, Spring,* 1–3, University of Minnesota, Minneapolis.

Eliason, M.J.(1993). Ethics and transcultual nursing care. *Nursing Outlook, 41*(5), 225–8.

Foster, G. M. (1962). *Traditional cultures and the impact of technological change.* New York: Harper.

Freidman, M. (1990). Transcultual family nursing: Application to Latino and black families. *Journal of Pediatric Nursing, 5*(3), 214–222.

Gagnon, A. T. (1983). Transcultural nursing: Including it in the curriculum. *Nursing and Health Care, 4*(3), 127–31.

Hall, E. T. (1959). *The silent language.* Garden City, N.Y.: Doubleday.

Holm, C. (1991). Deafness: common misunderstandings. In B. Spradley, *Readings in Community Health Nursing,* (4th ed.). Philadelphia:Lippincott pp 544–49.

Kark, S. L. (1974). *Epidemiology and community medicine.* New York: Appleton-Century-Crofts.

Landy, D. (1977). *Culture, disease, and healing: Studies in medical anthropology.* New York: Macmillan.

Leininger, M. (1991). *Culture care diversity and universality: A theory of nursing.* New York: National League for Nursing Press.

Leininger, M. (1991b). Transcultural care principles, human rights, and ethical considerations. *Journal of Transcultural Nursing, 3,* 21–23.

Leininger, M. (1994a). *Transcultural nursing: concepts, theory, research and practice,* (2nd ed). Columbus, OH: McGraw Hill and Greyden Press.

Lin-Fu, J.S. (1991). Population characteristics and health care needs of Asian Pacific Americans. In B. Spradley, *Readings in Community Health Nursing,* (4th ed.). Philadelphia: Lippincott.

Magar, V. (1990). Health care needs of Central American refugees. *Nursing Outlook, 38*(5), 239–42.

Martin, M.E. & Henry, M. (1989). Cultural relativity and poverty. *Public Health Nursing, 6*(1), 28–34.

McAuley P., et al (1992). A trichinosis outbreak among Southeast Asian refugees. *American Journal of Epidemiology, 135*(12), 1404–10.

Mead, M. (1960). Cultural contexts of nursing problems. In F. C. MacGregor (Ed.), *Social science in nursing.* New York: Wiley.

Meisenhelder, J. B. (1982). Boundaries of personal space. *Image, 14*(1), 16–19.

Muecke, M.A. (1983). Caring for Southeast Asian refugee patients in the U.S.A. *American Journal of Public Health, 73*(4), 431–38.

Murdock, G. (1972). The science of culture. In M. Freilich (Ed.), *The meaning of culture: A reader in cultural anthropology,* (pp. 252–66). Lexington, MA: Xerox College Publishing.

National Center for Health Statistics (1993). *Health, United States, 1992.* Hyattsville, MD: U.S. Public Health Service.

Orque, M. S. (1983). Orque's ethnic/cultural system: A framework for ethnic nursing care. In M. S. Orque, B. Bloch, & L. S. Montroy (Eds.), *Ethnic nursing care.* St. Louis: C. V. Mosby.

Pesznecker, B. L. (1984). The poor: A population at risk multidimensional model of poverty . . . practice implications. *Public Health Nursing, 1*(4), 237–49.

Pickett, G.E. & Hanlon, J. (1990). *Public Health Administration and Practice,* (9th ed.). St. Louis: Times Mirror/ Mosby.

Porter, C. & Villarruel, A. (1993). Nursing research with African American and Hispanic people: Guidelines for action. *Nursing Outlook, 41*(2), 59–67.

Primeaux, M., and Henderson, G. (1981). American Indian patient care. In G. Henderson & M. Primeaux (Eds.), *Transcultural health care.* Philadelphia: F. A. Davis.

Robertson, H. R. (1969). Removing barriers to health care. *Nursing Outlook, 17,* 43–46.

Robertson, M. J., & Cousineau, M.R. (1986). Health status and access to health services among the urban homeless. *American Journal of Public Health, 76*(5), 561–63.

Seideman, R., Williams, R., Burns, P., Jacobson, S., Weatherby, F., & Primeauz, M. (1994). Culture sensitivity in assessing urban Native American parenting. *Public Health Nursing, 11*(2), 98–103.

Sich, D. (1988). Childbearing in Korea. *Social Science and Medicine, 27,* 497–504.

Spradley, J. P. (1979). *The ethnographic interview.* New York: Holt.

Spradley, J. P. (1980). *Participant observation.* New York: Holt.

Spradley, J. P. (1988). *Your owe yourself a drunk: An ethnography of urban nomads.* Lanham, MD: University Press of America.

Spradley, J. P. & McCurdy, D.W. (1994). *Conformity and Conflict: Readings in cultural anthropology,* (8th ed.) New York: Harper Collins.

Stehr-Green, J. K. & Schantz, P.M. (1986). Trichinosis in Southeast Asian refugees in the United States, *American Journal of Public Health, 76*(10), 1238–39.

Strauss, A. L. (1967). Medical ghettos. *Trans-Action, 4*(62), 7–15.

Taylor, C. (1973). The nurse and cultural barriers. In D. Hymovich and M. Barnard (Eds.), *Family health care,* (pp. 119–27). New York: McGraw-Hill.

Thernstrom, S., et al. (Eds.). (1980). *Harvard encyclopedia of American ethnic groups.* Cambridge: Harvard University Press.

Tripp-Reimer, T. (1982). Barriers to health care: Variations in interpretation of Appalachian client behavior by Appalachian and non-Appalachian health professionals. *Western Journal of Nursing Research, 4*(2), 179–91.

Tripp-Reimer, T. (1985). Cultural assessment. In J. Bellack & P. Bamford (Eds.), *Nursing assessment.* North Scituate, MA: Duxbury.

Tripp-Reimer, T., Brink, P.J., & Saunders. J.M. (1984). Cultural assessment: Content and process. *Nursing Outlook, 32*(2): 78–82.

U.S. Bureau of the Census.(1990). The 1990 Census. U.S. Department of Commerce. Washington, D.C.: U.S. Government Printing Office.

U.S. Bureau of the Census.(1992). *Current Population Reports.* Washington, DC: U.S. Government Printing Office.

U.S. Bureau of the Census.(1993). *Current Population Reports.* Washington, DC: U.S. Government Printing Office.

U.S. Immigration and Naturalization Service. (1993). *Statistical Yearbook of the Immigration and Naturalization Service.* Washington, DC: U.S. Government Printing Office.

Watkins, E., Larson, K., Harlan, C., & Young, S., (1990). A model program for providing health services for migrant farmworker mothers and children. *Public Health Reports, 105*(6), 567–75.

West, E.A. (1993). The cultural bridge model. *Nursing Outlook, 41*(5), 229–34.

SELECTED READINGS

Alvarez, W. F., Doris, J., & Larson, O., III. (1988). Children of migrant farm work families are at high risk for maltreatment: New York state study. *American Journal of Public Health, 78*(8), 934–36.

Braithwaite, R. & Lythcott, W. (1989). Community empowerment as a strategy for health promotion for black and other minority populations. *Journal of the American Medical Association, 261*(2):282–3.

De Santis, L. & Thomas, J. (1992). Health education and the immigrant Haitian mother: cultural insights for community health nurses. *Public Health Nursing, 9*(2), 87–96.

Dyck, I. (1989). The immigrant client: issues in developing culturally sensitive practice. *Canadian Journal of Occupational Therapy, 56*(5), 248–54.

Eliason, M. & Macy, N. (1992). A classroom activity to introduce cultural diversity. *Nursing Education, 17*, 32–6.

Feraca, S.E. (1990). Inside the Bureau of Indian Affairs. *Society, 27*, 29.

Fingerhut, L. & Makuc, D. (1992). Mortality among minority populations in the United States. *American Journal of Public Health, 82*(8), 1168–70.

Fox, P.G., Cowell, J.M., & Montgomery, A.C. (1994). The effects of violence on health and adjustment of Southeast Asian refugee children: an integrative review. *Public Health Nursing, 11*(3), 195–201.

Gordon, A.J. (1991). Alcoholism treatment services to Hispanics: an ethnographic exam of a community's services. *Family & Community Health, 13*(4), 12–24.

Haraldson, S. (1988). Health and health services among the Navajo Indians. *Journal of Community Health, 13*(3), 129–42.

Henkle, J.O. & Kennerly, S. (1990). Cultural diversity: a resource in planning and implementing nursing care. *Public Health Nursing, 7*(3), 145–49.

Iskander, R. (1987). Developing a black consciousness health needs of black communities. *Nursing Times, 83*(42), 66, 69.

Jonas, S. (1986). On homelessness and the American Way. *American Journal of Public Health, 76*(9), 1084–86.

Kemp, C. (1985). Cambodian refugee health care beliefs and practices. *Public Health Nursing, 2*(1), 41–52.

Koch, D. (1988). Migrant day care and the health status of migrant preschoolers: a review of the literature. *Journal of Community Health Nursing, 5*(4), 221–33.

Leininger, M. (1992). Self-care ideology and cultural incongruities: some critical issues *Journal of Transcultual Nursing, 4*(11), 2–5.

Leininger, M. (1992). Strange myths and inaccurate facts in transcultural nursing. *Journal of Transcultural Nursing, 4*(2), 39–40.

Leininger, M. (1992). Transcultural nursing education: a world wide imperative. *Nursing and Health Care, 15*(5), 254–7.

Lyon, J.L., et al. (1988). Mormon health. *Health Values, 12*(3), 37–44.

Mahon, J., McFarlane, J., & Golden, K. (1991). De Madres a Madres: A community partnership for health. *Public Health Nursing, 8*(1), 15–19.

Malone, R.E. (1990). The challenge of third world nursing. *American Journal of Nursing, 90*(7), 32–7.

Nugent, K., Linares, A., Brykczynski, K., Crawford, F.,Fuller, S., & Riggs, H. (1988). A model for providing health maintenance and promotion to children from low-income, ethnically diverse backgrounds. *Journal of Pediatric Health Care, 2*(4), 175–80.

Nutting, P.A., Helgerson, S., Welty, T., Kileen, M., & Jackson, M.Y. (1990). A research agenda for Indian health. Part 5: Researchable questions in chronic disease. *The Indian Health Service Primary Care Provider,* March, 29–38.

Office of Minority Health (1994). Pocket Guide to Minority Health Resources. Washington, DC: U.S. Department of Health and Human Services, Public Health Service, Publication No. 94-019.

Pletsch, P.K. (1990). Hispanics: at risk for adolescent pregnancy? *Public Health Nursing, 7*(2), 105–10.

Reinert, B.R. (1986). The health care beliefs and values of Mexican-Americans. *Home Healthcare Nurse, 4*(5), 23–31.

Russell, K., et al. (1992). Cultural impact of health care access: challenges for improving the health of African Americans. *Journal of Community Health Nursing, 9*(3), 161–9.

Smith, K. G. (1986). The hazards of migrant farm work: An overview for rural public health nurses. *Public Health Nursing 3*(1), 48–56.

Spector, R. (1991). *Cultural diversity in health and illness.* Norwalk, CT: Appleton-Century-Crofts.

Spector, R. (1993–94). Diversifying your approach. *Minority Nurse,* Winter-Spring, 28–31, 49, 51.

Thomas, S. (1990). Community health advocacy for racial and ethnic minorities in the United States: issues and challenges for health education. *Health Education Quarterly, 17*(1), 13–19.

Thompson, J.L. (1991). Exploring gender and culture with Khmer refugee women: Reflections on participatory feminist research. *Annals of Nursing Science, 13*(3), 30–48.

Wing, D.M. (1989). Community participant-observation: issues in assessing diverse cultures. *Journal of Community Health Nursing, 6*(3), 125–133.

CHAPTER

8 Values and Ethical Decision Making in Community Health

LEARNING OBJECTIVES

Upon completion of this chapter, readers should be able to:

- Describe the nature of values and value systems and their influence on community health.
- Identify personal and professional values that they bring to decision making with and for community clients.
- Articulate the impact of key values on professional decision making.
- Discuss the application of ethical principles to community health nursing decision making.
- Use a decision-making process with and for community clients that incorporates values and ethical principles.
- Participate in discussions about ethical aspects of community health nursing practice as a member of an agency ethics committee.

KEY TERMS

- Autonomy
- Beneficence
- Distributive justice
- Egalitarian justice
- Equity
- Ethics
- Ethical decision making
- Ethical dilemma
- Fidelity
- Instrumental values
- Justice
- Moral

- Moral evaluations
- Nonmaleficence
- Respect
- Restorative justice
- Self-determination
- Terminal values
- Values
- Values clarification
- Value systems
- Veracity
- Well-being

Barbara Walton Spradley and Judith Ann Allender
COMMUNITY HEALTH NURSING: CONCEPTS AND PRACTICE, 4th ed.
© 1996 Barbara Walton Spradley and Judith Ann Allender

Today's community health nurses, together with other health care professionals, face an expanding number of ethical, or moral, dilemmas. Scientific and technological advances have created many of these dilemmas. Computerized record-keeping systems, for instance, make client information readily accessible and raise issues of confidentiality and clients' rights. Organ transplants and who should receive them raise additional ethical questions. Numerous other issues, such as informed consent, inadequate care of elderly at home, lack of access to health care, euthanasia (facilitating a painless or easy death for untreatable patients), or individual rights versus the common good, force nurses to deal with an endless barrage of ethical conundrums. Underlying every issue and influencing every ethical (and professional) decision are values. In fact, ethics and values are inextricably intertwined in professional decision making.

Values serve as the criteria or standards by which judgements and decisions are made. In order to understand the relationship between values and health and the influence of values on ethical decision making, it is necessary to describe the nature or function of values and value systems in human behavior. Once it is clear how values and value systems affect behavior, then one can understand the role of values in choices related to health. This chapter explores (1) the nature and function of values and value systems, (2) the role of values and value systems in ethical decision making, (3) the central values related to health care choices and their potential conflicts, and (4) the implications of values and ethics for community health nursing decision making and practice.

Values

What are values? A **value** is something one perceives as desireable or ought to be (Carey, 1989: Preister, 1992) and motivates people to act or behave in certain ways that are personally or socially preferable. As we saw in Chapter 7, a group's culture is often defined by its members' common or shared values.

STANDARDS FOR BEHAVIOR

In general, values function as standards that guide actions and behavior in daily situations. Once internalized by an individual, a value such as honesty becomes a criterion for that individual's personal conduct. Values may function as criteria for developing and maintaining attitudes toward objects and situations or for justifying one's own actions and attitudes. Values also may serve as the standard by which we pass moral judgment on ourselves and others (Rokeach, 1968).

Values have a long-term function in giving expression to human needs. The strong motivational component of values help people adjust to society, defend egos against threat, and test reality (Priester, 1992). In addition, values are employed as standards to guide presentation of the self to others, to ascertain whether one is as moral and as competent as others, and to persuade and influence others by indicating which beliefs, attitudes, and actions of others are worth trying to reinforce or change.

QUALITIES OF VALUES

The nature of values can be described according to five qualities: endurance, hierarchical arrangement, prescriptive-proscriptive belief, reference, and preference.

Endurance

Values remain relatively stable over time and persist to provide continuity to personal and social existence. Enduring religious beliefs, for example, offer stability to many people. This is not to say that values are completely stable over time; one's values do tend to change throughout one's life. Yet social existence in community requires standards within the individual as well as an agreement on standards among groups of individuals. As Kluckhohn (1951, p. 400) points out, without values, "the functioning of the social system could not continue to achieve group goals; individuals . . . could not feel within themselves a requisite measure of order and unified purpose." A group's culture, as discussed in the previous chapter, provides such a set of enduring values. Thus, by adding an element of collective purpose in social life, values guarantee endurance and stability in social existence.

Hierarchical System

Isolated values are usually organized into a hierarchical system in which certain values have more weight or importance than others. For instance, in a team sport such as baseball, values regarding individual performance, batting and running records, speed, throwing and catching, all fall into a hierarchy with the values of team and winning being at the top. As an individual confronts social situations throughout life, isolated values learned in early childhood come into competition with other values, requiring a weighing of one value against another (see Fig. 8.1). Concern for others' welfare, for instance, competes with self-interest. Through experience and maturation, the individual integrates values learned in different contexts into systems in which each value is ordered relative to other values.

Prescriptive-Proscriptive Beliefs

Rokeach (1973) describes values as a subcategory of beliefs. He argues that some beliefs are descriptive or capable of being true or false (eg: the chair I am sitting on will hold me up). Other beliefs are evaluative involving judgments of good and bad (eg: that was an excellent lecture). Still other beliefs are prescriptive-proscriptive determining whether an action is desirable or undesirable (eg: that music is too loud; or those baseball fans shouldn't yell when the pitcher is winding up). Values, he says, are prescriptive-proscriptive beliefs. They are concerned with desireable behavior or what ought to

be. Parents' values about child behavior, for example, determine how they choose to discipline their children. Values have cognitive, affective, and behavioral components. According to Rokeach to have a value one must (1) know the correct way to behave or the correct end-state to strive for (cognitive component), (2) feel emotional about it, be affectively for or against it (affective component), and (3) take action based on it (behavioral component).

Reference

Values also have a reference quality. That is, they may refer to end-states of existence called **terminal values**, such as spiritual salvation, peace of mind, or world peace. Or they may refer to modes of conduct called **instrumental values**, such as confidentiality, keeping promises, and honesty. The latter can have a moral focus or a nonmoral focus, and these values may conflict. For example, a nurse may experience a conflict between two moral values such as whether to act honestly (tell a client he or she has a fatal diagnosis) or to act respectfully (honor the family's request not to tell the client). Similarly, the nurse can experience conflict between two competence or nonmoral values such as whether to plan logically (design a traditional group intervention for mental health clients) or to plan cre-

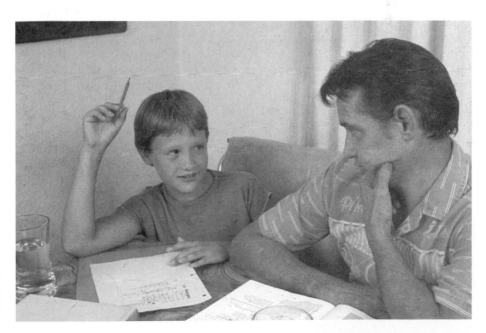

FIGURE 8.1. The value of mastering academics may compete with peer social values later in this youngster's life.

atively (design an innovative field experience). The nurse can also experience conflict between a competence value and a moral value such as whether to act efficiently or to act fairly when establishing priorities for funding among community health programs.

Preference

A value shows preference for one mode of behavior over another, such as exercise over inactivity. Or it may be a preference for one end-state over another, such as trimness over obesity. The preferred end-state or mode of behavior is located higher in one's personal value hierarchy.

Value Systems

Value systems are generally considered organizations of beliefs that are of relative importance in guiding individual behavior (Priester, 1992; Rokeach, 1973). Instead of being guided by single or isolated values, however, behavior at any point in time (or over a period of time) is influenced by multiple or changing clusters of values. Thus, it is important to understand how values are integrated into a person's total belief system, how values assume a place in a hierarchy of values, and how this hierarchical system changes over time.

HIERARCHICAL SYSTEM OF VALUES

Learned values are integrated into an organized system of values and each value has an ordered priority with respect to other values (Rokeach, 1973). For example a person may place a higher value on physical comfort than on exercising. This system of ordered priority is stable enough to reflect the continuity of one's personality and behavior within culture and society, yet it is sufficiently flexible to allow a reordering of value priorities in response to changes in the environment, or social setting, or based on one's personal experiences. Behavioral change would, of course, be regarded as the visible response to a reordering of values within an individual's hierarchical value system.

Adults generally possess only a few, perhaps a dozen and a half, terminal values, such as peace of mind or achievement. These are influenced by complex physiological and social factors. The physiological needs of security, love, self-esteem, and self-actualization, proposed by Maslow (1969), are believed to be the greatest influences on terminal values. While a person may have only a few terminal values, the same person may possess as many as 50 to 75 instrumental values. Any single instrumental value or several combined may also help determine terminal values. For example, instrumental values of acceptance, taking it easy, living one day at a time, or not being concerned about the future, can help to shape the terminal value of peace of mind. Or instrumental values of hard work, driving oneself to compete, or not letting anyone get in one's way, can influence one's terminal value of achievement. Figure 8.2 illustrates the influence of instrumental values as well as human needs on the development of terminal values.

CONFLICT RESOLUTION AND DECISION MAKING

When an individual encounters a social situation, several values within his or her value system are activated rather than just a single value. All the activated

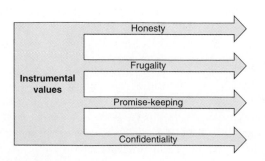

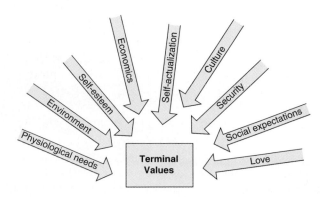

FIGURE 8.2. Factors influencing personal values.

values will not be compatible with one another. Thus, conflict between values occurs. This conflict between values is a part of the decision-making process and resolving these value conflicts is crucial in order to make good decisions. Community health nurses face conflicting values when they seek to promote the well-being of certain individuals, a result that may come at the expense of the public good (Aroskar, 1990). Even within a single community agency nurses may find that they prioritize client service or programming values differently.

Some values seem to consistently triumph over others and seem to be stronger directives for individual behavior, such as the value placed on high achievement in the United States. It is this persistence on the part of some values, like individualism versus community, that make universal coverage and other issues so controversial in health care reform (Priester, 1992). Other values do, of course, lose their positions of importance in a value hierarchy. It is this changing arrangement of values in a hierarchical system that determines, in part, how conflicts will be resolved and decisions will be made. Thus, people's value systems function as a learned organization of principles and rules that help them choose between alternative courses of action to reach decisions (see Figure 8.3).

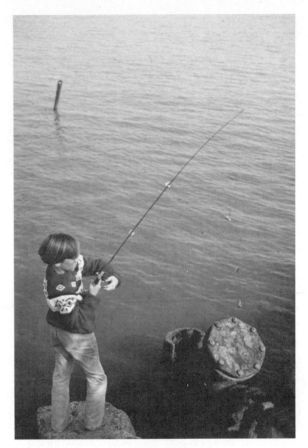

FIGURE 8.3. Pursuing a recreational activity overpowers this young man's values about authority.

Values Clarification

One way to understand the influence and priority of values in one's own, as well as community clients', behavior is to employ various values clarification techniques in decision making. **Values clarification** is a process that helps one identify the significant values that guide one's actions by examining what one believes about the worth, truth, or beauty of any object, thought, or behavior (Davis and Aroskar; 1991). Since individuals are largely unaware of the motives underlying their behavior and choices, values clarification is important for understanding and shaping the kind of decisions people make. Only by understanding one's own values and their priority or importance can one be certain that one's choices are more the result of rationality and less the result of other influences, such as cultural, social, or other kinds of previous conditioning. Values clarification by itself does not yield a set of rules for future decision making and does not indicate the rightness or wrongness of alternative actions. Values clarification

does, however, help guarantee that any course of action chosen by people is consistent and in accordance with their beliefs and values.

PROCESS OF VALUING

Before values clarification can take place, one must understand how the process of valuing occurs in individuals. Uustal (1977) lists the following seven steps.

1. One chooses the value freely and individually.
2. One chooses the value from among alternatives.
3. One carefully considers the consequences of the choice.
4. One cherishes or prizes the value.
5. One publicly affirms the value.
6. One incorporates the value into behavior so that it becomes a standard.

Name Tag

Take a piece of paper and write your name in the middle of it. In each of the four corners, write your responses to these four questions:

1. What two things would you like your colleagues to say about you?
2. What single most important thing do you do (or would you like to do) to make your nurse-client relationships positive ones?
3. What do you do on a daily basis that indicates you value your health?
4. What are the three values you believe in most strongly?

In the space around your name, write at least six adjectives that you feel best describe who you are.

Take a closer look at your responses to the questions and to the ways in which you described yourself. What values are reflected in your answers?

FIGURE 8.4. Values clarification strategy 1.

Patterns

Which of the following words describe you? Draw a circle around the seven words that best describe you as an individual. Underline the seven words that most accurately describe you as a professional person. (You may circle and underline the same word.)

ambitious reserved assertive opinionated
concerned generous independent
easily hurt outgoing reliable indifferent
capable self-controlled fun-loving
suspicious solitary likable dependent
intellectual argumentative dynamic unpredictable
compromising thoughtful affectionate obedient
logical imaginative self-disciplined
moody easily led helpful slow to relate

Reflect on the following questions:

1. What values are reflected in the patterns you have chosen?
2. What is the relationship between these patterns and your personal values?
3. What patterns indicate inconsistencies in attitudes or behavior?
4. What patterns do you think a nurse should cultivate?

FIGURE 8.5. Values clarification strategy 2.

---

7. One consciously employs the value in decision making.

These steps provide specific actions for the discovery and identification of people's values. They also assist the decision-making process by explicating the process of valuing itself. For example, some people may choose to value honesty in a presidential candidate. They choose this over other values, like knowledge of foreign affairs or public speaking ability, because, considering the consequences, they want a leader who will deliver on promises made and be the person she represents herself to be. They prize this value of honesty, affirm it publicly, and consciously employ it as a standard in deciding whom to vote for and whom to reject based on the candidate's record of honesty.

VALUES CLARIFICATION STRATEGIES

Uustal (1978) offers several strategies of values clarification that are ultimately useful to the decision-making process in community health nursing practice. Strategy 1 is a means by which nurses can come to know themselves and their values better (see Figure 8.4). Strategy 2 assists in discovering value clusters and the priority of values within personal value systems (see Figure 8.5). Strategy 3 can be used to examine one's responses to selected issues in nursing practice. Each response helps establish priorities of values by asking the nurse to choose among the alternatives presented or to indicate degree of agreement or disagreement (see Figure 8.6).

Other values clarification strategies are included in the critical thinking activities at the end of this chapter to assist nurses in understanding their ordering of values and to help them consider directions for change. These strategies may also help nurses assist community clients to become clearer about their own values.

All of these strategies can be used to analyze and understand how values are meaningful to people and ultimately influence their choices and behavior. Clarification of one's values is the first step in the decision-making process and affects the ability of people to make ethical decisions. Values clarification also promotes understanding and respect for values held by others, such as community clients and other health care providers. As pointed out by Uustal (1977, p.10), "Nurses cannot hope to give optimal, sensitive care to any patient without first under-

---

Forced Choice Ranking

How do you order the following alternatives by priority? (There is no correct set of priorities.) What values emerge in response to each question?

1. With whom on a nursing team would you become most angry? The nurse who
   _____ never completes assignments.
   _____ rarely helps other team members.
   _____ projects his or her feelings on clients.

2. If you had a serious health problem, you would rather
   _____ not be told.
   _____ be told directly.
   _____ find out by accident.

3. You are made happiest in your work when you use
   _____ your technical skills in caring for adults with complex needs.
   _____ your ability to compile data and arrive at a nuring diagnosis.
   _____ your ability to communicate easily and skillfully with clients.

4. It would be most difficult for you to
   _____ listen to and counsel a dying person.
   _____ advise a pregnant adolescent.
   _____ handle a situation of obvious child abuse.

FIGURE 8.6. Values clarification strategy 3.

standing their own opinions, attitudes, and values." This values clarification process provides a backdrop for next exploring the role of values in ethical decision making.

Ethical Decision Making

Values are central to any consideration of ethics or ethical decision making. Yet it is not at first obvious what counts as an ethical problem in health care or in the practice of community health nursing. Most nurses easily recognize the moral crisis in some kinds of decisions, for example, whether to let seriously deformed newborn infants die, whether to terminate pregnancies resulting from rape, or whether to provide universal health care coverage. Yet there are other less obvious moral dilemmas that are faced in the routine practice of community health nursing that are not often considered ethical in nature. What is "ethics" and what is "ethical"? *Merriam-Webster* defines **ethics** as "the discipline deal-

ing with what is good and bad and with moral duty and obligation" (1993, p. 398). Ethics, Bandman and Bandman explain, "is concerned with doing good and avoiding harm" (1985, p.4). **Ethical decision making**, then, means making a choice that is consistent with a moral code or that can be justified from an ethical perspective. Of necessity the decision maker must exercise moral judgment. It is important to remember that the term **moral** refers to conforming to a standard that is right and good. Aroskar points out that all nurses, "as moral agents, make decisions that have direct and indirect consequences for the welfare of themselves and others" (1995, p. 135). The next section examines how a nurse makes these moral decisions or judgments.

IDENTIFYING ETHICAL SITUATIONS

Ethics involves making evaluative judgments. In order to be ethically responsible in the practice of nursing, it is important to develop the ability to recognize evaluative judgments as they are made and implemented in nursing practice. One must be able to distinguish between evaluative and nonevaluative judgements. Evaluative statements involve judgments of value, rights, duties, and responsibilities. Examples are, "parents should never strike their children" or "it is the duty of every citizen to vote". Among the words to watch for are verbs such as want, desire, refer, should, or ought and nouns such as benefit, harm, duty, responsibility, right, or obligation.

Sometimes the evaluations are expressed in terms that are not direct expressions of evaluations but are clearly functioning as value judgments. For example, the American Nurses Association (ANA) Code for Nurses (1985, p.5) states that "the nurse provides services . . . unrestricted by considerations of social or economic status, personal attributes, or the nature of health problems." In this statement the ANA could be describing the facts about the way all nurses behave. It is not the case, however, that all nurses behave in this manner. Rather, this statement prescribes that nurses ought to provide services without discrimination as an ethical ideal or goal.

Another important step is to distinguish between moral and nonmoral evaluations (Thompson & Thompson, 1992; Veatch, 1977). **Moral evaluations** refer to judgements that conform to standards of what is right and good. Moral evaluations assess human actions, institutions, or character traits rather than inanimate objects such as paintings or architectural structures. They are prescriptive-proscriptive beliefs having certain characteristics that separate them from other evaluations such as aesthetic judgments, personal preferences, or matters of taste.

Moral evaluations also have distinctive characteristics.

1. The evaluations are ultimate. They have a preemptive quality, meaning that other values or human ends cannot, as a rule, override them (Beauchamp and Childress, 1989; Fried, 1978).
2. They possess universality or reflect a standpoint that applies to everyone. They are evaluations that everyone in principle ought to be able to make and understand, even if some individuals, in fact, do not (Baier, 1958; Rawls, 1971).
3. Moral evaluations avoid giving a special place to one's own welfare. They have a focus that keeps others in view, or at least considers one's own welfare on a par with that of others (Beauchamp and Childress, 1989; Rawls, 1971).

RESOLVING MORAL CONFLICTS AND ETHICAL DILEMMAS

When judgments involve moral values, conflicts are inevitable. In clinical practice the nurse may be faced with moral conflicts such as the choice between preserving one set of clients' welfare over that of others' welfare. For example, the nurse may have to choose whether to keep a promise of confidentiality to persons who are HIV positive when these individuals continue to have unprotected sex with unknowing partners. Nurses may have to choose between protecting the interests of colleagues or the interests of the employing institution. They may have to decide whether to serve future clients by striking for better conditions or to serve present clients by refusing to strike. Each decision involves a potential conflict between moral values and is called an **ethical dilemma**. An ethical dilemma occurs when "moral claims conflict with one another" (Davis & Aroskar, 1991, p.7), causing the nurse to face a choice with equally unsatisfying alternatives. It can create a decision-making problem even in quite ordinary nursing situations. See the Research in Community Health Nursing display on ethical dilemmas below.

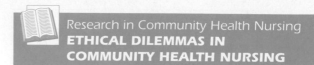

Research in Community Health Nursing
ETHICAL DILEMMAS IN COMMUNITY HEALTH NURSING

(Source: Aroskar, M.A. (1989). Community health nurses: their most significant ethical decision-making problems. *Nursing Clinics of North America, 24*(4), 967–75).

A survey of community health nurses was conducted to identify the ethical problems they confronted and to determine how they handled these problems. Their most significant problems fell into three categories of conflict between ethical principles. First was conflict between autonomy and beneficence. These problems arose when clients' choices conflicted with what the nurse thought was best for them, for example, situations where the nurse thought certain actions would promote client health that were against clients' wishes. Second was conflict between veracity and nonmaleficence. Here, nurses were forced to choose between telling the truth or choosing an action that might jeopardize clients' welfare. An example was exposing questionable professional practice or allowing it to continue at clients' expense. The third area involved issues of distributive justice. Here nurses confronted dilemmas such as lack of community resources to meet poor families' needs, and inadequate funds and staff to provide quality services.

The nurses handled these dilemmas by consulting with nursing colleagues and other community resource people. The nurses personal values and professional standards of conduct also helped to guide their decision making.

DECISION-MAKING FRAMEWORKS

In attempts to resolve ethical dilemmas, or the conflict between moral values in community health nursing practice, and to provide morally accountable nursing service, several frameworks for ethical decision making have been proposed. Among these frameworks three key steps are considered fundamental to choosing alternative courses of action that reflect moral reasoning: (1) separate questions of fact from questions of value, (2) identify both clients' and nurse's value systems, and (3) consider ethical principles and concepts. See the case study below.

The identification of clients' values and those of other persons involved in conflict situations is an important part of ethical decision making. For example, what are Mr. Bell's values, what are the values of neighbors who are concerned but feel they can no longer care for him, what are the nurse's values, and values of the nurse's employing agency? An ethical decision-making framework that includes the identification and clarification of values impinging on the making of ethical decisions is outlined below:

CASE STUDY

MR. BELL

Community health nurses encounter value differences every day, and value differences, in turn, create ethical problems. Consider, for example, the dilemma one nurse in Seattle faced on her first home visit to an elderly man whom we shall call Mr. Bell. Referred by concerned neighbors, this 78-year-old gentleman was homebound and living alone with severe arthritis under steadily deteriorating conditions. Overgrown shrubs and vines covered the yard and house, making access impossible except through the back door. A wood-burning stove in the kitchen was the sole source of heat and that room plus a corner of the dining room were Mr. Bell's living quarters. The remainder of the once lovely three-bedroom home, including the bathroom, was layered with dust, unused. His bed was a cot in the dining room, his toilet a two-pound coffee can placed under the cot. Unbathed, unshaven, and existing on food and firewood brought in by neighbors, Mr. Bell seemed to be living in deplorable and unsafe conditions. Yet he prized his independence so highly that he adamantly refused to leave.

The conflict in values between Mr. Bell's choice to live independently and the nurse's value of having him in a safer living situation raises several ethical questions. When do health practitioners or family members have the right or duty to override an individual's preferences? When do neighbors' rights (Mr. Bell's home was an eyesore and his care was a source of anxiety for his neighbors) supersede one homeowner's rights? Should the nurse be responsible when family members can help but won't take action? Mr. Bell had one son living in a neighboring state.

In this case, the nurse entering Mr. Bell's home applied her values of respect for the individual and his right to autonomy even at the risk of his physical safety. Not until he fell and broke a hip did he reluctantly agree to be moved into a nursing home.

1. Review the situation.
   a. What health problems exist?
   b. What decisions need to be made?
   c. Separate ethical components of the decisions from those decisions that can be made solely on a scientific knowledge base.
   d. Identify all individuals/groups affected by the decision.
2. Decide what further information is needed before a decision can be made.
3. Identify ethical issues. Discuss historical, philosophical, and religious bases for these issues.
4. Identify your own values and beliefs. Identify professional responsibilities dictated by the ANA Code for Nurses.
5. Identify values and beliefs of other people involved in the situation.
6. Identify value conflicts, if any.
7. Decide who should make the decision. Determine nurse's role in making the decision.
8. Identify range of decisions or actions that are possible. Determine implications for all people involved. Identify how suggested actions conform to the Code for Nurses.
9. Decide on a course of action and follow through.
10. Evaluate the results of the actions or decisions and what has been learned for use in reviewing and resolving similar future situations. (Thompson and Thompson, 1992)

Another framework displayed in Figure 8.7 summarizes a number of views in the field on ethical decision making. This framework advocates keeping multiple values in tension before resolution of conflict and action on the part of the nurse. It suggests that value conflict is not capable of resolution until all possible alternative actions have been explored. Final resolution of the ethical conflict occurs through conscious choice of action even though some, or even many, values would be overridden by other stronger, presumably moral values. The triumphant values would be those values located higher in the decision maker's hierarchy of values.

BASIC VALUES THAT GUIDE DECISION MAKING

When applying a decision-making framework, certain values influence community health nursing deci-

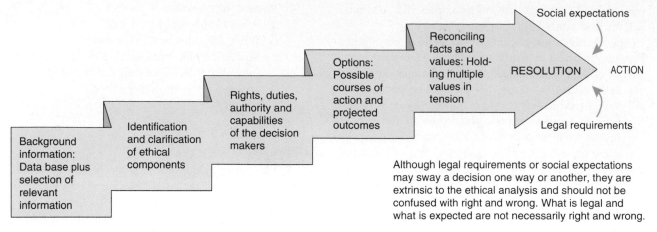

FIGURE 8.7. An ethical decision-making framework.

sions. Three basic human values are considered key to guiding decision making in the provider-client relationship and can be used with the Thompson and Thompson (1992) framework. They are self-determination, well-being, and equity (Davis and Aroskar, 1991; President's Commission, 1983).

Self Determination

The value of **self-determination** or individual autonomy is a person's exercise of the capacity to shape and pursue personal plans for life. Self-determination is instrumentally valued because self-judgment about one's goals and choices is conducive to an individual's sense of well-being. Thus, respecting self-determination is based on the belief that better outcomes will result when self-determination is respected. Those outcomes that could be maximized by respecting self-determination include enhanced self-concept, enhanced health-promoting behaviors, and enhanced quality of care. Self-determination is a major value in the United States but does not receive the same emphasis in all societies or ethnic groups.

In health care contexts the desire for self-determination has been of such high ethical importance in United States' society that it actually overrides practitioner determinations in many situations. An early survey undertaken by the President's Commission (1982) showed that 72% of those surveyed said they would prefer to make decisions jointly with their physicians after treatment alternatives had been explained. Physician re-

sponses in the same survey, however, indicated that the majority of physicians (88%) believed that patients wanted doctors to make decisions for them. The wide difference between patient expectations regarding self-determination and physician beliefs indicated that self-determination on the part of patients was at high risk in most health care contexts. Although the situation has improved in recent years, many physicians and other health providers still fail to recognize the high value attributed to self-determination by many consumers.

Priester (1992) sees this conflict between provider self-determination or autonomy versus consumer autonomy as posing a major road block to health care reform in the United States. An emphasis on individualism and provider autonomy, he says, is a hindrance to promoting the dignity and well-being of all persons and the welfare of society as a whole (community-oriented values) seen in social welfare systems in western European countries.

Self-determination and taking personal responsibility for health care decisions should be nourished in the provision of health care. This includes informing clients of options and of the reasoning behind all recommendations (Davis and Aroskar, 1991; President's Commission, 1982). Yet there are times when self-determination and personal autonomy is impermissible or even impossible. For example, society must impose restrictions on acceptable client choices, such as child abuse or situations when clients are not competent to exercise self-determination, as is true for certain levels of mental illness or dementia. There are two situations in which self-determination should be restricted: (1) when some objectives of individuals are contrary to the public interest or the interests of others in society, and (2) when a person's decision making is so defective or mistaken that the decision fails to promote the person's own values or goals. In these situations, self-determination is justifiably overridden on the basis of the promotion of one's own well-being or the well-being of others, another important value in health care decision making.

Well-Being

Well-being is a state of positive health or people's perceptions concerning positive health. Although all therapeutic interventions by health care professionals are intended to improve clients' health and promote well-being, sometimes well-intended interventions may fall short if they are in conflict with clients' preferences and needs. Determining what constitutes health for people and how their well-being can be promoted often requires a knowledge of clients' subjective preferences. It is generally recognized that clients may be inclined to pursue different directions in treatment procedures based on individual goals, values, and interests. Community health nurses, who are not only committed to helping clients but to respecting their wishes and avoiding harming them, must understand each client group's needs and develop reasonable alternatives for service from which clients may choose. See the case study below. In addition, when individuals are not capable of making a choice, the nurse or other surrogate decision maker is obliged to make health care decisions that promote the value of well-being. This may mean that the alternatives the nurse presents for choice are only the alternatives that will, in fact, promote well-being. With shared decision making, the nurse not only seeks to understand clients' needs and develop reasonable alternatives to meet those needs but also to present the alternatives in a way that enables clients to choose those they prefer. Well-being and self-determination are therefore two values that are intricately related in the provision of community health nursing service.

Equity

The third value important to decision making in health care contexts is the value of **equity** which means being treated equally or fairly. The principle of equity implies that it is unjust (or inequitable) to treat people the same if they are in significant respects unalike. In other words, different people have different needs in health care but all must be served equally and adequately. Equity generally means that all individuals should have the same access to health care according to benefit or needs.

The major problem with this definition of equity, of course, is that it assumes that an adequate level of health care can be economically available to all citizens. In times of limited technical, human, and financial resources, however, it may be impossible to fully respect the value of equity. Choices must be made and resources allotted while the value obligations of professional prac-

CASE STUDY

WELFARE FAMILY

Contrasting value systems may be seen in many community health practice settings. Andrea, a community health nurse, experienced such a contrast on her first home visit to a welfare family. Referred by a school nurse for recurring problems with head lice and staphylococcal infections, the family was living in the worst conditions the nurse had ever seen. Papers, moldy food, soiled clothing, and empty beer cans covered the floor. The nurse recoiled in dismay. The children, home from school, were clustered around the television. Their mother, a divorced, single parent, unkempt and obese, sat smoking a cigarette with a can of beer in her hand. Although she worked as a waitress part-time, she had been unable to earn enough money to support herself and the children, so the family was now on welfare. Her main pleasure in life was television soap operas. The nurse interpreted the situation through the framework of her own value system in which health and cleanliness were priorities. Yet the mother, who might have shared those values in the past, appeared to prize freedom and pleasureable diversion, perhaps as a way to cope with her situation. In this instance it is possible that environmental influences reordered the family's value system priorities. Rather than imposing her own values, the nurse chose to determine what the families' priorities were, assessed their needs, and began where they were.

tice create conflicts of values that seem impossible to resolve. Many of these conflicts are reflected in current health care reform efforts that focus on access of services, quality of services, and the way to control rising costs.

To promote the achievement of equity, self-determination, and clients' well-being, certain conclusions drawn from the literature can enhance community health nursing's practice (Preister, 1992; President's Commission, 1983).

1. Society has an ethical obligation to ensure equitable access to healthcare for all. This obligation rests on the special importance of health care and is derived from its role in relieving suffering, preventing premature death, restoring functioning, increasing opportunity, providing information about an individual's condition, and giving evidence of mutual empathy and compassion.

2. The societal obligation is balanced by individual obligations. Individuals ought to pay a fair share of the cost of their own health care and take reasonable steps to provide for such care when they can do so without excessive burdens.

3. Equitable access to health care requires that all citizens be able to secure an adequate level of care without excessive burdens. Equitable access also means that the burdens borne by individuals in obtaining adequate care ought not to be excessive or to fall disproportionately on particular individuals.

4. When equity occurs through the operation of private forces, there is no need for government involvement. But the ultimate responsibility for ensuring that society's obligation is met, through a combination of public and private sector arrangements, rests with the Federal government.

5. The cost of achieving equitable access to health care ought to be shared fairly. The cost of securing health care for those unable to pay ought to be spread equitably at the national level and not allowed to fall more heavily on the shoulders of particular practitioners, institutions, or residents of different localities.

6. Efforts to contain rising health care costs are important but should not focus on limiting the attainment of equitable access for the least well-served portion of the public. Measures designed to contain health care costs that exacerbate existing inequities or impede the achievement of equity are unacceptable from a moral stand point.

Ethical Decision Making in Community Health Nursing

The key values described in this chapter of self-determination, well-being, and equity influence nursing practice in many ways. The value of self-determination has implications for how community health nurses (1) respect the choices of clients, (2) protect privacy, (3) provide for informed consent, and (4) protect diminished capacity for self-determination. The value of well-being has implications for how community health nurses (1) reduce or prevent harm and provide benefits to client populations, (2) measure the effectiveness of nursing services, and (3) balance costs of services against real client benefits. The value of equity has implications for community health nursing in terms of its priorities for (1) broadly distributing health goods which are macroallocation issues and (2) deciding which populations will obtain available health goods and services—microallocation issues.

Decisions based on one value mean that this value will often come in conflict with other values. For example, deciding primarily on the basis of client well-being may conflict with deciding on the basis of self-determination or equity. How community health nurses balance these values may even conflict with their own personal values or the values of the nursing profession. In these situations, values clarification techniques used with an ethical decision-making process may assist community health nurses in making decisions that promote the greatest well-being for clients without substantially reducing their self-determination or ignoring equity.

ETHICAL PRINCIPLES

Seven fundamental ethical principles should guide community health nurses when making decisions: respect, autonomy, beneficence, nonmaleficence, justice, veracity, and fidelity (Aroskar, 1995; Jenkins, 1989).

Respect

The principle of **respect** refers to treating people as unique, equal, and responsible moral agents. This principle emphasizes people's importance as members of the community and of the health services team. To apply this principle in decision making is to acknowledge community clients' as valued participants in shaping their own and the community's health outcomes. It includes treating them as equals on the health team and holding them and their views in high regard.

Autonomy

The principle of **autonomy** means freedom of choice and the exercise of people's rights. Individualism and self-determination are dominant values in this principle where people are free to make self-directed choices. As nurses apply this principle in community health they promote individuals' and groups' rights to and involvement in decision making (see the Issues in Community Health Nursing display). This is true, however, only as long as those decisions enhance these people's well-being and do not harm the well-being of others

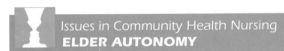

Issues in Community Health Nursing
ELDER AUTONOMY

Frequently community health nurses face an ethical dilemma when clients' autonomy conflicts with families' or professionals' judgements for the best course of action. One population group whose autonomy is often jeopardized is the elderly. Decisions about life style, nursing home placement, type and length of treatment protocols, or the right to die are examples of value conflicts with this age group. As elderly persons experience increased dependency and diminished physical, mental, and financial resources, how can their autonomy be preserved? Gale argues, "Elderly persons should have the personal liberty to choose and decide on their own actions from plans or alternatives that are available" (1989, p. 192). She posits that elderly people can be taught self-determination and skills in adaptive problem solving. The community health nurse's role should be one of advocate for this population to determine their values and wishes and to provide them with adequate information to make decisions. As advocate, the nurse can also speak on their behalf to influence family and community actions and legislation impinging on elder autonomy.

(Aroskar, 1989). It becomes especially important in applying this principle for nurses to make certain that clients are fully informed and that the decisions are deliberate with careful consideration of the consequences.

Beneficence

The ethical principle of **beneficence** means doing good or benefitting others. It is the promotion of good or taking action to ensure positive outcomes on behalf of clients. In community health the nurse applies the principle of beneficence by making decisions that actively promote community clients' best interests and well-being. Examples would be developing a senior's health program that ensures equal access to all in the community who need it or supporting enforcement of mandatory preschool immunizations.

Nonmaleficence

The principle of **nonmaleficence** means avoiding or preventing harm to others as a consequence of one's own choices and actions. This involves taking steps to avoid negative consequences from happening to people. Community health nurses can apply this ethical principle in decision making by such actions as promoting legislation to protect women and children against domestic abuse or by supporting lead-free environmental efforts.

Justice

The principle of **justice** refers to treating people fairly. It means the fair distribution of both benefits and costs among society's members. Decisions about equal access to health care, equitable distribution of services to rural as well as urban populations, not limiting amount or quality of service because of income level, and fair distribution of resources all draw on the principle of justice.

Within this principle are three different views on allocation, or what constitutes the meaning of "fair" distribution. One, **distributive justice**, says that benefits should be given first to the disadvantaged or those who need them most. See Levels of Prevention display. Decisions based on this view particularly help the needy even though it may mean witholding good from others who are also deserving but less in need. The second view, **egalitarian justice**, promotes decisions based on equal distribution of benefits to everyone, regardless of need.

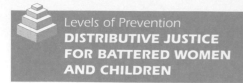

Levels of Prevention
DISTRIBUTIVE JUSTICE FOR BATTERED WOMEN AND CHILDREN

GOAL
To change the proposed law in your state that would eliminate funding for battered women's and children's shelters to a law preserving resources for this population.
PRIMARY PREVENTION
Early advocacy through active lobbying against the bill and garnering community support in favor of the revised law.
SECONDARY PREVENTION
Advocate for ammendments to the proposed law to preserve limited funding for shelters.
TERTIARY PREVENTION
After the proposed law has passed and funding is eliminated, seek private resources to fund shelters (such as a private foundation or a women's coalition) and propose a new bill to match private funding for shelters at the next legislative session.

The third, **restorative justice**, says that benefits should primarily go to those who have been wronged by prior injustice such as victims of crime or racial discrimination. The principle of justice seeks to promote equity, a value that was discussed in the previous section.

Veracity

The principle of **veracity** refers to telling the truth. Community clients deserve to be given accurate information in a timely manner. To withold information or not tell the truth can be self-serving to the nurse and hurtful as well as disrespectful to clients. Truth-telling treats clients as equals, expands the opportunity for greater client involvement, and provides needed information for decisions.

Fidelity

The final ethical principle of **fidelity** means keeping one's promises. People deserve to count on commitments being met. This principle involves the issues of trust and trustworthiness. Nurses who follow through on what they have said they will do earn their clients' respect and trust. In turn, this influences the quality of the nurse's relationship with clients who will more likely share information leading to improved decisions. Conversely, when a promise such as a commitment to institute child care during health classes is not kept, community members may lose faith and interest in participation.

ETHICAL STANDARDS AND GUIDELINES

As the number and complexity of ethical decisions in community health increase, so too does the need for ethical standards and guidelines to help nurses make the best choices possible. The American Nurses Association's Code for Nurses with Interpretive Statements (1985) provides a helpful guide. Some health care organizations and community agencies, using the ANA Code or some other similar document, have developed their own specific standards and guidelines. More and more health care organizations are using ethics committees or ethics rounds to deal with ethical aspects of client services (Abel, 1990).

Summary

Values strongly influence community health nursing practice and ethical decision making. Values are lasting beliefs that are extremely important to individuals as well as groups and cultures. A value system organizes these beliefs into a hierarchy of relative importance which motivates and guides human behavior. Values function as standards for behavior, as criteria for attitudes, as standards for moral judgments, and give expression to human needs. One can understand the nature of values by examining their qualities of endurance, their hierarchical arrangement, as prescriptive-proscriptive beliefs, and by examining them in terms of reference and preference.

The nurse is often faced with decisions that affect client's values and involve conflicting moral values and ethical dilemmas. Understanding what personal values are and how they affect behavior assists the nurse in making ethical evaluations and addressing ethical conflicts in practice. There are various strategies available to guide the nurse which can help in making these decisions such as values clarification, which helps make clear what values are important, and several frameworks for ethical decision making. Two frameworks described in this chapter include the identification and clarification of values impinging on the making of ethical decisions.

Three key human values influence client health and nurse decision making: the right to make decisions regarding one's health (self-determination), the right to health and well-being, and the right to equal access and quality of health care. Seven fundamental principles guide community health nurses in making ethical decisions: respect, beneficence, nonmaleficence, justice, veracity, and fidelity.

Activities to Promote Critical Thinking

1. Describe where you stand on the following issues. For each statement, decide whether you strongly agree, agree, disagree, strongly disagree, or are undecided.
   a. Clients have the right to participate in all decisions related to their health care.
   b. Nurses need a system designed to credit self-study.
   c. Continuing education should be mandatory.
   d. Clients should always be told the truth.
   e. Standards of nursing practice should be enforced by state examining boards.
   f. Nurses should be required to take relicensure examinations every five years.
   g. Clients should be allowed to read their health record when they request to do so.
   h. Abortion should be an option available to every woman.
   i. Badly deformed newborns should be allowed to die.
   j. There should be laws guaranteeing desired health care for each person in this country.

2. In a grid similar to the one below, write a statement of belief in the space provided and examine it in relation to the seven steps of the process of valuing. Areas of confusion and conflict in nursing practice that you might want to examine are peer review, accountability, confidentiality, euthanasia, licensure, clients' rights, abortion, informed consent, and terminating treatment.

   To the right of your statements, check the appropriate boxes indicating when your beliefs reflect one or more of the seven steps in the valuing process. Is your belief a value according to the valuing process?

Statement	Freely chosen	Alternatives	Consequences	Cherished	Affirmed	Incorporated	Employed
	1	2	3	4	5	6	7

Activities to Promote Critical Thinking (continued)

3. Rank in order the following 12 potential nursing actions by using 1 to indicate the choice that you feel is most important in a nurse-community client relationship and 12 to indicate the choice you believe is least important.

_____ Touching people.

_____ Empathetically listening to clients.

_____ Disclosing yourself to clients.

_____ Becoming emotionally involved with clients.

_____ Teaching clients.

_____ Being honest in answering clients' questions.

_____ Seeing that clients conform to professionals' advice.

_____ Helping to decrease clients' anxiety.

_____ Making sure that clients are involved in decision making.

_____ Following legal mandates regarding health practices.

_____ Remaining "professional" with clients.

_____ Choice. (Add an alternative of your own.)

Examine the way in which you have ordered these options. What values can you identify based on your responses in this exercise? How do these values emerge in your behavior?

4. Request to attend two or three sessions of a community health agency ethics committee meeting. Observe and make notes on (a) what values are evident in the discussion, (b) what ethical principles are used, (c) what decision-making framework is used, and (d) if you were a member of the committee, what would you have liked to contribute?

REFERENCES

Abel, P.E. (1990). Ethics committees in home health agencies. *Public Health Nursing, 7*(4), 256–59.

American Nurses Association. (1985). *Code for nurses with interpretive statements.* Kansas City, Mo.: Author.

Aroskar, M.A. (1989). Community health nurses: their most significant ethical decision-making problems. *Nursing Clinics of North America, 24*(4), 967–75.

Aroskar, M.A. (1995). Envisioning nursing as a moral community. *Nursing Outlook, 43*(3),134–138.

Aroskar, M.A. (1990). Ethical issues and dilemmas in community health. In S. Wold *Community health nursing: issues and topics.* East Norwalk, CT: Appleton & Lange.

Baier, K. (1958). *The moral point of view.* Ithaca, NY: Cornell University Press.

Bandman, E.L. & Bandman, B. (1985). *Nursing ethics in the life span.* Norwalk, CT: Appleton-Century-Crofts.

Beauchamp, T. L. & Childress, J.F. (1989). Principles of biomedical ethics (3rd ed.). New York: Oxford.

Carey, R. (1989). How values affect the mutual goal setting process with multiproblem families. *Journal of Community Health Nursing, 6*(1), 7–14.

Davis, A. & Aroskar, M.A. (1991). *Ethical dilemmas and nursing practice* (3rd ed.). Norwalk, CT: Appleton & Lange.

Fried, C. (1978). *Right and wrong.* Cambridge, MA: Harvard University Press.

Gale, B.J. (1989). Advocacy for elderly autonomy: a challenge for community health nurses. *Journal of Community Health Nursing, 6*(4), 191–197.

Jenkins, H.M. (1989). Ethical dimensions of leadership in community health nursing. *Journal of Community Health Nursing, 6*(2), 103–112.

Kluckhohn, C. (1951). Values and value-orientations in the theory of action: An exploration in definition and classification. In T. Parsons & E. A. Shils (Eds.), *Toward a general theory of action* (p. 388–433). Cambridge, MA: Harvard University Press.

Maslow, A. (1969). *Toward a psychology of being.* (2nd ed.). New York: Van Nostrand.

Merriam-Webster. (1993). *Merriam-Webster's collegiate dictionary* (10th ed.). Springfield, MA: Author

President's Commission for the Study of Ethical Problems in Medicine and Biomedical and Behavioral Research. (1982). *Making health care decisions: Volume one report.* Washington, DC: U.S. Government Printing Office.

President's Commission for the Study of Ethical Problems in Medicine and Biomedical and Behavioral Research. (1983). *Summing up.* Washington, DC: U.S. Government Printing Office.

Priester, R. (1992). A values framework for health system reform. I Spring, 84–107.

Rawls, J. (1971). *A theory of justice.* Cambridge, MA: Harvard University Press.

Rokeach, M. (1968). Beliefs, attitudes and values: A theory of organization and change. San Francisco: Jossey-Bass.

Rokeach, M. (1973). The nature of human values. New York: Free Press.

Thompson, J.E. & Thompson, H.O. (1992). *Bioethical decision making for nurses.* Lanham, MD: University Press of America.

Uustal, D.B. (1977). The use of values clarification in nursing practice. *Journal of Continuing Education in Nursing 8,* (May-June), 8–13.

Uustal, D.B. (1978). Values clarification in nursing. *American Journal of Nursing, 78,* 2058–63.

Veatch, R.M. (1977). *Case studies in medical ethics.* Cambridge, MA: Harvard University Press.

SELECTED READINGS

Allen, D.G. (1987). Critical social theory as a model for analyzing ethical issues in family and community health. *Family and Community Health, 10*(1), 63–72.

Anderson, R.C., et al. (1987). Ethical issues in health promotion and health education. *American Association of Occupational Health Nurses Journal, 35*(5), 220–23, 246–48.

Armstrong, M. (1987). Ethics in community nursing. *Recent Advances in Nursing, (15),* 52–73.

Aroskar, M.A. (1993). Ethical issues: politics, power, and policy. In D.J.Mason, S.W. Talbott, & J.K. Leavitt. *Policy and politics for nurses.* Philadelphia: Saunders.

Beauchamp, D.E. (1985). Community: The neglected tradition of public health. *Hastings Center Report, 15,* 28–36.

Beauchamp, D.E. (1976). Public health as social justice. *Inquiry, 13,* 3–14.

Beauchamp, T.L. & Childress, J.F. (1994). *Principles of Biomedical Ethics* (4th ed.). New York: Oxford.

Benjamin, M. & Curtis, J. (1992). *Ethics in nursing* (3rd ed.). New York: Oxford.

Collopy, B., et al (1991). New directions in nursing home ethics. *Hastings Center Report, 21*(2), 1–15.

Cunningham, N. & Hutchinson, S. (1990). Myths in health care ethics. *Image, 22,* 235–38.

Danis, M. & Churchill, L.R. (1992). Autonomy and the common weal. *Hastings Center Report, 21*(1), 25–31.

Erickson, G.P. (1988). Ethical dilemmas in home care of chronically ill elderly persons. *Home Healthcare Nurse, 6*(6), 19–23.

Ewing, W. A. (1987). Domestic violence and community health care ethics: Reflection on systemic intervention . . . AMEND, Abusive Men Exploring New Directions. *Family and Community Health, 10*(1), 73–82.

Fowler, M. (1990). *Nursing ethics.* Philadelphia: Lippincott.

Husted, G. & Husted, J. (1991). *Ethical decision making in nursing.* St. Louis: Mosby Year Book.

Kanoti, G.G. (1988). The ethical implications of AIDS. In K.D.Blanchet, (Ed.). *AIDS: A health care management response.* Rockville, MD: Aspen.

Lanik, G. & Webb, A. (1989). Ethical decision making for community health nurses. *Journal of Community Health Nursing, 6*(2), 95–102.

Last, J. M. (1987). Ethical issues in public health. In *Public Health and Human Ecology.* East Norwalk, CN: Appleton & Lange.

Last, J. M. (1987). Ethics, mores and values—and AIDS. *Canadian Journal of Public Health, 78*(2), 75–76.

McElmurry, B.J., et al. (1989). Ethical concerns in caring for older women in the community. *Nursing Clinics of North America 24*(4), 1041–50.

Reinhardt, U.E. (1990). Rationing the health-care surplus: an American tragedy. In P.R. Lee and C.L.Estes (Eds.). *The nation's health,* (3rd ed.) Boston: Jones and Bartlett.

Roemer, R. (1987). Public health ethics and the law. *The Nation's Health,* May/June, 2.

Rogers, B. (1988). Ethical dilemmas in occupational health nursing. *American Assocction Occupational Health Nursing Journal, 36*(3), 100–104.

Schultz, R.C. (1987). Ethics and community health: philosophical traditions and recent turnings. *Family & Community Health, 10*(1), 1–7.

Sciegaj, M., Wade, T.E., Dever, G.E.A., & Alley, J.W. (1987). A framework for applying ethical theory to public health practice. *Family & Community Health, 10*(1), 15–23.

UNIT

II

Applying the Tools of Community Health Nursing Practice

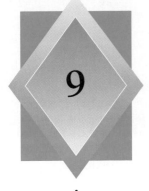

CHAPTER

9

The Community as Client: Assessment and Planning

LEARNING OBJECTIVES

Upon completion of this chapter, readers should be able to:

- Explain why nurses must move beyond an individualistic focus to practice population-based community health nursing.
- Describe the meaning of community as client.
- Articulate specific considerations of each of the three dimensions of the community as client.
- Express the meaning and significance of community dynamics.
- Explain four types of community needs assessment.
- Discuss community needs assessment methods.
- Describe characteristics of a healthy community.
- Identify the steps in planning for the health of a community.

KEY TERMS

- Client myth
- Community
- Community as client
- Community needs assessment
- Community subsystem assessment
- Comprehensive assessment
- Descriptive epidemiological study
- Familiarization assessment
- Individualism
- Location myth
- Location variables
- Population variables
- Problem-oriented assessment
- Skills myth
- Social class
- Social system variables
- Survey

Barbara Walton Spradley and Judith Ann Allender
COMMUNITY HEALTH NURSING: CONCEPTS AND PRACTICE, 4th ed.
© 1996 Barbara Walton Spradley and Judith Ann Allender

Acentral theme of this book is community health nursing's involvement in promoting the health of aggregates of people. This idea has been emphasized because, in both subtle and direct ways, American culture works against it. The value of individualism is one of the greatest barriers to carrying out the mission of community health nursing.

Every society has a small number of core values that give meaning to life. United States culture, for example, values success and material rewards. Such values provide motivation for millions of people. They uphold the work ethic; they become the measures by which successful and wealthy people are elevated to the status of popular heroes. The very existence of our society and its way of life depends on a deep commitment to such values. People learn them early in life and come to take them for granted as the way things ought to be. One value that most Americans hold as God-given, a value that profoundly influences the entire practice of nursing, is individualism. **Individualism** refers to a "doctrine that the interests of the individual are or ought to be ethically paramount" (Merriam-Webster, 1993, p. 593).

Nearly every social observer who has written about American society has identified this value. A cornerstone of civilization, this basic premise underlies most American institutions. "Protect the rights of the individual"; "Equal justice for all under the law"; "Life, liberty, and the pursuit of happiness for all individuals" are familiar cries. More than 50 years ago, the sociologist Robert Lynd described this value: "Individualism, 'the survival of the fittest,' is the law of nature and the secret of America's greatness; and restrictions on individual freedom are un-American and kill initiative" (Lynd, 1939, p. 60).

Individual effort and success is rewarded in schools and in the workplace. The criminal justice system punishes individual crimes far more harshly than corporate crimes. A woman who stole five dollars in a southern state was punished by several years in prison whereas a large oil company that stole millions by overcharging customers paid a relatively small fine. Health care too in American society is dominated by a commitment to the treatment of individuals. The vast majority of researchers, personnel, and health care institutions focus on the care of individual illness rather than promotion of community health.

How does this value of individualism affect community health nursing? All nurses are first educated to focus on the individual client in clinical nursing. But in community health practice the focus must shift to the community as client. This can include families, groups, organizations, populations, and communities (Campbell, 1988; McKnight & Van Dover, 1994; *Redesigning Nursing Education,* 1973).

Myths Perpetuated by an Individualistic Focus

Three pervasive myths seem to hinder the nurse from focusing on aggregates or community: the location myth, the skills myth, and the client myth.

LOCATION MYTH

The **location myth** defines community health nursing by describing it in terms of where it is practiced—in a specific setting or location such as outside of the hospital. This myth silently influences nurses to define their practice based not on the nature of the service given but on the location of its delivery. This myth promotes the belief that community health nursing emphasizes care of individuals. Instead, community health nursing focuses on assessing and treating the health needs of population groups and aggregates wherever that might occur—in the hospital, at home, in the workplace, or in the community (McKnight & Van Dover, 1994; Williams, 1985, 1992).

SKILLS MYTH

The **skills myth** states that community health nurses employ only the skills of basic clinical nursing when working with community clients. This myth leads many nurses to assume that their clinical skills are completely adequate for population-focused practice. It can lead them to overlook a large and sophisticated body of knowledge and competencies required for defining problems and developing solutions for populations (Williams, 1985, 1992). Community health nurses need skills drawn from the public health sciences in measurement and analysis (epidemiology and biostatistics), skills in social policy based on the history and philosophy of public health, and skills in management and organization for public health (McKnight & Van Dover, 1994; Milbank, 1976). At the baccalaureate level, nurses can begin to build these skills; they can strengthen and refine them at the masters and doctoral levels.

CLIENT MYTH

Community health nursing involves working with populations, but the **client myth** says that the primary clients are individuals and families. This myth can hinder the nurse from a broader focus on the health of aggregates and groups at risk which is central to community health nursing practice. It is population-focused practice that distinguishes community health nursing from other nursing specialties (APHA, 1981; Dunn, et al, 1990; Williams, 1992).

Levels of Community Health Nursing Practice

To envision the broad scope of community health nursing, there are six levels of clients with which the nurse might work: individuals, families, groups, subpopulations, populations, and communities. Table

9.1 presents the characteristics of these clients and describes typical nursing involvement with each level.

Although community health nurses work at all six levels of practice, working with communities is a primary mission and is of considerable significance for two important reasons. First, the **community** directly influences the health of individuals, families, groups, subpopulations, and populations who might be a part of it. When the city of Los Angeles failed to take aggressive action to stop air pollution, it adversely affected the health of millions of people. Second, working with communities is important because it is at this level that most health service provision occurs. Community agencies help develop specific health programs and disseminate health information to many types of groups and populations.

The community health nurse, then, must work with the community as the client (Anderson et al., 1986; Hanchett, 1988; McKnight & Van Dover, 1994). The **community as client** refers to the concept of a community-wide group of people as the focus of nursing ser-

TABLE 9.1. *Variations in Scope of Community Health Nursing Practice*

	Client	Example	Health Characteristics	Nursing Assessment	Involvement
Individual	Individual	Kim Murphy	One person with various needs	Individual health assessment	A dyad; interaction with the individual
	Family	Murphy family (seven members)	A small group based on kin ties; specific roles	Family health assessment	Family visits; interaction with members as a group
	Group	Parenting group; Alanon club	Two or more people; face-to-face communication; interdependency	Assessment of group effectiveness in fulfilling its functions	Group participation; having a role in meetings
	Subpopulation	Unmarried pregnant adolescents in a school district	Large group sharing one or more characteristics (subset of a larger group)	Assessment of collective health problems and needs	Study of and planning for meeting specific health needs
Aggregate	Population	Homeless people in Chicago	An aggregate of people who share one or more personal or environmental characteristics	Study of health needs and vital statistics	Membership in organizations such as a health planning council
	Community	East Harlem; New York City; gay community in the United States	A large aggregate sharing geographic location or special interests	Study of community health characteristics and competence	Researching the community; planning and setting up services

vice. Understanding the concept of the community as client is a prerequisite for effective service at every level of community nursing practice.

Dimensions of the Community as Client

Chapter 1 defined a community as having three features: (1) a location, (2) a population, and (3) a social system (Lynd, 1939). This three-dimensional view (Fig. 9.1) especially suits the idea of a local community which can vary by expanding or constricting the geographic boundary. For example, one might define the community of Seattle, Washington, as all the people living within the city limits or the community of greater Seattle, as the city, its suburbs, and other small towns located on its perimeter. A community health nurse might want to restrict the size of the community to a specific district within Seattle for study or services. Regardless of size or geographic boundaries, all these communities still share the three common denominators of an identified location, population, and social system. It is useful to think of these three dimensions of every

community as a rough map one can follow for assessing needs or planning for service provision. In considering each dimension, one should pay particular attention to the questions that must be asked to assess the health of a community.

LOCATION

Every community carries out its daily existence in a specific geographic location. The health of a community is affected by this location, including the placement of health services, the geographic features, climate, plants, animals, and the human-made environment (Allor, 1983). The location of a community places it in an environment that offers resources and also poses threats (Barker, et al, 1994; Neuman, 1982; West, 1984). The healthy community is one that makes wise use of its resources and is prepared to meet threats and dangers. In assessing the health of any community, it is necessary to collect information not only about these location variables, but also about how the community relates to them. Do groups cooperate to identify threats? Do health agencies cooperate to prepare for an emergency such as flood or earthquake? Does the community make certain that its members are given available information about resources and dangers?

Guiding the nurse in assessing the health of any community is a Community Profile Inventory divided into three parts, location, population, and social system (Tables 9.2, 9.3, 9.4, respectively). Table 9.2 covers the location perspective including the six **location variables** of community boundaries, location of health services, geographic features, climate, flora and fauna, and the human-made environment.

Community Boundaries

In order to talk about the community in any sense, one must first describe its boundaries (Shamansky & Pesznecker, 1981). All measurements of wellness and illness within a community depend on defining the outer limits of the unit under consideration. Nurses need to be clear, for example, that a target community of the elderly includes a description of age and location (e.g., all persons 65 and older in a city or county). Some communities are distinctly separate, such as an isolated rural town, while others are closely situated to one another, such as suburbs of a large metropolis. Thus it is important for the nurse to know the nature of each one's location and explicitly define its parameters.

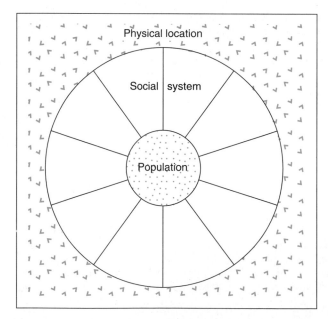

FIGURE 9.1. A community has (1) a physical location, represented here by the square boundary; (2) a population, shown here by the central circle; and (3) a social system, divided here into subsystems.

TABLE 9.2. *Community Profile Inventory: Location Perspective*

Location Variables	Community Health Implications	Community Assessment Questions	Information Sources
Boundary of community	Community boundaries serve as basis for measuring incidence of wellness and illness, and for determining spread of disease.	Where is the community located? What is its boundary? Is it a part of a larger community? What smaller communities does it include?	Atlas State maps County maps City maps Telephone book City directory Public library
Location of health services	Use of health services depends on availability and accessibility.	Where are the major health institutions located? What necessary health institutions are outside the community? Where are they?	Telephone book Chamber of commerce State health department County or local health departments Maps Public library
Geographic features	Injury, death, and destruction may be caused by floods, earthquakes, volcanoes, tornadoes, or hurricanes. Recreational opportunities at lakes, seashore, mountains promote health and fitness.	What major landforms are in or near the community? What geographic features pose possible threats? What geographic features offer opportunities for healthful activities?	Atlas Chamber of commerce Maps State health department Public library
Climate	Extremes of heat and cold affect health and illness Extremes of temperature and precipitation may tax community's coping ability.	What are the average temperature and precipitation? What are the extremes? What climatic features affect health and illness? Is the community prepared to cope with emergencies?	Weather atlas Chamber of commerce State health department Maps Local government Weather bureau Public library
Flora and fauna	Poisonous plants and disease-carrying animals can affect community health. Plants and animals offer resources as well as dangers.	What plants and animals pose possible threats to health?	State health department Poison control center Police department Emergency rooms Encyclopedia Public library
Human-made environment	All human influences on environment (housing, dams, farming, type of industry, chemical waste, air pollution, etc.) can influence levels of community wellness.	What are the major industries? How have air, land, and water been affected by humans? What is the quality of housing? Do highways allow access to health institutions?	Chamber of commerce Local government City directory State health department University research reports Public library

Location of Health Services

If the members of a town must travel 300 miles to the nearest clinic or dental office, the health of the community will be affected. When assessing a community, the community health nurse will want to identify the major health centers and know where they are located. In one city, for example, the alcoholism treatment center for indigent alcoholics was located 30 miles outside the city. This location presented transportation problems and profoundly affected who volunteered for treatment and how long they remained at the center. If a well-baby clinic is located on the edge of a high-crime district, this location may deter parents from using it. It is often enlightening to plot the major health institutions, both inside and outside the community, on a map that shows their proximity and relation to the community as a whole.

Geographic Features

Communities have been constructed in every conceivable physical environment and that environment certainly can affect the health of a community (see further discussion in Chapter 6 on environmental health). A healthy community takes into consideration the geography of its location, identifies the possible problems and likely resources, and responds in an adaptive fashion (Neuman, 1982). For example, both Anchorage, Alaska, and San Francisco, California, are located on a geologic fault line and subject to major earthquakes. In such places, the health of the community is partly determined by its preparedness for an earthquake and its ability to cope when such a crisis occurs. In Ontario, Canada, a series of lakes called the Lac la Croix is a valuable food resource for the Ojibway Indian communities as they depend on fish from the lakes for their livelihood. In recent years acid rain generated from coal-burning power plants in the United States and Canada has begun to affect the lakes and the fish. A major food supply has thus become contaminated for the Ojibway Indian communities.

Climate

The climate also has a direct influence on the health of a community (Green & Anderson, 1986). When Buffalo, New York, is blanketed with deep winter snows, members of this community are sometimes immobilized for days. Deaths from coronary occlusions increase as people attempt to shovel their walks and uncover their cars. The intense summer heat of another location, such as Phoenix, Arizona, can create other health problems. Skin cancer, for example, is highest in states that constitute the Sun Belt. A healthy community will encourage physical activity among its members, but the climate, in turn, affects this activity. Although long cold winters can restrict activity, one community, St. Paul, Minnesota, holds an annual Winter Carnival, which includes sporting events. Parades, ice sailing, dogsledding, a treasure hunt, and hot air balloon races bring thousands of Minnesotans outdoors at a time when they might otherwise be confined by the weather.

Flora and Fauna

Plant and animal populations in a community are often determined by location. The way a community responds to these populations, whether wild or domesticated, can affect the health of the community. In the Sierra foothill communities of central California, black widow and tarantula spiders, scorpions, and rattlesnakes form insect and reptile populations which pose potential health threats. The poison from a single bite may cause injury and death. In western Washington state, a bushy, attractive plant, known as Deadly Nightshade, grows in yards and vacant lots and its appealing black berries are extremely poisonous. The community health nurse will want to know about the major sources of danger from plants and animals affecting the community under study. Are there community agencies that provide educational information about these dangers? Does the populace understand their significance? Are emergency services, such as a poison control center, available to community members?

Human-Made Environment

Every community is located in the midst of an environment created and transformed by human ingenuity. People build houses and factories; they dump wastes into streams or vacant lots; they fill the air with gasses; they build dams to control streams. All these human alterations of the environment have important implications for community health (Blumenthal, 1985). (See Fig. 9.2). A community health nurse might improve the health of a community by working for legislation to prevent disposing of waste chemicals into water or landfills. Such legislation could have avoided the disaster at New York State's Love Canal, where toxic wastes continued to seep into residential areas for many years severely affecting the community's health.

Agricultural activity can alter the environment through chemical fertilizers and pesticide applications creating potential health hazards to the community. Many farm communities attract migrant workers whose economic and health needs often pose a challenge to community resources. Thus a community's physical location has many health implications.

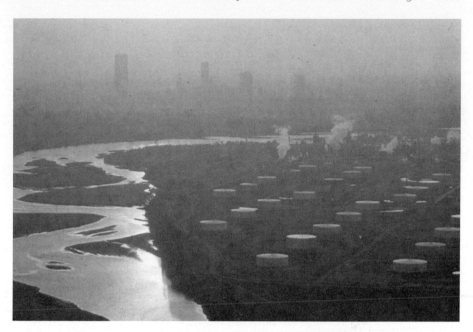

FIGURE 9.2. Air and water pollution result from environmental alteration typical of the 20th century life style.

POPULATION

When one considers the community as the client, the second dimension to examine is the population of the total community. Population consists not of a specialized aggregate, but of all the diverse people who live within the boundaries of the community.

The health of any community is greatly influenced by the population that lives in it. Different features of the population suggest health needs and provide a basis for health planning (Dever, 1980). A healthy community has leaders who are aware of the population's characteristics, know its different needs, and respond to those needs. Community health nurses can better understand any community by knowing about it's **population variables** which are its size, density, composition, rate of growth or decline, cultural characteristics, social class, and mobility. Table 9.3 presents the population perspective section of the Community Profile Inventory.

Size

The town of Dover, Delaware, with approximately 10,000 people, and the city of Los Angeles, California, have radically different health problems. If a single case of salmonella poisoning occurred in Dover, health officials would likely learn of it. It would be relatively easy to trace the course, check the few restaurants in town, and interview people about sanitation practices. However, many cases might occur in Los Angeles without the health department's knowledge. Moreover, if these cases were discovered, tracing the source of contamination might involve a long and complicated search. This is only one small way in which population size might affect the health of a community, but it also would influence the presence of slums, heterogeneity of the population, and almost every conceivable area of health need and service. Knowing a community's size provides community health nurses with important information for planning.

Density

In some communities, thousands of people are crowded into high-rise apartments. In others, such as farm communities, people live at great distances from one another. We do not yet know the full impact of living in high-density communities, but some research has already shown that crowding affects individual and community health. A classic study of Ohio farmers, living in low-density communities, suggested that the absence of stress from crowding may have contributed to their reduced rate of coronary artery disease (Nagi, 1959).

A low-density community may have other problems. When people are spread out, health care provision may

TABLE 9.3. *Community Profile Inventory: Population Perspective*

Population Variables	Community Health Implications	Community Assessment Questions	Information Sources
Size	The number of people influences number and size of health care institutions. Size affects homogeneity of the population and its needs.	What is the population of the community? Is it an urban, suburban, or rural community?	State health department Census data Maps City or town officials Chamber of commerce
Density	Increased density may increase stress. High and low density often affect the availability of health services.	What is the density of the population per square mile?	Census data State health department
Composition	Composition of the population often determines types of health needs.	What is the age composition of the community? What is the sex composition of the community? What is the marital status of community members? What occupations are represented and in what percentages?	Census data State health department Chamber of commerce U.S. Department of Labor Statistics
Rate of growth or decline	Rapidly growing communities may place excessive demands on health services. Marked decline in population may signal a poorly functioning community.	How has population size changed over the past two decades? What are the health implications of this change?	Census data State health department
Cultural differences	Health needs vary among subcultural and ethnic populations. Utilization of health services varies with culture. Health practices and extent of knowledge are affected by culture.	What is the ethnic breakdown of population? What racial groups are represented? What subcultural populations exist in the community? Do any of the subcultural groups have unique health needs and practices? Are different ethnic and cultural groups included in health planning?	Census data State health department Social and cultural research reports Human rights commission City government Health planning boards
Social class	Class differences influence the utilization of health services. Class composition influences cost of public health services.	What percentage of the population falls into each social class? What do class differences suggest for health needs and services?	State health department Census data Sociological reports
Mobility	Mobility of the population affects continuity of care. Mobility affects availability of service to highly mobile population.	How frequently do members move into and out of the community? How frequently do members move within the community? Are there any specific populations, such as migrant workers, that are highly mobile? How does the pattern of mobility affect the health of the community? Is the community organized to meet the health needs of mobile groups?	State health department Census data Health agencies serving migrant workers Farm labor offices Program serving transients and the homeless

become difficult. There may not be enough resources in the form of taxes to support public health services. Rural communities often suffer from inadequate distribution of health care personnel, ranging from private physicians to community health nurses. A healthy community will take into consideration the density of its population. It will organize in ways to meet the differing needs created by its density levels; for example, it will recognize differences in density between the inner city and the suburbs and allocate services accordingly.

Composition

Communities differ in the types of people who live within their boundaries. A retirement community in Florida whose members are mostly over 65 years of age has one set of interests and concerns. A city with a large number of women in the childbearing years will have another set of concerns. A healthy community is one that takes full account of, and provides for, differences in age, sex, educational level, and occupation of its members all of which may affect health concerns. For example, in a town where 75% of the workers are employed by a textile mill, the community lives under the threat of brown lung disease, caused by cotton dust. Understanding a community's composition is an important early step in determining its level of health.

Rate of Growth or Decline

Community populations change over time. Some grow rapidly, thus placing extreme demands on the provision of health services. Others, because of economic change, may decline. Any significant fluctuation in population size can affect the health of the community. As people leave to find new employment or better living conditions, overall consumption of goods and services drops. Community morale may suffer, and community leadership may decline. Even a stable community may have problems; for instance, members may resist needed change because they see little fluctuation in their population.

Cultural Characteristics

A community may be composed of a single cultural group such as an Ojibway Indian reservation in Wisconsin or a community may be made up of many cul-

tures or subcultures. If a city has a large Hispanic population, a grouping of Native Americans living in the inner city, and a cluster of Vietnamese refugees, the cultural differences among these members will influence the health of the community. These differences, for example, can create conflicting or competing demands for resources and services or create intergroup hostility. A healthy community is aware of such cultural differences and acts to promote understanding between subcultural groups.

Social Class and Educational Level

Social class refers to the ranking of groups within society by income, education, occupation, prestige, or a combination of these factors (Goode, 1977). There is no absolute agreement on the income amounts or other criteria used to designate social class categories (upper, middle, lower) other than the government formula used to compute poverty level. Although class distinctions are not clearly defined, class rankings based on occupation, education, and wealth (income plus assets) seem to correlate with many different social patterns and are used frequently in research. Occupational level, in particular, has proven to be a reliable measure with extraordinarily similar rankings among all societies for which there are data. It appears that people with higher occupational levels experience higher incomes; have more education; exert more political influence; and are more highly esteemed by others.

Educational level, which is closely associated with social class, "is the most powerful determinant . . . with regard to influence on health-related behavior" (Green & Anderson, 1986, p. 35). People with higher educational attainment tend to be healthier, respond more readily to health professionals' interventions, and are more likely to modify their behavior in positive, health-enhancing ways. These modifications may include smoking cessation, weight control, exercise, dental care, and use of immunizations. Persons in the lower economic strata of society frequently have the worst health and are more difficult to reach with health information; they also tend to have a higher incidence of communicable diseases. "In general, preventive health services and health promotion activities are most needed by members of low-income groups and individuals of less educational attainment, but all people in a community will benefit from an overall community health program" (Ibid., p. 35).

TABLE 9.4. *Community Profile Inventory: Social System Perspective*

Social System Variables	Community Health Implications	Community Assessment Questions	Information Sources
Health system Family system Economic system Educational system Religious system Welfare system Political system Recreational system Legal system Communication system	Each system must fulfill its functions for a healthy community. Collaboration among the systems to identify goals and problems affects health of community. Undue influence of one system on another may lower the health of the community. Agreement on the means to achieve community goals affects community health. Communication among organizations in each system affects Community health.	What are the functions of each major system? What are the major subsystems of each system? What are the major organizations in each subsystem? How well do the various organizations function? Are the subsystems in each major system in conflict? Is there adequate communication among the major systems? Is there agreement on community goals? Are there mechanisms for resolving conflict? Do any parts of the total system dominate the others? What community needs are not being met?	Chamber of commerce Telephone book City directory Organizational literature Officials in organizations Community self-study Community survey Local library Key informants

It is generally known that social classes have different health problems, resources for coping with illness, and ways of using health services (Freeman, et al, 1979). A healthy community recognizes these differences and creates health care services to meet these varied needs.

Mobility

Americans are a mobile population. People move to go to college, take new jobs, or seek new climates upon retirement. This mobility has a direct effect on the health of communities. If the population turnover is extensive, continuity of services may suffer. Leadership for improving the health of the community may change so frequently that concerted action becomes difficult. High turnover may require special attention to health education about local conditions.

Population groups may arrive and depart in seasonal swings; migrant farm workers, tourists, and college students can affect a community. The community health nurse will want to identify those populations that are seasonally mobile. They not only present special health needs, but may place an added burden on a community. If a town of 3000 people has an annual influx of 10,000 students who disappear in the summer, residents must prepare to meet this population change. A healthy community neither ignores nor overreacts to this kind of mobility. Rather, it identifies the nature of population change, determines the needs created by such change, and organizes to meet those needs.

SOCIAL SYSTEM

In addition to location and population, every community has a third dimension: a social system. The various parts of a community's social system that interact and influence the system, are called **social system variables.** These variables include the health system, family systems, economic system, educational system, religious system, welfare system, political system, recreational system, legal system, and communication system (Anderson et al., 1986; Dever, 1991). Whether assessing a community's health, developing new services for the mentally ill within the community, or promoting the health of the elderly, the community health nurse needs to understand the community as a social system. A community health nurse working in a tiny village in Alaska needs to grasp the social system of that village no less than a nurse working in New York City. Table 9.4 guides the nurse in assessing a community's social system variables.

A social system is an abstract concept and can be more readily understood by first considering the people who make up the community's population. Each person enacts multiple roles, such as parent, spouse, employee, citizen, church member, or political volunteer. Certain roles tend to be more closely connected, such as supervisor and staff nurse or customer and sales clerk, and the patterns and interactions that emerge among roles form the basis of organizations. Some organizations are informal, an example is the interactions among an extended family group. Other organizations are formal such as the city police department or a local business. However all organizations are constructed from roles that are enacted by individual citizens. Organizations, in turn, interact with one another forming linkages, for example, a medical equipment company and a laboratory establish contracts (linkages) with a home care agency. When a group of organizations are linked and have similar functions, such as all those providing social services, they form a community system or subsystem. See Figure 9.3. It is important to remember that the various community systems have a profound influence on one another. Because this interaction among parts determines the health of the whole, it is the total social system that concerns community health nurses. See the case study that follows.

The Health System as Part of a Community

Although community health nurses must examine all the systems in a community and how they interact, the health system is of particular importance. Studying the health system in a community can be compared to assessment of an individual client. The latter involves a head-to-toe examination looking for indications of wellness and illness in the respiratory, musculoskeletal, glandular, skin, and circulatory systems, among others. Initial assessment of a community also begins with a survey of its ten major systems. Before asking about how well the specific parts are functioning such as whether the police doing their job, or whether the mayor an effective leader, the nurse would inquire first about the political system as a whole: What are its constituent parts? Are there gross signs of health or illness? In order to answer questions about a system's level of functioning, one must first know its function—that is, the job it has to do as part of the larger system. The nurse might ask, for example, "How well does the communication system keep citizens informed about important matters?" This question implies that this system

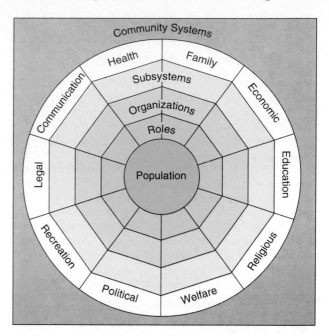

FIGURE 9.3. The community as a social system. Each of the ten major systems of a community includes a number of subsystems that are made up of organizations. Members of the community occupy roles in these organizations.

has a basic function, information dissemination. The nurse might also ask, "Does the educational system offer equal education to all children of the community?" This question implies that this system's function is to offer learning opportunities to everyone in a particular age group.

The major function of the health system is to promote the health of the community. Community assessment does not merely ask if, but also how well, the system is functioning. What is the level of health promotion as carried out by the health system of a community? In order to answer this question, which can be applied to any system, one needs a clear notion about the subsystems, organizations, and roles that make up the system. Any evidence of inadequate functioning becomes a warning signal for more careful assessment. For example, a high rate of teenage pregnancies in a city may signal inadequate functioning of several systems; perhaps the family, educational, religious, and health systems. Thus, a closer look is in order. What community values influence sexual behavior among adolescents? What sex education programs are available to this population? Does the health system provide information and counseling?

CASE STUDY: CENTERVILLE

INTERACTION OF SOCIAL SYSTEM VARIABLES

The health department of the city of Centerville reported more than 75 pregnancies in one year among teenage girls, a large number for the size of this community. The situation placed a marked strain on the families of the girls and caused increased demands for services from the health system. Because the vast majority of these pregnancies were unwanted, they presented a problem for the unwed teenage parents, their families, and eventually, the community. What would happen to the babies of these girls? Evidence from research suggested that, in the future, the girls were likely to have larger families, depend more frequently on the welfare system, and have a higher number of health problems than women who were not teenage mothers (Pickett & Hanlon, 1990).

How should the community respond to this situation? The way it did respond gave clues to the overall health of the community. For one thing, the problem had been ignored, a sign of defense rather than adaptation. When it came to public attention, it divided various groups. Families blamed the schools; school officials in turn blamed the changing sexual mores represented in motion pictures and television shows. Some members of the health system asked Planned Parenthood to set up a clinic in the town to provide family planning education and services as a preventive measure. Almost immediately, however, the religious system entered the picture with groups forming to picket Planned Parenthood facilities because of the association's stand on abortion. Planned Parenthood set up its clinic in an old restaurant on the edge of the business district. Individuals from the religious and economic system (local businessmen) joined to file suit to prevent Planned Parenthood from occupying the old building. Within months, every major system of this community was involved in the problem, yet it was as far from solution as ever. Indeed, the original problem had almost fallen by the wayside as community members fought over the issues of abortion and the Planned Parenthood headquarters. Vandals set several fires that destroyed part of the building. Pickets daily called attention to what they considered to be an unwanted health agency. Moreover, in the midst of the trouble, more teenagers, some with parents who were deeply involved in the conflict, became pregnant.

What were the signs that this was an unhealthy community? How should the situation be handled? What role could community health nursing play in helping to resolve the problem of teen pregnancies?

The components of the health system, described in Figure 9.4, include eight major subsystems, each with one or more organizations. Although the community health nurse must be aware of all the systems in a community, the health system is of central importance.

Community Dynamics

The discussion to this point may have suggested that the community is a rigid structure composed of a geographic location, a population, and a social system. Yet every community has a dynamic or changing quality. Think of the diagram in Figure 9.3 as a wheel that turns as the community changes. Two factors in particular affect community dynamics: (1) citizen participation in community health programs and (2) the power and decision-making structure of the community (Lynd, 1939; Green & Anderson, 1986).

CITIZEN PARTICIPATION

In some communities, citizens show little concern about public health issues and rely on health officials to take the entire responsibility. When such apathy abounds, community health nurses will need to promote community education and awareness. In other communities, participation may be widespread but either uninformed or obstructive as when citizens hamper or block the development of some programs. It is much more difficult to work in a community where groups have become polarized by issues such as abortion and fluoridation. Assessing the type and extent of citizen participation will be a necessary first step in community work.

The goal of encouraging responsible participation touches on the concept of self-care discussed in earlier chapters. One goal of community nurses when working with families or groups is to encourage people to participate and take responsibility for their own health care. They have the right to make decisions, to have adequate information, and to consult widely about their own health. The nurse's role is to encourage the full development of a self-care attitude. On a community level, self-care occurs when citizens become committed to the goal of a healthy community (see Fig. 9.5). Such a commitment includes responsible involvement in assessing, planning, conducting, and evaluating programs to meet community needs (Kinlein, 1978). Community self-care is community health nursing's goal.

POWER AND DECISION MAKING STRUCTURE

The second dynamic factor, the power and decision-making structure of a community, is a central concern to anyone wishing to bring about change. The descrip-

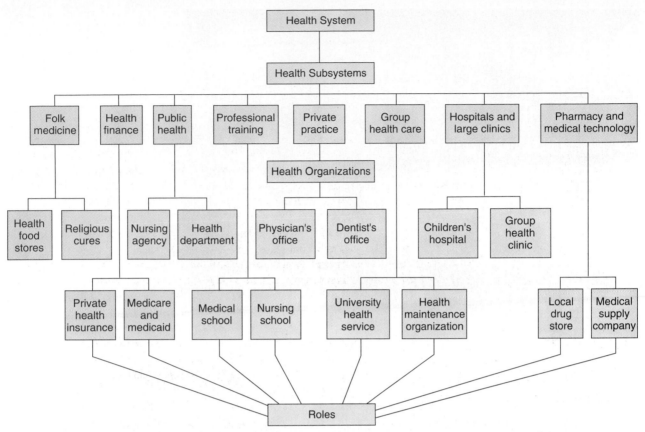

FIGURE 9.4. Components of the health system. This figure shows some representative types of organizations for each of the major subsystems. In turn, each of these organizations also has members with many different roles, and the health of the entire system depends, in part, on how well these roles are carried out.

tion of the community as a social system may suggest that power and decision making reside primarily in the political system, but that is not the case. Sanders and Brownlee have argued against oversimplifying the decision-making process: "In its naivest, simplest terms this [oversimplification] blandly states that (1) every community has an identifiable power clique and (2) that if you get the members on your side, all of your problems will be solved" (1979, p. 421).

Decision making in any community is much more complex than this description. Sanders and Brownlee suggest that power is distributed unevenly among members of organizations in various community systems. A key leader may have influence in more than one system, but that power will be diffuse. Seldom does a public health official have power in the religious system or a member of the clergy in the legal system. A dominant

leader is one who has specific power, but only within a single community system. An organizational leader will have power, but generally within a single organization, not often in the entire system. Sanders and Brownlee also say that key and dominant leaders will often work through other, less powerful leaders, called functionaries, issue leaders, and spokesmen. This text returns to the topic of leadership and types of leaders in Chapter 25.

Although power and decision making in any community are complex, Sanders and Brownlee do suggest several propositions to use as general guidelines for understanding this aspect of a community's dynamics.

1. Because communities differ widely in their power structures, do not assume that what is known about one community will be true of another.

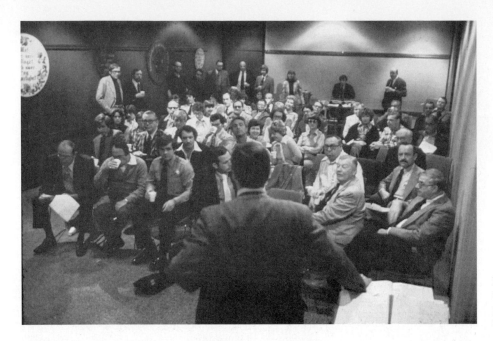

FIGURE 9.5. This community meeting demonstrates active participation and self care by the residents.

2. The leaders within the health system have different degrees of power and varying spheres of influence; a knowledge of these differences is prerequisite to effective community work.
3. Those leaders whose power is limited to the health system or organizations often have a network of contacts with similar leaders in other systems. Many of the decisions are made informally through this network.
4. Power does not automatically flow through the established bureaucratic channels. Locate the informal patterns of power and decision making.
5. Beware of leaders who speak authoritatively on issues outside their sphere of power. Their power may be more apparent than real.
6. Leaders from the health system may become key leaders with power that extends far beyond the health system.
7. Learn to distinguish between political, economic, and social power; then use the appropriate combination needed to promote community health issues.
8. Do not overestimate the support of key leaders or power cliques; their support may be helpful but still leave much organizational work to be done.
9. Try to encourage participation in the decision-making process at every level, from average citizen to key leader.

10. One can assume that leaders in one part of a community are ignorant of needs and problems in other parts of the system. When one contacts such leaders, recognize that they will have to be educated in community health issues.

Types of Community Needs Assessment

Community needs assessment is the process of determining the real or perceived needs of a defined community of people. In some situations, an extensive community study becomes the first priority. In others, all that is needed is a study of one system or even one organization. At other times community health nurses may need to familiarize themselves with an entire community without going into any depth—in other words, to perform a cursory examination. The type of assessment will depend on variables such as the needs that exist, the goals to be achieved, and the resources available for carrying out the study. Although it is difficult to determine the type of assessment needed in advance, the decision will be facilitated by understanding several different types of community assessment.

COMPREHENSIVE ASSESSMENT

The **comprehensive assessment** seeks to discover all relevant community health information. It begins with a review of existing studies and all the data presently available on the community. A survey would compile all the demographic information on the population, such as its size, density, and composition. Key informants would be interviewed in every major system—education, health, religious, economic, and others (Neuber et al., 1980). Then more detailed surveys and intensive interviews would yield information on organizations and the various roles in each organization. A comprehensive assessment would not only describe the systems of a community but also how power was distributed throughout the system, how decisions were made, and how change occurred (Green & Anderson, 1986; Hanchett, 1988).

Because comprehensive assessment is an expensive, time-consuming process, it is seldom performed. Indeed, in many cases such a thorough research plan might be a waste of resources and might repeat, in part, other studies. Performing a more focused study based on prior knowledge of needs is often a better strategy. Yet knowing how to conduct a comprehensive assessment has an important influence over the approach to a more focused study.

FAMILIARIZATION

A second type of community assessment, familiarization, is also the most necessary. **Familiarization assessment** involves studying data already available on a community, and gathering a certain amount of firsthand data, in order to gain a working knowledge of the community. Such an approach, sometimes called a "windshield survey," has been used in nursing students' community assessment courses (Caretto, et al, 1991; Campbell, 1988; Flynn et al., 1978; Ruybal, et al, 1975; Smith & Barton, 1992; White & Valentine, 1993). Nurses drive around the community, find health, social, and governmental services, obtain literature, introduce themselves as working in the area, and generally become familiar with the community. This type of assessment is needed whenever the community health nurse works with families, groups, organizations, or populations Familiarization provides a knowledge of the context in which these aggregates exist and may enable the nurse to connect clients with the community and its resources as with the case study of the Angelo family below.

CASE STUDY: THE ANGELO FAMILY

COMMUNITY ASSESSMENT USING FAMILIARIZATION

A community health nurse named Jean visited the Angelo family on the outskirts of Philadelphia. During the initial visit, she gathered information, learning that the family was Italian American and that there were four children. The father had been out of work for six months; the oldest boy had been in trouble with the juvenile authorities; a younger child was deaf; their house appeared run-down to Jean. She assessed this family, trying to determine its coping ability, its level of health. Furthermore, because community health nursing is population-focused, her concern was not only for the Angelo family but for the population of families with similar problems that this family represented.

However, the nurse's assessment was almost impossible without further knowledge of the community. Was theirs an Italian-American neighborhood with specific cultural influences? What was the extent of unemployment in this city? What were the services for the deaf? Were all the houses in this part of town old and in need of repair? Once the nurse began working with the family, familiarity with the community became even more imperative. She discovered that as a result of the Angelos' low income, family conflicts were intense. The family members seldom got out; they made almost no use of the community's recreational system. Before she could help them make use of it, however, the nurse had to find out what resources were available. As she familiarized herself with the community, she discovered Friends of the Deaf, which sponsored a group for parents of deaf children. The nurse could now help Mr. and Mrs. Angelo become part of that group. A quick survey of the religious system in the community revealed two job transition support groups, one of which would welcome Mr. Angelo. In the meantime, the nurse chose to find out about the welfare system and how this family and other similar families could benefit from its services. Even her own attitude changed as she studied the community. For instance, she discovered that a strike closed down the plant where Mr. Angelo worked for 20 years, and so could view his and others' unemployment from a broader perspective. Using a familiarization assessment helped this nurse to enhance her practice.

Whatever role nurses play in community health promotion, they will want to be making a continuous study, an ongoing assessment. Whether nurses become client advocates, work with the local government, or operate from a nursing agency serving the elderly, a familiarization assessment is prerequisite for their work.

PROBLEM-ORIENTED ASSESSMENT

A third type of community assessment is **problem-oriented assessment** which begins with a single problem and then assesses the community in terms of that problem. Suppose that Jean, the nurse who explored services available for the Angelos' deaf child, had discovered that there were none. Confronted with this problem, one family with one deaf child, she could make a problem-oriented community assessment. Her first step would be to seek to discover the incidence of childhood deafness, both in the community and in the state. Second, the nurse might begin interviewing officials in the schools and health institutions to find out what had been done in the past with such problems. She could check the local library to locate available resources on the subject of deafness. Do they subscribe to *The Deaf American*? Are there interpreters available for adults who use sign language? How do hospitals and courts approach deafness? Are there any clubs or other organizations for deaf adults? Are there school programs for the deaf and where are they located?

The problem-oriented assessment is commonly used when familiarization is not sufficient and a comprehensive assessment is too expensive. This type of assessment responds to a particular need. For an example see Research in Community Health Nursing below. The data collected will be useful in any kind of planning for a community response to the problem.

COMMUNITY SUBSYSTEM ASSESSMENT

In the **community subsystem assessment**, the community health nurse focuses on a single dimension of community life. For example, the nurse might decide to survey churches and religious organizations to discover their roles in the community. What kinds of needs do the leaders in these organizations believe exist? What services do these organizations offer? To what extent are services coordinated within the religious system and between it and other systems in the community?

Research in Community Health Nursing
PROBLEM-ORIENTED COMMUNITY NEEDS ASSESSMENT

Barker, J., Bayne, T., Higgs, Z., Jenkin, S., Murphy, D., & Synoground, G. (1994). Community analysis: a collaborative community practice project. *Public Health Nursing, 11*(2), 113–118.

A concern in many communities is lack of access to health care. To determine the factors that adversely affect access to care, a group of nurses and community members in Washington State conducted a community analysis. Focusing on the problem of access they developed a questionnaire to obtain information from providers regarding barriers to access. As a result four community diagnoses were formulated. One was an "insufficient data base for community-wide planning" due to lack of certain specified data. Two was "inadequate low-income housing" in the county caused by certain specified conditions. Three was "insufficient community resources for low income clients". And four was "lack of use of existing community services" by low-income clients due to certain specified barriers. Analysis of this data will be combined with data derived from a subsequent survey of consumers to be used in community wide planning (Ibid. p.116).

The community subsystem assessment can be a useful way for a team to conduct a more thorough community assessment. If five members of a nursing agency divided up the ten systems in the community, and each person did an assessment of two systems, they could then share their findings and create a more comprehensive picture of the community and its needs.

Community Assessment Methods

Community health needs may be assessed through a variety of methods. Two important methods are surveys and descriptive epidemiological study.

SURVEYS

A **survey** is an assessment method in which a series of questions is used to collect data for analysis of a specific group or area. Surveys are commonly used and provide a broad range of data which is helpful when used in conjunction with other sources or when other sources are not available (Urrutia-Rojas & Aday, 1991). According to Dever (1980, p. 147), "The basic objective of planning and conducting community health surveys is to determine the occurrence and distribution of selected environmental, socioeconomic, and behavioral conditions important to disease control and wellness promotion." Thus, the nurse may choose to conduct a survey to determine such things as health care use patterns, immunization levels, demographic characteristics, or health beliefs and practices. The survey method involves nine steps needed to ensure an adequate design and appropriate collection of data.

1. Establish objectives.
   a. What information is needed?
   b. Why is it needed?
   c. How accurate does it need to be?
2. Define the study population.
   a. What groups will be studied?
   b. What are their distinguishing characteristics (i.e.,age, occupation, location)?
3. Determine data to be collected.
   a. What specific data will be collected (i.e., behavior, opinions, beliefs)?
   b. What sources will provide this data (i.e., records, people)?
   c. How will you measure this data?
4. Select sampling unit.
   a. Will it be an individual, a household, a city block?
   b. What sample size is needed?
   c. What sampling method is most appropriate and feasible?
5. Select contact method.
   a. What will the data gathering method/instrument be (i.e., interviews, telephone calls, questionnaires)?
   b. Will you exclude any types of organizations or facilities (i.e., omit interviews in businesses)?
6. Develop the instrument (i.e., construct questionnaire or interview guide).
7. Organize and conduct the survey.
   a. Identify and train data collectors (i.e., interviewers).
   b. Pretest and adjust instrument.
   c. Supervise actual collection.
   d. Plan for nonresponses or refusals.
8. Process and analyze data.
   a. Code, keypunch, tabulate?
   b. Apply appropriate statistical methods, as indicated.
   c. Determine relationships and significance.
9. Report the results. Include implications and recommendations (Ibid., p. 147).

DESCRIPTIVE EPIDEMIOLOGICAL STUDIES

A second assessment method is a **descriptive epidemiological study** which examines the amount and distribution of a disease or health condition in a population by person (who is affected?), place (where does the condition occur?), and time (when do the cases occur?). In addition to their value in assessing the health status of a population, descriptive epidemiological studies are useful for suggesting what persons may be at greatest risk and where and when the condition might occur. They are also useful for health planning purposes and for suggesting hypotheses of disease etiology. Their design and use are detailed in Chapter 12.

Choice of assessment method varies depending upon the reasons for data collection, goals and objectives of the study, and available resources (see Issues in Community Health Nursing below).It also varies with the theoretical framework the nurse uses to view the community (Hanchett, 1988). That is, the community health nurse's theoretical basis for approaching community assessment will influence her or his purposes and the selection of methodology for conducting the assessment. For example, Neuman's health care systems model forms the basis for the "community-as-client" assessment model developed by Anderson, McFarlane and Helton (1986). Additional methodology resources for assessing community health are available in the list of references and selected readings at the close of this chapter.

What is a Healthy Community?

What is a healthy community? If health practitioners are going to assess a community, set goals for community health, plan to improve the health of a community, and work toward goals, they require some criteria of a

Issues in Community Health Nursing
MAKING COMMUNITY NEEDS ASSESSMENT MANAGEABLE

Community needs assessment is essential in planning services for the community as client. Nonetheless, for many nurses the job can seem formidable. Conducting community assessments can be time consuming, complex, and involve major effort. Two solutions make the entire assessment process, from collection to analysis, manageable and enriching.

The first is collaboration. When assessing the health of communities, nurses operate most effectively and efficiently as members of a community team. A collaborative community practice model (Barker, et al, 1994) provides an opportunity to pool perspectives and ideas, share the work, and enhance the quality of the assessment.

The second solution is to make better use of technology for the entire process of community needs assessment. Faculty and students from the University of Colorado School of Nursing used a computer program format called "The Ethnograph" to code and enter community assessment data from interviews. Other computer applications facilitated the merging of secondary data with primary data, analysis, and presentation of community needs findings. They found that the use of this technology improved the accuracy of their needs analysis, enhanced the richness of the data, increased the ease of the process, and improved the nurses' facility with community needs assessment (Smith and Barton, 1992).

healthy community. Just as health for individuals is relative and changes, all aggregates exist in a relative state of health. New needs emerge every day; the system is threatened or weakened and must respond to maintain equilibrium.

Because of their complexity, criteria for healthy communities must be discussed cautiously. At present, there is not wide agreement on such criteria but four important characteristics of a competent or healthy community are outlined by Cottrell (1976):

1. They can collaborate effectively in identifying community needs and problems.

2. They can achieve a working consensus on goals and priorities.
3. They can agree on ways and means to implement the agreed-upon goals.
4. They can collaborate effectively in the required actions.

These general requirements take one closer to an understanding of a healthy community. However, one must still determine the factors that enable a community's systems to work together in these ways. Cottrell suggests several essential conditions for community competence: (1) commitment of members, (2) self-awareness and awareness of others among groups, (3) clarity of situational (positional) definitions, (4) articulateness of various subgroups, (5) effective communication, (6) conflict containment and accommodation, (7) participation (community involvement), (8) management of relations with the larger society, and (9) machinery for effective decision making. Drawing from this list and other sources (Goeppinger & Baglioni, 1986; Goeppinger, et al, 1982; Muecke, 1984; Klein, 1986), the following descriptors can serve as a guide for assessing a healthy community:

1. A healthy community is one in which members have a high degree of awareness that "we are a community."
2. A healthy community uses its natural resources while taking steps to conserve them for future generations.
3. A healthy community openly recognizes the existence of subgroups and welcomes their participation in community affairs.
4. A healthy community is prepared to meet crises.
5. A healthy community is a problem-solving community; it identifies, analyzes, and organizes to meet its own needs. (See Fig. 9.6)
6. A healthy community has open channels of communication that allow information to flow among all subgroups of citizens in all directions.
7. A healthy community seeks to make each of its systems' resources available to all members of the community.
8. A healthy community has legitimate and effective ways to settle disputes that arise within the community.
9. A healthy community encourages maximum citizen participation in decision making.
10. A healthy community promotes a high level of wellness among all its members.

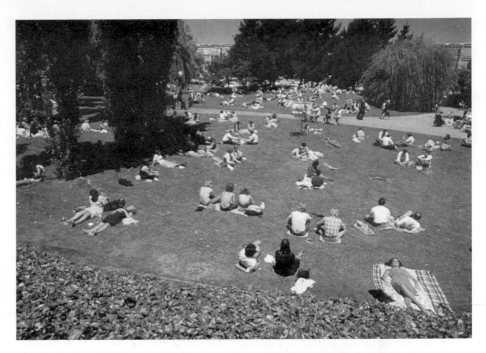

FIGURE 9.6. Neighbors in this northern urban environment worked together to create a local park to enjoy the outdoors during the summer.

Planning for the Health of a Community

Planning for community health is based on assessment of the community. Once community health nurses have this essential information, they can determine needs, rank them, establish goals and objectives, and develop a plan of action (See Levels of Prevention below).

The nursing process, detailed in Chapter 11, again becomes an important tool to facilitate nursing practice, this time with the community as the client. The health planning process reflects most planning methods. Four stages in the health planning process have been proposed (Blum, 1981; Nutt, 1984).

1. Assessment stage
   Determine data needed and collect data.
   Interpret data and identify needs.
   Set goals based on needs.
2. Analysis and design stage
   Analyze findings and set specific objectives.
   Design alternative interventions.
   Analyze and compare pros and cons of various solutions.
   Create a plan.

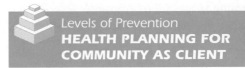

Levels of Prevention
HEALTH PLANNING FOR COMMUNITY AS CLIENT

GOAL

To reduce the incidence of child abuse in a given community by 50% within two years.

PRIMARY PREVENTION

Assess factors contributing to child abuse; identify families in the community at greatest risk (parents with history of child abuse, families under great stress, etc.); institue family life education programs through schools and community groups; develop community resources to support health promtion and protection programs.

SECONDARY PREVENTION

Develop early detection programs through schools, clinics, and physicians' offices; promote enforcement of child protection laws; establish programs to provide prompt treatment for abused children and abusing parents.

TERTIARY PREVENTION

Establish rehabilitation programs for abused children including safer home placement, physical and emotional treatment, self-esteem building.

3. Implementation stage
   Describe how to operationalize the plan.
   Design a method for monitoring progress.
4. Evaluation stage
   Examine costs and benefits of proposed solution.
   Judge the potential outputs, outcomes, and impact of plan.
   Modify to achieve the best plan.
   Present plan to sponsoring group or agency.
   Obtain acceptance (and funding).

Planning for community health programs can be enhanced by the use of conceptual frameworks and models. A model helps to identify target population characteristics for intervention, clarify program goals, and specify nursing interventions and client outcomes (Ervin & Kuehnert, 1993). A planning model also enables the nurse to test ideas and adjust solutions before actual implementation. Ervin and Kuehnert apply a model proposed by McLaughlin (1982) to develop a childhood lead poisoning program. They assert that use of the model enhances the planning process and promotes effectiveness of services as well as professional standards of practice.

A further health planning consideration is that aggregate-level nursing practice requires teamwork. The job of planning for the health of an entire community or a community subsystem requires that the nurse collaborate with other professionals. "Community-wide programs require, above all, more planning and coordination than do small-scale programs" (Green & Anderson, 1986, p. 40). Working with a health board task force to recommend methods for improved communication between health care agencies is one way the nurse works as a team member in serving the community as the client. All sound public health practice depends on pooling resources, including people, in ways that will best serve the public. Whether health service is aimed at families, a group, subpopulation, population, or community, the consumers of that service are equally important members of the team. In planning for a community's health, the community (represented by appropriate individuals and agencies) must be involved. Community health nurses cannot lose sight of the need for client involvement at all levels and in all stages of community health practice.

Summary

A major mission of community health nursing practice is to promote the health of aggregates of people. This focus conflicts with the strong value of individualism in the United States which often distracts nurses from a broad focus. An individualistic focus has led to three pervading myths: (1) that community health nursing involves only clinical nursing in the community setting; (2) that community health nursing employs only the skills of basic nursing; and (3) that the primary client in community health nursing is the individual. In reality, community health nursing is practised in many settings, employs not only basic nursing expertise but adds many important concepts and skills from public health, and focuses primarily on promoting the health of populations and aggregates, not only individuals.

Any geographic community has three important dimensions to consider when assessing its health needs: location, population, and social system. Location may be further analyzed by considering such variables as its boundary, location of health services, geographic features, climate, flora and fauna, and human-made environment. Population, the second dimension, should be analyzed by determining population size, density, composition, rate of growth or decline, cultural differences, social class, and mobility, to help better understand the community. The third important dimension of a community is its social system which includes ten major systems (health, family, economic, education, religious, welfare, political, recreation, legal, and communication) and many subsystems. Each subsystem is composed of organizations whose members assume various roles. A Community Profile Inventory guides the community health nurse in making thorough assessments of all these important facets of a community.

Initial assessment of a community begins with a survey of the major systems to determine how well they are functioning. Evidence of malfunctioning in any part becomes a stimulus for further and more detailed analysis.

Community dynamics, the driving forces that govern a community's functioning, also must be considered when assessing community health. Two factors, in particular, affect community dynamics: citizen participation in community health programs, and the power and decision-making structure. Community health nurses need to encourage community self-care by promoting the community's involvement in, commitment to, and responsibility for, its own health. Nurses also need to recognize the sources of community influence in order to use the system effectively to promote community health.

There are primarily four different types of community assessment: (1) comprehensive assessment which surveys the entire community in depth, (2) familiarization assessment which studies available data, perhaps adding some firsthand data, to gain a general understanding of the community, (3) problem-oriented assessment which focuses on a single problem and studies the community in terms of that problem, and (4) community subsystem assessment which examines a single facet of community life. There are many methods for assessing a community's health. Two important ones are surveys and descriptive epidemiologic studies.

A healthy community has a number of characteristics that health practitioners look for when assessing its health. Among them are a sense of unity, ability to collaborate and communicate effectively, a problem-solving orientation, ability to utilize yet conserve resources, and ability to handle crises and conflict.

Planning for community health draws on a thorough assessment and utilizes the nursing process. Five health planning stages include (1) formulation, (2) conceptualization, (3) detailing, (4) evaluation, and (5) implementation. It involves a team effort by professionals and community personnel.

Activities to Promote Critical Thinking

1. Explain to a colleague why it is important to understand and work with the community as a total entity.

2. How does defining community as client change the community health nurse's practice? List some specific examples of how this concept can be applied.

3. If you were part of a health planning team concerned about the health needs of the elderly in your community, what are some location, population, and social system variables you would want to assess? Name some of the sources from which you might collect the data.

4. Discuss under what circumstances you might choose to conduct a problem-oriented community health assessment? What method would you consider using to conduct this assessment, and how would you carry it out.

5. Interview someone from your state or local health department who has recently conducted a community needs assessment survey. Analyze the process they used comparing that with the nine steps for conducting a survey described in this chapter.

REFERENCES

Allor, M.T. (1983). The "community profile." *Journal of Nursing Education, 22*(1), 12–17.

American Public Health Association. (1981). *The definition and role of public health nursing in the delivery of health care: A statement of the Public Health Nursing Section.* Washington, DC: Author.

Anderson, E., McFarlane, J., & Helton, A. (1986). Community-as-client: A model for practice. *Nursing Outlook, 34*(5), 220–24.

Barker, J., Bayne, T., Higgs, Z., Jenkin, S., Murphy, D., & Synoground, G. (1994). Community analysis: a collaborative community practice project. *Public Health Nursing, 11*(2), 113–118.

Blum, H.L. (1981). *Planning for Health.* New York: Human Sciences Press.

Blumenthal, D. (1985). *Introduction to environmental health.* New York: Springer Publishing.

Campbell, B.F. (1988). Program attunes students to population-focused care. *Nursing and Health Care, 9*(1), 42–45. Caretto, V.A., et al. (1991). Community as client: a "hands on" experience for baccalaureate nursing students. *Journal of Community Health Nursing, 8*(3), 179–189.

Cottrell, L.S., Jr. (1976). The competent community. In B. H. Kaplan, R.N. Wilson, and A. H. Leighton (Eds.). *Further explorations in social psychiatry* (pp. 195-209). New York: Basic Books.

Dever, G.E.A. (1980). *Community health analysis: A holistic approach.* Germantown, MD: Aspen Systems.

Dever, G.E.A. (1991). *Community health analysis: Global awareness at the local level* (2nd ed.). Gaithersburg, MD: Aspen.

Dunn, A.M. & Decker, S. (1990). Community as client: appropriate baccalaureate- and graduate-level preparation. *Journal of Community Health Nursing, 7*(3), 131–139.

Ervin, N.E. & Kuehnert, P.L. (1993). Application of a model for public health nursing program planning. *Public Health Nursing, 10*(1), 25–30.

Flynn, B., Gottschalk, J., Ray, D., Selmanoff, E. (1978). One masters curriculum in community health nursing. *Nursing Outlook, 26*, 633–37.

Freeman, H.E., Levine, S., & Reeder, L.G. (Eds.). (1979). *Handbook of medical sociology* (3rd ed.). Englewood Cliffs, NJ: Prentice-Hall.

Goeppinger, J., Lassiter, P., & Wilcox, B. (1982). Community health is community competence. *Nursing Outlook, 30,* 464–67.

Goeppinger, J. & Baglioni, J.P., Jr. (1986). Community competence: A positive approach to needs assessment. *American Journal of Community Psychology, 13,* 507–23.

Goode, W. J. (1977). *Principles of sociology.* New York: McGraw-Hill.

Green, L. & Anderson, C.L. (1986). *Community health.* St. Louis: Times Mirror/Mosby.

Hanchett, E. S. (1988). *Nursing frameworks and community as client: Bridging the gap.* East Norwalk, CT: Appleton and Lange.

Kinlein, L. (1978). Nursing and family and community health. *Family and Community Health, 1*(1), 57–68.

Klein, D. C. (1986). Assessing community characteristics. In B. Spradley (Ed.), *Readings in community health nursing* (3rd ed.). Boston: Little, Brown.

Lynd, R. (1939). *Knowledge for what? The place of social science in American culture.* Princeton: Princeton University Press.

McKnight, J. & Van Dover, L. (1994). Community as client: a challenge for nursing education. *Public Health Nursing, 11*(1), 12–16.

McLaughlin, J.S. (1982). Toward a theoretical model for community health programs. *Advances in Nursing Sciences, 5*(1), 7–28.

Merriam-Webster. (1993). Merriam-Websterr's Collegiate Dictionary (10th ed.). Springfield, MA: Author.

Milbank Memorial Fund Commission. (1976). *Higher education for public health: A report.* New York: Prodist.

Muecke, M.A. (1984). Community health diagnosis in nursing. *Public Health Nursing, 1,* 23–33.

Nagi, S.Z. (1959, October). Factors related to heart disease among Ohio farmers. *Ohio Agricultural Experiment Station Research Bulletin,* p. 842.

Neuber, K.A., Atkins, W.T., Jacobson, J.A., & Reuterman, N.A. (1980). *Needs assessment: A model for community planning.* Beverly Hills: Sage.

Neuman, B. (1982). *The Neuman systems model: Application to nursing education and practice.* Norwalk, CT: Appleton-Century-Crofts.

Nutt, P. (1984). *Planning methods for health and related organizations.* New York: Wiley.

Pickett, G. & Hanlon, J. (1990). *Public Health: Administration and practice* (9th ed.). St. Louis: Times/Mirror Mosby.

Redesigning nursing education for public health: Report of the conference (Pub. No. 75-75). (1973). Bethesda, Md.: U.S. Department of Health, Education and Welfare.

Ruybal, S.E., Bauwens, E., & Fasla, M. (1975). Community assessment: An epidemiological approach. Nursing Outlook 23:365-68.

Sanders, I.T. & Brownlee, A. (1979). Health in the community. In H. E. Freeman, S. Levine, & L.G. Reeder (Eds.), *Handbook of medical sociology* (3rd ed., pp. 412-33). Englewood Cliffs, NJ: Prentice-Hall.

Shamansky, S. & Pesznecker, B. (1981). A community is... *Nursing Outlook, 29,* 182–85.

Smith, M.C. & Barton, J.A. (1992). Technologic enrichment of a community needs assessment. *Nursing Outlook, 40*(1), 33–37.

Urrutia-Rojas, X. & Aday, L.A. (1991). A framework for community assessment: Designing and conducting a survey in a Hispanic immigrant and refugee community. *Public Health Nursing, 8*(1), 20–26.

West, M. (1984). Community health assessment: The man-environment interaction. *Journal of Community Health Nursing, 1*(2), 89–97.

White, J.E. & Valentine, V.L. (1993). Computer assisted video instruction and community assessment. *Nursing and Health Care 14*(7), 349–353.

Williams, C.A. (1992). Community-based population-focused practice: the foundation of specialization in public health nursing. In M. Stanhope and J. Lancaster (Eds.), *Community health nursing: process and practice for promoting health.* St.Louis: Mosby.

Williams, C.A. (1985). Population-focused community health nursing and nursing administration: A new synthesis. In J.C. McCloskey & H. K. Grace (Eds.), *Current issues in nursing* (2nd ed.). Boston: Blackwell Scientific Publications, Ltd.

SELECTED READINGS

Archer, S.E., Kelly, C.D., & Bisch, S.A. (1984). *Implementing change in communities: A collaborative process.* St. Louis: C. V. Mosby.

Balacki, M.F. (1988). Assessing mental health needs in the rural community: a critique of assessment approaches. *Issues in Mental Health Nursing, 9*(3), 299–315.

Barton, J., Smith, M., Brown, N., & Supples, J. (1993). Methodological issues in a team approach to community health needs assessment. *Nursing Outlook, 41*(6), 253–261.

Dean, D., et al. (1988). Local health planning: a report of a collaborative process between a university and a church. *Family & Community Health, 10*(4), 13–22.

Ekstrand, C., et al. (1992). Using public health nursing data for program advocacy. *Journal of Nursing Administration, 22*(4), 32–36.

Finnegan, L. & Ervin, N.E. (1989). An epidemiological approach to community assessment. *Public Health Nursing, 6*(3), 147–151.

Goeppinger, J. (1988). Challenges in assessing the impact of nursing services: A community perspective. *Public Health Nursing, 5*(4), 241–245.

Green, L. & Kreuter, M. (1991). *Health promotion planning: An educational and environmental approach.* Mountain View, CA: Mayfield.

Hamilton, P. (1985). Community nursing diagnosis. *Advances in Nursing Science, 5,* 21–36.

Jewell, M.L., et al. (1989). An assessment guide for community health nurses. *Home Healthcare Nurse, 7*(5), 32–36.

Kuehnert, P. (1991). The public health policy advocate: Fostering the health of communities. *Clinical Nurse Specialist, 5*(1), 5–10.

McKnight, J., et al. (1991). The delphi approach to strategic planning. *Nursing Management, 22*(4), 55–57.

Milio, N. (1975). *The care of health in communities: Access for outcasts.* New York: Macmillan.

Nettle, C., Laboon, P., Jones, N., Pavelicch, J., Pifer, P., & Beltz, C. (1989). Community health nursing diagnosis. *Journal of Community Health Nursing, 6*(3), 135–145.

Powell, M, Faghfoury, N., Hill, K., & Nyenhuis, P. (1989). Fostering public participation. *Health Promotion, 27*(2), 5–8.

Rivera, S.J. & Palmer-Willis, H. (1991). County nursing ser8(4), 264–266.

Rogers, S. (1984). Community as client: A multivariate model for analysis of community aggregate health risk. *Public Health Nursing, 1,* 210–22.

Ruffing-Rahel, M.A. (1985). Qualitative methods in community analysis. *Public Health Nursing, 2,* 130–37.

Thomas, E. (1990). Mapping community health. *Community Outlook 6,* 8.

Wickizer, T., Von Korff, M., Cheadle, A., Maeser, J., Wagner, E., Pearson, D., Beery, W., & Psaty, B. (1993). Activating communities for health promotion: a process evaluation method. *American Journal of Public Health, 83*(4), 561–567.

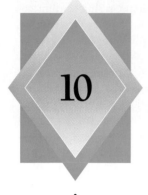

CHAPTER

10

Working with Populations and Groups

LEARNING OBJECTIVES

Upon completion of this chapter, readers should be able to:

- Differentiate between five different kinds of groups with whom community health nurses work.
- Identify essential group needs.
- Describe the elements to be considered in starting a group.
- Explain the significance of group cohesiveness.
- Identify the phases of group development.
- Describe and practice group leader and member roles and functions.
- Assist a group through termination.
- Design both process and outcome evaluation of group goals.
- Differentiate between groups and populations.
- Articulate strategies for working with populations.
- Compare similarities in working with groups and populations.

KEY TERMS

- Conflict
- Counterdependence phase
- Dependence phase
- Group
- Group cohesiveness
- Interdependence phase
- Learning group
- Maintenance roles

- Outcome evaluation
- Population
- Process evaluation
- Psychotherapy group
- Socialization group
- Support group
- Task-oriented group
- Task roles

Barbara Walton Spradley and Judith Ann Allender
COMMUNITY HEALTH NURSING: CONCEPTS AND PRACTICE, 4th ed.
© 1996 Barbara Walton Spradley and Judith Ann Allender

Community health offers nurses a considerable challenge: to promote the health of groups and populations. Outside public health, no other health discipline has aggregates as its primary concern or the entire community's health as its trust. For the community health nurse, then, the challenge is two-fold—first, to adopt an aggregate orientation for practice and second, to develop skills in working with aggregates.

How do nurses work with aggregates? The purpose of this chapter is to explore how the community health nurse works with populations and groups of all sizes. The chapter begins by examining how to work with small groups because they are more familiar. Then knowledge of groups is applied to subpopulations and larger aggregates in the community.

Understanding and Working with Small Groups

Small groups are an important part of community health nursing service. Nurses meet the collective needs of many elements of the community population through work with groups. Each collection of people—a parenting group, a mastectomy club, a group of Southeast Asian refugees learning a new culture, a school health committee, or a group of developmentally disabled clients—has different needs. Some groups function for the purpose of problem solving, others for sharing, support, learning, or therapy. Whatever the reason for the group and regardless of whether the nurse serves as leader or member, basic knowledge and skill with groups enables the nurse to facilitate group process and outcomes.

All nurses have had experience with groups. One's first group encounter is with the family, which is known as a primary group because it is one of several basic, informal social groups to which people belong during their lifetime (Sampson & Marthas, 1981). As individuals grow, their primary groups extend to include childhood peer groups, associations with neighbors, friendship groups, and other social affiliations. Informal and generally social in nature, primary groups function with spontaneous and unstructured communication.

In addition to primary groups, people also experience secondary, or formal, group relationships (Robbins, 1993). These groups usually exist for a specific purpose and include professional associations, therapeutic groups, work-related relationships, educational gatherings, and community affiliations. Examples are a student council, an exercise group, a patients' rights committee, and an assertiveness training class. These groups emphasize completing a job and accomplishing specific goals.

Although nurses spend much of their adult lives participating in formal and informal groups, how well do they understand such groups and how they function? With an increasing number of the community health nurse's activities taking place in and for groups—client groups, community groups, work groups, and others—the nurse's need for group skills becomes ever more important. Before considering groups and ways in which nurses can work more effectively with them, it is important to understand what a group is.

DEFINITION OF A GROUP

Robbins defines a group as "two or more individuals, interacting and interdependent, who have come together to achieve particular objectives" (1993, p. 285). A **group** is a collection of persons who engage in repeated, face-to-face communication, identify with each other, experience interdependence, and share a common purpose or purposes. This definition suggests several characteristics of groups. A group must consist of at least two people, but it can never be so large that members cannot maintain direct communication with one another (Clark, 1994; Veninga, 1982). Because their collective social interaction influences the way they think, members assume similar values and norms and establish a sense of belonging to each other. Konopka (1954) refers to this characteristic as the development of "bonds," the links that connect individuals and create a group from a mass of loosely related people. Furthermore, the members of a group are interdependent; that is, they need and help each other. As Konopka points out, human beings need to belong to groups: "group life . . . gives the individual security and nourishment so that he can fulfill his greatest promise while helping others to fulfill theirs too" (1954, p. 22). At the same time, the group molds its members' behavior and attitudes, thus developing its own personality, or identity (Veninga, 1982). Finally, group members share one or more common purposes. They have a reason for being a group. Whether a group forms to lobby for new playground equipment, to support persons experiencing a crisis, to exercise together, or to promote parenting skills, its members share a common purpose. This characteristic becomes clearer in discussing types of groups.

Consider some examples of how these group characteristics influence the health of clients. Steve discovered when he was 15 years of age that he had epilepsy. The fact was difficult to accept, particularly because he had just been elected captain of his swim team. He was afraid that epilepsy meant an end to his future in swimming. After a seizure at work, his boss fired him. A period of several months of bitterness and frustration followed, and then he was invited to attend an epilepsy club recently formed in his high school. All members of this group knew what it was like to be epileptic. Many of them had undergone experiences similar to Steve's and could truly empathize with him. They helped him see that others shared his same problems and fears and that he could look forward to living a near normal life. They gave him a new sense of hope. The attitudes and behavior of the group gradually helped shape his feelings about himself so that he could accept his diagnosis and start developing constructive plans for his life.

Not all groups influence people positively. Some groups generate negative peer pressure and influence. For example, Nancy, once a good student, became a hard drug user. Her group of friends used drugs and made fun of anyone who did well in school. In order to be accepted in this group, Nancy began taking drugs too.

Groups are powerful. Although groups meet basic individual needs for belonging, security, safety, and the opportunity to help others, they also shape their members' thinking and behavior through internal processes of acceptance and rejection (see Fig. 10.1). They can be either a constructive or destructive force in people's lives. Nurses' concern in community health is to facilitate the constructive use of groups for client health.

As the nurse prepares to work with a group, she or he will need to know the answers to three important questions. First, what types of groups are there? Second, what are the essential needs of groups? Third, what are the major functions of a group?

TYPES OF SMALL GROUPS

Community health nurses work with many different kinds of small groups. Since each group forms for some purpose, they can be categorized according to their primary goals. There are five types of small groups with which community health nurses work: learning groups, support groups, socialization groups, psychotherapy groups, and task-oriented groups.

Learning Groups

The primary goal of a **learning group** is to have its members gain understanding in order to effect behavioral change in some specified area of need. Many community health nurses lead prenatal groups. The parents-

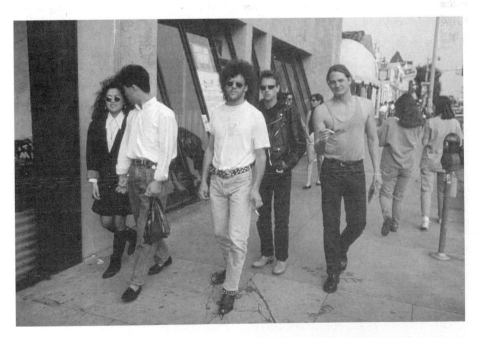

FIGURE 10.1. Peer pressure is a powerful influence on dress and behavior.

to-be have many practices to learn, such as exercises, diet, breathing techniques, and what to do during labor and delivery. For each topic, nurses leading these groups make certain that the needed information is covered and, when appropriate, they demonstrate its application. The parents-to-be practice their new skills regularly at home, and the nurse-leader may ask them to display their understanding by demonstrating what they have learned to the group. This learning group will have met its goals when the members have assimilated knowledge to the point that it changes their behavior (See Fig. 10.2).

A class can be considered a learning group if it meets certain criteria of a group. That is, the members of a group have repeated interaction and communication, identify with each other, and are interdependent. The function of a learning group is to use the benefits of group identity and interaction to accomplish learning and behavioral change (Payne, 1993). In the cases of both classes and learning groups, the nurse is giving information to a number of people at once. However, learning groups, in contrast to most lecture classes, use group commitment and reinforcement to produce desired behavior changes. Group members may actually practice natural childbirth, control hypertension, or maintain a postcoronary diet and exercise program. Individuals in these groups not only learn what to do and how to do it (the limit of most classes), but also have the advantage of group influence to promote and stabilize their practices at a healthier level.

The composition of a learning group varies widely and depends upon the group's goals. Some groups may be gender-related, such as one with a goal of teaching assertiveness to females, or age-related, such as a group goal aimed at preparing people for retirement which would probably include members at midlife or approaching retirement. Other learning groups are determined by their members' shared interest in a topic, such as those concerned with weight loss, leadership training, or learning how to manage diabetes. The chief common denominator of most learning groups, however, is that the members are people who desire to gain information about some subject and to better themselves as a result.

The nurse's role will vary depending upon whether she or he initiates and leads the group, participates as a member, or participates as an outside consultant, such as with self-help groups like Weight Watchers or Alcoholics Anonymous. Nevertheless, the nurse's role in any learning group includes providing some degree of structure and focus to the group's activities. The nurse also uses the basic teaching-learning principles described in Chapter 14 to encourage client interest in, and application of, the information presented.

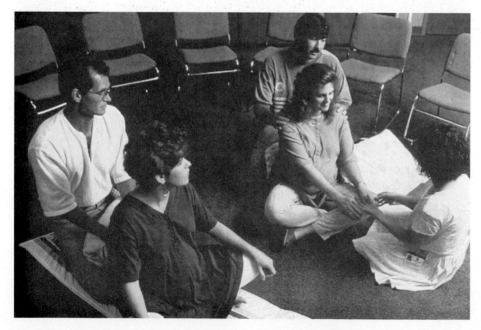

FIGURE 10.2. These expectant parents are learning techniques to promote relaxation and comfort during labor.

Support Groups

The primary goal of a **support group** (sometimes called a therapeutic group) is to promote healthy behaviors and prevent maladaptive coping patterns among its members (Balk, et al., 1993). These groups are composed of emotionally healthy people (not needing psychiatric help) caught in some change or crisis, such as divorce or post-partum depression. In community health, nurses encounter many people who already have good health practices but who need help during these times of stress. The support of other people enables them to adapt and preserve their healthy behaviors (Olson, et al., 1991; Pesznecker & Zahlis, 1986). Support groups meet this need. For example, a woman undergoing the ordeal of a mastectomy often experiences feelings of loss, disfigurement, and fear, in addition to physical weakness and discomfort. Members of mastectomy clubs share feelings and concerns and offer comfort and support to each other. Their shared experiences and the support and acceptance of the group often give members the courage they need to face the future and go on with their lives.

Other examples of support groups include parenting groups for the purpose of reassurance and reinforcement of personal resources (Booth, 1990; Kagey et al., 1981) and job transition support groups with a primary goal of giving emotional support to those undergoing the stress of major job changes. Sometimes these groups may have secondary learning goals to help members learn strategies to change their situation such as a lecture on the interview process for those in job transition. A support group for relatives coping with mentally ill family members (Kane, et al., 1990) or for family caregivers experiencing stress and burnout (Lindgren, 1990) are other examples. Support groups seek to maintain and use their members' existing strengths, help them cope successfully, and regain their equilibrium (see Fig. 10.3).

Support groups sometimes serve an advocacy role as well. They can plead the cause of their members whose physical and emotional health, job security, or social status may be threatened because of their current problem. Alcoholics Anonymous, while primarily a support group, represents a strong social force working in favor of its members' rehabilitation and constructive participation in the community. The Gray Panthers, a senior citizens' lobbying group, promotes the causes of the elderly while providing them with a group with which they can identify and from which they can derive sustenance.

Nurses working with support groups aim to facilitate group interactions, but their most important role is to model acceptance and caring. Demonstrating a warm, understanding attitude with, for example, a smoking cessation group or a group of individuals grieving the

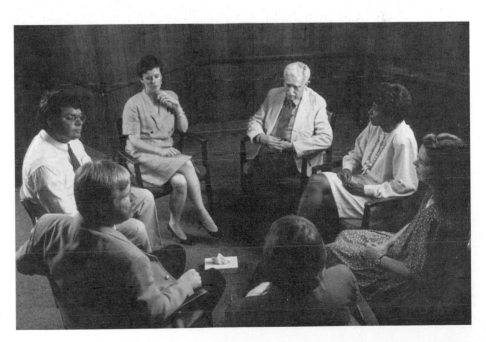

FIGURE 10.3. Members of a support group share common experiences and strengths to facilitate healthy coping behaviors.

loss of spouses encourages members to assume these same caring feelings and to create a supportive climate. This approach energizes individuals to resume responsible, healthy behaviors.

Socialization Groups

A **socialization group** is composed of people who meet together to learn new social roles in order to achieve a positive level of health. Their old patterns of behavior are inappropriate, nonfunctional, sometimes detrimental, or at least a source of uneasiness in the larger society. Some Native Americans, accustomed to living on a remote reservation, have difficulty adjusting to urban living. Latino refugees, flocking to American cities in increasing numbers, experience even greater culture shock. Contrasting patterns of food preparation, eating, living, rearing children, and health practices, as well as language barriers and value differences, all call for adaptation in order for these clients to function in the new culture. Even armed services veterans returning from overseas experience some degree of culture shock upon re-entry to the United States. They must adjust to new values, clothing styles, social relationships, as well as political and economic changes. Some individuals in our society have lived in a confined subculture, such as a mental hospital, a prison, or a school for the deaf, and upon discharge must learn new ways of behaving. All of these individuals can benefit from a socialization group.

A socialization group should not be confused with a purely social group in which members come together for friendship, enjoyment, and support, such as a bridge club, bowling league, or bird-watching group. The elderly often need information about such social activity groups in their area and encouragement, even assistance, to participate. But social activity groups are not considered a socialization group in which the community health nurse works.

The primary goal of a socialization group is to help its members learn new social roles. The nurse's role in a socialization group is first to demonstrate caring and acceptance of the group's members, to respect their present values and behaviors. The nurse also provides structure and focus to the group process. For example, with discharged mental patients or a refugee enculturation group, the nurse can encourage members to share their experiences and help them learn ways of coping with their new life-style. The mental patients may discuss how to interview for a job, how to meet people, or how to behave at parties. Topics such as shopping in a supermarket, how to ride a bus, or what to expect when one goes to a health clinic might be discussed in the refugee group. The nurse uses group support to give these people courage to give up their familiar practices and group influence to help them learn new roles.

Psychotherapy Groups

Psychotherapy groups are formed to promote the health of people with an emotional disturbance. Many clients in community health have emotional problems ranging from minor neuroses to severe maladjustments. Psychotherapy groups can serve a variety of needs including, those families in which child abuse or parent abuse occurs, married couples in conflict, chemically dependent persons, and those with suicidal impulses. These individuals may be referred by a family member, neighbor, professional worker, or agency. They may also refer themselves. Some receive group therapy following individual counseling; others are able to gain all the help they need from a psychotherapy group alone.

The primary goal of psychotherapy groups is to provide members insight into themselves and to help members change their behavior. The group focuses on how its members relate to themselves and to each other; it becomes a "social microcosm" (Loomis, 1979, p. 10). That is, the group serves as a minisociety, allowing members to display their negative feelings and behaviors in an accepting and corrective milieu. An occasional group member may not be ready or willing to participate in this method of self-change and may need to be counseled in some other setting.

Some nurses in community health have advanced training and experience in group psychotherapy and serve as therapists for these groups. More often, the community health nurse is a cotherapist working with a psychiatrist, psychologist, or psychiatric social worker. For example, a nurse and psychiatric social worker, working together, led a psychotherapy group for delinquent adolescent girls. They considered many behaviors, but they focused on the girls' tendency to "run away," to avoid anything perceived as unpleasant. The nurse's role included demonstrating acceptance and caring, encouraging the girls to share their feelings, helping them to understand the reasons behind their feelings and behavior, and providing structure and focus to the group process.

Task-Oriented Groups

A final category of small groups with which community health nurses work includes **task-oriented groups** whose purpose is to accomplish certain tasks toward meeting specified goals (Robbins, 1993). In community health there are many complex problems to solve, decisions to make, and tasks to accomplish that require a collaborative effort (Callahan, 1980). Examples of task-oriented groups include a nursing team in a public health agency trying to determine the proper method for supervising home health aides; a day-care center seeking to develop new health and safety policies; a community task force developing a proposal for new jogging and bicycle trails; and a local elementary school planning a health fair. Each of these tasks can be accomplished by people contributing their unique perspectives and skills, and working together as a group. Community health nurses play a significant part in this process.

Membership in task-oriented groups varies but generally encompasses clients, community residents, and health-related professionals. Client task-oriented groups often form spontaneously out of a desire to improve an existing situation, such as retirees becoming involved in a foster grandparenting program. The community health nurse may work with a group of clients whose goal is to accomplish some task but whose collaboration also serves other health-related functions. One such group was made up of mothers who wanted to redecorate the waiting room of a well-child clinic. The nurse helped them plan and implement a fundraising rummage sale and worked as a group member during the redecoration. Group cohesiveness developed as a result of the many hours spent together, and the nurse was able to form an ongoing mothers' support group with these women.

Community residents frequently initiate task-oriented groups in which community health nurses participate. For example, two community health nurses served on a local community council's planning committee to develop a hypertension screening program. In contrast, a nurse may initiate a task-oriented group involving community residents such as convening a group to develop a friendly visitor program for elderly shut-ins.

Professional task-oriented groups are a frequent part of community health nursing practice (see Fig. 10.4). They might include an agency nursing work group (Hernandez, et al, 1988), a state nursing association subcommittee, a state health planning commission, or an environmental safety task force. In these groups, the nurse, whether leader or member, works with other

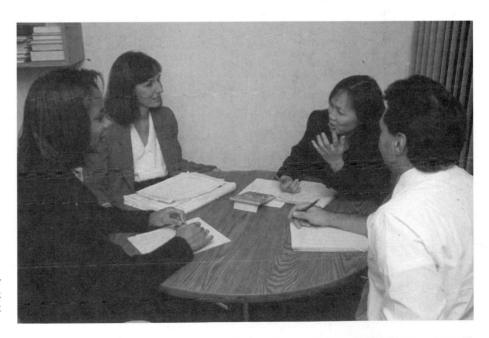

FIGURE 10.4 A community health nurse serves on a task force discussing ways to prevent gang violence.

health-related professionals to accomplish specific tasks (Rankin, et al., 1993). For example, a community health nurse in St. Paul, Minnesota, chaired a subcommittee of the Metropolitan Health Board to study ways and means of facilitating greater collaboration between health care agencies. In addition to consumer members, the committee included health care administrators from public and private agencies, nurses, physicians, and health planners.

The nurse's role in task-oriented groups varies depending upon whether the nurse is the leader or a member of the group. Later, this chapter examines group leader and member roles in more detail. In either case, however, the nurse works to facilitate group progress toward goal achievement.

Table 10.1 summarizes the five types of small groups with which community health nurses work by listing each type's primary goal, membership, and nurse's role.

ESSENTIAL GROUP NEEDS

A group, as an entity, has a different set of needs that must be satisfied and maintained in order to allow optimal group functioning. Four essential small-group needs are shared goals, consistent norms, motivation, and communication (Clark, 1994; Veninga, 1982; Sampson & Marthas, 1981).

Shared Goals

First, a group needs an agreed-upon goal and a shared understanding about the means for its achievement. No purposeful small group can function for long if its members have different ideas about what it is trying to accomplish. A group learning about family planning, for instance, can make little progress if some members define it as a sex education class, others join to help influence people against abortion, and some use it as a social outlet. The group must be solidly behind its stated goals if members are to work together and accomplish desired results.

Consistent Norms

Second, a group needs consistency in its norms. That is, there must be some continuity and stability in the internal rules and policies, spoken and unspoken, that govern the group's actions (Loomis, 1979; Veninga, 1982). Every group has to establish ground rules for operating. These rules govern areas such as membership eligibility, attendance requirements, whether or not new members can join after the group is in progress, what kind of participation is expected of each member, and what is expected of the leader. If rules and policies are ignored or frequently broken, the structure of the

TABLE 10.1. Types of Small Groups in Community Health

Type of Group	Primary Goal	Membership	Nurse's Role
Learning	Develop and apply knowledge	People desiring information and improvement in their lives	Provide structure and focus for group process
Support	Maintain healthy behavior and prevent maladaptive coping	Emotionally healthy people needing support during change or crisis	Present role model of acceptance and caring Facilitate group interaction
Socialization	Learn new social roles	People adapting to a new culture or subculture	Offer acceptance and caring Provide structure and focus for group process
Psychotherapy	Gain insight into self and change behavior	People needing treatment of an emotional disturbance	Offer acceptance and caring Encourage sharing of feelings Help members understand the reasons behind their feelings and behavior Provide structure and focus for group process
Task-oriented	Accomplish task	People assigned to or volunteering to complete a job	Facilitate progress toward goal achievement

group is weakened, members do not feel secure, and the group eventually is unable to function.

Motivation

Third, a group needs members motivated to do their various jobs. Many variables influence motivation; among them are leader power and charisma, degree of member commitment to group goals and group success, how well individual needs are being met, group cohesiveness, and members' sense of belonging. Group goals can be accomplished only through collaborative effort; unless members do their share of the work, the job does not get done. Nor can the group function if members are lazy or morale is low. Each member has a unique role to play and, as for any system, the group's viability depends on the proper functioning of all its parts.

Communication

Fourth, every group needs stable communication channels among the members (Veninga, 1982). No group can function without a dependable system for giving and receiving information. The effectiveness of a divorce support group depends on members' ability to share their feelings of anger, rejection, or loneliness freely and to receive accepting, understanding responses in return. The work of a committee to study safety hazards in a summer camp cannot be done without an active exchange of ideas. Were it not for demonstrated acceptance and caring and constant two-way communication to help members gain insight into their feelings and behavior, a psychotherapy group would have minimal success. In order to function, all groups require viable lines of communication.

GROUP FUNCTIONS

Every small group serves two types of functions: a task-related function and a group maintenance function (Robbins, 1993; Veninga, 1982). The task function focuses on completing the job, while the maintenance function deals with how members are interacting. The former is goal-related and instrumental; the latter is member-related and interpersonal.

Consider how a student council operates. Part of the group's focus will be on the task dimension. Members will explore ideas, make plans, decide on jobs to be done, keep discussions on target, and make certain that members have done their delegated tasks. The other part of the group's concentration is on the maintenance dimension, which includes responsibilities such as keeping up group morale, making certain that individual members' needs are met, encouraging and praising members' accomplishments, and mediating conflicts.

A well-functioning group emphasizes both task and maintenance concerns. You may have experienced membership in a group that focused so heavily on tasks that the interpersonal dimension was neglected. This situation happens most often in task-oriented groups, such as committees, where the job to be done becomes so important that it is accomplished at the expense of members' feelings. Internal dissatisfaction develops, resulting in poor attendance, disruptive behavior, or withdrawal. Everyone expects and needs to get something from group membership; if they do not, they will either drop out or possibly disrupt the group in some way. On the other hand, a group that concentrates too heavily on the interpersonal dimension may have happy members but not accomplish its goals. An appropriate balance between task and maintenance functions is needed.

The Process of Working with Groups

How can community health nurses work more effectively with groups? The following are the six major processes in which a community health nurse will be involved while working with small groups:

1. Preparing for small-group work occurs before the group begins, but may continue after the group forms. Preparation involves knowing the nature of groups, types of groups, and their functions and needs.
2. Starting a group involves specific activities to help the group begin work.
3. Building group cohesiveness is essential during the early growth of a group.
4. Working with a group involves recognizing its developmental phases, assuming appropriate leader and member roles, and solving various sorts of problems that arise.
5. Terminating a group begins early in the group's life and requires specific interventions.
6. Evaluating a group occurs in two dimensions: one examines group process as well as the outcomes of the group's work.

STARTING A GROUP

When any group is about to be formed, certain questions must be answered. First, does a group need or wish to form, and who initiates that process? In some instances, several people may come together because they have identified a reason for meeting. Their common concern prompts the group's formation. Sometimes an outside person or agency, such as Alcoholics Anonymous, starts a new group in the community. On other occasions, a nurse, having identified a need, may be the initiator. For example, a community health nurse with several postpartum clients in her caseload may suggest that they meet as a group for mutual support and shared information. Or a nurse may contact several local churches and offer to form a group of interested volunteers who would begin making friendly visits to shut-ins. Initial formation of a group is based on identifying a need—determining a reason or reasons for people to get together—then convening the group. Once the decision is made to form the group, other questions must be addressed. Who should the members be? What is the best size for this group? What are the group's needs, and what should its goals be? Where should it meet, and what type of physical arrangements would best suit its purpose? How can members be oriented to facilitate effective group development and group process? The following section considers the answers to each of these questions separately.

Selecting Members

A group's membership is determined by several factors. One is the group's general purpose. If it is task-oriented, its members should be people who have expertise or skills pertinent to accomplishing the task. If its purpose is support, the members will be people who are experiencing change or crisis and need emotional reinforcement. In other words, the members should have something in common that relates to the group's primary goal.

Members should also exhibit similarities relative to the group's specific goals. Sometimes age- or sex-specific membership is necessary. For example, a support group for men in midlife crisis would limit its membership to middle-aged men. A preschoolers' mothers' group aiming to understand early childhood growth and development and learn appropriate mothering responses would limit its membership to young mothers. In other groups, the members may be very dissimilar in age, sex, or social

role, but have some other common denominator. A weight-loss group, for instance, might be composed of members of a variety of ages and both sexes since obesity is their shared concern. The epileptic support group mentioned earlier included young people from grade school through high school. Their variant ages and sexes gave a broader range of perspectives to group discussion and further enhanced the group's value. Their common denominator was epilepsy.

Members should choose to be part of the group. Any group member who does not participate willingly is not likely to benefit from or contribute positively to the group. If, for example, a client is coerced into a psychotherapy group or a professional is drafted reluctantly to serve on a health committee, they may be passive or absent, cause conflict, or disrupt the group process.

One should also select members on the basis of their commitment to the group's success. People who are genuinely interested in the group's goals and motivated to work for their accomplishment will gain more from the group experience and make a greater contribution to its process and outcomes. There is strong evidence of this contribution particularly in self-help groups, such as Alcoholics Anonymous, where group loyalty and commitment accomplish significant results.

Finally, leaders are helped by selecting members with whom they enjoy working and are more likely to be effective. Some leaders enjoy working with challenging groups, such as drug addicts, while groups with a strong commitment to change may be more satisfying for others. As Loomis points out, "Therapists should be encouraged to become familiar with their own personal characteristics and preferences in the selection of clients" (1979, p. 52). This factor clearly affects a group's success.

Determining Group Size

Group size affects performance (Robbins, 1993; Veninga, 1982). The larger the group, the longer it takes to reach decisions, especially if consensus is required. In addition, the subgroups that almost always develop within larger groups can polarize interests, create conflicts, and impede group progress.

Group size also influences satisfaction. Research shows that as a group expands, the individual member's satisfaction declines (Sampson & Marthas, 1981). The larger the group, the less likely is the opportunity for all members to participate. In a large group, a few people usually do most of the talking while the rest are either intimidated, bored, or dissatisfied to the point of choosing not to participate.

Large groups do exist; examples are professional nursing groups, parent-teacher-student associations, student bodies, and older adults' clubs. In order to meet specific group needs, however, formal, purposeful groups must divide into smaller units of workable size. Loomis emphasizes: "It is not good clinical practice to remain with too large a group simply because there are not enough funds available to start a second group. Client needs and group task should be the primary consideration in determining group size" (1979, p. 61).

The ideal number of members in a group varies, depending upon the situation and the group goals. To allow an appropriate mix of members and enough people to promote good interaction, a group should have at least five or six members. Ten to twelve members is considered the maximum size before subgroups start to form. The optimal size for any talk-oriented group that aims at problem solving, support, learning, insight, or behavior change is six to ten members (Loomis, 1979; Veninga, 1982). The choice of seven members is often preferred for providing the best balance of variety of ideas with opportunity for all members to participate.

Setting Group Goals

Goals and objectives for the group are established on the basis of need. Assessment, that important step in the nursing process, must be taken to determine needs. Every group must identify its needs before setting goals. The process involves collecting and interpreting data, and then making a diagnosis and developing a plan for making needed changes. A detailed discussion of needs assessment, diagnosis, and goal setting is provided in Chapter 11. A community health nurse, working with an interpreter, started a socialization group for deaf students graduating from a state residential school for the deaf to help prepare them for reentry into the hearing world. The nurse's assessment showed that they were concerned about functioning in a hearing world, getting jobs, developing a social life, applying to colleges, and planning careers. On the basis of these needs, the group established its goals and objectives.

Setting goals is a group activity involving all members. Unless members participate in this process, it is possible that their expectations for the group will differ (Callahan, 1980). Members and leader together need to agree on the group's major goals and its specific objectives, the activities that will ensure the desired out-

comes. It is often helpful to negotiate a group contract in which the nurse-leader and members mutually agree on their expectations for the group and the manner in which the outcomes will be achieved. Negotiating a fee for service with some groups is an important element in the contract and contributes to group commitment (Loomis, 1979).

Making Physical Arrangements

Where, how, and when a group meets influences its productivity significantly. The meeting place must be conveniently located, perhaps near a bus line, in order to be accessible to members. It must also have appropriate facilities, such as wheelchair access or parking space, to accommodate members' needs.

Space is another consideration. Some groups, such as an exercise group or a first-aid demonstration class, need a larger meeting area in order to accomplish their goals. Other groups function best in a more intimate setting that is conducive to sharing and expressing feelings; for them, a smaller room works best.

Seating arrangements can influence group process. If chairs are set in classroom style, there is a tendency for members to direct their comments only to the leader. Many task-oriented groups, such as committees, work around long tables. It is difficult for members along the sides of the tables to have eye contact with others along the same side. As a result, communication is inhibited and group cohesiveness is slower to develop. A circular seating pattern in which every member can see every other member facilitates communication in all directions.

A comfortable atmosphere, compatible with group goals, is important. A group dealing with feelings may find softer chairs or even sitting on the floor relaxing, informal, and conducive to free expression, while a "think" group may need firmer seating. Background noise, a room that echoes, distracting posters, or distasteful decorations may often detract from group productivity.

Finally, the time when a group meets is also important. Dates and times should fit members' schedules so that all can attend, and length and frequency of meetings should enhance group goals. A support group, for instance, may find it most helpful to meet weekly to receive frequent reinforcement. Other groups, such as some learning or task groups, may need more time between sessions to practice new skills or research a problem.

Orienting Group Members

Three conditions must be met to ensure smooth functioning as a group starts. First, members must agree on the group's goals. Members should agree as early as possible in the life of the group to erase misconceptions and to help solidify the group behind its purpose.

Second, new group members need to know how the group will function; they must begin to establish its structure and rules for operating. Structure refers to the way a group defines and regulates its members' behavior in terms of roles, communication patterns, and power relationships within the group (Sampson & Marthas, 1981). It must be clear from the beginning of any group who, if anyone, is leader and what that person is expected to do. Expectations for the members should be clearly spelled out, and special roles, such as a timekeeper in a discussion group or a referee for debates, should be assigned. More specific leader and member roles will emerge during the life of the group; they will be discussed shortly. Communication patterns evolve as group members work together, but awareness from the start of how members communicate is important. The interaction networks tend to be most effective in groups whose members are all free to communicate with each other as well as with the nurse-leader (Clark, 1994).

Power structure in informal groups often fluctuates, depending upon which members have the most influence, while formal groups, such as an agency's nursing organization, generally have a stable, clear-cut structure of power, influence, and authority. In any group, however, decisions can be made to designate who has power to do what. For example, the leader of a learning group may have absolute power over all decisions, or the group may choose a completely democratic format with decision-making power distributed among the members. Rules governing group action also need to be established early. The group must decide on matters such as attendance, physical arrangements, and whether smoking will be permitted.

Third, members need to hold the same expectations for the group's outcomes. The anticipated final product of the group can be restated and discussed to make certain that everyone understands and agrees that this is the desired outcome. Part of this discussion should include how the group members will evaluate the group's final product. How will they know when their goals have been met? Some groups will find evaluation easier than others will. A smoking cessation group or a weight-loss group, for instance, will have clear standards for measuring success. An assertiveness training group for women may decide that its outcome is the ability of every member to assert herself appropriately in public and will evaluate this outcome by having each member describe one such experience. A divorce support group may have more difficulty agreeing on outcomes but perhaps will choose to measure them in terms of each member's satisfaction, feelings of comfort, or self-confidence.

BUILDING GROUP COHESIVENESS

Group cohesiveness is the sum of all the forces that influences members to stay in a group including (1) meeting members' needs, (2) group goals consistent with members' needs, (3) group is actually beneficial to members, and (4) members perceptions that the group is benefitting them (Daum, 1993; Veninga, 1982). These are positive forces that attract members toward the group. In some instances, negative or outside pressures may also promote group cohesiveness. External competition or fear of some threat, for instance, can cause group members to develop stronger bonds.

Cohesive groups display certain characteristics that begin early in the group's development and increase over time. There is an attraction of members to the group and a sense of pride in membership, which intensifies as the group becomes more successful. Pride is usually accompanied by an emotional commitment of the members to the group and manifests itself in increasing loyalty and high morale. The members feel good about one another and their group identification. They are loyal to each other and to the group's goals and values and, in some instances, may talk, dress, or act in similar ways. They work well together and enjoy spending time together, even outside of the regular group meetings.

During the life of every group there are times of internal problems and external threats. Group cohesiveness helps a group to weather these times (Kagey, et al., 1981). When the members of a parenting group disagreed among themselves over ways to discipline children, their closeness and unity as a group helped them over this period of conflict and prevented the group from disintegrating. The members of a chemical dependency group discovered that their funding source had been cut off and that there would be no more money for medications or consultation. Because of the members' commitment to remaining together, they sought and found new resources and continued working on their goals.

Group cohesiveness is as important to the group as the nurse-client relationship is in one-on-one interactions. Research demonstrates that there is a positive correlation between group cohesiveness and positive group therapy outcomes. Robbins states, "highly cohesive groups are more effective than those with less cohesiveness" (1993, p.312). Thus it becomes essential to foster group cohesiveness in the small groups with which nurses work.

Nurse-leaders build cohesiveness in a group by making certain that its four basic needs are met:

1. There must be agreement among all members on the group's goals and the means by which these goals will be achieved. No group will be cohesive if members disagree on or misunderstand the goals. To avoid misunderstanding, members need to know exactly what the goals mean, have a clear (preferably written) statement of them, agree on the methods and actions to use in implementing them, and have a sense of hope that they are attainable.

2. Group norms, the standards for acceptable behavior in the group, must be continuous and stable to help the group function (Clark, 1994). These norms are developed through discussion between leader and members about what is expected and acceptable behavior. Formal groups tend to define norms at the start. Norms often develop more gradually in informal groups.

3. There must be group motivation. Clarity and feasibility of goals can help members feel that working for the group is worthwhile. The leader can be a strong motivator by giving individual members recognition and positive reinforcement and by promoting each member's participation and sense of belonging.

4. Communication channels within the group must remain viable. It is often up to the leader to monitor communication networks and make certain that they function effectively. Members, too, can help to facilitate a good exchange of information and feelings, but the group may need an outside process observer to make objective recommendations for improving its communication patterns.

Several factors can block group cohesiveness from developing or remaining (Daum, 1993; Veninga, 1982). Open membership, particularly with an unlimited number of sessions, sometimes makes it difficult for a group to stabilize its norms. Some groups, such as Alcoholics Anonymous or Weight Watchers, overcome this difficulty by having established goals and norms for the group that essentially do not change as new members join. In a less formal group with open membership, such as an ostomy club, the nurse-leader can help the founding members to develop a charter or written statement describing the group's general purpose and policies. Then, as new members enter and old ones leave, there can be some flexibility within this structure to allow specific goals and norms to reflect the changing membership's needs. That is, both goals and norms would have to be renegotiated depending on the rate of member turnover. When members move into and out of a group very rapidly, it is almost impossible to establish cohesiveness. In general, the more stable the membership, the more likely is the achievement of group cohesiveness.

Other blocks to group cohesiveness include members who do not conform to norms or agree with goals, the formation of competitive subgroups, or a leader-centered group. Deviant members can sometimes be persuaded to change their behavior or perhaps to leave the group. Strong group agreement on goals and norms prevents competition and allows the formation of positive subgroups that enhance cohesiveness. One can also minimize splintering by keeping the subgroups task-specific and time-limited. Responsible group leadership focuses on uniting the group behind its goals and maximizing its potential to meet client needs.

Some groups need cohesiveness more than others. Without a close working relationship, a support group, for example, will probably not be able to function while a learning group may be able to accomplish its goals; however, the learning group's full potential cannot be realized without group cohesiveness.

PHASES OF GROUP DEVELOPMENT

Groups, like individuals, go through predictable growth phases. It is easiest to observe these phases in groups whose membership is constant; it is more difficult to distinguish the phases in groups whose membership or goals frequently change. The phases are dependence, counterdependence, and interdependence (Guthrie & Miller, 1978).

Dependence Phase

The **dependence phase** refers to the early period of group formation when members depend on the leader for guidance and direction. They are still sorting out why they are there and what their roles will be. They generally do not question the leader's authority. It is during this phase that members are most concerned with inclusion in the group. It is a time of personal contact and encounter. Members want to be part of the group but still feel some conflict in giving up their personal identity. Dependence has been called the "childhood" stage of group development (Ibid.).

Counterdependence Phase

In the **counterdependence phase** of group development, members become more comfortable in their roles, become more assertive, and begin to question the leader's authority. Conflict and power struggles develop. The major issue in the counterdependent phase is control. Who has power and authority? Who will influence and control? Who will be controlled? This is an "adolescent" stage of group development.

Interdependence Phase

The **interdependence phase** is the final and mature phase of group development in which group members learn to work out their relationships with one another. They make decisions together, engage in open communication, manage conflict sucessfully, and experience satisfaction in the entire group's accomplishments. During this phase, the issues revolve around communicating and meeting individual needs to express and receive affection. Subgroups develop and members pair to handle intimacy needs. Interdependence is a "mature" phase of group development that may take weeks, months, or even years for a group to reach, depending on the stability of the membership. Some groups never achieve interdependence.

Working Through Group Phases

While monitoring a group's development, leaders notice that as each new issue arises the group will again progress through the developmental phases with regard to that issue. According to Sampson and Marthas, "A particular developmental stage . . . is never fully completed for all time; rather, as circumstances change, the same developmental [stage] may crop up again and again"(1981, p. 196). For example, a nursing team in a community health agency has been working on solving case problems. For five months the team members have worked through their dependence on the team leader

and their conflicts over different ways to manage family problems; now they are communicating well and assuring everyone the opportunity to express ideas. They are experiencing the interdependent phase on this issue. Recently the team was told that it would have to redistribute members' geographic work boundaries. Feeling insecure and uncertain about how to accomplish this task, members initially looked to the team leader for suggestions (dependent phase). Soon they recognized advantages and disadvantages of various proposals for redefining work boundaries, ignored the leader, and began arguing among themselves over how to decide. Power struggles signal that they are currently in the counterdependent phase on this issue.

Knowing the phases of group development helps one to recognize at what stage a group is and what to expect from the members. Groups must be allowed to progress through each phase at their own pace; this progress can be greatly enhanced by an understanding and facilitative leader.

GROUP ROLES

Leadership Roles

The group leader has a specific responsibility: to help the group achieve its goals (Robbins, 1993). Sometimes a formal, designated leader assumes this role; at other times, an informal leader emerges to help focus the group's energy on its business. The nurse may be either a formal leader, an informal leader, or simply a member. All the members, including the leader, must be committed to working together to accomplish the group's goals. Leadership style influences this task. Whether the leader should assume an autocratic (leader-centered, persuasive) style, a democratic (member-centered, problem-solving) style, or a laissez-faire (noncentered) style depends on the group's needs. Each style has advantages as well as disadvantages, although the democratic style works best in most situations. Leadership styles are presented in more detail in Chapter 25. During the group process, the leader exercises some unique functions and employs certain techniques.

A leader performs a variety of activities designed to strengthen the group's ability to achieve its purpose. These are the leader's functions. Important ones are the following (Sampson & Marthas, 1981):

1. Obtain and receive information;
2. Help diagnose group goals, obstacles, and consequences of decisions;

3. Facilitate communication;
4. Help integrate varying perspectives and alternate possibilities for action;
5. Test and evaluate proposals and decisions.

To carry out these functions, the leader needs skill in the use of certain techniques or leader interventions (Clark, 1994; Rankin, et al, 1993):

1. By *offering support* the leader helps create an encouraging climate that reinforces positive behaviors and makes members feel secure and accepted. A leader could use this technique by telling the group, "You have made real progress today. Several people shared feelings as well as ideas, and you have all listened attentively and accepted these comments without judging them."

2. *Confrontation* is a technique that counters negative behavior through constructive feedback. The leader may direct it toward an individual member or the group as a whole. It consists of making direct, honest, reflective statements about how behaviors appear to one. People do not always want to hear these statements, but they may be necessary to facilitate group progress. It is helpful to combine support with confrontation.

3. *Offer advice and suggestions* only when leader expertise or perspective is needed. Leaders should be careful to offer it only when members are unable to solve problems for themselves.

4. *Summarizing* is used to provide the group with a concise, descriptive review. The leader may wish to summarize the group's actions to date, its progress in relationship to goals, its unresolved issues, and other areas of functioning. The value of this technique is to refocus group attention for future planning.

5. *Clarification* is used to prevent confusion or distortion of ideas. A leader could use this technique by saying, "From the comments I've heard, it seems to me that the group would like to switch to Tuesdays. Is that correct?"

6. *Questioning* is a useful technique for gaining information and greater understanding. By asking questions, leaders help members explore ideas in greater depth.

7. *Reflection* is a technique used to clarify people's ideas, feelings, or behaviors and facilitate communication. The leader does this by repeating, paraphrasing, or highlighting the client's statements or behaviors. For example, when a member says, "I don't agree," a reflective response is, "You don't agree?"; which promotes an opportunity to discuss why they don't agree. Reflecting feelings means restating to the group or member the feelings the leader thinks are being conveyed. If a learning group complains, "We've never had to do anything like this before," the leader may reflect back, "You seem to be a little frightened of doing this." To reflect behavior, leaders simply describe the behavior they see, which allows the group to clarify the meaning. The leader can say to the group, "I notice that you've become silent since I made that last suggestion."

8. *Interpretation and analysis* may be used as a technique to uncover the underlying meaning of group comments and behaviors. In using this technique, leaders summarize observations of the group and then offer an analysis of the behavior's deeper meaning or reason. The leader might say, "I notice that several of you who are usually active have not participated in the past two sessions. I wonder if the decisions about this issue seem to be a foregone conclusion, and you feel it's useless to say anything?"

9. *Listening attentively* shows the group that the leader is interested in them and what they have to say. It also provides a positive model for group members to use with each other. Attentive listening helps sharpen the focus of the conversation by allowing specific responses to the comments being made.

Member Roles

Every group needs its members to perform specific roles. There are two types of roles, either task-related which help the group accomplish its goals or maintenance-related which help promote member participation. The most common roles of group members are listed in Table 10.2 (Mill & Porter, 1976; Kelly et al., 1989). All of these roles are needed for a group to function effectively (Kelly et al., 1989). Some members will play several overlapping roles; others will play only one or two. A leader can determine the roles the group's members are playing by having an outside observer evaluate the group or by using one of various member participation checklists (Clark, 1994; Hill, 1977). Should a vital role, such as gatekeeper, be missing from a group, the leader and the group may wish to ask someone to assume this role.

TABLE 10.2. *Role and Functions of Group Members*

Type of Role	Role	Functions Performed
Task Roles	Initiator	Proposes tasks, goals, or actions; defines group problems; suggests procedures
	Information Seeker	Asks for factual clarification; requests facts pertinent to the discussion
	Opinion Seeker	Asks for a clarification of the values pertinent to the topic under discussion; questions values involved in alternative suggestions
	Informer	Offers facts; expresses feelings; gives opinions
	Clarifier	Interprets ideas or suggestions; defines terms; clarifies issues before the group; clears up confusion
	Summarizer	Pulls together related ideas; restates suggestions; offers a decision or conclusion for the group to consider
	Reality Tester	Makes a critical analysis of an idea; tests an idea against some data to see if the idea would work
	Orienter	Defines the position of the group with respect to its goals; points to departures from agreed-upon directions or goals; raises questions about directions that the group discussion is taking
	Follower	Goes along with movement of group; passively accepts ideas of others; serves as audience in group discussion and decision
Maintenance Roles	Harmonizer	Attempts to reconcile disagreements; reduces tension; gets people to explore differences
	Gatekeeper	Helps to keep communication channels open; facilitates the participation of others; suggests procedures that permit sharing remarks
	Consensus Taker	Asks to see if the group is nearing a decision; sends up a trial balloon to test a possible solution
	Encourager	Is friendly, warm, and responsive to others; indicates by facial expression or remark the acceptance of others' contributions
	Compromiser	Offers a compromise that yields status when his own idea is involved in a conflict; modifies in the interest of group cohesion or growth
	Standard Setter	Expresses standards for the group to attempt to achieve; applies standards in evaluating the quality of a group process

A new mothers' group has been meeting weekly now for a month and a half. As their leader, you notice that each person's behavior is unique in some way. Susan, for instance asks many questions and also tends to agree with whoever is speaking. She performs two different task roles of information-seeker and follower. Diane, on the other hand, is full of ideas and frequently offers suggestions or proposes some new plan of action. She, too, performs a task role by initiating ideas. Maureen's friendly, warm responses seem to always make the others feel better. Maureen performs a maintenance role of showing acceptance and support to others. Verona has been especially helpful by keeping the group on track, helping to smooth out differences, and encouraging others to participate in the discussion. Verona performs a maintenance role of gatekeeper, helping to keep communication open and facilitating member involvement.

Task Roles. Task roles are behaviors that help the group accomplish its goals and they fall into two categories: process roles and content roles (Clark, 1994; Kelly et al., 1989). Process roles include activities such as setting agendas, keeping records, leading the group, coordinating activities, delegating tasks, and managing information needed for and resulting from group decisions. Content roles include behaviors that contribute to the group's decision making, such as offering opinions, providing new information, summarizing discussions, or disagreeing with ideas.

Maintenance Roles. Maintenance roles are behaviors that promote a climate of cohesiveness and effective working relationships among group members. Maintenance roles include activities such as encouraging other members, providing supportive comments, and mediating conflicts. (See Table 10.2.)

Dysfunctional Roles. Dysfunctional roles hinder the group from reaching its goals. An example is a member who constantly complains, inhibits communication, and demoralizes the group. Other behaviors, such as being aggressive, blocking, dominating, distracting, or seeking recognition or sympathy, are also dysfunctional. These roles cannot be ignored. The group must identify and deal with them. If someone disrupts the group meeting, the leader may redirect the focus back to the topic by saying, for example, "I'd like to hear other people's ideas, too." When disruptive behavior is persistent, a technique such as reflection or interpretation and analysis may be a constructive way to deal with it. Confrontation should be used with discretion, particularly in front of the group, since it may be too threatening and counterproductive.

SOLVING GROUP PROBLEMS

Many difficulties arise during the life of a group. Some have been described, such as how to start the group, avoid blocks to group cohesiveness, and deal with dysfunctional behavior. Three group problems in particular are worthy of further discussion. They are interpersonal conflict, dominance, and nonparticipation.

Resolving Conflicts

Conflict has been defined as a process that begins when one person perceives that another person has negatively affected, or is about to negatively affect, something the first person cares about (Robbins, 1993, p.445). There may be sharp disagreement, arguing, tension, and impatience. Conflict may occur because one or more members is seeking special status or making a power play, because some members have vested interests in or loyalty to another conflicting organization, or because members have overinvested in the group's productivity.

Conflict, by itself, is neither good nor bad. It is a form of tension frequently found in groups that may be used constructively by broadening the group's outlook and sharpening its problem-solving skills, or destructively by dissolving group cohesiveness. See the Issues in Community Health Nursing display on managing group conflict below.

Managing conflict means taking neither the extreme of flight (avoidance) or of fight (head-on confrontation), but rather a realistic attitude aimed at maximum

 **Issues in Community Health Nursing
MANAGING CONFLICT
IN GROUPS**

The potential for conflict to arise is always present when community health nurses work with groups and populations. When conflict promotes group performance it is constructive or functional. Dissenting views can lead to better ideas for planning or implementing a program. Conflict that hinders group performance is destructive or dysfunctional. Community health nurses can manage both the stimulation of conflict as a tool to enhance program development as well as manage the resolution of conflict. Robbins (1993, p.454) suggest techniques for both.

Conflict stimulation techniques include:
- Raise questions that challenge the status quo and current ideas.
- Bring in outsiders to present differing views.
- Realign work sub-groups to shift polarities.
- Assign critics to argue against majority positions.

Conflict resolution techniques include:
- Arrange face-to-face meetings of conflicting parties.
- Emphasize common goals and interests, deemphasize differences.
- Expand needed resources if scarcity contributes to conflict.
- Find compromise solutions to achieve win-win results.

gain for all those concerned. It is called a Win/Win approach (Robbins, 1993; Veninga, 1982):

Lose/Lose (you lose/I lose)
Win/Lose (you win/I lose)
Lose/Win (you lose/I win)
Win/Win (you win/I win)

Using the Win/Win approach encourages people to work together to benefit all parties. Group members examine all the issues at stake and maximize the opportunity for everyone to satisfy at least some of their desires. Win/Win refocuses energy into problem solving instead of competition.

There are four steps to take to resolve conflicts.

(1) Acknowledge that there is a conflict and clarify what the conflict is in the group. People may not be ar-

guing different points, after all. (2) Identify possible areas of agreement. There are nearly always some points that are not mutually exclusive. (3) Determine the changes each party in the dispute must make to resolve the problem satisfactorily. (4) Keep the focus of the conflict on issues rather than people. Personal attack will stalemate any attempt at resolution and may even strengthen the conflict (Veninga, 1982).

Dealing with Difficult Situations in Groups

Excessive Participation. Excessive participation of members in the form of monopolizing conversation can produce feelings of anger and frustration for the leader and the group. Most groups need relatively equal member participation for group work to be effective. To allow a full diversity of views, to foster cohesiveness through members' self-expression, and to make best use of the group's time, each member should have a fair share of the group's attention. Dominant members may be trying to cover up anxiety or to seek attention, recognition, and approval. However, their compulsive talking and apparent insensitivity to others in the group create dislike and disrespect. Other members feel cheated out of their share of the group's time, and the group cannot benefit from a complete range of member contributions.

The leader copes with a dominant member by first trying supportive interruption: "Your point is well taken, but, in the interest of time, we need to allow others to express their views." If the member is not responsive to this approach, the leader may try another technique, such as reflection with the individual privately: "You seem to be doing most of the talking today." The leader might offer an interpretation: "I wonder if you are talking so much because you feel a little anxious about something, perhaps about how the group sees you?" Even confrontation may be necessary. It is also possible that the group is permitting the dominant member to monopolize as a way of avoiding its own responsibility. In that case, confrontation of the member by the group may be needed.

Nonparticipation. A member may refuse to participate as a result of apathy, lack of commitment to the group's goals, anger, fear of ridicule, timidity, or poor self-image. When other members do not know why this person is quiet, they begin to feel uncomfortable (is this person judging us, ridiculing us, or not liking us?) and resentful (it is unfair of members not to carry their share of the group's work). The silence of several members may indicate an angry reaction to a few who are

dominating or it may indicate discomfort in the presence of conflict. When the entire group is silent or apathetic, they may be responding to the leader's style or the current task, which may seem unimportant or too difficult.

Nonparticipation must be diagnosed before the leader can intervene. Diagnosis can be made by offering a reflective or interpretive statement such as, "I've noticed that there is very little participation in the group today. Are people uncomfortable with this topic or perhaps with the way I'm leading the group?" or "Susan, you haven't said much in the last few sessions. Are the rest of us not giving you a chance?" From member responses and discussion, the leader learns the reasons behind the silence and then can take appropriate action. Nonintervention is sometimes best if it appears that too much group time and energy will be spent on the problem or if nonparticipation is infrequent. Occasional silence, particularly in one individual, may only be temporary. As the group becomes increasingly supportive and accepting, such individuals may gradually feel secure enough to start participating on their own.

Emotional Expressions. Emotional expressions, such as crying or hostile reactions, occur occasionally in client groups. The client who cries unexpectedly during the group session needs to feel comfortable enough to continue to express feelings. Equally important, the nurse must recognize how this may be affecting the rest of the group. Supportive statements acknowledge client feelings, such as, "We can see how touched you are by this discussion and you are expressing how many others here may feel about . . . ;" or "Talking about . . . can make one remember a personal tragedy, something only a few here can even imagine. Is there something we can do for you?" While offering supportive statements, walk near the client and give a moment of personal attention, touch the person's hand or offer to take a short break. Each gesture demonstrates recognition of the pain the person is feeling. Acknowledging the person's feelings helps to relieve the tension of the moment that others may be feeling and gives them the "OK" to also express a variety of feelings.

Dealing with the hostile client takes a different kind of approach and fortunately these people do not appear too often. The most important thing to remember is not to argue. This leads to more argument (Clark, 1994). Instead say, "I understand your beliefs but the current information on this recommends . . ." or "I can see that you have strong feelings about this, could we discuss it privately after the group session is over?" If the nurse's attempts to diffuse the situation fail, the person may have to be asked to leave the group. This can be done by saying, "I don't think the group is meeting your needs. Perhaps we could talk after the group session and find a more suitable group for you." Or "This group focuses on . . . , if this doesn't fit with your values then perhaps another group would be better for you." At this point the hostile person will either calm down and participate more appropriately or leave. Whichever happens the change will benefit the group and facilitate group process and outcomes.

TERMINATING A GROUP

Termination is an extremely important phase in the life of a small group (Loomis, 1979). Like any ending, including death, termination involves a mixed set of feelings that the group must face, explore, and resolve. Members must cope with feelings of loss and grief at leaving people to whom they have become attached. They must deal with a sense of success or failure, depending on whether their goals were met. They must recognize that they will no longer experience the group's support and other benefits. Termination is important because it is a time in the group's life when members have an opportunity to analyze the meaning of the group experience, which they can build on when planning for the future. Successful termination creates a sense of completion and a positive attitude toward future group experiences.

Termination is an issue that must be dealt with in every group. Most health care groups mark a beginning to their work and an ending when that work is complete. For these groups, the entire group will terminate. Other groups have an open-ended membership; thus the group, such as an ongoing support group, remains while members come and go. In these instances, the individual member terminates. Leaders, too, sometimes leave a group, perhaps for health reasons or a job change. Whether it is the entire group or an individual who is terminating, all the group members are affected. Positive leader intervention can make the difference in whether or not a group terminates successfully.

Preparing for Termination

Ideally, criteria for termination are established at the onset of the group. If the criteria are built into individual and group goals, clients know that, upon completion of their goals, it will be time to terminate. A failure

on the part of many leaders, however, is not to explain these criteria fully to clients. The subject of termination is even avoided by some leaders, which suggests they may be denying its reality because they do not want to face the pain of separation. Part of the leader's responsibility, as early as possible in the life of the group, is to clarify with the group the exact conditions and date for termination.

Termination may be defined in terms of time (number of sessions or specific target date), behavior (when specific behavior changes have occurred), or circumstances (moving, job change, health). For example, a parenting group may choose to meet for 12 sessions and then terminate. If additional needs are identified at the end of that period, the group can renegotiate for more time. The members of a psychotherapy group will most likely decide that termination is appropriate when they see the desired changes in their behavior. Circumstances, such as moving or job change, are usually known far enough in advance to allow the group time to prepare adequately for termination.

Working Through Termination

When facing termination, group members may experience a mixture of feelings, such as sadness, anger, joy, or fear. They may deny the possibility of termination altogether. Members' behavior gives the leader clues about their reactions to termination. For instance, members who were formerly open in sharing feelings may become defensive and superficial. Others may appear angry and upset for no apparent reason. People may start to make plans for getting together beyond the termination date. Some may withdraw, come late, or act as if the group were no longer important to them. Most of these are unhealthy responses and require intervention.

Leader intervention during the termination process includes the following. First, the leader helps the group to identify and acknowledge that termination is occurring. Members must accept its reality. Second, the leader assists group members in finding appropriate alternatives for meeting the needs that the group has met. Fear of having to function without the group drives some members to return to old, unhealthy behaviors such as smoking or overeating after not having smoked or gone off their diets for months. Instead, the leader should encourage members to assess what the group has been providing for them and identify other ways to meet these needs outside of the group. For instance, one woman who was leaving an assertiveness training group decided to meet weekly with a friend for continued reinforcement of her new behaviors. The leader should allow enough time before termination for members to accomplish this task. Third, the leader gives group members an opportunity to express and deal with their feelings, which need to be worked through until the group senses that its business is finished. Finally, the leader facilitates termination by having the group evaluate its progress. "Here is where we were when we started. Look how far we have come" is a message that helps people leave with a sense of accomplishment and a positive outlook on the future.

EVALUATING A GROUP

Group evaluation includes two important areas, process measurement and outcomes measurement. The first examines ongoing group interaction, and the second looks at the group's final product.

Process Evaluation

Process evaluation is an assessment of how well a group or project is functioning. It is important for groups to conduct periodic self-examinations. Leaders and members both need to hear reactions to their performances. Are they conducting their roles effectively? Are they making progress toward their goals? This information is vital to making improvements in the way members work together.

Process evaluation can be done in several ways. One useful method is to have an outside observer sit in on the group, watch for specific behaviors, and then give reactions to the group. The observer can use one of several guides available for this purpose (Sampson & Marthas, 1981). Another method is to have a group member act as an impartial observer during a session in which the member only observes and refrains from participating. The group itself may diagnose its health by periodically or even regularly using some form of checklist or questionnaire, followed by discussion (Clark, 1994; Guthrie & Miller, 1978; Hill, 1977). The kinds of behaviors to observe will vary with each group; generally, however, a group needs to examine all of the roles listed earlier and ask questions pertaining to areas such as communication skills and patterns, responses to leadership style, group climate, stage of group development, and progress on group objectives. Sweeney (1975) has developed a useful set of criteria that appraise the strength and effectiveness of groups in terms of their physical, interpersonal, intrapersonal, and community dimensions.

Outcome Evaluation

Outcome evaluation is a measurement of the end results or consequences of a program or intervention. Determining the effectiveness of any group means measuring its outcomes. Did the group accomplish its objectives? Are the group members different now from how they were when the group started? Clear goals and specific objectives are the keys to unlocking the answers to these questions. Goals are broad statements of the overall purpose of the group. Objectives are statements of measureable behaviors that describe specific steps toward accomplishment of goals. For example, the group's goal may be to learn the techniques of natural childbirth. Objectives should describe separate behaviors, such as demonstrating specific breathing techniques or exercises. Thus, objectives that describe outcome behaviors become criteria for measuring the group's performance. If members can and do demonstrate ability in the breathing techniques and the exercises (or any other behaviors outlined in the objectives), then one can say that the group goal has been accomplished.

Some groups' goals are more difficult to evaluate than others, but all can be measured to some degree. A group of women with mastectomies may have a goal of learning to accept their own bodies. They identify specific behaviors that indicate they have met this goal such as looking in the mirror without wincing, admitting to having undergone a mastectomy to another person outside the group, or wearing form-fitting clothing and not feeling overly self-conscious.

The group should participate equally with the leader in the evaluation process. Group members' own observations, insights, and feedback are essential to collecting the necessary data for evaluating the objectives. If specific behavior changes, such as staying on a special diet or exercising daily at home, are part of the objectives, then further supporting data can be solicited from family members or friends.

Working with Populations

Concern for populations and communities is a basic public health value but one that tends to be foreign to an individualistic or even small-group orientation and customary provision of health services. Enlarging that view requires adopting a new mind set, a new way of perceiving community health needs. For an example of this new mindset, see the case study below.

IDENTIFYING POPULATIONS

What is a population? A **population** is the total of individuals occupying an area or making up a whole, based on having a quality or characteristic in common (Merriam-Webster, 1993). In contrast to a small group, a population is a looser collection of people. As a whole these people do not interact directly or have face-to-face contact. They may or (more often) may not be aware of common problems or share similar goals. Members share a set of defining criteria but do not participate in a structure. That is, when one designates a special population, one identifies one or more environmental or personal characteristics that the group of people have in common (Williams, 1977, 1992; Shamansky & Pesznecker, 1981). They might share the feature of age, as in a pediatric population or a population group of the elderly. The defining characteristic might involve spoken language such as the Spanish-speaking population. Some population groups, such as blue-collar workers or farmers, are defined in terms of their common type of employment (see Fig. 10.5). Other populations share a common diagnosis. One may speak of the diabetic population, or the populations of stroke or automobile accident victims. Often populations are defined in terms of their potential vulnerability to health problems; for instance, one might identify populations at risk for coronary heart disease, home accidents, or family violence. The special population groups of unwed teenage mothers in a city, managers demonstrating stress symptoms in a specific corporation, and farm workers in the state who have sustained injuries with machinery in the past year all share a clear set of defining criteria. These criteria describe the population group.

The purpose for designating a population group arises from some special need residing in that collection of people. When a number of school children in the same school district contract measles, the nurse may

CASE STUDY

AGGREGATE LEVEL NURSING

To broaden nursing practice from small group to aggregate level it is helpful to hear one nurse's description of her experience. She was employed by a county public health nursing agency:

"I received a referral to see a family whose 15-year-old daughter, Mary Jo, had run away from home for the third time. She was obese (215 pounds) and flunking out of school. There were so many problems in that family—unemployment, poor diet, stress, family conflict, another daughter's recent delivery of a sick, illegitimate baby, and the obesity of the mother and all three daughters—that I hardly knew where to begin, but the parents were willing to work with me. We discussed their concerns and started with their biggest worry—Mary Jo's running away. We finally found her. She and another girl who was also flunking out of school had hitchhiked to the city to find jobs but had no luck and ended up at the YWCA. When they got home, we had some long talks, and she agreed to stay and give it another try.

Up to this point, I felt some success in working with this family, and Mary Jo in particular. Then, an offhand comment made by Mary Jo shifted my attention to a larger aggregate.

'I know a lot of other girls at school in the same boat as me,' she said. I asked her what she meant. 'Well, there's a lot of others who don't give a damn about school and feel that life is pretty worthless.' I should have followed up on that remark right away, but I didn't. Then a girl committed suicide in that same school, one of my schools. I felt terrible. If some kind of effort had been made to reach those kids who were hurting emotionally, maybe that girl would be alive today. I had spent a lot of time with Mary Jo and her family, but it wasn't too late to work with other girls. I formed a task force of school personnel, students, and parents and we started to look at the needs of the whole population of adolescent girls. Then we went into both of my schools and started working with their organizations. We did something about those other students and, would you believe, we now have 35 girls coming to our Teen Topics meetings after classes on Tuesdays in one school and 22 on Thursdays in the other."

Because nurses have traditionally worked with individuals and families, it was not surprising that this nurse focused on Mary Jo. Here was a family that needed and, in fact, asked for help. The nurse understandably provided service where a need had been clearly identified. In contrast, a whole population of girls appeared to be an amorphous mass of people, too indistinct to be assessed, too nebulous to treat as a whole, and too large for one nurse to serve. But was it? Belatedly, this nurse discovered that she could assess and meet the needs of aggregates. In this case, the aggregate was a population of high school girls.

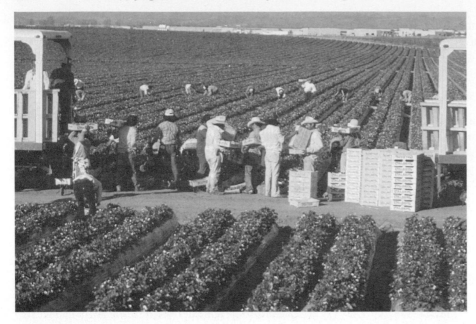

FIGURE 10.5. A group of migrant workers is defined by their common occupation and life style.

study all the children of that district as a population group to determine immunization levels and institute preventive immunization programs. There may be a large group of elderly people living alone in a community who are at risk of developing physical and emotional health problems because they do not make use of available resources. A significant number of employees with hypertension in an organization may attempt to function with their problem unrecognized and untreated. Community health professionals, therefore, single out population groups for the purpose of meeting health needs. The larger groups themselves become units for study and service.

STRATEGIES FOR WORKING WITH POPULATIONS

Populations, in contrast to small groups, require a different orientation and set of strategies for use by community health nurses. Despite the differences, however, there are many similarities in the approaches the nurse can apply.

Work with populations still employs the nursing process, but its application is on a larger scale. The nurse may work alone with a small group; aggregate work involves the expertise and input of a collaborating interdisciplinary team of which the nurse is a part. With small groups, every member is expected to participate to accomplish group goals. Work with populations

should also involve people in the decisions that affect them, but that involvement, of necessity, means that representatives of the group speak for the rest. Small groups have a collective identity or personality, as do population groups, and one needs to respect each group's uniqueness. Even as small groups go through stages of development, so do population groups' needs change over time. Both require ongoing assessment. Different tools are employed, such as epidemiologic research, when working with aggregates to facilitate systematic assessment and health planning on a larger scale. Finally, external determinants of health, such as social, biological, organizational, and environmental factors, must be considered in working with groups of any size. Their significance in the context of the total community is greater, however, when applied to work with populations.

Assessment and Diagnosis

Populations as clients in community health have needs that are just as real as those identified for families or small groups (McGrath, 1986). See the World Watch display about children in war that follows. The community health nurse assesses those needs through a combination of various methods including observation, interviewing, epidemiologic survey, and examination of existing data.

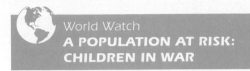

World Watch

A POPULATION AT RISK: CHILDREN IN WAR

While the main casualties of war in previous eras has been soldiers, this is no longer true. According to UNICEF (1994), an estimated 1.5 million children were killed in wars in the last decade alone. Four million more were disabled, maimed, blinded, or brain-damaged as a result of rape, torture, crippling by land mines, and other atrocities. At least 5 million children became refugees of war and an additional 12 million were uprooted from their communities. Even greater numbers of children suffer poor health, inadequate nutrition, and loss of education because of the effects of war. "Uncounted millions of these young people are suffering from post-traumatic stress disorders, a new and chilling term in the international lexicon" (Ibid. p.5).

In response to this problem, there is a growing international commitment to protect children in war. At the 1990 World Summit for Children a declaration was signed by the world's political leaders asking for protection of children during war. Furthermore, the Convention on the Rights of the Child ratified calls for specific protection for children during war as well as declaring their right to basic health services, nutrition, and education in 1994 by a vote of 150 of the 184 members of the United Nations. Activation of these protection principles during recent wars has occurred on a small scale in El Salvador, Lebanon, the Sudan, and Sarajevo through such actions as immunization days and other protective measures. Much work remains to be done to protect this at-risk population.

Observation. Observation can provide valid information about aggregates. It is often one of the best ways to begin any assessment (Spradley, 1980). In the course of daily practice, nurses can watch for evidence of existing or potential problems. For example, after a community health nurse noticed symptoms of malnutrition in some migrant children, she broadened her observations to include the entire migrant community. Many of these hard-working people showed evidence of being undernourished. A nurse at an automobile manufacturing plant observed that several workers acted tense and fatigued. She began to pay attention to these symptoms when she walked through the plant.

Interviewing. Interviewing, a second assessment strategy, can offer detailed information about a population group (Spradley, 1979). The nurse assisting migrant workers prepared a set of questions about diet and eating practices. She interviewed several families in their shacks and discovered they ate no meat or dairy products, but only white bread, potatoes, and occasional vegetable scraps stolen from the fields. Their income was too meager to allow purchase of better foods. At the automobile plant, the nurse interviewed several selected workers and discovered that they had frequent headaches and nausea. These symptoms were most evident at the end of the day after long hours of exposure to the chemicals they were using in their work.

An Epidemiologic Survey. An epidemiologic survey, a third assessment strategy, studies the distribution and determinants of disease or other health condition in a population (Dever, 1991). In an organization such as the automobile manufacturing plant mentioned earlier, it is also possible to conduct an epidemiologic survey. In her role as part of the company's middle management, the nurse pointed out the symptoms among workers on this unit. Others agreed that they had noticed them, too, and had seen them in workers in other units as well. She then helped develop a study to determine the plant's chemical hazards and their impact on employees' health. (Epidemiologic research as an aggregate assessment tool is discussed in Chapter 12.)

Examine Existing Data. Examine existing data is a fourth assessment strategy. Nurses can learn a great deal about a population group by examining information that has already been collected for other purposes. Census records, community demographic data, or surveys done by other community organizations can often provide needed information for assessment and health planning for population groups. Statistics on infant morbidity and mortality from automobile accidents, for example, as well as records describing infant car seat use could assist in a study of the safety of the infant car-riding population. Other sources of existing data are described in Chapters 11 and 12.

Collaborative Needs Assessment. Collaborative needs assessment is a final assessment strategy. Thorough needs assessment at the aggregate level usually requires an interdisciplinary team effort to ensure proper data collection and analysis. Community-wide needs assessment is discussed in Chapter 9.

The determination of health problems among population groups, then, depends on careful analysis and interpretation of this collected data. At the aggregate level diagnosis becomes a more complex task, and the community health nurse seldom does it alone. As during needs assessment, the nurse requires the expertise and collaborative input of other public health professionals, such as epidemiologists, statisticians, health planners, and environmentalists. There must be a clear and accurate diagnosis of the problem to be addressed.

Planning and Implementation

Interventions at the aggregate level are on a larger scale and generally more complex than working with small groups. They are often what we know as community health programs. Nonetheless, many group principles apply. A clear goal and set of objectives are needed (Blum, 1981). There must be agreement among the planning team members (Nutt, 1984). Nurses cannot easily communicate with an entire aggregate to gain each person's input and cooperation; therefore, they ask representatives of that population to serve on the planning team along with an appropriate mix of health professionals. Because the planning is done by a team, the nurse can apply principles of small-group interaction to enhance the group's functioning. Health planning and implementation for aggregates follow the same general process as any kind of nursing care planning. For population groups, however, health planners must also be concerned about factors in the external environment, such as health policy, economic conditions, legislation, other programs competing for service to the same population, or funding, that may influence planning decisions. A family planning education program for Southeast Asian refugees, for example, was being considered by a local public health nursing agency. However, state funding for refugees' programs was drying up, and the nurses had to seek other sources of financial backing before the program could be implemented.

Evaluation

Most often one evaluates aggregate-level health care in terms of four types of results depending on specified goals. They are outputs, outcomes, impact, and efficiency (Churgin, 1981). *Output evaluation* describes results in terms of what is produced. That is, if a family planning program aims to teach a certain number of people in the population, then the evaluation effort measures how many people were served. *Outcome evaluation*, as discussed earlier, measures the consequences of the program or intervention. Were the desired end re-

sults accomplished? For example, did the family planning program accomplish fewer unwanted pregnancies or were health practices changed as a result of health promotion (Ruffing-Rahal, 1994)? See the Research in Community Health Nursing discussion below. *Impact evaluation* looks beyond the immediate results of the intervention and determines the long range effects on the rest of the community. Did this program meet the needs of one population but overlook other populations' needs? Should more extensive programs be developed? Finally, *efficiency evaluation* examines the cost-benefit and cost-effectiveness of the program results. It asks if the resources (costs in money, time, and personnel) were used as effectively as possible, or if the resources produced as much as could reasonably be expected (Churgin, 1981).

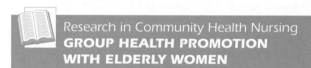

Research in Community Health Nursing
GROUP HEALTH PROMOTION WITH ELDERLY WOMEN

Ruffing-Rahal, M.A. (1994). Evaluation of group health promotion with community-dwelling older women. *Public Health Nursing, 11*(1), 38–48.

Among older populations, more small group interventions could be used. In particular, low-income, non-Caucasion elderly women seldom receive "either preventive or health-promotion interventions that endeavor to facilitate optimum functioning and quality in everyday life" (p. 38). Nursing research was conducted to evaluate the effectiveness of a six-month group project with elderly minority women. The project was designed to promote health and quality of well-being through weekly nurse-conducted health education meetings and group exercises.

Evaluation of the group project was done by means of pre and post one-on-one interviews with a control group and the intervention group. While the findings showed no significant increases in outcomes for the intervention group, there were significant contrasts among controls in terms of "well-being, health practices, and life satisfaction, suggesting a preventive-maintenance effect for the participants" (p.38). Conclusions from this study were that health promotion using small group process is a useful vehicle for the high-risk elderly.

Evaluation of community health programs follows five steps (Ibid.). (1) Develop a list of criteria to be used to determine successful completion of the objectives. This is best done during the planning stage. (2) Devise ways to measure these criteria. The measures should be objective, reliable, and valid. For example, if the group is evaluating a child health promotion program, one criterion may be fewer school absence days, measured in number of days missed. (3) Collect data. (4) Analyze and interpret the data. (5) Present the findings to relevant groups or organizations for future planning decisions.

Evaluation may be formative or summative. Formative evaluation is conducted to give feedback during the development of the health program. It examines the program while it is forming, as one might wish to do with a new health education effort. Is the program process working effectively? Is the program generating the desired outcomes as it goes along? Summative evaluation is conducted after the program is complete. It assesses the sum of the program's final product.

Summary

Groups of all sizes are an important focus for community health nursing service. A small group consists of a collection of persons who engage in repeated, face-to-face communication, identify with each other, are interdependent, and share a common purpose or purposes.

In preparing to work with small groups, the community health nurse must understand their different types, their essential needs, and their primary functions. There are five major types of small groups encountered by community health nurses: (1) learning groups, (2) support groups, (3) socialization groups, (4) psychotherapy groups, and (5) task-oriented groups.

Like individuals, groups have needs. The small groups with which community health nurses work need clear, shared goals and an agreement about how to reach those goals. They need consistent group norms and members who are motivated to participate in the group. Finally, every group needs stable communication channels among the members. Groups have two primary types of functions: task-related functions and group maintenance functions.

Starting a small group involves determining the criteria for membership and then selecting people who are committed to the goals of the group. It is important to determine the optimal size of the group, set clear group goals, make physical arrangements for the group, and orient the members.

Every small group varies in terms of the degree of cohesiveness experienced by members. The community health nurse can build a cohesive group by assuring that its four basic needs are met and by avoiding certain barriers such as open membership. Building group cohesiveness must be an ongoing process in any group.

Working with a small group is enhanced by recognizing the phases of group development: dependence, counterdependence, and interdependence. The group leader has specific functions and ways to carry out those functions. Every group also needs its members to carry out specific roles such as initiator, information seeker, informer, and clarifier. The community health nurse must be alert to resolving conflicts, dealing with difficult situations such as those who monopolize the group, handling members who do not participate, or members who are emotional or hostile.

Every small group must deal with the issue of termination, the last phase in the life of a group. It is important to prepare members for termination early in the life of a group and to work through the feelings generated by termination. Group evaluation involves assessing the ongoing group interaction as well as the final outcomes.

Working with aggregates involves a different orientation and some different strategies from those employed for small-group work. A population is a total of individuals occupying an area or making up a whole based on having a quality or characteristic in common, such as age, ethnic background, or vulnerability to a health problem.

Assessment strategies for working with population groups include observation, interviewing, conducting epidemiologic studies, and use of existing data. The community health nurse works collaboratively with other public health professionals to assess needs, diagnose, plan, implement, and evaluate interventions on behalf of population groups. Evaluation efforts address four primary types of results: outputs, outcomes, impact, and efficiency.

Work with populations shares similarities as well as differences with small-group work. Community health nurses use the nursing process on a larger scale in work with populations. They work on a team. They seek input from population group representatives. They respect the group's unique features and recognize that its needs change. They employ epidemiologic research and other assessment and planning tools applicable for macro-level use. They consider the impact of external health determinants on the health of population groups.

Activities to Promote Critical Thinking

1. Select a small group (not social) of which you are currently or have recently been a member. Which of the three phases of group development is it in? Would you describe this group as a healthily functioning one? Why or why not?

2. Compare and contrast a socialization group with a social group. Is socialization a health-promoting activity? Justify your answer.

3. Normally in groups we each tend to play certain typical roles. Analyze your own role behavior in groups. What roles do you commonly play as a member, and are they task- or maintenance-focused?

4. Imagine yourself to be the community health nurse in the case study of the Wilford County Public Health Nursing Service. You have just become a member of a planning team newly formed to assess and plan for the needs of these adolescent girls. What are some assessment strategies you could use and suggest to the group? Discuss some specific actions you might take to begin the assessment.

5. Write goals and objectives for the adolescent girls project mentioned in exercise number four. Now design a process evaluation plan and an outcomes evaluation plan. Is your outcome evaluation measuring output, outcome, impact, or efficiency? State a rationale for your choice.

REFERENCES

Balk, D. E., et al. (1993). Social support as an intervention with bereaved college students. *Death Studies, 17*(5), 427–50.

Blum, H. L. (1981). *Planning for health: Generics for the eighties* (2nd ed.). New York: Human Sciences Press.

Booth, K.E. (1990). Bringing support groups to the community. *Oncology Nursing Forum, 17*(4), 619.

Callahan, J., et al. (1980). Processing a task group: A continuing education committee at work planning a conference. *Journal of Continuing Education in Nursing, 11,* 8.

Churgin, S. (1981). Evaluation. In H. L. Blum (Ed.), *Planning for health: Generics for the eighties* (2nd ed.). (pp. 270–99). New York: Human Sciences Press.

Clark, C. C. (1994). *The nurse as group leader* (3rd ed.). New York: Springer.

Daum, A. L. (1993). Cohesion vs collusion: Maintaining group direction. *Nursing Management, 24*(11), 90–1.

Dever, G. E. A. (1991). Community health analysis, 2nd ed. Gaithersburh, Md.: Aspen.

Guthrie, E. & Miller, S. (1978). *Making change: A guide to effectiveness in groups.* Minneapolis: Interpersonal Communication Programs.

Hernandez, S.R., Kaluzny, A., Parker, B., Chae, Y., & Brewington, J. (1988). Enhancing nursing productivity: a social psychologic perspective . . . Public health nursing work groups. *Public Health Nursing, 5*(1), 52–63.

Hill, W. F. (1977). *Learning through discussion: Guide for leaders and members of discussion groups.* Beverly Hills: Sage.

Kagey, J. R., et al. (1981). Mental health primary prevention: The role of parent mutual support groups. *American Journal of Public Health, 71,* 166.

Kane, C., DiMartino, E., & Jimenez, M. (1990). A comparison of short-term psychoeducational and support groups for relatives coping with chronic schizophrenia. *Archives Psychiatric Nursing, 4,* 343–353.

Kelly, L., Lederman, L.C., & Phillips, G.M. (1989). *Communicating in the workplace: A guide to business and professional speaking.* New York: Harper.

Konopka, G. (1954). *Group work in the institution.* New York: Whiteside.

Lindgren, C. (1990). Burnout and social support in family caregivers. *Western Journal of Nursing Research, 12,* 469–487.

Loomis, M. E. (1979). Group process for nurses. St. Louis: Mosby.

McGrath, B. B. (1986). The social networks of terminally ill skid row residents: An analysis. *Public Health Nursing, 3,* 192.

Merriam-Webster, (1993). *Merriam-Webster's Collegiate Dictionary* (10th ed.). Springfield, MA: Author.

Mill, C. R. & Porter, L.C. (1976). What to observe in a group. In C. Mill and L. Porter (Eds.), *Reading book for human relations training* (pp. 28–30). Washington, DC: National Training Laboratories Institute for Applied Behavioral Science.

Nutt, P. C. (1984). *Planning methods for health and related organizations.* New York: Wiley.

Olson, M.R., et al (1991). Bittersweet: A postpartum depression support group. *Canadian Journal of Public Health 82*(2):135–136.

Payne, J. A. (1993). The contribution of group learning to the rehavilitation of spinal cord injured adults. *Rehabilitation Nursing, 18*(6), 375–9, 427–8.

Pesznecker, B., and E. Zahlis. (1986). Establishing mutual-help groups for family-member caregivers: A new role for community health nurses. *Public Health Nursing, 3,* 29.

Rankin, C. et al. (1993). Learning to lead . . . How to collaborate by committee. *American Journal of Nursing,* March, Suppl:16–9.

Robbins, S. P. (1993). *Organizational behavior* (6th ed.). Englewood Cliffs, NJ: Prentice Hall.

Ruffing-Rahal, M.A. (1994). Evaluation of group health promotion with community-dwelling older women. *Public Health Nursing, 11*(1), 38–48.

Sampson, E. & Marthas, M. (1981). *Group process for the health professions.* Somerset, NJ: Wiley.

Shamansky, S. & Pesznecker, B. (1981). A community is . . . *Nursing Outlook, 29,* 182.

Spradley, J. (1979). *The ethnographic interview.* New York: Holt.

Spradley, J. (1980). *Participant observation.* New York: Holt.

Sweeney B. (1975). Learning groups: Survival level, growth level. *Journal of Nursing Education, 14*(3), 20–26.

UNICEF (1994). *The state of the world's children 1994.* New York: Oxford.

Veninga, R. (1982). *The human side of health administration: A guide for hospital, nursing, and public health administrators.* Englewood Cliffs, NJ: Prentice-Hall.

Williams, C. (1992). Community-based population-focused practice: The foundation of specialization in public health nursing. In M. Stanhope & J. Lancaster (Eds.), *Community Health Nursing.* St.Louis: Mosby Year Book.

Williams, C. (1977). Community health nursing—What is it? *Nursing Outlook, 25,* 250–53.

SELECTED READINGS

Abdellah, F.G. (1990). Self-help groups offer prime areas for nurse researchers. *Journal of Professional Nursing, 6*(5), 257.

Bailey, B., et al. (1994). An educational support group. *Nursing Standard,* (Apr 20–26) 8(3), 65–7, 69, 71.

Birkinshaw, W., Darby, P., & Strasser, S. (1991). The parents' group: A multidisciplinary project. *Health Visitor, 64*(8), 259–261.

Carpenter, A. (1990). Sleep problems: a group approach. *Health Visitor, 63*(9), 305–307.

DesRosier, M.B., et al. (1989). Focus groups: a program planning technique. *Journal of Nursing Administration, 19*(3):20–25.

Dhooper, S. S., et al. (1993). Efficacy of a group approach to reducing depression in nursing home elderly residents. *Journal of Gerontological Social Work, 20*(3/4), 87–100.

DiSogra, L., et al (1990). Working with community organizations for nutrition intervention. *Health Education Research, 5*(4), 459–465.

Edwards, R. & Ramsey, S. (1992). Health visiting on a playbus: a community approach. *Health Visitor, 65*(5):169–170.

Ehrenfeld, M., et al. (1993). Small groups in Israeli education programmes. *Nursing Standard,* (Dec 8–14) 8(12): 33–7.

Goodman, R.M., et al. (1989). A model for the institutionalization of health promotion programs. *Family and Community Health, 11*(4):63–78.

Mallick, M. J. (1985). A community-based support group for families and patients with acute coronary disease. *Public Health Nursing, 2,* 43.

McLemore, M. K. M. (1980). Nurses as health planners. *Journal of Nursing Administration, 1*(9), 13–17.

McMurray, A. (1991). Advocacy for community self-empowerment. *International Nursing Review, 38*(1), 19–21.

Ochoco, L. & Shimamoto, Y. (1987). Group work with the frail ethnic elderly . . . new focus and spirit. *Geriatric Nursing, 8*(4), 185–187.

Remocker, A.J., et al. (1993). *Actions speak louder: a handbook of structured group techniques* (5th ed.). New York: Churchill Livingston.

Schneider, W.J., et al. (1989). Health promotion in a scheduled cyclical format. *Journal of Occupational Medicine, 31*(5), 443–446.

Smith, G. B., et al. (1994). Quality work improvement groups: from paper to reality. *Journal of Nursing Care Quality, 8*(4), 1–12.

Sorensen, J. L., et al. (1994). Psychoeducational group approach: HIV risk reduction in drug users. *AIDS Education Prevention, 6*(2), 95–112.

Volaitis, R., et al. (1994). A local community's approach to breastfeeding promotion. *Journal of Human Lactation, 10*(2), 113–8.

Wenckus, E.M. (1994). Storytelling: using an ancient art to work with groups. *Journal of Psychosocial Nursing and Mental Health Services, 32*(7), 30–2, 44–5.

11

Using the Nursing Process to Promote the Health of Aggregates

LEARNING OBJECTIVES

Upon completion of this chapter, readers should be able to:

- Describe each of the nursing process components as they apply to community health nursing.
- Identify data sources for assessing aggregate health.
- Formulate nursing diagnoses for aggregates.
- Develop a plan, including measurable goals and objectives, for addressing an identified aggregate health need.
- Describe the process of evaluating aggregate health interventions.
- Discuss characteristics of the nursing process affecting nursing practice with the community as client.

KEY TERMS

- Assessment
- Data base
- Evaluation
- Goals
- Implementation
- Interaction
- Needs
- Nursing diagnosis
- Nursing process
- Objectives
- Planning
- Setting priorities

Barbara Walton Spradley and Judith Ann Allender
COMMUNITY HEALTH NURSING: CONCEPTS AND PRACTICE, 4th ed.
© 1996 Barbara Walton Spradley and Judith Ann Allender

Underlying all community health nursing practice flows one of its essential dynamics—the nursing process (White, 1982). Consisting of a systematic, purposeful set of interpersonal actions, the nursing process provides the active, driving force for change that is the first and most important tool employed by the community health nurse.

Three characteristics emphasize the importance of this tool for community health nursing. First, the nursing process is a problem-solving process that addresses community health problems at all aggregate levels and aims to prevent illness and to promote the public's health. Second, it is a management process that requires analysis of a situation, making decisions, planning, organizing, directing and controlling service efforts, and evaluating outcomes. As a management tool the nursing process addresses all aggregate levels. Third, it is a change process that works to improve various levels of health-related systems and the way people behave within those systems.

This chapter examines the nursing process: its components and dynamics for solving problems, managing nursing actions, and improving community health nursing practice.

Nursing Process Components Applied to Community as Client

Process, the moving element of this tool, means forward progression in an orderly fashion toward some desired result. In community health, the nursing process involves a series of components, or steps, that enable the nurse to work with clients to achieve their optimal health. Nursing theorists attach different labels to these components, but all agree on the basic sequence of actions. The **nursing process** is a systematic, purposeful set of nursing actions that includes assessment, diagnosis, planning, implementation, and evaluation. All of these depend on a sixth component—interaction. Nursing literature and practice give increasing emphasis to this element of the process (Capers & Kelly, 1987; Goldmann, 1990; Kemp, 1994). Nurse-client interaction is often an implied or assumed element in the process; for community health nurs-ing, particularly, it is an essential first consideration.

INTERACTING WITH AGGREGATES

Community health nursing practice involves assisting community clients to help themselves. Listening to a group of elderly persons, teaching a class of expectant mothers, lobbying in the legislature for the poor, or working with parents to set up a dental screening program for children—all involve relationships. The nurse may establish an initial relationship, maintain an existing one, or redefine a previous one. Relationships involve reciprocal exchange and influence between people or **interaction**. This mutual give and take between nurse and clients, whether a family, a group of mothers on a Native American reservation, or a population of school children, is the first step in the nursing process.

Need for Communication

Interaction requires communication. When a community health nurse initially contacts a group of expectant parents, for example, any information she may have in advance can give only partial clues to that group's needs and wants. Unless they begin by talking and listening, the later steps in the nursing process will go awry. By open, honest sharing, the nurse (and possibly others on the health team) will begin to develop trust and establish lines of effective communication. For instance, the nurse will explain who she is and why she is there. She will encourage the group members to talk about themselves. Nurse and group members together will discuss their relationship and clarify the desired nature of that alliance. Does the group want help to identify and work on its health needs? Would its members like this nurse to continue regular contacts? What will their respective roles be? Effective communication, as a part of interaction, is essential to develop understanding and facilitate a free exchange of information between nurse and clients.

Interaction is reciprocal. It is a two-way sharing of information, ideas, feelings, concerns, and self. Nurses must avoid the temptation either to do all the talking or merely to listen while group members monopolize the conversation. There is a dynamic exchange between two systems, with the community health nurse (and, when appropriate, other collaborating health professionals) representing one system and the client group the other. Whether the client is a parent group, a homeless population, or an entire community, this exchange involves a two-way sharing between the nurse and client group. The key elements of interaction are mutuality and cooperation.

Consider the following example: A dozen junior high school boys, most of whom were on the football team, met for several weeks with the school nurse to discuss physical fitness, nutrition, and other health topics. After their agreed-upon goals had been accomplished, the nurse wondered whether further meetings were needed. She raised the question and offered several topics, such as taking drugs and preventing injuries, for possible future sessions. The boys were not interested in these suggestions but, after more discussion, said they did want help with talking to girls. Renewed interaction was necessary as a first step in reapplying the nursing process and redefining the goals for the group.

Interaction paves the way for a helping relationship. As nurse and client interact, each is learning about the other. There is a period of testing before trust can be fully established. For the school nurse, establishing interaction had been more difficult at the time of her initial contact with the boys. They had been reluctant to talk, felt embarrassed to discuss personal subjects with a woman, and yet had strong interests in bodybuilding and personal appearance, strong enough to attract them to these optional sessions. Interaction began with a friendly exchange on nonthreatening topics and gradually deepened as the boys seemed ready to discuss personal subjects. Now it was relatively simple to talk about a new "problem" (to start the nursing process over again) because a helping relationship had already been developed. The nurse had a track record. The boys trusted, respected, and liked her, so they were happy to interact around a newly stated need.

Aggregate Application

Because community health practice focuses largely on the health of population groups, interaction goes beyond the one-to-one approach of clinical nursing (Williams, 1977, 1992). The challenge that the community health nurse faces is a one-to-aggregate approach. A group of parents concerned about teenage alcoholism, handicapped persons needing access ramps, and a neighborhood's elderly frightened by muggings and theft are all aggregates of people with different concerns and opinions. As defined in previous chapters, an aggregate refers to a mass or grouping of distinct individuals who are considered as a whole. Each person in an aggregate is influenced by the thinking and behavior of the other group members. Nursing interaction with a group or aggregate as the client, demands an understanding of group behavior and group-level decision making and it requires interpersonal communication at the group level. Thus, the task of interacting becomes more complex with a group than with an individual, but it also can be challenging and rewarding. Once community health nurses address themselves to understanding aggregate behavior, they can capitalize on the potential of group influence in order to make a far-reaching impact on the health of the total community. During this phase of the nursing process, however, the challenge lies with learning to interact effectively at the aggregate level. Other chapters examine communicating and working with groups more closely.

Interaction is more than a first step; it is an integral, ongoing part of the nursing process (see Fig. 11.1). It is central to the process because nurse-client interaction forms the core of the relationship and information exchange. The effectiveness of each successive step—assessment, diagnosis, planning, implementation, and evaluation—depends on nurse-client interaction.

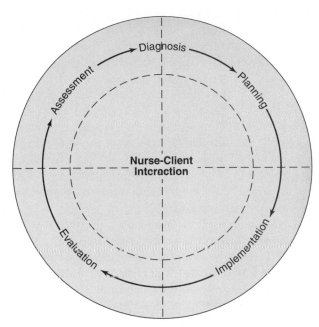

FIGURE 11.1. Nursing process components. Nurse-client interaction, a permeable structure, forms the core of the process. As nurse and client maintain a reciprocal exchange of information and trust through interaction, they can effectively assess client needs; diagnose needs; and plan, implement, and evaluate care.

ASSESSING AGGREGATE HEALTH

After establishing ongoing interaction, the community health nurse is ready to determine the client group's needs. The next step of the nursing process is **assessment** which for nurses means to collect and evaluate information about clients' health status in order to discover existing or potential needs as a basis for planning future action (Aggleton & Chalmers, 1986; Barton, et al, 1993).

Assessment involves two major activities: (1) collection of pertinent data and (2) analysis and interpretation of data. These actions overlap and are repeated constantly throughout the assessment. Thus, while assessing a group of overweight individuals' need for nutritional counseling, the nurse may simultaneously collect data on life-style behaviors and interpret previously collected data about dietary habits.

Data Collection

Data collection in community health requires the exercise of sound professional judgment, effective communication techniques, and special investigative skills. See Issues in Community Health Nursing below. The nurse can collect a wide range of data in the process of assessing community clients. What information and how much to collect depends on the initial reason for nurse-client contact. A specific health problem, such as chemical dependency among workers, depression within a nursing home population, or widespread pediculosis in a grade school, focuses the data collection on information related to the present problem and its resolution. If the initial reason for nurse-client contact is health promotion, as for normal postpartum mothers, data collection can be broadened to include information such as family coping abilities, support systems, and parenting skills.

A second consideration in data collection involves existing (actual) needs versus potential needs. Assessment of clients, such as a group of homeless men, with multiple problems may force the community health nurse to focus only on the existing needs of trying to provide food, shelter, and basic health care because of limited time and resources. When possible, however, the community health nurse tries to collect data aimed at uncovering potential needs in order to prevent problems from occurring (see Fig. 11.2). Preventive assessment with the homeless men might include health and nutrition screening and job skills assessment.

Issues in Community Health Nursing
METHODOLOGICAL ISSUES DURING ASSESSMENT

Assessment of the needs of a population or community is a complex task. Accuracy of the assessment influences the quality and relevance of community health programs. A team of nurse faculty and graduate students at the Unversity of Colorado analyzed the issues encountered in previous community health needs assessment projects and identified six major problem areas and proposed solutions to address them.Barton, et al, 1993)

1. *Data generation* problems were encountered in finding complete and accurate data. Solutions proposed included cross checking data with local officials, ongoing analysis and communication within the needs-assessment team, making certain that views of both insiders and outsiders were obtained.

2. *Data analysis* problems were had with handling volume and variety of data and assessors' disagreements on data interpretation. Solutions proposed included conformity in data coding, representative sampling, involving consumers in data interpretation.

3. *Conceptual framework* problems focused on philosophic disagreement among the study team. Solution proposed was to use conceptual framework with secondary data but let themes "emerge" from primary data.

4. *Dissemination of findings* problems arose around adequate sharing of findings with the community. Solutions proposed included timely presentation of written reports and adequate public notification.

5. *Rigor* problems focused on competency, integrity, and experience of investigating team. Solutions proposed included closer team communication and consistency of team members' data collection and computer entry.

6. *Group process* problems related to work load distribution, time constraints, member commitment and computer skills. Solutions proposed included team-building skills and communication, plus training team members in computer use.

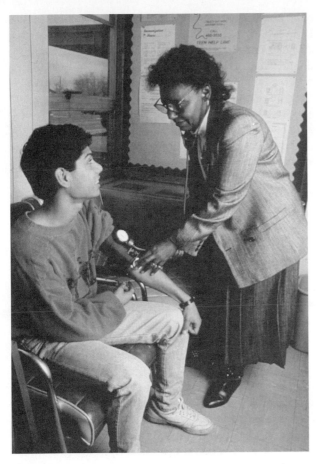

FIGURE 11.2. Collecting data to assess a member of an at-risk population for a potential health problem.

Primary and Secondary Data. Community health nurses make use of many sources in data collection. They begin by talking with the clients because they can frequently offer the most accurate insights and comprehensive information. This is primary data because it is obtained directly from clients. A secondary source of data is people who know the client group well. In working with a family, the extended family members, friends, neighbors, and work associates may all be potential sources of information, pending client permission. Additional secondary sources include health team members, client records, community health statistics, census bureau data, reference books, research reports, and community health nurses themselves. Secondary data may not totally describe the client group or reflect client self-perceptions. Thus, secondary data may need augmentation or further validation.

Methods for Gathering Data. Observation is a basic method for gathering primary data. Seeing people in their environment tells the nurse something about their resources and coping abilities. Hearing interpersonal conflict among the members of a weight control group can give the nurse clues about possible client concerns and levels of stress. Noticing the absence of a caring atmosphere in a nursing home may suggest a need for intervention. Observation, as a data-gathering method, depends largely on nonverbal communication. The tone of a conversation may be friendly, hostile, or passive. Clinic clients may fail to keep appointments. A group's body language and a neighborhood's appearance convey a message. All offer information about clients.

Another method for data collection is the interview. The interview involves a series of questions designed to elicit needed information. The community health nurse may conduct formal interviews during an early phase to gather background information and elicit clients' perceptions (Ruffing-Rahal, 1994). Informal directed questioning can sometimes provide even more data about clients' health status and needs. Communicating with clients serves as an important follow-up. If the nurse observes children with bruises that suggest possible abuse, carefully planned informal interviews may be useful. The nurse may discover mothers who are isolated and under emotional stress. Then cooperative nurse-client planning can be undertaken for dealing with the problem.

Listening is an important data collection method. It is a skill that must be acquired through discipline and concentration. Too often one listens inattentively while formulating a next question or allowing one's mind to wander. Good listening involves eye contact (in American culture). It assures clients of sincere interest and encourages greater expression of ideas and feelings. The community health nurse who is a good listener can gain a wealth of information about clients.

Direct examination is still another method for collecting data. When assessing individuals, the nurse uses percussion, auscultation, palpation, inspection, and measurement as means of direct examination. Applied to community groups and aggregates, direct examination assumes different forms such as surveys, screening instruments, epidemiologic research, or environmental testing for pathological determinants. Surveys, like interviews, provide specific information in response to selected questions. Surveys can be especially useful for gathering data such as patterns of behavior among teenage alcoholics or needs of immigrants (Urrutia-Rojas & Aday, 1991). Community health nurses use surveys to assess neighborhood and community needs. Many kinds of standard screening instruments, including blood pressure apparatus, audiometers, scales, neurologic appraisal guides, and developmental tests, are useful for collecting data about client groups. Epidemiologic research and environmental measurements add further data for community health analysis.

Data Analysis and Interpretation

This stage of assessment requires analyzing the information gathered, drawing inferences or possible conclusions about the data's meaning, and validating those inferences to determine their accuracy. First, the nurse separates the data into categories such as physical, mental, social, and environmental. In many instances, data base sheets used in community agencies provide a structure for gathering and analyzing data. Second, the nurse examines each category to determine its significance. At this point the nurse may need to search for additional information to clarify the meaning of the present data. Next, inferences are made. The nurse has analyzed the data base and come to a tentative conclusion about its meaning. But before making a diagnosis, the nurse must validate those assumptions. Are they accurate? Are they sound? Clients should participate actively in data interpretation by clarifying perceptions, explaining the circumstances surrounding the situation, and acting as sounding boards for testing assumptions. The nurse also uses other resources, such as other health team members, to explore and confirm inferences.

The following example illustrates how the nurse interprets data. A community health nurse collected data about a group of mothers who regularly attended a well-child clinic. Their responses to child health information and parenting classes had been considerably less than enthusiastic, yet when questioned, they expressed no dissatisfaction with the teaching program. The nurse observed that the women spent most of their time talking among themselves and appeared to be enjoying one another's company. Their facial expressions were most animated outside of class sessions. After examining the observed data, the nurse concluded that their social and supportive needs were far greater than their need for child care information. Merely gathering weekly at the clinic served an important function for them. She sat down with the mothers and discussed her findings. All agreed that they needed to get out of the house and be with people who had similar kinds of problems and interests. Data analysis led to drawing an inference that the mothers needed socialization and support with other mothers more than they needed specific parenting classes. This inference was validated when the nurse questioned the mothers.

There is an ever-present danger in data interpretation, however, of making inaccurate assumptions and diagnoses. Many nursing care plans and activities have been based on false ideas of clients' needs, resulting in wasted and sometimes detrimental efforts. Thus, the importance of validation cannot be overemphasized. Data collection and data interpretation are sequential activities, with validation serving as a bridge between them (see Fig. 11.3). When performed thoroughly, these steps lead to an accurate diagnosis.

DIAGNOSING AGGREGATE HEALTH

The next step in the nursing process is **nursing diagnosis** which is the conclusion the nurse draws from interpretation of collected data and is a statement de-

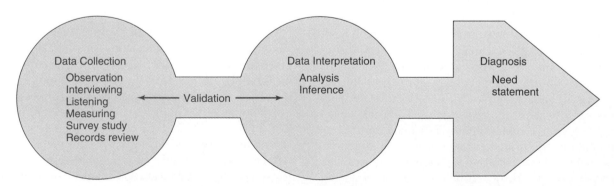

FIGURE 11.3. Assessment and diagnosis phases of the nursing process. Interpretation of data leads to diagnosis of clients' needs.

scribing clients' healthy or unhealthy responses that can be influenced or changed by nursing interventions. A nursing diagnosis is often called a problem statement.

Wellness and Deficit Diagnoses

In community health, a nursing diagnosis can focus on either a wellness response or a deficit response on the part of clients (Neufeld & Harrison, 1990). In community health, nurses do not limit their focus to problems; they consider the client group as a total system and look for evidence of all kinds of responses that may influence the members' level of wellness (Lee & Frenn, 1987; Neufeld & Harrison, 1990). Responses encompass the whole length of the health-illness continuum from a specific deficit behavior, such as chemical dependency, all the way to opportunities for maximizing client health by promoting improvement of parenting skills or successful aging. See the Research in Community Health Nursing discussion concerning diagnosis of wellness below. Thus the statement of client response, the diagnosis, can focus on a wide range of topics.

Aggregate Nursing Diagnoses

Diagnostic categories for individuals, such as impaired coping ability or risk of injury, can sometimes be applied to aggregates. Kneeshaw and Lunney (1989) describe diagnoses applied to a community of elders such as altered coping related to fear of crime. They also caution that *nursing* diagnoses must represent situations in which nurses can intervene.

Aggregate level nursing diagnoses consist of several parts. Since the focus of community health nursing is promoting health as well as preventing illness, Neufeld and Harrison (1990) propose that nursing diagnoses should include both emphases. They state that whether writing a nursing diagnosis for a wellness response or a deficit response, it should consist of three parts. (1) Identify the specific target aggregate or group, (2) describe the healthful, or actual, or potential, unhealthful response, and (3) list related factors. The related factors include host factors (such as the group's knowledge, motivation, and skills) and environmental factors (such as cultural, social, physical, or political characteristics of their environment). These should only be factors that nursing can influence for change.

Example: Wellness Nursing Diagnosis for an Elderly Group. The senior residents of a local retirement center have the potential for achieving optimal functioning related to (host factors) their expressed interest

Research in Community Health Nursing
DIAGNOSING A WELLNESS RESPONSE

Laferriere, R. H. & Hamel-Bissell, B. (1994). Successful aging of oldest old women in the Northeast Kingdom of Vermont. *IMAGE, 26*(4), 310–23.

In addition to studying problems, community health nurses also examine wellness responses to learn more effective health promotion interventions. One population with a clear wellness response is that segment of the elderly who have aged successfully. A nursing study conducted in rural northeast Vermont focused on "oldest old" women (over 85 years of age) to determine why, despite certain health problems, they maintained a high level of morale and adjusted successfully to the challenges of aging.

Using ethnographic methodology the researchers obtained life histories from six of these women (ages ranged from 87 to 93 years) by means of participant observation and extensive interviewing. All lived alone and remained in their own homes with limited assistance. From the data four dominant themes were identified with successful aging: (1) "Being a woman with family and friends" which emphasized close and supportive relationships, (2) "living off the land" which emphasized their enjoyment of raising their own food and the outdoors, (3) "dealing with the difficult times" which showed their ability to face hardships of all sorts with practicality and self-reliance, and (4) "working hard and staying active" which emphasized the purpose and meaning that work gave to their lives as well as a sense of accomplishment and control over their lives.

The researchers concluded that the ingredients for successful aging with these women were challenge, commitment, control, and resiliency, combined with an adequate social support system. They recommended that nursing health promotion with this age group emphasize maximizing independence and self-reliance while encouraging strong social support systems.

in exercise, diet, and meaningful activities, and to (environment factors) their access to exercise opportunities, nutritional information, and social outlets.

Example: Deficit Nursing Diagnosis for Farm Worker Population. Farm workers in a particular state are at risk for injuries related to (host factors) lack of motivation to add or use safety devices on farm machinery, lack of safety knowledge, choice to take unnecessary risks, and to (environment factors) lack of family income to purchase newer equipment, plus long hours leading to stress and exhaustion.

The above examples illustrate that a broad statement, such as the well-child clinic mothers' lack of emotional support, must be further broken down to understand underlying factors influencing the situation and to make it useful for planning services. The community health nurse in the clinic mothers example did further data collection and interpretation to determine related factors affecting their need for emotional support. Together, she and the mothers identified their feelings of inferiority as housewives, feelings of limited sexual satisfaction, and feelings of powerlessness about family decision making and spending of family money. A broad statement is useful as a starting point. It can serve as a summary, as in a diagnosis of culture shock, nonsupportive parenting, or an unsafe school playground. Using the broad statement as a base, the nurse can ask further questions, examine the data, and with the clients develop a complete diagnosis on which to act (Porter, 1987; Wright, 1985).

The nursing diagnosis changes over time because it reflects changes in client health status; therefore, diagnoses need to be periodically reevaluated and redefined. The changing diagnosis can be a useful means of encouraging clients toward improved health because it gives them a clear standard against which to measure their progress.

PLANNING TO MEET AGGREGATE HEALTH NEEDS

The purpose of the planning phase is to determine how to satisfy clients' needs. Assessment and diagnosis disclose needs but do not prescribe the specific actions necessary to meet them. Knowing that the group of mothers at the well-child clinic needed emotional support did not tell the nurse what further action was indicated. A diagnosis of culture shock (adjustment deficit to a contrasting culture) for a family newly arrived from Cuba does not reveal what action to take. The nurse must plan.

Planning is a logical, decision-making process of designing an orderly, detailed program of action to ac-

complish specific goals and objectives. There is a systematic approach to planning that guides the community health nurse during this phase of the nursing process: (1) list needs in order of priority, (2) establish goals and objectives, and (3) write an action plan. As they do in the rest of the nursing process, community health nurses collaborate with clients and other appropriate professionals in each of these planning activities.

Setting Priorities

Setting priorities involves assigning rank or importance to clients' needs to determine the order in which goals should be addressed (Vilnius, et al., 1990). One way to order needs is to group them into three categories—immediate, intermediate, and long-range—and then assign a priority to those in each group. Immediate needs are more urgent but not necessarily more important. For example, a community health nurse and a group of senior citizens wanted a class on exercise techniques yet did not have a place to meet. Obviously their goal, to learn about appropriate exercises, was more important than finding a place to meet; however, they had to first find a place to meet (immediate need) in order to accomplish their long-range goal. Some needs are ranked as immediate because they are potentially hazardous or life-threatening, such as lack of eye protection in a school welding class. Other needs are ranked first because they are of the greatest concern to clients, such as a group of elderly persons who were fearful of crime selected that focus as their highest priority although they had identified many other needs.

Establishing Goals and Objectives

Goals and objectives are crucial to planning. The diagnosis which identifies needs must be translated into goals to give focus and meaning to the nursing plan. **Goals** are broad statements of desired end results and **objectives** are specific statements of desired outcomes stated in behavioral terms that can be measured and include target dates. Objectives, as used here, are like stepping stones to help one reach the end results of a larger goal. For the elderly group concerned about crime in their neighborhood, their need, goal, and objectives were defined in the following manner:

Need: The group of elderly has altered coping ability related to their fear of crime.
Goal: Within six months, this group of elderly persons will be free to walk the streets of their neighborhood without any incidence of criminal assault.

Objectives:

1. By the end of the first month, a safety committee (composed of seniors, nursing, police, and other appropriate community members) will be established to study the crime patterns in the neighborhood.
2. The safety committee will develop strategies for crime reduction and elder protection to be presented to the city council for approval by the end of the third month.
3. Safety strategies, such as increased police surveillance and escort services, will be implemented by the end of month five.
4. By the end of the sixth month, nursing assessment of the seniors will demonstrate that they report feeling free to walk the streets.
5. Within the sixth month there will be no reported incidence of criminal assault.

Development of objectives depends on a careful analysis of all the ways one could accomplish the larger goal. One should first select the courses of action best suited to meeting the goals, and then build objectives. For the group of elderly, other alternatives, such as staying indoors, or always walking in pairs, were considered and rejected. Their choice was to find a way to make their environment safe and enjoyable.

Some rules of thumb are helpful when writing objectives. (1) Each objective should state a single idea. When more than one idea is expressed, as in an objective to obtain equipment and learn procedures, completion of the objective is much more difficult to measure. (2) State each objective so that it describes one specific behavior that can be measured. For instance, the fourth objective describes that the seniors will report feeling free to walk outdoors within six months. It describes a behavior that can be measured at some point in time. One can more readily evaluate objectives that include specifics such as *what* will be done, *who* will do it, and *when* it will be accomplished. Then everyone knows exactly what has to be done and within what time frame. Writing measurable objectives makes a tremendous difference in the success of planning.

Planning means thinking ahead. The nurse looks ahead toward the desired end product and then decides on all the intermediate actions necessary to meet that goal. Sometimes an objective itself describes the intermediate actions. At other times the nurse may wish to break down an objective further into several activities. For example, with the second objective, the safety committee was charged with developing strategies, presenting them to the city council, and gaining approval. Good planning requires this kind of detail.

Decision making is an important part of planning. Decisions must be made while establishing priorities.

Selecting goals and, from a variety of possible solutions, choosing the best courses of action to meet the goals requires decisions. Further decision making is involved in selecting objectives and, when indicated, the specific actions to accomplish the objectives.

To facilitate planning and decision making, the community health nurse involves other people. Clients, of course, must be included at every step. They, after all, are the ones for whom the planning is being done and without whose insights and cooperation the plan may not succeed. At times the involvement of other nurses is important. Team meetings, nurse-supervisor conferences, or nurse-expert consultant sessions are all useful resources for planning. In addition, the community health nurse will frequently wish to confer with members of other health and professional disciplines. Interdisciplinary team conferences are valuable for gaining a broader perspective and enlisting wider support for the evolving plan.

Recording the Plan

Recording the plan is the next step. Up to this point, the planning phase has been a series of intellectual exercises done jointly with clients and perhaps with other health team members. The nurse has probably written notes on the decisions made about priorities, goals, objectives, and actions but now the nurse needs to clearly record the plan. One way to record the plan is to list items in columns with space for the nurse to record specifics. It is also helpful to share copies of the plan with clients. In many instances, having copies of the plan promote clients' sense of being equal partners in the responsibility of meeting goals.

Regardless of the type of plan format used, certain items must be included in the written plan:

1. **Data base** comprises all the subjective and objective information collected about clients—physical, psychological, social, and environmental. It includes background health information (past and present); aggregate health assessment; and group history or group systems review. The data base is best kept with a format that allows space for ongoing entries and analysis. Various computer programs and applications can assist this process (McHugh, 1989).
2. Aggregate **needs** are the specific areas related to clients' health that have been identified for intervention. Preferably, they are areas that both clients and nurse agree require action. They are drawn

from the nursing diagnosis. Goals are statements that describe the resolution of needs. For clarity in planning, both a written need statement and a written goal statement are helpful.

3. Objectives are the specific statements that describe in behavioral and measureable terms what the nurse and clients hope to accomplish. It is often necessary to construct several objectives, sometimes around different categories of needs, to achieve comprehensive results. These objectives provide the nurse planner with specific targets at which to aim and around which to design actions.

4. Planned actions are the specific activities or methods of accomplishing the objectives or expected outcomes. Plans should include appropriate actions by nurse, clients, and other persons.

5. **Evaluation** is the process of measuring and judging the effectiveness of goal attainment. How and when was each objective met, and if not, why not? It is essential to include evaluation in the written plan. Progress notes are *not* the same as an evaluation. Progress notes are useful, periodic summaries which give a running account of what is occurring but evaluation requires analysis of these occurrences and conclusions to be drawn. Progress notes and evaluation may be combined if space is allowed on the plan format. Generally, it is best to enter progress notes on a separate space.

IMPLEMENTING PLANS FOR AGGREGATE HEALTH

Implementation is putting the plan into action and actually carrying out the activities delineated in the plan, either by the nurse and other professionals, or by clients. Implementation is often referred to as the action phase of the nursing process. In community health nursing, implementation includes not just nursing action or nursing intervention but collaborative implementation by the clients. Certainly, the nurse's professional expertise and judgment provide a necessary resource to the client group. The nurse is also a catalyst and facilitator in planning and activating the action plan. But a primary goal in community health is to help people learn to help themselves toward their optimal level of health. (See the following World Watch discussion about implementing a program for youth in Mexico.) To realize this goal, the nurse must constantly involve clients in the deliberative process and encourage their sense of responsibility and autonomy. Other health

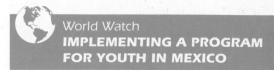

World Watch
IMPLEMENTING A PROGRAM FOR YOUTH IN MEXICO

Low income youth in Mexico's overcrowded cities face significant health and social problems. Many have poor relationships with their families, are unable to find work, and spend all day in the streets. Some have turned to selling drugs or joined gangs, often because they have no positive ways to channel their energy. Poor nutrition, dental caries, sexually-transmitted diseases, drug addiction, violence and crime are among this population group's problems. Starting in 1982, an organization called Centro Juvenil Promocion Integral (CEJUV) offered programs and activities for young people between 14 ands 28 years of age in Mexico City, Cuernavaca, and Juarez (Kellogg, 1994). Using an integrated approach, CEJUV continues to provide young people assistance with such things as studies and homework, career counseling, vocational training, sports activities, health education programs, and community celebrations to promote intergenerational dialogue. CEJUV's purpose is to provide alternative educational experiences for low-income youth by involving them in volunteer activities in their neighborhoods. Many young Mexicans are discovering new capabilities and building bridges to a more promising future.

team members, too, may participate in carrying out the plan. Therefore, all are partners in implementation.

Preparation

The actual course of implementation, outlined in the plan, should be fairly easy to follow if goals, expected outcomes, and planned actions have been designed carefully. Professionals and clients should have a clear idea of the who, what, why, when, where, and how. Who will be involved in carrying out the plan? What is each person's responsibilities? Do all understand why and how to do their parts? Do they know when and where activities will occur? As implementation begins, nurses should review these questions for themselves as well as clients. This is the time to clarify any doubtful areas and thus facilitate a smooth implementation phase.

Even the best planning, though, may require adjustments. For example, some nurses offering a Senior health fair discovered that the target group of seniors did not have transportation to the site because the volunteering bus company had withdrawn its offer. Instead, the nurses arranged for volunteers from local churches to pick up the seniors and deliver them afterwards to their homes. Thus, implementation requires flexibility and adaptation to unanticipated events.

Activities or Actions

The process of implementation requires a series of nursing actions or activities to be taken. (1) The nurse applies appropriate theories, such as systems theory or change theory, to the actions being performed. (2) The nurse helps to facilitate an environment that is conducive for carrying out the plan, such as a quiet room in which to hold a group teaching session or engaging local officials' support for an environmental clean up project. (3) The nurse, along with other health team members, prepares clients for the service to be received by assessing the clients' knowledge, understanding, and attitudes and carefully interpreting the plan to clients. This interaction nurtures open communication and trust between nurse and clients. Professionals and clients (or if a larger aggregate, its representatives) form a contractual agreement about the content of the plan and how it is to be carried out. (4) The plan is carried out or modified and carried out by professionals and clients. Modification requires constant observation and interchange during implementation since these actions determine the success of the plan and the nature of needed changes. (5) The nurse and the team monitor and document the progress of the implementation phase by process evaluation which measures the ongoing achievement of planned actions.

EVALUATING AGGREGATE HEALTH PLANS

Evaluation, the final component of the nursing process, is the last in a sequence of actions leading to the resolution of client health needs. As described before, evaluation refers to measuring and judging the effectiveness of that goal attainment. The nursing process is not complete until evaluation takes place. Too often emphasis is placed primarily on assessing client needs and planning and implementing service. But how effective was the service? Were client needs truly met? Pro-

fessional practitioners owe it to their clients, themselves, and to other health service providers to evaluate.

Evaluation is an act of appraisal in which one judges value in relation to a standard and a set of criteria (Mitchell, et al., 1989). For example, when eating dinner in a restaurant, diners evaluate the dinner in terms of the standard of a satisfying meal. Their criteria for "a satisfying meal" may include qualities such as a wide variety of choices on the menu, reasonable price, tasty food, nice atmosphere, and good service. They also evaluate the meal for a purpose. Does this restaurant serve their purpose of providing a satisfying meal at reasonable prices for future dining experiences? Evaluation requires a stated purpose, specific standards and criteria by which to judge, and judgment skills.

Purpose

The ultimate purpose of evaluating interventions in community health nursing is to determine whether planned actions met client needs; how well they were met; and if not, why not. For example, an evaluation was conducted to determine the effectiveness of a group health promotion program with elderly low income women (Ruffing-Rahal, 1994). Criteria for evaluation focused on health practices, psychologic and spiritual well being, and social integration. No significant increases in outcomes were demonstrated for the intervention group over the six-month period of weekly interventions. However, the evaluation suggested that the program had a preventive-maintenance effect for the participants by shielding them against factors that might otherwise cause erosion of beneficial health outcomes.

Criteria

Sometimes plans may include individual goals and criteria and group goals and criteria. For example, several diabetic women attending a clinic had a problem with obesity. A community health nurse working in the clinic helped them form a weight-loss group. Each member developed individual weight loss goals and objectives to accomplish within a year. The women planned ways to meet their individual objectives, such as specific daily calorie limits (i.e. 2000 calories per day) and regular exercise programs (i.e. exercise 20 minute sessions, 3 times a week). They evaluated their individual goals by determining whether they met these criteria.

To maximize group support and encourage healthy behavior patterns during weight loss, the nurse suggested having a group goal and objectives to measure group success:

Group Goal
   The group will stay healthy while accomplishing 90% of member weight loss goals.
Group Criteria
   1. By the end of the year the group will lose at least 90% of the sum of the expected individual weight losses.
   2. The group will have no diabetes-related infections during the year.
   3. All of the group members will be exercising at least once a week by the end of the year.
   4. No more than 10% of the group will have had an illness that kept them in bed more than one day during the year.
   The prepared set of criteria helped the group evaluate its success.

The above examples emphasize the relationship of good planning to evaluation. When nurse and clients prepare clear, specific goals and objectives, then there is no question about how or what to evaluate. It will be obvious that the goal is either met or not met (see Fig. 11.4).

Judgment Skills

Evaluation requires judgment skills by which the nurse compares real outcomes with expected outcomes and looks for discrepancies (Hegyvary, et al., 1987).

When actual client behavior matches the desired behavior, then the goal is met. If goals are not met the nurse will need to examine several possible explanations for the failure. They may include inadequate data collection, incorrect diagnosis, unrealistic plan, or ineffective implementation. Circumstances, clients' motivation, or both may have changed. There may not have been enough client participation in one or more parts of the process. After determining the cause of the failure, the nurse can reassess, plan, and initiate corrective action.

Quality Assurance

In community health nursing, evaluation is also performed to measure the quality of services, programs, and nurse performance (Ingram, 1987; Newman, et al., 1990; Schmele, et al., 1989). These systems of measuring quality of services, programs, and nurse performance are called *quality assurance* and reflect nursing's increasing concern with quality improvement. A sound quality assurance system includes the following:

1. An organizational entity created for assessing quality;
2. Establishment of standards or criteria against which quality is assessed;
3. A routine system of gathering information;
4. Assurance that such information is based on the total population or representative sample of clients or potential clients;

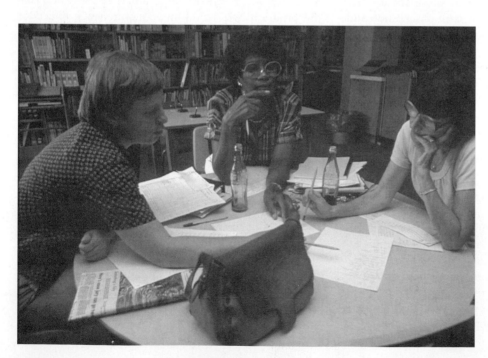

FIGURE 11.4. A community health nurse works with clients to develop specific measurable goals.

5. A process that provides the results of review to clients, the public, providers, and sponsoring organizations, as well as methods to institute corrective actions.

With the burgeoning emphasis on accountability in health services, community health nursing is being challenged to devise better ways of documenting service effectiveness and cost efficiency. A variety of methodologies and tools exists and is constantly being broadened to facilitate these evaluative processes (Martin & Scheet, 1988; Pearson, et al, 1991). One method is the nursing audit (Stewart, et al., 1987–1988), which evaluates quality of nursing care by analyzing client records. Another is peer review (American Nurses Association, 1988). All of these methods, however, operate on the same basic principle discussed earlier, that is, that evaluation requires a clear purpose as well as a standard and specific criteria against which outcomes are measured. Quality management is discussed in depth in Chapter 27.

Nursing Process Characteristics Applied to Community as Client

The nursing process provides a framework or structure upon which community health nursing actions are based. Application of the process varies with each situation, but the nature of the process remains the same. Certain elements of that nature are important for community health nurses to emphasize in their practice (see Fig. 11.5).

DELIBERATIVE

The nursing process is deliberative—purposefully, rationally, and carefully thought out (Weidenbach, 1964). It requires the use of sound judgment based on adequate information. Community health nurses often practice in situations that demand independent thinking and making difficult decisions. Furthermore, thoughtful, deliberative problem solving is a skill needed for working with the community health team to address the needs and problems of aggregates in the community. The nursing process is a decision-making tool to facilitate these determinations.

ADAPTABLE

The nursing process is adaptable (Lewis, 1988). Its dynamic nature enables the community health nurse to adjust appropriately to each situation, to be flexible in applying the process to aggregate health needs. Furthermore, it's flexibility is a reminder to the nurse that each client group, each community situation is unique. The nursing process must be applied specifically to that situation and that group of people. Based on assessment

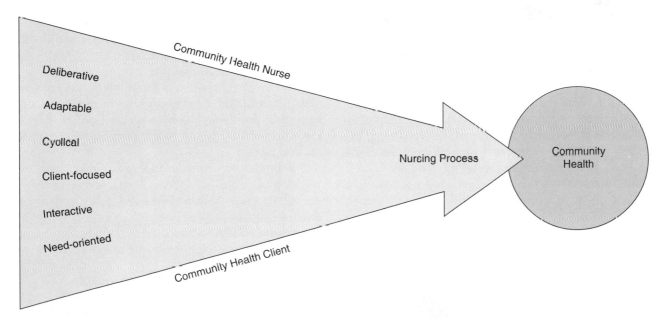

FIGURE 11.5. Nursing process characteristics emphasized in community health nursing practice.

and sound planning, the nurse adapts and tailors services to meet the identified needs of each community client group.

CYCLICAL

The nursing process is cyclical or in constant progression (Henley, 1986). Steps are repeated over and over in the nurse-aggregate client relationship. The nurse in any given situation engages in continual interaction, data collection, analysis, intervention, and evaluation. As interactions between nurse and client group continue, various steps in the process overlap with one another and are used simultaneously. The cyclical nature of the nursing process enables the nurse to engage in a constant information feedback loop. That is, information gathered and lessons learned at each step of the process promote greater understanding of the group being served, the most effective way to provide quality services, and the best methods of raising this group's level of health.

CLIENT FOCUSED

The nursing process is client focused; it is used for and with clients. Community health nurses use the nursing process for the express purpose of addressing the health of populations (Koch, et al., 1994). They are helping aggregate clients, directly or indirectly, to achieve and maintain health (Cooper, 1986). Clients as total systems, whether groups, populations, or communities, are the target of community health nursing's use of the nursing process.

INTERACTIVE

The nursing process is interactive wherein nurse and clients are engaged in a process of ongoing interpersonal communication. Giving and receiving accurate information is necessary to promote understanding between nurse and clients and foster effective use of the nursing process. Furthermore, as the consumer movement, client's rights, and the self-care concept have gained emphasis, client groups and community health nurses have increasingly joined forces to assume responsibility for promoting community health. The aggregate client-nurse relationship can and should be a partnership (Yura & Walsh, 1988). Called "peer practice" by some (Bayer & Brandner, 1977, p. 86), use of this tool can be a shared experience by professionals (nurses and others) and client groups.

NEED-ORIENTED

The nursing process is need-oriented (Clark, 1985). Long association with problem solving has tended to limit the nursing process's focus to the correction of existing problems. Although problem solving is certainly an appropriate use of the nursing process, the community health nurse can also use the nursing process to help anticipate clients' needs and prevent problems. The nurse should think of nursing diagnoses as ranging from health problem identification to primary prevention and health promotion opportunities. This focus is needed if the goals of community health, "to protect, promote, and restore the people's health," are to be realized (Sheps, 1976, p. 3).

Summary

The effectiveness of community health nursing practice depends on how well the nursing process is used as a tool for enhancing aggregate health. The nursing process means appropriately applying a systematic series of actions with the goal of helping clients achieve their optimal level of health. These actions or components of the process include interaction, assessment, diagnosis, planning, implementation, and evaluation.

Interaction is the first component, because nurse and clients must first establish a relationship of reciprocal influence and exchange before any change can take place. Effective communication is essential in assessing needs and establishing trust between nurse and clients as partners in the nursing process.

The second step, assessment, includes appraising aggregate client health status to determine existing or possible future needs. Community health nursing is not limited to identifying problems but can also help clients focus on prevention and health promotion to achieve optimal health.

The third step, formulating nursing diagnoses, involves analyzing the collected data and identifying client responses, both wellness and deficit responses, that nursing can help influence or change. Nursing diagnoses are written statements that include three parts: a broad statement identifying the target aggregate or group, a description of the healthy or unhealthy response, and a list of related environmental factors.

The fourth step, planning, includes designing a specific course of action to address the target group's diagnosis. It involves ranking group or aggregate's needs, establishing goals and measureable objectives, designing activities to meet the objectives, and developing a plan. The plan also includes a means to evaluate each objective.

The fifth step, implementation, activates the plan and sees it through to completion. During implementation, the nurse applies appropriate theory; provides a facilitative environment; prepares clients for service; carries out or modifies and carries out a plan (with clients); and documents the implementation.

The last and very important step is evaluation which measures and judges the effectiveness of the plan. Well-prepared goals and objectives are essential for adequate evaluation. If goals are not met, the failure may result from inadequate assessment or planning. Determining the cause of the failure can lead to corrective action.

Evaluation does not end the nursing process; rather, it documents what has been accomplished and what yet needs to be done in order that the process, a continuing cycle, can start again.

Certain characteristics are important to the nursing process and should be emphasized by community health nurses in their practice: the process is deliberative, requiring and aiding the exercise of judgment in decision making. It is adaptable, encouraging flexibility in practice. It is cyclical, fostering a constant, ongoing use of the process. It is client focused, helping the nurse to keep the proper target of clients' health in view. It is interactive, promoting nurse-client communication and client participation. Finally, it is need oriented, focusing on the clients' current and future needs including prevention and health promotion to help clients achieve optimal health.

Activities to Promote Critical Thinking

You have been practicing the nursing process with individuals to effect change in their health status. Now consider how you can expand that application to aggregates. Select a population group in your community, such as preschoolers, unwed mothers, a group of refugees, or elderly homebound persons.

1. As potential clients, how might you start the interaction phase with them?

2. What specific areas would you want to assess? Make a list of hypothetical indicators that suggest a need.

3. Invent a diagnosis for this group that would be supported by the data you collected in your assessment.

4. What alternative courses of action should you consider for addressing this need? Select the most appropriate one.

5. Start a plan for implementation including an overall goal and at least one objective.

6. List the activities needed to meet your objective(s), and describe how you might carry them out.

7. How would you evaluate your nursing interventions with this population group?

REFERENCES

Aggleton, P. & Chalmers, H. (1986). Nursing research, nursing theory, and the nursing process. *Journal of Advanced Nursing, 11*(2), 197–202.

American Nurses Association. (1988). *Peer review guidelines.* Kansas City, MO: Author.

Barton, J., Smith, M., Brown, N., & Supples, J. (1993). Methodological issues in a team approach to community health needs assessment. *Nursing Outlook, 41*(6), 253–261.

Bayer, M. & Brandner, P. (1977). Nurse/patient peer practice. *American Journal of Nursing, 77*, 86–90.

Capers, C.F. & Kelly, R. (1987). Neuman nursing process: A model of holistic care. *Holistic Nursing Practice, 1*(3),19–26.

Clark, J. (1985). Delivering the goods   the nursing process in health visiting. *Community Outlook,* (Jan.), 23–24,26–28.

Cooper, I. (1986). The nursing process at work . . . Occupational health nurses. *Nursing Times, 82*(1), 32–35.

Goldmann, R.C. (1990). Nursing process components as a framework for monitoring and evaluation activities. *Journal of Nursing Quality Assurance, 4*(4), 17–25.

Hegyvary, S., et al. (1987). *Outcome measures in home health care: Research.* National League for Nursing Publication #21-2194, 29–37.

Henley, M. (1986). The health visiting process . . . based on the nursing process. *Senior Nurse, 4*(5), 23–24.

Ingram, H. H. (1987). Quality assurance in a public health agency. *Quarterly Review Bulletin, 12*(11), 372–76.

Kellogg Foundation (1994). *International Journal of the W.K. Kellogg Foundation, 5*(2), 27.

Kemp, C. (1994). Community health clinical experiences: The primary care setting. *Public Health Nursing, 11*(1), 2–6.

Kneeshaw, M.F. & Lunney, M. (1989). Nursing diagnosis: not for individuals only. *Geriatric Nursing, 10*(5), 246–247.

Koch, C. K., et al. (1994). Population-oriented nursing: preparing tomorrow's nurses today. *Journal of Nursing Education, 33*(5), 236–7.

Lee, H. & Frenn, M.D. (1987). The use of nursing diagnoses for health promotion in community practice. *Nursing Clinics of North America, 22*(4), 981–986.

Lewis, T. (1988). Leaping the chasm between nursing theory and practice. *Journal of Advanced Nursing, 13*(3), 345–51.

Marriner, A. (1979). *The nursing process* (2nd ed.). St. Louis: Mosby.

Martin, K.S. & Scheet, N.J. (1988). The Omaha system: providing a framework for assuring quality of home care. *Home Healthcare Nurse, 6*(3), 24–28.

McHugh, M.L. (1989). Computer support for the nursing process. *Health Matrix, 7*(1), 57–60.

Mitchell, M.K., et al (1989). *Standards of excellence for community health organizations . . . Community Health Accreditation Program (CHAP).* NLN Publication, Community Health Accreditation Program #21-2328:various paging.

Neufeld, A. & Harrison, M.J. (1990). The development of nursing diagnoses for aggregates and groups. *Public Health Nursing, 7*(4), 251–255.

Newman, D.L., et al. (1990). What is evaluation: nurse decision-makers' perceptions of program evaluation. *Journal of New York State Nurses Association, 21*(3), 10–14.

Pearson, M.A., et al. (1991). Progam evaluation application of a comprehensive model for a community-based respite program. *Journal of Community Health Nursing, 8*(1), 25–31.

Porter, E.J. (1987). The nursing diagnosis of population groups. In R.M. Carroll-Johnson (Ed.), *Classification of Nursing Diagnoses, Proceedings of the Eighth Confer-ence.* North American Diagnosis Association. Philadelphia: Lippincott.

Ruffing-Rahal, M.A. (1994). Evaluation of group health promotion with community-dwelling older women. *Public Health Nursing, 11*(1), 38–48.

Schmele, J.A. (1989). A process method for clinical practice evaluation in the home health setting. *Journal of Nursing Quality Assurance, 3*(3), 54–63.

Sheps, C. G. (1976). *Higher education for public health: Report of the Milbank Memorial Fund Commission.* New York: Neale, Watson.

Stewart, M.J., et al. (1987–1988). Adaptation of the nursing audit to community health nursing. *Nursing Forum, 23*(4), 134–153.

Urrutia-Rojas, X. & Aday, L.A. (1991). A framework for community assessment: designing and conducting a survey in a Hispanic immigrant and refugee community. *Public Health Nursing, 8*(1), 20–26.

Vilnius, D., et al. (1990). A priority rating system for public health programs. *Public Health Reports, 105*(5), 463–470.

Weidenbach, E. (1964). *Clinical nursing: A helping art.* New York: Springer.

White, M. S. (1982). Construct for public health nursing. *Nursing Outlook, 30,* 527–30.

Williams, C. A. (1977). Community health nursing—What is it? *Nursing Outlook, 25,* 250–53.

Williams, C. A. (1992). Community-based population-focused practice: The foundation of specialization in public health nursing. In M. Stanhope & J. Lancaster (Eds.), *Community health nursing: Process and practice for promoting health.* St.Louis: Mosby.

Wright, C. (1985). Computer-aided nursing diagnosis for community health nurses. *Nursing Clinics of North America, 20*(3), 487–95.

Yura, H. & Walsh, M.B. (1988). *The nursing process: Assessing, planning, implementing, evaluating* (5th ed). Norwalk, CT: Appleton and Lange.

SELECTED READINGS

American Nurses' Association (1986). *Standards for community health nursing practice.* Kansas City, MO: Author.

Barker, J. B., et al. (1994). Community analysis: A collaborative community practice project. *Public Health Nursing, 11*(2), 113–8.

Barriball, K., et al. (1992). The demand for measuring the impact of nursing interventions: a community perspective. *Journal of Clinical Nursing, 1*(4), 207–12.

Brooking, J. (1989). A scale to measure use of the nursing process. *Nursing Times,* Apr 12–18, 85(15), (Occasional Paper, 44,46,48–9).

Burns, J. (1993). Caring for the community. *Modern Health Care, 23*(45), 30–3.

Caretto, V.A., et al. (1991). Community as client: a "hands on" experience for baccalaureate nursing students. *Journal of Community Health Nursing, 8*(3), 179–189.

Carpenito, L.J. (1989). *Nursing diagnosis: Application to clinical practice* (3rd ed). Philadelphia: Lippincott.

Chambers, L.W., et al. (1991). New approaches to addressing information needs in local public health agencies. *Canadian Journal of Public Health, 82*(2), 109–114.

Glick, D. F., et al. (1994). Grant writing: An innovative project for teaching community health program planning. *Journal of Nursing Education, 33*(5), 238–40.

Goeppinger, J. (1988). Challenges in assessing the impact of nursing service: A community perspective. *Public Health Nursing, 5*(4), 241–245.

Halbert, T.L., et al. (1993). Population-based health promotion: a new agenda for public health nurses. *Canadian Journal of Public Health, 84*(4), 243–5.

Lambert, M.A., et al. (1989). Nursing diagnoses recorded in nursing situations encountered in a department of public health. *Classification of Nursing Diagnoses, Proceedings of the Eighth Conference*, 234–238.

McKnight, J. & Van Dover, L. (1994). Community as client: a challenge for nursing education. *Public Health Nursing, 11*(1), 12–16.

Meyers, J. & Stull, M. (1989). The use of nursing diagnoses in community-based nursing agencies. *Classification of Nursing Diagnoses, Proceedings of the 7th Conference.*

Peckham, S., et al. (1994). Community development approaches to health needs assessment. *Health Visitor, 67*(4),124–5.

Penner, S. (1994). HIV/AIDS and mental illness: the case for community health planning. *Psychosocial Rehabilitation Journal, 17*(4), 127–36.

Schmele, J.A. & Allen, M.E. (1990). A comparison of four nursing process measures of quality in home health. *Journal of Nursing Quality Assurance, 4*(4):26–35.

Veney, J.E. & Kaluzny, A.D. (1991). *Evaluation and decision making for health services* (2nd ed.). Ann Arbor, MI: Health Administration Press.

Wickizer, T., VonKorff, M., Cheadle, A., Maeser, J., Wagner, E., Pearson, D., Beery, W., & Psaty, B. (1993). Activating communities for health promotion: a process evaluation method. *American Journal of Public Health 83*(4), 561–567.

Zielstorff, R.D., et al (1988). Computer design criteria for systems that support the nursing process. American Nurses Association Publication NS-30:1–40.

Epidemiological Assessment of Community Health Status

LEARNING OBJECTIVES

Upon completion of this chapter, readers should be able to:

- Explain the host, agent, and environment model.
- Describe theories of causality in health and illness.
- Define immunity and explain passive, active, cross, and herd immunity.
- Explain how epidemiologists determine populations at risk.
- Explain the four stages of a disease or health condition.
- List the major sources of epidemiologic information.
- Distinguish between incidence and prevalence in health and illness states.
- Use epidemiologic methods to describe an aggregate's health.
- Distinguish between types of epidemologic studies useful for researching aggregate health.

KEY TERMS

- Agent
- Analytic epidemiology
- Causality
- Cohort
- Descriptive epidemiology
- Environment
- Epidemiology
- Experimental epidemiology
- Host

- Immunity
- Incidence
- Morbidity rate
- Mortality rate
- Prevalence
- Prospective study
- Rates
- Retrospective study
- Risk

Barbara Walton Spradley and Judith Ann Allender
COMMUNITY HEALTH NURSING: CONCEPTS AND PRACTICE, 4th ed.
© 1996 Barbara Walton Spradley and Judith Ann Allender

Epidemiology is the study of the determinants and distribution of health, disease, and injuries in human populations. It is a specialized form of scientific research which can provide health care workers, including community health nurses, with a body of knowledge on which to base their practice and methods for studying new and existing problems. The term is derived from the Greek words *epi* (upon) *demos* (the people) and *logos* (knowledge), thus meaning the knowledge or study of what happens to people. Epidemiologists ask such questions as, What is the occurrence of health and disease in a population? Is there an increase or decrease in a health state over the years? Does one geographic area have a higher frequency of disease than another? What characteristics of persons with a particular condition distinguish them from those without the condition? Is one treatment or program more effective than another in changing the health of affected individuals? Why do some people recover from a disease when others do not? The ultimate goal of epidemiology is to search for causes of health problems and identify solutions to prevent disease and improve the health of the entire population (Dever, 1991).

Epidemiology offers community health nurses a specific methodology for assessing the health of aggregates (see Fig. 12.1). Furthermore, it provides a frame of reference for investigating and improving clinical practice in any setting. For example, if a community health nursing goal is to lower the incidence of sexually transmitted diseases (STDs) in a given community, such a prevention plan requires information about population groups. How many cases of STDs have been reported in this community in the past year? What is the expected number of STD cases (the morbidity rate)? What members of the community are at highest risk of contracting STDs? Any program of screening, treatment, or health promotion regarding STDs must be based on this kind of information about population groups in order to be effective. Whether the community health nurse's goals are to improve a population's nutrition, to control the spread of HIV, to deal with health problems created by a flood, or to protect and promote the health of battered women, epidemiologic data is essential.

The author is indebted to Drs. Shirley J. Thompson and Sara L. Turner, who contributed the epidemiology chapter for the second edition of this text and whose ideas have influenced the development of this chapter.

Historical Roots of Epidemiology

The roots of epidemiology can be traced to Hippocrates (460–477 B.C.). Sometimes referred to as the first epidemiologist, Hippocrates believed that disease not only affected individuals but was a mass phenomenon. He was one of the first to associate the occurrence of disease with lifestyle and environmental factors. However, it was not until the late nineteenth century that modern epidemiology actually came into existence.

Some of history's greatest disasters that led to the development of epidemiology as a science were epidemic diseases. An epidemic refers to a disease occurrence that clearly exceeds normal or expected frequency in a community or region. In past centuries epidemics of cholera, bubonic plague, and smallpox swept through community after community, killing thousands of people, changing the community structure, and altering the life-style of masses of people. When an epidemic, such as the plague or AIDS, is worldwide in distribution it is called a pandemic. Epidemiology became a distinct branch of medical science through its concern with epidemics and pandemics of infectious diseases. In 1348, the Black Death swept through continental Europe and England, killing millions of people. In England alone, approximately one-fourth of the population died from the plague. The plague continued in Europe, but with less force, for three centuries and then waned, only to

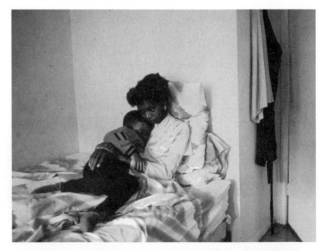

FIGURE 12.1. Developmental difficulties among children in foster homes can be assessed from an epidemiological perspective.

reappear in an epidemic in Hong Kong in 1896. Kitasato, a Japanese bacteriologist, discovered the plague bacillus during this Hong Kong epidemic; within ten years, epidemiologists had traced its life cycle from rats to their infected fleas that bit humans. Now intervention was possible, and public health officials declared war on rats, seeking to make ships and wharf buildings rat-proof. The first major campaign against rats which took place in California after an outbreak of plague in 1900 was successful. However, wild rodents, especially ground squirrels, remain a natural reservoir of the plague bacillus as well as rabbits and domestic cats. Cases still occur occasionally in western United States with periodic outbreaks in various African, Asian, and South American countries (Benenson, 1990). The continuing presence of a disease or infectious agent in a given geographic area, such as plague in Vietnam and malaria in the tropics of Brazil and Indonesia, means the disease is endemic to that area.

As the threat of the great epidemic diseases declined, epidemiologists began to focus on other infectious diseases such as diphtheria, infant diarrhea, typhoid, tuberculosis, and syphilis. They also gathered data pertaining to host characteristics, agent, and environmental factors in diseases such as scurvy among sailors and the occupational disease of scrotal cancer among chimney sweeps. In recent years, epidemiologists have turned to the study of major causes of death and disability, such as cancer, cardiovascular disorders, AIDS, mental illness, accidents, arthritis, and congenital defects.

Nursing's epidemiologic roots can be traced back to Florence Nightingale (1820–1910) (Cohen, 1984). Miss Nightingale often obtained advice on issues related to hospital statistics and disease classification from her close friend William Farr, who was chief statistician of England's General Register Office for health and vital statistics. Her detailed records, morbidity (sickness) statistics, and careful description of the health conditions among the military in the Crimean War represents one of the first systematic descriptive studies of the distribution and patterns of disease in a population. Changes made according to her suggestions brought dramatic proof of the authenticity of her observations and knowledge. Forty out of every 100 British troops (40%) were dying in the Crimea before Miss Nightingale instituted environmental and nutritional changes in the hospital and field. When her work in the Crimea was finished, the mortality (death) rate was only 2%.

Florence Nightingale's use of statistical data along with her commitment to environmental reform strongly influenced nursing's evolution into a profession whose service addressed public health problems as well as hospital care (Kopf, 1978). As nursing has evolved, community health nurses have been increasingly challenged to intervene at the aggregate level, using epidemiologic approaches to address the needs of high-risk groups and populations.

Concepts Basic to Epidemiology

The science of epidemiology draws on certain basic concepts and principles to analyze and understand patterns of occurrence among aggregate health conditions.

HOST, AGENT, AND ENVIRONMENT MODEL

Through their early study of infectious diseases, epidemiologists began to consider disease states generally in terms of the epidemiologic triad, or the host, agent, environment model. Interactions among these three elements explained infectious and other disease patterns.

Agent

An **agent** is the causative factor contributing to a health problem or condition. Causative agents can be factors that are present, such as the presence of bacteria causing tuberculosis, or factors that are lacking, such as lack of iron in the body which causes anemia.

Agents vary considerably and include five types: biological, chemical, nutrient, physical, and psychological. Biological agents include bacteria, viruses, fungi, protozoa, worms, and insects. Some biological agents are infectious, such as influenza virus or HIV. Chemical agents may be in the form of liquids, solids, gases, dusts, or fumes. Examples are poisonous sprays used on garden pests and industrial chemical wastes. The degree of toxicity of the chemical agent influences its impact on health. Nutrient agents include essential dietary components, which if deficient or taken in excess can produce illness conditions. For example, a deficiency of niacin can cause pellagra, and too much Vitamin A can be toxic. Physical agents might be anything mechanical (a chainsaw or an automobile), material (rockslide), or atmospheric (ultraviolet radiation or earthquake), or genetically transmitted that cause injury to humans. The shape, size, and force of physical agents influence the degree of harm to the host. Psychological agents are events producing stress that lead to health problems.

Agents may be classified as either infectious or non-infectious. Infectious agents cause diseases, such as AIDS or tuberculosis, that are communicable. That is, the disease can be spread from one person to another. Certain characteristics of infectious agents are important for community health nurses to understand. Extent of exposure to the agent, the agent's pathogenicity (disease causing ability), infectivity (invasive ability), virulence (severity of disease), and the infectious agent's structure and chemical composition all influence its effects on the host. Chapter 23 examines the subject of communicable disease in greater depth. Noninfectious agents have similar characteristics in that their relative abilities to harm the host vary with type, intensity, duration, and exposure of agent.

Host

The **host** is a susceptible human or animal who harbors and nourishes a disease-causing agent. Many physical, psychological, and life-style factors influence the host's susceptibility and response to an agent. Physical factors include such things as age, sex, race, and genetic influences on the host's vulnerability or resistance. Psychological factors, such as people's outlook and response to stress, can strongly influence host susceptibility. Life style factors also play a major role. Diet, exercise, sleep patterns, healthy or unhealthy habits—all contribute to either increased or decreased vulnerability to the disease-causing agent.

The concept of resistance is important for community health nursing practice. People sometimes have an ability to resist pathogens that is called inherent resistance. They may have inherited or acquired characteristics that make them less vulnerable. The various factors mentioned above play a role in this inherent resistance. People who are healthy and maintain a healthful life style may be exposed to the flu virus or some other pathogen but not contract the disease. Resistance can be promoted through preventive interventions, a point that will be discussed further under levels of prevention.

Environment

The **environment** refers to all the external factors surrounding the host that might influence vulnerability or resistance. The physical environment includes factors like geography, climate, weather, safety of buildings,

and water and food supply, presence of animals, plants, insects, and microorganisms which have the capacity to serve as reservoirs (storage sites for disease-causing agents) or vectors (carriers) for transmitting disease. The psychosocial environment refers to social, cultural, economic, and psychological influences and conditions which affect health, such as access to health care, cultural health practices, poverty, and work stressors that can all contribute to disease or health.

Host, agent, and environment interact with each other to effect a disease or health condition. For example, the agent responsible for Lyme disease is the spirochete, *Borrelia burgdorferi*; humans of all ages are susceptible hosts, along with dogs, cattle, and horses. Ticks that feed on wild rodents and deer transfer the spirochete to human hosts after feeding on them for several hours. Environmental factors, such as working or playing in tick-infested areas, influence host vulnerability. The host, agent, and environment model, shown in Figure 12.2, offered the epidemiologist a plan for intervention. As soon as the agent was identified, measures could be taken to keep the spirochete from infecting human hosts, such as wearing protective clothing or tick repellent in tick-infested areas and prompt removal of surface or attached ticks (Benenson, 1990).

CAUSALITY

The concept of **causality** refers to the relationship between a cause and its effect. A purpose of epidemiologic study has been to discover causal relationships in order to understand why conditions develop and offer effective prevention and protection. Over the years, as sci-

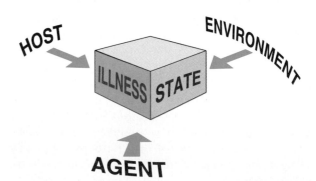

FIGURE 12.2. Epidemiologic Triad. Epidemiologists study the causal agent, the susceptible host, and environmental factors that contribute to an illness state (or a wellness state). Intervention may focus on any of these three to prevent the spread of illness or to improve health in a population.

entific knowledge of health and disease has expanded, epidemiology has changed its view of causality.

Early Theories

Early causal thinking was dominated by Sydenham's miasma theory. This theory held that "foul emanations from impure soil and water cause disease" (Susser, 1973, p.12). Prevention based on this theory attempted to eliminate the sources of the miasma or polluted vapors. Despite its faulty reasoning, this type of prevention has had positive consequences in our awareness that decaying organic matter can be a source of infectious diseases.

A contagion theory of disease had developed by the mid-eighteenth century. This theory inspired various concepts of immunity and even some initial attempts at vaccination against smallpox. Late in the nineteenth century, following the work of Jacob Henle, Louis Pasteur, and Robert Koch (Dever, 1991), the germ theory of disease was established. Epidemiologic efforts then began to focus on identifying the microorganisms that caused disease as a first step in prevention. Once an agent had been identified, measures could be taken to contain its spread. Fumigating ships to kill rats, protecting wharf buildings and human habitations against rats, and removing rat food supplies from easy access were all measures to protect the public by further preventing the spread of plague bacilli.

Up to this point, epidemiologists viewed disease in terms of a simple cause-and-effect relationship. Finding a single cause (plague bacilli) and attacking it (eliminating rats) seemed the solution for preventing many diseases. In the case of bubonic plague, this approach appeared quite effective. However, scientific research revealed that disease causation was much more complex than was first suspected. For example, although most members of a group might be exposed to the plague, many did not contract the disease. With bubonic plague, as with many other infectious diseases, the characteristics of the host can determine the spread of the disease. Not everyone in a population is at risk; it is now known that "untreated bubonic plague has a case fatality rate of about 50%; rarely, it is no more than a localized infection of short duration (pestis minor). Plague organisms have been recovered from throat cultures of asymptomatic contacts of pneumonic plague patients" (Benenson, 1990, p. 324). Clearly, such evidence makes it difficult to speak of a single cause for plague and many other disease states.

Furthermore, even the agent and course of transmission can be quite complex. Although it is a flea that carries the bacilli from rat to human in bubonic plague, pneumonic plague can spread directly from one human being to another. The environment must also be considered as part of the cause in nearly every disease and health state. Considering the plague again, evidence suggests that it originated in the high steppes of Asia and spread to other parts of the world. But questions remain as to whether the bacillus spread from rats to ground squirrels or whether it had always been part of the squirrels' ecology. Although isolated cases continue to occur, epidemics have not occurred and are quite unlikely since squirrels usually live in an environment somewhat separated from that of humans.

Chain of Causation

As the scientific community's thinking about disease causation has grown more complex around the tripartite model of host, agent, and environment, epidemiologists have used the idea of a chain of causation (see Figure 12.3). The chain begins by identifying the reservoir, that is, where the causal agent can live and multiply. With plague, that reservoir may be other humans, rats, squirrels, and a few other animals. With malaria, humans are the major reservoir for the parasitic agents, although certain nonhuman primates also act as reservoirs but transmission is very rare (Benenson, 1990). Next, the agent must have a portal of exit from the reservoir as well as some mode of transmission. The next link in the chain of causation is the agent itself. Malaria, for instance, actually consists of four distinct diseases caused by four kinds of tiny microorganisms called protozoa. These agents spend part of their life cycle in the body of the Anopheles mosquito, which acts as a mode of transmission. The mosquito bite provides a portal of exit as well as a portal of entry into the human host.

The circle surrounding this chain of causation in Figure 12.3 represents the environment, which can have a profound influence at almost any point along the chain. Consider the impact of environmental factors in the malaria epidemic of Ceylon in the Indian Ocean off South India in 1934–1935. Two or three million cases occurred, resulting in eighty thousand deaths. Malaria occurred frequently in the dry northern area where sparse vegetation allowed pools of water to be exposed to the sun, providing excellent breeding grounds for the Anopheles mosquito. The more populous southwestern

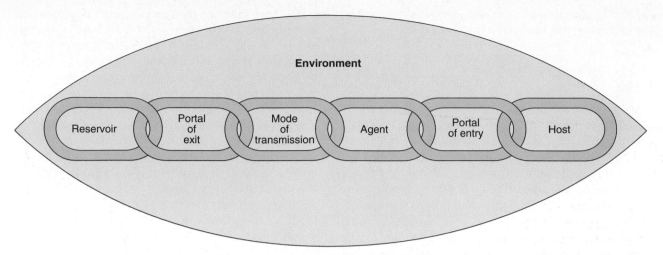

FIGURE 12.3. Chain of causation in infectious disease.

area had heavy monsoon rains and was relatively free from malaria. In 1934 a severe drought changed this environment drastically; rivers almost dried up, leaving stagnant pools of water for mosquito breeding. Widespread crop failure caused the population to become badly undernourished, which added to the conditions that would foster a malaria epidemic. The epidemic hit in October 1934 with devastating results for the population, and the environment must certainly be seen as a major part of the causal chain (Burnet, 1962). A similar tragedy occurred in the African country of Rwanda in July of 1994. Civil war caused a large percent of the population to flee an unfriendly regime. Hundreds of thousands of people filled refugee camps to overflowing. Conditions of squalor and poor sanitation led to contaminated water and resulted in a large scale epidemic of cholera, a severe form of bacterial dysentery. Relief workers had limited supplies of intravenous or oral rehydration solutions and could do little to help. Uncounted thousands lost their lives. The unstable political environment, unsanitary conditions, and malnourishment were all part of the causal chain.

Multiple Causation

Recently, a more advanced concept of multiple causation has emerged to explain the existence of health and illness states and to provide guiding principles for epidemiologic practice (Dever, 1991). Sometimes discussed as a "web of causation," this model attempts to identify all the possible influences on the health and illness processes (Friedman, 1994). Figure 12.4 shows the web of causation for myocardial infarction; such a health problem cannot be explained in single causal terms, even if that cause represents part of a larger chain. Recognition of multiple causes provides many points of intervention for prevention, health promotion, and treatment. For example, examination of Figure 12.4 suggests interventions such as directly attacking significant coronary atherosclerosis (bypass surgery), reducing the incidence of obesity, helping people stop smoking, developing an exercise program, and making dietary modifications.

A concept helpful in determining multiple causality is called association. Events are associated when they appear together more often than they would appear by chance alone. These events may include risk factors or other characteristics affecting disease or health states. Examples are the frequent association of cigarette smoking with lung cancer or obesity with heart disease. Thus study of frequently appearing associated factors suggests possible causality and points for intervention. Contemporary epidemiologists continue to explore new and more comprehensive ways of viewing health and illness. Life-style, behavior, environment, and stress of all kinds affect health states.

In the model of host, agent, and environment, one can note a shifting emphasis over time. Early epidemiologists worked to identify and manage the causative agent; the focus of concern was disease states. The emphasis then shifted to the host. Who was susceptible? What characteristics led to susceptibility? Through immunization and health promotion, efforts were made to improve hosts' resistance. Increasingly, however, com-

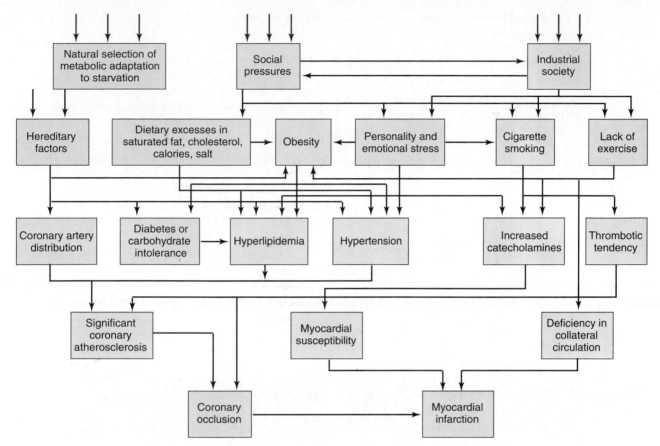

FIGURE 12.4. Web of causation for myocardial infarction. (Adapted from G. D. Friedman, *Primer of Epidemiology.* New York: McGraw-Hill, 1987.) Reprinted by permission.

munity health workers have come to realize the limitations imposed on individual control of health. Even those in the best of health cannot withstand toxic agents in the workplace, nuclear wastes in the atmosphere from power plant accidents, or other debilitating conditions created by modern society. More and more, public health professionals are turning to a study of the environment and looking for methods to change environmental conditions that contribute to illness.

IMMUNITY

The concept of **immunity** refers to the host's ability to resist a particular infectious disease-causing agent. This occurs when the body forms antibodies and lymphocytes that react with the foreign antigenic molecules and render them harmless. For community health nursing, this concept has significance in determining which individuals and groups are protected against disease and

which may be vulnerable. Four types of immunity are important in community health. They are passive, active, cross, and herd immunity.

Passive Immunity

Passive immunity refers to short term resistance that is acquired either naturally or artificially. Newborns, through maternal antibody transfer, have natural passive immunity lasting about six months. Artificial passive immunity is attained through inoculation with a vaccine that gives temporary resistance. Such immunizations must be repeated periodically to maintain immunity levels.

Active Immunity

Active immunity is long term and sometimes life long resistance that is acquired either naturally or artifically. Naturally acquired active immunity comes through host infection. That is, a person who contracts a disease develops long-lasting antibodies that provide immunity against future exposure. Artifically acquired active immunity is attained through vaccine innoculation. Such vaccines are prepared from killed, living-attenuated, or living-virulent organisms administered to artificially produce or increase immunity to a particular disease. The concept of active immunity underlies public health immunizations programs that have successfully kept polio, diphtheria, small pox, and other major diseases under control world wide.

Cross Immunity

A third type, cross immunity, refers to a situation in which a person's immunity to one agent provides that person with immunity to another related agent. The immunity can be either passive or active. Sometimes infection with one disease, such as cow pox, gives immunity to a related disease, such as small pox. The concept of cross immunity has also been useful in the development and administration of vaccines. Innoculation using a vaccine made from one disease organism can provide immunity to a related disease-causing organism. An example is the administration of BCG vaccine, used to prevent tuberculosis, to people who have been exposed to Hansen's disease (leprosy). This provides them with cross immunity to the related infectious agent, *Mycobacterium leprae*, and prevents their contracting the disease (Benenson, 1990).

Herd Immunity

Herd immunity describes the immunity level present in a population group (Benenson, 1990). A population with low herd immunity is one that has few immune members and is consequently more susceptible to the disease. Nonimmune persons are more likely to contract the disease and spread it throughout the group, placing the entire population at greater risk. Conversely, high herd immunity means that the number of immune persons in the group outnumber the susceptible persons, thus reducing the incidence of disease. High herd immunity (80% or more) provides the population with greater overall protection because nonimmune persons are at less risk of disease exposure. Mandatory preschool immunizations and required travel vaccinations are applications of the herd immunity concept.

RISK

To determine the chances that a disease or health problem will occur, epidemiologists are concerned with **risk** or the probability that a disease or other unfavorable health condition will develop. For any given group of persons, risk of developing a health problem is directly influenced by their biology, environment, lifestyle, and the system of health care. Situations or factors in these four areas can negatively affect health and increase the likelihood that a health problem will occur. These negative influences are called risk factors. For example, low birth weight babies (health status) tend to be at greater risk for health problems and people whose lifestyles are very stressful are more prone to illness. The degree of risk is directly linked to people's susceptibility or vulnerability to a given health problem.

Epidemiologists study populations at risk. A population-at-risk means a collection of people among whom a health problem has the possiblity of developing because certain influencing factors are either present (such as exposure to HIV) or absent (such as lack of childhood immunizations). A population-at-risk has a greater probability of developing a given health problem than other groups. Epidemiologists measure this difference using relative risk ratio which statistically compares the disease occurrence in the population-at-risk with the occurrence of the same disease in persons without that risk factor.

$$\text{Relative risk ratio} = \frac{\text{Incidence in exposed group}}{\text{Incidence in unexposed group}}$$

The risk is the same for both groups if the relative risk ratio is 1:1. When the ratio is greater than 1:0 the exposed group is at greater risk. An example is the difference between the incidence of heart disease among smokers (risk factor) as compared to the incidence of heart disease among nonsmokers. Relative risk ratio assists in determining the most effective points for community health intervention with health problems.

NATURAL PROGRESSION OF DISEASE OR HEALTH CONDITION

Any disease follows a progression known as its natural history which refers to events preceeding its development, during its course, and its outcomes. This process involves the interaction between host, agent, and environment. The natural progression of a disease occurs in four stages as they affect a population. They are susceptibility, exposure, onset, and culmination. (See Fig. 12.5).

1. In the *susceptibility stage*, also called the stage of prepathogenesis, the disease is not present nor have individuals been exposed. However, host and environment factors could very likely influence people's susceptibility to a causative agent and lead to development of the disease. For example, in 1994 the overcrowded conditions and poor sanitation of Rwandan refugee camps in Africa (described earlier in this chapter) as well as refugees' stress, fatigue, and malnutrition made them extremely vulnerable to contracting cholera and other diseases.

2. The *exposure stage* occurs when individuals have been exposed but are asymptomatic. This stage has also been called early pathogenesis because the disease is present in an early form and has begun its work. Vulnerable children who have been exposed to chicken pox but do not yet display signs of fever or lesions are an example.

3. During the *onset stage*, signs and symptoms of the disease or condition develop. In the early phase of this period, the signs may only be evident through laboratory tests, such as tubercular lesions on x-ray or premalignant cervical changes evident on Pap smears. Later in this stage acute symptoms are clearly visible as in the case of widespread enterocolitis in a salmonellosis (food poisoning) outbreak. Other names for this stage are the clinical stage or early discernible lesions stage since evidence of the disease or condition is now present.

4. In the *culmination stage* the disease or health condition is fully advanced and concludes either in a return to health, a residual or chronic form with some disabling limitations, or death. This is also called the advanced disease stage because the disease or condition has completed its course.

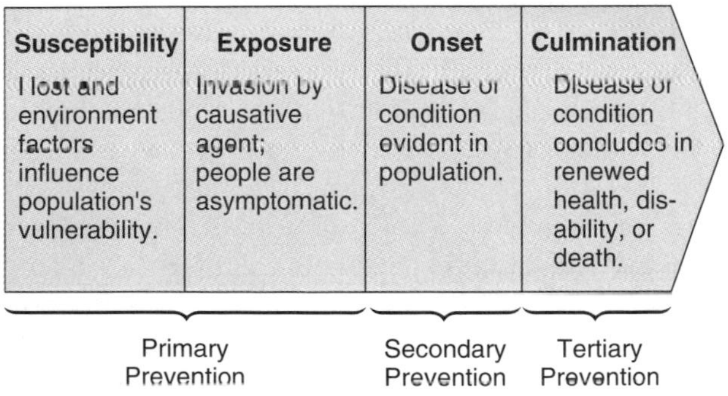

Community health nurses can intervene at any point during these four stages to delay, arrest, or prevent the progress of the disease. Primary, secondary, and tertiary prevention can be applied to the stages and are depicted in the Levels of Prevention discussion below.

EPIDEMIOLOGY OF WELLNESS

The concepts discussed thus far refer primarily to disease; epidemiology, however, is also turning its attention to the study of wellness. See Issues in Community Health Nursing below. Epidemiology has moved from concentrating only on illness to examining how agent, host, and environment are involved in wellness at various levels. In response to an escalating need for improved methods for health planning and health policy analysis, epidemiology has developed more holistic models of health. These newer epidemiologic models are organized around four attributes that influence health: (1) the physical, social, and psychological environment, (2) lifestyle with its self-created risks, (3) human biology and genetic influences, and (4) the system of health care organization (Blum, 1981; Dever, 1991). Wellness models that at first focused on individual behavior now include approaches that encompass aggregates. Such a model was used by nurse researchers to study the substance abuse pandemic (Talashek, et al, 1994). Societal changes, such as the growing elderly population, communication revolution, global economy, environmental threats, technology development, holism and wellness movements, are driving these new approaches.

The natural history stages of disease can apply to one's understanding of any health condition including wellness states. In stage one, susceptibility, people can become amenable to healthier practices and improved health system organization. In stage two, exposure, a community can learn about these health promoting behaviors. Stage three, onset, could be a period of trying out the beneficial policies and activities, and stage four, culmination, could be full adoption and a higher level of well being for the community. This fact has important implications for community health nursing preventive and health promotive practice.

Susceptibility	Exposure	Onset	Culmination
Host and environment factors influence population's vulnerability.	Invasion by causative agent; people are asymptomatic.	Disease or condition evident in population.	Disease or condition concludes in renewed health, disability, or death.

Primary Prevention   Secondary Prevention   Tertiary Prevention

FIGURE 12.5. Natural history stages of a disease or health condition.

Levels of Prevention
PREVENTION DURING NATURAL HISTORY STAGES OF DISEASE

GOAL

Since the events leading to a disease or health condition generally develop over time, there are a number of instances where preventive measures can alter or stop their progress. Community health nurses have a prime opportunity to apply the three levels of prevention, primary, secondary, and tertiary, discussed in Chapter 1, to the natural history progression of a health condition.

PRIMARY PREVENTION

Primary prevention, which keeps a health problem from ever occurring, can be applied in both the susceptibility and exposure stages. Susceptible and exposed people are at risk. The number and type of risk factors can be eradicated or reduced through health promotion and protection measures. Health promotion measures might include nutritional counseling, sex education, and smoking cessation. Protective measures might address such areas as improved housing and sanitation, immunizations, and removal of environmental hazards.

Public health efforts using primary prevention have been very successful in reducing disease occurrence with its associated mortality and morbidity. This can be attributed, in particular, to mandatory immunization programs and environmental management.

SECONDARY PREVENTION

Secondary prevention seeks to find and treat existing health problems as early as possible. Sec-

ondary preventive measures are used to address the third stage in the natural history of disease, the onset stage, through early detection, diagnosis, and timely treatment. When an illness exists, screening programs can detect such conditions as breast and testicular cancer, hypertension, hearing problems, tuberculosis, and diabetes. Screening tests and early case-finding provide opportunities to diagnose and treat conditions in the early stage of the disease or illness condition's progress. The aim of secondary prevention is to remove the health problem, cure the disease, or at least arrest its progression and prevent associated disability.

TERTIARY PREVENTION

Tertiary prevention seeks to reduce the extent and severity of a health problem in order to minimize disability and restore or preserve function. This level addresses the culmination stage of the natural history of disease process. At this stage the health condition is advanced, thus tertiary preventive measures include treatment to arrest further progression of the disease and rehabilitative efforts to limit disability. At the aggregate level, an example of tertiary prevention is providing food, shelter, health services, and training for employment with a homeless population. Another example is group treatment and rehabilitation for adolescent drug users.

Community health nurses apply all three levels of prevention but concentrate their efforts especially on the primary and secondary levels.

Current Epidemiologic Study: Causal Relationships

One of the main challenges to epidemiology today is to identify causal relationships in disease and health conditions in populations. As has been suggested in previous sections, the assessment of causality in human health is difficult at best; no single study is adequate to establish causality. Causal inference is based on consistent results obtained from many studies. Frequently the accumulation of evidence begins with a clinical obser-

vation or an educated guess that a certain factor may be causally related to a health problem. A cross-sectional study (exploring a health condition's relationship to other variables in a specified population at a certain point in time) can show that the factor and problem co-exist. An example is a study of never smokers, former smokers, and current smokers to examine the association of smoking with facial wrinkling (Ernster, et al, 1995). Results of the study showed that risk of facial wrinkling was greater in cigarette smokers than in never smokers. A **retrospective study** (looking backward in time to find a causal relationship) allows a fairly quick

The public health science of epidemiology has traditionally studied the occurrence of disease and health problems. Because of their devastating effect on the health of populations, infectious diseases like plague, cholera, and AIDS as well as chronic illnesses like heart disease and cancer and fatal or debilitating injuries all require a continued epidemiologic focus. Nonetheless, the need to examine the epidemiology of wellness grows increasingly urgent. In the United States, establishment of health objectives for the year 2000 (*Healthy People*, 1991) and greater recognition of the importance and cost effectiveness of illness prevention and health promotion are driving new efforts at developing policy and research initiatives for public health.

Community health nursing can play a primary role in the investigation and identification of factors that not only prevent illness but also promote health. This means sharpening skills in epidemiologic research to uncover the factors that contribute to a full measure of healthful living. The time for an epidemiology of wellness has come.

crease the probability of occurrence of the disease or condition as observed in many studies in different populations; and (2) there is evidence that a reduction in the factor decreases the frequency of the given disease (Hennekens & Buring, 1987). The synthesis of data begins by selecting as many as possible of all the various types of epidemiologic studies on the problem. After discarding those studies that are not methodologically sound, the studies are reviewed. The better the data meet the following six criteria, the more likely the factor of interest will be one of several causes of the disease:

1. Temporal relationship: Exposure to the suspected factor must precede the onset of disease.
2. Strength of the association: This refers to the ratio of disease rates in those with and without the suspected causal factor. A strong association would be noted when disease rates are much higher in the group with the factor than in the group without it.
3. Dose-response relationship: This relationship is demonstrated if, with increasing levels of exposure to the factor, there is a corresponding increase in occurrence of disease.
4. Consistency: Association is demonstrated in varying types of studies among diverse study groups.
5. Biological plausibility and coherence of the evidence: The hypothesized cause makes sense based on current biological knowledge.
6. Lowering of disease risk: Interventions that decrease the exposure or factor result in a lowering of disease risk (relative risk).

The goal of any epidemiologic investigation is to identify causal mechanisms that meet the above criteria and to develop measures for preventing illness and promoting health. The community health nurse may need to gather new data for this type of investigation, but should thoroughly examine existing, pertinent data before doing so. This type of information can be obtained by the community health nurse from a variety of sources, discussed in the next section.

assessment of whether or not an association exists. Nonepidemiologic animal studies may suggest a biologic mechanism whereby the factor could cause the disease or condition. At this point, a **prospective study** (looking forward in time to find a causal relationship) is crucial to assure that the presumed causal factor actually antedates the onset of the health problem. The prospective approach is concerned with current information and provides a direct measure of the variables in question. And finally, if ethically possible, an experimental study (when the investigator controls or changes factors suspected of causing the condition and observes results) is used to confirm the associations obtained from the observational studies. Thus, it often requires many years to accumulate enough evidence to provide adequate information for developing a health intervention strategy or for changing a current practice.

Epidemiologically, one can accept that a causal relationship may exist when two major conditions are met: (1) the factor of interest (causal agent) is shown to in-

Sources of Information for Epidemiologic Study

Epidemiologic investigators may draw data from three major sources or a combination of these sources. They are (1) existing data, (2) informal investigations, and (3) scientific studies. The community health nurse will find all three sources useful in efforts to improve the health of aggregates.

EXISTING DATA

A variety of information is available nationally, by states, and by sections, such as counties or urbanized areas. This information includes vital statistics, census data, and morbidity statistics on certain communicable or infectious diseases. Local health departments often can provide this data upon request. Community health nurses seeking information on near by communities may find local health system agencies helpful. These agencies work to collect health information for groups of counties within states and interact with health planning authorities at the state level. They have access to many types of information and can give advice on specific problems raised by nurses.

Vital Statistics

Vital statistics is a term used for the information gathered from ongoing registration of "vital" events relating to births, deaths, adoptions, divorces, and marriages. Certification of births, deaths, and fetal deaths are the vital statistics most useful in epidemiologic study. The community health nurse can obtain blank copies of a state's birth and death certificates to become familiar with the information contained in each. It will become apparent that much more information is recorded than the fact and cause of death on the death certificate. Birth certificates also can provide helpful information. For example, the weights of infants and the amount of prenatal care received by their mothers have been used to identify high-risk mothers and infants.

Census Data

Data from population censuses taken every ten years in many countries are the main source of population statistics. This information can be a valuable assessment tool for the community health nurse taking part in health planning for aggregates. These population statistics can be analyzed by age, sex, race, ethnic background, type of occupation, income gradient, marital status, or educational level, as well as by other standards, such as housing. Analysis of population statistics can provide the community health nurse with a better understanding of the community and help identify

specific areas that may warrant further epidemiologic investigation.

Reportable Diseases

Each state has developed laws or regulations that require health organizations and practitioners to report to their local health authority cases of certain communicable and infectious diseases that can be spread through the community (Benenson, 1990). This reporting enables the health department to take the most appropriate and efficient action. All states require that the diseases subject to international quarantine regulations be reported immediately. These diseases (plague, cholera, yellow fever, and small pox) are virtually unknown now in developed countries. The World Health Organization announced the eradication of smallpox in 1979 after more than ten years of international effort (Henderson, 1980). In addition, the diseases under surveillance by the World Health Organization (louse-borne typhus fever and relapsing fever, paralytic poliomyelitis, malaria, and viral influenza) must be reported. The other reportable diseases (varying between 20 and 40 by state) are usually classified according to the speed with which the health department should be notified. Some should be reported by phone or electronic mail, others weekly by regular mail. They vary in potential severity from chicken pox to rabies and include AIDS (acquired immune deficiency syndrome), encephalitis, meningitis, syphilis, and toxic shock syndrome. Community health nurses should obtain the list of reportable diseases from their local or state health department offices. Following up on occurrences of these diseases is a task frequently assigned to community nursing services.

Disease Registries

In some areas or states there are disease registries or rosters for conditions with major public health impact. Tuberculosis and rheumatic fever registries were more common in past years when these diseases occurred more frequently. Cancer registries provide useful incidence, prevalence, and survival data and assist the community health nurse in monitoring cancer patterns within a community.

Environmental Monitoring

State governments, sometimes through health departments and sometimes through other agencies, now monitor health hazards found in the environment. Pesticides, industrial wastes, radioactive or nuclear materials, chemical additives in food, and medicinal drugs have joined the list of pollutants. (See Chapter 6, Environmental Health and Safety, for detailed discussion). Concerned community members and leaders view these as risk factors that affect health at both the community and individual levels. Community health nurses can also obtain data from federal agencies such as the Food and Drug Administration, the Consumer Product Safety Commission, and the Environmental Protection Agency.

National Center for Health Statistics Health Surveys

On the national level (published data are frequently available also for regions), the National Center for Health Statistics (NCHS) furnishes valuable health prevalence data from surveys of Americans (Pickett & Hanlon, 1990). The Health Interview Survey includes interviews from approximately 40,000 households each year and provides information about the health status and needs of the entire country. The Health Examination Survey reports physical measurements on smaller samples of the population and augments the information provided by interviews. This survey provides prevalence information on injuries, diseases, and disabilities that appear frequently in the population. A third type of NCHS survey is of health records. This survey samples institutional records of hospitals and nursing homes, primarily. This survey provides information on those who are using services from these institutions along with diagnoses and other characteristics. Other NCHS surveys focus on fertility and family planning, follow-back studies on vital statistics events, and characteristics of ambulatory patients in physicians' community practices.

Each of these nationally sponsored efforts suggests ways in which community health nurses can examine health problems or concerns affecting their communities. Interviews, physical examinations of samples of community members, and surveillance of institutions, clinics, and private physicians' practices can be carried out locally when needs are identified and funds made available. Other sources may be found in data kept routinely but not centrally on the health problems of workers in local industry or health problems of school children, a key issue to many community health nurses. Existing epidemiologic data can be used to plan parent education programs, health promotion among students, and almost any other type of service.

INFORMAL OBSERVATIONAL STUDIES

A second information source in epidemiologic study comes through informal observation and description. Almost any client group encountered by the community health nurse can trigger such a study. If, for example, the nurse encounters an abused child at a clinic, screening the clinic's records for possible further instances of child abuse and neglect could lead to more case finding. If several cases of diabetes come to the attention of a nurse serving on a Navaho reservation, a widespread problem might come to light through conducting informal inquiries about the incidence and age of onset of the disease among this Native American population. A nurse working with several elderly widows living alone learned by questioning them that being independent was secondary to staying in their own homes. Interview data revealed that these older widows had learned to accept their aloneness, exercised freedom and delegation in getting things done, practiced safety measures, and took good care of themselves thus enabling them to continue to live at home (Porter, 1994). Collecting such information, complemented with existing data, could lead to improved understanding and service to the broader population of elderly widows living alone. Informal observational study often raises questions and suggests hypotheses that form the basis for designing larger scale epidemiologic investigations.

SCIENTIFIC STUDIES

The third source of information used in epidemiologic inquiry involves carefully designed scientific studies. Nursing, as a profession, has recognized the need to develop a systematic body of knowledge on which to base nursing practice. Already, systematic research is becoming an accepted part of the community health nurse's role. Findings from epidemiologic studies conducted by or involving nurses are appearing more frequently in the literature. For example, concern about a large number of infant injuries led a nurse and physician research team to study sociodemographic and psychosocial risk factors causing unintentional infant injuries in the home (Harris & Kotch, 1994). They learned that family conflict and maternal unemployment were among predictors for unintentional injury. They also learned that use of social support to alleviate maternal stress resulted in fewer unintentional infant injuries. In another study, three nurses in Houston wanted to prevent the battering of pregnant women

(Helton, et al., 1987). They conducted a scientific study and discovered that 36% of the study population (14,047 prenatal patients served by area clinics) had been battered or were at risk for battering and none had been assessed for abuse by their health care providers. The nurses started an educational program and successfully increased (to 75%) health care providers' knowledge of and routine assessment for abuse. Part of their study was a scientific evaluation of the outcomes of their nursing interventions. Systematic studies such as these, as well as informal studies and existing epidemiologic data, can provide the community health nurse with valuable information that can be used to positively affect aggregate health.

Methods in the Epidemiologic Investigative Process

The goal of epidemiologic investigation is to identify the causal mechanisms of health and illness states and to develop measures for preventing illness and promoting health. Epidemiologists employ an investigative process that involves a sequence of three approaches that build on one another: descriptive, analytic, and experimental studies. All three approaches have relevance for community health nursing.

DESCRIPTIVE EPIDEMIOLOGY

Descriptive epidemiology includes investigations that seek to observe and describe patterns of health-related conditions which naturally occur in a population. For example, a community health nurse might seek to learn how many children in a school district have been immunized for measles, how many home births occur each year in the county, or how many cases of sexually transmitted diseases have occurred in the city in the past month. At this stage in the epidemiologic investigation one seeks to establish the occurrence of a problem. Data from descriptive studies suggest hypotheses for further testing. Descriptive studies almost always involve some form of broad-based quantification and statistical analysis.

Counts

The simplest measure of description is a count. For example, an epidemiologic study of childhood drownings was conducted to provide data for prevention ef-

forts in Harris County, Texas (Warneke & Cooper, 1994). One of the first steps in the research was to make a simple count of the number of child and adolescent (newborn through 19 years) drownings that occurred. The investigators gathered data from death certificates (1983 through 1989) and medical examiner data (1983 through 1990); most of the 196 unintentional drownings occurred in swimming pools, half of which were in apartment pools and a third in private home pools (See Fig. 12.6). Obtaining a count of this type always depends on the definition of what one counts. This count, for example, does not represent all drownings occurring in the county, but only those in this age group. As in most kinds of research, availability of data influences the count. Before making use of any statistics, whether from official state offices, the census bureau, or a health agency, it is necessary to determine what the information represents.

The count of reported drownings describes one population group in Harris County. If one wishes a count to be descriptive of a group it must be seen in proportion to that group. That is, it must be divided by the total number in the group, in this case the childhood popu-

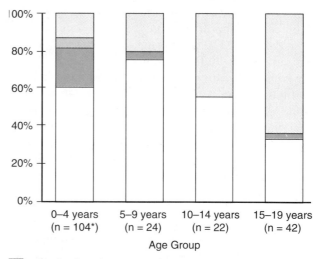

FIGURE 12.6. Percentage distribution for location of submersion, by age group, for unintentional drownings that, according to medical examiner files, occurred in Harris County, Texas, 1983 through 1990, among persons newborn through 19 years (Warneke & Cooper, 1994, p.595). Reprinted by permission.

lation of Harris County. The 196 drownings would have quite a different significance if the total childhood population in the county were 1,000 on the one hand, or 500,000 on the other.

Rates

Rates are a statistical measure expressing the proportion of persons with a given health problem among a population at risk. The total number of persons in this group serves as the denominator for various types of rates. In order to express a count as a proportion, or rate, one must first decide on the population to be studied. If 196 drownings are considered in relation to the total number of children in Harris County, there will be one rate; if they are considered in relation to the total population of children in the state, there will be a different proportion.

In epidemiology, the population represents the universe of people defined as the objects of one's study. Because it is often difficult, if not impossible, to study an entire population, most epidemiologic studies draw a sample to represent that group. For example, in the Houston study dealing with prevention of battering during pregnancy, the nurse investigators selected a random sample of 290 pregnant women to interview out of a population of 14,047 prenatal clients served by area clinics (Helton, et al., 1987). Sometimes it is important to seek a random sample (when everyone in the population has an equal chance of selection for study and choice is made without bias); at other times, a sample of convenience (when study subjects are selected because of their avaliablity) is sufficient. In many small epidemiologic studies it may be possible to study nearly every person in the population, thus eliminating the need for a sample.

Several proportions have wide use in epidemiology. Those most important for the community health nurse to understand include prevalence rate, period prevalence rate, and incidence rate.

Prevalence refers to all people with a health condition existing in a given population at a given point in time. The prevalence rate describes a situation at one point in time (Friedman, 1994). If a nurse discovers 50 cases of measles in an elementary school, that is a simple count. If that number is divided by the number of students in the school, it describes the prevalence of measles. For instance, if the school has 500 students, the prevalence of measles on that day would be 10% (50 measles/500 population).

$$\text{Prevalence Rate} = \frac{\text{Number of Persons with a Characteristic}}{\text{Total Number in Population}}$$

In the study of reported drownings, on the other hand, the investigators had a count for a seven-year period, 1983 to 1990. Rather than portraying only one day, this number covered an extended period of time. Calculating the prevalence rate over a period of time is called a period prevalence rate.

$$\text{Period Prevalence Rate} = \frac{\text{Number of Persons with a Characteristic During a Period of Time}}{\text{Total Number in Population}}$$

Not everyone in a population is at risk for developing a disease, incurring an injury, or having some other health-illness characteristic. The incidence rate recognizes this fact. **Incidence** refers to all new cases of a disease or health condition appearing during a given time. Incidence rate describes a proportion in which the numerator is all new cases appearing during a given time and the denominator is the population at risk during the same period of time. For example, some childhood diseases give lifelong immunity. The children in a school who have had such diseases would be removed from the total number of children at risk in the school population. The incidence rate, after three weeks of a measles epidemic in a school, was

$$\frac{200}{1000} \text{ or } \frac{200 \text{ New Cases}}{1000 \text{ Persons at Risk}}$$

during the three-week time period. The health literature is not always consistent in the use of the term incidence; sometimes this word is used synonymously with prevalence rates and the reader must take this into consideration.

$$\text{Incidence Rate} = \frac{\text{Number of Persons Developing a Disease}}{\text{Total Number at Risk}} \text{ per Unit of Time}$$

Another rate describing incidence is called an attack rate. An attack rate describes the proportion of a group or population that develops a disease among all those exposed to a particular risk. This term is used frequently in investigations of outbreaks of infectious diseases such as influenza. When the attack rate changes, it may suggest an alteration in the population's immune status or that the disease-causing organism is present in a more virulent strain.

Computing Rates

In order to make comparisons between populations, epidemiologists often use a common base population in computing rates. For example, instead of merely saying that the rate of an illness is 13% in one city and 25% in another, the comparison is made per 100,000 persons in the population. This population base can vary for different purposes from 1000 to 100,000. To describe the **morbidity rate**, which is the relative incidence of disease in a population, one would describe the ratio of the number of sick individuals to a total given population. The **mortality rate** refers to the relative death rate or the sum of deaths in a given population at a given time. The following are formulas for computing rates commonly used in community health:

$$\text{Mortality Rate} = \frac{\text{Number of Reported Deaths}}{\text{Estimated Population as of July 1 of Same Year}} \times 100,000$$

$$\text{Infant Mortality Rate} = \frac{\text{Number of Deaths Under 1 Year of Age for Given Year}}{\text{Number of Live Births Reported for Same Year}} \times 1000$$

$$\text{Case Fatality Rate} = \frac{\text{Number of Deaths from a Particular Disease}}{\text{Total Number with the Disease}}$$

The goal of descriptive studies is to identify the patterns of occurrence of any health-related condition. They can be retrospective (identify cases and controls, then go back to review existing data) or prospective (identify groups and exposure factors and follow them forward in time). In a descriptive study of child abuse, for example, the investigator would note the age, sex, race or ethnic group, and physical and emotional conditions of the children affected. In addition, data would be collected that described the economic status and occupation of parents, the location and setting of abusive behavior, and the time and season of the year when abuse occurred. In the study on reported drownings in Harris County, Texas (retrospective design), the investigators described the age, sex, and ethnic background of victims and other features such as location and time of drowning. Describing facets of these health conditions provided information for further study as well as suggested avenues for intervention or prevention.

ANALYTIC EPIDEMIOLOGY

A second type of epidemiologic investigation is analytic. **Analytic epidemiology** goes beyond simple description or observation and seeks to identify associations between a particular human disease or health problem and its possible cause(s). Analytic studies tend to be more specific than descriptive studies in their focus. They test hypotheses or seek to answer specific questions and can be retrospective or prospective in design. As an example of an analytic study of prospective design, several nurses set out to address the question, are paper diapers more effective in controlling fecal contamination than cloth diapers in a day care environment by studying children and providers in four licensed day care centers in Davidson County, Tennessee (Holaday, et al., 1995). A total of 104 children and 25 caregivers participated in the study over a period of eight weeks. The centers were supplied with cloth and paper diapers and two centers used cloth diapers for the first four-week period while the other two used paper, each then switching to the other diaper type for the second four-week period. The investigators monitored selected rooms twice weekly in each center for the presence of fecal bateria by sampling of play/sleep area, diaper changing area, and caregivers' and children's hands. (See Fig. 12.7) No significant differences were found between cloth and paper diapers in the frequency or intensity of fecal contamination. However, the study revealed that sink faucets and caregivers' and children's hands were often contaminated suggesting the need for further study of handwashing and diapering techniques, use of disinfectant hand creams, and altering the environment by installing automatic, faucet-free hand-washing sinks. Like many analytical studies, this one gathered a great deal of descriptive data as well.

Analytic studies fall into three types—prevalence studies, case-control studies, and cohort studies.

Prevalence Studies

When one examines prevalence it is helpful to remember that the health condition may be new or have affected some persons for many years. Prevalence studies describe patterns of occurrence, as in the study of reported drownings in Texas and in the Research in Community Health Nursing display below. They may examine causal factors, but these are always from the same point in time and the same population. Hypothesized causal factors are based on inferences from a sin-

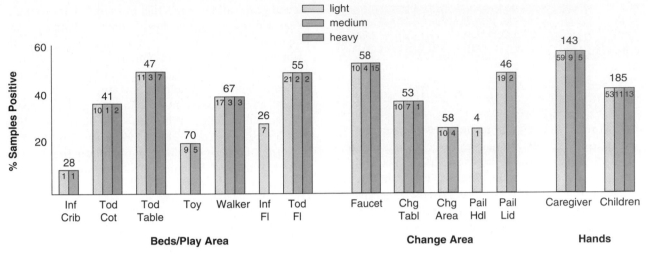

FIGURE 12.7. Cloth vs. paper diaper study. Total fecal cultures by collection site and location: percentage of positive samples from all four centers in both time periods (Holaday, et al, 1995, p. 31). Reprinted by permission. Note: Above each bar is the total number of specimens collected at each site. Within each bar is the number of positive samples that are classified as light, medium, or heavy growth. Inf crib = infant crib; tod cot = toddler cot; tod table = toddler table; inf fl = infant floor; tod flr = toddler floor; chg table = diaper change table; chg are = diaper change area; hdl = diaper pail handle; lid = diaper pail lid.

gle examination and most likely need further testing for validation.

Case-Control Studies

Case-control studies make a comparison between persons with a health-illness condition (cases) and those who lack this condition (controls). These studies begin with disease (case) and look back over time for presence or absence of the suspected causal factor in both cases and controls. In the study of battered wives, the 20 women who had been beaten by their husbands represented the cases, the 30 who had not experienced violence were the controls. This study then reviewed the history of cases and controls for the presence of wife battering in the woman's nuclear family. In a case-control study, both groups should share as many characteristics as possible in order to isolate possible causes. Comparison between one group of women in their early twenties with another group in their late seventies would have invalidated the conclusion in the study of the battered wife syndrome.

Cohort Studies

A **cohort** is a group of people who share a common experience in a specific time period. Examples are a group of school children or the employees of an indus-

try. In epidemiology, a cohort of people often becomes a focus of study. Cohort studies, rather than measure the relationship of variables in existing conditions, study the development of a condition over time. A cohort study begins by selecting a group of persons who display certain defined characteristics before the onset of the condition being investigated. In studying a disease, the cohort might include individuals initially free of the disease but known to have been exposed to a particular factor. They would be followed over time to evaluate what variables were associated with the development or nondevelopment of the disease. An example is the prospective study of unintentional infant injuries, mentioned earlier (Harris & Kotch, 1994). The subjects, a cohort of 367 mothers, were interviewed six to eight weeks following the newborns' hospital discharge and then again approximately one year later. Investigators were able to identify injury predictors (family conflict and maternal unemployment) and also interventions (social support) for reducing the number of injuries.

In actual practice, the various types of studies just discussed are frequently mixed. A case-control study may include description and analysis with a retrospective focus; a cohort study may be conducted prospectively or retrospectively. Flexibility is essential to allow the investigator as much freedom as possible in choosing the most useful methodology.

Research in Community Health Nursing
PREVALENCE OF TECHNOLOGY-ASSISTED CHILDREN

Palfrey, J. et al., (1994). Prevalence of medical technology assistance among children in Massachusetts in 1987 and 1990. *Public Health Reports, 109*(2), 226–233.

A research team that included two nurses conducted two statewide surveys of children using medical technology in 1987 and 1990. The children, aged 3 months to 18 years, were using one or more of the following: respirator, tracheostomy, suctioning, oxygen, gastrostomy, jejunal or nasogastric feedings, urethral catherizations, ureteral diversion, ostomies, dialysis, or intravenous access. The number of technology-dependent children remained stable during the three year period. However, the pattern of technology use changed to an increase in use of gastrostomy and oxygen and a decrease in use of urostomy. The children's age distribution also changed from mostly 12 to 24 months using technology in 1987 to mostly children in the first year of life in 1990.

Based on study findings, the researchers calculated a prevalence estimate of 101,800 children nationwide who were being assisted by medical technology. "This information will facilitate policy analysis and program planning on regional and nation levels for this medically complex group of children" (p.226).

EXPERIMENTAL EPIDEMIOLOGY

Experimental epidemiology follows and builds on information gathered from descriptive and analytic approaches. It is used to study epidemics, the etiology of human disease, the value of preventive and therapeutic measures, and the evaluation of health services (Lilienfeld & Stolley, 1994). In an experimental study the investigator actually controls or changes the factors suspected of causing the health condition under study and observes what happens to the health state. In human populations, experimental studies should focus on disease prevention or health promotion rather than testing the causes of disease, which is primarily done on animals.

Experimental studies are carried out under carefully controlled conditions. The investigator uses an experi-mental group and exposes them to some factor thought to cause disease, improve health, prevent disease, or influence health in some way. Simultaneously, the investigator uses a control group which is similar in characteristics to the experimental group but without the exposure factor. An example is a study conducted by several nurses to examine the influence of case management approaches on client use of preventive child health services (Erkel, et al., 1994). An experimental group of infants received continuity of care provided by a single public health nurse who integrated case management and preventive services. The control group of infants received the customary pattern of services which were fragmented and delivered by multiple public health nurses. Findings showed that continuous, integrated public health nursing case management was significantly more effective in achieving client use of preventive child health services and was also one-fifth the cost of the control group's fragmented services.

The community health nurse should be alert for opportunities to conduct experimental studies in the course of working with groups. The study need not be elaborate and can provide important data for future nursing practice. For example, a study conducted in Albuquerque, New Mexico, compared 17 schoolboys with violent behavior with a control group of 27 carefully matched students (second through fifth grades) who were not overtly violent at school (Sheline, et al., 1994). Data were gathered through questionnaires completed by all students and in-home interviews with parents or guardians. Findings showed that boys from families with absent fathers, divorced parents, or numerous siblings were at higher risk for violent behavior. Lack of parental affection and expression of pride and use of spanking as discipline were parenting practices most strongly associated with violent behavior. The findings suggested the need for programs in parental education and encouragement to show affection and to use other methods of discipline. Similar experimental studies could be done with almost any small group within the community health nurse's practice.

An expanding area of experimental epidemiology involves the use of computers to simulate epidemics. With mathematical models it is possible to determine the probability of various aspects of disease occurrence. This approach is making an increased contribution to epidemiologists' knowledge of etiology and prevention.

Occasionally, an experiment occurs naturally in which conditions offer the researcher the chance to make important discoveries. John Snow discovered such a "natural experiment" in London in 1854 (Pickett & Hanlon, 1990). In his seminal study of an epidemic of cholera, he observed one group that contracted the disease and another that did not. Closer inspection revealed that the major difference between these groups was their water supply. Eventually the spread of cholera was traced to the water supply of the group with the high morbidity rate.

Community Trials

A community trial is a type of experimental study done at the community level (Hennekens & Buring, 1987). In this type of study geographic communities are assigned to intervention (experimental) or non-intervention (control) groups and compared to determine whether the intervention produces a positive change in the community. Community trials can be extremely expensive and are not undertaken unless there is substantial evidence that the intervention will make a difference at the aggregate level.

The Minnesota Heart Health Program was one such community trial conducted in the Minneapolis/St. Paul area (Mittlemark, et al., 1989). This study compared three sets of paired communities in the Upper Midwest. Each pair had one community in the intervention group and one in the non-intervention group. The intervention communities received multiple intervention techniques such as dietary instruction, smoking cessation intervention, and risk factor instruction. Myocardial infarction, stroke, and mortality rates along with other measurements were done at regular intervals to evaluate whether the interventions were improving the health in the communities that received them. Another example was an earlier Kingston/Newberg, New York study in which two towns on opposite sides of a river, one whose water system was flouridated and the other was not, compared dental records and learned that there was an association between flouridated water and reduced dental caries. One consequence of this study was the development of flouridated toothpaste

Conducting Epidemiologic Research

The community health nurse who engages in an epidemiologic investigation becomes a detective. First there is a problem to solve, a puzzle to unravel, or a question to answer. Then one begins to search for basic information, clues that might help answer the question. But information is never self-explanatory and, like a detective, one must analyze and interpret every additional clue. Slowly there is a narrowing of possible suspects until the causes of a disease, the consequences of a prevention plan, or the results of treatment are identified. On the basis of this investigation, one can then draw further conclusions and make new applications to improve health services.

As discussed previously, epidemiologic studies are a form of research. The steps outlined below are similar to those discussed later in Chapter 26. Epidemiologic research involves seven steps. Both an informal study in the course of nursing practice and the most comprehensive epidemiologic research project can be undertaken with these steps:

1. Identify the problem.
2. Review the literature.
3. Design the study.
4. Collect the data.
5. Analyze the findings.
6. Develop conclusions and applications.
7. Disseminate the findings.

Each of these steps will be considered in the context of a single nursing study examining stress in Cambodian refugee families.

IDENTIFY THE PROBLEM

Community health nurses are constantly confronted with threats to the health and well-being of the community. Almost daily, questions are raised, puzzles presented, and problems identified. Pregnant women who smoke or use cocaine threaten the health of their unborn children; what can be done to reduce this behavior? Rape is increasing; what can be done to bring aid to victims? Children are injured and die from bicycle accidents; why do these occur and how can they be prevented? Many farm workers have been killed or injured in farm equipment accidents; what can be done to prevent them? Any threat to the health of a group offers fertile ground for epidemiologic investigation.

One team of nurse researchers identified a problem of severe stress-related disorders among Cambodians living in the United States (D'Avanzo, et al., 1994). This group of refugees was at particularly high risk for stress related disorders because of traumatic experiences associated with war in their home country.

REVIEW THE LITERATURE

All too often, after identifying a problem, health professionals rush to take immediate action without reviewing solutions that have been tried previously. Every epidemiologic investigation should begin with a review of the literature. Even discovering that little research has been done on the problem can be valuable information. Conversely, if many studies have already been conducted on the area, this information can help narrow the study to areas not previously investigated or allow researchers to replicate earlier studies to confirm findings in a different setting. One of the most valuable sources in the literature is the review article which essentially summarizes all the research that has been conducted on a subject.

A review of the literature often suggests hypotheses from discoveries made in other studies. In the Cambodian refugee study a review of the literature did provide helpful background information but also revealed that little research had been done to study this group, furthermore their sources of stress and coping strategies had not been well documented.

DESIGN THE STUDY

The first step in designing a study is to formulate a specific question(s) to answer or perhaps a hypothesis to test. Sometimes this question or hypothesis may emerge from the review of literature but at other times it will have to be developed through the researcher's own analysis and hunches. It is a good idea to write out one or more hypotheses to test or questions to answer. The researchers in the Cambodian study formulated several research questions whose purpose was to "improve understanding of the beliefs of Cambodian refugee women about stressors that affect their families, and how the resulting stress is handled" (D'Avanzo, et al., 1994, p.102).

The next step is to plan what type or combination of study types will best suit the goals of the research (descriptive, analytic, or experimental) and how the study will be conducted. Will the data be collected retrospectively from existing records or will new data be collected? Who will conduct interviews? What kinds of data will be needed to measure the outcomes of intervention?

The Cambodian study involved a comparative descriptive design: two groups, one in Long Beach, California and the other near Lowell, Massachusetts and each with 60 Cambodian refugee women, were selected for comparison. Data was to be collected by means of in-home interviews with a translator whom the women trusted.

COLLECT THE DATA

Data in the Cambodian study were collected using structured two-hour interviews conducted in the Cambodian language and then translated and clarified for the researchers.

Often it is useful to perform a pilot study that pretests an interview guide or questionnaire. If one wishes to interview women about battering during pregnancy, it might be useful to prepare a guide and interview one or two persons, then revise the guide on the basis of one's experience. If developing a questionnaire to assess the nutritional needs of elderly persons living alone, it would be helpful to test the survey on some volunteers to determine its clarity and relevance.

In community health nursing, data collection often can occur as part of ongoing practice. Unless the study has been carefully designed, however, one may collect data for months or years, only to discover that important questions have been omitted.

ANALYZE THE FINDINGS

In most epidemiologic studies, data analysis will consist of summarizing the findings, computing rates and ratios, and displaying the findings in tables and graphs. It is at this stage that the data is used to address the original questions or test the original hypothesis. Was the hypothesis supported or not supported by the data? Summarized data can also generate more questions or indicate areas that warrant further investigation.

One study compiled findings from existing national data on leading causes of injury mortality in children ages 14 and under in the United States. (See Fig. 12.8) By compiling and categorizing this data, the researchers were able to identify geographic and subgroup injury problems that are often masked in larger, less specific categories. This identification increases the likelihood that specific injury problems will be targeted and given higher priority in prevention programs, eventually leading to a reduction in injury mortality (Waller, et al., 1989).

Analysis of the Cambodian study findings revealed that memories of war; financial concerns; family problems including infidelity, loneliness; and grief over ex-

<1 Year Old (33.9 deaths/100,000)

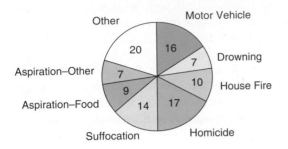

Ages 1–4 (25.4 deaths/100,000)

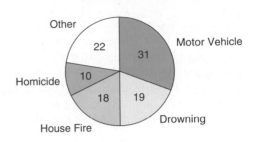

Ages 5–9 (14.4 deaths/100,000)

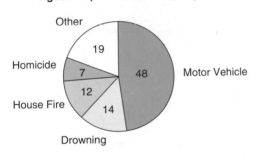

Ages 10–14 (16.2 deaths/100,000)

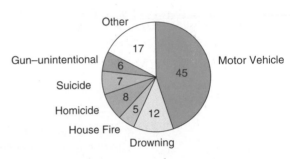

FIGURE 12.8. Pie charts showing percentages of childhood injury deaths by cause and age groups (Waller, et al., 1989, p. 311). Reprinted by permission. Since these figures, homicide has increased in children.

tended family and cultural losses; and language problems were major sources of stress for the refugee women. Their stress-related symptoms were mostly somatic including headaches, feeling sick, excessive sleep, chest pain, and shortness of breath and their coping strategies consisted of avoiding sad thoughts and avoiding being alone as well as keeping busy.

DEVELOP CONCLUSIONS AND APPLICATIONS

Stating conclusions is an outcome of analysis and interpretation. The investigators summarize the results and their meaning for the purpose of making it useful to other health services providers. Many times the research will have direct practical application for improving health services, continuing or discontinuing services, and conducting future research. It is also important to describe mistakes made and lessons learned about study

design and other aspects of the research to assist future investigators.

The researchers' conclusions from the Cambodian study were that these women had a general sense of inability to cope with stress and that nurses and other health care providers need to be sensitive to their culturally based responses and many unstated problems.

DISSEMINATE THE FINDINGS

Finally, research findings should be shared. Information gained from epidemiologic study must be disseminated throughout the professional community to strengthen the knowledge base for improved practice and to promote future research. The Cambodian study was published in *IMAGE: Journal of Nursing Scholarship* in the summer of 1991 and provided useful information for future work with the Cambodian refugee population.

Summary

Epidemiology is the study of the distribution and determinants of health, health conditions, and disease in human population groups. It shares with community health nursing the common focus of the health of populations. It is a specialized form of scientific research which can provide public health professionals with a body of knowledge on which to base their practice and methods for studying new and existing problems. To understand epidemiology, one must first understand some basic epidemiologic concepts: the host-agent-environment model, causality, immunity, the natural history of disease or health conditions, risk, and prevention strategies.

Community health nurses can use three sources of information when conducting epidemiologic investigations: existing epidemiologic data, informal investigations, and carefully designed scientific studies.

Epidemiology employs three investigative approaches: descriptive studies, analytic studies, and experimental studies. Although studies can be either retrospective or prospective, some merely describe existing conditions (descriptive studies) while others seek to explain causes (analytic studies). Experimental studies seek to confirm causal relationships identified in descriptive and analytic studies. Analytic studies can be of three types—prevalence, case-control, or cohort. In practice, all these types of studies often become combined in various ways. They also make use of quantitative concepts such as count, prevalence rate, incidence rate, mortality rate, and various types of morbidity (sickness) rates.

Epidemiologic research includes seven steps:

1. Identify the problem, which is usually some threat to the health of a population.
2. Review the literature to determine what other studies have found.
3. Carefully design the study.

Activities to Promote Critical Thinking

1. Identify an aggregate-level health problem in your community. Using the host-agent-environment model explain who is the host, what is the causative agent(s), and the environmental factors that have promoted or delayed the development of the problem.

2. Select an aggregate health (wellness) condition, such as preschoolers' normal growth and development or elders' healthy aging, and list all the causal factors that might contribute to this healthy state. Now plot these schematically in a diagram (such as Fig. 12.4) to show the web of causation for this condition.

3. Using the same health condition that you selected in the previous exercise, describe the natural history of this condition, outlining its four stages. Identify three preventive nursing interventions, one for each level of prevention, that could apply to this condition.

4. Select an article that reports an epidemiologic study from a recent nursing or public health journal and record your responses to the following questions:
   a. What prompted the study and what was its purpose?
   b. Was it descriptive, analytic, or experimental research?
   c. Was the study design retrospective or prospective?
   d. Why did the investigators choose this design?
   e. What existing sources of epidemiologic data did this study use? List all sources specifically, such as morbidity and mortality weekly report or incomes by household in census data.
   f. What were the study findings? Identify the population group that will benefit from this research.

5. Interview one or more practicing public health nurses in your community and identify an aggregate-level problem that needs epidemiologic investigation. Propose a rough draft study design to research this problem.

4. Collect the data.
5. Analyze the findings.
6. Develop conclusions and applications.
7. Disseminate the findings.

Thinking epidemiologically can significantly enhance community health nursing practice. Epidemiology provides both the body of knowledge—information on the distribution and determinants of health conditions—and methods for investigating health problems and evaluating services.

REFERENCES

Benenson, A. S. (1990). *Control of communicable disease in man* (15th ed.). Washington, DC: American Public Health Association.

Blum, H.L. (1981). *Planning for health* (2nd ed.). New York: Human Sciences Press.

Burnet, M. (1962). *Natural history of infectious diseases.* (3rd ed.). Cambridge, England: Cambridge University Press.

Cohen, I. (1984). Florence Nightingale. *Scientific American, 250*(3), 128–33.

D'Avanzo, C. E., Frye, B., & Froman, R., (1994). Stress in Cambodian refugee families. *IMAGE, 26*(2), 101–5.

Dever, G.E.A. (1991). *Community Health Analysis* (2nd ed.). Gaithersburg, MD: Aspen.

Erkel, E., Morgan, E., Staples, M., Assey, V., & Michel, Y. (1994). Case management and preventive services among infants from low-income families. *Public Health Nursing, 11*(5), 352–60.

Ernster, V., Grady, D., Miike, R., Black, D., Selby, J., & Kerlikowske, K. (1995). Facial wrinkling in men and women, by smoking status. *American Journal of Public Health, 85*(1), 78–82.

Friedman, G. D. (1994). *Primer of epidemiology* (4th ed.). New York: McGraw-Hill.

Harris, M.J. & Kotch, J.B. (1994). Unintentional Infant Injuries: Sociodemographic and psychosocial factors. *Public Health Nursing, 11*(2), 90–97.

Healthy People 2000: National Health Promotion and Disease Prevention Objectives. (DHHS publication PHS 91-50213.) (1991). Washington, D.C.: U.S. Department of Health and Human Services.

Helton, A., McFarlane, J., & Anderson, E. (1987). Prevention of battering during pregnancy: Focus on behavioral change. *Public Health Nursing, 4*(3), 166–74.

Henderson, D. A. (1980). Smallpox eradication. *Public Health Reports, 95*, 422–26.

Hennekens, C.H. & Buring, J.E. (1987). *Epidemiology in medicine.* Boston: Little, Brown.

Holaday, B., Waugh, G., Moukaddem, V., West, J., & Harshman, S. (1995). Fecal contamination in child day care centers: cloth vs paper diapers. *American Journal of Public Health, 85*(1), 30–3.

Kopf, E.W. (1978). Florence Nightingale as statistician. *Research in Nursing and Health, 1*(3), 93–102.

Lilienfeld, D. E. & Stolley, P. (1994). *Foundations of epidemiology* (3rd ed.). New York: Oxford.

Mittlemark, M., Luepker, R., Jacobs, D., Bracht, N., Carlaw, R., Crow, R., Finnegan, J., Grimm, R., Jeffrey, R., Kline, G., Mullis, R., Murray, D., Pechacek, T., Perry, C., Pirie, P., & Blackburn H. (1989). Prevention of cardiovascular disease: Education strategies of the Minnesota Heart Health Program. *Preventive Medicine, 15*, 1–17.

Palfrey, J., Haynie, M., Porter, S., Fenton, T., Cooperman-Vincent, P., Shaw, D., Johnson, B., Bierle, T., & Walker, D. (1994). Prevalence of medical technology assistance among children in Massachusetts in 1987 and 1990. *Public Health Reports, 109*(2), 226–233.

Pickett, G. & Hanlon, J. (1990). *Public Health: Administration and Practice.* St. Louis: Times Mirror/Mosby.

Porter, E. J. (1994). Older widows' experience of living alone at home. *IMAGE, 26*(1), 19–24.

Sheline, J. L., Skipper, B.J., & Broadhead, W.E. (1994). Risk factors for violent behavior in elementary school boys: Have you hugged your child today? *American Journal of Public Health, 84*(4), 661–3.

Susser, M. (1973). *Causal thinking in the health sciences: concepts and strategies of epidemiology.* New York: Oxford.

Talashek, M., Gerace, L., & Starr, K. (1994). The substance abuse pandemic: determinants to guide interventions. *Public Health Nursing, 11*(2), 131–139.

Waller, A., Baker, S., & Szocka, A. (1989). Childhood injury deaths: National analysis and geographic variations. *American Journal of Public Health, 79*, 310–15.

Warneke, C. L. & Cooper, S.P. (1994). Child and adolescent drownings in Harris County, Texas, 1983 through 1990. *American Journal of Public Health, 84*(4), 593–8.

SELECTED READINGS

Allen J. R. & Curran, J.W. (1988). Prevention of AIDS and HIV infection. Needs and priorities for epidemiologic research. *American Journal of Public Health, 78*, 381–86.

Brown, J. S. & Semradek, J. (1992). Secondary data on health-related subjects: Major sources, uses, and limitations. *Public Health Nursing, 9*(3), 162–71.

Cappelleri, J., Eckenrode, J., & Powers, J. (1993). The epidemiology of child abuse: findings from the second national incidence and prevalence study of child abuse and neglect. American Journal of Public Health 83(11):1622–1624.

Celentano, D. D. (1987). The epidemiology of alcohol consumption and hypertension with special reference to stroke. *Public Health Review, 15*(2), 83–119.

Copp, L. (1987). Implications of epidemiological research. *Recent Advances in Nursing, *(17), 94–107.

Davies, A.M. (1988). Epidemiology and services for the aged. *Public Health Reports, 103*(5), 516–520.

Duffy, M. E. (1988). Statistics: Friend or foe? *Nursing and Health Care, 9*, 73–75.

Ehrenberg, R.L. (1989). Use of direct surveys in the surveillance of occupational illness and injury. *American Journal of Public Health* (Supplement), 79, 12–14.

Erickson, G.P. (1992). Epidemiology and biostatistics content in baccalaureate education for community health nursing. *Public Health Nursing, 9*(1), 45–52.

Gleavey, D. (1990). The nursing role in epidemiology, risk management, and patient-public education. *Journal Opthalmic Nursing Technology, 9*(5), 215–219.

Harper, A.C. & Lambert, L. (1993). *The health of populations* (2nd ed.). New York: Springer.

Helgerson, S.D., Jekel, J., & Hadler, J. (1988). Training public health students to investigate disease outbreaks—examples of community service. *Public Health Reports, 103*(1), 72–76.

Johnson, C.C. (1987). The epidemiology of cancer. *Family and Community Health, 10*(3), 1–7.

Kent, G., Greenspan, J., Herndon, J., Mofenson, L., Harris, J., Eng, T., & Waskin, H. (1988). Epidemic giardiasis caused by a contaminated public water supply. *American Journal of Public Health, 78*(2), 139–143.

Landrigan, P.J. (1989). Improving the surveillance of occupational disease. *American Journal of Public Health, 79*(12), 1601–1602.

Lee, P.R. & Toomey, K.E. (1994). Epidemology in public health in the era of health care reform. *Public Health Reports, 109*(1), 1–3.

Massanari, R. M. (1987). Risk management: An epidemiologic approach. *Infection Control, 8*, 3–6.

Misener, T.R., Watkins, J.G., & Ossege, J. (1994). Public health nursing research priorities: a collaborative delphi study. *Public Health Nursing, 11*(2), 66–74.

Robitaille, Y., Legault, J., Abbey, H., & Pless, B. (1990). Evaluation of an infant car seat program in a low-income community. *American Journal of Diseases of Children, 144* (1),74–78.

Salsberry, P. J., Nickel, J.T., & Mitch, R. (1994). Immunization status of 2-year olds in middle/upper- and lower-income populations: a community survey. *Public Health Nursing, 11*(1), 17–13.

Sheps, S.B., et al. (1987). Epidemiology of school injuries: a two-year experience in a municipal health department. *Pediatrics, 79*(1), 69–73.

Toughill, E., Mason, D., Beck, T., & Christopher, M.A. (1993). Health, income, and postretirement employment of older adults. *Public Health Nursing, 10*(2), 100–107.

Turner, J. G. & Chavigny, K.H. (1988). *Community Health Nursing: An Epidemiologic Perspective.* Philadelphia: Lippincott.

Valanis, B. (1986). *Epidemiology in nursing and health care.* East Norwalk, CT: Appleton-Century-Crofts.

Venter, M.H. (1989). Family-oriented prevention of cardiovascular disease: a social epidemiological approach. *Social Science and Medicine, 28*(4), 309–314.

Vredevoe, D. L., Brecht, M., Shuler, P., & Woo, M. (1992). Risk factors for disease in a homeless population. *Public Health Nursing, 9*(4), 263–9.

Yankauer, A. (1990). What infant mortality tells us. *American Journal of Public Health, 80*(6), 653–654.

Communication and Collaboration in Community Health

LEARNING OBJECTIVES

Upon completion of this chapter, readers should be able to:

- Identify the seven parts of the communication process.
- Describe four barriers to effective communication in community health and how to deal with them.
- Explain three sets of skills necesary for effective communication in community health nursing.
- Discuss four techniques for enhancing group decision making.
- Describe five characteristics of collaboration in community health.
- Identify four features of community health contracting.
- Develop an aggregate level contract in community health.

KEY TERMS

- Active listening
- Brainstorming
- Channel
- Collaboration
- Communication
- Contracting
- Decoding
- Delphi technique
- Electronic meetings
- Empathy

- Encoding
- Feedback loop
- Formal contracting
- Informal contracting
- Message
- Nominal group technique
- Nonverbal messages
- Receiver
- Sender
- Verbal messages

Barbara Walton Spradley and Judith Ann Allender
COMMUNITY HEALTH NURSING: CONCEPTS AND PRACTICE, 4th ed.
© 1996 Barbara Walton Spradley and Judith Ann Allender

Communication and collaboration are primary tools for community health nurses. They form the basis for effective relationships that contribute both to the prevention of illness and to the protection and promotion of aggregate health. In order to use communication and collaboration skillfully in community health practice, one must understand the meaning and value of these concepts. For the nurse accustomed to communicating one-on-one with clients, communication with aggregates and a host of professionals requires new skills. Unlike ordinary social relationships, collaborative relationships are based on a team approach with shared responsibilities and mutual participation in establishing and carrying out goals. Clients and health professionals enter into a working agreement or contract tailored to address specific client needs. The concept of contracting can further assist the collaborative process. This chapter examines these tools and discusses their integration into community health nursing practice.

Communication in Community Health Nursing

Groups cannot exist without communication. Nor can nurses practice without communication. It is a fact too often taken for granted since most people spend close to 70% of their waking hours communicating—speaking, listening, reading, writing. Yet the quality of people's communcation has far reaching effects. Lack of effective communication can lead to misunderstanding, poor performance, interpersonal conflict, ineffective programs, weak public policy, and many other undesireable outcomes. To communicate, people must "construct shared realities—create shared meanings" (Shockley-Zalabak, 1994, p. 2). In other words, they must engage in an exchange that is both understood and meaningful. **Communication**, then, can be defined as "the transference and understanding of meaning" (Robbins, 1993, p. 327).

Communication is the lifeblood of effective community health nursing practice. It provides a two-way flow of information that nourishes professional-client and professional-professional relationships. It also establishes the base of information upon which health planning decisions are made and programs developed. For communication to take place, clients and professionals send and receive messages. As participants in the communication process, community health nurses play both roles—sender and receiver (Veninga, 1982). The nurse working with a group of abused women must learn to "read" the messages these women send. Similarly, as a member of a health planning team, the nurse must be able to elicit ideas as well as contribute to the planning process by speaking and acting in ways that communicate effectively.

Communication serves several functions in community health nursing. It provides information for decision making at all levels of community health. From the choice of goals for a small group to health policy affecting a population at risk, decisions are enhanced through effective communication. It functions as a motivator by clarifying information so that consensus is reached and the people involved can move forward with commitment to shared goals. Effective communication facilitates expression of feelings and promotes closer working relationships. It also controls behavior by providing clear expectations and boundaries for group-member actions.

THE COMMUNICATION PROCESS

Communication occurs as a sequence of events or a process. The process is made up of seven parts that need to work together to result in the transference and understanding of meaning. They are: (1) the message, (2) a sender, (3) a receiver, (4) encoding, (5) a channel, (6) decoding, and (7) a feedback loop.

The first part of the communication process is a **message** which is an expression of the purpose of communication. Without the message there can be no communication. The next two parts are a sender and a receiver. The **sender** is the person (or persons) conveying a message and the **receiver** is the person (or persons) to whom the message is directed and who is its actual recipient. The fourth step is the act of **encoding** which refers to the sender's conversion of the message into symbolic form. This involves how the sender will translate the message to the receiver. It can be accomplished through verbal or nonverbal means. For example, a nurse teaching breathing techniques to a prenatal class may explain verbally while also demonstrating the correct procedures. The degree of the sender's success in encoding is influenced by her or his communication skills, knowledge about the topic of the message, attitudes related to the message and the receiver, and by the beliefs and values that the sender holds. The fifth part involves a **channel** which refers to the medium through which the sender conveys the message. The channel may be a written, spoken, or nonverbal expression. Examples could include a letter stating a request, a report providing information, a written health plan, a verbal message for clarification, or facial expression indicating confusion. Communication channels may be formal such as a written grant proposal, or informal like a face-to-face verbal statement.

Once the sender has conveyed a message via a channel, the receiver must translate the message into an understandable form, called **decoding**, which is the sixth part of the communication process. Receivers' ability to decode the message is influenced by their knowledge about the topic, skills in reading and listening, attitudes, and sociocultural values. The seventh and final part is a **feedback loop** which refers to the receiver indicating that the message has been understood (decoded) in the way that the sender intended (encoded). It requires feedback from the receiver to the sender serving as a check on the success of the transference of meaning. Figure 13.1 portrays the seven parts of the communication process.

COMMUNICATION BARRIERS

Community health nurses should be aware of the barriers that block effective communication. This section discusses four that pose particular problems: selective perception, language, filtering, and emotions (Robbins, 1993).

Selective perception

Receivers in the communication process interpret a message through their own perceptions which are influenced by their own experience, interests, values, motivations, expectations, and other influences. They project this perceptual screen onto the communication process as they decode a message. They might distort or misinterpret meaning from the sender's original intent. For example, the nurse may propose a class session on nutrition to a group of elderly persons who may translate that message to mean a focus on dieting—which is not the intended meaning. Nurses can overcome this barrier by using the feedback loop to ask clients or others involved to restate their understanding of the message, such as asking the elderly clients in the example above what the term nutrition means to them. This provides an opportunity for clarification and correction of misunderstandings.

Language Barriers

People interpret the meaning of words differently depending on many variables, such as age, education, cultural background, and primary spoken language. An adolescent would understand the terms "cool" and "with it" to mean that something is fashionable or desireable while an eighty year old woman might not undertand the current slang terms. In community health, nurses work with a wide range of clients and professionals whose disparate ages, education, and cultural backgrounds lead to different speech patterns. Some health professionals' use of scientific terminology or jargon can be confusing as in the case of the Hmong refugee woman who was asked if her son had experienced enuresis. These can become barriers to communication unless the differences are taken into consideration during the communication process.

Filtering Information

A third barrier to communication is filtering, which means manipulation of information by the sender to influence the receiver's response. One purpose might be

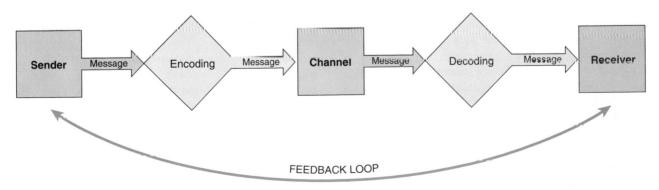

FIGURE 13.1. The communication process

to gain favor with the receiver to say what one thinks they want to hear, rather than the whole truth (Robbins, 1993). Clients sometimes use filtering during a needs assessment process, giving only partial or distorted information because they think this is what health professionals want to hear. Another intent of filtering is to slant information in a certain way. Prepared minutes from a meeting or a department's quarterly report can emphasize some points and omit or deemphasize others giving (sometimes unintentionally) false impressions that influence decision making.

Emotional Influence

How one feels at the time a message is sent or received will influence its meaning. Senders can distort messages when emotionally upset and receivers can interpret messages incorrectly when emotions cloud their perception. Emotions can interfere with rational and objective reasoning, thus blocking communication. Nurses need to be aware of their own emotions as they send messages. They also need to ascertain the emotional status of clients or health professionals with whom they are communicating to avoid misunderstandings.

CORE COMMUNICATION SKILLS

Overcoming the barriers to effective communication described above requires the development of sound communication skills. Community health nurses need to cultivate three sets of communication skills: sending skills, receiving skills, and interpersonal skills.

Sending Skills

Sending skills enable nurses to transmit messages effectively. Through these skills nurses convey information to clients and other persons. Two important considerations will influence clarity and effectiveness of message sending. First, the extent of the nurse's self-awareness will affect the communication. Does she or he feel anxious, angry, tired, impatient, or concerned? Does the nurse find certain individuals irritating or offensive? What motives and interests prompt the communication? Second, the nurse's awareness of the receivers will influence the sending of messages. What do clients or the professionals with whom the nurse is interacting want or need? Is the message suited to their cultural backgrounds and level of understanding? Does the message have significance for them? How are re-

ceivers responding as the nurse sends the message? (See Research in Community Health Nursing below.)

Two main channels are used to send messages: nonverbal and verbal. **Nonverbal messages** are those conveyed without words and constitute nearly two-thirds of the messages transmitted in normal communication (Brill, 1973). People send messages nonverbally in many

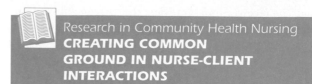

Research in Community Health Nursing
CREATING COMMON GROUND IN NURSE-CLIENT INTERACTIONS

Kristjanson, L. & Chalmers, K. (1990). Nurse-client interactions in community-based practice: Creating common ground. (4), 215–223, December.

Communication between nurses and community clients has not been extensively studied. Yet knowledge of this process has significant bearing on improving practice effectiveness. These researchers conducted a pilot study in a Canadian public health nursing department of nurses' interactions with clients in a variety of settings and contexts. A random sample of five experienced (two or more years of experience) nurses was observed for a total of 19 nurse-client interactions. Videotaping was done of five home visits with families across the life span, two school children's consultations, three classroom presentations, a prenatal class, five well baby clinics, a school eye-screening clinic, a meeting with two community health workers, and a consultation session with a day care worker. Data were also collected through field notes and semistructured interviews with clients and nurses.

Based on content analysis, the researchers developed a conceptual map of nurse-client interactions in community health practice. The conceptual schema, called "creating common ground," examined three interaction phases (social, working, closing), content of the interaction, assessment approaches, nursing interventions, control of information flow, nursing style, context or setting, and continuing evaluation. Findings revealed that nurse communication varied with the setting and the nurses' overall style and that these, in turn, affected the quality of the interventions.

ways. Personal appearance, dress, posture, facial expression, and physical distance between sender and receiver all communicate messages. These nonverbal statements may enhance or discredit what someone says verbally (Robbins, 1993). Body language often speaks louder than words. Facial expressions convey acceptance or rejection, interest or boredom, anger or patience, fear or confidence. Gestures and bodily movements such as clenched hands, crossed arms, tapping a finger, or a turned shoulder all communicate messages. Eye contact or lack of it carries additional meaning. Tone of voice and use of silence also send nonverbal messages. Accepting food in certain situations may communicate acceptance and the desire to be friendly. Nonverbal messages may have different cultural meanings or social interpretations. Nurse self-awareness and validation of meaning can save considerable misunderstanding.

Verbal messages are communicated ideas, attitudes, and feelings transmitted by speaking or writing (Veninga, 1982). Nurses cannot assume that the intent of their words is always understood by clients or other professionals. Effective sending skills depend on asking for feedback to make certain that receivers have understood the verbal message's intent. Communication is more effective if speakers avoid using jargon that is unfamiliar to clients. Like all occupations, nursing has its own vocabulary or jargon which clients do not understand and may make them feel ignorant or inferior. For example, the terms "critical pathways" or "case management approach" might have little meaning to a community group. Nurses must make special effort to avoid using jargon that is part of everyday speech. The basic rules for effective sending can be summarized in this manner:

1. Keep the message honest and uncomplicated;
2. Use as few words as possible to state it; and
3. Ask for reactions (feedback) to make certain that it is understood.

Receiving Skills

Receiving skills are as important to communication as sending skills and involve not only listening to what people say but also observing their behavior. They enable nurses to receive accurate and complete messages. If members of a seniors' exercise class agree to certain exercises but do not participate in them, they are sending a message. What message is their behavior sending? Were the proposed exercises too difficult? Did they mis-

understand the nurse's instructions on how to perform the exercise? Are they resisting in other areas of the program? Effective receiving skills require attention to nonverbal as well as verbal messages and seeking feedback to understand their meaning.

An essential skill to develop for receiving messages is **active listening**, the skill of assuming responsibility for and seeking understanding of the meaning of the sender's message (Wismer, 1978). Instead of expecting clients or others to help the nurse understand, the nurse should actively work to discover what they mean. Understanding the message from the sender's perspective demands careful attention. It arises from a genuine interest in what the speaker has to say. Active listeners demonstrate their interest, perhaps by sitting forward, sustaining eye contact, nodding the head, and asking occasional questions for clarification. They concentrate in order to avoid daydreaming or the pretense of listening, both of which block communication.

Nurses can also listen actively by asking reflective questions which attempt to restate what clients or others have said to clarify the received meaning. Reflective questions have a twofold purpose: to show a sincere attempt to understand senders' messages, and to make clear that the messages and the people who send them are important to the nurse. An example of a reflective question follows:

> Class members state: "Quitting smoking is impossible." Reflective question by nurse: "You feel you can't quit smoking?"

Active listening helps communicate acceptance and increase trust, especially when the listener refrains from making any negative judgements of the message or the way it is delivered (Veninga, 1982). A critical response to the message on the part of the listener cuts off communication. Active listening enables nurses to encourage clients to deliberate carefully and to exercise problem-solving skills; it avoids the pitfall of telling receivers what to do.

Interpersonal Skills

Effective communication in community health nursing also requires interpersonal skills. Three types of interpersonal skills build on sending and receiving skills but go beyond the mere exchange of messages. They are showing respect, empathizing, and developing trust.

Showing Respect. Showing respect means conveying the attitude that clients and others have importance, dignity, and worth. Community health nurses can express respect by treating ideas and comments as valuable and worthy of attention. Nurses can demonstrate an interest in wanting to understand the situation from other persons' points of view. Nurses show respect by the manner in which they address people—for instance, by using the courtesy titles of "Mr." or "Mrs." until permission is granted to use first names. On a more subtle level, the tone of voice can either show respect or make people feel inferior and insignificant. Clients, community members, and other professionals need to feel respected if they are to enter fully into the mutual exchange necessary for effective communication. See Issues in Community Health Nursing below.

Empathizing. Empathizing is another important interpersonal skill. **Empathy** is the ability to understand and vicariously experience the feelings and thoughts of others while maintaining one's own identity (Kalisch, 1973; La Monica & Karshmer, 1978). Nurses show empathy by reflecting another person's feelings and expressing that message in the receiver's language. The same terms and, if possible, the same tone of voice as the other person's should be used. For example, the nurse should assume a serious manner if the speaker seems serious. Empathy conveys the message, "This is the way it seems to me. Is that correct?" The nurse should attempt to keep validating the speaker's true feelings so the nurse makes certain that she or he is interpreting correctly. Empathy focuses attention on receivers and their feelings and reduces clients' anxiety and defensiveness (Veninga, 1982). It shows that the nurse shares their concerns, and it makes them feel that their contributions are valued.

Developing Trust. Developing trust is necessary for effective communication. Clients and others will not express their true feelings if they do not fully trust the nurse. Many times clients will say what they think the nurse wants to hear. They may agree to a plan of action simply because they do not want to displease the nurse or may hide true feelings because they think that the nurse is eager for a decision.

Nurses develop trust in the communication process by showing that they truly accept others, that they believe in them as people. Trust generates trust; as the nurse shows confidence in clients and the other professionals with whom the nurse is communicating, they will respond in kind. Treating people as fully participating partners in the communication process means demonstrating that they are trustworthy and responsible. Trust is also developed through an open, honest, and patient approach with others. Candid discussion in a flexible time frame encourages people to share their real feelings and to move at their own pace. As trust develops, communication becomes more free flowing and productive (see Fig. 13.2).

FACTORS INFLUENCING COMMUNICATION

Effective communication, both sending and receiving, is strongly influenced by three factors: previous experiences, culture, and relationships.

Previous experiences of both sender and receiver influence their perceptions and the meanings they attach to messages. For example, adolescents who are having difficulty with parents' authority, may hear the nurse's suggestion to "learn more about STDs" as a command

---

Issues in Community Health Nursing
LOW LITERACY HEALTH COMMUNICATION

Most poorly educated populations, those with lowest literacy levels, have the highest mortality and morbidity rates. Yet it has been well documented that most "health information materials cannot be read or comprehended by low literacy adults" (Plimpton & Root, 1994, p. 83). Communication with these high risk groups needs to be simplified and include easy-to-read materials. At the same time there is the danger of communication being too simple to the point of being insulting. Low literacy does not necessarily mean low intelligence. How does the nurse find the right balance?

The goal of communication is to achieve understanding. If clients are to understand health communication, whether the messages are spoken or written, they must be given ample opportunities to provide feedback. Pamphlets and other written health information should be reviewed by their intended audiences before final printing and distribution. Proposed users should comment on readability and acceptability of both text and graphics. With spoken communication, nurses should solicit feedback regularly to make certain that messages are understood.

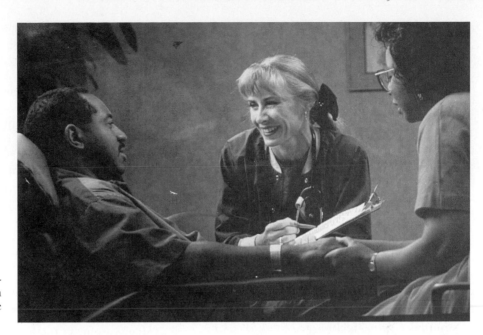

FIGURE 13.2. Nonverbal behavior of a community health nurse and family demonstrate respect and trust.

or effort to control them. Requests for clarification will help verify that messages are being received as intended.

The respective cultures of sender and receiver influence understanding and acceptance of messages. A nervous laugh, appropriate as an outlet in one culture, may appear rude and disrespectful to someone from another culture. Silence, which in Native American cultures indicates patience and thoughtfulness, may be interpreted as weakness or indifference to someone not familiar with their cultural practices. With many clients, the nurse will have to communicate cross-culturally, which requires patience and constant effort to ensure accurate and inoffensive messages (Kreps & Kunimoto, 1994).

Since much of community health nursing involves groups, the relationships among group members can significantly influence communication effectiveness. When a large number of people are involved, group communication patterns can be quite complex and interaction requires skill on the nurse's part to elicit feedback from all members and generate a common understanding among the group.

GROUP DECISION MAKING

An important aspect of communicating with groups in community health is group decision making. Community health nurses are actively involved in this activity. Thus nurses need to understand how groups function as they make decisions and to learn techniques for facilitating group decision making.

Group Functions in Decision Making

Groups, regardless of size, perform many functions (See details in Chapter 10, Working with Populations and Groups). Four functions are of particular relevance to group decision making.

1. Group members share information. In community health groups often include clients, health professionals, and community members who share their experience and expertise to help arrive at solutions and decisions
2. Groups present diverse views that lend richness to generation of alternatives and the problem-solving process.
3. Groups influence their members' thinking by broadening their perspectives and presenting new ways of thinking about the issues. This influencing function can improve the quality of the group decision making.
4. Groups progress toward consensus and/or resolution by discussing a set of alternatives and arriving at solutions. Time pressures and desire for completion help move this process along.

Techniques for Enhancing Group Decision Making

As a member of many decision-making groups in the community, the community health nurse can facilitate the process through certain techniques. Robbins (1993) describes four useful strategies: brainstorming, nominal group technique, delphi technique, and electronic meetings.

Brainstorming. Brainstorming is an idea-generating process that encourages group members to freely offer suggestions in which members sit around a table if group size permits and take turns presenting ideas. They are encouraged to be creative and unusual; thus no idea is too bizarre. Furthermore, no criticism or discussion is allowed until all ideas have been exhausted and recorded. This technique is helpful for generating creative possibilities and is most useful in the early stages of decision making.

Nominal Group Technique. Nominal group technique is a group decision making method that pools face-to-face group ideas after members initially think and write down their ideas independently. In this approach, members meet together but spend time silently writing down their ideas first. Following that, members take turns presenting one idea at a time to the group without discussion until all ideas have been recorded. Discussion then follows for clarifying and judging. Next members independently and silently rank-order the ideas and read these rankings to the group. This allows the decisions to be narrowed down to one with the highest aggregate ranking

Delphi Technique. Delphi technique is a method of arriving at group consensus through a systematic pooling of separate individuals' judgments by written questionnaire and suggestions. Members do not need to be physically present to participate. It follows a series of steps:

1. Identify problem or topic and design questionnaire to elicit responses from members.
2. Members respond independently and anonymously and return questionnaire.
3. Compile responses centrally, send results and a new questionnaire to members.
4. Members offer new responses or solutions based on earlier results and return these.
5. Repeat steps 3 and 4 as needed until consensus is reached.

This process is useful for polling experts who may be geographically distant from one another. It also provides a way to reach a decision without group members unduly influencing each other. Its disadvantages are that it is time consuming and can be expensive.

Electronic Meetings. Electronic meetings provide a fourth group decision-making method. This method, currently used more in business settings, applies nominal group technique combined with computer technology. Group members sit around a large table furnished with a computer terminal for each person. As issues are presented, members enter their responses into their computers which are anonymously displayed on a large projection screen. Group decisions are also displayed for group viewing. This method promotes greater honesty and speed; in fact, experts claim that electronic meetings are 55% faster than face-to-face meetings (Robbins, 1993).

In community health, availability of such technology may be limited in many settings. Nonetheless, computer-assisted decision making will become increasingly useful in the future. Computers can be used in conjunction with other group decision-making techniques for recording ideas, tabulating rankings, conducting simulations, and other applications.

Collaboration in Community Health

Collaboration for community health nurses means a purposeful interaction between nurses, clients, other professionals, and community members based on mutual participation and joint effort. This definition highlights two basic features of collaboration: it has a goal, and it involves several parties assisting one another to achieve that goal. The overriding purpose or goal of collaboration in community health practice is to benefit the public's health. To that end many players must work together.

Addressing the needs of aggregates requires a variety of team players. Community health nursing practice draws on the expertise and assistance of numerous individuals. The list includes health planners and policy makers, epidemiologists, biostatisticans, community citizens, demographers, environmentalists, educators, politicians, housing experts, safety professionals, industrial hygienists, and numerous others in addition to physicians, social workers, psychologists, physical therapists, and most of the other professionals involved in health services. Depending on the need to be addressed, community health nurses may work with many of these people on a single project. Furthermore, perhaps the most important team players are community clients—those populations and groups who are the targets of community health services. Clients' perspectives and expressions of need provide important information for the planning and delivery of services. Their participation, either collectively or through representatives, ensures more comprehensive and accurate information as well as commitment to fully using the health programs designed for their benefit. Stevens and Hall emphasize the importance of gaining the community's perspective and add, "To facilitate dialogue with communities, we must form alliances and build coalitions with community groups" (1992, p. 6).

CHARACTERISTICS OF COLLABORATION

In order to explore the meaning of collaboration in the context of community health nursing, this section will examine four characteristics that distinguish collaboration from other types of interaction: shared goals, mutual participation, maximized resources, and clear responsibilities.

Shared Goals

First, collaboration in community health nursing is goal-directed. The nurse, clients, and others involved in the collaborative effort recognize specific reasons for entering into the relationship. For example, a lumber company with 150 employees seeks to develop a wellness program. The community health nurse, company representatives, a safety expert, an industrial hygienist, a health educator, an exercise therapist, a nutritionist, and a psychologist might work together to develop specific physical and mental health goals. The team enters into the collaborative relationship with broad needs or purposes to be met and specific objectives to accomplish.

Mutual Participation

Second, in community health nursing, collaboration involves mutual participation; all team members contribute (Jones, et al., 1993). Collaboration involves a reciprocal exchange in which each team player discusses what her or his involvement and contribution will be. The lumber company representatives may out-

line assessed areas of need such as back strengthening exercises to facilitate lifting and reduce strain. Each of the professionals, including the nurse involved in the collaboration, will offer their own specific ideas and expertise to help design the wellness program.

Maximized Use of Resources

A third characteristic of collaboration is that it maximizes the use of community resources. That is, the collaborative effort is designed to draw on the expertise of those most knowledgeable and in the best positions to influence a favorable outcome. If the lumber company team has identified a need for health education materials, the nurse and other members of the collaborating team may seek use of health education resources through the local health department.

Clear Responsibilities

Fourth, the collaborating team members assume clearly defined responsibilities. Like a football team, each member in the collaborative effort plays a specific role with related tasks. The nurse may play a case-management or group-leadership role while others assume roles appropriate to their areas of expertise. Effective collaboration clearly designates what each member will do to accomplish the identified goals. The nurse, for example, might coordinate the planning effort for the lumber company wellness program and work with the health educator to develop classes on various topics. The psychologist might advise on a chemical dependency program and the industrial hygienist provide assistance with safety measures. Each member of the team develops an understanding of individual responsibilities based on realistic and honest expectations. This understanding comes through effective communication. The collaborating group explores necessary resources, assesses their capabilities, and determines their willingness to assume tasks.

Set Boundaries

Fifth, collaboration in community health practice has set boundaries with a beginning and an end. An important part of defining collaboration is determining when and under what conditions to terminate it. The temporal boundaries are determined sometimes by progress toward the goal, sometimes by the number of team member contacts, and often by setting a time limit. The collaborating group might target six months as a completion date for the lumber company wellness program and establish a time line with designated activities to reach the goal. Once the purpose for the collaboration has been accomplished, the group as a formal entity can be terminated.

FOSTERING CLIENT PARTICIPATION IN COLLABORATION

This text has stressed that communication and collaboration are based on mutual participation. The extent of clients' involvement in that participation varies, however, depending on their readiness and ability to participate. Clients' level of wellness at the time of initial professional-client encounter directly influences participation. Some people are not physically or emotionally well enough to assume an active role in the relationship. Women recently discharged from the hospital following a mastectomy, for example, have many physical and emotional adjustments with which to cope. Their families, too, must expend additional energies to provide needed support and to cope with the temporary loss of each woman's usual role in the family. They may find it difficult to engage actively in identifying their needs and goals at the start of the collaborative process. The nurse may have to take stronger initial leadership; however, the goals of collaboration are not abandoned. Gradually, as clients' wellness levels improve, the nurse can encourage more active participation.

Sometimes clients' previous experiences with health personnel limit participation in collaboration. Clients from poverty areas, from different cultural backgrounds, or with little education may need extensive encouragement to participate actively (Kreps & Kunimoto, 1994). Clients, regardless of income or educational level, who were not previously encouraged to participate in decision making by physicians, nurses, or other professionals may follow the pattern of a passive role in collaboration. Unless the nurse persists in efforts to reduce the dependence of clients, the relationship can fall short of the therapeutic goals.

The nurse's own view of collaboration will also influence the degree of client participation. Those nurses accustomed to relating to clients in an adult-to-child manner will restrict client involvement. If nurses see their position as more informed and the clients' position as one of complete ignorance and need, a paternalistic relationship may develop. All clients have resources on which to build, and the community health nurse helps clients discover them and use them to enhance collaboration and to attain health goals.

Clients who initiate or seek service are frequently best able to assume an active participant role, such as abused women seeking protection or elderly widowed persons seeking support. They have already demonstrated a sense of responsibility for their health by identifying a need and asking for assistance. The nurse must still work carefully to build mutual participation and respond with concern and caring to foster continued interest and participation by clients.

STRUCTURE OF COLLABORATIVE RELATIONSHIPS

Effective collaboration occurs within a particular structure and sequence. During this process, the work of identifying and meeting client needs takes place. Because the relationship is bound by time, the structure involves several phases: (1) a beginning phase when the team relationship is just being established; (2) a middle, working phase; and (3) a termination phase when the relationship ends.

The first phase is a period of establishing and defining the team relationship. All the team members, including clients, are getting to know each other; they seek to establish communication patterns and develop trust. From these bases, they identify the clients' needs and determine the goals toward which they will work.

The middle phase occurs when team members start working together to accomplish desired goals. Their work may include assessment and planning as well as implementation and evaluation. The cycle of the nursing process will be repeated as needed during this working phase until goals are satisfactorily accomplished.

The termination phase occurs when the need for team members to work together has ended. When team members have grown close in the relationship, termination can be difficult. Termination should never be abrupt or without participation. It often requires careful advance preparation to make certain that all parties understand when and why it is taking place. Termination helps to ensure a clear-cut end to the collaborative relationship. For example, nurse, physician, social worker, psychologist, and nutritionist collaborated with a refugee group for nearly a year. As the group's multiple needs declined, the professionals began to taper off their assistance. Two months before ending the relationship, they discussed termination with the group. At first group members were frightened at the loss of help, but slowly they came to accept it and assumed more and more responsibility for their health needs.

Contracting in Community Health Nursing

Contracting means negotiating a working agreement between two or more parties in which they come to a shared understanding and mutually consent to the purposes and terms of the transaction. Some kinds of contracts are familiar, such as when one signs a contract agreeing to pay a certain amount for a car over a certain period of time. Paying tuition for an education still involves a form of contracting although a formal document is not signed. A student agrees with an educational institution on a purpose (to obtain a degree) with the terms of the contract being regular tuition payments and regular learning opportunities over a specified period of time.

In contrast to legal contracts that are written and legally binding, contracts in a collaborative relationship are flexible and changing and based on mutual understanding and trust. Sloan and Schommer (1991) describe the community nursing contract as a working agreement that may be renegotiated continuously between clients and health professionals. The flexibility built into contracting makes it a valuable tool for community health nurses.

CHARACTERISTICS OF CONTRACTING

The concept of contracting as used in the collaborative relationship incorporates four distinctive characteristics: partnership, commitment, format, and negotiation.

Partnership

All aspects of contracting involve shared participation and agreement between team members; they become partners in the relationship. For example, a parenting group of 15 couples requested community health nursing involvement. The group entered into a partnership with the nurse and came to an agreement on what they needed and what the nurse could provide. Together they developed goals, outlined methods to meet those goals, explored resources to help achieve them,

defined the time limits for the contract, and outlined their separate responsibilities. The contract involved reciprocal negotiation and shared evaluation. A partnership means that all parties are responsible for setting up and carrying out the terms of the agreement.

Commitment

Second, every contract implies a commitment. The involved parties make a decision that binds them to fulfilling the purpose of the contract. In community health collaboration, contracting does not mean making a binding agreement in the legal sense; rather, it is a pledge of trust and dedication. Accompanying that sense of dedication is a strong motivation to see the contract through to completion. All parties feel responsible for keeping promises; all want to achieve the intended outcomes. When the nurse and the parenting group identified their separate tasks, they committed themselves: "Yes, we will do thus and so."

Format

Format is the third distinctive feature of contracting, it involves outlining the specific terms of the relationship. Clients and professionals gain a clear idea of the purpose of the relationship, of their respective responsibilities, and of the specific limits within which they will work. The format of contracting provides the framework for collaboration. Once the terms of the contract have been spelled out, there is no question about what has to be done, who is to do it, or within what time frame it is to be accomplished. This format helps to avoid the difficulty of terminating long-term relationships and helps shift health care responsibilities from the professionals to the group (Helgeson & Berg, 1985).

Negotiation

Finally, contracting always involves negotiation. The nurse and other team members propose to accept certain responsibilities, and then ask if the clients agree. The nurse might ask, "What do you feel you can do to achieve this goal?" A period of give-and-take occurs in which ideas are discussed and conclusions and consensus reached. Team members may find over time that terms or goals they had agreed upon need modification. For example, perhaps clients have assumed more responsibility than they can realistically handle at that point in time and need to redefine their specific responsibilites. Perhaps the nurse feels a need to involve another professional in the collaborative process. Kreps and Kunimoto (1994) emphasize the importance of effective interpersonal communication between clients and professionals in order to keep contracts updated. Negotiation during contracting allows for changes that facilitate the ultimate achievement of goals. It provides built-in flexibility and encourages ongoing communication among all team members. Negotiation gives contracting a dynamic quality (see Fig. 13.3).

VALUE OF CONTRACTING

The value of contracting has been demonstrated in many settings and disciplines. Contracts have been used for many years in psychiatric and other nursing settings to promote client self-respect, problem-solving skills, autonomy, and motivation (Brockenshire, 1987; Rosen, 1978). Other disciplines, such as social work, have used contracting as a tool in the helping relationship to enhance realistic planning and emphasize partnership (Sauer, 1973). Educational contracts between nursing students and instructors have proven valuable for facilitating learning (Brown et al., 1987; Gross et al., 1986).

Community health nursing also has used the concept of contracting for many years. Without always labeling it as contracting, community health nurses have used these techniques with clients who, for example, wanted to lose weight. In this case the contract involved mutually agreeing to certain exercise and eating patterns for clients and teaching and support responsibilities for the nurse. Often they have set a time limit, such as six months, within which to achieve the intended weight loss. In each case, a partnership developed, with agreement about the purpose of the relationship and the conditions under which it would be carried out. Nurses and clients were, in effect, contracting.

As more and more nurses seek to promote client autonomy and self-care, contracting's wide applicability to nursing practice is being increasingly recognized (Brockenshire, 1987; Helgeson & Berg, 1985; Larson, et al., 1987; Wandel, et al., 1991). Community health nurses have entered into wellness and behavior contracting (Kittleson, et al., 1988), or contracted with diabetics (Wilson, et al., 1988; Morgan, et al., 1988), chronically ill children (Wesolowski, 1988), infants on total parenteral nutrition (Cady, et al., 1991), chemotherapy outpatients (Hiromoto, et al., 1991), prenatal groups, postpartum mothers, and many others.

Potential Problems with Contracting

Emphasis on contracting as a method rather than a concept can create problems. If one's experiences with contracts have all been business agreements, it is possible to carry the stereotype of a cold, formal arrangement

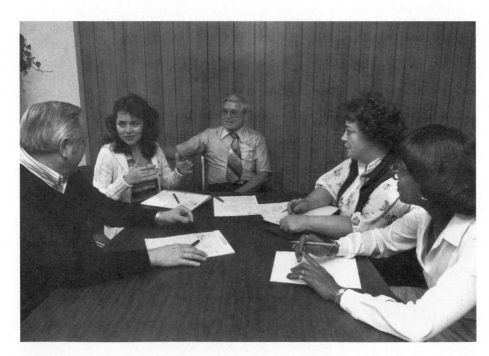

FIGURE 13.3. Skillful interpersonal communication facilitates negotiation.

into the nursing practice setting. Some nurses fear that asking clients to negotiate a contract will place clients under stress, impede the development of trust, and negatively influence the relationship (Lindell, 1986). Others have found that some clients may prefer to have the nurse make decisions for them and are not ready to enter into any kind of negotiation. These potential problems in contracting can be ovecome by nurses understanding the true concept of contracting.

Advantages of Contracting

Contracting applies basic principles of adult education: self-direction, mutual negotiation, and mutual evaluation (Gustafson, 1977). It need not be a formal, written, or complex negotiation. Sloan and Schommer (1991) demonstrate that contracting can be formal or informal, written or verbal, simple or detailed, and signed or unsigned by clients and nurse. It should be adapted to the particular clients' abilities to assess, plan, implement, and evaluate which can greatly vary from situation to situation. Like all nursing tools, contracting will enhance client health only if adapted to each particular set of client needs and abilities.

The advantages of contracting in community health nursing can now be summarized:

1. It involves clients in promoting their own health.
2. It motivates clients to perform necessary tasks.
3. It focuses on clients' unique needs, regardless of aggregate size.
4. It increases the possibility of achieving health goals identified by collaborating team members.
5. It enhances all team members' problem-solving skills.
6. It fosters client participation in the decision-making process.
7. It promotes clients' autonomy and self-esteem as they learn self-care.
8. It makes nursing service more efficient and cost-effective.

PROCESS OF CONTRACTING

Contracting follows a sequence of steps. As a working agreement it depends on knowing what clients want, agreeing on goals, identifying methods to achieve these goals, knowing the resources that collaborating members bring to the relationship, using appropriate outside resources, setting limits, deciding on responsibilities, and providing for periodic reviews. Each of these tasks requires discussion among members of the contractual group. The tasks are incorporated into the contracting process described as eight phases by Sloan and Schommer (1991):

1. *Exploration of needs*: Assessment of clients' health and needs by clients, nurse, and other relevant persons.
2. *Establishment of goals*: Discussion and agreement between contracting members on goals and objectives.
3. *Exploration of resources*: Defining what each member has to offer and can expect from the others; identifying appropriate resources and agencies.
4. *Development of a plan*: Identifying methods, activities, and a time line for achieving the stated goals.
5. *Division of responsibilities*: Negotiating the activities for which each member will be responsible.
6. *Agreement on time frame*: Setting limits for the contract in terms of length of time or number of meetings.
7. *Evaluation*: Periodic and final assessment of progress toward goals occurring at agreed-upon intervals.
8. *Renegotiation or termination*: Agreement to modify, renegotiate, or terminate the contract.

As community health nurses use this process to negotiate a contract, they must adapt it to each situation. The exact sequence of phases may change and some steps may overlap. Nevertheless, the basic elements remain important considerations for successful contracting. They are depicted in Figure 13.4.

LEVELS OF CONTRACTING: FORMAL AND INFORMAL

Community health nurses use contracts at levels ranging from formal to informal. The degree of formality depends on the demands of the situation. To fund a community health program for preventing child abuse, for example, a formal contract in the form of a written grant proposal may be needed. Or to conduct a wide-scale homeless population needs assessment, the services of an epidemiologist, statistician, and others may necessitate a formal contract to clarify roles and expec-

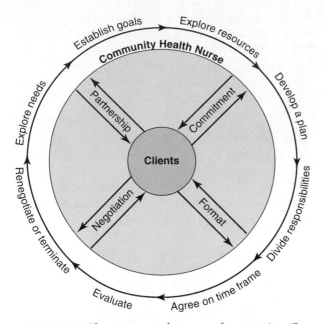

FIGURE 13.4. The concept and process of contracting. Contracting is based on four distinctive features shown here as spokes that support a wheel. These features form the basis for a reciprocal relationship between clients, nurse and other persons. This relationship is not static; it is a dynamic process that moves through phases, represented here as the outer rim of the wheel. The process moves forward, focused on meeting clients' needs, and enables the collaborating group to facilitate ultimate achievement of clients' goals.

tations. **Formal contracting** involves all parties negotiating a written contract by mutual agreement, signing the agreement, and sometimes having it witnessed or notarized. This level of contract has sometimes been used with mental health or substance abusing clients where the seriousness of the working agreement and the need to involve clients actively were important aspects of therapy.

Some situations lend themselves best to a modified and less formal use of contracting in which the nursing plan becomes the written contract. For example, a school nurse formed a support group for pregnant adolescents. The nurse used modified contracting by discussing with the girls the purpose of the group and the number of sessions needed and by obtaining their agreement to attend all sessions.

Informal contracting involves some form of verbal agreement about relatively clear cut purposes and tasks. A client group may agree to prioritize their list of needs,

the nurse may agree to conduct health teaching sessions, the social worker to obtain informational materials, and so on. Sometimes nurses use contracting informally without realizing it. They conclude a session with clients by agreeing with them about the purpose and time of the next meeting. Conscious use of contracting, however, is a more effective way to provide structure for the relationship and foster client involvement, regardless of the level at which it is applied.

The level of contracting may also change during the development of communication and collaboration. Clients often need education about their options. Initially they may have difficulty in identifying needs and making choices. The professional team can work to promote clients' self-confidence and help them assume increasing responsibility for their own health (Larson et al., 1987). See the World Watch discussion on international contracting below. Through these efforts, contracting becomes a consciously recognized part of the relationship. Clients can become fully participating partners.

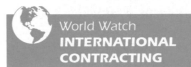

World Watch
INTERNATIONAL CONTRACTING

International organizations have engaged in a form of health contracting for many years. Agencies like the World Health Organization, The American Refugee Committee, or the Peace Corps have established agreements with authorities in third world countries to develop health programs and provide services that will prevent health problems and promote the health of at-risk populations. Sanitation programs, mass immunization efforts, flood and famine relief, and treatment and prevention of such diseases as tuberculosis, HIV, and cholera are examples. The concept of contracting applies equally at the international level. Needs must be explored, goals established, resources explored, a plan developed, responsibilities assigned, a time frame agreed upon, progress and outcomes evaluated, and interventions renegotiated or terminated. As a part of the collaborative team, community health nurses can play an important role in international contracting.

Summary

Communication and collaboration are important tools for community health nurses to use in promoting aggregate health. Communication involves the transfer and understanding of meaning between individuals. The communication process is made up of seven parts: a message, a sender and receiver, encoding, a channel, decoding, and a feedback loop. Barriers to effective communication include selective perception, language barriers, clients filtering out parts of the message, and emotional influence. Core skills essential to effective community health nursing communication include sending skills which allow the nurse to transmit messages effectively, receiving skills which allow the nurse to receive accurate and complete messages, and interpersonal skills which allow the nurse to interact and respond to the messages from clients. These skills include special techniques of active listening, ability to show respect regardless of the message whether positive or negative, ability to empathize with clients' thoughts and feelings, and ability to develop trust. There are many factors which can influence the quality of communication such as negative previous experiences, cultural in-

fluences, and relationships among the people involved. The community health nurse must be able to take all these factors into consideration when trying to foster good communication.

In community health, nurses frequently need to promote communication in groups and in group decision making. Decisions made by groups have many advantages including the sharing of experience and expertise of members, diversity of opinions, potential for broadening members perspectives and focus on arriving at consensus solutions. These are several methods of enhancing group decision making, including brainstorming, nominal group technique, delphi technique, and electronic meetings.

Collaboration is a purposeful interaction between nurse, clients, community members, and other professionals based on mutual participation and joint effort. It is characterized by shared goals, mutual participation, maximized use of resources, clear responsibilities, and set boundaries. Clients play an important role in the collaborative relationship.

Contracting can also be a helpful tool in promoting clients' participation, independence, and motivation. It is used at all levels in community health nursing to promote partnership in the collaborative process, to encour-

Activities to Promote Critical Thinking

1. Discuss how you would handle the communication barrier of selective perception with a group of clients.

2. Practice active listening with a colleague and analyze the factors that interfered with your total concentration. Identify three actions to take to improve your active listening and apply them during the next week, keeping a log of your progress.

3. Use nominal group technique with a group of classmates to arrive at a rank-ordering of barriers to cross-cultural communication. What did you learn about arriving at a quality decision in the process?

4. Organize a group of classmates to represent a group of clients, professionals, and community members that are collaborating to address the needs of an inner city homeless population. Analyze how well you integrated the five characteristics of collaboration into your activity.

5. Explain the concept of contracting as it applies to aggregates. Discuss its four distinctive characteristics and the advantages that contracting offers to the community health nurse.

6. Develop a hypothetical contract with a group of elderly widows who need support and outlets for their loneliness. What other community members and professionals might be helpful as part of a collaborative team to address the widows' needs?

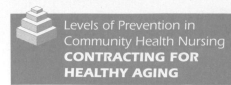

Levels of Prevention in
Community Health Nursing
**CONTRACTING FOR
HEALTHY AGING**

GOAL

Population of elderly will experience healthful living to the full extent of their ability.

PRIMARY PREVENTION

Objective: Group of healthy elderly will maintain or raise their level of well-being and ability to function.

Method:

1. Assess group members' current health status.
2. Identify specific activities that will improve healthy elderly persons' current health status and functional ability.
3. Implement and evaluate identified activities.

SECONDARY PREVENTION

Identify factors contributing to resolution of elderly group's existing health limitations and functional status

TERTIARY PREVENTION

Identify factors that prevent recurrence of health problems or that restore the elderly to a healthful level of functioning within their limitations.

---

age commitment to health goals, and to ensure a format and a means for negotiation among the collaborating group. Contracts can be formal or informal, written or verbal, simple or complex. The nurse must know the needs and abilities of clients and tailor-make the type of contracting that best suits the clients' particular situation.

REFERENCES

Brill, N. I. (1973). *Working with people: The helping process*. Philadelphia: Lippincott.

Brockenshire, A. (1987). Therapeutic contracts: A nursing tool. *Perspectives, 11*(1), 13–14.

Brown, S. T., et al. (1987). Contract learning: A leadership experience for the RN student in a BSN program. *Nurse Manager 18*(4), 66–68, 70.

Cady, C., et al. (1991). Using a learning contract to successfully discharge an infant on home total parenteral nutrition. *Pediatric Nursing, 17*(1), 67–71, 74.

Gross, J. W., et al. (1986). Modified contractual grading. *Nursing Outlook, 34*(4), 184–87.

Gustafson, M. B. (1977). Let's broaden our horizons about the use of contracts. *International Nursing Review, 24*(1), 18–19.

Helgeson, D. M. & Berg, C. (1985). Contracting: A method of health promotion . . . more clearly define a purpose for home visiting. *Journal of Community Health Nursing, 2*(4), 199–207.

Hiromoto, B.M., et al. (1991). Contract learning for self-care activities: a protocal study among chemotherapy outpatients. *Cancer Nursing, 14*(3), 148–154.

Jones, A., et al. (1993). Collaboration in coronary heart disease prevention. *Health Visitor, 66*(7), 257–9.

Kalisch, B. (1973). What is empathy? *American Journal of Nursing, 73*, 1548–52.

Kittleson, M. J., et al. (1988). Wellness and behavior contracting. *Health Education, 19*(2), 8–11.

Kreps, G. L. & Kunimoto, E.N. (1994). *Effective communication in multicultural health care settings*. Thousand Oaks, CA: Sage.

Kristjanson, L. & Chalmers, K. (1990). Nurse-client interactions in community-based practice: creating common ground. *Public Health Nursing, 7*(4), 215–23.

La Monica, E. & Karshmer, J. (1978). Empathy: Educating nurses in professional practice. *Journal of Nursing Education, 17*(2), 3–11.

Larson, E., et al. (1987). Effect of a written nurse/patient contract on the practice of primary nursing. *Nurse Manager, 18*(11), 113.

Lindell, A. R. (1986). Clinical contractual agreements: Liability or blessing? *Journal of Professional Nursing, 2*(3), 138.

Morgan, B.S., et al. (1988). A closer look at teaching and contingency contracting with Type II diabetes . . . In a home setting. *Patient Education Counseling, 12*(2), 145–158.

Plimpton, S. & Root, J. (1994). Materials and strategies that work in low literacy health communication. *Public Health Reports, 109*(1), 86–92.

Robbins, S.P. (1993). *Organizational Behavior* (6th ed.). Englewood Cliffs, NJ: Prentice-Hall.

Rosen, B. (1978). Contract therapy. *Nursing Times, 74*, 119–21.

Sauer, J. K. (1973). The process of contracting in the helping relationship. *Minnesota Welfare,* (Summer), 12–14, 23.

Shockley-Zalabak, P. (1994). *Understanding organizational communication*. New York: Longman.

Sloan, M. & Schommer, B.T. (1991). The process of contracting in community nursing. In B. W. Spradley (Ed.), *Readings in community health nursing* (4th ed.). Boston: Little, Brown.

Stevens, P.E. & Hall, J.M. (1992). Applying critical theories to nursing in communities. *Public Health Nursing, 9*(1), 2–9.

Veninga, R. (1982). *The human side of health administration*. Englewood Cliffs, NJ: Prentice-Hall.

Wandel, J.C., et al. (1991). Case report . . . The care of patients with behavioral problems . . . Including commentary by Mian P. and Danis D. *Journal of Professional Nursing, 7*(2), 126–135.

Wesolowski, C.A. (1988). Self-contracts for chronically ill children. *Maternal Child Nursing, 13*(1), 20–23.

Wilson, M., et al. (1988). A contract for change in diabetes self-management: Case report. *Diabetes Education, 14*(1), 37–40.

Wismer, J. (1978). Communication effectiveness: Active listening and sending feeling messages. In J. W. Pfeiffer and J. Jones (Eds.), *The 1978 annual handbook for group facilitators.* La Jolla, CA: University Associates.

SELECTED READINGS

Burghardt-Fitzgerald, D.C. (1989). Pain-behavior contracts: effective management of the adolescent in sickle-cell crisis. *Journal of Pediatric Nursing, 4*(5), 320–324.

Butterfoss, F. D., et al. (1993). Community coalitions for prevention and health promotion. *Health Education Research, 8*(3): 315–30.

Douglas, G., Robbins, W., & Sullivan-Paal, C. (1994). Beyond rhetoric: building and achieving community consensus in planning and developing an innovative public health nurse-midwifery education program. *Public Health Nursing, 11*(3), 181–187.

Farley, S. (1993). The community as partner in primary health care. *Nursing and Health Care, 14*(5), 244–249.

Fay, P. (1986). Contracting: A collaborative approach. *Journal of Nursing Staff Development, 2*(4), 157–61.

Fisher, D. (1993). *Communication in organizations* (2nd ed.). Minneapolis/St. Paul, MN: West Publishing.

Fontana, S.A. (1991). Applying marketing concepts to promote health in vulnerable groups. *Public Health Nursing, 8*(2), 140–143.

Froner, G. & Rowniak, S. (1989). The health outreach team: taking AIDS education and health care to the streets. *AIDS Education and Prevention, 1*(2), 105–18.

Johnson, R. A. (1993). *Negotiation basics: concepts, skills, and exercises.* Newbury Park, CA: Sage.

Katzenbach, J. R. & Smith, D.K. (1993). *The wisdom of teams: Creating the high performance organization.* Boston, MA: Harvard Business School Press.

Ovretveit, J. (1992). Fulfilling the need for a coordinated approach: case management and community nursing. *Professional Nurse, 7*(4), 264–266, 268–269.

Petosa, R. (1984). Using behavioral contracts to promote health behavior change: Application in a college-level course. *Health Educator, 15*(2), 22–26.

Wright, J., Henry, S., Holzemer, W., & Falknor, P. (1993). Evaluation of community-based nurse case management activities for symptomatic HIV/AIDS clients . . . California pilot care and waiver projects for HIV/AIDS. *Journal of Association of Nurses in AIDS Care, 4*(2), 37–47.

CHAPTER

14

Educational Interventions to Promote Community Health

LEARNING OBJECTIVES

Upon completion of this chapter, readers should be able to:

- Examine the community health nurse's role as teacher in promoting health, and preventing or postponing morbidity.
- Choose selected learning theories that are applicable to an individual, family, or aggregate client.
- Select teaching methods and materials that facilitate learning for clients at different developmental levels.
- Develop teaching plans focusing on primary, secondary and tertiary levels of prevention for clients of all ages.
- Identify teaching strategies the nurse can use when encountering the "hard to help" client.
- Locate appropriate audio-visual and printed material resources to enhance client learning.

KEY TERMS

- Accommodation (Piaget)
- Adaptation (Piaget)
- Affective domain
- Anticipatory guidance
- Assimilation (Piaget)
- Cognitive domain
- Deductive
- Gestalt-field

- Learning
- Levels of prevention
- Operant conditioning
- Operationalize
- Primary prevention
- Psychomotor domain
- Secondary prevention
- Teaching

Barbara Walton Spradley and Judith Ann Allender
COMMUNITY HEALTH NURSING: CONCEPTS AND PRACTICE, 4th ed.
© 1996 Barbara Walton Spradley and Judith Ann Allender

The rationale for health promotion and client education is to equip people with the knowledge, attitudes, and behaviors to live the fullest life possible for the greatest length of time. Infirmity, due to ill health, needs to be compressed into the very late years of life (Lorig, 1992). Ideally even the later years will be healthy and full of vigor.

Clients anticipate achieving their maximum life span. However, without knowledge of and implementation of necessary health information they may fall short of their goal by years, even decades. How many times has a nurse seen a client die prematurely from a preventable or manageable illness state? The implementation of vital health education can help prevent such situations from occurring. Teaching has been an important part of the community health nurse's role since the origins of the profession and is frequently the primary role function. The nurse develops partnerships with a client to achieve a behavior change that promotes, maintains, or restores health. This partnership focuses on self-care and the learning is measured by the degree of behavior change. Nurses cannot assume that imparting knowledge will guarantee understanding or change a client's health practice. Thus, the need for the nurse to know about the nature of learning becomes essential to effective community health practice.

When the community health nurse identifies a need that is best met through health education, the nurse is faced with a series of questions: How can nurses teach effectively? What content should they cover? What method of presentation will communicate most effectively? What written material or audio-visual aids can nurses use as teaching tools? How do they know when the client has grasped the information or mastered the skills? What does a nurse do with the "hard to help" client? In other words, what makes teaching effective, how are teaching skills acquired, and how is mastery measured? This chapter addresses these questions and discusses teaching as a basic intervention tool in community health nursing practice.

The Nature of Learning

Teaching is a specialized communication process in which desired behavior changes are achieved. The goal of all teaching is **learning**. However, learning involves far more than the simple sharing of information. It is a process of assimilating new information which promotes a permanent change in behavior. All people have been presented with information that was not interesting, relevant to their needs, or comprehensible. In such situations, learning was difficult if not impossible. The nurse as a teacher seeks to transmit information in such a way that the learner understands and some change in behavior results. Effective teaching is a cause; learning becomes the effect. To teach effectively, especially in the community where teaching is the focus of care, nurses need to understand the various domains of learning and related learning theories.

The Domains of Learning

Learning occurs in several realms or domains, cognitive, affective, and psychomotor. In this section, these domains are described followed by examples of each. Understanding the differences among the domains and the related role of the nurse gives the nurse the background necessary to teach effectively.

COGNITIVE DOMAIN

The **cognitive domain** of learning involves the mind and thinking processes. When the meaning and relationship of a series of facts is grasped, cognitive learning is experienced. The cognitive domain deals with the recall or recognition of knowledge and the development of intellectual abilities and skills (Bloom, 1956). There are six major levels in the cognitive domain (Gronlund, 1970): knowledge, comprehension, application, analysis, synthesis, and evaluation. When **operationalizing** these levels, that is putting these ideas or concepts into words that can be used, think of verbs. As the behavioral objective changes, so do the verbs indicating the learning to be accomplished within that particular level of the cognitive domain. A representative sample of behavioral objectives focusing on nutrition and appropriate cognitive level verbs follows.

Knowledge

Knowledge, the lowest level of learning, involves recall. If students can remember material previously learned, they have acquired knowledge. This level may be used with clients who are unable to understand underlying reasons or rationales such as people who have had strokes or very young children. Stroke clients may need to remember that medication should be taken daily, that regular exercise restores function, and not to drink alcohol, even though they may not grasp the reasons behind these measures. Five year olds may need to be able to identify healthy foods rather than understand why they are healthy.

A knowledge-level behavioral objective might be: The client can *recall* the names of six fruits to eat as healthy snacks. Other knowledge level verbs include: define, repeat, list, and name.

Comprehension

The second level of cognitive learning, comprehension, combines remembering with understanding. When possible, teaching aims at instilling at least minimum understanding. Nurses want clients to grasp the meaning and to recognize the importance of suggested health behaviors.

An example of a comprehension-level behavioral objective might be: the pregnant client will *describe* a well balanced diet during pregnancy. Other appropriate verbs at the comprehension level include: discuss, explain, identify, tell, and report.

Application

Application is the third level of cognitive learning in which the learner not only is able to understand material but also apply it to new and actual situations. Application approaches the possibility of self-care in which clients use their knowledge for improvement of their own health. The test of application is a transfer of understanding into practice. To encourage application, the nurse can design teaching plans that show clients how to put knowledge into practice. A tobacco elimination study using this approach resulted in decreased use of tobacco products among the adolescents in the study (Sussman, et al., 1993). A nurse may suggest that a diabetic client write down glucometer readings on a sheet of paper to show the nurse at the next visit or ask adolescents in a weight-loss group to keep a diet record for a week, draw up a diet plan, and share this plan with the group at the next meeting. The construction worker who understands on-the-job hazards but seldom wears a protective hat in the work area has yet to transfer comprehension into practice.

An example of an application-level behavioral objective might be: the client will *practice* eating well balanced meals at least two times a day (see Fig. 14.1). Other verbs at this level include: apply, use, demonstrate, and illustrate.

Analysis

The fourth level of cognitive learning is analysis in which the learner can break material down into parts, distinguish between elements, and understand the relationships among the parts. This level of learning becomes a preliminary step toward problem solving. The learner carefully scrutinizes all the variables or elements and their relationships to each other in order to explain the situation. A family that studies its own communication patterns for the purpose of identifying sources of conflict is using analysis. A mother analyzes when she seeks to determine the cause of an infant's crying. After viewing the total situation, she breaks it down into variables such as hunger, pain, loneliness, type of crying, and intensity of crying. She examines these parts and draws conclusions about their relationships. In health teaching, community health nurses foster clients' analytic skills by demonstrating how to isolate the parts in a situation and then encouraging them to consider the relationship of the parts and draw conclusions from their thinking.

An analysis-level behavioral objective for senior citizens trying to learn more about low fat foods might be: the seniors should be able to *compare* the fat content in a variety of packaged foods. Other verbs at the analysis

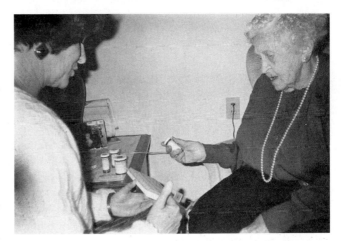

FIGURE 14.1. Teaching methods and tools vary with clients' learning needs. On this home visit, the nurse uses a weekly medication container to help an elderly woman with limited vision devise a plan for taking her medications.

level include: differentiate, contrast, debate, question, and examine.

Synthesis

Synthesis, the fifth level of cognitive learning, is the ability to not only break down and understand the elements of a situation but to form elements into a new whole. Synthesis combines all the earlier levels of cognitive learning to culminate in the production of a unique plan or solution. Clients who achieve learning at this level will not only analyze their problems but also find solutions for them. For example, a nurse may assist mental health clients in a therapy group to examine their frequent depression and then to generate their own plan for alleviating it. A young couple who want to toilet train their two-year-old child learns the physiological and psychological dimensions of toilet training, analyzes their own situation, and then develops strategies (their own plan) for training the child. Nurses facilitate synthesis by assisting and encouraging clients to develop their own solutions with specific plans. When a problem is identified, the client should be asked, "What are some possible causes? Do you see anything that has been overlooked about the problem?" If the client asks for a solution, the nurse should encourage synthesis by asking, "What are some possible solutions to this problem that you might carry out?"

An example of a synthesis-level behavioral objective for a client on a sodium restricted diet might be: the client will be able to *prepare* an enjoyable meal using low sodium foods. Other verbs at this level include: compose, design, formulate, create, and organize.

Evaluation

The highest level of cognitive learning is evaluation in which the learner judges the usefulness of new material compared with a stated purpose or specific criteria (Gronlund, 1970). Clients can learn to judge their own health behavior by comparing it with standards established by others such as abstinence from smoking, maintenance of normal weight, regular exercise, or clients may establish their own criteria. A parent support group designs activities to enhance parent-child communication, and judges their performance by using their desired outcomes as evaluation criteria. When nurses aim for this level of client learning, they have made self-care a concrete objective. Evaluation, because it goes beyond attempts at problem solving, enables the

client to judge the adequacy of solutions, to critique life-style and health-related behavior, and to anticipate needed improvements.

An example of a behavioral objective at the evaluation level might be: the clients in a nutrition class will be able to *measure* the cholesterol content in one portion of the low cholesterol dish they brought to share. Other verbs at this level include: judge, evaluate, rate, choose, and estimate.

How to Measure Cognitive Learning

Cognitive learning at any of the levels described can be measured easily in terms of learner behaviors. Nurses know, for instance, that clients have achieved teaching objectives for application of knowledge when their behavior demonstrates actual use of the information taught. Client roles in cognitive learning range from relatively passive (at the knowledge level) to active (at the evaluation level). Conversely, as clients become more active, the nurse's role becomes less directive. It is important to point out that not all clients need to be brought through all levels of cognitive learning. Nor does one client need to reach the evaluation level for each aspect of care. For some clients and situations, comprehension is an adequate and effective level. For others, the application level is the level of achievement the nurse focuses on. Table 14.1 illustrates client and nurse behaviors for each cognitive level.

AFFECTIVE DOMAIN

The **affective domain** in which learning occurs involves emotion, feeling, or affect. This kind of learning deals with changes in interest, attitudes, and values (Bloom, 1956). Here nurses face the task of trying to influence what clients' value and feel. Nurses want them to develop an ability to accept ideas that promote healthier behavior patterns even though those ideas may conflict with their own values.

Attitudes and values are learned (Bigge, 1982). They develop gradually over time as the way an individual feels and responds is molded by family, peers, experiences, and societal influences. These feelings and responses are the result of imitation and conditioning. In this way, clients acquire their health-related beliefs and practices. Because attitudes and values become part of the person, they are difficult to change unless the nurse is aware of how they develop.

TABLE 14.1. *Cognitive Learning: Case Study in Controlling Diabetes*

Level	Illustrative Client Behavior	Illustrative Nurse Behavior
Knowledge (recalls, knows)	States that insulin, if taken, will control own diabetes	Give information
Comprehension (understands)	Describes insulin action and purpose	Explains information
Application (uses learning)	Adjusts insulin dosage daily to maintain proper blood sugar level	Suggests how to use learning
Analysis (examines, explains)	Discusses relationships between insulin, diet, activity, and diabetic control	Demonstrates and encourages analysis
Synthesis (integrates with other learning, generates new ideas)	Develops a plan, incorporating above learning, for controlling own diabetes	Promotes client formulation of own plan
Evaluation (judges according to a standard)	Compares degree of diabetic control (outcomes) with desired control (objectives)	Facilitates evaluation

Affective learning occurs on several levels as learners respond with varying degrees of involvement and commitment. At the first level, learners are simply receptive; They are willing to listen, show awareness, and be attentive. The nurse aims at acquiring and focusing learners' attention (Gronlund, 1970). This limited goal may be all that clients are ready for at the early stages of the nurse-client relationship.

At the second level, learners become active participants by responding to the information in some way. Some examples might be willingness to read educational material, participate in discussion, complete assignments such as keeping a diet record, or voluntarily seek out more information.

At the third level, learners attach value to the information. Valuing ranges from simple acceptance through appreciation to commitment. For example a nurse taught members of a therapy group a number of principles concerning group effectiveness. An explanation of the importance of a democratic group process and ways to improve group skills was given. Members showed acceptance when they acknowledged the importance of these ideas. They showed appreciation of the ideas by starting to practice them. Commitment came when they assumed responsiblity for having their group function well.

The final level of affective learning occurs when learners internalize an idea or value. The value system now controls learner behavior. Consistent practice is a crucial test at this level. Clients who know and respect the value of exercise but only occasionally play tennis or do an aerobic activity have not internalized the value. Even several weeks of enthusiastic jogging is not evidence of an internalized value. If the jogging continues for six months, a year, and longer, learning may have been internalized.

Affective learning often remains elusive, difficult to measure. Indeed, this quality may influence community health nurses to concentrate their efforts on cognitive learning goals instead. Yet client attitudes and values have a major effect on the outcome of cognitive learning—desired behavioral changes. For this reason, both cognitive and affective domains must remain linked in teaching; otherwise, results may quickly fade.

Attitudes and values can change in the same way they were first learned, that is, through imitation and conditioning (Redman, 1988). Role models, particularly those from the client's peer group who practice the desired health behaviors, can be a strong influence. Support groups like mastectomy clubs or chemical dependency support groups can have a powerful role model effect. Frequently the nurse may be viewed as a role model by clients, thus nurses should be careful to demonstrate healthy behaviors.

Attitudes often change when the nurse provides clients with a satisfying experience during the learning process. The nurse who recognizes clients' participation in a group, praises them for completing assignments, or commends them for sticking to diet plans will have more success than the nurse who only criticizes failures. Another point to keep in mind is that clients can develop a close relationship with the nurse during the teaching-learning process and some sharing of the nurse's ability to manage personal health promotion issues lets clients know that the nurse too, is human. This can be an effective addition to teaching strategies for the nurse, if it feels comfortable and is used wisely. Table 14.2 shows client and nurse behaviors for each level of affective learning.

To influence affective learning requires patience. Values and attitudes will seldom change overnight. Keep in mind that other forces will continue to reinforce former values. For example, a middle-aged housewife may want to pursue a career for self-fulfillment but does not because she has children in college and feels their education comes first. A young man can verbalize the importance of safe sex but is uncomfortable discussing the subject, making it difficult to assess compliance with the nurse's instruction.

PSYCHOMOTOR DOMAIN

The **psychomotor domain** includes visible, demonstrable performance skills that require some kind of neuromuscular coordination. Clients in the community need to learn skills such as infant bathing, temperature taking, breast or testicular self-examination, prenatal breathing exercises, range-of-motion exercises, catheter irrigation, crutch-walking, and a variety of dressing changes.

For psychomotor learning to take place, three conditions must be met: (1) learners must be capable of the skill, (2) learners must have a sensory image of how to perform the skill and, (3) learners must practice the skill. The nurse must be certain the client is physically, intellectually, and emotionally capable of performing the skill. An elderly diabetic man with tremulous hands and fading vision should not be expected to give his own insulin injections; it could frustrate and possibly harm him. An accessible person more physically capable should be enlisted and taught the skill. Clients' intellectual and emotional capabilities also influence their capacity to learn motor skills. It may be quite inappropriate to expect persons of limited intelligence to learn complex skills. The degree of complexity should match the learners' level of functioning. However, the nurse should never equate educational level with intelligence. Many clients may have had limited formal schooling but are able to learn complex skills for themselves or as a caregiver after thorough instruction. Developmental stage and abilities is another point to consider in determining whether it is appropriate to teach a particular skill. For example, most children can put on some article of clothing at two years of age but are not ready to learn to fasten buttons until well past their third birthday.

Learners must also have a sensory image of how to perform the skill through sight, hearing, touch, and sometimes taste or smell. This sensory image is gained by demonstration. In order to teach clients motor skills effectively, the nurse has to provide them with an adequate sensory image. The nurse must demonstrate and explain slowly, one point at a time, and sometimes repeatedly, until clients understand the proper sequence or combination of actions necessary to carry-out the skill.

The third necessary condition for psychomotor learning is practice. After acquiring a sensory image, clients can start to perform the skill. Mastery will come over time as clients repeat the task until it is smooth, coordinated, and unhesitating. During this process the nurse should be available to provide guidance and encouragement. In the early stages of practice the nurse may need to use hands-on guidance to give clients a sense of how the performance should feel. When clients give a return demonstration, the nurse can make suggestions, give encouragement, and thereby maximize the learning. For example, a nurse demonstrates passive range-of-motion exercises on a client's wife to show her how the

TABLE 14.2. *Affective Learning: Case Study in Family Planning*

Level	Illustrative Client Behavior	Illustrative Nurse Behavior
Receptive (listens, pays attention)	Attentive to family planning instruction	Directs client's attention
Responsive (participates, reacts)	Discusses pros and cons of various methods	Encourages client involvement
Valuing (accepts, appreciates, commits)	Selects a method for use	Respects client's right to decide
Internal consistency (organizes values to fit together)	Understands and accepts responsibility for limiting number of children	Brings client into contact with role models
Adoption (incorporates new values into life-style)	Consistently practices birth control	Positively reinforces healthy behaviors

exercises should feel (giving her a sensory image). Then the wife learns to do them for her husband. During practice, feedback from the nurse will enable the wife to know if the skill is being performed correctly.

The psychomotor domain, like the cognitive and affective domains, ranges from simple to complex levels of functioning. It is necessary to exercise judgment in assessing clients' ability to perform a skill. Even clients with limited ability can often move on to higher levels once they have mastered simple skills. Nurse behaviors that influence psychomotor learning are shown in Table 14.3.

Learning Theories

What is a learning theory? A learning theory is a "systematic, integrated outlook in regard to the nature of the process whereby people relate to their environments in such a way as to enhance their ability to use both themselves and their environments more effectively" (Bigge, 1982, p. 3). Nurses, whether they are conscious of it or not, have and use a theory of learning and that theory, in turn, dictates the way they teach. It is useful to discover what that learning theory is and how it affects the nurse's role as health educator.

Learning theories can be grouped into three categories; behavioral, cognitive, and humanistic. More recently the adult learning theory of Malcolm Knowles (1980; 1984) has influenced client teaching. A brief examination of these categories and the specific theories of each follows.

BEHAVIORAL THEORIES

Behavioral theory (also known as stimulus-response or conditioning theory), approaches the study of learning by focusing on behaviors that can be observed, measured, and changed. Developed early in the twentieth century, behaviorial theory work is primarily associated with three famous names, Ivan Pavlov, Edward Thorndike, and B.F. Skinner. Essentially, to a behav-

ioralist, learning is a behavioral change—a response to certain stimuli. Thus the behaviorialistic teacher seeks to significantly change learners' behaviors through a series of selected stimuli.

The stimulus-response "bond" theory proposes that with conditioning, certain causes (stimuli) evoke certain effects (responses). The teacher promotes acquisition of the desired stimulus-response connections so that transfer of learning can occur in another situation with the same stimulus-response elements present. Pavlov's early work with stimulus-response and involuntary reflex actions is perhaps the best known application of this theory. Pavlov conditioned a dog to anticipate food by ringing a bell at feeding time. Initially, the dog would salivate as the food was brought to the cage. However after time, the dog would salivate at hearing the bell, before seeing or smelling the food. Two other behavioral theories are conditioning with no reinforcement (Thorndike) and conditioning through reinforcement (Skinner). No-reinforcement theorists focus on the learner's innate reflexive drives to accomplish the desired response after conditioning, such as when the nurse repeatedly emphasizes to a group of pregnant women that the prenatal classes they are attending promote a positive delivery experience and healthy newborns. The reinforcement theorists use successive, systematic changes in the learner's environment to enhance the probability of desired responses such as a nurse giving attendance rewards (balloons, coloring books, crayons) to children who attend each class on safety. Skinner's work with **operant conditioning**, a form of learning whereby a person is rewarded for right behavior and punished for wrong behavior, made a major contribution to stimulus-response theory (Hergenhahn, 1982; Sprinthall & Sprinthall, 1990).

COGNITIVE THEORIES

Jean Piaget is probably the most widely known cognitive theorist. His theory of cognitive development has contributed to the theories of Kohlberg (moral development) and Fowler (development of faith). Piaget (1966)

TABLE 14.3. *Nurse Behaviors in Psychomotor Learning*

Determining Capability	Providing Sensory Image	Encouraging Practice
Nurse assesses client's physical, intellectual, and emotional ability	Nurse demonstrates and explains	Nurse uses guidance and positive reinforcement

Research in Community Health Nursing
THE EFFECTS OF EDUCATION ON BSE WITH OLDER WOMEN

Lerman, L.M., Young, H.M., Powell-Cope, G., Georgiadou, F., & Benoliel, J.Q. (1994). Effects of education and support on breast self-examination in older women. *Nursing Research*, 43(3), 158–163.

This study was designed to determine the effects of education and structured support on breast self-examination (BSE), frequency, proficiency, and perceived control in women over the age of 50 who were subscribers of a health maintenance organization (HMO). One year of follow-up at 6 and 12 month intervals was planned. The women received one-on-one instruction and supervised practice of SBE. They were also randomly assigned to a control group of no support, peer support group, or selected partner support group. BSE performance was measured by self-report of frequency and proficiency in addition to an expert rating of demonstrated behavior. Research assistants conducted interviews in the participants home on three occasions, initially, at 6 months, and at 12 months.

Results indicate no significant differences across the three support groups on any variables on all three occasions using a variety of tests including analysis of variance, chi-square, the Wilcoxon Z test and the Kruskal-Wallis test. There were significant positive findings with BSE frequency, proficiency, and perceived skill. Frequency increased to 98% at the 6 month interval and 63% at 12 months. Self-report proficiency doubled at six month and continued to increase by one year, as did perceived skill.

The results led the researchers to conclude that the motivation of the women to change their behavior and the strong teaching program all women received contributed most to the changes in behavior. The strong internal motivation and intense teaching may have reduced the need for external motivation in the form of a support partner initially. Perhaps the support partner would have helped the waning internal motivation at a later time during the follow-up period.

believed that cognitive development is an orderly, sequential, and interactive process in which a variety of new experiences must exist before intellectual abilities can develop. His work with children led him to develop five phases of cognitive development from birth to 15 years:

Age	Stage	Behavior
Birth to 2 years	Sensorimotor stage	The child moves focus from self to the environment (rituals are important)
2 to 4 years	Preconceptual stage	Language development is rapid and everything is related to "me"
4 to 7 years	Intuitive thought stage	Egocentric thinking diminishes and words are used to express thoughts
7 to 11 years	Concrete operations stage	Child can solve concrete problems and recognize others' viewpoints
11 to 15 years	Formal operations stage	Child uses rational thinking and can develop ideas from general principles (**deductive** reasoning) and apply them to future situations

Each stage signifies a transformation from the previous one and a child must move through each stage sequentially. The three abilities of **assimilation** (reacting to new situations by using skills already possessed), **accommodation** (being sufficiently mature so that previously unsolved problems can now be solved), and **adaptation** (the ability to cope with the demands of the environment) are used to make the transformation. It is important for the nurse to know which stage their audience is in to ascertain how to approach teaching for that developmental stage. The nurse can see how the use of puppets with 3 year olds may be a beneficial addition to a presentation on safety, whereas a group of young teens with diabetes can respond to the consequences of taking or not taking their insulin.

The **Gestalt-field** family of cognitive theories assumes that people are neither good nor bad—they simply interact with their environment, and their learning is related to perception. Thus, this theory defines learning as a "reorganization of the learner's perceptual or psychological world—his psychological field" (Bigge, 1982, p. 57).

The first Gestalt-field family is called insight theory which regards learning as a process in which the learner develops new insights or changes old ones. Learners sense their way intuitively but intelligently through problems. The "insight" is useful only if the learner understands its significance. The second theory, goal-insight, is very similar to insight theory but goes beyond intuitive hunches to tested insights. Teachers subscribing to this theory promote insightful learning but assist learners in developing higher-quality insights. In the third theory, cognitive-field theory the learner is seen as purposive and problem-centered. Teachers seek to help learners gain new insights and restructure their lives accordingly.

HUMANISTIC THEORIES

Humanistic theories assume that there is a natural tendency for people to learn and that learning flourishes in an encouraging environment. There are several notable humanists, but two of the most notable are Abraham Maslow and Carl Rogers. Abraham Maslow developed the classic hierarchy of human needs in the 1940's. It suggests that man's first need is physiologic (air, food, water, etc.), second in the hierarchy are safety and security needs, third comes love and belonging, then self-esteem needs (positive feelings of self-worth), and lastly the need for self-actualization, or becoming all that one can be (Maslow, 1970).

In community health nursing the clients' needs must be considered when planning health education programs. For example, it would be difficult for a group of young mothers to concentrate on learning about proper nutrition if they are worried about their babies crying in the next room. Their need to care for their children (need of love and belonging) would be greater than the need to learn about future health considerations (self-esteem/self-actualization). Likewise, it is impossible to learn if the room is so warm that the participants are falling asleep (physiological needs not being met).

Carl Rogers developed the client-centered counseling approach that has long been important in the guidance and counseling arena. He believed the role of therapist should be nondirective and accepting and proposed approaching clients in a warm, positive, and empathetic manner to get in touch with the client's feelings and thoughts. Rogers (1969, 1989) soon applied his beliefs to education, suggesting that the learning environment

be learner-centered. The outcome of a learner-centered educational environment is that the students become more self-directed and guide their own learning. Clients who are self-directed in learning are more apt to follow through with the material, personalizing it to their own situation. It is the client who is best able to decide how to find the solutions to his, or her, problems. The client identifies the problem, and given time and space, can find a way through the problem to solution. The nurse acts as a facilitator in this learning process.

For the community health nurse the client-centered approach has many possibilities. A group of parents are looking for ways to communicate more effectively with their teenagers. A 55-year-old man wants to quit smoking after a prolonged upper respiratory infection, aggravated by his habit, and has come to a "Stop Smoking" class conducted by a nurse in the county health department. Several older adults realize they need to increase daily activity and are looking for direction from the nurse working in their senior center.

Teaching at Three Levels of Prevention

Nurses should develop teaching programs that coincide with the level of prevention needed by the client. The three levels (defined in Chapter 1) of primary, secondary, and tertiary prevention are shown in Table 14.4.

Ideally the nurse focuses teaching at the primary level. If nurses were able to reach more people at this level it would help to compress the years of morbidity and limit subsequent infirmity. There are many people who suffer from preventable disabilities that might not have happened if they had incorporated primary prevention behaviors into their daily activities. The primary level of prevention is not possible in all cases, so a significant share of the nurse's time is teaching at the secondary or tertiary level. An example of this is an 88-year-old woman with a fractured hip who has returned home after three weeks of physical therapy at an extended care facility. The nurse would assess her environment, gait, functional limitations, safety, and initiate any referrals needed. The teaching focuses on rehabilitation and prevention of a secondary problem that may affect the healing process and the client's health in general.

TABLE 14.4. *Levels of Prevention*

Level	Focus	Examples
Primary prevention	Health teaching, specific protection	Health education, immunizations
Secondary prevention	Early diagnosis and treatment	Screening, case-finding, prompt treatment
Tertiary prevention	Maintenance and rehabilitation	Restore function, prevent a secondary problem, alternative house, retraining

Effective Teaching

Teaching is an art. It can be performed with such skill and grace that the client becomes a part of a well-orchestrated event with learning as the natural outcome. Instead of relying on prescribed teaching methods, the skillful nurse can make judgements based largely on client qualities, situations, and needs that guide the experience to fruition. When teaching has developed to the form of being an art, the nurse is able to take this form of human interaction to a level of change that emerges in the course of interaction rather than at a preconceived level prior to the teaching (Eisner, 1985). Before the community health nurse can reach this level there is much to learn about being an effective teacher.

TEACHING-LEARNING PRINCIPLES

Teaching lies at one end of a continuum. At the other end is learning. Without learning, teaching becomes useless in much the same way that communication does not occur unless a message is both sent and received (Lorig, 1985). Both the teacher and the learner have responsibilities on that continuum. Learners must take responsibility for their own learning (Levin, 1978). Teachers obstruct that process if they assume complete responsibility for bringing about changed behavior. Clients can be directed toward health knowledge, but will not learn unless they have the desire to learn. Teaching, then, becomes a matter of facilitating both the desire and the best conditions for satisfying it. Teaching in community health nursing means to influence, motivate, and act as a catalyst in the learning process. Nurses bring information and learner together and stimulate a reaction which leads to a change (Douglass & Bevis, 1974). Nurses facilitate learning when they make it as easy as possible for clients to change. To do

this, the nurse needs to understand the basic principles underlying the art and science of the teaching-learning process and the use of appropriate materials to influence learning as displayed in Table 14.5.

Client Readiness

Clients' readiness to learn influences teaching effectiveness (Miller, 1985; Johnson & Jackson, 1989). Two facets of client readiness have been identified. Emotional readiness or receptiveness to learning and experimental readiness, the learner's knowledge and understanding, need to be assessed by the nurse (Nobel, 1991). For instance, one community health nurse found that a young primipara was not ready for prenatal teaching on fetal growth and development. She had strong fears, the nurse discovered, that "losing her figure" would make her sexually unattractive to her husband. Until these anxieties had subsided, the teaching would remain ineffective. Clients' needs, interests, motivation, stress, and concerns determine their readiness for learning.

Another factor that influences readiness is educational background. If a group of women who never completed grade school meet to learn how to care for a sick person in the home, material should be presented simply, factually, and in terms that they understand. To discuss complex concepts of health, illness, and scientific research would be above their level of readiness. However, increasingly complex concepts can be introduced as the nurse works with the women and assesses their readiness to assimilate advanced concepts.

Maturational level also affects readiness. An adolescent mother who is still working on normal developmental tasks of her age group, such as seeking independence or selecting a career path, may not be ready to learn parenting skills. Readiness of the client will determine the amount of material presented in each teaching

TABLE 14.5. *Seven Principles for Maximizing the Teaching-Learning Process*

Teaching Principles	Learning Principles
1. Adapt teaching to clients' level of readiness.	1. The learning process makes use of clients' experience and is geared to their level of understanding.
2. Determine clients' perceptions about the subject matter before and during teaching.	2. Clients are given the opportunity to provide frequent feedback on their understanding of the material taught.
3. Create an environment that is conducive to learning.	3. The environment for learning is physically comfortable, offers an atmosphere of mutual helpfulness, trust, respect, and acceptance, and allows for free expression of ideas.
4. Involve clients throughout the learning process.	4. Clients actively participate. They assess their needs, establish goals, and evaluate learning progress.
5. Make subject matter relevant to clients' interest and use.	5. Clients feel motivated to learn.
6. Ensure client satisfaction during the teaching-learning process.	6. Clients sense progress toward their goals.
7. Provide opportunities for clients to apply material taught.	7. Clients integrate the learning through application.

Source: Adapted from Knowles (1980), pp. 57–58.

session. The pace or speed with which information is presented must be manageable. A moderate amount of anxiety will often increase client receptivity to learning; however, high or low levels of anxiety can have the opposite effect.

Client Perceptions

Clients' perceptions affect their learning. People's perceptions, the way they see the world, serve as a screening device through which all new information must pass (Marriner, 1979). Individual perceptions help people interpret and attach meaning to things. A wide range of variables affects human perception. These variables include values, past experiences, culture, religion, personality, developmental stage, educational and economic level, surrounding social forces, and the physical environment. In community health nursing, one client may view the experience of parenting as a positive, growth-producing relationship; another may see it as a conflict-ridden, unhappy experience to avoid. Each kind of perception has a different consequence for teaching and learning. The nurse, working with adolescents to educate them about the dangers of taking drugs should understand that adolescents seeking independence need to feel they have options and choices, and not to be told what to do.

Frequently clients use selective perception. They screen out some statements and pay attention to those that fit their values or personal desires. For example, a nurse is teaching a client the various risk factors in coronary disease; the individual screens out smoking and obesity, paying attention only to factors that would not require a drastic change in life-style. Nurses must know their clients, understand their backgrounds and values, and learn what their perceptions are before health teaching can influence their behavior. (See the Levels of Prevention display below.)

Educational Environment

The setting in which the educational endeavor takes place has a significant impact on learning. All nurses have had the experience of sitting in a cold room and trying to concentrate during a lecture, or of being distracted by noise, heat, uncomfortable seating, or some other nuisance. Ventilation, lighting, decor, room temperature, view of the speaker, whispering, and other physical conditions need to be controlled so as to provide the environment most conducive to learning.

Equally important for learning is an atmosphere of mutual respect and trust. The nurse needs to convey this attitude through both verbal and nonverbal means. The way clients are addressed, courtesies are shown, and recognition is given will make a considerable difference in establishing respect and trust. Both nurse and clients need to be mutually helpful and considerate of one another's needs and interests. All participants in the

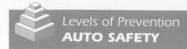

Levels of Prevention
AUTO SAFETY

GOAL

To prevent auto accidents, provide immediate and adequate response at the scene of accidents, and provide appropriate rehabilitative services to injured passengers

PRIMARY PREVENTION

Use passive restraints, air bags

Drivers education programs

Public education: drinking and driving, fatigue, mechanical failures, emergency actions

Driving safe speeds for road and traffic conditions

Regular checks of vehicle for safety, equipment, lights, brakes

Suspension of license when appropriate

Retesting drivers for knowledge of laws and auto handling, vision tests at intervals and as driver ages

SECONDARY PREVENTION

Cellular phones, early reporting of accidents by passing motorists

Emergency medical services for treatment at the scene

Professional specialites in emergency medical services

Public education in first-aid

Cross training of ambulance drivers, police and fire fighters as paramedics

Develop and upgrade trauma centers and reporting systems

Teach necessary care to family members

TERTIARY PREVENTION

Develop or use existing rehabilitation programs with physical therapy, occupational therapy, speech therapy

Educate industry on the employment of disabled individuals(Americans with Disabilities Act)

Develop community services for disabled, job retraining programs

Financial assistance during rehabilitation and job training

Aid to totally disabled and partial aid to those unable to support self totally but still able to work part-time

educational experience should feel free to express ideas, know that their views will be heard, and feel accepted despite differences of opinion and perspective. According to Knowles, this requires that the nurse refrain from seeming judgmental or inducing competitiveness among learners. Knowles adds that the teacher shares her or his own feelings and knowledge "as a colearner in the spirit of inquiry" (1980, p. 58).

Client Participation

The degree of client participation in the educational process directly influences the amount of client learning (Murray & Zentner, 1985). One nurse discovered this principle while working with a group of people nearing retirement. After talking to them about the changes they would face and receiving little response, the nurse shifted to a different method of teaching. Pamphlets were distributed and everyone was asked to read them during the week and come prepared for discussion. This was enough to have the group slowly began to participate in their own learning. Whenever the nurse works with clients in a learning context, one of the first questions to discuss is what does the client want to learn? As Carl Rogers (1969, p. 159) has said:

> Learning is facilitated when the student participates responsibly in the learning process. When he chooses his own directions, helps to discover his own learning resources, formulates his own problems, decides his own course of action, lives with consequences of each of these choices, then significant learning is maximized.

The amount of learning is directly proportional to the learners' involvement. A group of senior citizens attended a class on nutrition and aging, yet still made almost no changes in diet or eating patterns. It was not until the members became actively involved in the class, encouraged by the nurse to present problems and solutions for food purchasing and preparation on limited budgets, that any significant behavioral changes occurred.

Contracting, in which the client participates in the process as a partner to determine goals, content, and time for learning, can contribute to the nurse's teaching goals. Contracting in the context of teaching can develop a great sense of accountability in clients for their own learning. Contracting is discussed in Chapter 13.

Subject's Relevance to Client

Subject matter that is relevant to the client is learned more readily and retained longer than information that is not meaningful. Learners gain the most from subject matter immediately useful to their own purposes. This is particularly true of adult learners who have more life experiences to which to relate learning and tend to see the immediate relevance of material taught (Knowles, 1980).

Consider two middle-management men taking a physical fitness course offered by their employer. One, the father of a boy scout, has agreed to co-lead his son's troop on a two-week backpacking trip in the mountains. He wants to get in shape. The second man is taking the course because it is required by the company. Its only relevance to his own purposes is that it keeps him from gaining his boss's disfavor. There can be little question about which man will learn and retain the most. The course has considerable relevance and meaning to the first man and almost none to the second.

Relevance also influences the speed of learning. Diabetics who must give themselves daily injections of insulin to live learn that skill very quickly (see Fig. 14.1). When clients see considerable relevance in the learning, they accomplish it with great speed. According to Rogers (1969) 65 to 85% of the time alloted for learning various subjects could be deleted if the material was perceived by the learner as related to his or her own purposes. This is seen in the short period of time it takes for families to learn the skills they need to provide home care for a family member in need.

When subject matter is relevant to the learner, there is also greater retention of knowledge. The learner, upon seeing the usefulness of the material, develops a strong motivation to acquire it, use it, and will be less likely to forget it. Even in instances when a previously learned motor skill has not been used for many years, it is often quickly recaptured when it is needed.

Client Satisfaction

Clients must derive satisfaction from learning to maintain motivation and increase self-direction (Redman, 1988). Learners need to feel a sense of steady progress in the learning process. Obstacles, frustrations, and failures along the way discourage and impede learning. Many stroke clients with potential for rehabilitation give up trying to regain speech or move paralyzed limbs because they become too frustrated, discouraged, and dissatisfied. On the other hand, clients who experience satisfaction and progress in their speech and muscle retraining maintain their motivation and work on exercises without prompting. Nurses can promote client satisfaction through support and encouragement.

Realistic goals contribute to learner satisfaction. Objectives should be set within the learner's ability, thereby avoiding the frustration that comes from a too-difficult task and the loss of interest that results from a too-easy one. Setting objectives requires agreement on goals, periodic reviews, and revision of goals if they become too easy or too difficult. Nurses further promote clients' learning satisfaction by designing tasks with rewards. One nurse led a class for obese adolescents, and together they set the goal of a weekly two-pound weight loss. The school nurse helped the group design a plan that included counting calories, measuring fat in their diets, increasing physical activity, and a buddy system as ways to help bring about a behavior change. As members in the group achieved monthly goals, they were encouraged to reward themselves with a pair of earrings, new nail polish, or a special outing as a group. These students found this learning experience satisfying because goals were attainable and their progress was rewarded. Instead of competing with one another, the group set out to help each member achieve the goal. As a result, most kept the weight off after the class had finished.

Client Application

Learning is reinforced through application (Shropshire, 1981). Learners need as many opportunities as possible to apply the learning in daily life. If such opportunities arise during the teaching-learning process, clients can try out new knowledge and skills under supervision. Learners are given an opportunity to begin integrating the learning into their daily lives at a time when the teacher is there to help reinforce that pattern. Take a prenatal class as an example. The learning only begins with explanations of proper diet, exercise, breathing techniques, hygiene, avoidance of alcohol and tobacco, and so on. More learning occurs as the group members discuss these issues and apply them intellectually, exploring ways they could practice them at home. Additional reinforcement comes by demonstrating how to do these activities. Sample diets, demonstrations of exercises, display of posters, pamphlets, or models may be used. The group can begin application in the classroom by making diet plans, exercising, role-playing parenting behavior, or engaging in group problem solving. Then the members can be encouraged to apply these activities on a daily basis at home and prepare to share their results at future sessions.

Frequent use of newly acquired information fosters transfer of learning to other situations. The major goal of prevention and health promotion depends on such a transfer. For instance, mothers who learn and practice a well-balanced diet, free of nonnutritious snacks, can be encouraged to offer more nourishing foods to other family members. A family that practices asepsis and good hand-washing techniques when caring for a post-surgical wound can learn to transfer this same principle to prevention of infection in daily living.

TEACHING PROCESS

The process of teaching in community health nursing follows steps similar to those of the nursing process:

1. Interaction: Establish basic communication patterns between clients and nurse.
2. Assessment and diagnosis: Determine clients' present status and identify clients' need for teaching (keeping in mind that clients should determine their own needs).
3. Setting goals and objectives: Analyze needed changes and prepare objectives that describe the desired learning outcomes.
4. Planning: Design a plan for the learning experience that meets the mutually developed objectives; include the content to be covered, sequence of topics, best conditions for learning (place, kind of environment), methods, and materials (visual aids, exercises, etc.). A written plan is best; it may or may not be part of the written nursing care plan.
5. Teaching: Implement the learning experience by carrying out the planned activities.
6. Evaluation: Determine whether learning objectives were met and if not, why not. Evaluation measures progress toward goals, effectiveness of chosen teaching methods, or future learning needs.

Interaction

Reciprocal communication must take place between the nurse and client. It is essential in the helping rela-

tionship and requisite to effective use of the nursing process. Community health nurses need to develop good questioning techniques and listening skills to determine clients' learning needs and levels of readiness. (See discussion on interaction in Chapter 11.)

Assessment and Diagnosis

Identifying clients' learning needs presents a challenge to the nurse. Too often teaching occurs based on the nurse's assumption of what the learner needs to know. In client education, nurses have a serious responsibility to tailor teaching to clients' real and perceived needs. Knowles (1980; 1984) describes educational needs as gaps between what people know and what they need to know to function effectively. He goes on to say that the potential learners, the sponsoring organization, and the community may all help determine the needs to be addressed in the teaching-learning situation.

Assessing educational needs may be accomplished in several ways. The nurse can use surveys, interviews, open forums, or task forces that include representative clients as members. The important principle to remember is that clients should be involved in identifying what they want to learn. When a "need" to learn something, such as the importance of getting children immunized, is identified by the nurse rather than clients, then the nurse may need to "sell" clients on the importance of the topic. Nurses need to use approaches that assist clients toward their own awareness of the need.

Setting Goals and Objectives

Once a need has been clearly identified, then nurse and clients can establish mutually agreed-upon goals and objectives. Goals are broad statements of intent, and objectives are more specific descriptions of intended outcome (Mager, 1975). Sometimes in a teaching situation a goal may be stated as short term goals and long term goals. For example, the nurse may have identified a group's need to stop smoking. The need and teaching goals might be stated thus:

Need

A group of smokers wish to stop their addiction to nicotine.

Short Term Goal

All members of the group will stop smoking within one month.

Long Term Goal

90% of the group members will remain tobacco free for six months.

Objectives should be stated in measurable behavioral terms, using a grammatical structure that contains a subject, verb, condition/criteria and a time frame. That is, each objective should include a single idea that describes an outcome that can be measured within a certain timeframe. To accomplish the short- and long-term goals of smoking cessation, educational objectives are developed from the levels of cognitive learning covered earlier in this chapter. Each behavioral objective is stated in measurable terms and includes a verb that coincides with one of the six levels within the cognitive domain. Objectives might appear like this:

At the end of the program all clients should be able to:

1. *List* three reasons why smoking is unhealthy.
2. *Identify* at least two factors that have influenced their smoking habit.
3. *Apply* a series of action steps that will lead to smoking cessation within one month.
4. *Examine* the steps as they contribute to living tobacco free.
5. *Design* a way to live a fulfilled tobacco free life.
6. *Evaluate* success in remaining tobacco free for six months.

Each of the above objectives, (1) refer to a subject, (2) can be readily measured because each describes a specific outcome, condition, criteria, or expected behaviors, (3) uses a verb for stating cognitive outcomes, and (4)includes a specific timeframe. Well-written objectives meet these four criteria and greatly enhance evaluating the success of the educational effort.

Planning

Teaching preparation can be done formally or informally. Generally, it is best to have a written plan when teaching groups than include: (1) subject, (2) intended audience, (3) date(s), time, and place, (4) short and long term goal statements, (5) teaching-learning methods, (6) activities and assignments, (7) course outline of topics, and (8) evaluation method and criteria.

Teaching

The class or workshop should be conducted according to the plan prepared above. Using a variety of teaching methods addresses unique needs of the learners and makes the teaching more interesting. Include and combine such methods as lectures, discussions, role playing, demonstrations, and videos (see teaching methods and materials discussed later in this chapter).

If necessary, make assignments such as readings, presentations, journals, practice experiences, or return demonstrations designed to reinforce and synthesize the learning. The teaching methods used and activities selected are important parts of the teaching plan. The nurse will find that a well-designed plan will greatly enhance the smoothness and effectiveness of the actual teaching situation; problems in teaching can often be related back to a poorly developed plan.

Evaluation

This final step is a critical one in the teaching-learning process. At this point the nurse determines whether the goals and objectives for the educational experience have been met, and if not, why not. Clear, measurable objectives will facilitate evaluation. For example, to measure the third objective in the stop-smoking program previously noted, "Apply a series of action steps that will lead to smoking cessation within one month," the nurse may ask group members to share the steps they will employ and then have a group discussion about the ideas shared. To measure the fifth objective, "evaluate success in remaining tobacco free for six months" would require follow-up contacts and relying on self-reporting. Sussman et al (1993) found upon evaluation, that a combined intervention of refusal skills, and awareness of social misperceptions was the most effective in reducing tobacco use in a school-based prevention project with teens. Each intervention alone was not effective. A well-developed evaluation component revealed this important finding. According to Tyler (1949, p.106), "evaluation is the process for determining the degree to which changes in behavior are actually taking place."

If objectives have not been met, or have been met only partially, this too requires attention. The nurse should explore this outcome with the clients to determine what hindered their success and what action, if any, might be helpful. Partially met objectives gives the nurse a place to begin with the group at follow-up sessions and should not be considered a failure. See the Issues in Community Health Nursing display below.

TEACHING METHODS AND MATERIALS

Teaching occurs on many levels and incorporates various types of activities. It can be formal or informal, planned or unplanned. Formal presentations, such as lectures with groups, are generally planned and fairly structured. Some teaching is less formal but still planned and relatively structured, as in group discussions in which questions stimulate exploration of ideas and guide thinking. Informal levels of teaching, such as counseling or **anticipatory guidance** (the client is assisted in preparing for a future role or developmental stage), require the teacher to be prepared but no defined plan of presentation. All nurses use one or a combination of methods and a variety of materials to facilitate the teaching-learning process. It is important, however, for nurses to expand their repertoire of teaching methods and not rely on one or two methods. Generating a

variety of teaching methods stimulates creative thinking (Seigal, 1991). Nurses use knowledge from physiology, pathology, sociology, and psychology in their practice and when teaching, nurses can benefit from using concepts, principles and teaching methods from education, especially adult education (Gessner, 1989). This chapter will close by discussing four commonly used teaching methods (lecture, discussion, demonstration, and role playing), teaching materials for enhancing learning and how to more effectively teach the "hard to help" client.

Lecture

There are times when the community health nurse will present information to a large group, such as a local PTA, a women's club, or a county board of commissioners. Under such circumstances, the lecture method, a formal kind of presentation, may be the most efficient means of communicating general health information. However, lecturers tend to create a passive learning environment for the audience unless strategies are devised to involve the learners. Many individuals are visual rather than auditory learners. To capture their attention, slides, overhead projections, or videotapes can supplement the lecture. Allowing time for questions and discussion after a lecture will also involve the learners more actively. This method is best used with adults but even they have a limited attention span and a break at least midway through a presentation longer than one hour will be much appreciated. Distributing printed material that highlights and summarizes the content shared, or supplements it, will also help to reinforce important points.

Discussion

Two-way communication is an important feature of the learning process. Learners need an opportunity to raise questions, make comments, reason out loud, and receive feedback in order to develop understanding. When discussion is used in conjunction with other teaching methods such as demonstration, lecture, and role playing, it will improve their effectiveness. In group teaching, discussion enables clients to learn from one another as well as from the nurse. The nurse must exercise leadership in controlling and guiding the discussion so that learning opportunities are maximized and objectives are met. Discussion organized around specific questions or topics make the discussion most fruitful (Bavaro, 1980).

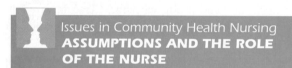

Issues in Community Health Nursing
ASSUMPTIONS AND THE ROLE OF THE NURSE

A nurse was visiting a family in a section of town with many families from Mexico. This family had olive skin, dark hair and eyes and had a Spanish surname. The nurse assumed they were from Mexico, especially when a heavy accent colored the halting English. They were asked if they spoke Spanish and the nurse was baffled when they promptly replyed, "oh no!." Nevertheless, the visit continued hesitantly in English. It was on the third visit that the nurse quite accidently found out that the family was from the Philippines and spoke Tagalog. The family had four grown sons who eventually helped their parents achieving the home visit goals. Much time was lost, however, because the nurse assumed, and thus did not ask where the family was from. The nurse could then have drawn upon the expertise of appropriate other family or community members earlier. Most certainly the nurse should have asked the family their native language.

Demonstration

The demonstration method is often used for teaching psychomotor skills and is best accompanied by explanation and discussion with time set aside for return demonstration by the client or caregiver. It can give clients a clear sensory image of how to perform the skill. Because a demonstration should be within easy visual and auditory range of learners, it is best to demonstrate in front of small groups or one-to-one. Use the same kind of equipment that clients will use in order to show exactly how the skill should be performed, and provide learners with ample opportunity to practice until the skill is perfected.

This is an ideal method to use in the client's home as well as in groups. The actual materials and supplies that the client will be using when the nurse is not there should be used. This might be the time when the nurse uses improvising skills. Helping families figure out ways to accomplish goals with materials found at home often becomes the hallmark of an experienced community health nurse. The new mother learns how to bathe her baby safely in the kitchen sink. The nurse assists several low income parents in using household items to make inexpensive toys (mobiles from coat hangers, string, and pictures from a magazine or bean bags using dry beans and scraps of material). The husband learns how to change dressings over his wife's central line site using sterile technique while conserving supplies that he has to buy on a fixed income. Each activity takes a different type of psychomotor skill and ingenuity on the part of the nurse (See Fig. 14.2).

Role Playing

There are times when having clients assume and act out roles maximizes learning (Wise, 1980). A parenting group, for example, found it helpful to place themselves in the role of their children; their feelings about various ways to respond became more apparent. Reversing roles can effectively teach spouses in conflict about better ways to communicate. In order to prevent role playing from becoming a game with little learning, plan the proposed drama with clear objectives in mind. What behavioral outcomes do you hope to achieve? Define the context, the "stage," clearly so that everyone shares in the situation. Then define each role ahead of time, making sure everyone understands his or her performance. Emphasize that no wrong or right performance exists, and that participants should merely behave the way people behave in everyday life. Avoid having people

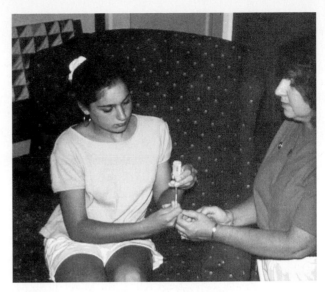

FIGURE 14.2. An adolescent with diabetes readily learns injection technique.

play themselves; it can embarrass them and make it difficult for them to achieve objectivity. After the drama has concluded, elicit discussion with carefully prepared questions. This technique can be used with staff, co-workers, young children and teens, as well as adults. However, this technique can be a risk-taking experience for people and they may be reluctant to particpate. The nurse needs to use judgement, begin with volunteers, and not push this technique on unwilling or nonreceptive people. Build up to full participation.

Teaching Materials

Many different kinds of teaching materials are available to the nurse. They are often used in combination and are useful during the teaching process. Visual images—pictures, slides, posters, chalkboards, videotapes, bulletin boards, flash cards, pamphlets, flyers, charts, and even gestures—can enhance almost any learning. Some tools such as tapes and compact discs provide an auditory stimulus. Americans readily learn from television; it appeals to sight and sound and grabs attention. Education via television can be more effective and efficient than traditonal teaching methods (Schoenbeck, 1992). There are many programs on educational television channels and network channels that can be recommended by the nurse. Other tools, such as anatomical models, improvised or purchased equipment, allow clients both visual and tactile learning. Still others, such as interactive computer games, or instruction, actively involve learners.

The choice of teaching materials varies with clients' interests, abilities and depending on what resources are available. Teaching often occurs in casual conversations, spontaneously in situations in which clients raise unexpected questions, or when a crisis arises. In these instances, nurses draw on their background of knowledge and exercise professional judgment in their selection of content, methods, and materials.

There are several different types of printed educational support materials available. Pamphlets, brochures, booklets, flyers, and informations sheets are but a few. Each should be evaluated for its appropriateness and effectiveness with particular individuals, families, or groups. Many come from state and local official sources. Others come from nonprofit national agencies such as the American Diabetes Association, the March of Dimes, and the American Heart Association. Materials from these sources can be acquired in large numbers free or at a nominal cost to the agency. Major manufacturers of infant formulas, foods, diapers, and toys are good sources for literature on growth and development, safety, and caring for infants and children. Pharmaceutical companies develop educational material for the public along with the manufacturers of in-home supplies and equipment. Usually these are excellent sources of information for families or groups, however, the nurse needs to assess the material for appropriateness. Factors to be considered include the material's content, complexity, reading level, and cultural sensitivity (Anderson, 1993; American Red Cross, 1985). At times the commercial message in the literature outweighs the educational impact making it not useful or confusing to the client.

Finally, nurses teach by example. Actions usually speak louder than words. If a nurse teaches the importance of washing hands to reduce disease transmission and then begins a dressing change without hand washing, the message of observed actions will carry more impact than the words. Nurses who exhibit healthy practices use themselves as tools and serve as role models as well as health teachers.

The "Hard to Help" Client

At times the nurse will experience a challenging teaching situation with an individual, a family, or a group. The difficulties may involve cultural or language differences, distracting personality characteristics, or demonstrations of stress or emotions. Regardless of the situation the nurse will feel most comfortable and confident if prepared to deal with these situations before experiencing them.

Before beginning to teach a client, family, or aggregate, thorough preparation is of utmost importance for successful learning. This includes finding out if teaching in English is possible or if any other modifications will need to be made as the teaching plan is being developed. Nurses should never assume anything, including the primary language spoken by clients, their visual or hearing ability, or capacity to understand. When teaching unfamiliar groups, a center manager, or program director can give information regarding the interests and abilities of the members. These human resources are invaluable in planning any teaching where English may be a second language or where other barriers exist that may impede success if they are not known by the nurse. The phases of the nursing process continue to guide the nurse as a teacher.

Another difficulty that can arise is unexpected behavior from a client which affects the group process in a variety of ways. The client may monopolize the discussion, answer questions asked of others, burst out with personal experiences that have no relevance to the topic, become irate by the comments of others, sit silently and never speak, or any other possible form of behavior that could become disruptive. This can be unnerving to even the most experienced nurse. Any behavior that has the potential to distract the other learners needs to be diffused by the nurse. This is accomplished caringly by giving the recognition the person is seeking, while also setting limits (see Chapter 10 for specific strategies for handling the uncooperative or disruptive client in groups).

Summary

A large part of community health nursing practice involves teaching. Far more than simply giving health information to clients, the purpose of teaching is to change client behavior to healthier practices. When these practices are internalized and implemented regularly, years of morbidity and premature mortality can be avoided, contributing to the quality and length of the human lifespan.

Understanding the nature of learning contributes to the effectiveness of teaching in community health. Learning occurs in three domains: cognitive, affective, and psychomotor. The cognitive domain refers to learning that takes place intellectually. It ranges in levels of learner functioning from simple recall to complex evaluation. As learners move up the scale of cognitive learning, they become more self-directed; the nurse assumes a more facilitative role.

Affective learning involves the changing of attitudes and values. Learners may experience several levels of affective involvement from simple listening to adopting the new value. Again, as the client increases involvement, the nurse becomes less directive.

Psychomotor learning involves the acquisition of motor skills. Clients who learn psychomotor skills must meet three conditions: they must be capable of the skill; they must develop a sensory image of the skill; and they must practice the skill.

Learning theories can be grouped into three broad categories: (1) behavioristic theories, views learning as a behavioral change through stimulus-response or conditioning, (2) cognitive learning theories which seek to influence learners' understanding of problems and situations through promoting their insights, and (3) humanistic theories which assume that there is a natural tendency for people to learn and that learning flourishes in an encouraging environment.

Teaching in community health nursing is the facilitation of learning that leads to behavioral change in the client. Ideally this is done at the primary level of prevention. However, much of the nurse's work is done at the secondary and teritary level. The nurse uses several teaching-learning principles which can facilitate the learning process, such as clients' readiness for learning, clients' perceptions, learners' physical and emotional comfort within an educational setting, degree of client participation, relevant subject matter, allowing clients to derive satisfaction from learning, and reinforcing learning through application.

The teaching process in community health nursing is similar to the nursing process including steps of interaction, assessment and diagnosis, goal setting, planning, teaching, and evaluation. The actual teaching may be formal or informal, planned or unplanned and methods may range from structured lecture presentations to demonstration and role playing. Selection of teaching materials depends on how well they suit learners and helps to meet the desired objectives. Sources of teaching materials that are free or inexpensive can enhance the nurses' teaching but need to be evaluated for effectiveness. The nurse needs to know how to help the "hard to help" client such as those from a different culture or who speak a different language, those who monopolize the discussion, become emotional, or even hostile. The nurse must be prepared for each situa-tion in order to teach the individual, family, or group effectively.

Activities to Promote Critical Thinking

1. What learning theory or theories discussed in this chapter most closely reflect your own position? How would you apply it or them in your practice.

2. A children's day-care center is located in your service area. What populations in this setting could be potential recipients of health teaching? How would you assess each group's learning needs?

3. Your city governmental officials often makes decisions that appear to reflect a lack of knowledge regarding health and health care. How might you "educate" them using the concepts and principles described in this chapter?

4. Discuss the differences between cognitive, affective, and psychomotor learning. Why do cognitive and affective learning need to be linked in health teaching?

5. Explore the possible use of role models as teaching tools for community health nursing practice. What examples exist in your community? What new ones might you develop?

6. You are teaching an aggregate of middle aged women about menapause. One woman monopolizes the class time by telling stories and talking negatively about her husband. The other women are getting upset with her. What would you do?

REFERENCES

Anderson, J. & Yuhos, R. (1993). Health promotion in rural settings: A nursing challenge. *Nursing Clinics of North America, 28*(1), 145–155.

American Red Cross. (1985). *Instructor Specialist Manual, Nursing and Health Services.*

Bavaro, J. A. (1980). Questioning: The key to learning. *Supervisor Nurse, 11*(6), 26.

Bigge, M. L. (1982). *Learning theories for teachers* (4th ed.). New York: Harper.

Bloom, B. (Ed.). (1956). *Taxonomy of educational objectives: The classification of educational goals. Handbook I: Cognitive domain.* New York: Longman.

Douglass, L. M. & Bevis, E.O. (1974). *Nursing leadership in action: Principles and application to staff situations.* St. Louis: C. V. Mosby.

Eisner, E.W. (1985). *The educational imagination* (2nd. ed.). New York: MacMillan.

Gessner, B.A. (1989). Adult education, The cornerstone of patient teaching. *Nursing Clinics of North America, 24*(3), 589–593.

Gronlund, N. E. (1970). *Stating behavioral objectives for classroom instruction.* New York: Macmillan.

Hergenhahn, B. R. (1982). *An introduction to theories of learning* (2nd ed.). Englewood Cliffs, NJ: Prentice-Hall.

Johnson, E.A. & Jackson, J.E. (1989) Teaching the home care client. *Nursing Clinics of North America, 24*(3), 687–693.

Knowles, M. (1980). *The modern practice of adult education: Androgogy versus pedagogy* (2nd ed.). Chicago: Follett.

Knowles, M. (1984). *The adult learner: A neglected species* (3rd ed.). Houston: Gulf Publishing.

Levin, L. S. (1978). Patient education and self-care: How do they differ? *Nursing Outlook, 26,* 170–75.

Lorig, K. (1992). *Patient education: A practical approach.* St. Louis: Mosby Year Book

Lorig, K. (1985). Health education: Beyond health teaching. In S. Archer and R. Fleshman (Eds.), *Community health nursing* (3rd ed.). Monterey, CA: Wadsworth.

Mager, R. F. (1975). *Preparing instructional objectives* (2nd ed.). Belmont, CA: Pitman Learning.

Marriner, A. (1979). Health teaching. In A. Marriner (Ed.), *The nursing process* (2nd ed.). St. Louis: Mosby.

Maslow, A.H. (1970). *Motivation and personality* (2nd.ed.). New York: Harper and Row.

Miller, A. (1985). When is the time ripe for teaching? *American Journal of Nursing, 85*(7), 801.

Murray, R. & Zentner, J. (1985). *Nursing concepts for health promotion* (3rd ed.). Englewood Cliffs, NJ: Prentice-Hall.

Nobel, C. (1991). Are nurses good patient educators? *Journal of Advanced Nursing, 16,* 1185–1189.

Piaget, J. (1966). *The origin of intelligence in children.* New York: Norton.

Redman, B.K. (1988). *The process of patient teaching in nursing* (6th ed.). St. Louis: Mosby.

Rogers, C. (1969). Freedom to learn. Columbus, Ohio: Merrill Publishing Co.

Rogers, C. (1989). *Freedom to learn for the eighties.* Columbus, OH: Merrill Publishing Co.

Schoenbeck, S.B. (1992). Teaching the nurse to teach with health information videos. *Journal of Nursing Staff Development, 8*(2), 66–71.

Seigal, H. (1991). Innovative approaches to inservice education. *Journal of Continuing Education in Nursing, 22,* 147–151.

Shropshire, C. D. (1981). Group experiential learning in adult education. *Journal of Continuing Education in Nursing, 12*(6), 5.

Sprinthall, N.A. & Sprinthall, R.C. (1990) *Educational psychology: A developmental approach* (5th ed.). New York: McGraw Hill.

Sussman, S., Dent, C.W., Stacy, A.W., et al. (1993). Project towards no tobacco use: 1-year behavior outcomes. *American Journal of Public Health, 83*(9), 1245–1250.

Tyler, R.W. (1949). *Basic principles of curriculum and instruction.* Chicago: University of Chicago Press.

Wise, P. (1980). Methods of teaching—revisited. Character play and role play. *Journal of Continuing Education in Nursing, 11*(1), 37.

SELECTED READINGS

Bethea, C., Stallings, S., Wolman, P., & Ingram, R. (1989). Comparison of conventional and videotaped diabetes exchange list instructions. *Journal of the American Dietetic Association, 89*(3), 405–406.

Bortz, W.M., II. (1991). *We live too short and die too long.* New York: Bantum Books.

Burnard,P. (1992). *Counselling: a guide to practice in nursing.* Oxford:Butterworth-Heinemann Ltd.

Cummings, K. M., Sciandr, R., & Markello, S. (1987). Impact of a newspaper-mediated quit smoking program. *American Journal of Public Health, 77*(11), 1452–53.

Dachs,R.J., Garb, J.L., White, C., et al. (1989). Male college students' compliance with testicular self-examination. *Journal of Adolescent Health Care, 10,* 295–299.

Dailey, C. (1985). Teaching parents and children preventive health behaviors. *Family and Community Health,* (7), 34–43

Falvo, D.R. (1994). Effective patient education: A guide to increased compliance. (2nd ed.). Gaithersburg, MD: Aspen.

Flay, B. R.(1987). Mass media and smoking cessation: A critical review. *American Journal of Public Health, 77*(2), 153–60.

Fleming, V.E.M. (1992). Client education: A futuristic outlook. *Journal of Advanced Nursing, 17,* 158–163.

Freire, P. & Shor, I.(1987) *A pedagogy for liberation. Dialogues on transforming education.* Basingstoke, Hampshire: MacMillan Education.

Gagliano,M.(1989).A literature review on the efficacy of video in patient education. *Journal of Medical Education, 63,* 785–792.

Goldenging,J.M.(1992). Testicular self-exam: A lifesaver. *Patient Care, 26*(17), 62–76.

Gould, J.E. & Bevis, E.O.(1992). Here there be dragons: Departing the behaviorist paradigm for state board regulation. *Nursing and Health Care, 3*(3), 126–133.

Jackson,J. & Johnson, E. (1988). *Patient education in home care.* Rockville, MD: Aspen.

Jewell, M.L. (1994) Partnership in learing: Education as liberation. *Nursing and Health Care, 15*(7), 360–364.

Job, R.F.S. (1988). Effective and ineffective use of fear in health promotion campaigns. *American Journal of Public Health 78*(2), 163–67.

Kick, E. (1989). Patient teaching for elders. *Nursing Clinics of North America, 24*(3), 681–686.

Knowles, M. (1975). *Self-directed learning: A guide for learners and teachers.* New York: Associated Press.

Lewin, K. (1951). *Field theory in social science.* New York: Harper Publishing Co.

Luker, K. & Caress, A.L. (1989). Rethinking patient education. *Journal of Advanced Nursing, 14*, 711–718.

Macleod Clark, J., Haverty, S., & Kendall, S. (1990). Helping people to stop smoking: A study of the nurse's role. *Journal of Advanced Nursing, 16*, 357–363.

Miller, A. (1985). When is the time ripe for teaching? *American Journal of Nursing, 85*(7), 801.

O'Donnell, L.N., San Doval, A., Duran, R. & O'Donnell, C. (1995). Video-based sexually transmitted disease patient education: Its impact on condom acquisition. *American Journal of Public Health 85*(6):817–822.

Pender, N. (1987). *Health promotion in nursing practice.* Norwalk, CT: Appleton and Lange.

Rankin, S. & Stallings, K. (1990). *Patient education: Issues, principles, practices.* Philadelphia: Lippincott.

Richardson, S. & Petrarca, D. (1990) Educating nurses in health promotion. *Journal of Nursing Education, 29*, 351–354.

Schonfeld, D.J., O'Hare, L.L., Perrin, E.C., Quackenbush, M., Showalter, D.R., & Cicchetti, D.V. (1995). A randomized, controlled trial of a school-based, multi-faceted AIDS education program in the elementary grades: The impact on comprehension, knowledge and fears. *Pediatrics 95*(4): 450–486.

Sheridan-Leos, N. (1995). Women's Health Lotería: A new cervical cancer education tool for Hispanic females. *ONF 22*(4):697–700.

Tanner, G. (1989). A need to know. *Nursing Times, 85*(31),54–56.

Timmreck, T. C., et al. (1987). The health education and health promotion movement: A theoretical jungle. *Health Education, 18*(5), 24–28.

Tones, B. K. (1986). Health education and the ideology of health promotion: A review of alternative approaches. *Health Education Research, 1*(1), 3–12.

Tuazon,N.C.(1992) Taking Charge. Discharge teaching: Use this MODEL. *RN, 55*(4) 19–20,22.

Warner, K. E. (1987). Television and health education: Stay tuned. *American Journal of Public Health, 77*(2), 140–42.

15

Community Crisis: Prevention and Intervention

LEARNING OBJECTIVES

Upon completion of this chapter, readers should be able to:

- Define crisis.
- Describe the phases of a crisis.
- Explain the difference between developmental crisis and situational crisis and give several examples of each.
- Plan strategies to prevent situational crisis and developmental crisis at each level of prevention.
- Describe the role of a community health nurse in crisis intervention during each phase of the crisis.

KEY TERMS

- Bargaining
- Coping
- Crisis
- Crisis theory

- Developmental crisis
- Post-crisis phase
- Pre-crisis phase
- Situational crisis

Barbara Walton Spradley and Judith Ann Allender
COMMUNITY HEALTH NURSING: CONCEPTS AND PRACTICE, 4th ed.
© 1996 Barbara Walton Spradley and Judith Ann Allender

All human beings, individually and collectively, experience periods of crisis. Some are personal family events: a teenager discovers she is pregnant; a father and sole breadwinner in a family loses his job; a worker faces retirement. Others are larger in scope and more random, such as a drive-by shooting which kills a child, or a community devastated by a fire which causes several deaths and millions of dollars in property damage. A flood can damage, even destroy, homes and farms for miles along a major river. An accident at a nuclear power plant threatens the lives and health of a community. These events have the potential to affect many people, producing stress and anxiety. Each requires varying periods of time for adjusting and coping by those directly or indirectly affected. Each event results in changes to a person's behavior.

A **crisis** is a stressful and disruptive event that comes with or without warning and disturbs the equilibrium or balance of a person, group, or community. People respond to crises differently. Some approach them as a challenge, an event to be reckoned with; others are overwhelmed and feel defeated or give up. Some seek help if needed and come through the experience unscathed, perhaps even stronger than before. Others who are unable to cope with the crisis may suffer severe, sometimes permanent, damage.

Regardless of their responses, people in crisis need help. Yet, not all people realize they are in need of help. For example, an older woman is barely surviving on her limited income, cannot afford enough food to eat adequately, and must ration medications to last each month rather than taking the proper prescribed dose. This woman may be so accustomed to this way of life that she does not view it as a crisis-in-the-making and may not seek help. But her situation is a potential crisis; this woman is at risk of becoming seriously ill because of malnutrition or improper use of medication.

On the other hand, if the crisis is disruptive enough to life, safety, and security, for instance, a natural disaster (earthquake, flood, tornado) or a major illness, people may react in more predictable ways and seek help. Community health practitioners have a unique opportunity to provide assistance to clients in a broad variety of situations. Not only can they provide direct assistance during times of crisis, more importantly, they can help prepare people by teaching the tools needed for crisis management and prevention. In particular, community health nurses are concerned about crises or potential crises that affect groups or aggregates. For example, when floods inundated the Midwest in the summers of 1993 and 1994, and parts of California in the winter of 1995, they provoked a crisis for families, groups, communities—indeed, society as a whole. With these floods came the loss of homes, farmland, crops, and a multiplicity of related jobs affecting agricultural production and the economy of the nation. Some of a community health nurse's major professional challenges are to prevent crises and to help people during a crisis. This chapter examines how nurses can sharpen their knowledge and skills in the practice of crisis prevention and intervention in order to promote the health of the community.

Crisis Theory

Our understanding about crises has grown considerably. At one time, crisis was equated only with disaster; it might have been a natural disaster such as a hurricane, an economic disaster such as a recession, a political disaster such as a presidential assassination, an environmental disaster such as water polluted with hazardous chemicals, or a personal disaster such as the death of a loved one. But today it is known that any event that has the potential to disrupt the dynamic equilibrium between a person and the environment can be considered a crisis. A crisis can also result when problem-solving methods fail. Researchers have studied the nature of crisis and have developed a body of knowledge called **crisis theory**. Initially limited to the field of mental health, crisis theory now influences every field of health care (Lawler & Yount, 1987). It is recognized, for example, that a crisis is not an event per se, but rather a person's perception of the event, and there are different kinds of crises that can occur. Crisis theory helps explain why people respond in certain ways to a crisis and explains predictable phases that people go through in a crisis of any kind. These are important ideas for the community health nurse to understand before crises can be prevented or managed.

Dynamics and Characteristics of a Crisis

How does a crisis occur? People as dynamic and living systems behave in certain ways. How people behave and react is generally unconscious and gauged to maintain a balance within themselves and in their relations with others. When some internal or external force disrupts the system's balance and alters its functioning, loss of equilibrium occurs. A person will attempt to restore equilibrium by using whatever resources they have available to them, in an effort to cope with the situation. **Coping** refers to the actions and ways of thinking that assist people in dealing with and surviving difficult situations. Coping and problem-solving behaviors become habitual through repeated use, even if they are not always successful.

There are five key characteristics of crises (France, 1989). Crises are *precipitated* by specific identifiable events that become too much for the usual problem-solving skills of those involved. Often, a single distressing event follows a host of previous difficulties and becomes the "straw that broke the camel's back." For example, a wife who suffers years of spousal abuse finally becomes unable to cope and shoots her husband during a violent attack. Occasionally single tragic and distressing events occur suddenly without previous stressors—a father is killed in a plane crash or, as another example, four teenagers working late one evening in a fast food restaurant who are shot and killed.

Crises are *normal* in that all people feel overwhelmed occasionally. It is very possible that a person who intervenes in today's crisis will be tomorrow's crisis victim. No individual or group is immune from sudden overwhelming difficulties. For example, the community health nurse assists families through crisis states as part of his/her job. But, suddenly the nurse learns that community rezoning for a highway makes it necessary to move his/her own family.

Crises are *personal* in that each person reacts in their own individual way. A situation that throws one person off course may merely create an interesting detour for another (see the Case Study, Two Families' Reaction to Crisis). It is the individual's perception and interpretation of the event, rather than the event itself, that is crucial. The same principle applies to an aggregate or community. One community welcomes the newly proposed prison on the outskirts of town, viewing it as a source of new jobs, revenue, and growth. Another community may protest, perceiving that the prison will increase crime, hinder tourism, and not be a desirable addition to their community.

Crises are *resolved,* either positively or negatively, within a brief period of time. Crisis is a temporary condition too intense to last long or become chronic. In the family of the wife who shot her abusive husband, as shocking as the event might seem, life returns to a recognizable pattern in a few weeks. Although the members will feel the change for years, the crisis will soon disappear. The wife's case goes to trial, followed by a prison term; the children stay with relatives and attend school. People's strong need to regain homeostasis or balance means that the disequilibrium of a crisis cannot continue indefinitely. Most crises last from four to six weeks (Aguilera, 1993). Refer to the case study that follows.

CASE STUDY

TWO FAMILIES' RESPONSE TO CRISIS

The Rallys and the Fosters will be moving to a town in another state, 900 miles away, because of a job change. The Rallys are in crisis over the move. They have never lived in any other town. They will have to leave relatives and lifelong friends who live near by and a community in which they have been very involved. Mrs. Rally is the secretary at her family's church. Their teenage daughter, a cheerleader, just started high school. Their son is in kindergarten; Grandma happily watches him in the mornings before school. Everyone is upset because of how the move will affect them. The family is stressed and argues each evening. They don't want to put their house up for sale or even to visit the new community to which they will be moving. Mr. Rally is second guessing his decision to move, but his choices were limited as his company is relocating. The Rallys, in crisis, are not exploring alternatives that may allow them to stay in their present community. One possible alternative might be for Mrs. Rally to work while Mr. Rally looks for another job. When people perceive they are in crisis, decision making and solving problems becomes more difficult.

The Fosters, however, are excitedly looking forward to their move. They have two young children who are not yet in school. The move will bring them only 50 miles from old college friends. They hope to realize a significant profit on their house which they recently remodeled. They can't wait to go "house hunting" in the new town. Everyone is enjoying planning the anticipated move; their two children, aged three and four, have been playing "moving day" with their favorite toys.

Both families are experiencing the same event. The difference is each person's perception of the event. The Rallys' equilibrium is being disrupted. They have not developed previous coping skills and do not see the move as a positive experience. They are at a different time in their family life cycle than are the Fosters. For the Fosters, although the move upsets their equilibrium, too, it is experienced as an exciting event that conjures positive feelings; they are passing these feelings on to their children. They see this move as an opportunity.

Crisis resolution can be an *adaptive* process in which growth and improved health occur or it can be *maladaptive* resulting in illness or even death. The battered wife reevaluates her life, gets divorced, learns employment skills in jail, becomes more assertive with stronger self-esteem, pays her debt to society, and returns to her children able to support them financially and emotionally when she is paroled. She finds growth and health while successfully resolving the crisis. The children settle into their aunt's home with minimal difficulty, start a new school, and visit their mother and father regularly. When their mother is released, she finds an apartment near her sister's home so the children can continue in the same school district. The husband recovers from his wounds, gets counseling, relocates to another town, and sees his children frequently. This crisis situation was resolved at a higher level of wellness for all members than existed before the crisis. In this example, the members were determined to improve their situation by working with skilled health care professionals. By using the resources within the community, this family is healthier after their crisis.

Phases of a Crisis

Regardless of the kind of crisis, it has been observed that people follow a fairly predictable pattern when reacting to crisis situations as they seek to regain balance or normalcy. Several authors define steps or phases of crisis resolution that correspond to Kubler-Ross' stages of dying: shock, denial, anger, bargaining, and acceptance (Kubler-Ross, 1969). However, an important phase is missing from these models—the pre-crisis phase.

PRE-CRISIS PHASE

The **pre-crisis phase** is the time before a potentially unhealthy situation reaches a crisis or before a crisis occurs. For an event to have potential for crisis, the individual must perceive the alteration to be a problem. This is an important concept for the community health nurse to be aware of when planning teaching during the pre-crisis phase. For nurses this is an extremely important period because they can intervene before the crisis, at the primary prevention level.

It is important to recognize how people respond at the pre-crisis phase as well as the other phases. For example, a family living in an earthquake zone would perceive their situation and risk depending upon the frequency with which they have personally experienced earthquakes and the damage they have seen near their neighborhood. In another example several families refuse to leave their homes in low lying areas after the community is warned of continued rain and a rising river. The families perceive that they are not at risk and don't prepare. If people do not perceive their situation as risky, they probably will not welcome or respond to teaching on the subject initially. In another example, however, parents of pre-teen children who are friends with parents having trouble with their teenagers may be more likely to welcome anticipatory guidance to prevent problems later. They perceive this as a potential crisis. At this pre-crisis phase, the receptiveness to teaching is only as great as the individual or group perceives that this may be a *real* situation for them. These concepts are depicted in Table 15.1.

CRISIS PHASE

During the crisis phase, acute emotional upset arises from situational, developmental, or social sources, which results in a temporary inability to cope (Hoff, 1989). A person, family, or aggregate in crisis is at a turning point; there is the potential for either heightened maturity and growth or for deterioration and greater vulnerability to future stress (Caplan, 1964). Variables that determine the reaction to a crisis include the following: (1) severity of the event precipitating the crisis, (2) resources of the individual, family, or aggregate, and (3) social or community resources available (Johnson & Mattson, 1992).

Early Crisis Phase

The shock, or impact, occurs when clients first encounter the crisis situation. This phase can last a few moments, hours, or sometimes days during which people first react to a crisis. It is primarily an emotional reaction. Feelings of shock and disbelief are expressed. The client is thinking or saying, "This cannot be happening to me." The impact of the shock may leave some feeling numb or indifferent, unable to *do* anything. Then a period of realization follows when panic sets in with feelings of distress, anxiety, and helplessness. Perception of reality becomes clouded, and it becomes difficult to think logically, understand the situation, or

TABLE 15.1. **Phases of Crisis**

	Pre-crisis	Crisis	Post-crisis
Duration	Years-seconds	Seconds-hours	Hours-months
Perception	Unaware, infalable	Clear, then clouded, avoidence, depression	Gradually faces reality
Emotional Response	"It won't happen to me"	"Not me!" "What, me!" "Why me!" "Woe is me!"	"Yes me" "I'll be OK"
Cognitive ability	Norm for client	Unable to comprehend situation disorganized, rigid, resistant to change	Reorganized effective reconstruction
Behavior	Norm for client	Numb, anxious, helpless, overwhelmed, disoriented, unable to cope, fight or flight	Decreasing anxiety, more optimistic, reoriented, purposeful, mastery and stabilizing efforts

make plans. Sometimes clients respond by performing some unimportant or routine task that seems inappropriate to the situation. For example, clients might explain, "While I was waiting for the rescue squad after my son fell, I made the bed. I didn't want the paramedics to find the bed unmade," or "When the policeman asked me my daughter's name I couldn't think of it—nothing would come out of my mouth."

During this early crisis phase, clients may try usual problem-solving means, but without success. Self-esteem is threatened, and behavior is disorganized and disoriented. Clients at this point are usually receptive to suggestions and assistance, which sometimes makes them vulnerable to being exploited by others. This is not the time to settle insurance claims or make other legal decisions that have long-term ramifications. The community health nurse has an important role as a client advocate during this phase.

Late Crisis Phase

During the late crisis phase, clients begin to use coping strategies such as defensive mechanisms of retreat, denial, anger, and bargaining. Their chief efforts are aimed at reducing the stress and tension of the moment. How someone reacts to a crisis often depends on their previous experiences and problem-solving techniques in crisis situations. At first, they may directly confront the problem with previously effective strategies. They may react by saying, "This is tough, but we've handled this before and we can do it again." However, the stress remains until the situation is successfully resolved. Attempts to resolve the situation may be unsuccessful or

the magnitude of the problem may be so great, the stress and tension continues and may increase. If unable to immediately or adequately resolve a crisis, some people may begin to use defense mechanisms such as denial (denying that the crisis exists) or anger (attacking and blaming others for the crisis). Avoidance of reality, wishful thinking, denial, and bargaining represent typical attempts by people in this phase of the crisis to escape the situation. A man whose wife has been severely injured in an auto accident may use **bargaining** by saying, "Let my wife live and I will never miss a Sunday church service again." A bereaved person may refuse to believe that their loved one is dead. A man with a new diagnosis of cancer may ignore it and avoid treatment. Victims of the great floods in the Midwest during the summers of 1993 and 1994, and in California in 1995, in some cases had to wait days or weeks before the flood waters subsided enough to reenter their homes. Emotional expressions in this phase fluctuate between indifference, apathy, euphoria, and anger. People may display extremes of emotions. They may show no emotion, as if they were numb (apathy), or they may inappropriately express well-being and elation (euphoria).

Initially, these defense mechanisms can be helpful emotionally by allowing clients to avoid the harshness of reality. It also offers a brief respite, a time for recouping energy needed to regain equilibrium. In this sense, denial, retreat, and coping mechanisms of anger and bargaining may be useful as stepping stones toward healthy adaptation. But, extended denial or anger is a maladaptive response and leads to poor physical, mental, spiritual, and psychological health. (See the World Watch discussion.)

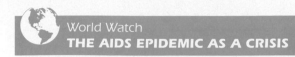

At the beginning of the acquired immune deficiency syndrome (AIDS) epidemic, in the early 1980's, it was centered among people with high risk life style behaviors—the gay community, bisexuals, IV drug users, and large communities of people in African countries. There was much resistance on the part of the United States government to recognize that there was a health care crisis. By the late 1980's the disease had spread across the world population to babies and children of people with AIDS, people with hemophilia, people who received blood from contaminated sources during surgery, and health care workers exposed to HIV infected clients. Barbara Fassbinder, a registered nurse, represents the first known case of occupational transmission of HIV to a health care worker. She went public with her infection in 1990. Ms. Fassbinder became an advocate for using universal precautions to protect health care workers from bloodborne pathogens. She died from the HIV infection on September 20, 1994.

By the time the 1990s were underway, no one was immune from contracting the disease. Sexually active teenagers and the heterosexual population as a whole were the new victims. AIDS cannot be considered a disease of a certain population group. Everyone has heard of someone who has died of the complications of AIDS. Most nurses have cared for HIV positive or AIDS clients. More nurses will care for AIDS clients in the future. Panic and fear spread quickly in the early years of the epidemic. Who would contract the rapidly developing symptoms next and perhaps die? An overwhelming feeling of helplessness arose as worldwide public health agencies struggled to control the disease and identify its cause. The situation is clearly a crisis for the individuals and families affected, and society as a whole. This pandemic event threatens the nation's health and the survival of the world itself.

POST-CRISIS PHASE

The **post-crisis phase** is the time after the crisis event when clients gradually begin to recognize and accept the situation and begin efforts to resolve the crisis successfully. This phase ends when those involved have adapted to a new life.

Early Post-crisis Phase

The actual crisis event is over, and the early post-crisis phase is entered. Assessing the situation's significance and planning for its management can now begin. However, realistic assessment for some leads to depression and withdrawal expressed in apathy, agitation, remorse, or bitterness. A divorced person may feel guilty and at fault or, conversely, might be angry or bitter over being treated unfairly. The pain of rejection, loss of relationships, and anxiety about how to cope with the present and future can create severe depression. Acknowledgment during this phase is often a time of mourning, self-deprecation (being critical of self), and emotional decline. Although difficult and stressful, anger and sadness often must be experienced before healing and restructuring. The early post crisis phase is a necessary step before people can move from disorganized and negative emotions to redefine and attempt to solve the problem. Tension, though still felt, is converted into a constructive energy force. Behavior becomes more purposeful and planning more realistic.

Again, maladaptive responses can occur when people do not successfully work through this phase. The news often reports stories of disgruntled former employees whose problems mounted until they suffered an emotional breakdown and randomly shot co-workers. Most unresolved crises do not make national news, however, such as the lonely widower who passively commits suicide by not taking his medications, or the teenager who drives at high speed and is killed in an auto accident after a girlfriend breaks off their relationship. Obviously these people failed to resolve their crises successfully during the early post-crisis phase when they were so vulnerable. Most people, however, discover that healing and growth from the crisis situation is possible with the help and support of others.

Late Post-crisis Phase

The late post-crisis phase is recognized when people successfully resolve problems and adapt to a new life. They not only acknowledge, face, and accept reality but test it by restructuring their lives to make them workable. This adaptation is marked by feelings of hope and a positive approach to problem solving. The level of anxiety diminishes as people gain a new sense of identity and self-worth. They can talk about the situation openly. They reorganize their thinking toward effective reconstruction, making the best use of their own and other available resources. Their behavior is directed toward mastering the situation and stabilizing the change. People who successfully complete the post-crisis phase, which may last for days to months, and occasionally longer, have developed new coping abilities. They have grown stronger, more mature, and better equipped to deal with future crises.

Types of Crises

There are many different kinds of crises but all crises can be categorized as situational or developmental. These two categories of crises have several major differences (see Table 15.2).

DEVELOPMENTAL CRISES

Developmental crises are periods of disruption that occur at transition points in a person's normal growth and development. During developmental crises, people feel threatened by the demands placed on them and

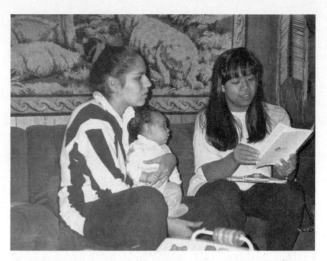

FIGURE 15.1. A young woman who has experienced the developmental crisis of childbirth and motherhood is being taught infant care by a community health nurse on a home visit.

they have difficulty making the changes necessary to fit the new stage of development (see Fig. 15.1).

During the process of normal biopsychosocial growth, people go through a succession of life cycle stages from birth through old age. Each stage is quite different from the previous one and transitions from one stage to the next require changes in roles and behavior. There are periods of upset and disequilibrium. Popular writers like Sheehy (1976) and Levinson (1978) have called these periods "passages" and "transitions." They are the times when developmental crises occur.

Groups and communities, too, develop through successive stages that frequently parallel the birth-to-old-age pattern. Theorists have variously described the stages of group growth (Schwartz, 1994), which are summarized in Chapter 10, as dependence, counterdependence, and interdependence. Community development may be less easily distinguished. Nonetheless, anthropologists, sociologists, philosophers, historians, and other social scientists have observed and recorded the birth, rise, decline, and sometimes renewal of societies, communities, and other aggregates of people. Groups and communities, like most living systems, encounter stages of growth with accompanying transitions that require adaptation and lead to what can be described as "developmental" crises. For example, a new community may find that its growing population of young children lacks adequate playgrounds and recre-

TABLE 15.2. *Major Differences Between Types of Crises*

DEVELOPMENTAL CRISIS

Part of normal growth and development which can upset normalcy
Precipitated by a life transition point
Gradual onset
Response to developmental demands and society's expectations

SITUATIONAL CRISIS

Unexpected period of upset in normalcy
Precipitated by a hazardous event
Sudden onset
Externally imposed "accident"

ational activities. The community is experiencing a developmental transition that requires adaptation.

Most developmental crises have a gradual onset. The change is evolutionary rather than revolutionary. People anticipate and even prepare to start school, enter adolescence, leave home, marry, have a baby, retire, or die. They move into and through each transitional period knowing in advance that some kind of change will be required. So, too, with communities. A new town needs to develop its schools, businesses, city ordinances, recreational areas, hospitals, law enforcement, and churches. As the town grows, its needs change to maintenance and controlling expansion. In many instances, people have already seen others or whole communities experience these transitions. As a result, developmental crises have a degree of predictability. They offer the possibility of a period of time for anticipation and adjustment.

Developmental crises arise from both physical and social changes. Each new life stage confronts people with changed relationships, responsibilities, and roles. The transition to parenthood, for example, demands a change in role from caring for oneself and one's mate to include nurturing, caring for, and protecting a completely helpless infant. Relationships with adults, children, and even one's own parents also change. Parenthood is an entrance into a previously inexperienced part of the adult world. New parents may fear the unknown. Will this infant develop normally? Can I give adequate care? Parents often feel anxiety over the responsibility of shaping this new person's life and satisfying society's expectations for their child's proper education and training. They may worry about the increased financial burden and struggle with mixed feelings about giving up a large measure of freedom. At the aggregate level, a community may find it lacks adequate resources to cope with increasing law enforcement demands, or a small town may struggle with its identity as it increases in size and loses its unique intimacy. These transitions put people under considerable stress, which contributes to building tension, feelings of helplessness, and resultant crisis. Some people adapt quickly; others cannot cope, probably because earlier developmental crises went unresolved. When people lack a repertoire of adaptive skills, a crisis can become major and disastrous. One can easily see how abused children become abusive parents when most, if not all, of their developmental crises have been detrimental rather than growth producing and healthy.

CASE STUDY

A DEVELOPMENTAL CRISIS

Marcia Sand is 39 years old. Married for 22 years, she has been a capable homemaker and mother of four children. Her husband, Lou, a construction worker for the past 20 years, thinks Marcia does a "super job at home." In the past, Marcia's time was filled with cooking, laundry, cleaning, shopping, and meeting the endless demands of the family. Their limited income prompted her to adopt many money-saving strategies. She made most of her own and the children's clothes, did all her own baking, and raised vegetables in her backyard garden. Now the youngest of the children, Tommy, has just left home to join the Navy. Her husband spends much of his spare time at the local bar with his friends, leaving Marcia alone. With a nearly empty house and little need for cooking, baking, and sewing, Marcia has lost her sense of usefulness. She thinks of taking a job, but knows her choices are limited because she has only a high school education. Marcia has not slept well in weeks; she wakes up tired and drags through the day barely able to manage the simplest task. She cries frequently but does not know why. Her hair, always neat and attractive in the past, looks bedraggled, and her shoulders slump. "I just can't seem to get on top of things anymore," she complains.

Marcia has entered a developmental crisis that is sometimes called the "empty nest syndrome." She faces a turning point in her life, a time when parenting has seemingly ended. Leaving her satisfying homemaker role, she faces a new life stage filled with unknowns, changes, and a seeming lack of purpose. The transition came about gradually, almost imperceptibly, but now she must deal with it. Yet she feels unable to cope and wishes to turn to someone who would understand and lend her strength. She can be helped, but her crisis could also have been prevented at the pre-crisis phase. Anticipatory planning could have prevented the dilemma Marcia finds herself in now.

SITUATIONAL CRISES

A **situational crisis** is a stressful and disruptive event arising from an external event which occurs suddenly often without warning to a person, group, aggregate, or community. These events require behavioral changes and coping mechanisms beyond the abilities of the people involved.

Sudden events over which we have little or no control come in many forms (see Fig. 15.2). They are not predicted, expected, or planned. They occur to people because of where they are in time and space. For instance, the couple who, after 25 years of marriage, gets

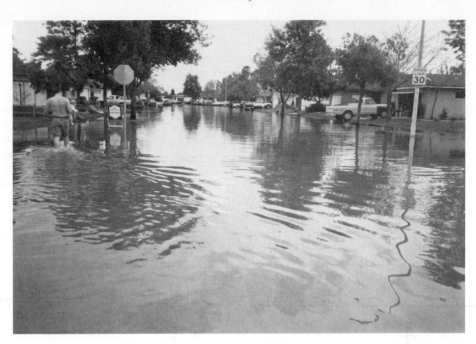

FIGURE 15.2. Members of this California neighborhood experienced a situational crisis during the winter floods of 1995.

divorced; the epidemic of influenza that strikes a skilled nursing facility; the train derailment where many are injured and killed; or the terrorist bomb that explodes in an office building injuring or killing hundreds of employees. These kinds of events, which involve loss or the threat of loss, represent life hazards to those affected. Some crisis-precipitating events can be positive, such as a significant job promotion or sudden news of acquiring great wealth; however, they still make increased demands on individuals who must make major life adjustments (Forman, 1993; Woolley, 1990). Even positive events involve a modified grieving process as individuals may be losing or giving up old familiar and comfortable situations and face stressful changes.

Situational crises arise from external sources, that is, events or conditions generally outside of people's normal life processes. They are extraordinary experiences. They create life changes and disrupt equilibrium by imposing stresses that are usually foreign to ordinary living. The result is overwhelming tension and incapacitation. Natural disasters, for example, are clearly an external cause of a situational crisis. Said one client, "I shall never forget my feelings when one of my high school classmates was killed instantly by lightning. Mel was a popular boy, and his death threw us all into crisis."

Community health nurses see an almost infinite variety of situational crises: included are debilitating dis-

CASE STUDY

A SITUATIONAL CRISIS

The Cooper family eagerly anticipated the birth of their first child. When they first learned that Danny had a harelip and cleft palate, Jan and Frank were numb. They were overwhelmed by the shock of seeing their disfigured baby and worried about the possibility of other defects. Then came the first painful days adjusting to Danny's appearance and trying to feed and care for him. Jan and Frank alternated between feelings of guilt ("Perhaps we didn't do something right during pregnancy!") and resentment ("Why did this have to happen to us?"). Added to these anxieties was the specter of several corrective surgeries. Each operation threatened them with the risk to Danny, the stress of hospitalization, the struggle to stay with Danny while juggling jobs, the consequences to home life, and the impossible financial costs. How could they handle it all? They felt unable to cope.

As with most situational crises, this one took the Coopers completely by surprise. It upset their normal pattern of living and disrupted their equilibrium. The onset was sudden, precipitated by an event that they perceived as threatening to their well-being. Unlike developmental crises that are brought on by normal demands of growth, their child's congenital defect was externally imposed. Also, it required behavioral changes and adjustments that the Coopers' usual coping abilities were not equipped to handle.

ease, economic misfortune, unemployment, physical abuse, divorce, unwanted pregnancy, chemical abuse, sudden death of a loved one, tragic accidents such as mine explosions, and many others. In each situation, people feel overwhelmed and need help to cope. Skilled intervention can make the difference between a healthy or unhealthy outcome.

MULTIPLE CRISES

Different kinds of crises can overlap in actual experience, compounding the stress felt by the persons involved. For example, a couple could experience a developmental crisis (birth) and a situational crisis (birth defect) simultaneously; with the resulting stress compounded. The developmental crisis of midlife may be complicated by situational crises such as divorce and job change. With older adults the developmental crisis of retirement may be compounded by the situational crisis of a fall causing a fractured hip. The transition a child faces entering school may occur at the same time the family moves to a new neighborhood and a new infant joins the family. The child must share his parents' attention and affection with a new sibling at a time when all the child's resources are needed to cope with starting school and adjusting to the new neighborhood. Classic research has shown that these accumulated stresses can lead to ill health (Holmes & Rahe, 1967). Those who might normally work through one crisis in a healthy way may find that compound events overwhelm them and cause more stress than they can handle.

Crisis Intervention

Many people unnecessarily go through crises that might have been prevented. Other crises could be shortened in length or diminished in intensity through preventive measures (Goetz, 1992). Because of the nature and philosophy of community health practice, nurses should place a high priority on crisis prevention. Community health nurses are in a unique position to prevent or detect potential crises. They encounter people in their own settings where direct observation, discussion, and intervention can occur. Also, through their participation in communities' communication networks, nurses can learn about family and community programs to assist in crisis prevention.

GOALS OF CRISIS INTERVENTION

Crisis prevention is considered on three levels: primary, secondary, and tertiary.

Primary Prevention

Primary crisis prevention means keeping the crisis from ever happening, taking actions to completely eliminate its occurrence. Primary prevention is obviously the most effective level of intervention both in terms of promoting clients' health and in terms of cost containment. Primary prevention can be practiced in all settings: in the work place with employee assistance programs; in the home with programs to teach nutrition, safety, interpersonal skills; and in the community through efforts to cut down pollution, or encourage health-promoting legislation. Primary prevention efforts are one area where the community health nurse should focus time and effort.

Primary prevention reflects a fundamental human concern for well-being and includes planned activities, undertaken by the nurse, to prevent an unwanted event from occurring, to protect current states of health and healthy functioning, and to promote desired states of health for the members of a particular community (Bloom, 1991). For the community health nurse, any activity that fosters healthful practices and counteracts unhealthful influences can help prevent a crisis. Health promotion should take into account physical, psychological, sociocultural, and spiritual needs.

The second aspect of primary crisis prevention is anticipatory guidance. Because developmental crises are often predictable, community health nurses can help clients prepare for these life changes. Clients can discuss with the nurse the kinds of adjustments and role changes the next transition period will require. The woman whose children have all left home and who has no career or any interests to fill the time might have avoided the "empty nest" depression by anticipating this time would come. She might have taken classes towards a career or worked part-time while her children were still at home.

Placing an aging parent in a nursing home is often very stressful for the entire family, an event that anticipatory planning can make less intense, averting the crisis phase. Even situational crises, like many "accidents," are often predictable. In a family history of myocardial infarctions, family members can change life-styles to prevent heart attacks such as making changes in diet, exercise patterns, choosing less stressful jobs, and learning coping skills.

Anticipatory work means experiencing some of the feelings of loss, tension, or anxiety before the crisis-precipitating event occurs (Wright & Leahy, 1994). It is much easier to do this at a time when energy and intellectual processes are at a high level of functioning. Anticipatory work dissipates the impact of the crisis event (Flanagan, 1990). One can help a family prepare for grief and loss before a terminally ill family member dies by talking about the impending death, talking with the ill family member, and assisting with final wishes the dying family member may have shared. If such preparations are made, a crisis of large proportions can often be prevented (Kubler-Ross, 1969).

Public health primary prevention interventions have led to the most spectacular health achievements in recorded history particularly in sanitation methods and mass immunizations to prevent dreaded diseases. Yet these primary prevention methods receive limited acknowledgment in contrast to clinical medicine, in the acute care setting, with its elaborate and expensive technology which has received the lion's share of public attention and support (Bloom, 1991). The role and benefit of primary prevention in community health nursing has been overlooked even though the literature indicates it is the most effective and cost-efficient level of prevention. Because primary prevention lacks the excitement and drama of secondary and tertiary prevention it has received little attention in the form of financial support in recent past years. However, the financial crisis of the health care delivery system dictates an increasing focus on primary prevention. Community health nurses can take the lead in directing the preventative work that needs to be done by being prepared academically, clinically, and politically. See the Levels of Prevention example that follows.

Secondary Prevention

Secondary crisis prevention focuses on early detection and treatment. It seeks to reduce the intensity and duration of a crisis and to promote adaptive behavior. Community health nurses often encounter clients in the crisis phase of an event. The nurse is visiting a family to follow up on three members with positive Mantoux tests. Six teens walking in a high school parking lot are injured by an auto out of control. A mobile home community is devastated by a tornado and the local health department's community health nurses work

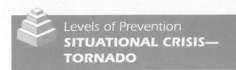

Levels of Prevention
SITUATIONAL CRISIS— TORNADO

GOAL
To prevent as much damage, injury, and death as possible from an uncontrollable event.

PRIMARY PREVENTION
Increase community awareness and preparation through education. Each person is as prepared as possible physically and emotionally and knows what to do and where to go whether at home, work, school, or elsewhere in the community.

SECONDARY PREVENTION
Get to safety before the impact—either the southwest corner of the basement or an interior room away from windows and under heavy furniture. Leave damaged residence cautiously if able and not seriously injured. Prevent a second disaster and do not return to house if it is damaged. Beware of hazards such as live wires, broken gas lines, fallen debris.

TERTIARY PREVENTION
Remain safe during immediate recovery period, accept help from others. Go to friends, family members and community services for support. Accept counseling and other services to get life stabilized physically, emotionally, and financially.

with the American Red Cross to provide emergency assistance. These are examples of situational crises, that are unexpected and occur, or are discovered, suddenly.

Developmental crises, if not prevented at the pre-crisis phase will continue into the crisis phase as do situational crises. However, developmental crises often are not recognized as easily as situational crises. For example, the quiet, shy teenager who slips into depression, or the parents with four small children who feel stressed and find themselves "punishing" their children constantly.

During the course of normal practice, community health nurses can watch for signs that individuals or aggregates may be entering a crisis. By suspecting any event that might potentially provoke crisis, the nurse can monitor clients' responses. Families or communities which experience several simultaneous or rapidly succeeding hazardous events may be at risk for crisis. A family might be able to handle the loss of the father's job, and even appear to cope adequately with the death of a grandparent a few weeks later. However, when these crises are further compounded by the mother needing surgery, the family reaches the breaking point. In such a situation nursing intervention should be at an early stage to offer support to the family and prevent the crises from overwhelming them.

A community was economically impacted by the closing of a chicken processing plant in April. In May, an abandoned building collapsed and killed a security guard. Just as the town was struggling to evaluate and overcome the effects of these two events, a tornado leveled a mobile home park on the edge of town, killing three children. The community is in crisis due to the unexpectedness and multiplicity of events affecting the town. If the occupational health nurse at the processing plant had provided the employees and their families the early support needed to cope with the plant closure, then they may have been better able to handle the other events.

Tertiary Prevention

Tertiary crisis prevention involves reducing the amount and degree of disability or damage resulting from crisis. Although it involves rehabilitative work, it can help clients recover and reduce the risk of future crises (France, 1989). In this sense, it is a preventive measure. Clients can easily become caught in a web of maladaptive responses. For instance, workers laid off from their jobs may remain bitter and hostile, and reinforce one another's heavy drinking. A grieving widower, who continues for months or years to deny his wife's death, withdraws socially, and develops chronic physical problems. An older woman, who cannot accept aging and subsequent limitations due to impaired vision and hearing, insists on driving and has a major accident that injures several people. Tertiary crisis prevention involves helping clients like these face the reality of their present situations and develop improved coping skills.

Working with individuals in groups is a particularly effective means of providing support, reality orientation, and the prevention of further disability (Roberts, 1991). However, tertiary levels of care are the most expensive and least productive form of care. They are often delivered to clients who have suffered potentially irreversible damage from events such as cerebral vascular accidents or spinal cord injuries that result in paraplegia. The long term rehabilitation may be for comfort or to increase independence in activities of daily living. In many cases lives have been permanently altered.

METHODS OF INTERVENTION

People in crisis need help. They often desperately want help. The crisis and its associated disequilibrium has a two-fold effect on the individuals involved: (1) It renders them temporarily helpless, unable to cope on their own, and (2) it makes them especially receptive to outside influence. There are crisis resolution models that community health nurses could use to help clients at the secondary level. The following steps (Roberts, 1991: Aguilera, 1993) have been used successfully by people in the mental health field working on crisis hot lines, mental health centers, and emergency rooms. The steps are (1) assess the individual and the problem for lethality, (2) establish rapport, (3) identify major problems and intervene, (4) deal with feelings, (5) explore alternatives and coping mechanisms, (6) develop action plan, and (7) follow up including anticipatory planning for coping with future crises. People in crisis will seek and generally receive some kind of help, but the nature of that help can rule in favor of or against a healthy outcome where the participants can grow and evolve (Shaw & Halliday, 1992). Clients' desires for assistance give the helping professional a prime opportunity to intervene; this opportunity also presents a challenge to make that intervention as effective as possible.

One goal of crisis intervention should be to help clients reestablish a sense of safety and security while allowing them to ventilate their feelings and be validated (Young, 1991). This will help to reestablish equilibrium at as healthy a level as possible and can result in change and growth within clients (Dean, 1994). Minimally that goal involves resolving the immediate crisis and restoring clients to their pre-crisis levels of functioning. Ultimately, however, intervention seeks to raise that functioning to a healthier, more mature level that will enable them to cope with and prevent future crises. As discussed earlier, crises tend to be self-limiting, which causes intervention time to last from four to six weeks with resolution, one way or another within two to three months (Roberts, 1991; Aguilera, 1993). The urgency of the situation represents a window of opportunity that invites the prompt, focused attention of clients and nurse working together to achieve intervention goals.

Crisis intervention in community health may use one or both of two approaches: generic and individual. For the majority of crisis encounters, the generic approach is more appropriate.

Generic Approach

The generic approach designs interventions to fit a particular type of crisis focusing on the nature and course of the crisis, rather than on the psychodynamics of each client (Aguilera, 1993). Crisis intervention using the generic approach is tailored to a specific kind of crisis, situational or developmental, and comprises four important elements: (1) encouraging use of adaptive behavior and coping strategies, (2) support, (3) preparation for the practical and emotional future, and (4) anticipatory guidance.

An example of the generic approach is used with all mastectomy clients. The nurse encourages discussion and analysis of feelings, teaches exercises to regain physical functioning, and creates a supportive, caring atmosphere especially through self-help groups like "Reach for Recovery." The nurse can help in the fitting and use of prostheses, rebuilding self-image, and strengthening self-esteem by encouraging positive interpersonal relationships. The community health nurse also prepares people to handle future feelings of depression and anxiety related to bodily disfigurement, and the possibility of metastasis.

The generic approach does not require advanced professional psychotherapy skills. More important for community health practice, it works well with families, groups, and even communities in crisis. The community health nurse may work with a group of cancer clients, grieving spouses, adolescents struggling with developmental crisis, or an entire community recovering from some natural or man-made disaster. The generic approach allows the nurse to intervene with any group of people who have a crisis in common. It offers a broad base of support, since such a group can offer resources for the members beyond those brought by the nurse.

Individual Approach

The individual approach is used when clients do not respond to the generic approach or when they need special therapy. Individual crisis intervention should not be confused with individual psychotherapy which tends to focus on clients' developmental past. In contrast, crisis intervention directs treatment toward the immediate state of disequilibrium, identifying its causes and developing coping mechanisms. Family members or significant others are included during the process of crisis resolution. An entire group may need this type of intervention. When this approach is needed, clients are usually referred to a professional with specialized training.

(See the Issues in Community Health Nursing display that follows.)

INTERVENTION STEPS USING THE NURSING PROCESS

Crisis intervention in community health assumes that clients have resources. If their potential for managing stressful events can be tapped, people in crisis will need minimal direct assistance. In accordance with the self-care concept, crisis intervention seeks to identify and build on client strengths. Aguilera (1993) outlines a series of four steps for intervention during crisis: assessment, planning, intervention, and resolution. Interventions to promote crisis resolution are presented using the three levels of prevention in Table 15.3.

Assessment and Nursing Diagnosis

Initially, the nurse must assess the nature of the crisis and the clients' response to it. How severe is the problem, and what risks do the clients face? Are other peo-

Issues in Community Health Nursing
PRACTICAL APPLICATION OF CRISIS THEORY

In a time of economic and social change the traditional biomedical model of teaching nursing is clearly inadequate. Nurses today need to be prepared not only to deliver care to clients suffering consequences of the social ills of substance abuse and violence, but also to intervene creatively to promote healthy lifestyles. One RN to BSN nursing program developed a senior-level clinical course, Nursing and Crisis Intervention for Victims of Family Violence, in response to this need. The course integrates theories of violence, grief, and crisis intervention with nursing theory. By the end of the course, students invariably report that their professional practice has been reshaped, with sharpened assessment skills, and increased empathy. Students also credited the new interventions with an increase in the scope of their daily practice—they were better able to treat clients currently ignored or unrecognized by the health care delivery system.

ple also at risk? Assessment must be rapid but thorough, focusing on certain specific areas.

First, the nurse concentrates on the immediate problem during the assessment. Why have clients asked for help right now? How do they define the problem? What precipitated the crisis? When did it occur? Was it a sudden accidental or situational event, or a slower developmental one?

Next, the nurse focuses on the clients' perceptions of the event. What does the crisis mean to them, and how do they think it will affect their future? Are they viewing the situation realistically? When crisis occurs to a family or group, some members see the situation differently from others. During intervention, all should be encouraged to express themselves, to talk about the crisis, and to share their feelings about its meaning. Acceptance of the range of feelings is important.

Determine what persons are available for support. Consider family, friends, clergy, other professionals, community members, and agencies. With whom are the clients close and who do they trust? One advantage of group intervention is that the members provide some of this support for each other. In subsequent sessions, the quality of support should be evaluated. Sometimes a well-meaning individual may worsen the situation or deter clients from facing and coping with reality.

Next, the nurse needs to assess the clients' coping abilities. Have they had similar kinds of experiences in the past? What techniques have they previously used to relieve tension and anxiety? Which ones have they tried in this situation, and if they have not worked, why not? Clients should be encouraged to think of other stress-relieving techniques, perhaps ones they have used in the past, and to try them.

Finally, and of crucial importance, the nurse needs to find out if there is a possibility of suicide or homicide. Ask directly and specifically about any plans or hints of anyone to hurt or kill himself or anyone else. If plans are specific and the threat appears real, psychiatric referral is indicated. Do not discount threats as idle talk (Kalafat, 1991).

The nurse gathers all of this data and mentally begins to form nursing diagnoses. As a plan of care is developed for the client these nursing diagnoses are formalized in writing. Standardized nursing diagnoses are available for reference or the agency for whom the nurse works may have a format of nursing diagnoses that it prefers. The development of these nursing diagnoses are effective tools as the nurse begins planning the care.

Planning Therapeutic Intervention

Several factors influence the clients' reaction to crises. Nurses should try to determine what factors are affecting clients before making intervention plans. The major balancing factors—clients' perceptions of the event, situa-

TABLE 15.3. *Interventions to Promote Crisis Resolution*

Phase	Goals	Interventions
		PRIMARY INTERVENTION
Precrisis	Health promotion Disease prevention Education	Anticipatory guidance Reduce factors that increase vunerability Reduce hazards in some events (safety and multiplicity of stressors) Reinforce positive coping strategies Mobilize social supports and other resources
		SECONDARY PREVENTION
Crisis	Reduction of stress load Cure or restoration of function	Assist with reaction to the event and functioning Allow behavior: dependence, grief Set goals with client Refer to resources
		TERTIARY PREVENTION
Postcrisis	Rehabilitation and maintenance	Promote adaptation to a changed level of wellness Promote interdependence Reinforce newly learned behaviors, lifestyle changes, coping strategies Explore application of learned behaviors to new situations Identification and use of additional resources

tional supports, human resources, and clients' coping skills—have been assessed in the first step (Aguilera, 1993). While continuing to explore these, the nurse now also considers the clients' general health status, age, past experiences with similar types of situations, sociocultural and religious influences, and the actual assets and liabilities of the situation. This helps to clarify the situation and gives the nurse the opportunity to further encourage clients' participation in the resolution process. If clients are defensive, resistant, and rigid, behaviors that are frequently seen in the late crisis stage, they are not processing clearly and can complete only simple tasks. As clients enter the post-crisis phase they are encouraged to begin to problem-solve the effects of the crisis on themselves and the loss they are experiencing.

The plan is based on the kind of crisis (situational or developmental, acute or chronically recurring), the effect the crisis is having on clients' lives (can they still work, go to school, keep house?), the phase of crisis clients are in, the ways significant others are affected and respond, and the clients' strengths and available resources.

Using the problem-solving process, nurse and clients develop a plan. They review the event that precipitated the crisis, obvious symptoms, and the disruption in the clients' lives. The plan may focus on one or several areas. For instance, clients may need to grasp intellectually the meaning of the crisis, to engage in greater expression of feelings, or both. Part of the plan may be directed toward finding appropriate replacement for material losses such as temporary housing, emergency financial aid, or physical care. Another part may focus on helping clients identify and use more effective coping techniques or locate supportive agencies and resource persons (Roberts, 1991). The plan will also include the development of realistic goals for the future.

Implementation

During implementation it is important for nurse and clients to continue to communicate. They should discuss what is happening, review the plan and the rationale behind its elements, and make appropriate changes when indicated. It is helpful to assign definite activities at the end of each session so that clients can try out different solutions and evaluate various coping behaviors.

The implementation step is enhanced by use of the guidelines below (Murray and Zentner, 1993; Roberts, 1991).

1. Demonstrate acceptance of clients. A crisis will often shatter the ego. Clients need to feel the support of a positive, caring person who does not judge their feelings or behavior. Some negative expressions such as anger, withdrawal, and denial are normal aspects of the crisis phase. Accept them as normal.

2. Help clients confront crisis. Clients need to face and discuss the situation. Expressing their feelings reduces tension and improves reality perception. Recounting what has actually occurred may be painful, but it helps clients confront the crisis. Do not assume that once clients have told about the event, no further recounting is necessary. Each time the story is told, they come closer to dealing realistically with the crisis.

3. Help clients find facts. Distorted ideas and unknown factors of the situation create additional tension and may lead to maladaptive responses. For instance, it would help the Coopers to know that their son's cleft palate was not preventable. Facts about surgical treatment and speech training would also be important for them to know.

4. Help clients express feelings openly. Suppressed feelings can be harmful. For instance, a widow may feel guilty that she is glad her husband is gone. Expression of such feelings as these helps reduce tension and gives clients an opportunity to deal with them.

5. Do not offer false reassurance. Clients need to face reality, not avoid it. A statement such as "Don't worry, it will all work out" is demeaning and meaningless. Rather, make positive statements about faith in their ability to cope: "It is a very difficult situation, but I believe you will be able to deal with it."

6. Discourage clients from blaming others. Clients often blame others as a way to avoid reality and the responsibility for problem solving. Withhold judgment when they blame others, but point out other causal factors and avenues for dealing with the situation.

7. Help clients seek out coping mechanisms. Explore and test old and new techniques to reduce stress and anxiety. Ask questions. What are all the things the client and nurse might do together to resolve the problem? What are the things that need to be done? What do clients think they can do? This assistance gives clients more adaptive energy to work toward resolution.

8. Encourage clients to accept help. Denial in the early phases of crisis cuts off help. Encouraging clients to acknowledge the problem is a first step toward acceptance of help. Often, however, clients fear the loss of their independence and the invasion of their privacy. They may say, "We ought to be able to handle this problem." At this point, the community health nurse can assure clients that people in a crisis of this sort almost always need help. Preparing people to accept help will enable them to make the best use of what others have to offer.

9. Promote development of new positive relationships. Clients who have lost significant persons through death or divorce should be encouraged to find new people to fill the void and provide needed supports and satisfactions.

Evaluation of Crisis Resolution and Anticipatory Planning

In the final step, clients and nurse evaluate, stabilize, and plan for the future. First, evaluate the outcome of the intervention. Are clients using effective coping skills and exhibiting appropriate behavior? Are adequate resources and support persons available? Is the diagnosed problem solved, and have the desired results been accomplished? Analysis of these outcomes gives a greater understanding for coping with future crises.

To stabilize the change, identify and reinforce all the positive coping mechanisms and behaviors. Discuss why they are effective and explore ways to use them in future stressful situations. Summarize the crisis experience, emphasizing the clients' successes with coping in order to reconfirm progress and reinforce self-confidence. Point to evidence that they have reached their pre-crisis, or an even higher, level of functioning.

Clients' plans for the future should include setting realistic goals and means for implementing them. Review with clients how their handling of the present crisis can help them cope with, minimize, or preferably prevent future crises. A similar crisis intervention model based on Aguilera and Messick's work is proposed by Lawler and Yount (1987). They call the four stages (1) analysis, (2) design, (3) intervention, and (4) anticipatory guidance. Applied to an organizational setting, their model holds considerable potential value for community health nurses working with organizations and communities.

Summary

Crisis is a temporary state of severe disequilibrium for persons who face a threatening situation. It is a state that they can neither avoid nor solve with their usual coping abilities. A crisis occurs when some force disrupts normal functioning and thus causes a loss of balance or normalcy in life. A crisis creates tension; subsequently, efforts are made to solve the problem and reduce the tension. When such efforts meet with failure, people feel upset, redefine the situation, try other solutions, and, if failure continues, eventually reach the breaking point.

There are two kinds of crises: developmental and situational. Developmental crises are disruptions that occur during transitional periods in normal growth and development. They usually have a gradual onset and are often predictable. Situational crises are precipitated by an unexpected external event and occur suddenly sometimes without warning.

There are three main phases of a crisis: pre-crisis, crisis, and post-crisis. A crisis can be prevented, or its frequency and intensity diminished, through primary crisis prevention. During this phase the nurse seeks to obstruct the occurrence of a crisis by promoting a high level of wellness and teaching people to anticipate and thus avoid a possible crisis. Secondary crisis prevention focuses on early detection and treatment. Tertiary crisis prevention seeks to reduce the degree of disability resulting from crisis and provide the follow up needed.

Crises tend to progress through the three stages of pre-crisis, crisis, and post-crisis before coming to resolution. People's perception of the crisis changes through these stages, as do emotional response, cognitive ability, and behavior.

People in crisis both need and seek help. Crisis intervention builds on these two phenomena to achieve its primary goal—reestablishment of equilibrium. The two major methods for crisis intervention are the generic and individual approaches. The generic approach deals with a single type of crisis, such as rape or mothers who have lost children from drunken driving, and often works with groups of people involved in the same type of crisis. The individual approach is used when clients do not respond to the generic approach or need additional therapy. Crisis intervention begins with assessment of the situation; then a therapeutic intervention is planned. Next, the nurse carries out the intervention, building on the strengths and self-care ability of clients. Crisis intervention concludes with resolution and anticipatory planning to avert possible future crises.

Activities to Promote Critical Thinking

1. What are the major differences between a developmental and a situational crisis? Give examples of each from personal experiences.

2. Describe a developmental crisis experienced by a community. What was this community's response? Describe some actions a community health nurse might have taken (alone or within an interdisciplinary team) to help the community cope with the crisis.

3. California communities are frequent victims of earthquakes. What preventive actions could the community health nurse take? Design actions at each level of prevention.

4. Watch a news station on the television. Listen for crises or disasters occurring in the world. Analyze the situations and anticipate what the role of a community health nurse would be during the crises selected.

5. Family violence is a significant public health problem. Assume that a battered wife becomes a community health nurses' client and the nurse suspects there may be more women with this problem in the community. Describe how the nurse might provide assistance using the crisis intervention steps. Then discuss how a three-level preventive program might be instituted in the community.

REFERENCES

Aguilera, D. C. (1993). *Crisis intervention: Theory and methodology* 7th ed.). St. Louis: Mosby.

Bloom, M. (1991). Primary prevention: Theory, issues, methods, and programs. In A.R.Roberts (Ed.), *Contemporary perspectives on crisis intervention and prevention* (pp. 150–160). Englewood Cliffs, NJ: Prentice-Hall.

Caplan, G. (1964). *Principles of preventive psychiatry*. New York: Basic Books.

Dean,C. (1994). Strengthening families: From "deficit" to "empowerment". *Journal of Emotional and Behavioral Problems, 2*(4), 8–11.

Flanagan, C.M. (1990). *People and change: An introduction to counseling and stress management*. Hillsdale, NJ: L. Erlbaum Associates.

Forman, S.G. (1993). *Coping skills interventions for children and adolescents*. San Francisco: Jossey-Bass.

France, K. (1989). *Crisis intervention: A handbook of immediate person-to-person help* (2nd ed.). Springfield, IL: Charles C. Thomas.

Goetz, K. (Ed.). (1992). Providing support for families in special circumstances. *Family Resource Coalition Report, 11,*3.

Hoff, L.A. (1989). *People in crisis: Understanding and helping* (3rd ed.). Redwood City, CA: Addison-Wesley.

Holmes, T. & Rahe, R. (1967). The social readjustment rating scale. *Journal of Psychosomatic Research, 11,* 213–17.

Johnson, L. & Mattson, S. (1992). Communication: The key to crisis prevention in pediatric death. *Critical Care Nurse, 12*(8), 23–27.

Kalafat, J. (1991). Suicide interventions in the schools. In A.R. Roberts (Ed.), *Contemporary Perspectives on Crisis Intervention and Prevention* (pp. 218–239). Englewood Cliffs, NJ: Prentice-Hall.

Kubler-Ross, E. (1969). *On death and dying.* New York: Macmillan.

Lawler, T. G. & Yount, E.H. (1987). Managing crises effectively: An intervention model. *Journal of Nursing Administration, 17*(11), 39–43.

Levinson, D. J. (1978). *The Seasons of a man's life.* New York: Knopf.

Murray, R. & Zentner, J. (1993). *Nursing assessment and health promotion strategies* (5th ed.). Englewood Cliffs, NJ: Prentice-Hall.

Roberts, A. (Ed.). (1991). Contemporary perspectives on crisis intervention and prevention. Englewood Cliffs, NJ: Prentice-Hall.

Schwarz, R.M. (1994). *The skilled facilitator: Practical wisdom for developing effective groups.* San Francisco: Jossey-Bass.

Shaw, M.C. & Halliday, P.H. (1992). The family, crisis and chronic illness: An evolutionary model. *Journal of Advanced Nursing, 17,* 537–543.

Sheehy, G. (1995). *New passages: Mapping your life across time.* New York: Random House.

Sheehy, G. (1976). *Passages: Predictable crises of adult life.* New York: Dutton.

Woolley, N. (1990). Crisis theory: A paradigm of effective intervention with families of critically ill people. *Journal of Advanced Nursing, 15*(21), 1402–1408.

Wright, L.M. & Leahey, M. (1994). Calgary family intervention model: One way to think about change. *Journal of Marital and Family Therapy, 20,* 381–395.

Young,M.A. (1991) Crisis intervention and the aftermath of disaster. In A.R. Roberts (Ed.), *Contemporary perspectives on crisis intervention and prevention,* (pp. 83–103). Englewood Cliffs, NJ: Prentice-Hall. .

SELECTED READINGS

Allinson, R.E. (1993). *Global disasters: Inquiries into management ethics.* New York: Prentice Hall.

Aptekar, L. (1994). *Environmental disasters in global perspective.* New York: G. H. Hall.

Benthall, J. (1993). *Disasters, relief and the media.* London: I.B. Tauris.

Berglin, S.L. (1990). Emergency nurses in community disaster planning. *Journal of Emergency Nursing, 16*(4), 290–292.

Caplan, G. (1990). Loss, stress, and mental health. *Community Mental Health Journal, 26*(2), 27–48.

Clarke,R.V. & Jones, P.R. (1989). Suicide and increased availability of handguns in the United States. *Social Science and Medicine, 28*, 805–809.

Cummings, E.M. & Davies, P. (1994). *Children and marital conflict: The impact of family dispute and resolution.* New York: Guilford Press.

Halm, M.A. (1990). Effects of support groups on anxiety of family members during critical illness. *Heart and Lung, 19*(1), 62–71.

Jaime, D. (1992). Managing the at-risk situation: Tales from the trenches. *Caring, 11*(2), 14–15.

Koller, P.A. (1991). Family needs and coping strategies during illness crises. *AACN Clinical Issues in Critical Care Nursing, 2*(2), 338–345.

Lane, P.S. (1994). Critical incident stress debriefing for health care workers. *Omega: Journal of Death and Dying, 28*(4), 301–315.

Long, N.J. (1992). Managing a shooting incident. *Journal of emotional and behavioral problems, 1*(1), 23–26.

Mandt, A.K. (1993). The curriculum revolution in action: Nursing and crisis intervention for victims of family violence. *Journal of Nursing Education, 32*(1), 44–46.

Moore, A.C. (1989). Crisis intervention: A care plan for families of hospitalized children. Pediatric Nursing. 15(3), 234–236.

Patel, C. (1991). *The complete guide to stress management.* New York: Plenum Press.

Pitcher, G.D. & Poland, S. (1992). *Crisis intervention in the schools.* New York: Guilford Press.

Roberts, A.R. (1990). *Helping crime victims: Research, policy and practice.* Newbury Park, CA: Sage

Roberts. A.R. (Ed.). (1990). *Crisis intervention handbook: Assessment, treatment, and research.* Belmont, CA: Wadsworth Publishing Co.

Sheehy, S.B. & Jimmerson, C.L. (1994). *Manual of clinical trauma care: The first hour* (2nd ed.). St. Louis: Mosby.

Smith, J.C. (1991). *Stress scripting: A guide to stress management.* New York: Praeger.

Sutherland, V.J. & Cooper, C.L. (1990). *Understanding stress: A psychological perspective for health professionals.* London: Chapman and Hall.

Uphold, C.R. & Graham, M.V. (1993). Schools as centers for collaborative services for families: A vision for change. *Nursing Outlook, 41*(5), 204–11.

Van Auken, E. (1991). Crisis intervention: Elders awaiting placement in an acute care facility. *Journal of Gerontological Nursing, 17*(11), 30–33.

Veninga, R. & Spradley, J. (1981). *The work-stress connection.* Boston: Little, Brown.

Waugh, W.L. (1990). *Terrorism and emergency management: Policy and administration.* New York: M. Dekker.

UNIT

III

Promoting and Protecting the Health of Families

16

Theoretical Bases for Promoting Family Health

LEARNING OBJECTIVES

Upon completion of this chapter, readers should be able to:

- Analyze changing definitions of family.
- Discuss characteristics all families have in common.
- List the traditional and nontraditional units that make up families.
- Describe the functions of a family.
- Identify the developmental tasks of a family as it grows.
- Analyze the role of the community health nurse in promoting the health of the family unit.

KEY TERMS

- Blended family
- Cohabitating couples
- Commune family
- Commuter family
- Energy exchange
- Family
- Family culture
- Family functioning
- Family map
- Family structure
- Family system boundary
- Foster families
- Gangs
- Group-marriage family
- Group-network family
- Homeless family
- Intrarole functioning
- Kin-network
- Multigenerational family
- Nontraditional family
- Nuclear-dyad family
- Nuclear family
- Primary relationship
- Roles
- Single-adult family
- Single-parent family
- Traditional family

Barbara Walton Spradley and Judith Ann Allender
COMMUNITY HEALTH NURSING: CONCEPTS AND PRACTICE, 4th ed.
© 1996 Barbara Walton Spradley and Judith Ann Allender

What is a **family**? Many different definitions exist, but most family theorists agree that a family consists of one or more individuals who share a residence, or live near one another; possess some common emotional bond; and engage in interrelated social positions, roles, and tasks (Friedmann, 1986; Duvall & Miller, 1985; Baranowski & Nader, 1985). Traditionally the **nuclear family** has been the family structure most often thought of—mother, father, and children living together, separate from others.

However, society is accepting nontraditional definitions of family. "With today's wide variety of family types and structures, the most advanced definition of family may be 'the family is who the client says it is' " (Bell & Wright, 1993, p. 391). The traditional characteristics of a family are summarized again as follows: A family consists of one or more persons who live in the same household (usually), share a common emotional bond, and perform certain interrelated social tasks.

As this definition suggests, families may assume many different types of structures. **Family structure** comprises the characteristics of individuals who make up a family unit (age, gender, and number). A growing body of research on family structure and function shows that families have changed dramatically since the nuclear family was the dominant form. Today's community health nurse needs to understand and work with many types of families. Each family will have different health problems and needs. For example, a young single mother seeks help in caring for her sick infant. Another family has an elderly parent recently discharged from the hospital after a Cerebral Vascular Accident (CVA). The third family, refugees from Vietnam, needs instruction on the purchase and preparation of food. In other families, the progress of a serious burn on the arm of a ten-year-old child will be checked and a contract developed for weight control with his mother; and a recently retired couple is assisted in adjusting to their new stage of life.

What kinds of things does the community health nurse need to know during a workday? The nurse has to deal with specific health problems such as CVAs, burns, and retirement. Infants, young adults, and the elderly (both ill and well) will be visited.

The nurse needs to know the goals of the visits—the promotion of health and self-care. The nurse must rely on knowledge of cultural differences when working with the Vietnamese family and other clients. The nurse needs to know how to use certain tools, such as problem solving and contracting. Understanding communication and knowing how to develop a helping relationship are also needed skills.

But does the nurse need to know something about the nature of families? What should the nurse know about the five families that will be visited, apart from their individual members and problems? Do families, as basic units of a community, have characteristics that affect community health nursing service? The answer is an unqualified yes. As a community health nurse, effectiveness depends on knowing how to work with a family as a unit of care. This chapter examines the nature of families and draws from various theories to strengthen the understanding of families as clients. This understanding gives the nurse the skills to intervene with families at the primary, secondary, and tertiary levels of prevention. (See the Levels of Prevention discussion that follows.)

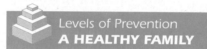

Levels of Prevention
A HEALTHY FAMILY

GOAL
The family will provide the emotional and material resources necessary for its members' growth and wellbeing.

PRIMARY PREVENTION
Adults well prepared for the responsibilities of marriage enter it with the personal resources necessary to promote the growth and development of their family unit.

SECONDARY PREVENTION
At the earliest possible moment of recognition that problems exist in the relationships among or between family members; or if one family member has personal problems which affects the family as a whole, the family seeks out the appropriate resources which brings the family to the highest level of wellness possible.

TERTIARY PREVENTION
After the family suffers a crisis, the members recognize the need for help and accept that help, drawing on personal resources to rebuild relationships and heal the family unit again bringing it to the highest level of wellness possible.

Characteristics of Families

Several observations can be made about families in general. First, each family is unique. The five families mentioned earlier each have their own distinct problems and strengths. As the nurse approaches the door of a house or pushes the buzzer of an apartment, the nurse cannot assume what the family inside will be like. Consequently, the nurse will have to gather information about each particular family in order to achieve nursing objectives.

Second, every family shares some universal characteristics with every other family. These universal characteristics provide an important key to understanding each family's uniqueness. Five of the most important family universals for community nursing are listed below:

1. Every family is a small social system.
2. Every family has its own cultural values and rules.
3. Every family has structure.
4. Every family has certain basic functions.
5. Every family moves through stages in its life cycle.

No matter how many families a nurse might visit in the course of a year, each one will have these universal features. It is important for community health nurses to know how the social system, cultural values, structure, function, and stage of development affect health care provision. These five universals of family life provide the framework of this chapter and are based on systems theory, sociological theories, and theories of family development.

Third, some families are more alike than others. Although unique, there are certain similarities among some families that allow them to be categorized into structural subtypes: **nuclear family** (husband, wife, children); **nuclear-dyad family** (husband and wife); **multigenerational family** (such as the aged mother of the husband, wife, teen age children and one teen's infant); and **single-parent family**, (mother or father, but not both, and children). Knowing the range of variation within these family universals will help prepare the nurse for the variety of families they may encounter. While considering the universals of family life, this chapter will also cover those family structural subtypes that characterize a changing society. If a worldwide perspective were taken, subtypes in family life would greatly proliferate, although the universals would still exist. (See the World Watch that follows.)

World Watch
SOUTHEAST ASIAN REFUGEE WOMEN: DISRUPTION TO FAMILY STRUCTURE AND FUNCTION

(Fox, P. G., Cowell, J. M. & Johnson, M. M. (1995). Effects of family disruption on Southeas Asian refugee women. *International Nursing Review*, 42(1). 26–30.)

Southeast Asia is an agricultural economy with a society that promotes strong family ties. Families are large and extended; its members have clearly defined roles and responsibilities. Religious roots in Budddism and Confucism also serve to maintain devotion and allegiance to the family as well as ancestors.

The Southeast Asian woman's dominant role is to meet the needs of her extended family, husband, and children. She is directed by cultural norms to accept the authority of her husband and the other men in her extended family. Since a woman's identity is attached to her family role, loss or separation from other family members, particularly their husbands is an emotionally stressful experience.

Over the past two decades over one million refugees have immigrated to the United States from Southeast Asia to escape war, economic, and political oppression. Many of these refugees are women who suffer profound grief and chronic stress from the loss of their husbands, and from lack of news of family members left behind. These women feel isolated in a foreign culture without their past supports and role identities. Adjustment for them is difficult and the stress may lead to illness.

The loss of family members forces women into new gender roles without the benefit of traditional family assistance that is so important to them. Nurses need to assess the importance of the loss of family members on the lives of refugee women and design intervention programs that encourage social support networks, family viability and ethnic community development.

Families as Social Systems

Many people fall into the trap of viewing families merely as collections of individuals. Caused partly by a strong cultural emphasis on individualism, this error also occurs because families are encountered through the individual members. Families are seldom thought of as a unit. When a community health nurse sits in a living room talking with a young mother about her new infant, it is difficult to realize that all the other family members are present by way of their influence. Systems theory offers some insights about how families operate as social systems. Understanding the attributes of living systems or open systems (discussed in Chapter 4) can help strengthen an understanding of family structure and function. There are five attributes of open systems that help explain how families function: (1) families are interdependent; (2) families maintain boundaries; (3) families exchange energy with their environment; (4) families are adaptive; and (5) families are goal-oriented.

INTERDEPENDENCE AMONG MEMBERS

All the members of a family are interdependent; each member's actions affect the other members (Schultz, 1987). For example, the changes a father makes to reduce his risk of coronary heart disease will affect the rest of the family. If he cuts back on working overtime, the family's income will be reduced. If he begins to eat different foods, food preparation and eating patterns in the family will be altered. If he starts a new exercise program three evenings a week, this may upset other family routines. Even his ability to carry out his usual roles as husband and father may be affected if, for instance, he has less time to spend on his children's activities or on to social events with his wife.

The interdependence of family members involves a set of internal relationships that influence the effectiveness of family functioning (Friedmann, 1986). **Family functioning** is defined as those behaviors or activities by family members that maintain the family and meet family needs, individual member needs, and society's views of family. There is a complex communication pattern among family members. It is possible to illustrate the communication network between members using a **family map** which diagrams the dyads (two-way), triads (three-way), and combinations of interactions that occur within families (Satir, 1972). The way parents relate to each other, for instance, influences the quality of their parenting. When the bond between them is strong and nurturing, they have more to offer their children. Marital, parent-child, and sibling relationships all significantly influence family functioning. They determine how well the family as a system handles conflict, provides a support system for its members, copes with crises, solves daily problems, and capitalizes on its own resources.

FAMILY BOUNDARIES

Families, as systems, do set and maintain boundaries: ego-boundaries, generation boundaries, and family-community boundaries (Barker, 1992). Family closeness, which results from shared experiences and expectations, links family members together in a bond that excludes the rest of the world. A greater concentration of energy exists within the family than between the family and its external environment, thereby creating a **family system boundary**. This boundary is demonstrated by the energy within a family that is greater than the energy between the family and its external environment. The Petrocelli's extended family gathers for a Sunday afternoon backyard picnic. The distinctiveness of this family from all the others in the neighborhood is noticeable, as would any other family be. The elders in the family were born in Italy and they sit together reminiscing in Italian. The food is traditional and plentiful. It is prepared and served by the women: aunt Rosa's lasagna, cousin Theresa's pasta, and tiramisu and cannoli for dessert prepared from grandma Maria's own recipes. While the women prepare the foods the men play Bocci ball and discuss the future of the family business, a large meat market in the old section of town. The children gather in small groups and play loudly. Several of them, prompted by their parents, will display their musical talent later in the day, by singing some old favorite songs. Because of the things they have in common, the Petrocelli's set and maintain boundaries that unite them and also differentiate them from others (see Fig. 16.1).

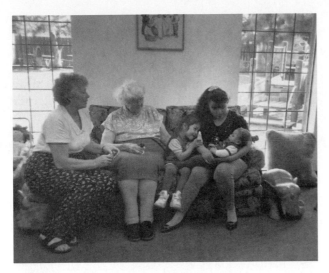

FIGURE 16.1. A family gathers to enjoy each others company, reminisce, and renew family bonds.

ENERGY EXCHANGE

Family boundaries are semi-permeable; they do provide protection and preservation of the family unit but they also allow selective linkage with the outside world. As open systems, in order to function adequately, families exchange materials or information with their environment. This process is called **energy exchange** (Kerr, 1988). All normally functioning living systems engage in such an input-output relationship. This information exchange serves to promote a healthy ecological balance between the family system and its environment, that is its immediate community.

A family's successful progress through its developmental stages depends on how well the family manages this energy exchange. For example, a child-bearing family, needs adequate food, shelter, and emotional support as well as information on how to accomplish its developmental tasks. The family also needs community resources such as health care, education, employment, all of which are forms of environmental input. In return, the family contributes to the community by working and by consuming goods and services. When a family does not have adequate income or emotional support or does not use community resources, that family is not experiencing a proper energy exchange with its environment (Clark, 1986). An inadequate exchange can lead to dysfunctioning and poor health (Neuman, 1989).

ADAPTIVE BEHAVIOR

Families are adaptive, equilibrium-seeking systems. In accordance with their very nature, families never stay the same. They shift and change in response to internal and external forces. Internally, the family composition changes as new members are added or members leave through death or divorce. Roles and relationships change as members advance in age and experience; normative expectations change as members resolve their tensions and differing points of view. Externally, families are bombarded by influences from sources such as school, work, peers, neighbors, church, and government; consequently, they are forced to accommodate to new demands. Adapting to these influences may require a family to change its behavior, goals, and even its values. Like any system, the family needs a state of quasi-equilibrium in order to function (Neuman, 1989). Thus, with each new set of pressures, the family shifts and accommodates to regain balance and a normal life-style.

There are times when a family's capacity for adaptation is stressed beyond its limits. At this point the system may be in danger of disintegrating; that is, family members will leave or become dysfunctional because of unresolved stress. This is an indication that families may need some form of intervention to help restore family equilibrium. These interventions may take the form of extended family mediation or external professional help.

Community health nurses play an influential role in family equilibrium-seeking. Neuman describes the major goal of nursing as keeping the individual and family client systems stabilized within their environment (Neuman, 1989; Ross & Helmer, 1988). Chapter 17 explores the community health nurse's stabilizing interventions with families in detail.

GOAL-DIRECTED BEHAVIOR

Families as social systems are goal directed. Families exist for a purpose—to establish and maintain a milieu that promotes the development of their members. In order to fulfill this purpose, a family must perform basic functions such as providing love, security, identity, a sense of belonging, assistance with preparation for adult roles in society, and maintenance of order and control. In addition to these functions, each family member engages in tasks to maintain the family as a viable unit. Duvall and Miller describe specific functions and tasks for each stage of the family's development (1985). These functions and tasks will be examined in more detail later in this chapter.

Family Culture

Family culture is the acquired knowledge that family members use to interpret their experiences and to generate behaviors that influence family structure and function. The concept of family culture arises from a significant body of literature in the social and behavioral sciences of cross-cultural comparisons and in-depth analyses that demonstrates that each family has a "culture" that strongly influences its structure and function. Culture explains why families behave as they do (Helman, 1990; Lancaster et al., 1987; Leininger, 1991; Pender, 1987; van den Berghe, 1979). Family culture also gives the community health nurse a basis for assessing family health and designing appropriate interventions.

Three aspects of family culture deserve special consideration: (1) family members share certain values that affect family behavior; (2) certain roles are prescribed and defined for family members; (3) a family's culture determines its distribution and use of power.

SHARED VALUES AND THEIR EFFECT ON BEHAVIOR

Although families share many broad cultural values drawn from the larger society in which they live, they also develop unique variants. Every family has its own set of values and rules for operation that we can speak of as family culture (Barker, 1992). Some values will be explicitly stated: "Family matters must always stay within the family." Such values may give rise to specific operating rules: "Don't tell anyone about our problems."

Like all cultural values, however, many family values remain outside the conscious awareness of family members. These values, often not verbalized, become powerful determinants of what the family believes, feels, thinks, and does. Family values include those beliefs transmitted by previous generations, religious influences, immediate social pressures, and the larger society. Values become an integral part of a family's life and are very difficult to change. A family that values free expression for every member engages comfortably in loud, noisy debates. Another family that values quietness,

order, and control will not tolerate its members raising their voices. One family uses birth control based on beliefs about human life and parental responsibility; another family chooses not to use birth control because it holds a different set of values. How a family views education, health care, life style, courtship, marriage, child rearing, sex roles, or any of the myriad other issues requiring choices depends upon the cultural values of that family.

PRESCRIBED ROLES

Roles, the assigned or assumed parts that members play during day-to-day family living, are bestowed and defined by the family (Constantine, 1986; O'Grady Winston, 1989). For instance, in one family the father role assigned to the male adult may be defined as an authoritative one that includes establishing rules, judging behavior, and administering punishment for violation of rules. In another family, the father role may be defined primarily as that of a loving benefactor. If there is an absence of an immediate male parent, a grandfather, uncle, friend, or mother may take over the father role. Selection of specific roles to be played in any given family will vary depending on the family's structure, needs, and patterns of functioning. In a single-parent family, for example, the parent may need to assume the roles of mother, father, and breadwinner, as well as other roles.

Families distribute among their members' roles all the responsibilities and tasks necessary to conduct family living. The responsibilities of breadwinner and homemaker, for example, with their accompanying tasks, may belong to husband and wife, respectively, or may be shared if both husband and wife hold jobs outside the home. Older children may help younger ones with homework or entertain them. This relieves parents for other tasks and increases the responsibility of older children (see Fig. 16.2).

Family members play several roles at the same time, known as **intrarole functioning**. Often balancing intrarole functioning can be exceptionally taxing (O'Grady Winston, 1989). A woman, for instance, may play the role of wife to her husband, daughter to her mother who lives with her, and mother to each of her children. The mother role may involve taking on several additional roles and responsibilities and will vary with each child's needs. A single-parent family often combines the roles of father and mother in one person but may distribute responsibilities and tasks more widely. A grandmother or child(ren) may assume responsibility for

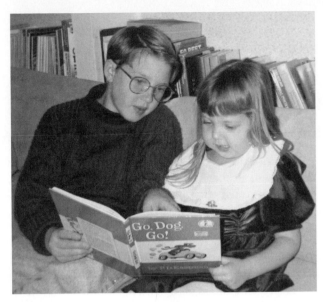

FIGURE 16.2. Family members all have assigned responsibilities. Older children often help with the care and training of their younger siblings. Here a young boy reads a story to his little sister.

some chores and thus relieve the demands placed on the single parent. Among families, there is great variation in expectations for each role and the degree of flexibility in role prescriptions. Consequently, a family may place great demands on some members, although those same members may interpret the expectations placed on them and their roles, differently. Confusion and conflict can develop unless roles are clarified.

Other roles of family members, extend beyond the immediate family. There may be extended family members nearby that interact with the family on a regular basis or only on special occasions such as birthdays. If both parents are employed, they may have an expansive social network from work or from within the neighborhood. Friendships are often made with the parents of the childrens' friends particularly if their children participate in the same extracurricular activities. Many families enjoy the fellowship of organized religious or cultural groups. This fellowship can be a source of support and comfort in addition to being an additional role function for the family members. Another intrarole function is that of community participant in activities separate from the family. These roles may revolve around local or regional politics, community improvement, volunteerism for non-profit agencies, or any

other service outside the home the community may offer. These diverse role relationships should enrich and energize the participants. However, many people may become over involved, thus creating an imbalance of role responsibilities that is draining and causes friction and stress. The community health nurse must work with families to achieve a balance of activities and roles to promote family health.

POWER DISTRIBUTION

Power, the possession of control, authority, or influence over others, assumes different patterns in each family. In some families, power is concentrated primarily in one member, while in others it is distributed on a more egalitarian basis. The traditional patriarchal family, in which the father holds absolute authority over the other members, is rare in American society. However, the pattern of husband as head of the household and dominant member of the family is still frequently seen. Whether male or female, the dominant partner holds the majority of the decision-making power, particularly over the more important family affairs, such as employment, financial matters, and sexual activity. Other areas of decision making, including choices about vacations, housing, leisure activities, household purchases, and child rearing, may be shared or delegated. With changing societal influences, however, the present trend among American families is toward egalitarian power distribution. Rudolf Dreikurs long ago advocated that families form a "family council" for shared decision making and distribution of tasks (1964). Today many families practice joint decision making and equal participation by all members. However, the community health nurse can suggest this activity for families not using such a method of shared decision making. Role playing this technique can be incorporated on a home visit or as a teaching technique with an aggregate group. Specific educational interventions are discussed in Chapter 14.

Roles often influence power distribution within the family. Along with the responsibilities attached to a role, a family may assign decision-making authority. The mother role frequently includes decision making regarding household management. A responsibility related to a son's role, such as lawn mowing, may empower him to decide when and how often he does the job.

Family power structure is also influenced by the amount of personal power residing in each member (Friedman, 1986). A mother or eldest son, for example, can exercise considerable influence over the family by virtue of personality and position rather than delegated authority. Even a child who throws temper tantrums can wield considerable power in a family.

Family Structures

Families are social systems with cultural dimensions, families are also tied biologically through kinship and socially through choice. This structure exists for a purpose. Duvall's definition nicely summarizes these aspects of the family: "The family is a unity of interacting persons related by ties of marriage, birth, or adoption, whose central purpose is to create and maintain a common culture which promotes the physical, mental, emotional, and social development of each of its members" (Duvall & Miller, 1985, p. 6). For many people, the term family evokes a picture of a husband, wife, and child(ren) living under one roof with the male as breadwinner and the female as homemaker.

This nuclear family was often seen as the norm for everyone. Variations from this pattern often were treated as deviant and abnormal even in studies of the family as recent as 1983 (Olson, et al.). However, unmarried people living together increased from 500,000 in 1970 to 2.8 million in 1989 (Saluter, 1992). There is every indication that this trend will continue into the 21st century. The traditional nuclear family has been a fundamental part of the European cultural heritage shared by many Americans, reinforced by religion, education, and other influential social institutions. But the pressures of changing social values and cultural lifestyles, such as women working outside the home, combined with the acceptance of alternative life-styles has changed the definition of family. Today definitions of family include a variety of households such as unmarried adults living together with or without children, single parent households, divorced couples who combine households with children from previous marriages (the blended family), and even homosexual couples with or without children. Each type of household requires recognition and acceptance by professionals who must help families achieve optimal health.

Families come in many shapes and sizes. The varying family structures or compositions fall into two general categories, traditional and nontraditional.

TRADITIONAL FAMILIES

Traditional family structures are those which are most familiar to us and which are readily accepted by society. They include the most familiar form of the nuclear family: husband, wife, and children all living together in the same household. In nuclear families, the workload distribution between the two adults can vary. Both adults can work outside the home; one adult can work outside the home and the other may stay at home and assume primary responsibilities for the household; or partners can alternate, constantly renegotiating work and domestic responsibilities. A nuclear-dyad family, consists of a husband and wife living together who have no children or who have grown children living outside the home. Traditional families also include **single-adult families** in which one adult is living alone either by choice to remain single or because of separation from spouse and/or children because of divorce, death, or distance from children. Some traditional families are **multigenerational families** in which several generations or age-groups live together in the same household, for example a household in which a widowed woman lives with her divorced daughter and two grandchildren, ages 7 and 3 (Jendrick, 1994). Sometimes, particularly in close-knit ethnic communities, we see families forming a **kin-network** in which several nuclear families live in the same household, or near one another, and share goods and services. They may own and operate a family business, sharing the work and child-care responsibilities, incomes and expenses, and maybe even meals. Variations of this trend are increasing among all groups as children postpone leaving home because of economic conditions, or educational plans; or an elderly parent may move into the adult child's home to recover from a recent illness.

Another deviation from the traditional nuclear family is the **blended family**. In this structure, divorced or widowed parents marry and raise the children from each of their previous marriages. They may be the custodial parents who have the children with them except for planned visits with the noncustodial parent or they may share custody so the children live in the blended arrangement only part-time. This couple may decide to have children from their union in addition to the children from each of their previous relationships.

Single-parent families include one adult (either father or mother) caring for a child or children as a result of separation, or divorce, from, or the death of, a spouse. In single-parent families, sometimes the parent is working and sometimes not, such as in situations where the wife has always stayed at home raising the children and is suddenly left alone with no job skills or career. There are other single-parent family situations that are nontraditional forms which are described in the next section.

One variant type of traditional family that is the **commuter family** in which both partners work but their jobs are in different cities. The pattern is usually for one partner (married or unmarried) to live and work and perhaps raise children in the "home" city while the second partner generally lives in the other city and commutes home for weekends or less frequent visits, depending on the distance. Sometimes this arrangement is short-term, as when one partner is transferred through work and the couple chooses not to move the rest of the family until the end of the school year. In other instances the commuting may continue for years. Clearly this arrangement influences family roles and functions, challenging a family's ability to maintain healthy relationships. A traditional family in which one partner is required to travel a great deal of the time for business or when one is caring for an ill family member at a distant location, may experience similar problems and stressors. Table 16.1 lists a number of traditional family structures.

NONTRADITIONAL FAMILIES

Families that do not fit the traditional nuclear model make up an increasing proportion of the American population. For instance, in 1960, legally married couples made up 75% of American households but by 1990 that number had dropped to nearly 50% (U. S. Bureau of Census, 1990). Fewer than 20% of American families now have a working father, a full-time homemaker mother, and one or more children. The number of couples who share a household without marrying increased more than five times between 1970 and 1989 (Saluter, 1992). As of 1990, approximately 25% (more than 20 million) of all families in the United States were headed by one adult, usually a woman. The number of single households headed by men has increased to 3% of all families, an increase from 2.1% in 1980. The proportion of children under 18 years of age who lived with one parent increased from 12% in 1970 to 25% in 1990 (U. S. Bureau of Census, 1990). Divorce is also changing family structures; half of all marriages now end in divorce (higher for teenage marriages) and the median duration of marriages is approximately seven years.

Nontraditional family structures include a variety of family forms; some of which are accepted by society and others are strongly questioned on the basis of illegitimate union. Table 16.1 lists some of the prominent nontraditional structures. One of the most common forms of nontraditional family seen today is the single-parent family headed by a woman. Sometimes this is by choice as in the cases of single women who decide to adopt or have children without being married. In most cases, though, this nontraditional form occurs when an unplanned pregnancy occurs and there is no marriage. Statistics indicate that the single-parent family is being headed more and more frequently by teenagers, with pregnancies in junior high school a common happening (U.S. Bureau of the Census, 1990). The implications for the role of community health nurse is greatest with this population.

Many adult couples form a family alliance outside of marriage or through a private ceremony not legally recognized as marriage. **Cohabitating couples** may range from young adults living together to an elderly couple sharing their lives outside of marriage to avoid tax penalties or inheritance issues. Cohabitating couples may be heterosexual or homosexual; they may or may not share a sexual relationship. In some instances, these couples have their own biological or adopted children.

Another nontraditional family form is the **commune family**, a group of unrelated, monogamous (married or committed to one person) couples living together and collectively rearing their children. A **group-marriage family** involves several adults who share a common household and consider that all are married to each other; they share everything, including sex and child rearing. This is different from polygamy were a spouse of either sex has more than one mate at a given time. These group-marriage families usually center around one main male patriarch who designates responsibilities and dictates to the other members some religious or social ideology. The Branch Davidians in Waco, Texas, and their group self-destruction in 1993 is an example of this family type that can become a negative experience for members.

A **group-network family** is made up of nuclear families, not related by birth or marriage, but bound by a common set of values such as a religious system who live close to each other and share goods, services, and child-rearing responsibilities. Some commune and

TABLE 16.1. *The Traditional and Nontraditional American Family*

Structure	Participants	Living Arrangements
TRADITIONAL		
Nuclear dyad	Husband Wife	Common household
Nuclear family	Husband Wife Children	Common household
Commuter family	Husband Wife Children (sometimes)	Household divided between two cities
Single-parent family	One adult (separated, divorced, widowed) Children	Common household
Divorced family (shared custody of children)	One adult parent, children part-time	Two separate households
Blended family	Husband Wife (His and/or hers, and possibly their children)	Common household
Single adult	One adult	Living alone
Multigenerational family	Any combination of the first four traditional family structure	Common household
Kin network	Two or more reciprocal households (related by birth or marriage)	Close geographic proximity
NONTRADITIONAL		
Unmarried single-parent family	One parent (never married) Children	Common household
Cohabitating couple	Two adults (heterosexual, homosexual, or "just friends") Children (possibly)	Common household
Commune family	Two or more monogamous couples Shared children	Common household
Group marriage commune family	Several adults "married" to each other Shared children	Common household
Group network	Reciprocal nuclear households or single members	Close geographic proximity
Homeless families	Any combination of "family members" previously mentioned	The streets and shelters
Foster families	Husband and wife or single adult Natural children (possibly) Foster children	Common household
Gangs	Males and Females usually of same cultural or ethnic background	Close geographic proximity (same neighborhood)

group-network families select one of their members, usually a male, to be their leader, or head.

Many children are removed from their homes of origin due to family stresses of abuse, violence, or neglect. In most communities these children are housed with families known as **foster families**. These families, may take a variety of forms, but all foster families have had formal training to accept unrelated children into their home on a temporary basis while the parent(s) of the foster child(ren) receive the help necessary to reunify the original family. While this arrangement is not ideal, most foster families provide a safe and loving home for these children in transition. Often the foster children have emotional and physical health problems; and they may never have experienced the structure foster families provide. These issues can cause stress for everyone involved, representing another area in which the community health nurse can intervene.

Some families, due to their lack of marketable skills, negative economic changes, or chronic mental health problems, including substance abuse, find themselves without permanent shelter. These **homeless families** are increasing in numbers and their characteristics are changing (Blau, 1992; Berg, 1994). More and more of the homeless population is made up of nuclear families or single parent families. This is different from the homeless population, as characterized years ago, by the single adult male who was "down on his luck"; or the war veteran who could not reenter society at a productive level. Frequently the community health nurse provides services to shelters or drop-in clinics frequented by the homeless. Since this population is increasing, it has many implications for the nurse.

A destructive form of "family" occurring in many major cities is the power and influence of gangs. **Gangs** are formed by young people searching for the emotional ties of family as a substitute for an absent or dysfunctional family. Gang members consider themselves family and go to each other or the group for support that they are not receiving from members of their family of origin. Obviously gangs are a dysfunctional and destructive form of family often drawing members into drugs and violence with frequent injury and even death to gang members and innocent bystanders (Bell & Jenkins, 1991). Many nurses serving the inner city may be working with families and groups who are involved with gangs and should be prepared to deal with the issues gangs create. (See the Issues in Community Health Nursing discussion that follows.)

IMPLICATIONS FOR THE COMMUNITY HEALTH NURSE

The variety of family structures raises three important issues for consideration. First, community health nurses can no longer hold to a myth that idealizes the traditional nuclear family. They must work with all these types of families and accept them as valid. Unless the community health nurse is able to accept both traditional and nontraditional family lifestyles and address the special problems and needs these lifestyles may present, the nurse may create more problems for those families.

Issues in Community Health Nursing
FACTS AFFECTING FAMILIES OF TODAY—SOCIETAL TRENDS

Families may be dealing with any of these issues, they all can impacts the stress level of the family unit and affect the role of the nurse.

- Five hundred thousand children are missing each year.
- There are 800,000 homeless single-head-of-household families (Berg, 1994).
- Two and a half million homeless persons exist in the United States; many of the "new homeless" include runaway teens, people with AIDS, and the aged displaced from their homes (Berg, 1994).
- More than three million children (3.3 million) live with their grandparents (Jendrek, 1994).
- There are increasing numbers of gay and lesbian couples co-parenting children (Wismont & Reame, 1989).
- Four hundred and sixty thousand children were in foster homes in 1991 (Chira, 1994).
- Violence is the third leading cause of death of children ages 5 to 14 (National Center for Health Statistics, 1993).
- Significant numbers of children are victims and perpetrators of violence through their connections with gangs; an increasing social problem just beginning to affect rural, as well as urban areas (Bell & Jenkins, 1991).
- Single Room Occupancy tenants in old hotels in deterioriating neighborhoods remain an underserved population, often with many physical and mental health needs (Rollinson, 1991)
- Spousal abuse is the leading cause of injury for women. One in every three women is assualted by her husband or male companion at least once during the relationship. (Grisso, et al., 1991)

Second, the nurse must realize that the structure of an individual's family may change several times over a member's lifetime. A girl may be born into a kin-network, shift to a nuclear family when her parents move and become part of a single-parent family when her parents are divorced. As she matures, she may become a single adult living alone, then become a part of a cohabitating couple, and still later, marry and have children in a nuclear family. For the individual, each variant family form involves changes in roles, interaction patterns, socialization processes, and linkages with external resources. The implications for the community health nurse are that the nurse must learn to address the client's needs throughout these life changes, equipping people with the flexibility needed to deal with the inevitability of changing structures.

Finally, the nurse must realize that each type of family structure creates different issues and problems that, in turn, influence a family's ability to perform its basic functions. Each particular structure determines the kind of support needed from nursing or other human service systems (Eliopoulos, 1993). A single adult living alone, for instance, may lack companionship or a sense of being needed by other family members. A kin-network family provides broad, extended family support and security but may have problems in power distribution and decision making. An unmarried couple raising a child may be parenting well but may feel isolated from other married couples in the community and need more peer support and socialization. Variations in structure create varitions in family strengths and needs, an important consideration for community health nurses.

Family Functions

Families in every culture throughout history have engaged in the same basic functions. In different societies these tasks have been performed in different ways. Nonetheless, families always have produced children, physically maintained their members, protected their health, given emotional support and acceptance, and provided supportive and nurturing care during illness (Johnson, 1987). Some societies have experimented with separation of these functions, allocating activities such as child care, socialization, or social control to a larger group. The Israeli kibbutz and Chinese commune are examples. Yet, for most peoples, the individual family unit (in its variant forms) persists, accompanied by most of the same basic functions. In American society, certain social institutions help perform some aspects of traditional family functions. Schools, for example, help socialize children; professionals supervise health care;

and churches influence values. Thus we see some modifications and overlap in patterns of functioning. Six functions are typical of American families today and are essential for maintenance and promotion of family health: (1) affection, (2) security, (3) identity, (4) affiliation, (5) socialization, and (6) controls (Duvall & Miller, 1985). Table 16.2 explains the families developmental tasks associated with these functions. These tasks help promote the growth and development of members.

AFFECTION

The family functions to give members affection and emotional support. Love brings couples together initially in our society and later produces children. In some cultures affection comes after marriage. Continued affection creates an atmosphere of nurturance and care for all family members that is necessary for health, development, and survival (Whitbourne, 1986; Grace, 1995). It is common knowledge that infants require love to thrive. Indeed, human beings of any age require love as sustenance for growth and find it most often in the family. Families, unlike many other social groups, are bound by affectionate ties whose strength determines family happiness and closeness. Consider how the sharing of gifts on a holiday or the loving concern of a family for a sick member draws the family together. Positive sexual identity and sexual fulfillment are also influenced by a loving atmosphere. Early students of the family emphasized sexual access and procreation as basic family functions. Now we recognize that families exist not only to regulate the sex drive and perpetuate the species but also to sustain life and foster human potential through a strong affectional climate (Lancaster et al., 1987).

PROVIDES SECURITY AND ACCEPTANCE

Families meet their members' physical needs by providing food, shelter, clothing, health care, and other necessities; in so doing, they create a secure environment. Members need to know that these basics will be available and that the family is committed to providing them.

The stability of the family unit also gives members a sense of security. The family offers a safe retreat from the competition of the outside world, a place where its members are accepted for themselves. They can learn, make mistakes, and grow in a secure environment.

TABLE 16.2. *Family Functions and Tasks*

Family Functions	Associated Developmental Tasks
Affection	Establishment of climate of affection Promotion of sexuality and sexual fulfillment Addition of new members
Security and acceptance	Maintenance of physical requirements Acceptance of individual members
Identity and satisfaction	Maintenance of motivation Self-image and role development Social placement and satisfying activities
Affiliation and companionship	Development of communication patterns Establishment of durable bonds
Socialization	Internalization of culture (values and behavior) Guidance for internal and external relationships Release of members
Controls	Maintenance of social control Division of labor Allocation and utilization of resources

Where else does the toddler, after repeated falls, receive the encouragement to keep trying to walk; or the child, teased by a bully, regain his courage; or a parent, feeling burned out on a job, find comfort and renewal? The dependability of the family unit promotes confidence and self-assurance among its members. This contributes to their mental and emotional health and equips them with the skills necessary to cope with the outside world.

INSTILLS IDENTITY AND SATISFACTION

The family functions to give members a sense of social and personal identity. From infancy on, the individual gains a sense of identity and worth from the family. Like a mirror, the family reflects back to its members a picture of who they are and how valuable they are to others. Positive reflections provide the individual with a sense of satisfaction and worth, such as that experienced by a girl when her family applauds her efforts in a swimming meet. Needs fulfillment in the home determines satisfaction in the outside world; it particularly affects other interpersonal relationships and career choices. Roles learned within the family also give members a sense of identity. A boy growing up and learning his family's expectations for the male role quickly develops a sense of the kind of person he must strive to

be; often, he is expected to be strong, competitive, successful, and unemotional (see Fig. 16.3). Families influence their members' positions in society by instilling values and goals. For some families the emphasis may be on higher education; for others it may be to work at a skill or trade. Still other families may be influenced by religious or political affiliations. Whatever the family influence, it is certain to shape each member's identity.

PROVIDES AFFILIATION AND COMPANIONSHIP

The family functions to give members a sense of belonging throughout life. Because families provide associational bonds and group membership, they help satisfy their members' needs for belonging. Each person knows that they are integral—that they belong—to their family. However, the quality of a family's communication influences its closeness. If communication patterns are effective, then affiliation ties are strong and needs for belonging are met. One family handles conflict over financial expenditures, for instance, by discussing differences and making compromises. Another family never resolves its financial conflicts because members keep spending selfishly and never discuss or reach compromises.

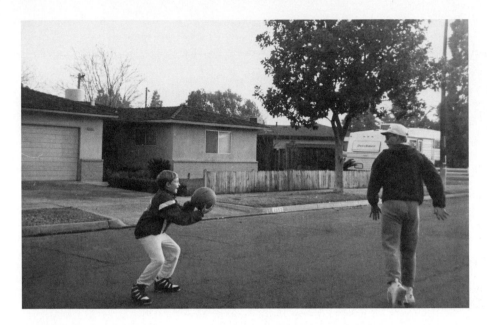

FIGURE 16.3. This boy has learned that sports are an important part of the male role.

The family, unlike other social institutions, involves permanent relationships. Long after friends from school, the old neighborhood, work, or church have come and gone, there is still the family. The family provides its members with affiliation and fellowship that remains unbroken by distance or time. Even when scattered across the country, family members will gather to support each other and to share in a holiday, wedding, graduation, or funeral. It is to the family that its members turn in times of happiness, tragedy, or need. This family affiliation remains a resource for life.

PROVIDES SOCIALIZATION

The family functions to socialize the young. Families transmit their culture—their values, attitudes, goals, and behavior patterns—to their members. Members, socialized into a way of life that reflects and preserves that family's cultural heritage, pass that heritage on, in turn, to the next generation. From infancy on, children learn to control their bowels, eat with utensils, dress themselves, manage emotions, and behave according to sociocultural prescriptions for their age and sex. Through this process, members also learn their roles in the family. Life-styles, the foods preferred, relationships with other people, ideas about child rearing, and attitudes about religion, abortion, equal rights, or euthanasia are all strongly influenced by the family. Although experiences outside of the family also have a strong influence on roles, those experiences are filtered through the perceptions acquired during early socialization.

The socialization process also influences the degree of independence experienced by growing children. Some families release their maturing members by degrees, preparing them early for adult roles. Other families promote dependent roles and find release painful and difficult.

ESTABLISHES CONTROLS

The family functions to maintain social control. Families maintain order through establishment of social controls both within the family and between family members and outsiders. Members' conduct is controlled by the family's definition of acceptable and not acceptable behaviors. From minor etiquette rules such as keeping elbows off the table to larger issues, such as standards of home cleanliness, appropriate dress, children's behavior towards adults, or a teenager's curfew, the family imposes limits. Then it maintains those limits by a system of rewards for conformity and punishments for violations. Children growing up in a family quickly learn what is "right" and what is "wrong" by family standards. Gradually family control shifts to self-control as members learn to discipline their own behaviors; later on, they will adopt or modify many of the same standards to use with their own children.

Division of labor is another aspect of the family's control function. Families allocate various roles, responsibilities, and tasks to their members in order to assure provision of income, household management, child care, and other essentials. Families also regulate the use of internal and external resources. The family identifies and directs the use of internal resources, such as member abilities, financial income, or material assets. For instance, if the man has artistic skills he may be chosen to landscape the yard, and if a woman has more mechanical aptitude she may be designated to repair appliances. One family may choose to drive an old car rather than buy a new one in order to spend more on entertainment.

Families also determine the external resources used by their members. Some families take advantage of the religious, health, and social services available to them in the community. They seek regular medical care, encourage their children to participate in scouting programs, become involved in church activities, or join a bowling league. Other families, either because they don't know about potential external resources available to them, or because they don't recognize those resources as having any value, limit their members' use of them.

Stages of the Family Life Cycle

Many of the characteristics and defined developmental stages of individual growth also apply to families. For example, it is known that families, while maintaining themselves as entities, change continuously. Families inevitably grow and develop as the individuals within them mature and adapt to the demands of successive life changes. A family's composition, set of roles, and network of interpersonal relationships change with the passage of time (Friedman, 1986). Family structures, too, vary with each stage of the family life cycle.

Consider the following example. The Jordans, a young married couple, concentrated on learning their respective roles of husband and wife and building a mutually satisfying marriage. With the birth of their first child, Scott, the family composition and relationships changed, and role transitions occurred. The Jordans were not only husband and wife but also father, mother, and son; the family had added three new roles. Within the next four years, two daughters, Lisa and Tammy, were born. The introduction of each new member not only increased family size but significantly reorganized family living. As Duvall and Miller (1985) point out, no

two children are ever born into precisely the same family. The children entered school; Mrs. Jordan went to work for a florist; and soon Scott was leaving for college. The Jordans, like every family, were moving through the family life cycle and, in so doing, were experiencing a series of developmental changes.

Changes in families tend to occur in a predictable and sequential pattern of stages known as the *family life cycle* (Ibid.). There are two broad stages: one of *expansion* as new members are added and roles and relationships are increased, and one of *contraction* as family members leave to start lives of their own. Within this framework of the expanding-contracting family are more specific stages that mark changing patterns in family growth and development. Family theorists describe similar stages in the family life cycle, which begins when two people become committed to each other, thereby forming their own family. This life cycle continues through the years of having, rearing, and launching children, to the empty nest stage, retirement years, and finally the death of one and then both partners (see Fig. 16.4).

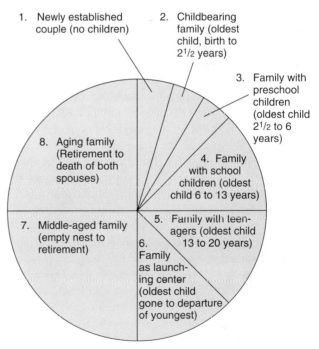

FIGURE 16.4. Duvall's eight stages of the nuclear family life cycle. Size of wedge reflects relative percent of total life cycle spent in each stage.

Duvall's model is most applicable to the traditional nuclear family structure. In this model the age of the oldest child serves as a criterion for demarcation between stages. A family enters the preschool stage, for instance, when the oldest child is 2 1/2 years of age and moves into the school stage when the oldest child is 6 years of age, even though the family may have other younger children. The size of each wedge in the circle reflects that stage's relative length. As a result of societal changes such as families postponing child rearing, having fewer children, and the elderly living longer, the child-rearing portion of life may be shrinking relative to the other of Duvall's stages. In addition, with the increasing numbers of divorces, remarriages, and blended families, many families do not conform to these sequential stages. There is an increase in the number of single young teens who are having babies. These child-mothers often stay with their parents who serve as primary caregivers. The young mother may prolong or perhaps never establish her own separate family. The grandparent(s) re-enter the child-rearing stages as they begin to care for grandchildren. One additional change in the Duvall stages has to do with increased longevity; elderly couples are living longer and thus spending a longer portion of their lives together alone.

FAMILY DEVELOPMENTAL TASKS

To progress through the stages of the life cycle, a family must carry out its basic functions and the developmental tasks associated with those functions (see Table 16.2). Unlike individual developmental tasks, which are specific to each age level, family developmental tasks are ongoing throughout the life cycle. All families, for instance, must provide for the physical needs of their members at every stage. The manner and degree to which each function is carried out will vary, however, depending on how well members are meeting their individual developmental tasks and on the demands of each particular stage. Physical maintenance, for example, will be affected by parents' ability to accept responsibility and seek out the necessary resources to provide food, clothing, and shelter for their children. At early stages, children will usually be dependent on their parents for meeting these needs; at the school, teenage, and launching stages, however, children may increasingly contribute to home management and family income. The responsibility for these tasks shifts from parents to other family members as well.

Some functions require greater emphasis at certain stages. Socialization, for example, consumes much of a family's time during the early years of member development. These same functions and their associated developmental tasks can be further broken down into actions specific to certain stages. A family, for example, while carrying out its function of maintaining controls, sets clearly defined limits for children at the preschool stage: "Do not cross the street." "You may have dessert only after you finish your vegetables." "Bedtime is at eight." During the school stage, control activities may center around allocating responsibilities and division of labor within the family: "Feed the dog." "Clean your room." "Take out the trash." When a family reaches the teenage stage, its control function increasingly focuses on the relationships between family members and outsiders. The family may regulate some activities by setting limits such as, "be home by midnight." In areas such as moral conduct, controls may involve family values and thus be more subtle. A family at this stage must recognize the need for young people to assume increasing responsibility for their own behavior with the complementary recognition of its own diminishing control over members. Duvall and Miller (1985) describe these activities as "stage-critical" family developmental tasks as seen in Table 16.3.

Emerging Family Patterns

Up to this point, the discussion of the family life cycle has focused primarily on the nuclear family. Since the nurse encounters many nuclear families in community health, the family life cycle provides a useful means for analyzing their growth and development.

Because of recent societal changes, today's community health nurses are facing increasing numbers of adolescent unmarried mothers, blended families, and elderly individuals living alone. Adolescent mothers are still undergoing emotional development themselves. They have limited parenting skills and need a tremendous amount of education and support. Merged or blended families require considerable adjustment and relearning of roles, tasks, communication patterns, and relationships (Settles, 1987). Elderly couples, or elderly individuals living alone or even those moving to a retirement center often feel isolated and cut off from meaningful contacts with friends and family. Many of

*TABLE 16.3. **Selected Stage-Critical Family Developmental Tasks***

Stage of Family Life Cycle	Family Position	Stage-Critical Family Developmental Tasks
Married couple	Wife Husband	Establishing a mutually satisfying marriage Adjusting to pregnancy and the promise of parenthood Fitting into the kin network
Childbearing	Wife-mother Husband-father Infant child(ren)	Having and adjusting to infants, and encouraging their development Establishing a satisfying home for both parents and infant(s)
Preschool-age	Wife-mother Husband-father Child, siblings	Adapting to the critical needs and interests of pre-school children in stimulating, growth-promoting ways Coping with energy depletion and lack of privacy as parents
School-age	Wife-mother Husband-father Child, siblings	Fitting into the community of school-age families in constructive ways Encouraging children's educational achievement
Teenage	Wife-mother Husband-father Child, siblings	Balancing freedom with responsibility as teenagers mature and emancipate themselves Establishing outside interests and careers as growing parents
Launching center	Wife-mother-grandmother Husband-father-grandfather Child, sibling, aunt or uncle	Releasing young adults into work, military service, college, marriage, etc., with appropriate rituals and assistance Maintaining a supportive home base
Middle-aged parents	Wife-mother-grandmother Husband-father-grandfather	Rebuilding the marriage relationship Maintaining kin ties with older and younger generations
Aging family members	Widow or widower Wife-mother-grandmother Husband-father-grandfather	Adjusting to retirement Coping with bereavement and living alone Closing the family home or adapting it to aging

these aging families do not understand or practice the appropriate stage-specific functions and developmental tasks that would help them adjust and experience positive aging. The community health nurse needs to understand the complex dynamics of such situations and offer support and encouragement as family members work through these problems.

Family theorists have yet to describe nonnuclear family stages in any systematic fashion. Even definitions of a family eludes many researchers because of the many variances and exceptions to traditional definitions. The approach used by Scanzoni, et al, (1989) is to consider the **primary relationship** of two or more persons interacting in a continuing manner within the greater environment. This primary relationship encompasses all the possible family structures. Stein (1981) suggests the notion of a "life-spiral" rather than a life-

cycle pattern to more realistically describe the fluctuations of contemporary nontraditional families. The spiral more realistically depicts the fluid-like movement within family structures than a cycle which provides a picture of a continuous linear movement along a path. Traditional functions and structures of the family continue to evolve as new combinations of people live together and consider their relationship that of a "family" (Macklin, 1987).

Divorce and remarriage are more frequent occurrences today than in previous generations. Many children living in these merged or blended families are required to master another set of roles. There are identifiable phases that occur in divorce, remarriage, and the blending of families; each phase has its own emotional transitions and developmental issues. Tables 16.4 and 16.5 show these phases.

*TABLE 16.4. **When Families Divorce***

Phase	Emotional Responses	Transitional Issues
1. Stressors leading to marital differenced	Reveal the fact that the marriage has major problems	Accepting fact that marriage has major problems
2. Decision to divorce	Accepting the inability to resolve marital differences	Accepting one's own contribution to the failed marriage
3. Planning the dissolution of the family system	Negotiating viable arrangements for all members within the system	Cooperating on custody visitation, and financial issues Informing and dealing with extended family members and friends
4. Separation	Mourning loss of intact family Working on resolving attachment to spouse	Develop coparental arrangements/relationships Restructure living arrangements Adapt to living apart Realign relationship with extended family and friends Begin to rebuild own social network
5. Divorce	Continue working on emotional recovery by overcoming hurt, anger or guilt	Giving up fantasies of reunion Staying connected with extended families Rebuild and strengthen own social network
6. Post-divorce	Separate feelings about ex-spouse from parenting role Prepare self for possibility of changes in custody as child(ren) get older, be open to their needs Risk developing a new intimate relationship	Make flexible and generous visitation arrangements for child(ren) and non-custodial parent and extended family members Deal with possibilities of changing custody arrangements as child(ren) get older Deal with child(ren)s reaction to parents establishing relationships with new partners

Summary

Community health nurses' effectiveness in working with families depends on their understanding of family theory and characteristics, in addition to the changing family structures of today.

Every family is unique; its needs and strengths are different from those of every other family. At the same time, each family is alike because of certain shared universal characteristics. Five of these universals have particular significance for community health nursing.

Every family is a small social system. All the members within a family are interdependent; what one does affects the others and, ultimately, influences total family health. Families, as social systems set and maintain boundaries that unite them and preserve their autonomy while also differentiating them from others. Because these boundaries are semipermeable, families engage in an input-output energy exchange with external resources. Families are equilibrium-seeking and adaptive systems that strive to adjust to internal and external life changes. Also, like other systems, families are goal directed. They exist for the purpose of promoting their members' development.

Every family has its own culture, its own set of values and rules for operation. Family values influence member beliefs and behaviors. These same values prescribe the types of roles that each member assumes. A family's culture also determines its power distribution and decision-making patterns.

TABLE 16.5. *Remarriage and Blending Families*

Phases	Emotional Responses	Developmental Issues
1. Meeting new people	Allowing for the possibility of developing a new intimate relationship	Dealing with child(ren) and exfamily members reactions to a parent "dating"
2. Entering a new relationship	Completing an "emotional recovery" from past divorce Accepting one's fears about developing a new relationship Working on feeling good about what the future may bring	Recovery from loss of marriage is adequate Discovering what you want from a new relationship Working on openness in a new relationship
3. Planning a new marriage	Accepting one's fears about the ambiguity and complexity of entering a new relationship such as: New roles and responsibilities Boundaries; space, time, and authority Affective issues: guilt, loyalty, conflicts, unresolvable past hurts	Recommitment to marriage and forming a new family unit. Dealing with stepchild(ren) as custodial or non-custodial parent Planning for maintenance of coparental relationships with ex-spouses Planning to help child(ren) deal with fears, loyalty conflicts and membership in two systems Realignment of relationships with exfamily to include new spouse and child(ren)
4. Remarriage and blending of families	Final resolution of attachment to previous spouse Acceptance of new family unit with different boundaries	Restructuring family boundaries to allow for new spouse or stepparent Realignment of relationships to allow intermingling of systems Expanding relationships to include all new family members Sharing family memories and histories to enrich members lives

Every family has structure that can be categorized as either traditional or nontraditional. The most common traditional family structure is the nuclear family, consisting of husband, wife, and children living together. Other traditional structures include husband and wife living as a couple alone, single-parent families, single-adult families, multigenerational families, kin networks, and blended families. Nontraditional family structures incorporate many family forms, some accepted by society and others not easily accepted. These variations include commune families, group marriages, group networks, unmarried single-parent families, and unmarried gay or straight couples living together with or without children. Variant family structures remind us that the nuclear family is no longer the only viable family form, that people experience many family structures during their lifetimes, and that a family's ability to perform its basic functions is influenced by its structure.

Every family has certain basic functions: (1) provides its members affection and emotional support; (2) promotes security by providing an accepting, stable environment in which physical needs are maintained; (3) provides its members a sense of social and personal identity, and influences their placement in the social order; (4) provides members with affiliation, a sense of belonging; (5) socializes its members by teaching basic values and attitudes that determine their behavior; and (6) establishes social controls to maintain order.

Every family moves through stages in its life cycle. Families develop in two broad stages: a period of expansion when they add new members and roles and a period of contraction when members leave. More specific developmental stages within this expanding-contracting framework for the nuclear family include eight stages ranging from the newly established couple through childbearing, child rearing, and child launching, to middle and old age.

While advancing through each developmental stage in the life cycle, a family must continue to perform all of its basic functions. It must also accomplish certain tasks specific to each stage. Life cycle stages and developmental tasks vary for families with differing structures.

There are emerging family patterns that influence the role of the community health nurse. More complex liv-ing arrangements are created by divorce, remarriage, and the blending of families. The single adolescent par-ent needs the community health nurse's knowledge of family developmental theory; as do older adults who are living longer, and whose population is growing.

Activities to Promote Critical Thinking

1. Within a small group of your colleagues, individually define "family" and then compare each of your definitions. How alike and how different is each definition? What in each persons background contributes to the differences in the definitions?

2. Select two families (other than your own), one traditional and the other nontraditional, that you know well and analyze them, answering the following questions:
   a. If the major breadwinner in this family became permanently disabled and unable to work, or lost their source of income, how would the family most likely respond—im-mediately and in the long run?
   b. What are some of this family's rules for operating and the values underlying those rules?
   c. Structurally, what kind of family is it?
   d. What are the strongest and weakest functions performed by this family and why do you think so?
   e. In what developmental stage is this family and how does that affect its functioning?

3. Talk with the members of a blended family and discuss with each member their rela-tionships with step-children or siblings, half-siblings, and step-parent. What problems do they identify? What are the positive elements of the union as they see it?

4. Gay and lesbian couples often seek parenting opportunities. How do you feel about this? What makes you feel this way? What are the positive and negative aspects of a child being raised by a homosexual couple?

REFERENCES

Baranowski, T., & Nader, P. (1985). Family health behavior. In D. Turk & R. Kerns (Eds.), *Health, illness, and families.* New York: Wiley.

Barker, P. (1992). *Basic Family Therapy* (3rd ed.). New York: Oxford University Press.

Bell, C.C. & Jenkins, E. J. (1991). Traumatic stress and chil-dren. Third national conference: Health care for the poor and underserved "Children at risk" (1991, Nashville). *Jour-nal of Health Care for the Poor and Underserved, 2*(1), 175–185.

Bell, J. M. & Wright, L.M. (1993). Flaws in family nursing ed-ucation. In G. Wegner & R. Alexander (Eds.), *Readings in Family Nursing.* (pp. 390–4) Philadelphia: Lippincott.

Berg, M. A. (1994). Health problems of sheltered homeless women and their dependent children. *Health and Social Work, 19*(2), 125–131.

Blau, J. (1992). *The visable poor: Homelessness in the United States.* New York: Oxford.

Chira, S. (1994). Starting point: Meet needs of our young chil-dren. *Capitol Bulletin,* #635: The Minnesota Women's Con-sortium, May 4, 1994

Clark, J. (1986). Supporting the family . . . heading off a breakdown. *Nursing Times, 82*(32), 33–34.

Constantine, L. L.(1986). *Family paradigms: The practice of theory in family therapy.* New York: Guilford.

Dreikurs, R. (1964). *Children: The challenge.* New York: Meredith.

Duvall, E. M., & B. Miller. (1985). *Marriage and family devel-opment* (6th ed.). New York: Harper & Row.

Eliopoulos, C. (1993). *Gerontological Nursing* (3rd ed.). Philadelphia: Lippincott.

Friedman, M. M. (1986). *Family nursing: Theory and as-sessment* (2nd ed.). Norwalk, CT: Appleton-Century-Crofts.

Grace, J.J. (1995). Families and nurses: Building partnerships for growth and health. *Journal of Obstetric, Gynecologic, and Neonatal Nursing 24*(4), 298–300.

Grisso, J.A., Wishner, A.R., Schwarz, D.F., Weene, B.A., Holme, J.H., & Sutton, R.L. (1991). A population-based study of injuries in inner-city womrn. *American Journal of Epidemiology, 134,* 59–68.

Helman, C. G. (1990). *Culture, health, and illness* (2nd ed.). Kent, England: Wright.

Jendrick, M. P. (1994). Grandparents who parent their children: Circumstances and decisions. *The Gerontologist, 34*(2), 206–216.

Johnson, R. (1987). Family developmental theories. In Stanhope, M. & Lancaster, J. (Eds.). *Community health nusing: Process and practices for promoting health* (2nd ed.). St. Louis: The C.V. Mosby Co.

Kerr, M. (1988). *Family Evaluation: An approach based on Bowen theory.* New York: Norton.

Lancaster, J. B., Altmann, J., Rossi, A.S., & Sherrod, L.R. (1987). *Parenting across the life span.* New York: Aldine de Gruyter.

Leininger, M. (1991). *Culture, care, diversity, and university: A theory of nursing.* Pub. #15-2402. New York: National League for Nursing.

Macklin, E. D.(1987). Nontraditional family forms. In M.B. Sussman & S.K. Steinmetz (Eds), *Handbook of marriage and the family* (pp. 317–345). New York: Plenum Press.

National Center for Health Statistics (1993) Public Health Service, U.S. Department of Health and Human Services Advance report of final mortality statistics, 1991. *Monthly Vital Statistics Report, 42*(2), 21.

Neuman, B. (1989). *The Neuman systems model: Application to nursing education and practice* (2nd ed.). Norwalk, CT: Appleton and Lange.

O'Grady Winston, K.(1989) Family roles. In P.J. Bomar (Ed.) *Nurses and Family Health Promotion: Concepts, Assesment, and Interventions.*(pp. 55–66). Baltimore: Williams and Wilkins.

Olson, D., McCubbin, H.I. & Associates. (1983). *Families: What makes them work.* Beverly Hills, CA: Sage.

Pender, N. J.(1987). *Health promotion in nursing practice* (2nd ed.) Norwalk, CT: Appleton and Lange.

Rollinson, P. A. (1991). Elderly single room occupancy (SRO) hotel tenants: Still alone. *Social Work, 36*(4), 303–308.

Ross, M. M. & Helmer, H. (1988). A comparative analysis of Neuman's model using the individual and family as the units of care. *Public Health Nursing, 5*(1), 30–36.

Saluter, A. F. (1992). Marital status and living arrangements: March 1991. In *Current Population Reports, Population Characteristics.* Washington, DC: U.S.Bureau of the Census, series P-20, No.461.

Satir, V. (1972). *Peoplemaking.* Palo Alto: Science and Behavior Books.

Scanzoni,J., Polonko, K., Teachman, J., & Thompson, L. (1989). *The sexual bond· Rethinking family and close relationships.* Newbury Park, CA: Sage Publications.

Schultz, P. R. (1987). When client means more than one: Extending the foundational concept of person. *Advances in Nursing Science, 10*(1), 71–88.

Settles, B. H. (1987) A perspective of tomorrow's families. In M.B. Sussman, & S.K. Steinmetx (Eds.). *Handbook of marriage and the family* (pp. 157–80). New York: Plenum Press.

Stein, P. J. (Ed.). (1981). *Single life: Unmarried adults in social context.* New York: St. Martin's.

U.S. Bureau of Census. (1990). *Current population reports: Marital status and living arrangements.* Washington, DC: U.S. Department of Commerce.

van den Berghe, P. L. (1979). *Human family systems: An evolutionary view.* New York: Elsevier North Holland.

Whitbourne, S. K. (1986). *Adult development.* New York: Praeger.

Wismont, J.M. & Reame, N.E. (1989). A lesbian childbearing experience: Assessing developmental tasks. *Image: Journal of Nursing Scholarship, 21,* 137–141.

SELECTED READINGS

Ahrons, C. R. & Rodgers, R.H. (1987). *Divorced families: A multidisciplinary developmental view.* New York: W.W. Norton Company.

Benner, P. & Wrubel, J. (1989) *The primacy of caring.* Menlo Park, CA: Addison-Wesley.

Burton, L. M. (1992). Black grandparents rearing chldren of drug-addicted parents: Stressors, outcomes and the social service needs. *The Gerontologist, 32,* 744–751.

Combrinck-Graham, L. (1985). A developmental model for family systems. *Family Process, 24*(2), 139–50.

Deevey, S. (1989). When mom or dad comes out, helping adolescents cope with homophobia. *Journal of Psychosocial Nursing, 27*(10), 33–36.

Duvall, E. M. (1988). Family development's first forty years. *Family Relations, 37,* 127–134.

Erikson, E. (1963). *Childhood and society* (2nd ed.). New York: Norton.

Forchuk, C. & Dorsay, J.P. (1995). Hildegard Peplau meets family system nursing: Innovation in theory-based practice. *Journal of Advanced Nursing 21,* 110–115.

Hairston, C. F. (1988). Family ties during imprisonment: Do they influence future criminal activity? *Federal Probation, 52,* 48–52.

Havighurst, R. J. (1972). *Developmental tasks and education* (3rd ed.). New York: McKay.

Jendrek, M. P. (1993). Grandparents who parent their grandchildren: Effects on lifestyle. *Journal of Marriage and the Family, 55,* 609–621.

Kiesler, C.A. (1991). Homelessness and public policy priorities. *American Psychologist, 46,* 1245–52.

Keshet, J. K. (1988). The remarried couple: Stresses and successes. In W.R. Beer (Ed). *Relative strangers: Studies of stepfamily processes.* Totowa, NJ: Rowman and Littlefield.

Kowal, K. A. & Schilling, K. M. (1985). Adoption through the eyes of adult adoptees. *American Journal of Orthopsychiatry, 55,* 354–362.

Kozol, J. (1988). *Rachel and her children: Homeless families in America.* New York: Crown Publishers.

Leavitt, M. (1982). *Families at risk: Primary prevention in nursing practice.* Boston: Little, Brown.

Mathabane, G. (1992). Our biracial family. *American Baby, 54*(7), 58,86,88.

Mills, D. (1984). A model for stepfamily development. *Family Relations, 33,* 365.

Phillips, J. R. (1993). Changing family patterns and health. *Nursing Science Quarterly, 6*(3), 113–4.

Piaget, J. (1973). *The psychology of intelligence.* Totowa, NJ: Littlefield, Adams.

Sachdev, P. (1989). *Unlocking the adoption files.* Lexington, MA: Lexington Books.

Spradley, J.P. & McCurdy, D.W. (1980). *Anthropology: The cultural perspective* (2nd ed.). New York: Wiley.

Family Health: Assessment and Practice

LEARNING OBJECTIVES

Upon completion of this chapter, the student should be able to:

- Describe the effect of family health on individual health and community health.
- Describe individual and group characteristics of a healthy family.
- Describe three conceptual frameworks that can be used to assess a family.
- Describe the 12 major assessment categories for families.
- List the five basic principles the community health nurse should follow when assessing family health.

KEY TERMS

- Developmental framework
- Eco-map
- Family health
- Family nursing
- Genogram
- Interactional framework
- Social support network map
- Strengthening
- Structural functional framework

Barbara Walton Spradley and Judith Ann Allender
COMMUNITY HEALTH NURSING: CONCEPTS AND PRACTICE, 4th ed.
© 1996 Barbara Walton Spradley and Judith Ann Allender

Community health nursing has a long history of concern for family health. During the nineteenth century, public health nurses became aware through home visits of the significant influence that the family had on individual's health and on the health of the larger community. For example, many of the sick poor failed to recover because they lacked resources and support from their families, and these needy families, in turn, drained existing community resources. Nurses began to view client care from the more holistic perspective of family care. Nursing educators, as early as 1919, were introducing concepts of family care into the curricula (Ford, 1973). By 1932, the National Organization of Public Health Nursing strongly declared that family health was the cardinal concern of all public health nursing practice. *Healthy People 2000: National Health Promotion and Disease Prevention Objectives* identified families as the bedrock of our society (USPHS, 1990). The report focuses on promoting the health of and preventing diseases in individuals within families; health within that setting is a priority for all ages (infants, children, adolescents, adults, and older adults) and in all settings (work, school, and at home).

Although community health nursing continues to emphasize the family as a unit of service, a gap exists between family nursing theory, development, and practice (Kristjanson & Chalmers, 1991). The problem derives in part from a health care system that fosters an individualistic orientation, often to the exclusion of the family. There is a proliferation of programs geared to individuals in specific age groups or with specific health problems. Many third-party payers and reimbursement policies impose limits on the kinds of services funded, most of which are for individuals. Even public health agencies tend to organize their services around individuals. Often in response to governmental requirements, they must keep statistical records on specific disease or service categories, thus reflecting an individual, rather than family or aggregate, orientation. Family-level problem solving techniques are needed to deal with many important health issues including health promotion, pregnancy and childbirth, acute life threatening illness, chronic illness, substance abuse, and terminal illness (Cox & Davis, 1993). Community health nurses need to focus their practice on a family and aggregate approach, an approach that has proved to be more beneficial both to individual clients and the community-at-large.

Impact of Family Health and Nursing

Family health is how well the family functions together as a unit and involves not only the health of each member and how they relate to other members but how well they relate and cope with the community outside the family. In fact, family health, like individual health, ranges along a continuum from wellness to illness. A family may be at one point on that continuum now and at a much different point six months from now. Family health refers to the health status of a given family at a given point in time.

Family nursing is practice or intervention that focuses on the family as a unit; the family is the client. Much research has demonstrated that families behave as units and need to be viewed in totality for therapy to be effective (Whall, 1987; Cox & Davis, 1993). The family (as discussed in Chapter 16) is a separate entity with its own structure, functions, and needs. In every society throughout history, the family is the most basic unit; so too in community health (Kristjanson & Chalmers, 1991). It is the family, more than any other societal institution, that nurtures and shapes a society's members (see Fig. 17.1).

EFFECTS OF FAMILY HEALTH ON INDIVIDUAL HEALTH

The health of each family member affects the other members and contributes to the total family's level of health. Following her husband's stroke, for example, a woman may cope successfully with the resulting physical and emotional demands of his care but have inadequate reserves to effectively meet the needs of her children. The level at which a family functions—how well it is able to solve problems and help its members reach their potential—significantly affects the individual's level of health (Gillis, et al., 1989). A healthy family will foster individual growth and resistance to ill health and sustain its members during times of crisis such as serious illness, emotional dilemmas, divorce, or death of a family member. On the other hand, a family with limited capacity for problem solving and self-management is often unable to promote the potential of its members or assist them in times of need.

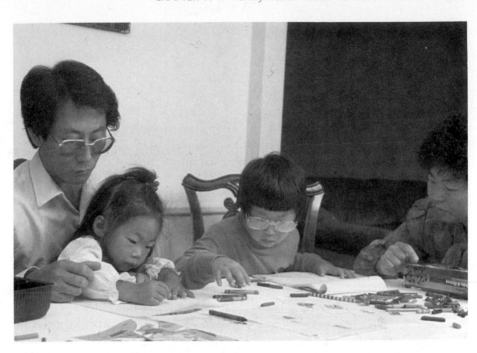

FIGURE 17.1. The family, as the most basic societal unit, profoundly affects its members.

Family health standards and practices influence each member's health. For instance, many individuals, even as adults, adhere to family patterns of eating, exercise, and communication. Family values influence decisions about health services such as whether or not a child receives immunizations or uses preventative measures such as regular visits to the doctor or birth control. Family health patterns also dictate whether members participate in their own health care and follow through and comply with professional advice. It is clear that individuals influence family health and that the family can either obstruct or facilitate individual health. The family, then, becomes an important focus for community health nursing assessment and intervention.

EFFECTS OF FAMILY HEALTH ON COMMUNITY HEALTH

Rarely do families live in isolation from one another. Even in the most uncommunicative of neighborhoods, one family's noisy children, another family's trash-littered yard, and another's barking dog all have an impact on the surrounding families. The level at which each family functions determines whether or not it can promote a healthier community and support other families and groups rather than merely remain a liability (Fox, 1989).

Healthy families influence community health positively. Some families, for example, have temporarily housed Southeast Asian or Cuban refugees and assisted them in finding employment. Others have formed community groups to encourage neighborhood safety and beautification. Many families are regularly involved in church, scouting programs, or various civic activities, such as parent-teacher-student associations, all of which work toward the common good.

Conversely, families with a low level of health have a negative influence on community health. Because they lack the resources to manage their own affairs, frequently they create problems and even health hazards for others. Garbage left to accumulate in a backyard, for example, attracts rats; abandoned appliances may become death traps for playing children. Regardless of socioeconomic level, a poorly functioning family becomes a drain on community resources and a threat to community health. Consider the large proportion of tax dollars and private funds that go into remedial programs for children with learning and behavior difficulties caused by problems at home, for adults with mental health problems, for the chemically dependent, and for victims of family violence—groups significantly influenced by unhealthy families. Since family health affects the health of other families, groups, and communities, nurses who help families develop and maintain positive health patterns and practices are also promoting community health.

Characteristics of Healthy Families

How does the community health nurse determine family health status? Analysis of a family in terms of how it meets its basic functions does not give a satisfactory picture of its health status. More definitive criteria are needed. Although it is difficult to define a "normal" family, studies have given some standards to determine if a family is healthy (Barker, 1992). Over the years, research on families, and particularly on family health behavior, has produced a growing body of data with which to assess family health.

Some researchers believe if couples have a healthy relationship they are likely to have healthy families. Beavers (1985) observed the following behavior patterns in healthy couples: a modest overt power difference, the capacity for clear boundaries, operating mainly in the present, respect for individual choice, skill in negotiating, and sharing positive feelings.

In looking at families, researchers have found many similar characterisitcs. Otto (1973) found characteristics of family unity, loyalty and interfamily cooperation, support and security, role flexibility, and constructive relationships with community. Becvar and Becvar (1988) found characteristics of (1) a legitimate source of authority that is supported and consistent over time, (2) a stable and consistent system of rules, (3) consistent and regular nurturing behaviors, (4) effective child rearing practices, (5) stable and well-maintained marriages, (6) a set of agreed-upon goals toward which the family and individual work, and (7) sufficient flexibility to change in the face of both expected and unexpected stressors. Olson, McCubbin, and Associates (1983) identified seven major family strengths important for family functioning and coping with crises: family pride, family support, cohesion, adaptability, communication, religious orientation, and social support.

Other researchers have identified various characteristics, such as showing respect and appreciation for one another (Stinnett, 1981), spending time together, having a strong religious orientation, dealing with crises positively (McCubbin, et al., 1982), having a sense of unity and commitment to one another (Peitze, 1984), and good communication patterns (Gilliss, et al., 1989).

Results from a White House Conference on Families survey defined "strong" families as (1) families that highly value their relationships and (2) families whose members support each other through good and bad times (Tanner-Nelson & Banonis, 1981). Hanson (1986) investigated the characteristics of healthy single-parent families and found that good communication, social support, and spirituality correlated with physical and mental health of the parent and children.

The recent literature on families concludes that healthy families have the following six important characteristics (Duffy, 1988; Duvall & Miller, 1985; Friedman, 1986; Gillis, et al., 1989; Olson, et al., 1983; Olson, 1991; Otto, 1973):

1. There is a facilitative process of interaction among family members.
2. They enhance individual member development.
3. Their role relationships are structured effectively.
4. They actively attempt to cope with problems.
5. They have a healthy home environment and lifestyle.
6. They establish regular links with the broader community.

HEALTHY INTERACTION AMONG MEMBERS

Healthy families communicate. Their patterns of interaction are regular, varied, and supportive. Adults communicate with adults, children with children, and adults with children. These interactions are frequent and assume many forms. Healthy families use frequent verbal communication. They discuss problems, confront each other when angry, share ideas and concerns, and write or call each other when separated. They also communicate frequently through nonverbal means, particularly those families from cultural or subcultural groups that are less verbal. There are innumerable ways—smiling encouragingly, embracing warmly, frowning disapprovingly, being available, withdrawing for privacy, doing an unsolicited favor, serving refreshments, giving a gift—to convey feelings and thoughts without words. The family that has learned to communicate effectively has members who are sensitive to each other. They watch for cues and verify messages in order to assure understanding. This kind of family recognizes and deals with conflicts as they arise. Its members have learned to share and to work collaboratively with each other (see Fig. 17.2).

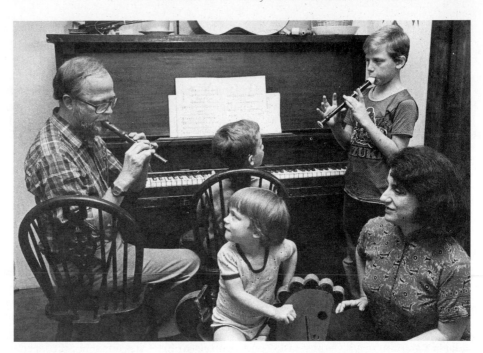

FIGURE 17.2. Healthy families share hobbies and leisure activities.

Effective communication is necessary for a family to carry out its basic functions. To demonstrate affection and acceptance, to promote identity and affiliation, and to guide behavior through socialization and social controls, family members must communicate. Like the correlation between a high degree of communication and a high degree of effectiveness in organizational functioning, families' facilitative communication patterns promote the health and development of their members (Schwebel & Fine, 1994). Huntley and Konetsky (1992) found that healthy families were more likely than unhealthy families to negotiate topics for discussion, use humor, show respect for differences of opinion, and clarify the meaning of each others' communications.

ENHANCEMENT OF INDIVIDUAL DEVELOPMENT

Healthy families are responsive to their individual members' needs and provide the freedom and support necessary to promote each member's growth. If a father in a healthy family loses his job, his family will work to support his ego and help him use his energy constructively to adjust and find new work. The healthy family recognizes the growing child's need for independence, and fosters it through increasing opportunities for the child to try new things alone. This kind of family can tolerate differences of opinion or life-style. It is able to accept each member unconditionally and respect each one's right to be his or her own self. Within an appropriate framework of stability and structure, the healthy family encourages freedom and autonomy for its members (Friedman, 1986).

Patterns for promoting individual member development will vary from one family to another, depending on its cultural orientation. The way autonomy is expressed in an Italian-American family will differ from its expression in a Native American family, yet each family can promote freedom and autonomy. The result is an increase in competence, self-reliance, social skills, intellectual growth, and overall capacity for self-management among family members (Gillis, et al., 1989; Wright & Leahey, 1994).

EFFECTIVE STRUCTURING OF RELATIONSHIPS

Healthy families structure their role relationships to meet changing family needs over time (Olson, 1991). In a stable social context, some families may establish member roles and tasks, such as breadwinner, primary decision maker, and homemaker, that are maintained as workable patterns throughout the life of the family. Families in rural areas, isolated communities, or religious and subcultural groups are more likely than others to retain role consistency because they face few, if any, external pressures or needs to change. The Amish communities in the midwest have maintained marked differentiation in family roles for more than 100 years.

In a technologically advanced industrial society such as the United States has, however, most families must adapt their roles to be consistent with changing family needs created by external forces. As women enter the work force, for instance, family roles, relationships, and tasks must change to meet the demands of the new situation. Many husbands assume more homemaking responsibilities; fathers engage in child rearing; children, along with the adults in their families, share decision making and a more equal distribution of power. The latter may be essential for the survival of a single-parent family in which the children must assume adult responsibilities while the parent is working to support the family (Hanson, 1986; Hetherington, 1989).

Changing life cycle stages require alterations in the structuring of relationships. The healthy family recognizes its members' changing developmental needs and adapts parenting roles, family tasks, and controls to fit each stage (Huntley & Konetsky, 1992). Household chores of increasing complexity and responsibility are assigned as children become capable of handling them. Rules of conduct relax as members learn to govern their own behavior.

ACTIVE COPING EFFORT

Healthy families actively attempt to overcome life's problems and issues. When faced with change, they assume responsibility for coping and seek energetically and creatively to meet the demands of the situation (Olson, et al., 1983).

Sometimes coping skills are needed for families to deal with emotional tragedies such as substance abuse problems, serious illness, or death. When it is known that a family member has a substance abuse problem the family will seek counseling and treatment opportunities involving all family members. If a family member is seriously ill, the family will ask for and accept assistance from extended family members or community health care workers. In the event of a death in the family, receiving consolation and support from one another and from relatives and friends is an important step in the healing process after a loss. The healthy family recognizes the need for assistance, accepts help, and pur-sues opportunities to eliminate or decrease the stressors which affect them.

More frequently healthy families cope with less dramatic, day to day changes. One family may cope with the increased cost of food by cutting down on meat con-

sumption, substituting other protein foods, and eating less frequently at restaurants. Healthy families are open to their innovative members and support new ideas and ways to solve problems. One family may try to solve the problem of spending too much on transportation by cutting down on daily travel; this may cause additional problems if three members have jobs in different areas of town, or need to go to school functions and meetings. Another family, responding to environmental concerns and a personal need for a healthier life style, may explore and arrive at new ways to reach their destinations by walking, bicycling, skating, or car pooling to school or work. Healthy coping may go beyond finding a simple obvious solution. Members may try to rearrange schedules to avoid frequency of trips to regular destinations; and plan ahead to avoid last-minute trips to stores. Healthy families actively seek and use a variety of resources to solve problems. They may discover these resources within the family or they may find them externally; they engage in self-care. For example, a professional couple faced with the unaffordable expense of daytime baby-sitting arranged their work schedules so that they could share child-care during the first two years and later joined a cooperative preschool that allowed their child to attend daily but required parental participation only one day a week. In another example, a single parent of five children who was also a full time nursing student was able to finance two or three family outings each year by recycling aluminum cans that everyone in the family collected.

HEALTHY ENVIRONMENT AND LIFE-STYLE

Another sign of a healthy family is a healthy home environment and life-style. Healthy families create safe and hygienic living conditions for their members. For instance, a healthy family with young children will child-proof their home by removing the potential hazards of exposed electric outlets and cleaning solvents out of a child's reach. In families where there are older adults prone to falls, the family will install good lighting and sturdy hand-rails. A healthy home environment is one that is clean and reduces the spread of disease-causing organisms.

A healthy family life-style encourages appropriate balance in the lives of its members. In an ideal family, there is activity and rest sufficient for the energy needs of daily living; the diet offered is varied and nutritionally sound; physical activity maintains ideal weight while promoting cardiac health; preventative hygiene habits are taught and followed by family members; the emotional and mental health is encouraged through a supportive network of caring others; family members seek out and use health care services and demonstrate compliance with recommended regimes (see Fig. 17.3).

The emotional climate of a healthy family is positive and supportive of member growth. Contributing to this healthy emotional climate is a strong sense of shared values, often combined with a strong religious orientation (Olson, et al., 1983). Such a family demonstrates caring, encourages and accepts expression of feelings, and respects divergent ideas. Members can express their individuality in the way they dress or decorate their rooms. The home environment makes family members feel welcome and accepted.

REGULAR LINKS WITH THE BROADER COMMUNITY

Healthy families maintain dynamic ties with the broader community (Pesznecker & Zahlis, 1986). They participate regularly in external groups and activities, often in a leadership capacity. We may see them join in local politics, participate in a church bazaar, or promote the school's paper drive to raise money for science equipment. They use external resources suited to their family's needs. For example, a farm family with teenagers, recognizing the importance of peer group influ-

ence on adolescents, became very active in the local 4-H club. Another family, in which the father was out of work, joined a job transition support group. Healthy families also know what is going on in the world around them. They show an interest in current events and attempt to understand significant social, economic, and political issues. This ever-broadening outreach gives families knowledge of external forces that might influence their lives. It exposes them to a wider range of alternatives and a variety of contacts, which increases their options for finding resources and strengthens their coping skills.

An unhealthy family has not recognized the value of establishing links with the broader community. This may be because of (1) a knowledge deficit regarding community resources, (2) previous negative experiences with the broader community services, or (3) a lack of connection with the community related to family expectations or cultural practices.

It is important for the community health nurse to assess the family for information regarding their relationship with the broader community in addition to structural and developmental family variations, family interaction, coping strategies, and life-style. With a comprehensive family assessment the nurse has a base from which to begin a plan of care.

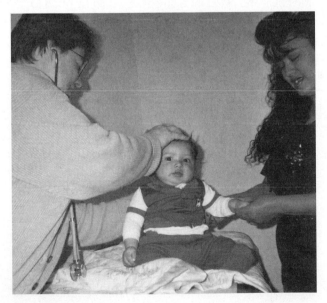

FIGURE 17.3. Healthy families seek out and use external resources such as regular health care.

Family Health Practice Guidelines

Family nursing is a kind of nursing practice in which the family is the unit of service (Friedman, 1986). It is not merely a family-oriented approach in which the family concerns affecting health of the individual are taken into account. Family nursing asks how one does provide health care to a collection of people. It does not mean that nursing must relinquish its service to individuals. On the contrary, one of the distinctive contributions of nursing as a profession is its holistic approach to individual needs. Community health nurses rise to the challenge of adding a service to population groups that include families.

Five guidelines can clarify an understanding of family nursing and enhance practice with families: (1) work with the family collectively, (2) start where the family is, (3) adapt nursing intervention to the family's stage of development, (4) recognize the validity of family structural variations, and (5) emphasize family strengths.

Research in Community Health Nursing
NURSING INTERVENTIONS WITH FAMILIES

Robinson, C.A. (1994). Nursing interventions with families: A demand or an invitation to change? *Journal of Advanced Nursing*, 19, 887–904.

From a review of the literature on family health, Robinson poses that nurses are adept at assessing individuals and families but lag behind on intervention skills, particularly in relation to the nursing of families. Three orientations or approaches to interventions can be conceptualized:

Traditional—a single truth or reality exists outside of us and must be sought and grasped. This is coupled with linear thinking as follows, A (intervention) causes B (the family response).

Transitional—a true or right experience or response exists but the nurse is partially linear and partially systematic. For example, a family member dies—the family is viewed as a whole—"the family is grieving." Reciprocal impact of member's responses is not assessed.

Nontraditional—focuses on a systems approach with attention on relationships, connections, and reciprocity. Predetermined judgements about "right" or "true" perspectives are avoided. For example, A (interventions) influences B (family response) and B influences A.

These views encourage the nurse to drift in the direction of a non-traditional systematic approach to interventions with families. Creating a context for change and offering families a different way to approach problems appears to hold promise for theraputically influencing changes in feelings and behaviors.

WORK WITH THE FAMILY COLLECTIVELY

To practice family nursing, nurses must set aside their usual focus on individuals and remind themselves that several people together have a collective personality, collective interests, and a collective set of needs. Viewing a group of people as one unit becomes less difficult when nurses examine the way they often think. An organization, for example, is often thought of as conservative or liberal. It is reported that a group has taken a stand on abortion or that a business needs to become better organized. In each case, the group is viewed collectively, as a single entity with attributes and activi-

ties in common. So it is with families. A family has its own personality, interests, and needs.

As much as possible, community health nurses want to involve all the members during nurse-client interaction (Miller & Janosik, 1980; Wright and Leahey, 1994). This approach reinforces the importance of each individual member's contribution to total family functioning. Nurses want to encourage everyone's participation in the work that the nurse and the family jointly agree to do. Like the coach, the nurse wants to help them work together as a team for their collective benefit (See Research in Community Health Nursing display).

Consider how a nurse might work with the family collectively in the following Case Study.

CASE STUDY

THE BECK FAMILY

A community health nurse had an initial contact with Mr. and Mrs. Beck and their youngest child at the well-baby clinic. The 9 month old child was over the 95th percentile for weight and at the 40th percentile for height. The nurse also noted that both parents were obese. The nurse asked about the eating patterns in the family and of the baby in particular and suggested a home visit to determine whether the Becks were interested in family nursing. The nurse explained the purpose of home visits (to assess all family members, coping patterns, eating patterns, and food purchasing choices) and the importance of including all family members and asked for a time that would be good for the family as a whole. The nurse explains that each person should be involved and committed to the agreed-upon goals; that, like a team of oarsmen, the family would have to pull together to accomplish the purpose of the visits. To help the Beck family improve its nutritional status, the nurse might suggest a session of brainstorming to uncover many causes of poor nutrition. More brainstorming might result in solutions and plans for action. On each visit the nurse would view the Becks as a group. Group responses and actions would be expected. Evaluation of outcomes would be based on what the family did collectively. The Becks were interested and a home visit date was made.

START WHERE THE FAMILY IS

When working with families, community health nurses begin at their present, not their ideal, level of functioning. To discover where a family is, the community health nurse first conducts a family assessment to ascertain the members' needs and level of health and then determines collective interests, concerns, and priorities. The Kegler family illustrates this principle.

ADAPT NURSING INTERVENTION TO THE FAMILY'S STAGE OF DEVELOPMENT

Although every family engages in the same basic functions, the tasks to accomplish these functions vary with each stage of the family's development. A young family, for instance, will appropriately meet its members' affiliation needs by establishing mutually satisfying relationships and meaningful communication patterns. As the family enters later stages, these bonds change with the release of some members into new families and the loss of others through death. Awareness of the family's developmental stage enables the nurse to assess the appropriateness of the family's level of functioning and to tailor intervention accordingly. Nurses are becoming adept at the assessment of families, however it is the intervention that needs to be focused on (Robinson, 1994). A nurse's work with the Roberts family illustrates this need.

RECOGNIZE THE VALIDITY OF FAMILY STRUCTURAL VARIATIONS

Many families seen by community health nurses are nontraditional in structure, such as single-parent families and unmarried couples (Hanson, 1986; Wright & Leahey, 1990). Other families are organized around nontraditional patterns; for example, both parents may have careers or a husband may care for children at home while his wife financially supports the family. These variant structures and organizational patterns have resulted from social change such as changes in employment practices, welfare programs, economic conditions, sex roles, status of women and minorities, birth control, incidence of divorce, even war. Such variations in family structure and organization lead to revised patterns of family functioning. Member roles and tasks often differ dramatically from our expectations, as in a family with a single parent who works full-time while raising children, or a dual-career marriage in which both partners have undifferentiated roles. Community health nurses, many of whom are accustomed to traditional family patterns, must learn to understand and accept these variations in family structure and organization in order to ad-

CASE STUDY

THE KEGLER FAMILY

Marcia Kegler brought her baby, Tiffany, to the well-child clinic once but failed to keep further appointments. Concerned that the family might be having other difficulties, Sara Villa, a community health nurse made a home visit. The mobile home was cluttered and dirty; the baby was crying in his playpen. Marcia seemed uninterested in the nurse's visit. She listened politely but had little to say. She repeated that everything was okay and that the baby was doing fine explaining that he was just fussy because he was teething. As they talked, Marcia's husband Bob, a delivery van driver, stopped by to pick up a sports magazine to read on his lunch hour. The three of them discussed the problems of inflation and how expensive it was to raise a child. Sara reminded them that the clinic was free, and that they could at least get good health care without extra cost. They agreed without enthusiasm. After Bob left, the nurse spent the remainder of the visit discussing infant care with Marcia, particularly emphasizing regular checkups and immunizations.

The next visit also focused on the baby, but Sara had an uncomfortable feeling that this family was not really interested in her help. After consulting her supervisor, the nurse did what she wished she had done in the first place. She asked to talk with Marcia and Bob together and explained frankly why she had first come to their home and what she could offer in the way of counseling, teaching, support, and referral to other community resources. She then asked them what problems or concerns they had. The Keglers were more than responsive and described their financial difficulties and feelings of isolation from family and friends. They were new in the city, and both their families lived some distance away on farms. The neighbors were friendly but not close enough to confide in. They believed they would eventually overcome their problems if they just had "someone to lean on," as they put it.

Now Sara could address the Keglers primary needs and concerns for friends and emotional support. The nurse began to address the Keglers' social needs first and introduced them to a young couples' group which met at the community center. Sara continued to make periodic home visits and shared additional information about community services that the Keglers might find helpful. She praised Marcia and Bob for following up on immunizations for Tiffany. Over time Sara saw differences in the family's interest in their relationship with the community and their connection to its services. Sara realized that before she could address the issue of Tiffany's health she needed to address the emotional health of the parents.

dress the needs of the families (see Chapter 16 for more information on changing family structure).

There are two important principles to remember. First, what is normal for one family is not necessarily normal for another. Each family is unique in its combination of structure, composition, roles, and behaviors. As long as a family carries out its functions effectively and demonstrates the characteristics of a healthy family, one must agree that its form, no matter how variant, is valid.

Second, families are constantly changing. Marriage transforms two people into a married couple without children. Adding children changes this family's structure. Divorce again alters structure and roles. Remarriage with the addition of children from another family changes the family again. Children grow up and leave the home while the parents, together or singly, are left to adjust to yet another family structure. And so it goes. Throughout the life cycle, a family seldom stays the same for very long. Each of these changes forces a family to adapt to its circumstances. Consider the young woman with a baby whose husband deserts her. She has no choice but to assume a single-parent role. Each change also creates varying degrees of stress, and demands considerable adaptive energy on the family's part. Many family changes are predictable; they are part of normal life cycle growth. Some are not. The nurse's responsibility is to help families cope with the changes while remaining nonjudgmental and accepting of the various forms encountered.

Homosexual unions may be difficult for some nurses to deal with particularly if they conflict with the nurse's own set of religious or cultural ideas. Yet the nurse's responsibility remains the same—to help promote the collective health. Consider the following referral.

CASE STUDY

THE ROBERTS FAMILY

The Roberts, a couple in their early seventies, had recently moved to a retirement complex. They had received nursing visits following Mrs. Roberts' stroke three years previously but requested service now because Mr. Roberts was feeling "poorly" all the time. He thought that perhaps his diet and lack of activity might be the cause and hoped the nurse would have some helpful suggestions. The couple had eagerly awaited Mr. Roberts' retirement from teaching, planning to be lazy, travel, visit all their children, and do all those things they had never had time to do when they were young. Now neither of them seemed to have enough energy or the capacity to enjoy their new life. The move from their home of 28 years had been difficult; they were still trying to find space in the tiny apartment for their cherished books and mementos, many of which they had given away.

The nurse recognized that the Roberts were experiencing a situational crisis (leaving their home of 28 years) and a developmental crisis (entering retirement and the aging stage). Many of the Roberts' expectations for this new life stage were unrealistic; they had not adequately prepared themselves for the adjustments that the loss of their home and retirement would demand. Through discussion, the nurse was able to help the Roberts understand their situation and express their feelings. The nurse also helped them join a support group of retired persons who were experiencing some of the same difficulties. Because this nurse was able to help the Roberts through their crisis in a supportive and nonjudgmental manner, she found them receptive later to discussing preparation for the inevitable loss and bereavement that would occur when one of them died. She was adapting her nursing intervention to this family's stage of development.

CASE STUDY

JAMES CUTLER AND BRIAN HOAG

James Cutler and Brian Hoag have a six-year monogamous relationship. A homosexual couple, they have been working with an attorney to privately adopt a child. The arrangements are completed and their two-week-old son, Adrian, arrived in their home last week. Helen Jeffers, a community health nurse, receives a referral from the county hospital where Adrian was born. The request is for an assessment of the home situation and parenting skills. The baby tested positive for cocaine with Apgar's of 6 and 8, with some initial difficulty sucking. Birth weight was 2900 gms. Discharge weight, at five days, was 2850 gms. At her first home visit, Helen finds a neat and orderly two bedroom condominium, well-equipped with baby supplies. The infant had gained 200 gms. and was being well cared for by two fatigued parents who have had limited contact with infants. James and Brian have many questions and are anxious learners. Helen plans with the couple to make weekly home visits to assess infant growth and development, provide support, and answer questions. She also suggests a neighborhood parenting class, finding a reliable babysitter, and helps James and Brian develop an infant care work schedule. After six weeks of intervention Adrian is thriving; Helen closes the case to home visits feeling confident that the parent's goal of becoming knowledgeable parents was achieved.

Nurses should view all families as unique groups, each with its own set of needs, whose interests can best be served through unbiased care. See the World Watch discussion that follows.

World Watch
CHRONIC PAIN AND ITS EFFECT ON THE FAMILY UNIT

Snelling, J. (1994). The effect of chronic pain on the family unit. *Journal of Advanced Nursing, 19,* 543–551.

A study conducted in England sought to explore the effect of chronic pain on the family unit. The researcher found that chronic pain caused social isolation, role tension, marital conflict, and reduced sexual activity among marital partners. Feelings of anger, anxiety, resentment, and despondency occurred in other family members. Additionally, it was found that the extent to which chronic pain negatively affected the partner and family members depended somewhat on how effective the family was in coping with a relative with chronic pain.

There are implications for community health nursing practice. Nurses seeing families in their homes or in outpatient settings are in a key position to enhance change. They are able to use and develop their knowledge of family dynamics to support and assist the family as it addresses unhealthy responses to the family member's pain. Helping the family members to share their knowledge and feelings may lead to more emotional stability and also to more realistic expectations of each other's behavior. Families need to be assessed for maladaptive coping techniques and taught effective coping techniques such as seeking information, seeking support from others, humor, laughter, and finding meaning in the experience.

EMPHASIZE FAMILY STRENGTHS

Too often, community health nurses tend to focus their attention on family weaknesses, looking for and referring to them as needs or problems. This negative emphasis can be devastating to a family and undermine any hopes of a truly therapeutic relationship between nurse and client. Instead, families need their strengths reinforced. Emphasizing a family's strengths makes people feel better about themselves. It fosters a positive self-image and promotes self-confidence and often helps the family to address other problems.

One helpful communication technique is **strengthening** in which the nurse, verbally or in writing, lists positive points about an otherwise negative situation. Examples include: the baby is kept warmly dressed (the clothing might be filthy, but the baby is warm); the two year old is taking a nap (albeit on the dirty floor), the five year old got to school three times last week (up from one to two times a week in the previous month), or the mother is awake with a robe on at 1 pm (not asleep like on other home visits made in the early afternoon). Each represents a positive change. If there is nothing positive the nurse can honestly say, the nurse may be able to say that the client seems to be managing as best she can. This strengthening technique helps the nurse approach clients positively rather than with a condescending or punative approach. This is not to say that nurses should ignore problems. On the contrary, their assessment should explore all aspects of family functioning to determine both strengths and weaknesses. The nurse needs a total picture to achieve adequate perspective in nursing care planning, and to know when the family is ready and chooses to begin work on problems. Yet, even as the nurse becomes more and more aware of a family's unhealthy behaviors, the emphasis should remain on the positive ones. Emphasizing strengths proves to the clients in effect that they are important to the nurse.

Family strengths are traits which facilitate the ability of the family to meet the members needs and the demands made upon it by systems outside the family unit. Not all traits that appear positive are necessarily strengths, however. Before the nurse selects a trait to emphasize, that trait should be examined closely to determine whether that behavior is actually facilitating family functioning. A strong work orientation may be a strength when balanced with play and relaxation, but a family obsessed by work is experiencing this trait as a weakness. The differentiating factor between whether a trait is a strength or a weakness is the amount of free choice, as opposed to compulsive drive, being exercised.

Some traits a nurse may consider possible strengths are basic family functions, family developmental tasks, and characteristics of family health. For instance, a nurse might wish to commend a family that meets its members' physical, emotional, and spiritual needs; shows respect for various members' points of view; or fosters self-discipline in its children.

A vivid illustration of this principle is found in the family nursing care of the Stevensons.

CASE STUDY

THE STEVENSONS

The community health nurse, Keith Dow, made an initial home visit after referral by an outpatient physician who was concerned about possible child abuse. Alice Stevenson had brought her baby to the emergency room for treatment of a laceration on the baby's forehead. He had fallen off the table while she was changing him, she claimed. A bruise on his arm made the physician suspicious, but Alice explained it was caused by his older brother's rough play. The nurse opened the visit by stating he was simply following up on the emergency room treatment and wanted to see how the baby was progressing. Keith made no mention of child abuse. He observed the mother and children closely, looking for small things to compliment Alice on (strengthening) while learning all he could about the family's background. Because the nurse appeared approving rather than suspicious or judgmental, Alice agreed to further visits. During a later visit Alice admitted to the nurse that she had slapped the baby and her ring cut his forehead. She could not get him to stop crying, no matter what she did; she just could not endure it any longer, she said. There had been other times when she grabbed him roughly to pull him away from things he wasn't allowed to touch, causing bruises on his arms. Alice told the nurse that she had not planned this baby; when her husband found out she was pregnant, he had left her shortly before the baby was born. Like many abusive parents, Alice had unrealistic expectations for her children's behavior as well as very inadequate self-esteem (Ryan, 1984; Herbert, 1989). Realizing that Alice would be particularly vulnerable to any criticism, the nurse concentrated on her strengths. Keith complimented her on how well she managed her home and dressed the children, on maintaining her job, and on reading to the three-year-old boy. It took many visits before Alice trusted the nurse, but in time they were able to discuss her feelings frankly and work toward improving this family's health. Keith got her to attend a support group for single parents and she began counseling. Emphasizing strengths had provided a bridge for Alice and helped to bring her into a helping relationship.

Family Health Assessment

To assess a family's level of health in a systematic fashion requires three tools: (1) a conceptual framework upon which to base the assessment, (2) a clearly defined set of assessment categories for data collection, and (3) a method for measuring a family's level of functioning.

CONCEPTUAL FRAMEWORKS

Several conceptual frameworks have been used historically to study families (Hill & Hansen, 1960; Kantor & Lehr, 1975; Reiss, 1981). More recently Beavers and Hampton (1990) and Olson (1991) have designed models to describe family functioning. Three, in particular, are mentioned here, as they are particularly useful in community health nursing : interactional, structural-functional, and developmental. The **interactional framework** describes the family as a unity of interacting personalities and emphasizes communication, roles, conflict, coping patterns, and decision-making processes. This framework focuses on internal relationships but neglects the family's interaction with the external environment.

The **structural-functional framework** describes the family as a social system relating to other social systems in the external environment, such as church, school, work, and health care system. This framework examines the interacting functions of society and the family, looks at family structures, and analyzes how a family's structure affects its functioning.

The **developmental framework** studies families from a life-cycle perspective by examining members' changing roles and tasks in each progressive life cycle stage. This framework incorporates elements from interactional and structural-functional approaches so that family structure, function, and interaction are viewed in the context of the environment through each stage of family development.

Others have combined these concepts in various ways to design family assessment and intervention models focusing on human-environmental interactions, interactional and structural-functional frameworks, self-care, responses to stressors, and a developmental framework.

The six characteristics of healthy families already discussed serve as an initial framework for assessing family health using a combination of interactional, structural-functional, and developmental concepts.

DATA COLLECTION CATEGORIES

Within a conceptual framework for assessing family health, the community health nurse selects specific categories for data collection. The amount of data that one can collect about any given family may be voluminous, perhaps more than necessary for the purposes of the assessment. Certain basic information is needed, however, to determine a family's health status and design appropriate nursing interventions. From many sources in the family health literature, particularly from Edelman and Mandle (1986), Friedman (1986), Turk and Kerns (1985), and Whall (1987), a list of twelve data collection categories have been generated. Table 17.1 lists the 12 categories grouped into three data sets: (1) family strengths and self-care capabilities, (2) family stresses and problems, and (3) family resources. The 12 assessment categories are explained below.

1. Family demographics refers to such things as a family's composition, socioeconomic status, and the ages, education, occupation, ethnicity, and religious affiliations of its members.
2. Physical environment data describe geography, climate, housing, space, social and political structures, food availability and dietary patterns, and any other elements in the internal or external physical environment that influence a family's health status.
3. Psychological and spiritual environment refers to information such as affectional relationships, mutual respect, support, promotion of members' self-esteem and spiritual development, and family members' life satisfaction and goals.
4. Family structure and roles includes family organization, socialization processes, division of labor, and allocation and use of authority and power.
5. Family functions refers to a family's ability to carry out appropriate developmental tasks and provide for its members' needs.

6. Family values and beliefs influence all aspects of family life. Values and beliefs might deal with raising children, making and spending money, education, religion, work, health, and community involvement.
7. Family communication patterns include the frequency and quality of communication within a family and between the family and its environment.
8. Family decision-making patterns refer to how decisions are made in a family, by whom are they made, and how are they implemented.
9. Family problem-solving patterns describe how a family handles its problems, who deals with them, the flexibility of a family's approach to problem solving, and the nature of its solutions.
10. Family coping patterns encompass how a family handles conflict and life changes, the nature and quality of family support systems, and family perceptions and responses to stressors.
11. Family health behavior refers to familial health history, current physical health status of family members, family use of health resources, and family health beliefs.
12. Family social and cultural patterns comprise family discipline and limit-setting practices; promotion of members' initiative, creativity, and leadership; family goal setting; family culture; cultural adaptations to present circumstances; and development of meaningful relationships within and without the family.

TABLE 17.1. *Categories of Data Collection for Family Health Assessment*

Assessment Categories	Family strengths and self-care abilities	Family stresses and problems	Family resources
1. Family demographics			
2. Physical environment			
3. Psychological and spiritual environment			
4. Family structure/roles			
5. Family functions			
6. Family values and beliefs			
7. Family communication patterns			
8. Family decision-making patterns			
9. Family problem-solving patterns			
10. Family coping patterns			
11. Family health behavior			
12. Family social and cultural patterns			

ASSESSMENT METHODS

Many different methods are used to assess families. These methods serve to generate information about selected aspects of family structure and function; thus the methods must match the purpose for assessment.

Three well-known graphic assessment tools are the eco-map, genogram, and the social support network map or grid (Tracy & Whittaker, 1990; Meyer, 1993). The **eco-map** is a diagram of the connections between a family and the other systems in its ecological environment, originally devised to depict the complexity of the client's story. Developed by Dr. Ann Hartman in 1975 to help child welfare workers study family needs, the tool visually depicts the dynamic family-environment interactions. The nurse involves family members in the map's development. They draw a central circle representing the family and then smaller circles on the periphery to represent people and systems, such as school or work, whose relationships with the family are significant. The map is used to discuss and analyze these relationships (Hartman, 1978; Meyer, 1993) (see Fig. 17.4).

The **genogram** displays family information graphically in a way that provides a quick view of complex family patterns and a rich source of hypotheses about a family over a significant period of time, usually three or more generations (McGoldrick & Gerson, 1985). It diagrams family relationships by listing the family genealogy accompanied by significant life events (birth, death, marriage, divorce, illness), identifying characteristics (race, religion, social class), occupations, and places of family residence (Meyer, 1993). Again, this tool is used jointly with the family. It encourages family expression and sheds light on family behavior and problems (see Fig. 17.5).

A **social network support map** or grid gives a detailed response regarding the quality and quantity of social connections. Strengths within the system can be elaborated with words, checks and/or numbers (Tracy & Whittaker, 1990). The nurse uses this tool to help the family understand its sources of support and relationships and to form a basis for nursing care planning and intervention. Figures 17.6 and 17.7 show samples of a social network support map and grid.

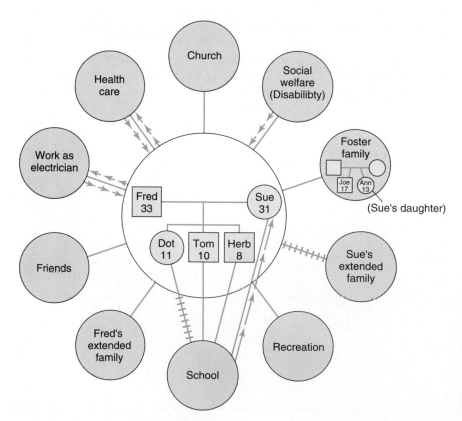

FIGURE 17.4. Ecomap of family's relationship to its environment. Lines indicate types of connections: solidline, strong; dotted line, tenuous; lines with cross bars, stressful. Arrows signify energy or resource flow, and absence of lines indicates no connection.

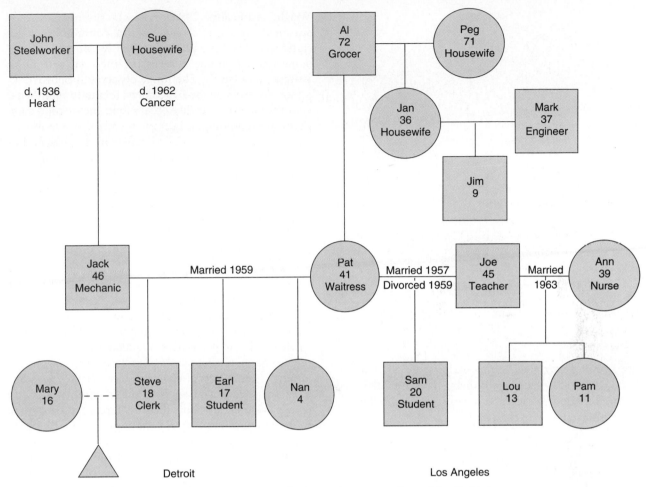

FIGURE 17.5. A genogram depicting three generations of family history.

Tapia (1972) depicted her concept of levels of family functioning through her model for family nursing. This model is based upon a continuum of five levels of family functioning. Levels of family functioning from infancy (Level I—a very chaotic family), childhood (Level II—an intermediate family), adolescence (Level III—the normal family with many conflicts and problems), the adult (Level IV—the family with solutions to its problems), and maturity (Level V—the ideal independent family). She gives specific behaviors of families at each level, the family's expectation from the nurse, and most importantly the nurse's specific skill needed at each level of family functioning to best meet the family needs and help them reach a higher level of functioning. This visualization of family strengths, weaknesses and expectations of the nurse and associated skills (see

Fig. 17.8) is a helpful tool for the novice nurse working with a variety of families in the community.

Community health nurses also use several different family assessment instruments to gather data on family structure, functions, development, or combinations of all three (Kandzari, et al., 1981). Public health nursing agencies generally develop their own tools, often in the form of questionnaires, checklists, or interview guides. The format varies to fit organizational needs. For example, most agencies have changed to computerized information management systems and adjusted data collection to be technologically compatible. Two sample assessment tools are shown in Figures 17.9 and 17.10.

Other methods, such as videotaping family interaction, structured observation, or analysis of life-chang-

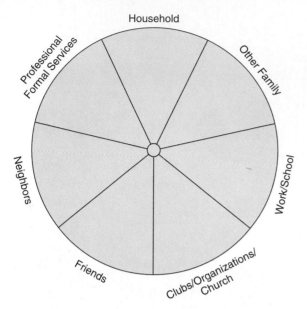

FIGURE 17.6. Social network support map.

ing events using the Holmes-Rahe scale (Holmes & Rahe, 1967) are all useful adjuncts. Tools are often used in combination to enhance breadth of data collection and understanding of the family.

Guidelines for Family Health Assessment

An assessment of family health will be most accurate if it incorporates the following five guidelines.

1. Focus on the family as a total unit.
2. Ask goal-directed questions.
3. Collect data over time.
4. Combine quantitative and qualitative data.
5. Exercise professional judgment.

FOCUS ON THE FAMILY, NOT THE MEMBER

Family health is more than the sum of its individual members' health. If the health of each person in a family was rated and those scores combined, it would not show how healthy that family was. To assess a family's health, the nurse must consider that family as a single entity and appraise its aggregate behavior (Whall, 1987;

Wright and Leahey, 1994). As each criterion in the assessment process is considered, the community health nurse asks, "Is this typical of the family as a whole?" Assume that the nurse is assessing the communication patterns of a family. The nurse observes supportive interaction between two members in the family. What about the others? Further observation shows good communication among all but one member. It may be decided that, in spite of that one person, the family as a whole has good communication. When individual member behavior deviates from the aggregate picture, the nurse will want to note these differences. They can influence total family functioning and will need to be considered in nursing care planning.

USE GOAL-DIRECTED QUESTIONS

The activities of any investigator, if fruitful, are guided by goal-directed questions. When solving a crime, a detective has many specific questions in mind. So, too, does the physician attempting a diagnosis, the teacher trying to discern a student's knowledge-level, or the mechanic repairing a car. Similarly, the nurse determining a family's level of health has specific questions in mind. It is not enough to make family visits and merely ask members how they are. If relevant data are to be gathered, relevant questions must be asked. Figure 17.9 provides a sample set of questions that community health nurses may use to assess a family's health. Built upon the framework of the characteristics of a healthy family, these questions guide thinking and observations. They direct attention to specific aspects of family behavior to facilitate the goal of discovering a family's level of health. Consider the characteristic, "active coping effort." When visiting a family the community health nurse watches for signs of their response to change and their problem-solving ability. The nurse asks, "Does this family recognize when it needs to make a change?" or "How does it respond when a change is imposed?" Perhaps a health problem has arisen, for instance, the baby has diarrhea. Does the family assume responsibility for dealing with the problem? Do family members consider a variety of ways to solve it? How do they respond to the nurses suggestions? Do they seek out resources on their own, such as reading about causes of infant diarrhea or consulting with the community health nurse, their doctor, or a nurse practitioner? How well do they use resources, once identified? Do they take a problem, try creative methods for solving it, and see it through to resolution? As the nurse

(*text continues on page 384*)

	Area of Life	Concrete support	Emotional support	Information/ advice	Critical	Direction of help	Closeness	How often seen	How long known
ID _____ Respondent _____ Name #	1. Household 2. Other family 3. Work/school 4. Organizations 5. Friends 6. Neighbors 7. Professionals 8. Other	1. Hardly ever 2. Sometimes 3. Almost always	1. Hardly ever 2. Sometimes 3. Almost always	1. Hardly ever 2. Sometimes 3. Almost always	1. Hardly ever 2. Sometimes 3. Almost always	1. Goes both ways 2. You to them 3. They to you	1. Not very close 2. Sort of close 3. Very close	0. Does not see 1. Few times/yr. 2. Monthly 3. Weekly 4. Daily	1. Less than 1yr. 2. 1–5 yrs. 3. More than 5 yrs.
01									
02									
03									
04									
05									
06									
07									
08									
09									
10									
11									
12									
13									
14									
15									
1-6	7	8	9	10	11	12	13	14	15

FIGURE 17.7. Social support network grid.

Social Support Network Grid. SOURCE: Tracy and Whittaker 1990.

381

Nursing activities	Trust	Counseling	Complex of skills	Prevention	None
Continuum of Nursing Skills	Nurse and Family Partners	Partnership	Partnership Stressing Family's Ability	Nurse—Expert and Partner	Family Independent / Nurse not Needed
	Acceptance and trust, maturity and patience, clarification of role, limit setting, constant evaluation of relationship and progress.	Based on trust relationship, uses counseling and interpersonal skills to help family begin to understand itself and define its problems. Nurse uses honesty and genuineness, and self-evaluation.	Information, coordination, teamwork, teaching; uses special skills; helps family in making decisions and finding solutions.	Anticipated problem areas studied, teaching of available resources, assistance in family-group understanding, maturity and foresight.	
Continuum of Family Functioning	Nurse—"Good Mother" to Family	Nurse and Family-Siblings	Nurse—Adult Helper to Family	Nurse—Expert and Partner with Family	
	Chaotic family, barely surviving, inadequate provision of physical and emotional supports. Alienation from community, deviant behavior, distortion and confusion of roles, immaturity, child neglect, depression-failure.	Intermediate family, slightly above survival level, variation in economic provisions, alienation with more ability to trust. Child neglect not as great, defensive but slightly more willingness to accept help.	Normal family but with many conflicts and problems, variation in economic levels, greater trust and ability to seek and use help. Parents more mature, but still have emotional conflicts. Do have successes and achievements, and are more willing to seek solutions to problems, future oriented.	Family has solutions, are stable, healthy with fewer conflicts or problems, very capable providers of physical and emotional supports. Parents mature and confident, fewer difficulties in training of children, able to seek help, future oriented, enjoy present.	Ideal family, homeostatic, balance between individual and group goals and activities. Family meets its tasks and roles well, and are able to seek appropriate help when needed.
Family Levels	I. Infancy	II. Childhood	III. Adolescence	IV. Adulthood	V. Maturity

FIGURE 17.8. Model of family nursing (Adapted from J. A. Tapia, 1972).

Family Assessment

Family Name _____

Family Constellation

Member	Birth Date	Sex	Marital Status	Education	Occupation	Community Involvement

Financial Status _____

Using the following scale, score the family based on your professional observations and judgement:

0 = Never   3 = Frequently
1 = Seldom   4 = Most of the time
2 = Occasionally   N = Not observed

	score	date	score	date	score	date	score	date

Facilitative Interaction among Members

  a. Is there frequent communication among all members?
  b. Do conflicts get resolved?
  c. Are relationships supportive?
  d. Are love and caring shown among members?
  e. Do members work collaboratively?

Comments _____

_____

Totals

Enhancement of Individual Development

  a. Does family respond appropriately to members' developmental needs?
  b. Does it tolerate disagreement?
  c. Does it accept members as they are?
  d. Does it promote member autonomy?

Comments _____

_____

Totals

FIGURE 17.9. Family assessment using questions based on characteristics of healthy families.

	score	date	score	date	score	date	score	date

Effective Structuring of Relationships
  a. Is decision making allocated to appropriate members?
  b. Do member roles meet family needs?
  c. Is there flexible distribution of tasks?
  d. Are controls appropriate for family stage of development?

Comments _____

_____ Totals

Active Coping Effort
  a. Is family aware when there is a need for change?
  b. Is it receptive to new ideas?
  c. Does it actively seek resources?
  d. Does it make good use of resources?
  e. Does it creatively solve problems?

Comments _____

_____ Totals

Healthy Environment and Life-style
  a. Is family life-style health promoting?
  b. Are living conditions safe and hygienic?
  c. Is emotional climate conductive to good health?
  d. Do members practice good health measures?

Comments _____

_____ Totals

Regular Links with Broader Community
  a. Is family involved regularly in the community?
  b. Does it select and use external resources?
  c. Is it aware of external affairs?
  d. Does it attempt to understand external issues?

Comments _____

_____ Totals

FIGURE 17.9. (*continued*)

focuses on these behaviors, he or she is asking goal-directed questions aimed at finding out the family's coping skills. This investigation will be one part of the nurse's assessment of the family's total health picture.

The set of questions presented in Figure 17.9 is one useful way to appraise family health. Another more open-ended format is used by some community health nursing agencies. This approach, displayed in Figure 17.10, proposes assessment categories as a stimulus for nursing questions. When exploring family support systems, for example, the nurse asks, "What internal resources or strengths does this family have?" "Who,

FAMILY ASSESSMENT

Family Name

Family Constellation

Member names   Occupation   Educational background

Significant change in family life

Coping ability of family

Energy level

Decision-making process within the family

Parenting skills

Support systems of the family

Use of health care (include plans for emergencies)

Financial status

Other impressions

Signature of Nurse   Date

FIGURE 17.10. Open-ended family assessment.

outside of the family, can they and do they turn to for help?" "What agencies, such as churches, clubs, or community services, do they use?" The open-ended style of this assessment tool allows a variety of questions to be raised aimed at determining family health.

ALLOW ADEQUATE TIME FOR DATA COLLECTION

Accurate family assessment takes time. An appraisal done on the first or second visit will most likely give only a partial picture of how a family is functioning. Time is needed to accumulate observations, make notes, and see all the family members interacting together in order to make a thorough assessment. To appraise family communication patterns, for instance, the nurse will want to observe the family as a group, perhaps at mealtime or during some family activity. They will need to feel comfortable in the nurse's presence in

order to respond freely; it takes time and patience for such rapport to develop.

Consider one nurse's experience. Joe Burns had talked with the Olson family twice, first in the clinic and then at home. Since Mr. Olson had not been present either time, Joe asked to see the family together and arranged an early evening visit. The Olsons were receiving nursing service for health promotion. They were particularly interested in discussing discipline of their young children and contracted with Joe for six weekly visits to be held in the late afternoon when Mr. Olson was home from work. Joe's assessment began on his first contact with the Olsons. He made notes on their chart and, guided by questions similar to those in Figure 17.9, he kept a brief log. After the fourth visit, he filled out an assessment form to keep as a part of the family record. It was not until then that Joe felt he had enough data collected to make valid judgments about this family's level of health.

COMBINE QUANTITATIVE WITH QUALITATIVE DATA

Any appraisal of family health must be qualitative. That is, the nurse must determine the presence or absence of essential characteristics in order to have a data base for planning nursing action. To guide planning more specifically, the nurse can also determine degrees of the presence or absence of these signs of health. This is a quantitative measure. The nurse is not just asking whether a family does or does not engage in some behaviors, but how often. Is this behavior fairly typical of the family, or does it occur infrequently? Figure 17.9 demonstrates one way to measure family health quantitatively. If the nurse were to use this tool to assess the Maxwell family's ability to enhance individuality, for example, the nurse could score their behavior on a scale from zero to four, zero meaning never and four meaning most of the time. After several observations, the nurse would probably conclude that they responded appropriately to the members' developmental needs (a. under "Enhancement of Individual Development") most of the time. Opposite a. on the assessment form, the nurse would write the numeral 4 and the date of assessment.

The value of developing a quantitative measure is to have some basis for comparison. The nurse can assess a family's progression or regression by comparing its present score with its previous scores. Had the nurse conducted a family health assessment six months ago on the Silvas, for instance, and compared it with their present level of health, the nurse would probably have discovered a drop in their scores in several areas. Many of their communication patterns, role relationships, and coping skills, in particular, would show signs of deterioration. A scored assessment gives a vivid picture of exactly which areas need intervention. For this reason, it is useful to conduct periodic assessments as a case is reopened or every three to six months if it is kept open longer. The nurse can monitor the progress of high-risk families through the early introduction of particular preventive measures, if a trend or regressive behavior in some area is seen. Periodic quantitative assessments also provide a means of evaluating the effectiveness of nursing action and can point to documented signs of growth.

Quantitative data serve another useful purpose. The nurse can compare one family's health status with that of another family as a basis for priority setting and nursing care planning. The difference in the levels of health between the Silvas and the Maxwells shows that the Silvas need considerably more attention right now.

EXERCISE PROFESSIONAL JUDGMENT

Although nurses seek to validate data, their assessment of families is still based primarily on their own professional judgment. Assessment tools can guide observations and even quantify those judgments, but ultimately any assessment is subjective. Even though it may be observed that a family makes good use of a community agency, the decision that the use of this external resource is contributing to their health is still a subjective one. This decision is not bad. Indeed, effective health care practice depends on sound professional judgment. However, nurses must, at the same time, be cautious about overemphasizing the value of an assessment tool. It is not infallible. It is only a tool and should be used as a guide for planning, not as an absolute and irrevocable statement about a family's health status. This caution is particularly important when dealing with quantitative scores, which may seem to be objective.

Ordinarily, it is best to conduct assessment of a family unobtrusively. The tool is not a questionnaire to be filled out in the family's presence; its purpose is to guide observations and judgments. Before going into a family's home, the community health nurse may wish to review the questions. The nurse may find it helpful to keep the assessment tool in a briefcase for easy reference during the visit. Depending upon the nurse's relationship with a family, notes may be made during or immediately after the encounter. Like Joe, the nurse may choose to keep a short log—an accumulation of notes—until enough data has been collected to complete the assessment form.

Occasionally, a family with high self-care capability may be involved in the assessment. The nurse will want to introduce the idea carefully and use professional judgment to determine when the family is ready to engage in this kind of self-examination.

Summary

The family as the unit of service has received increasing emphasis in nursing over the years. Today family nursing has an important place in nursing practice, particularly in community health nursing. Its significance results from recognition that the family itself must be a focus of service, that family health and individual health strongly influence each other, and that family health affects community health.

Healthy families demonstrate six important characteristics:

1. There is a facilitative process of interaction among family members.
2. They enhance individual member development.
3. Their role relationships are structured effectively.
4. They actively attempt to cope with problems.
5. They have a healthy home environment and lifestyle.
6. They establish regular links with the broader community.

To assess a family's health systematically, the nurse needs a conceptual framework upon which to base the assessment, a clearly defined set of categories for data collection, and a method for measuring the family's level of functioning. The six characteristics of a healthy family provide one assessment framework that community health nurses can use. There are also assessment tools to aid the nurse in appraising the health of families including the eco-map, genogram, and social support network map or grid. There are also 12 main categories of family dynamics for which the nurse must collect data: family demographics, physical environment, psychological/spiritual environment, family structure and roles, family functions, family values and beliefs, family communication patterns, family decision-making patterns, family problem-solving patterns, family coping patterns, family health behaviors, and family social and cultural patterns.

Community health nurses enhance their practice with families by observing five principles: (1) work with the family collectively, (2) start where the family is now, (3) fit nursing intervention to the family's stage of development, (4) recognize the validity of family structural variation, and (5) emphasize family strengths.

During assessment, the nurse should focus on the family as a total unit, use goal-directed assessment questions, allow adequate time for data collection, combine quantitative with qualitative data, and exercise professional judgment.

Activities to Promote Critical Thinking

1. Construct an eco-map of your family. Ask a peer to do the same thing. Assess the balance between your family and the resources in its environment. How does it compare with your peer? What changes are needed in each family system? Are you able to influence the changes that are needed?

2. Draw a genogram of your family and ask a peer to discuss it with you. Make your drawing of the genogram as complete as possible. Then analyze your thoughts and feelings: How did you feel while tracing your family history? Did you learn anything new about your family? Did any family trends or traits appear? Did any uncomfortable or suppressed information come to the surface? Do you have any new insights about your family?

3. Complete a social support network map or grid on yourself. Discuss it with a peer. Did any of the data surprise you? What areas need to be worked on?

4. Assess a family (other than your own) that you know well by completing a family assessment guide. You may use one of the forms in this chapter or a form available to you from some other source. Based on your assessment, determine as many nursing interventions that could be used to promote this family's health as practically possible.

REFERENCES

Barker, P. (1992). *Basic family therapy* (3rd.ed.). New York: Oxford.

Beavers, W.R. (1985) *Successful marriage: A family systems approach to couples therapy.* New York: Norton.

Beavers, W.R. & Hampton, R.B. (1990). *Successful families: Assessment and intervention.* New York: Basic.

Becvar, D. & Becvar, R. (1988). *Family therapy.* Newton, MA: Allyn and Bacon.

Cox, R.P. & Davis, L.L. (1993) Social constructivist approaches for brief, epiosodic, problem-focused family encounters. *Nurse Practitioner, 18*(8), 45–49.

Duffy, M. E. (1988). Health promotion in the family: Current findings and directives for nursing research. *Journal of Advanced Nursing, 13*(1), 109–17.

Duvall, E. & Miller, B. (1985). *Marriage and family development.* (6th ed.). New York: Harper & Row.

Edelman, C. & Mandle, C.L. (Eds.). (1986). *Health promotion throughout the life span.* St. Louis: Mosby.

Ford, L. C. (1973). The development of family nursing. In D. Hymovich & M. Barnard (Eds.), *Family health care*. New York: McGraw-Hill.

Fox, M.A. (1989). The community health nurse and multi-problem families. *Journal of Community Health Nursing, 6*(1), 3–5.

Friedman, M. M. (1986). *Family nursing theory and assessment* (2nd ed.). New York: Appleton-Century-Crofts.

Gillis, C., Highley, B., Roberts, B., & Martinson, I. (1989). *Toward a Science of Family Nursing*. Don Mills, Ontario: Addison-Wesley.

Hanson, S. M. (1986). Healthy single-parent families. *Family Relations, 35*(1), 125–32.

Hartman, A. (1978). Diagrammatic assessment of family relationships. *Social Casework, 59*(10), 59–64.

Herbert, M. (1989). *Working with children and their families*. Chicago, IL: Lyceum Books.

Hill, R. B. (1971). *The strengths of black families*. New York: Emerson Hall.

Hetherington, E.M. (1989). Coping with family transitions: Winners, losers, and survivors. *Child Development, 60*, 1–14.

Hill, R., and D. Hansen. (1960). The identification of conceptual frameworks utilized in family study. *Marriage and Family Living, 22*, 299–311.

Holmes, T. & Rahe, R. (1967). The social readjustment rating scale. *Journal of Psychosomatic Research, 11*, 213–17.

Huntley, D.K. & Konetsky, C.D. (1992). Healthy families with adolescents. *Topics in Family Psychology and Counseling, 1*, 62–71.

Kandzari, J. H., Howard, J.R., & Rock, M. (1981). *The well family: A developmental approach to assessment*. Boston: Little, Brown.

Kantor, D. & Lehr, W. (1975). *Inside the family: Toward a theory of family process*. San Francisco: Josey-Bass.

Kristjanson, L.J. & Chalmers, K.I.(1991). Preventative work with families: Issues facing public health nurses. *Journal of Advanced Nursing, 16*, 147–153.

McCubbin, H., A. Cauble, A., & Patterson, J. (Eds.). (1982). *Family stress coping and social support*. Springfield, IL: Charles C. Thomas.

McGoldrick, M. & Gersen, R. (1985). *Genograms in family assessment*. New York: Norton.

Meyer, C.H. (1993). *Assessment in social work practice*. New York: Columbia.

Miller, J. R. & Janosik, E.H. (1980). *Family-focused care*. New York: McGraw-Hill.

Olson, D.H. (1991, November). *Three-dimensional (3-D) circumplex model: Theoretical and methodological advances*. Paper presented at the Theory Construction and Research Methodology Workshop at the annual convention of the National Council on Family Relations, Denver.

Olson, D., McCubbin, H.I., and Associates. (1983). *Families: What makes them work*. Beverly Hills: Sage.

Otto, H. A. (1973). A framework for assessing family strengths. In A. Reinhardt and M. Quinn (Eds.), *Family-centered community nursing: A socio-cultural framework*. St. Louis: Mosby.

Peitze, C. F. (1984). Health promotion for the well family. *Nursing Clinics of North America, 19*(2), 229–37.

Pesznecker, B., & E. Zahlis. (1986). Establishing mutual help groups for family-member caregivers: A new role for community health nurses. *Public Health Nursing, 3*(1), 29–37.

Reiss, D. (1981). *The family's construction of reality*. Cambridge, MA: Harvard University Press.

Robinson, C.A. (1994). Nursing interventions with families: A demand or an invitation to change? *Journal of Advanced Nursing, 19*(5), 897–904.

Ryan, M. T. (1984). Identifying the sexually abused child. *Pediatric Nursing 10*, 419–21.

Schwebel, A.I. & Fine, M.A. (1994). *Understanding and helping families: A cognitive-behavioral approach*. Hillsdale, NJ: Lawrence Erlbaum Associates.

Stinnett, N. (1981). In search of strong families. In N. Stinnett, B. Chesser, and J. De Frain (Eds.), *Building family strengths: Blueprints for action*. Lincoln: University of Nebraska Press.

Tanner-Nelson, P. & Banonis, B. (1981). Family consensus and stress identified in Delaware's White House Conference on the family. In N. Stinnett, J. DeFrain, K. King, P. Knaub, & G. Rowe (Eds.), *Family strengths III: Roots of well being* (pp. 43–60). Lincoln: University of Nebraska Press.

Tapia, J.A. (1972). The nursing process in family health. *Nursing Outlook, 20*(4), 267–270.

Tracy, E.M. & Whittaker, J.J.(1990). The social network map: Assessing social support in clinical practice. *Families in Society, 71*, 461–470.

Turk, D. C. & Kerns, R.D. (Eds.). (1985). *Health, illness and families: A life span perspective*. New York: Wiley.

United States Public Health Service. (1990). *Healthy People 2000: National Health Promotion and Disease Prevention Objectives*. Department of Health and Human Services Publication No.(PHS) 91-50212. Washington, DC: U.S. Government Printing Office.

Whall, A. L. (1987). *Family therapy theory for nursing: Four approaches*. Norwalk, CT: Appleton-Century-Crofts.

Wright, L. M. & Leahey, M. (1990) Trends in nursing of families. Journal of advanced nursing. 15, 148–154.

Wright, L.M. & Leahey, M. (1994). *Nurses and families* (2nd ed.). Philadelphia: F.A. Davis.

SELECTED READINGS

Baranowski, T. & Nader, P. (1985). Family health behavior. In D. Turk & R. Kerns (Eds.), *Health, illness, and families*. New York: Wiley.

Berg, C. L. & Helgeson, D. (1984). That first home visit. *Journal of Community Health Nursing, 1*(3), 207–15.

Biller, H.B. (1993). *Fathers and families: Paternal factors in child development*. Westport, CT: Auburn House.

Choi, T., Josten, L., & Christiansen, M.L. (1983). Health-specific family coping index for noninstitutional care. *American Journal of Public Health, 73*, 1275–77.

Chin, S. (1985). Can self-care theory be applied to families? In J. Riehl-Sisca (Ed.), *The science and art of self-care*. Norwalk, CT: Appleton-Century-Crofts.

Clark, J. (1986). Supporting the family . . . heading off a breakdown. *Nursing Times, 82*(32), 33–34.

Crooks, C. E., et al. (1987). The family's role in health promotion. *Health Values, 11*(2), 7–12.

Duvall, E. M. & Miller, B.C. (1985). *Marriage and family development* (6th ed.). New York: Harper & Row.

Gillis, C.L. (1991). Family nursing research, theory and practice. *Image: The journal of nursing scholarship, 23*(1), 19–22.

Glasser, P. H. & Glasser, L.N. (1970). *Families in crisis.* New York: Harper and Row.

Holman, A. M. (1983). *Family assessment: Tools for understanding and intervention.* Beverly Hills, CA: Sage.

Jacobs, J. (1993). Families under siege. *Family Therapy Networker, 17*(1), 24–25.

Kaplan, L.(1986). *Working with multiproblem families.* Lexington, MA: Lexington Books.

Kaplan, L. & Hennon, C.B. (1992). Remarriage education: The personal reflections program. *Family relations, 41,* 127–134.

Johnston, R. L. (1987). Approaching family intervention through Rogers' conceptual model. In A. L. Whall (Ed.), *Family therapy theory for nursing: Four approaches.* Norwalk, CT: Appleton-Century-Crofts.

Lancaster, J. B., Altmann, J., Rossi, A.S., & Sherrod, L.R. (1987). *Parenting across the life span.* New York: Aldine de-Gruyter.

Loveland-Cherry, C. J. (1984). Family system patterns of autonomy and cohesiveness: Relationship to family members' health behavior. *Nursing Research, 33*(1), 51–52.

Marciano, T.D. & Sussman, M.B. (1991). Wider families: An overview. *Marriage and Family Review, 17,* 1–8.

Martin, E. P. & Martin, J.M. (1978). *The black extended family.* Chicago: University of Chicago Press.

McPhatter, A.R. (1991). Assessment revisited: A comprehensive approach to understanding family dynamics. *Families in Society, 71,* 236–245.

Mirvis, P.H. & Marks, M.L. (1992). *Managing the merger: Making it work.* Englewood Cliffs, NJ: Prentice-Hall.

Neuman, B. (1989). *The Neuman systems model* (2nd ed). Norwalk, CT: Appleton & Lange.

Pender, N. J. (1987). *Health promotion in nursing practice* (2nd ed.). Norwalk, CT: Appleton & Lange.

Ross, M. M. & Helmer, H. (1988). A comparative analysis of Neuman's model using the individual and family as the units of care. *Public Health Nursing, 5*(1), 30–36.

Simons-Morton, B.G., O'Hara, N.M., & Simons-Morton, D.G. (1986). Promoting healthful diet and exercise behaviors in communities, schools, and families. *Family and Community Health, 9*(3), 1–13.

Watson, W.L. (1992). Family therapy. In G.M. Bulechek & J.C. McCloskey (Eds.), *Nursing interventions: Essential nursing treatments* (2nd ed). Philadelphia: Saunders.

Weber, T., McKeever, J.E., & McDaniel, S.H. (1985). A beginner's guide to the problem-oriented first family interview. *Family Process, 24,* 357.

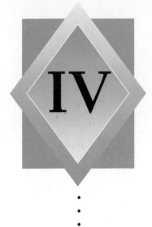

IV

Promoting and Protecting the Health of Populations

CHAPTER

18

Promoting and Protecting the Health of Maternal, Prenatal, and Infant Populations

LEARNING OBJECTIVES

Upon completion of this chapter, the student should be able to:

- Identify the health goals established by the U.S. Department of Health and Human Services in 1990 for the maternal-infant population.
- Discuss the major risk factors for pregnant women and infants.
- Describe the important considerations in designing good health promotion programs to fit the needs of diverse maternal-infant populations.
- List several features of a typical health promotion program for maternal-infant populations.
- Identify several methods of delivering services to maternal-infant populations.
- Describe the different roles of a community health nurse in serving the maternal-infant population.

KEY TERMS

- Continuous quality improvement
- Drug dependent
- Drug exposed
- Fetal alcohol effects
- Fetal alcohol syndrome
- High-risk infants
- Low birth weight
- Passive smoking
- Self-help group
- Smokeless tobacco products
- Very low birth weight

Barbara Walton Spradley and Judith Ann Allender
COMMUNITY HEALTH NURSING: CONCEPTS AND PRACTICE, 4th ed.
© 1996 Barbara Walton Spradley and Judith Ann Allender

Working with maternal and infant populations is a primary facet of community health nursing. More than 70% of nursing practice in official health agencies involves primary preventive work with mothers and infants, especially adolescent mothers and **high-risk infants**. The high-risk infant is one who has not received adequate nutrition or care during pregnancy due to a lack of proper prenatal care, economic disadvantage, or disease exposure.

Why should maternal and infant populations require this amount of attention from community health nursing? Despite the existence of advanced technology and availability of excellent perinatal services in our society, certain segments of the maternal and infant populations, particularly those which are economically disadvantaged, remain at high risk for disease, disability, and even death. While some women receive excellent prenatal care and benefit from the diagnostic capabilities of advanced technology, other women go without prenatal care and even without proper nutrition. Over four million women in the United States give birth each year, and 20% of these women have no medical insurance (Statistical Abstracts of U.S., 1993). Many of these women do not have the financial or social resources to sustain minimal health levels for themselves and their infants. A significant issue the community health nurse increasingly deals with is teenage pregnancy. In 1990 there were 10,700 live births to teens under the age of 15 and among the unmarried teens 15 to 19 years of age there were 350,000 infants born (Ibid.). These "children having children" will affect the health of society well into the future. Clearly these mothers and their babies need primary preventive services, but reaching them with well-designed programs presents a considerable challenge for community health nurses. This chapter addresses three major areas in the health of maternal and infant populations: (1) the health status and needs, (2) the design, implementation, and evaluation of maternal and infant health programs, and (3) the availability of community resources.

Health Needs and Goals for Pregnant Women and Infants

Community health nurses constitute a key group of health care workers involved in both the planning of programs and the actual delivery of services to mothers and babies. A solid understanding of vital statistics and other data regarding maternal-infant populations serves nurses as they determine both the appropriateness and the effectiveness of programs and services. Reviewing some of the vital statistics of the past decade provides insight into the problem areas in maternal-infant health.

In 1990, the U.S. Department of Health and Human Services established health goals for the year 2000. These goals were published as the *National Health Promotion and Disease Prevention Objectives* and include specific goals for the maternal and infant population (as presented in Table 18.1) along with significant vital statistics.

TABLE 18.1. *Selected Goals from National Health Promotion and Disease Prevention Objectives*

	1987	1990	2000 Target
Reduce the infant mortality rate to no more than seven deaths per 1,000 live births.	10.1	9.2	7.0
Reduce the black infant mortality rate to no more than 11 deaths per 1,000 live births.	17.9	17.0	11.0
Reduce the maternal mortality rate to no more than 3.3 per 100,000 live births.	6.6	8.2	3.3
Reduce the cesarean delivery rate to no more than 15 per 100 deliveries.	24.4	23.5	15.0
Reduce low birth weight to an incidence of no more than 5% of all live births.	6.9	7.0	5.0
Reduce low birth weight to an incidence of no more than 9% of black live births.	12.7	13.3	9.0

Source: *Healthy people 2000*, U.S. Dept. of Health and Human Services, 1990.

After years of working toward improving maternal-infant health, the United States has made very limited progress. Table 18.1 indicates both areas in which we have made progress and areas in which the country has fallen short of its goals. Although the infant mortality rate (deaths for all babies up to 1 year of age) has dropped substantially from the 20.0 per 1000 live births in 1970 to 9.2 per 1000 live births in 1990 the U.S. infant mortality rate remains higher than those of 21 other nations including Japan, France, Italy, and the countries of Scandinavia. A decade ago the Japanese reached the same goal the U.S. is trying to achieve. In 1993 the Japanese had an infant mortality rate of 4.5, a much more desirable rate than the 7 set by the United States for the year 2000 (Julnes, et al., 1994). The even higher infant mortality rate among African Americans is another area of great concern. Although progress has been made decreasing the rate from 32.6 per 1000 live births in 1970, to 17.0 per 1000 live births in 1990 (Statistical Abstracts of U.S., 1993) it is doubtful whether goals for the year 2000 will be met.

Low birth weight babies (less than 2500 gms but more than 1000 gms at birth) and a high rate of maternal mortality are two areas in which not only has there been no progress but the statistics have gotten worse. Statistics indicate a slight increase in number of low birth weight babies for the total population from 1987 to 1990 and also a slight increase in low birth weight babies in the black population as well. The maternal mortality rate has increased from 6.6 per 100,000 live births to 8.2 per 100,000 live births (see Table 18.1).

There are, however, several areas in which great progress has been made toward the year 2000 goals. The neonatal mortality rate (deaths for all infants up to 28 days old) decreased from 15.1 per 1000 live births in 1970, to 5.8 per 1000 live births in 1990—a considerable decrease. Also the number of women having Cesarean section deliveries decreased from 24.4 per 100 deliveries in 1987 to 23.4 per 100 deliveries in 1991. In these two areas, we are on the way to reaching the targeted goals (Statistical Reports of U.S., 1993).

Risk Factors for Pregnant Women and Infants

Most pregnant women in the United States are healthy, have normal pregnancies, and produce healthy babies. Nevertheless, there are many factors that contribute to the health problems of those mothers and babies who figure in the statistics on infant mortality and low birth weight. The factors associated with low birth weight and infant mortality can be grouped into three categories:

1. Lifestyle—smoking, inadequate nutrition, low prepregnancy weight, high alcohol consumption, narcotic addiction, environmental toxins, prolonged standing, strenuous work, stress, and lack of social support;
2. Sociodemographic—low maternal age, low educational level, poverty, and unmarried status; and
3. Medical and gestational history—primiparity, multiple gestation, premature rupture of the membranes, uterine abnormaly, febrile illness during pregnancy, abortion, genetic factors, gestational induced hypertension, and diabetes (Abrams & Newman, 1991; Pickering & Deeks, 1991; Stewart & Nimrod, 1993).

It is in the realm of life-style choices that the work of community health nurses can have the most significant impact. Data related to these factors are provided below.

DRUG USE

Cities, suburbs, and rural areas are being overwhelmed with drug-related problems. "Substance abuse during pregnancy is a problem of enormous scope and staggering social and medical implications" (Wheeler, 1993, p. 191). According to *Healthy People—2000* (U.S. Public Health Service, 1990) possible explanations for the recent slowed rate of progress in preventing infant mortality include changes in maternal characteristics. In the last decade when infant mortality rates should have been decreasing, an increasing number of women were using illicit drugs during their pregnancy. This increases the proportion of women entering pregnancy at a greater risk for poor pregnancy outcomes. Many of these women have unintended pregnancies, as outcomes of activities to support a drug habit, including prostitution. The focus on drug acquisition and use leaves everything and everyone else in their life a distant second. The important areas associated with narcotic addiction include limited prenatal care, inadequate nutrition, low prepregnancy weight, alcohol consumption, and smoking (Stewart & Nimrod, 1993).

All these factors contribute to low birth weight infants at a time when technological advancement is approaching maximum benefit from neonatal intensive care (Kleinman, 1990). There is only so much care that can be given extrautero for the **very low birth weight** infant (1000 gm or less at birth). All of these issues contribute to a slowing of the decrease in infant mortality. The year 2000 goals of 7 deaths per 1,000 live births most likely will not be realized (see Fig. 18.1).

In the United States it is estimated that up to 375,000 infants per year are born to **drug-exposed** women (a person who uses drugs intermittently) (U.S. General Accounting Office, 1990). Another 5000–10,000 infants each year are born to **drug dependent** women (those persons who physically and psychologically require use of drugs to function). Many pregnant addicts do not receive prenatal care, and it is not until their newborns exhibit signs of wthdrawal in the nursery that many of these women are identified (Sullivan, Boudreaux & Keller, 1993). The exposure to drugs is related to low birth weight; congenital anomalies; neonatal withdrawal characterized by abnormalities of the gastrointestinal tract, the central nervous system, and the respiratory system; poor feeding; abnormal sleep patterns; and long term learning disabilities in the infant (Givens & Wheeler, 1993; Holland, et al., 1990). Infants exposed to heroin or cocain prenatally are also more likely to succumb to sudden infant death syndrome (SIDS) (Durand, Espinoza & Nickerson, 1990). Although it is perceived that poor, inner-city women of color are more likely to be addicted to drugs, Chasnoff, Landress, and Barrett (1990) found that drug use among women is unrelated to race and socio-economic status.

A lifestyle choice which includes the use of drugs during pregnancy has placed millions, in fact, a generation of children at risk (Barry, 1991). These children are seen in neonatal intensive care units, the foster care system, special education programs in the public school system, and later in the juvenile court system. Family structure patterns are altered as grandparents, find themselves primary caregivers for their grandchildren. A woman who is an intravenous drug user introduces another public health problem, that of acquiring and possibly spreading the HIV virus to the fetus and possibly others (Goldstein, 1994). The primary, secondary, and tertiary prevention role of the community health nurse cannot be underestimated when the results of drug use demonstrate such a high toll on all aspects of society.

ALCOHOL USE

Use and especially addiction to alcohol as the substance of choice is another problem in society. "Because it is both legally and socially acceptable, alcohol is the substance most commonly abused by pregnant women" (Mercer, 1990, p. 128). When accompanied with pregnancy, alcohol use can cause devastating effects in the fetus, even with limited alcohol use early in the preg-

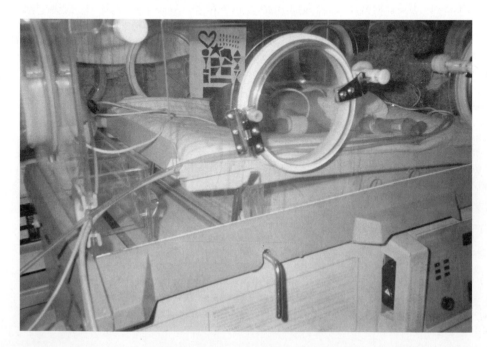

FIGURE 18.1. Low birth weight babies need special care and are at risk for neonatal mortality.

nancy and no addiction. **Fetal alcohol syndrome** (FAS) is a syndrome characterized by structural abnormalities of the head and face including microcephaly, flattening of the maxillary area, intrauterine growth retardation, decreased birth weight and length, developmental delays, intellectual impairment, hyperactivity, altered sleep pattern, feeding problems, perceptual problems, impaired concentration, mood problems, and language dysfuction. It is a national health problem that was only first identified in 1973 (Goldstein, 1994; Olson, 1994). This syndrome is seen in infants of 30% to 40% of the women who are chronic, heavy drinkers throughout pregnancy (Weiner & Morse, 1988). FAS is the number one cause of mental retardation in the Western world, with the estimated incidence of 1 to 3 per thousand live births, and is 100% preventable (Olson, 1994). **Fetal alcohol effects** (FAE) is a syndrome in which children suffer some but not all of the symptoms of fetal alcohol syndrome. It occurs in children whose mothers have used varying amounts of alcohol while pregnant, including those who engaged only in occasional binge drinking. FAE is seen three more times more often than fetal alcohol syndrome (Mercer, 1990; Robertson, 1993; Olson, 1994).

Alcohol use during pregnancy also increases the risk for abruptio placentae, stillbirth, spontaneous abortion, congenital anomalies, prematurity, postmaturity, and infections (Cook, et al., 1990; Robertson, 1993). Offspring of mothers who both drank heavily and smoked during pregnancy delivered babies that weighed 500 grams less than babies of non-drinking, non-smoking mothers. The combined effects of drinking and smoking are important factors in infant mortality and impaired mental and physical development (Edell, 1989; Wheeler, 1993). Eighty-three percent of women reporting alcohol consumption during pregnancy also smoked (Brooten et al., 1987).

TOBACCO USE

The nicotine in tobacco is a major addictive substance and smoking is considered an addiction which many people find difficult to stop. Although the risk factors of smoking are well documented many pregnant women continue to smoke (see Fig. 18.2). Smoking during pregnancy has been associated with stillbirths, spontaneous abortions, higher perinatal mortality, and low birth weights (Rienzo, 1993; Lawson, 1994). Infants, whose mothers smoked during pregnancy, weigh approximately 200 grams less at birth than infants whose mothers did not smoke (Brooten, et al., 1987).

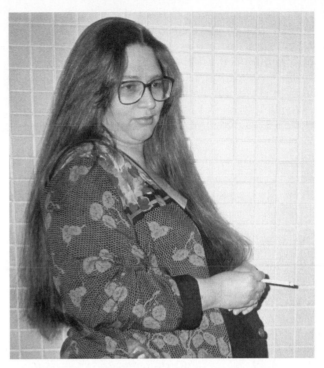

FIGURE 18.2. Pregnant women who smoke endanger their babies' lives as well as their own.

Passive smoking, which is exposure to tobacco smoke from other people smoking in one's environment, also puts a person at risk for smoking-related disease. It has been found that the smoke from a burning cigarette sitting on an ashtray, inhaled passively by the nonsmoker, contains a higher concentration of toxins and carcinogens than the smoke inhaled directly by the smoker (Rienzo, 1993). If a pregnant person lives with a smoker, she can be negatively affected by the other person's addiction.

The use of **smokeless tobacco products**, such as snuff and chewing tobacco, has led to an increase in oral cancers related to tobacco exposure, without exposure to smoke. Any form of tobacco is extremely hazardous to health (Ibid.). "The current trend to restrict smoking in public may induce the heavily addicted to turn to smokeless tobacco as a substitute, just as restrictions against public expectoration once contributed to the social acceptance of smoking instead of 'dipping' or chewing" (Rienzo, 1993, p. 26). At this time it is not known if passive smoke or smokeless tobacco have any direct adverse effects on the fetus.

The nurse must not only advise clients to quit smoking, they must offer methods or interventions to help.

The nurse may recommend available resources such as support groups where clients can get help, pharmacologic treatments such as nicotine patches or gum, and even a controlled-use of tobacco approach can be helpful. Any permanent reduction in the number of cigarettes smoked, amount of second-hand smoke inhaled, or smokeless tobacco used can only improve the health of the user and in the case of a pregnant user, the health of the fetus.

SEXUALLY TRANSMITTED DISEASES AND AIDS

Recently the public has been lulled into a sense of false security about the presence of sexually transmitted diseases (STDs) in the community. Because the major media has focused on HIV and AIDs for the last decade, information about the effects of other STDs has been ignored. However, "STDs are on the rise, jeopardizing the health and fertility of women and affecting the health and development of the fetus and newborn."(Killion, 1994. p. 156) Chlamydia is the most common sexually transmitted disease in the United States. Herpes affects 20 million Americans every year and there are nearly 2 million reported cases of gonorrhea. Other STDs include syphilis, chancroid, lymphogranuloma venereum, and granuloma inguinale. Two-thirds of all cases of STDs occur in persons aged 15–24 years old; the age group in which one-third of all births occur (Statistical Abstracts, 1993).

A positive HIV status is the tragedy of the last quarter of the 20th century. However, being pregnant or postpartum and HIV positive calls for special nursing management of the pregnancy and of the family after the birth of the newborn. There are many teaching opportunities for the community health nurse during a high-risk pregnancy such as helping the client identify, change, or curtail high-risk behaviors. Success in changing behaviors often requires an interdisciplinary approach of health care, social, emotional, and finacial resources. What follows is a discussion of some of the pregnancy management issues.

Antepartum Management. Evidence suggests that there is a higher rate of genitourinary tract infections and an increased incidence of STD's in HIV-positive women during pregnancy. In a study by Gloeb, O'Sullivan, and Efantis (1988) they followed 50 HIV positive women through pregnancy. One-third suffered a variety of STD's and only 15 (28.8%) had uncomplicated antenatal courses. The nurse should advise clients to see their health provider for an evaluation immediately if they develop fever, sweats, cough, or diarrhea. HIV positive clients should also receive nutritional counseling and be encouraged to gain weight appropriately (Minkoff, 1988). It should not be overlooked that a woman may be HIV negative at the beginning of a pregnancy and seroconvert, especially if she is continuing high risk behaviors, since HIV can be acquired at any time during pregnancy.

Postpartum Management. There is no clear evidence that an HIV positive woman experiences increased rates of postpartum or postoperative morbidity. However, the HIV-positive woman should be monitored for the development of any signs and symptoms of infections (Minkoff, 1988). If the community health nurse is doing a newborn assessment, a lochia check, or in some way coming into contact with maternal or infant blood, he or she should be wearing gloves. The importance of handwashing cannot be over stated. The use of universal precautions is no longer the "ideal to be achieved" but the standard under which all nurses *must* practice.

Breastfeeding. HIV can be cultivated from breastmilk and had been implicated in several documented cases of HIV transmission. Therefore HIV positive clients should be advised against breastfeeding (Ellerbrock & Rogers, 1990). The nurse focuses teaching on providing a safe, available form of infant formula. Additional information on the role of the community health nurse working with the HIV positive client is found in Chapter 23.

Women who discover that they have STDs often feel ashamed, betrayed, embarrassed, and angry. Those who are asymptomatic may deny the existence of the disease and not carry out the treatment plan. While educating the pregnant client about the effects of STDs is critical, providing information alone is not enough. The community health nurse has a pivotal role in enhancing the empowerment of women so they can act on the information. The nurse talks with the women and helps them understand that they have control over their bodies. Usually STDs are first discovered in pregnancy during routine prenatal screening which places the clinic nurse and the nurse who may make home visits in a position to take an affirmative approach to treatment and follow-up (Killion, 1994).

POOR NUTRITION AND WEIGHT GAIN

Research has demonstrated a positive correlation between weight gain during pregnancy and normal birth weight babies. (Stewart & Nimrod, 1993). Weight gains of 25 to 35 pounds during pregnancy are recommended. Obese women have a higher incidence of gestational hiatal hernia, diabetes, pre-eclampsia, primary cesarean section, gestational induced hypertension, and perinatal mortality if there are prenatal complications (Neeson & May, 1986; Johnston & Kandell, 1992). Community health nurses who work with morbidly obese pregnant women can help them most by emphasizing good nutrition and even maintaining prepregnant weight without reducing caloric intake. This can be accomplished primarily by a marked decrease in comsumption of "empty calories" from junk food. Pregnancy is never a time for dieting, but eating foods from the Food Guide Pyramid established by the U.S. Department of Agriculture will assure the proper servings and proportions of foods. Nutritional counseling, however, can have an additional benefit in that it may ultimately decrease the risk of obesity or eating disorders in the client's children.

Underweight women have twice as many low birth weight babies as women whose weight is within normal range. There is a correlation between poor weight gain in pregnancy and low birth-weight babies. Low birth weight is associated with higher incidences of growth problems, developmental delays, central nervous system disorders, and mental retardation (Brooten, et al., 1987; Johnston & Kandell, 1992). Two-thirds of infants who die before one year of age weighed less than 5 pounds 7 ounces at birth (Jacobson, 1987). Nutritional teaching, again is within the community health nurses' role with pregnant woman who had difficulty gaining weight. Finding ways to add calories to foods or increase the woman's desire to eat are effective methods to improve maternal weight gain. Insufficient caloric intake in pregnant adolescents (who themselves are still growing) is an additional concern (Brooten, et al., 1987).

TEENAGE PREGNANCY

Each year, more than one million American teenagers become pregnant. There is a strong association between young maternal age and high infant mortality rates, and infants born to teenagers are at increased risk for neonatal and postneonatal mortality (Nord, et al., 1992). Infants born to African-American adolescents are at higher risk of low birth weight than are white infants. Infants born to very young adolescents (aged 10 to 14 years) are at very high risk for neo-natal mortality. Since teen mothers disproportionately come from disadvantaged backgrounds, the markers for successful pregnancy outcomes and future life events are more complex. The mother's educational attainment, marital experiences, subsequent fertility behavior, labor force experience and occupational attainment, and her experiences with poverty and welfare are all directly related to the adolescent pregnancy (Nord, et al., 1992).

The issues of adolescent parenting are complex. The community health nurse may focus on one important and seemingly less complex issue of nutrition during pregnancy. However, it is a more difficult task to change the eating habits of teens than it is with adults. They are in a stage of development where they are more concerned with their body image than the growth and development of the fetus they are carrying. Fad dieting, peer pressure, and personal control are all issues with which the pregnant teen is struggling. If this teen is from the culture of poverty, multiple other issues impact her motivation to make dietary changes during the pregnancy. (See the Levels of Prevention discussion on a healthy pregnancy.)

Planning for the Health of Maternal-Infant Populations

Developing quality health care programs and services for specific populations does not happen by chance. Such programs are based upon identified needs and are organized and delivered in a thoughtful, logical fashion. Ideally, they result from coordinated community planning. Effective community health planning can save nurses valuable time and resources and can help prevent inappropriate distribution and duplication of services.

PLANS TO FIT THE NEEDS OF SPECIFIC POPULATIONS

To design programs and services for maternal-infant populations, planners need to have a sound understanding of the population they are attempting to serve. Specific aggregates of pregnant women have needs that the community health nurse should assess and incorporate into a prenatal program. Two important considerations include: (1) specific needs identified through data collection and client input, and (2) the developmental stage of the population being served.

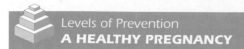

Levels of Prevention
A HEALTHY PREGNANCY

GOAL
A healthy full term infant comes into the world.

PRIMARY PREVENTION
(Planning a pregnancy) The parents plan the pregnancy at a time in life when it's "right." Pregnancies are spaced two years (or more) apart. Mother has a positive attitude going into the pregnancy. A health care provider is selected. The parents do not use alcohol, tobacco, or other mood-altering substances when planning to conceive. The mother attempts to have weight as close to ideal as possible, prior to conception. Family and significant others are supportive. There are financial resources to meet the expanding families needs.

SECONDARY PREVENTION
(The pregnancy) The mother starts prenatal care in the first trimester and it is continuous. She does not use alcohol, tobacco, or other mood altering substances. Parents avoid exposure to people with infectious diseases. Mother has adequate nutrition, rest, and exercise. Mother begins support services if eligible (AFDC, WIC). Family and significant others continue to be supportive. The parents attend labor preparation, infant care, and parenting classes. Name(s) are selected for the infant. Delivery method and location is selected. The home is prepared for the infant—adequate infant furnishings and supplies are acquired within the parents' budget. Preparations and plans are made regarding breast or bottle feeding. A pediatrician or pediatric nurse practitioner is selected. An infant car seat is acquired. Plan(s) are made to get to the health care facility when in labor.

TERTIARY PREVENTION
(After delivery) The parents and significant others begin to bond with the newborn. Parents get to know the newborn. Establish breast or bottle feeding routine. Infant returns home in an infant car seat which is used whenever traveling ina car. Exposure to people with infectious diseases is avoided. Infant's birth is celebrated according to cultural and religious preferences. Appointments are made and kept for post-partum and newborn visits to health care provider. Parents resume sexual intercourse using a family planning method of their choice. Infant immunization schedule begins on time. Enjoy the new life created!

Vital statistics assist planners to identify problems and pinpoint segments of the population where problems are more likely to occur, yet statistics alone cannot fully characterize the populations they represent. Society has witnessed numerous ineffective community, health care, and public works projects. Programs often have failed because the targeted populations were assessed incompletely or not involved in the planning process.

Most nurses realize that a predetermined, generalized plan may not meet the needs of any one specific client. To increase effectiveness, the nurse involves the client in designing a plan to meet individual needs and must consider the client's level of education, previous life experiences, level of motivation, culture, and developmental stage. A prenatal program would be very different when planned for a group of college-educated career women, pregnant adolescents, women in rural Appalachia, or female Hispanic migrant farm workers. The needs of the women in each of these subpopulations are very different and programs should be adjusted accordingly. The career women may want information on nurse-midwives, alternative birthing methods, and sources for literature on pregnancy, birthing, and newborn care. The pregnant teens may benefit by special teen pregnancy clinics, group classes on parenting, and assistance with selecting the supplies needed for the baby. The women living in rural Appalachia may respond best to a mobile health clinic staffed by a female nurse practitioner, a social worker to assist with completing the application process for social services, and someone to watch their other children during the appointments. The migrant workers may best be served by bilingual health care workers who offer a clinic in the evenings at a migrant camp or one that is mobile and can come to the workers in the fields. Women from each of these groups can provide valuable information to planners regarding their specific needs. As with individual clients, input from the targeted population increases the program's chances for success.

As individuals grow and mature, they continually experience physiological changes, personality changes as new psychosocial issues are met (Erikson, 1968), and increasingly sophisticated thought processes (Piaget, 1950). Consequently, a person's most pressing concerns at one stage in life may seem insignificant at the next stage of development.

When planning maternal-infant health programs, it is crucial that the community health nurse also consider the developmental stages of the women being served. For example, adolescents are in a stage of intellectual development in which their thinking processes are beginning to move from concrete thinking patterns to abstract thinking patterns (Ibid.). Concrete thinking is based on what the person has actually experienced or is experiencing. Abstract thinking involves the ability to hear or read something and be able to apply it to a future problem or dilemma. Some adolescents may have difficulty comprehending the complex psychosocial issues and problems with which they will be faced when caring for an infant and young child. Nurses must use innovative and creative approaches when helping adolescents to understand the complex and demanding nature of child care. Some maternal-infant health programs and high schools involve pregnant adolescents (and those judged at risk of becoming pregnant) in child day-care programs in which the adolescents participate in the day-to-day care of infants and toddlers. They experience first hand both the joys as well as the intense demands and heavy responsibility of being a parent.

The needs of pregnant women in the developmental stages of young adulthood and middle adulthood differ substantially from those of adolescents and will vary between individuals (Erikson, 1968). Women in young and middle adulthood more frequently have planned their pregnancy and make realistic decisions regarding their expanding responsibilites. The community health nurse's most valuable skills are teacher, coordinator, resource manager, counselor, and collaborator. The nurse uses these skills to design programs that meet the needs of the more mature prenatal client. Thorough understanding of the developmental tasks and the psychosocial issues confronting each population should be the cornerstone of solid, well-developed programs. Such programs can be adapted to the developmental needs of clients in adolescence, young adulthood, or middle adulthood.

Health Programs for Maternal-Infant Populations

For over a half century the federal government has been granting money to states for the promotion of maternal and child health. Through the Maternal and Child Health Block Grant Program millions of dollars come to individual states each year. This money supplements the state's own funds to meet the maternal and child health care needs for people at the local level. With this money each state provides basic services to its maternal-child population. An additional companion program provides services to special needs children. Community health nurses need to become familar with their state's Maternal and Child Health Program and the services provided by the program.

Program plans for maternal-infant populations across the country include many typical features. For example, there are concerted efforts to educate clients during the antepartum and postpartum periods and assess their specific needs. A major focus of community health nurses is teaching. Nurses introduce new information or reinforce existing knowledge of pregnancy, delivery, and postpartum health considerations (see Table 18.2). Through teaching, nurses help mothers adapt to the physiological and emotional changes they are experiencing and help them anticipate and plan for the impact their infants will have on their daily lives.

During the comprehensive, ongoing client assessments, in addition to considering their clients' physiological and emotional status, nurses must assess the clients' social support systems, access to medical care, financial status, housing needs, and ability to provide for their babies. If clients need assistance in any or all of these areas, nurses must intervene and refer them to other appropriate community resources (see Table 18.2). Nurses often must serve as advocate for the client in the referral process and should continue to work collaboratively with other professionals during follow-up services to meet clients' needs.

Implementation of Maternal-Infant Health Programs

Methods of delivering services to clients often are determined by the financial resources of the agency providing the services. The majority of maternal-infant

TABLE 18.2. *Typical Features of Maternal-Infant Health Programs*

I. Antepartum teaching
   a. Significance of prenatal care
   b. Self-responsibility
   c. Physiological changes during pregnancy
   d. Fetal growth and development
   e. Nutrition
   f. Proper exercise
   g. Hazards of substance use: drugs/alcohol/tobacco
   h. Breastfeeding techniques and problem solving
   i. Stages of labor
   j. Delivery—process and options available
   k. Future birth control
II. Introduction to community resources for prenatal care
   a. Childbirth classes
   b. Self-help groups (pregnant teens, parents of twins, etc.)
   c. WIC
   d. Department of Social Services
   e. Family planning services
   f. School-based clinics
   g. High-risk clinics
III. Postpartum teaching
   a. Newborn assessments
   b. Care of the newborn
   c. Growth and development of the infant
   d. Infant immunization schedule/health care follow-up
   e. Mother/infant bonding
   f. Postpartum physiological changes in the mother
   g. Breast/bottle feeding techniques
   h. Postpartum health care follow-up
   i. Exercise to regain muscle tone
   j. Family planning
   k. Returning to work (balancing home, family, and work)
   l. Child care
IV. Delivery of services for prenatal/postnatal care
   a. Clinic/private health care provider visits
   b. Home visits
   c. Formal classes
   d. Self-help groups
   e. Community education
V. Client advocacy and coordination with other community resources
   a. Physicians/nurse practitioners/nurse midwives
   b. Clinics
   c. Hospitals
   d. High schools
   e. Industries
   f. WIC
   g. Department of Social Services

health programs in the United States receive public funding through local tax dollars and through federal block grants given to each state for allocation by state officials.

Methods of delivering services will vary based upon the population and its specific needs. The geographical distribution of clients and the size of the nursing staff available to deliver the services also play significant roles. For example, in rural areas where clients are scattered over a large area, it may be appropriate to deliver services to the population on a one-to-one basis through nurse-run clinics (stationary or mobile) or home visits.

TYPES OF DELIVERY SERVICE

Clinic Programs

In the clinic setting each client receives an individualized examination, immunizations, and health teaching. Unfortunately, there are time constraints placed on the nurse and thus the actual time spent in teaching clients is relatively short. Clinics may be effective on Native American reservations where the population is centrally located and on sites where migrant farm workers and their families are temporarily located.

A motorhome, bus, or van converted to serve as a mobile clinic may be the resource needed in some rural or isolated areas that are populated by groups experiencing physical barriers to health care services. Often the community health nurse working in a mobile health clinic provides routine prenatal, postpartum, and newborn care including teaching and administering scheduled immunizations; a much needed service in some areas, and one met by no one other method as cost effectively. The recommended immunization schedule for children, which is started in infancy, is discussed in detail in Chapter 19.

Home Visits

Home visits also can provide clients with a one-to-one opportunity for teaching with the community health nurse. There are two major benefits to home visits. First, the client is in the comfortable, familiar surroundings of her own home. Second, the nurse's assessment is enhanced by observations in the home setting of such things as family interactions, values, and priorities. Home visiting to any client is costly for an agency. One-to-one delivery of service is becoming a luxury for some agencies with limited finances. In such agencies the nurses provide most of the routine care in clinic, or group settings. Home visits are made to the most serious of cases only. If clients are not at home at scheduled visit times and must be rescheduled this increases an already strained agency budget.

In metropolitan areas where community health nurses and clients are located near one another, nurse-run clinics and home visits may still be appropriate mechanisms for the delivery of services. In these cases, clients can visit the clinic frequently, and nurses can make more home visits with less distance to travel between clients. In addition, metropolitan areas afford community health nurses an opportunity to use a group approach with clients. This may include small, informal group discussions or larger, more formal classes. Whether small or large, groups can provide a vehicle for teaching by the nurse as well as a means for clients to teach and learn from one another. Group discussions can complement clinic and home visits and be ongoing at both neighborhood clinics and WIC clinics.

Self-help Groups

Self-help groups are usually formed by peers who have come together for mutual assistance to satisfy a common need, such as overcoming a handicap or life-disrupting problem. The group goal is to bring about specific desired behavior changes. While many groups are formed by peers, the community health nurse can often facilitate the formation, function, and direction of the group. The nurse's role is that of facilitator.

While many community health nurses may be unfamiliar with the concept of self-help groups, it is a concept that needs to be integrated into community health nursing practice more consistently. The role of the nurse will vary depending upon the size, interests, and level of sophistication of the group. For example, with a group of well-educated women who are effective problem solvers, the nurse may initiate the group and then serve primarily as a resource person. With a group of adolescents, on the other hand, the nurse may need to be present at each meeting to facilitate group process as well as to clarify information shared within the group. In Chapter 12 group work is described in greater detail.

Self-help groups provide many benefits to participants (see Fig. 18.3). Within the present health care system, clients often express feelings of insignificance and loss of control. However, in a self-help group environment, individuals regain their sense of identity and control. Acceptance of responsibility for health-promoting behaviors is a key concept supported by the majority of self-help groups. Members who lose sight of their responsibility are readily confronted by the group.

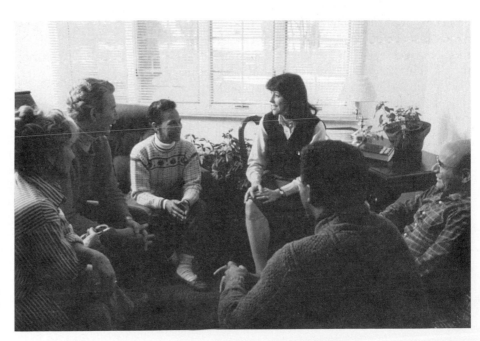

FIGURE 18.3. A self-help group fosters members' sense of identity and control.

Individuals reach out to help other members and in the process help themselves to become better informed and stronger in their own beliefs.

Self-help groups have been successfully developed for the prenatal population to address common concerns such as prenatal changes, adapting to pregnancy, fetal growth and development, and labor and delivery. For postpartum women, groups have been established for breastfeeding mothers, mothers of infants, mothers of toddlers, and mothers of twins. In each instance, members of healthy populations help one another to remain healthy and prevent potential problems.

The term peer counseling is used in some settings for the self-help group process. For instance in a high school, an informed and respected group of peers are identified, trained, and work with their classmates in small groups to discuss safe sex, saying no to drugs, self-esteem, or teen parenting. The topics vary to meet the needs of the peers. The concept of peer counselor and self-help groups can be initiated by the innovative and creative community health nurse.

School-based Programs

Delivering maternal and child health care programs in the school setting is a method of delivery that has been growing over the last ten years. Many high schools offer special courses for pregnant teens and at-home study programs after delivery, followed by on site day-care for the infants and toddlers of the postnatal teens. All of these services may be part of school-based programs. Some schools have initiated innovative programs that include additional health care services to their pregnant teens. This type of care may include family planning services, immunizations, and primary health care for illness and injury. Each community and school district needs to decide in consultation with community health nurses, school nurses, community leaders, parents, teens, and the board of education if these are services the community desires and/or needs.

High-Risk Clinics

High-risk clinics are established especially to meet the needs of pregnant women whose pregnancy is considered at high-risk. The pregnancy may be a multiple-pregnancy, a very young primapara client (under 15 years old), an older primapara client (over 40 years old), a grand multipara client, or the concern may be gestational diabetes or hypertension. The high-risk clinic is staffed by health care providers with special maternal-child health skills and advanced diagnostic equipment. They see clients experiencing a variety of conditions that might lead to fetal distress and so require special monitoring. In some communities, health care facilities have several types of high risk clinics. Some just see teens, or substance abusers. In smaller communities there may be one high-risk clinic meeting the needs of all those experiencing a special pregnancy. A community health nurse often becomes involved in the referral to such clinics, or may work in one as part of the job description in a small health department. The nurse needs to be knowledgeable about the clinic's services so potential clients can be referred if necessary.

THE ROLE OF COMMUNITY HEALTH NURSE

The maternal-child population makes up a major portion of a community health nurse's case load. There is a need for commitment to excellence in service for this special aggregate within the community. The reality is that the future health of the nation lies within each woman who is pregnant. The challenges are great for the nurses who work with this vulnerable group. Three areas/roles are especially focused on with the maternal-child population, (1) special professional qualities, (2) the role of educator, and (3) the role of client advocate and liaison.

Special Professional Qualities

Nurses working with maternal-infant health populations require special qualities and education. It is recommended that nurses have the following qualifications:

1. A sound educational background, minimally a baccalaureate degree in nursing.
2. A solid understanding of nursing process and ability to use it in working with individuals, families, and groups.
3. A knowledge of and willingness to work with other community resource offices.
4. Effective communication skills.
5. Effective organizational and leadership skills.
6. A sincere, nonjudgmental approach to clients.

Role of Educator

Because teaching is such an integral part of any maternal-infant program, nurses working in this area must possess good communication skills and teaching skills. In order for the teaching to be effective, however, the content and methods must vary depending on the needs, characteristics, and developmental stage of each population. For example, when teaching nutrition to pregnant women, the nurse must alter the recommended calorie intake according to the individual's height and weight and perhaps age group and life style. Nutrition information would be presented differently to groups who were college graduates and already familiar with the basics of the food guide pyramid, whereas information presented to pregnant teens may need to include the basic nutritional information.

In addition to tailoring subject matter to fit the client population, community health nurses should select teaching methodologies appropriate to clients. Some groups, such as couples attending childbirth education classes, may respond positively to structured classes; others, such as teens, may prefer a less formal discussion format. Peer-group counseling and self-help support groups may be appropriate formats for small groups who respond to the structure and support this format provides.

Teaching aids used should be appropriate for each audience. It is important to remember that many of the available teaching aids are in English and depict white, middle-class women and infants. While these will be appropriate for some populations, not all people will be able to identify with the mothers and babies portrayed. When at all possible, teaching aids should be congruent with the language, race, and culture of the population being served, so that clients can understand and identify. For example, pamphlets on infant care need to be made available in appropriate languages, with pictures portraying people from that cultural group and using supplies and equipment available in all homes. For instance, pamphlets that show infant room monitors, expensive educational toys, or fancy cribs with canopies may not depict the environment of the audience the nurse is trying to reach.

Teaching and motivating women to promote their own health and the health of their babies is a major challenge, and there is no single right way to approach the task. Community health nurses need to be innovative and creative in their approach to teaching, and to

also be aware that not all women are interested in their pregnancy. In Chapter 14 further information and resources, including appropriate teaching methods and materials for community health settings, are presented in more detail, and in Chapter 10 the hard-to-help client is also discussed.

Role of Client Advocate and Liaison with Community Resources

The maternal-infant population has complex needs. It is not unusual for community health nurses to see multiple personal and family problems in this group and, since community health nurses clearly cannot meet all these needs, it is essential that they act as client advocates in referring clients to other community resources. The nurse must have a working knowledge of available community resources for maternal and infant health which include family planning services, community childbirth education classes, those resources available through the Department of Social Services (state level), as well as the Special Supplemental Food Program for Women, Infants, and Children (WIC), a federal program administered by the states. A clear understanding of the services available and a positive working relationship between agency personnel will facilitate effective provision of services to this population group.

Department of Social Services. The Department of Social Services assigns each family a trained social worker. After interviewing the family, the social worker determines whether or not the family or individual members of the family meet eligibility criteria for programs administered by the Department of Social Services such as the Medicaid program (health insurance for low income families), the Food Stamp program (a program to increase low income families' buying power of most foods), and the Aid to Families with Dependent Children program (financial grants to low income and unemployed families with dependent children). If the social worker establishes family or individual eligibility, she or he starts the process of applying for benefits. These benefits are essential for the basic survival of many families, and it may be the community health nurse who first identifies a family in need of such social services and makes the initial referral. (See the Research in Community Health Nursing display that follows.)

Supplemental Food Program for Women, Infants, and Children (WIC). The Special Supplemental Food Program for Women, Infants, and Children (WIC) is a

Research in Community Health Nursing
A COST-BENEFIT ANALYSIS OF WIC PARTICIPATION

Buescher, P.A., Larson, L.C., Nelson, M.D., & Lenihan, A.J. (1993). Prenatal WIC participation can reduce low birth weight and newborn medical costs; A cost-benefit analysis of WIC participation in North Carolina. *Journal of the American Dietetic Association, 93*(2), 163–166.

This study linked Medicaid and WIC data files to birth certificates for live births in North Carolina for one year. Women who received Medicaid benefits and prenatal WIC services had substantially lower rates of low and very low birth weight infants than did women who received Medicaid but not prenatal WIC. Among white women, the rate of low birth weight was 22% lower for WIC participants and the rate of very low birth weight was 44% lower; among black women these rates were 31% and 57% lower, respectively. It was estimated that for each $1.00 spent on WIC services, Medicaid savings in costs for newborn medical care were $2.91. A higher level of WIC participation was associated with better birth outcomes and lower costs. The results indicate that prenatal WIC participation can effectively reduce low birth weight and newborn medical care costs among infants born to womem in poverty.

federal program that provides nutrition education for low-income women and children and vouchers for the purchase of specific supplemental foods and infant formula. Pregnant, breast-feeding, and postpartum women, infants, and children up to age 5 who are at medical or nutritional risk are eligible. The food provided by the program helps pregnant women to produce healthy, normal birth weight babies. WIC also refers participants to prenatal care, well-child care, and other services (Buescher, et al., 1993). Established in 1972 as a pilot program, WIC receives its funding from the Food and Nutrition Service of the U.S. Department of Agriculture.

Eligibility for WIC is based on income level, geographical area, and nutritional risk. Determining income eligibility is relatively uncomplicated, as guidelines are clearly defined by each state. Geographical eligibility varies, since many states offer services in all areas while others do not. Clients must live in an area that has been designated to receive funding. Nutritional risk is determined by the nurse or nutritionist through interviews with individual clients and by reviewing their previous medical and nutritional history (Mathematica, 1990). Eligibility factors for pregnant or postpartum women include age (i.e., adolescents or over 40); poor obstetrical history, such as previous low birth weight infants, miscarriages, short periods between pregnancies, and gestational diabetes; anemia; poor weight gain (low or high); and inadequate consumption of food. Risk factors for infants and children include poor growth, anemia, obesity, chronic illnesses, or nutrition-related diseases.

Based upon these risk factors, the health professional identifies areas of strength and areas for change. The program then offers supplemental food to clients. The food offered contains high-quality protein, iron, calcium, and Vitamins A and C. The specific foods offered tend to be combinations of fruit juice fortified with vitamin C, eggs, milk (lowfat or whole), cheese, beans, fortified cereals, and fortified infant formula. Distribution of food varies within states. In some states local dairies deliver the food to the home; in other states clients receive vouchers and exchange them for food at local grocery stores. The WIC program reevaluates clients at predetermined intervals. It reassesses needs, continues nutrition education, and recertifies food distribution if appropriate.

Family Planning Services. Family planning services may be an integral part of the comprehensive services of a local health department or community clinic. However in some communities these specialized services are provided by separate organizations, such as Planned Parenthood. Depending on the prevailing attitudes and needs in the community, the family planning services may include teen counseling, abortions, and long-term family planning methods such as administering Depo-Provera injections or inserting devices such as Norplant. Family planning service agencies provide counseling, gynecological examinations which include Pap smears and breast examinations, and mammograms. Some agencies may provide a broader range of services for which there is a need, such as genetic counseling, infertility counseling, and diagnosis and treatment of problems related to male and female sexual dysfunction.

Childbirth Education Classes. Most community clinics or health departments that provide maternal-child health care services also hold childbirth education classes. However, there are many community groups which develop and provide their own classes; possible sources include some churches, YWCAs, and hospitals. If the agency the nurse is working for does not provide such a service, it is the nurse's responsibility to know the community resources and refer interested women, and their siginificant others, to childbirth education classes. Women find these classes very helpful in preparing them for the birthing experience in addition to preparing them for the demands of parenthood. The group support effect from being in a class with other pregnant women is also rewarding. (See the Issues in Community Health Nursing display.)

Evaluation of Maternal-Infant Health Programs

Evaluation is a critical aspect of maternal-infant health program planning as it is with any health planning. Four questions, in particular, should be addressed: (1) Did the program meet the identified needs of this particular population? (2) Did the program meet its goals and objectives? (3) Was the program cost-effective? Did the outcomes justify the resources used? (4) What was the program's long-term impact on the health of this population?

Community health nurses find the answers to the above questions through a carefully designed, systematic evaluation plan. Program evaluation is discussed in detail in Chapter 11. For the purposes of this chapter, three useful methods for obtaining evaluation data are examined.

Vital statistics provide an important data base for evaluating maternal-infant programs. Local, state, or national figures can help agency personnel determine whether their own statistics are improving, remaining constant, or worsening. Using vital statistics, nurses can make comparisons between or within population groups. For instance, they might compare the incidence of low birth weight babies born to their clients with rates reported by similar agencies in other urban areas or in their agency the previous year. One disadvantage of using vital statistics is that the time required to compile this data can make it difficult to have the most current figures.

A second mechanism for evaluation within individual maternal-infant programs is assuring quality through **continuous quality improvement** (CQI) which is used by health professionals to monitor service and care of clients in order to maintain or improve delivery

Issues in Community Health Nursing
INFANT SLEEP POSITION AND SUDDEN INFANT DEATH SYNDROME

Approximately 6000 infants die each year with the diagnosis of Sudden Infant Death Syndrome (SIDS). SIDS is the leading cause of infant mortality between 1 month and 1 year of age in the United States. SIDS is defined as the sudden death of an infant under one year of age which remains unexplained after a thorough case investigation.

A variety of population characteristics were explored, such as families who had smokers, breast-feeding mothers, or side or back sleeping positions for the infant. The primary contributor to a 50% drop in SIDS deaths in seven countries, including the United States, during 1980 through 1992 was a decline in the prone sleeping position of infants.

The overwhelming opinion of the experts was that the evidence justified greater effort to reach parents with the American Academy of Pediatrics' recommendations that healthy infants, when being put down to sleep, be positioned on their side or back. (Willinger, M., Hoffman, H.J., & Hoarford, R.B. (1994). Sudden infant death syndrome. *Pediatrics, 93,* 814–819.)

of care. The CQI process (Akpunonu, et. al., 1994; Berwick, 1989) looks at maternal-infant program goals and raises questions such as the following:

How soon after receiving the referral were clients seen?
Was the data base complete?
Was the plan of care appropriate?
Were the established outcomes reasonable and achievable?
Were clients involved in the planning process?
Were appropriate referrals made?
Was there follow-up on the referrals?
Was discharge of the client appropriate?

Quality management systems use various methods to gather this type of information, such as feedback from clients through periodic questionnaires and personal interviews or telephone surveys. Disadvantages of these methods may be the time consumed, the expense for the agency, and the reliability of self-reported feedback rather than using more objective data obtained from client records and health outcomes. Chapter 27 discusses quality management and the role of the nurse in more detail.

A cost-effective mechanism for assessing a program and the client care delivered is by auditing client records. It is not feasible for an agency to review every client record, but random samplings can be done at predetermined times each year. If clearly defined criteria are established, then those conducting the audit can easily review a record and determine, in their professional judgment, whether or not the criteria have been met. Auditing client records can be a positive learning experience, and agency staff should be encouraged to participate in the process. Reading through another nurse's documentation can be a positive reminder of the impact that the community health nurse can have on the effectiveness of services delivered. (See the World Watch display.)

ROLE AS FACILITATOR TO INFLUENCE GOVERNMENT POLICIES

Another responsibility of the nurse in maternal-infant health programs is in the role of client advocate. This is done with clients at the local level on a daily basis, however changes are often needed at the state or federal level. The community health nurse can influence the legislation and policies which affect the services provided at the local level. Funding of maternal-child programs occurs through the state legislature. So, by giving testimony on behalf of the maternal-infant population, the community health nurse can attest to the needs of this population and promote the funding of additional programs at the local level. However, this takes time, and in the meantime, funding may begin to dwindle. Other sources for funding must be found.

The role of facilitator may include writing grants to obtain the funding for new projects or even to maintain existing programs. Writing grants and getting them funded is becoming a more important skill of the nurses in agencies which are experiencing fiscal constraints. Public and private grants, both large and small, can supplement the shrinking state funding. Limited funding and increasing client needs will continue into the 21st century, and the programs provided through local agencies may depend on grant monies generated by proposals written by community health nurses.

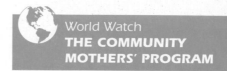

World Watch
THE COMMUNITY MOTHERS' PROGRAM

In Dublin, Ireland there is a large urban housing development rented by people who are largely unemployed and have problems with low self-esteem, alcoholism, depression, and anxiety. The incidence of violence against women and children and burglary is also high in the development. Against this background the community mothers' program was developed. It is a support program for first and second time parents with infants in the first year of life and occasionally up to the age of 2.

The model is one of parent enablement and empowerment. The program aims to recruit and train experienced mothers within the local community to give support and encouragement to parents in rearing their children. Emphasis of the program is on health care, nutrition, language, social, and cognitive development. Community mothers are expected to use patience, skill, and sensitivity to develop trust, empathy, and mutual respect with the parents taking part in the program. The community mothers are recruited, trained, and visited monthly by public health nurses, to provide support and discuss visits. Each "family development nurse" is responsible for up to 20 community mothers.

The program has contributed to the social and mental well-being of the community. An evaluation of the program revealed, in the families visited compared to a control group, more children completed immunizations, formula was used longer before switching to cow's milk or more mothers breast fed their infants, 98% of the parents read to their children, and the parents reported greater feelings of self-esteem. By 1991, 1100 families were in the program with 150 community mothers visiting. A shift in emphasis towards client involvement requires the families' acceptance that lay people can understand and implement activities previously carried out by professionals. The program also demonstrates how nurses can use their expertise and expand their scope of influence which reaches a widening circle of clients (Lloyd, 1993).

Summary

Vital statistics indicate that the status of maternal and infant health in the United States can be improved greatly when compared with that of other industrialized nations. Both the knowledge and the resources to improve the quality of life for mothers and babies is available in this country. However, the issues and importance of maternal and infant well-being extends beyond the borders of any single country.

Factors influencing the health of pregnant women and infants may be related to obstetrical history, genetics, socioeconomics, or life-style choices. The latter category is a prime target for community health nursing intervention. Life-style-related factors influencing the health status of pregnant women and infants include illicit drug, alcohol and tobacco use, presence of STD's during pregnancy, and weight gain during pregnancy. Pregnancy during adolescence, especially early adolescence, adds additional risk.

In planning effective maternal-infant programs, community health nurses must consider needs identified by the populations themselves as well as vital statistics. Maternal-infant programs across the country have certain features in common, including perinatal follow-up and teaching, client assessment, service delivery, coordination with other community resources, and client advocacy. These common features assist community health nurses in designing maternal and infant programs. Two other planning considerations include specific needs identified through data and client input

Activities to Promote Critical Thinking

1. What specific objectives has your local health department developed for mothers and infants to help achieve the U.S. Department of Health and Human Services goals for the year 2000? How do your county's statistics compare with those of others in your state on (1) infant death rates (collectively and by specific ethnic groups, e.g. Asian, black, white, Hispanic), (2) incidence of low birth-weight and very low birth-weight infants and (3) incidence of birth defects?

2. Describe three different maternal-infant populations in your county. What are their most pressing health needs? Do any existing services target these populations? How well, in your judgment, are clients' needs being met? Interview a city or county community health nurse as well as other public health professionals to help you find your answers.

3. Select one life-style related factor that affects pregnant women and infants (such as drug, alcohol, tobacco use, or nutritional status) and design a health program to deal with it. Be sure to include the main factors, discussed in this chapter, for planning and evaluating a maternal-infant program.

4. Sally, an 18-year-old woman, is single and 14 weeks pregnant. Her first prenatal visit was made at the urging of her aunt who uses the clinic. Sally reluctantly admitted to the clinic nurse that the pregnancy was unplanned, she consumes alcohol 2–3 times a week, frequently amounting to six 12 oz. cans of beer and 16 oz of wine, she smokes one pack of cigarettes a day, and has tried a variety of street drugs in the last three months, but does not use any regularly.

   The clinic nurse felt that the client might not return for regular prenatal care and made a referral to the community health nurse to make follow-up home visits to assess Sally's home environment and teach prenatal care and preparation for the infant. You were given the case. Design a plan of care to address Sally's needs. What specific services and programs might you recommend? What barriers might exist? How would the prenatal and postpartum teaching delivered to Sally differ from care needed by other single teens?

and the developmental stage of the population being served.

Creative and innovative methods of implementation such as discussion and self-help groups should be used more widely for teaching and working with maternal-infant populations. Effective implementation of health programs also depends on appropriately qualified staff members. The nature of the maternal-infant population is complex and diverse; thus, appropriate preparation of the community health nurse with highly developed professional skills and the knowledge and use of community resources provide important adjuncts to community health nursing services.

To evaluate the effectiveness of maternal-infant health programs, the community health nurse needs to ask the following questions: (1) Was the program relevant? (2) Did it meet identified goals and objectives? (3) Was the program cost-effective? (4) What was the program's long-term impact on the health of the population of mothers and infants? Three methods for obtaining evaluation data are collection of vital statistics, use of quality management processes, and the use of the auditing process.

There is an increasing need for the community health nurse to influence government policies and funding to the local level. More often the nurse will be called upon to acquire grant funding to maintain or promote needed programs that were once automatically funded or for the development of programs for a more complex client need now being experienced.

REFERENCES

Abrams, B. & Newman, V. (1991). Small-for-gestational-age birth: Maternal predictors and comparison with risk factors of spontaneous preterm delivery in the same cohort. *American Journal of Obstetrics and Gynecology, 164,* 785–790.

Akpunonu, B.E., Mutgi, A.B., Federman, D.J., et al. (1994). Enhancing faculty participation and interest in quality improvement in academic centers. *Journal of the American College of Medical Quality, 9*(1), 18–23.

Barry, E.M. (Winter, 1991). Pregnant, addicted, and sentenced. *Criminal Justice,* 23–27.

Berwick, D.M. (1989). Continuous improvement as an ideal in health care. *New England Journal of Medicine, 320,* 53–56.

Brooten, D., Peters, M.A., Glotts, M., Goffrey, S.E., Knapp, M., Cohen, S., & Jordan, C. (1987). A survey of nutrition, caffeine, cigarette, and alcohol intake in early pregnancy in an urban clinic population. *Journal of Nurse-Midwifery, 32*(2), 85–90.

Buescher, P.A., Larson, L.C., Nelson, M.D., & Lenihan, A.J. (1993). Prenatal WIC participation can reduce low birth weight and newborn medical costs: A cost-benefit analysis of WIC participation in North Carolina. *Journal of the American Dietetic Association, 93*(2), 163–166.

Chasnoff, I.J., Landress, H.J., & Barrett, M.E. (1990). The prevalence of illicit drug or alcohol use during pregnancy and discrepancies in mandatory reporting in Pinellas County, Florida. *New England Journal of Medicine, 322,* 1202–1206.

Cook, P.S., Peterson, R.C., & Moore, D.T. (1990). *Alcohol, tobacco, and other drugs may harm the unborn.* Rockville, MD: U.S. Department of Health and Human Services.

Durand, D.J., Espinoza, A.M., & Nickerson, B.G. (1990). Association between prenatal cocaine exposure and Sudden Infant Death Syndrome. *Journal of Pediatrics, 117,* 909–911.

Edell, D. (August, 1989). Smoking, drinking and nose sprays. *Edell Health Letter, 8,* 5.

Ellerbrock, T.V. & Rogers, M. (1990). Epidemiology of human immunodeficiency virus infection in women in the United States. *Obstetrics and Gynecology Clinics of North America, 17*(3), 523–544.

Erikson, E. H. (1968). *Identity, youth, and crisis.* New York: Norton.

Gloeb, D.J., O'Sullivan, M.J., & Efantis, J. (1988). Human immunodeficiency virus infection in women. The effects of human immunodeficiency virus on pregnancy. *American Journal of Obstetrics and Gynecology, 159,* 756–761.

Goldstein, A. (1994). *Addiction: From biology to drug policy.* New York: W.H. Freeman.

Holland, J.G., Graves, G.R., & Martin, J.N. (1990). Cocaine: A primer for providers of perinatal care. *Journal of Mississipi State Medical Association, 31*(9), 287.

Jacobson, H. N. (1987). Progress on key issues in maternal nutrition. *Public Health Reports,* July–August (Supp.), 50–52.

Johnston, C.S., & Kandell, L.A. (1992). Prepregnancy weight and rate of maternal weight gain in adolescents and young adults. *Journal of the American Dietetic Association 92*(12), 1515–1517.

Julnes, G., Konefal, M., Pindur, W., & Kim, P. (1994). Community-based perinatal care for disadvantaged adolescents: Evaluation of the resources mothers rogram. *Journal of Community Health, 19*(1), 41–53.

Killion, C. (1994). Pregnancy: A critical time to target STDs. *Maternal and Child Nursing, 19*(3), 156–161.

Kleinman, J.C. (1990). The recent slow down in the infant mortality decline. *Pediatric and Perinatal Epidemiology, 4,* 379–387.

Lawson, E.J. (1994). The role of smoking in the lives of low-income pregnant adolescents: A field study. *Adolescence, 29*(113), 61–77.

Lloyd, K. (1993). Mothering instinct. *Nursing times, 89*(26), 42–44.

Mathematica Policy Research Inc. (1990). *The savings in Medicaid costs for newborns and their mothers from prenatal participation in the WIC program.* Washington, DC: Food and Nutrition Service, U.S. Department of Agriculture.

Mercer, R.T. (1990). *Parents at risk.* New York: Springer.

Minkoff, H. (1988). Managing AIDS in pregnant patients. *Contemporary OB/GYN, 32*(3), 106–114.

Neeson, J. & May, K. (1986). Comprehensive maternity nursing. Philadelphia: Lippincott.

Nord, C.W., Moore, K.A., Morrison, D.R., Brown, B., & Myers, D.E. (1992). Consequences of teen-age parenting. *Journal of School Health, 62*(7), 310–315.

Olson, H.C. (1994). The effects of prenatal alcohol exposure on child development. *Infants and young children, 6*(3),10–25.

Piaget, J. (1950). *The psychology of intelligence.* London: Routledge and Kegan Paul, Ltd.

Pickering, R.M. & Deeks, J.J. (1991). Risks of delivery during the 20th to the 36th week of gestation. *International Journal of Epidemiology, 20*, 456–466.

Rienzo, P.G. (1993). *Nursing care of the person who smokes.* New York: Springer.

Robertson, B.E. (1993). *Alcohol disabilities primer: A guide to phychosocial disabilities caused by alcohol use.* Boca Raton: CRC Press, Inc.

Statistical Abstracts of U.S. (1993). no. 113, Washington, D.C.: U.S. Government Publishing Office.

Stewart, P.J. & Nimrod, C. (1993). The need for a community-wide approach to promote heathy babies and prevent low birth weight. *Canadian Medical Association Journal, 149*(3), 281–285.

Sullivan, J., Boudreaux, M., & Keller, P. (1993). Can we help the substance abusing mother and infant? *Maternal Child Nursing, 18*, 153–157.

U.S. General Accounting Office. (1990). *Drug exposed infants: A generation at risk.* Publication no. GAO/HRD-90-138.

United States Public Health Service. (1990). *Healthy people 2000: National health promotion and disease prevention objectives.* Washington, DC: U.S. Department of Health and Human Services.

Weiner, L. & Morse, B. (1988). F.A.S.: Clinical perspectives and prevention. In I.J. Chassnoff (Ed.), *Drugs, alcohol, pregnancy, and parenting* (pp. 127–148). United Kingdom: Kluwer Academic Publishers.

Wheeler, S.F. (1993). Substance abuse during pregnancy. *Primary Care, 20*(1), 191–208.

SELECTED READINGS

Balgopal, P., Pallassana, R., Ephross, P., & Vassil, T. (1986). Self-help groups and professional helpers. *Small Group Behavior, 17*(2), 123–27.

Bedics, B.C. (1994). Nonuse of prenatal care: Implications for social work involvement. *Health and Social Work, 19*(2), 84–92.

Cartwright, P.S., McLaughlin, F.J., et al. (1993). Teenagers' perceptions of barriers to prenatal care. *Southern Medical Journal, 86*(7), 737–741.

Catlett, A.T., Thompson, R.J., Johndrow, D.A., & Boshkoff, M.R. (1993). Risk status for dropping out of developmental follow-up for very low birth weigth infants. *Public health Reports, 108*(5), 589–594.

Cohen, F.L. & Durham, J.D. (Eds.).(1993). *Women, children, and HIV/AIDS.* New York: Springer.

Davis, B., et al. (1988). Implementation and preliminary evaluation of a community-based prenatal health education program. *Family and Community Health, 11*(1), 8–16.

Dodds, J. M. (1987). Nutrition and health: An individual responsibility. *Public Health Reports,* July–August (Supp.), 29–33.

Fleming, B.W., Munton, M.T., Clark, B.A., & Strauss, S.S. (1993). Assessing and promoting positive parenting in adolescent mothers. *The Journal of Maternal and Child Nursing, 18*, 32–37.

Freeman, E.W. & Rickles, K.(1993). Early childbearing: Perspectives of black adolescents on pregnancy, abortion, and contraception. Newbury Park, CA: Sage.

Gold, R. B., Kenney, A.M., & Singh, S. (1987). Paying for maternity care in the United States. *Family Planning Perspectives, 19*(5), 190–206.

Kieffer, E., Alexander, G.R., & Mor, J. (1992). Area-level predictors of use of prenatal care in diverse populations. *Public Health Reports, 107*(6), 653–658.

Killien, M.G. (1993). Returning to work after childbirth: Considerations for health policy. *Nursing Outlook, 41*(2), 73–78.

Kinsman, S.B. & Slap, G.B. (1992). Barriers to receiving adequate prenatal care. *American Journal of Obstetrics and Gynecology, 157*, 297–303.

MacDonald, D. I. (1987). An approach to the problem of teenage pregnancy. *Public Health Reports, 102*(4), 377–85.

McLemore, M.M. (1991). Nurses as health planners. In B.W. Spradley (Ed.), *Readings in community health nursing* (pp. 201–208). Philadelphia: Lippincott.

Olds, D.L., Henderson, C.R., & Kitzman, H. (1994). Does prenatal and infancy nurse home visitation have enduring effects on qualities of parental caregiving and child health at 25 to 50 months of life? *Pediatrics, 93*(1), 89–98.

Pearson, M.A., Hoyme, E., Seaver, L.H., & Rimsza, M.E. (1994). Toluene embryopathy: Delineation of the phenotype and comparison with fetal alcohol syndrome. *Pediatrics, 93*(2), 211 215.

Pesznecker, B. & Zahlis, E. (1986). Establishing mutual-help groups for family-member caregivers: A new role for community health nurses. *Public Health Nursing, 3*, 29.

Pollack, A.E. (1992). Teen contraception in the 1990's. *Journal of School Health, 62*(7), 288–293.

U.S.D.A. (1992). The food guide pyramid.

von Windeguth, B. & Urbano, M.T. (1989). Cocaine-Abusing mothers and their infants: A new morbidity brings challenges for nursing care. *Journal of Community Health Nursing, 6*(3), 147–153.

von Windeguth, B.,Urbano, M.T., Hayes, J.S., & Martyn, K., (1988). Analysis of infant risk factors documented by public health nurses. *Public Health Nursing, 5*(3), 165–69.

Zambrana, R.E., Dunkel-Schetter, C., & Scrimshaw, S., (1991). Factors which influence use of prenatal care in low-income racial-ethnic women in Los Angeles county. *Journal of Community Health, 16*, 283–295.

19

Promoting and Protecting the Health of Toddler, Preschool, School-Age and Adolescent Populations

LEARNING OBJECTIVES

Upon completion of this chapter, readers should be able to:

- Identify major health problems, and concerns for, toddler, preschool, school-age, and adolescent populations in the United States.
- Explain the programs that promote health and prevent illness and injury of toddler, preschool, school-age, and adolescent populations.
- State the recommended immunization schedule for children from birth through the teen years and give the rationale for the timing of each immunization.
- Describe the three functions of school nursing practice (health services, health education, and improvement of the school environment).
- Give examples of methods the community health nurse might use in working with toddlers, preschool, school-age, and adolescents to help promote their health.

KEY TERMS

- Anorexia nervosa
- Attention Deficit Disorder (without hyperactivity)(ADD)
- Attention Deficit Hyperactivity Disorder (ADHD)
- Bulimia
- Child abuse
- High risk families
- School nurse
- School nurse practitioner

Barbara Walton Spradley and Judith Ann Allender
COMMUNITY HEALTH NURSING: CONCEPTS AND PRACTICE, 4th ed.
© 1996 Barbara Walton Spradley and Judith Ann Allender

Healthy children are a vital resource to ensure the future well-being of the nation. They are the parents, workers, leaders, and decision makers of tomorrow, and their health and safety depend on today's decisions and actions. Their future lies in the hands of those people responsible for their well-being, including the community health nurse.

The well-being of children has been a subject of great concern in this country for many years. The nation has emphasized its importance through development of numerous laws and services, yet the needs of millions of children continue to go unmet. "Poor children are at risk in all kinds of ways. A small but growing proportion are homeless; many fall outside the medical care system and as a consequence suffer poor health; many endure poor quality, even dangerous child care; and the majority fail to make it through our educational system" (Hewlett, 1991, p. 56).

Furthermore, the many needs of America's 15 million poor children are only part of the picture. There are millions more children in moderate-income families who have inadequate child care, poor housing, limited health insurance, and limited access to higher education. Added to these are "a growing number of privileged youths (who) suffer from spiritual poverty, afflicted by what John Levy of the Jung Institute labels 'affluenza' " (Children's Defense Fund, 1988). Plagued with boredom, low self-esteem, and lack of motivation, children in wealthy homes are often insulated from challenge and risk. Many of the same problems exist for children of the rich as for those of the poor with the young people turning to drugs, alcohol, and indiscriminate sexual activity. Clearly there is a need for improvement in the nation's efforts to prepare children adequately for the future.

The loss of children's lives resulting from all injuries combined suggests a staggering number of years of productive life lost to society. Accidental trauma is the leading cause of death for children ages one to 14 (National Safety Council, 1990). Motor vehicle injuries are the most prevalent cause of death for children over one year old. Homicide is the most frequent cause of death for those under one year old. Drownings, house fires, and homicide are also leading causes of death in all children (U.S. Department of Commerce, 1993). Homicides have risen at a frightening rate. Homicide is the fourth leading cause of death among children aged 1 to 14 years and is the second leading cause of death for children ages 15–24 years. Homicides of children under the age of three most often result from family violence, but homicides involving children over the age of 12 generally involve violence outside the home.

Although childhood mortality rates have markedly decreased since the early 1900's, morbidity rates remain high. The most common types of acute conditions are respiratory illnesses (which account for the largest group), infectious and parasitic diseases, injuries, and digestive diseases (U.S. Bureau of Census, 1990).

Other child health problems, less easy to detect and measure but often as debilitating, are those of emotional, behavioral, and intellectual development. Although these problems are not new, awareness and concern for them have increased as the rates of occurrence for other life-threatening childhood diseases (measles, mumps, rubella, and polio) have diminished. Emotional disorders are quite prevalent in childhood; it is estimated that 10% to 12% of school-age children suffer from mental disorders, including autism, attention deficit-hyperactivity, and depression. Developmental delays and specific skill and conduct disorders are associated with additional cognitive, emotional, and behavioral dysfunctions (Ibid.).

Causes of learning disorders and emotional behavioral problems appear to have genetic, environmental, and cultural influences. Increased use of illicit drugs by pregnant women are producing a generation of children with developmental delays and learning disabilities. Immature, stressed, and dysfunctional families have high incidents of child abuse (physical and sexual) and neglect. The numbers of children affected by parental drug use has surpassed childhood disabilities caused by lead poisoning, which has, itself, been a major contributor to developmental problems in children.

Cultural and environmental influences include the violence to which children are exposed. Increased aggressive behavior among children has been attributed to violence in the environment, violence in the child's home (spousal and child abuse), to what the child sees in the community, on television, and in the movies. (See the Research in Community Health Nursing display.)

Health Problems of Toddlers and Preschool Children

The toddler (ages one and two) and preschool population (ages three and four years) have a low mortality rate that is becoming lower every year. Currently it is 0.47 deaths per 1,000 live births, compared with 20.0

Research in Community Health Nursing
EDUCATING INNER-CITY LOW LITERACY PARENTS

Berger, D., Inkelas, M., Myhre, S., and Mishler, A. (1994). Developing health education materials for inner-city low literacy parents. *Public Health Reports, 109*(2), 168–172.

Researchers from UCLA School of Public Health conducted a study in 1992, which included 200 mothers in a WIC program, to determine their interest in using health education materials. According to this study, the inner city mothers desired greater information on how to maintain the health of their children and treat common illnesses. After doing a literature review and interviewing key informants, the researchers met with women in a series of focus groups to identify health concerns. From this input an 18 page booklet, "Parents' Guide: When Your Child is Sick", was developed at the sixth grade level using the SMOG readability formula. The booklet is innovative because it is a health education tool that is pertinent, adaptable, and appropriate in a variety of settings, easy to understand, addresses the importance of self-care, helps parents make complex and accurate decisions, and is printed on heavy, colorful paper that makes it attractive and inexpensive. The cost of producing such a booklet is minimal if preventing even one unnecessary hosptialization or saving one life is the outcome.

per 1,000 at the beginning of the 20th century (U.S. Department of Commerce, 1993). This dramatic change can be credited to the prevention and control of acute childhood communicable diseases. The major cause of death in this population is unintentional injuries (motor vehicle accidents, falls, drownings, burns, poisonings), 0.17 per 1000; followed by malignant neoplasms, (0.3); congenital anomalies, (0.1); homicide, (0.15); and pneumonia and influenza, (0.04) (Ibid.).

A major cause of poisoning comes from lead. The primary sources of lead exposure in preschool children continue to be lead-based paint, lead-contaminated soil and dust, and drinking water from lead-soldered pipes (DeRienzo-DeVivio, 1992; U.S. Public Health Service, 1990). Children living and playing in substandard housing areas remain at risk for being directly exposed to significant sources of lead.

Toddlers and preschool children experience a high frequency of acute illnesses, more than any other age group. These account for a large number of days of restricted activity and disability requiring bed rest. Respiratory illness makes up over one half of acute conditions in toddlers and preschoolers (U.S. Department of Commerce, 1993). Toddlers and preschoolers are vulnerable to many types of accidents such as falls, burns, and poisonings. Their nutritional and dental health needs are great during this period of rapid growth, and their future mental health as adults will be influenced by how well their emotional needs are met during this phase of their development.

Health Problems of School-Age Children

The mortality rates of school-age children (5–14 years old) are low and decreasing; they have dropped from 4.0 per 1,000 in 1900 to 0.24 per 1,000 currently. Again, this reduction can be credited to effective prevention and control of the acute infectious diseases of childhood. Today motor vehicle accidents lead the list of causes of death for children aged 5 to 14, followed by all other accidents, malignant neoplasms, congenital anomolies, homicide, heart disease, and pneumonia and influenza (Ibid.).

COMMUNICABLE DISEASES

Morbidity in schoolchildren, however, is high. Children of this age group are most often affected by respiratory illness, followed by infectious and parasitic diseases, injuries, and digestive conditions. Among schoolchildren, the incidence of measles, rubella (German measles), pertussis (whooping cough), and infectious parotitis (mumps) has dropped considerably because of widespread immunization efforts. Yet cases of communicable diseases still occur, some with potentially serious complications, such as birth defects from rubella and nerve deafness from mumps. Vigorous campaigns have been undertaken by health departments to get children immunized. An immunization for mumps, measles and rubella (MMR) has been available for over 20 years and yet there has been a decreasing percent of children immunized ("Breaking Down the Barriers," 1994). Perhaps one reason is that many believe the threat of these diseases has been wiped out and young mothers have never seen disabling consequences of these diseases, such as polio. A chicken pox vaccine, Varivax, was recently developed and became available in 1995. It is now part of the childhood immunization schedule. Fewer cases of chicken pox should follow. Community health nurses need to inform clients about the vaccine.

BEHAVIORAL AND LEARNING PROBLEMS

Behavioral disorders and developmental disabilities are problems of this age group, often becoming exacerbated when the child enters school. The prevalence of these problems is difficult to measure epidemiologically, but approximately 10% to 15% of school-aged children have learning disabilities and behavioral problems. The cause is multifaceted and often difficult to identify.

Attention Deficit Hyperactivity Disorder (ADHD) is a cluster of problems related to hyperactivity and impulsivity. **Attention Deficit Disorder** (without hyperactivity)(ADD) is a cluster of problems related mainly to inattention, poor motivation, and disorganization. Both are seen in children and adults and it is estimated to affect 3% to 5% of all school-age children. These disorders are being diagnosed with increasing frequency in children, adolescents, and adults. Much confusion exists about the symptoms of both problems (Barkley, 1990; Shaywitz & Shaywitz, 1991). Descriptions of ADHD and ADD are displayed in Table 19.1 (Aust, 1994).

Children with disabilities, those with one or more chronic conditions that limit activities, make up approximately 12% of the school-age population (Zanga & Oda, 1987). Disabilities include speech, hearing, and visual defects, seizure disorders, asthma, cancer, AIDS, and partial or complete paralysis requiring a school nurse to provide such services as performing clean intermittent catheterizations (CIC) and tube feedings (Johnson-Russell and Anema, 1989).

POOR NUTRITION AND DENTAL HEALTH

Other health problems found in this age group are nutritional problems (primarily overeating and inappropriate food choices) and poor dental health. Obesity often begins in childhood and becomes a risk factor for heart disease, hypertension, and diabetes. As many as 15% to 20% of school-age children are overweight (Greenwood, et al., 1993). Obese children are three times more likely to become obese adults (Karp, 1993). School children's diets, often unreasonably high in sugar and fat, increase the incidence of coronary arteriosclerosis and dental caries in this population group. The practice of allowing infants to continue to bottle feed beyond 15–16 months, or to fall asleep with a bottle, can lead to "nursing bottle syndrome." This causes the decay of the front teeth and eventually the molars, requiring extraction of the affected teeth (Markowitz, 1993). The average American child between the ages of 5 and 17 has more than four decayed, missing, or filled teeth. Dental caries increase with age and are more prevalent in Native American poulations, in groups underserved by dentists, and in areas where there is no fluoridated water (Ibid.).

Health Problems of Adolescents

Adolescents, during the period roughly encompassing the teen years, encounter many complex changes, physically, emotionally, cognitively, and socially. Rapid

TABLE 19.1. **ADH and ADD: The Differences**

ATTENTION DEFICIT DISORDER WITH HYPERACTIVITY (ADHD)	ATTENTION DEFICIT WITHOUT HYPERACTIVITY (ADD)
A child with this diagnosis *often:*	A child with this diagnosis *often:*
has difficulty waiting turn in group situations.	has difficulty following through on instructions.
interrupts or intrudes on others.	has difficulty sustaining attention.
blurts out answers to questions.	seems not to listen.
has difficulty playing quietly.	loses things necessary for tasks.
leaves seat.	fails to give close attention to details.
runs about or climbs excessively.	is disorganized.
fidgets or squirms.	makes careless mistakes in schoolwork or work.
talks excessively.	is forgetful.
acts as if "driven by a motor" and cannot remain still.	daydreams when should be attending.
	is unmotivated to complete schoolwork or tasks.

and major developmental adjustments create a variety of stresses, with concomitant problems, that have an impact on their health.

Mortality and morbidity rates for adolescents are low overall and demonstrate considerable improvement over the early 1900s. However, people in this age group die 2.5 times more often than younger children, and since 1960, the adolescent death rate has been gradually increasing (U.S. Department of Commerce, 1993).

Violent death and injury lead the list of major threats to adolescent life and health. Accidents, homicides, and suicides together cause nearly 75% of all adolescent deaths. For whites (male and female), motor vehicle accidents cause the greatest number of deaths, followed by all other accidents, suicide, and homicide. For non-whites (male and female), homicides are the leading cause of death, with motor vehicle accidents second and all other accidents third (Ibid.).

EMOTIONAL PROBLEMS AND TEENAGE SUICIDE

The adolescent years are a time of rapid growth and change. Hormonal influences can cause a teen to be emotional and at times unpredictible. Peer pressure becomes more important than parental concerns. Teens test family rules and generally search for their own identity and individuality apart from the family. Most parents and teens ride out this period with love and understanding and no long term negative effects. However, for some teens there is a real or perceived lack of emotional support which can cause temporary or permanent emotional problems. In order to compensate, teenagers may experiment with and abuse a variety of substances which alter their judgement and place them at risk.

The suicide rate for adolescents has almost doubled in the last twenty years (1970 to 1990), but for the 10–14 year old child it has tripled. Suicide rates are higher among whites than blacks, with adolescent males 15 to 19 years of age at greatest risk in this population group. Their death rate is nearly five times higher than that of females. Suicide is the second leading cause of death among this age group (Ibid.).

VIOLENCE

An increasing threat for teenagers is firearm violence. Homicide from firearms is ten times more prevalent among black 15 to 19 year old youth than white youths (Ibid.). It is the leading cause of death for black males in

this age group. In some communities, children cannot play outside for fear of being hit by stray gunfire from gang warfare or random drive-by or walk-by shootings.

SUBSTANCE ABUSE

A study done by the U.S. Substance Abuse and Mental Health Services Administration shows that 20.3% of adolescents age 12–17 classify themelves as current users of alcohol; 4.3% use marijuana, 1.8% use inhalents, and 0.4% use cocaine (U.S. Department of Commerce, 1993). Many more report using the above substances at least once in the last month. Members of this age group tend to consume alcohol less frequently (an average of once monthly) than adults do, but when adolescents do drink they drink large quantities, and they experience more frequent episodes of intoxication than adults, thus increasing the chances of violent behavior and motor vehicle accidents.

Cigarette smoking continues to be the most significant preventable health problem of adolescents (Ibid.). The rates of cigarette smoking are decreasing among males and increasing among females but have been declining overall since 1974, when 25% of the adolescents in this age group classified themselves as current users of cigarettes, compared to 10.8% in 1990. White females age 12–17 smoke more than two times as frequently as black females.

An increasing number of adolescents today use heroin, inhalents, and analgesics (for non-medical use). Illegal use of all substances such as crack cocaine, hallucinogens, and prescription medications tends to be more common with older adolescents and young adults (18 to 25 years of age) than with younger adolescents, except for inhalents (Ibid.). Drug abuse among young people was almost unknown before 1950 and rare before 1962. Now, adolescent drug experimentation and use pose serious physical and psychological threats.

TEENAGE PREGNANCY

Increasing sexual activity among adolescents creates three other significant health problems for this age group. They are teenage pregnancies, sexually transmitted diseases (STDs), and HIV/AIDS. The United States leads most developed nations in rates of teenage pregnancy, abortion, and childbearing. Recently in the United States, 20% of all births were to adolescent females (U.S. Department of Commerce, 1993). Each year 10% of all teenage girls become pregnant (two-thirds of these are unmarried), and at least a third terminate their pregnancies. Babies born to teenage mothers are more likely to be premature and underweight (Ibid.). Young mothers are at high risk of bearing infants with low birth weight, less because of their biological age (except for preteen mothers whose youth increases their risk) than because of other associated factors, such as living in poverty, inadequate prenatal care, smoking, and alcohol consumption. They are also at risk for a greater number of physical, psychological, and social problems, including dropping out of high school, limited earning potential, social isolation, and child abuse related to unrealistic expectations of the infant, as a result of the pregnancy and subsequent birth (Mercer, 1990). Those who choose to end their pregnancies with abortion encounter other physical and psychosocial complications.

SEXUALLY TRANSMITTED DISEASES (STDS) AND HIV/AIDS

STDs, particularly chlamydia, gonorrhea, herpes, and syphilis, pose another threat to adolescent health. Nationally, 15–19 year olds have the highest rates of these diseases. About 2.5 million cases of STDs are reported among adolescents each year, representing about 25% of all reported STDs (Kipke, et al., 1990). Serious complications can result from these diseases, including sterility in young women who have pelvic inflammatory disease. Adolescents acquire HIV in the same ways as adults, primarily through risky sexual activities and injecting drugs. Despite AIDS prevention campaigns, more adolescents were initiating sexual intercourse at younger ages in 1988 than in 1982. The World Health Organization (Henson, 1995) reports that 60% of new HIV infections are among 15 to 24 year olds in many countries with a female to male ratio of 2 to 1. Among both men and women, young people are particularly at risk. Teens are risk takers and many are emotionally immature and have perceptions of personal invulnerability. The vast majority of adolescents are aware of the type of risk taking behaviors that lead to HIV transmission, but this knowledge does not necessarily translate into behavioral changes (Tucker & Cho, 1991).

POOR NUTRITION AND EATING DISORDERS

Poor nutrition and obesity are common among adolescents, whose diets often consist of snacks with limited nutritional value (see Fig. 19.1) and unhealthy meals. Among adolescent females, good nutrition is more at-risk than for males, for two reasons. First, female teens do more inappropriate dieting, have more finicky eating habits, and are less physically active than teen males. Girls as young as nine years old put themselves on diets. Even if teen males eat imbalanced meals, by the sheer quantity of food they consume, their diet becomes more balanced

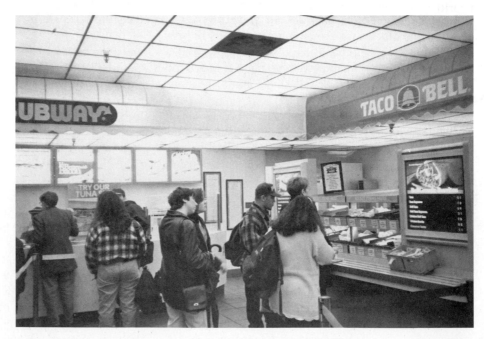

FIGURE 19.1. Fast food is popular with young people whose poor-eating habits frequently can lead to health problems.

and adequate than females. Additionally, the teen male is more involved in physical activity through organized sports, or on informal outings with friends for recreation than for females whose physical activity may only include walking in shopping malls (Schlicker, et al., 1994).

A second problem of mounting incidence and gravity are the diseases of anorexia nervosa and bulimia. **Anorexia nervosa** is an eating disorder with emotional etiology in which the person has a distorted self-image believing oneself to be overweight and refuses to eat, suffering marked weight loss, amenorrhea, and sometimes death from starving oneself (Herbert, 1989). **Bulimia** is an eating disorder in which the person engages in uncontrolled eating binges, often followed by purging (self-induced vomiting or ingesting large amounts of laxatives to cause diarrhea), then depression, and self-denial (Ibid.). These diseases have emotional etiologies that pose a complex challenge to treatment.

Health Services for Children

There are many ways in which the health of a child can be influenced. The goal is for their health to be influenced positively. A variety of programs now exist that directly or indirectly serve the health needs of children. Community health nurses play a major and vital role in delivering these services. In community health, they fall into three categories approximating the three practice priorities of community health nursing practice: preventive health programs, health protection, and health promotion.

PREVENTIVE HEALTH PROGRAMS

Quality Day Care

Quality child care provides a significant avenue for preventing illness and injury among young children. In the late 1980s, 64% of women with children were in the work force, with a predicted increase to at least 70% by 1990 (Bassoff & Willis, 1991). Today those figures are even higher, the result of economic necessity as family income is dropping steadily; in 1991 income growth lagged behind inflation for the first time since 1982 (Capitol Bulletin, 1992). The demand for child care has increased by more than 100% since 1970 (Children's Defense Fund, 1988).

Children in day care tend to contract a significantly higher number of illnesses (19% to 30% more) than children cared for at home (Johansen, et al., 1988). Many of these disease occurrences can be prevented through improved policies and adherence to those policies regarding sick children. Adhering to requirements for completed immunizations for all children and staff should be part of the community health nurse's role in services provided to aggregates in the community. Further preventive measures are needed to ensure cleanliness, good nutrition, proper ventilation, lighting, exercise, and a safe, emotionally secure environment (Bassoff & Willis, 1991; Belsky, 1990; Clark-Stewart, 1989; Cowan & Cowan, 1992). Many children suffer injuries and even death due to lack of safe child care; one important preventive measure is to ensure lower child-to-caregiver ratios (Children's Defense Fund, 1988). Community health nurses play a vital role in monitoring the quality of child care and educating parents, caregivers, and the public about appropriate preventive actions.

Immunizations

Health departments and the private sector continue to offer immunization against each of the major childhood infectious diseases—measles, mumps, rubella, chicken pox, polio, diphtheria, tetanus, pertussis, *haemophilus influenzae*, and hepatitis B—which can cause permanent disability and sometimes even death. Although their threat has been substantially reduced, vigilance cannot be relaxed. Low immunization levels in many areas, particularly among the poor, and increased disease rates signal the need for constant surveillance, outreach programs, and educational efforts. Community health nurses are deeply involved in each of these preventive activities. Health departments and schools often work collaboratively to provide immunization services (see Table 19.2 or Table 23.6 on p. 522). A compulsory immunization law, varying in its application from state to state, has enabled public health personnel to carry out these preventive services.

Education and Social Services

Parental support services, available through many public and private agencies including churches, have long-range effects on children's health. Emotionally healthy parents and stable families offer a healthful environment and support system for growing children. In most states community health nurses provide teaching and counseling services to parents in their homes and

*TABLE 19.2. **Recommended Childhood Immunization Schedule*—United States, January 1995***

Vaccine	Birth	2 Months	4 Months	6 Months	12[†] Months	15 Months	18 Months	4–6 Years	11–12 Years	14–16 Years
Hepatitis B[§]	HB-1	HB-2		HB-3						
Diphtheria, Tetanus, Pertussis[¶]		DTP	DTP	DTP	DTP or DTaP at ≥15 months			DTP or DTaP	Td	
H. influenzae type b[**]		Hib	Hib	Hib	Hib					
Poliovirus		OPV	OPV	OPV				OPV		
Measles, Mumps, Rubella[††]					MMR			MMR or MMR		

* Recommended vaccines are listed under the routinely recommended ages. Shaded bars indicate range of acceptable ages for vaccination.

† Vaccines recommended in the second year of life (i.e., 12–15 months of age) may be given at either one or two visits.

§ Infants born to hepatitis B surface antigen (HBsAg)-negative mothers should receive the second dose of hepatitis B vaccine between 1 and 4 months of age, provided at least 1 month has elapsed since receipt of the first dose. The third dose is recommended between 6 and 18 months of age. Infants born to HBsAg-positive mothers should receive immunoprophylaxis for hepatitis B with 0.5 ml Hepatitis B Immune Globulin (HBIG) within 12 hours of birth, and 0.5 ml of either Merck Sharpe & Dohme (West Point, Pennsylvania) vaccine (Recombivax HB®) or of SmithKline Beecham (Philadelphia) vaccine (Engerix-B®) at a separate site. In these infants, the second dose of vaccine is recommended at 1 month of age and the third dose at 6 months of age. All pregnant women should be screened for HBsAg during an early prenatal visit.

¶ The fourth dose of diphtheria and tetanus toxoids and pertussis vaccine (DTP) may be administered as early as 12 months of age, provided at least 6 months have elapsed since the third dose of DTP. Combined DTP-Hib products may be used when these two vaccines are administered simultaneously. Diphtheria and tetanus toxoids and acellular pertussis vaccine (DTaP) is licensed for use for the fourth and/or fifth dose of DTP in children aged ≥15 months and may be preferred for these doses in children in this age group.

** Three *H. influenzae* type b conjugate vaccines are available for use in infants: 1) oligosaccharide conjugate Hib vaccine (HbOC) (HibTITER®), manufactured by Praxis Biologics, Inc. [West Henrietta, New York], and distributed by Lederle-Praxis Biologicals, [Wayne, New Jersey]); 2) polyribosylribitol phosphate-tetanus toxoid conjugate (PRP-T) (ActHIB™, manufactured by Pasteur Mérieux Sérums & Vaccins, S.A. (Lyon, France), and distributed by Connaught Laboratories, Inc. [Swiftwater, Pennsylvania], and OmniHIB™, manufactured by Pasteur Mérieux Sérums & Vaccins, S.A., and distributed by SmithKline Beecham); and 3) *Haemophilus* b conjugate vaccine (Meningococcal Protein Conjugate) (PRP-OMP) (PedvaxHIB®, manufactured by Merck Sharp & Dohme). Children who have received PRP-OMP at 2 and 4 months of age do not require a dose at 6 months of age. After the primary infant Hib conjugate vaccine series is completed, any licensed Hib conjugate vaccine may be used as a booster dose at age 12–15 months.

†† The second dose of measles-mumps-rubella vaccine should be administered EITHER at 4–6 years of age OR at 11–12 years of age.

Source: U.S. Department of Health and Human Services, Public Health Service, Centers for Disease Control. *Morbidity and Mortality Weekly Report, General Recommendations on Immunizations: Recommendations of the Advisory Committee on Immunization Practices (ACIP)*, American Academy of Pediatrics and American Academy of Family Physicians, January 6, 1995.

in groups. Discussing parenting concerns and increasing parents' understanding of normal child growth and development allay fears and prevent problems. Through such efforts, family violence and abuse can be averted.

Family planning programs, often stationed strategically in inner cities, near schools, and in school-based clinics, provide birth control information and counseling to young people. In some communities the school-based clinic dispenses condoms. Community health nurses, in collaboration with an interdisciplinary team, are usually the primary care providers in these programs. Their major goals are to prevent teenage pregnancy, educate teenagers about reproduction and contraception, and encourage responsible sexual behavior.

Providing STD services and now HIV/AIDS education, has become more difficult. Young people with

STDs are often afraid or embarrassed to seek help. Others, exposed to the HIV virus, may not know they have been infected. Furthermore, community health professionals receive very little training in these areas and may be uncomfortable and judgmental in their approach. Vulnerable groups, particularly minority youths, inner-city residents, and homosexuals, are being reached, however. Quality services and nonjudgmental attitudes attract young people who need help, and such help is being offered through STD clinics, HIV testing sites in clinics and health departments, family planning clinics, private health care providers, schools, and employers. Community health nurses, available in most of these settings, are generally the professionals who deal most directly with these clients (Bocchino, 1991). Improved public awareness and education, screening of high-risk groups, appropriate antibiotic treatment of infected individuals, and identification and treatment of sexual contacts should reduce the threat of STDs. However, the numbers of young people with STDs are increasing even with new awareness. The threat to one's life if HIV/AIDS is acquired has not yet become a deterrent to sexual activity among the youth of today.

Treatment and prevention of alcohol and drug abuse is another difficult task. Many social and economic influences promote chemical abuse and dependency, complicating the reversal of these effects (Goldstein, 1994). Recommended strategies and areas in which community health nurses working with aggregates can be more involved include the following (Falco, 1993; Goldstein, 1994; U.S.Public Health Service, 1990):

1. Prevention through early and ongoing education.
2. Working to make the social climate less accepting of these behaviors.
3. Reducing stress factors contributing to chemical abuse.
4. Enforcing the law.

Educational efforts to discourage alcohol and drug use have often been ineffective, some have even back-fired and created an incentive to experiment with them. Educational strategies that have been most successful have focused on the young person's individual responsibility for daily decisions affecting his or her health (U.S.Public Health Service, 1990). Thus, programs such as youth service clubs and community activities that encourage children and adolescents to make wise choices that affect their well-being and promote self-worth, can serve as useful preventive measures.

HEALTH PROTECTION PROGRAMS

Safety and Injury Prevention

Accidents and injury control programs serve a critical role in protecting the lives of children. Efforts to prevent motor vehicle accidents, a major cause of death, include driver education programs, better highway construction, improved motor vehicle design and safety features, and continuing research into the causes of various types of crashes. Injury prevention and reduction has been addressed through strategies such as state laws requiring the use of safety restraints (see Figure 19.2), driver and front passenger air bags, substituting other modes of travel (air, rail, or bus), lower speed limits,

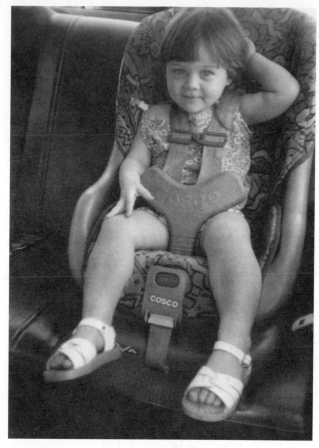

FIGURE 19.2. Appropriate use of restraints in motor vehicles can prevent many childhood injuries and deaths.

stricter enforcement of drunk driving laws, safer automobile design, and helmets for motorcyclists, bicycle riders, and skaters.

Falls, a major killer of toddlers and preschool children and the cause of deaths and injuries for millions of older children each year, occur mostly in the home. Here the community health nurse plays a major role in observing potential hazards, teaching safety measures, and reinforcing positive practices. Preventive and protective measures may be achieved through simple and inexpensive changes in the home. They include guards on windows and across stairways, safer walking surfaces, elimination of sharp objects or modification of surfaces that a child might fall against, securing of electrical outlets and toxic chemicals, and closer supervision of young children.

Child deaths and injuries from burns result primarily from house fires, but also from electrical burns, cigarette lighters, and scalds. Many local fire departments and public health programs offer safety education in this area, emphasizing the use of heat- and smoke-detecting systems, fire drills, and home evacuation plans; less flammable structural materials, furnishings, and clothing; and careful smoking or better, no smoking. Cigarette lighers are fascinating to young children and if left within their reach can be deadly. Scalds occur in kitchens and bathrooms most often. Adults can protect children by keeping pot handles turned toward the center of the stove, by not using their burners or ovens to heat their homes, by modifying water temperatures in water heaters, and by always testing bath water with an elbow before placing a child in the bath.

Safety programs also seek to protect children from the hazards of poisonings, ingestion of prescription and over-the-counter drugs, product-related accidents (unsafe toys, bicycles, skateboards, skates, playground equipment, and furniture), and recreational accidents, including drownings and sports injuries. Safety services assume various forms. Poison control centers in many localities offer information and emergency assistance. Toxic household substances, such as cleaning supplies, must be clearly labeled, and harmful drugs packaged with special seals and safety caps. Product safety is monitored by the Federal Consumer Product Safety Commission. Greater efforts are being made to reduce recreational injuries through improved boating and swimming regulations, water safety measures, teaching children to swim, team sports safety measures, and better protective equipment and playing fields for sports participants, including football helmets that don't injure other players and obstacle-free zones around playing fields. Generally, the community health nurse can educate families to recognize potentially hazardous situations and encourage efforts to eliminate them.

Programs to reduce environmental hazards begin at the federal level, where the government sets and enforces pollution standards and regulates environmental contamination that poses health risks. At the state and municipal government levels, enforcement of regulations occur. Measures include monitoring air and drinking water safety, carbon monoxide detection devices installed in housing units, providing proper sewage disposal, controlling ionizing radiation, asbestos, lead, and radon contamination and removal of barrier provisions installed, enforcing auto safety and emission standards, and controlling use of agricultural chemicals and pesticides. Locally, protective measures include educational programs warning against toxic agents in the environment, community surveillance, and enforcement of environmental health standards. At all levels, epi-

demiologic research probes the causes and seeks answers to provide better protection for the public. Community health nurses need to be alert to environmental hazards and work collaboratively with other members of the public health team to report problems and educate clients. Improved environmental control protects today's children against disease and disability and tomorrow's children against birth defects and the long-range hazards of environmental contamination.

It has been demonstrated in community health that infectious diseases can be controlled and in some cases eliminated. Witness the successful worldwide eradication of smallpox, the dramatic decline in paralytic polio, and the decreasing incidence of the other communicable diseases of childhood. Control of infectious diseases comes largely through a two-part effort. One part is wide-scale, persistent immunization programs, discussed earlier. The second part is rigorous monitoring and surveillance of communicable disease incidence. Such surveillance is done continuously in the United States by the federal Centers for Disease Control and Prevention in collaboration with state and local health departments. Surveillance involves four basic activities (U.S. Public Health Service,1990):

1. Case finding of disease or exposure to disease, done by community health professionals;
2. Case reporting to public health officials, by health care providers, schools, and industries;
3. Analysis and interpretation of communicable disease data to determine implications; and
4. Appropriate response with control measures.

Community health nurses do case finding and reporting and assist other health team members in carrying out control measures.

Programs protecting children against infectious diseases encompass efforts such as closing swimming pools with unsafe bacteria counts, conducting immunization campaigns in conjunction with influenza or measles outbreaks, and working with hospital pediatric units to reduce the incidence and threat of iatrogenic disease.

Child Abuse and Neglect

Child abuse and neglect has become a major concern for the United States. One and a half million children are reported as abused or neglected each year (Straus & Gelles, 1990). **Child abuse** is the maltreatment of children including any or all of the following: physical, emotional, medical or educational neglect; physical, emotional or sexual maltreatment and exploitation (see the Research in Community Health Nursing display).

It is believed many more children also suffer from forms of abuse and neglect, but thousands of cases are not reported and not reflected in the statistics. The problem is often difficult to detect and often under-reported (Browne, 1995). In recent years there has been an alarming increase in reported cases of physical and sexual abuse in day-care centers, nursery schools, children's organizations, and churches. It is alarming to note that regardless of race, culture, or socioeconomic origin, today's children run a high risk of suffering violence by their own caregivers.

Risk factors for abusive behavior include immaturity, stress, poverty, alcoholism, unstable employment, and physical and social isolation (Corby, 1992; Browne, 1993). Child abuse is seldom the result of any single factor, but rather a combination of stressful situations and parents who are unable to cope with problems and stress in a normal manner. Abusive adults often were abused, molested, or neglected themselves as children, carry low self-images into their adult lives, and are unable to cope with the demands of parenting. Other characteristics of abusive parents include immaturity, dependency, inability to handle responsibility, and low self-esteem. They often believe in the value of physical punishment, and misunderstand their children's ability to understand and perform certain tasks and frequently make unreasonable demands beyond their child's capability. During times of crisis, these parents often direct their anger and frustration at their children. These negative life patterns can continue for generations if intervention doesn't occur (Child Abuse Prevention Handbook, 1988).

Families at high risk for child abuse may be those which are chronically troubled or temporarily stressed. Teenage mothers and families with closely spaced children may also be more likely to engage in abusive behavior. Although poverty and lack of education are often linked with child abuse and neglect, no socioeconomic level is immune (Ibid.) (see Fig. 19.3).

Child Protective Services

Services to protect children from abuse are not as well developed or effective as safety and injury protection programs. A variety of factors account for this. Most child abuse occurs in the home; thus, only the most blatant situations become evident to outsiders.

Research in Community Health Nursing
CHILDREN IN THE UNITED STATES—FACTS

Chernoff, et al., 1994; Children's Defense Fund, 1991; Community Childhood Hunger Identification Project, 1991; Martin, 1992; McKay, 1994; Stark & Flitcraft, 1988; U.S. Bureau of Census, 1990; Urquiza, et al., 1994; U.S. Department of Health and Human Services, 1991; Wagner and Menke, 1991.

One in four children are born into poverty.

One third of poor children are black, and a black child is more likely to be poor than a white or Latino child.

Half of the children born into single-parent families are poor.

Minority children are disproportionately poor. (More than 45% of all black children and 39% of all Latino children are poor.)

One in eight children under the age of 12 (5.5 million) is suffering from hunger.

Twelve million children are uninsured with no access to health care.

Two-thirds of abused children are being parented by a battered woman.

One and a half million children are reported as abused and or neglected each year.

Thirteen thousand children are predicted to develop AIDS by the year 2000.

By the year 2000 there will be 125,000 motherless children due to the mother's death by AIDS.

One half million children are predicted to be in foster care in 1995.

One in five children is at risk of becoming a teen parent.

One in three children has never been to a dentist.

Poor children have higher rates of dental diseases.

One in seven children is at risk of dropping out of school.

Families with children make up 35% to 50% of America's homeless population.

Community health nurses and physicians who see injured children may find parents' explanations plausible and not suspect or want to believe that abuse might be responsible. Avoidance of legal involvement keeps others from reporting suspected cases. Fortunately this

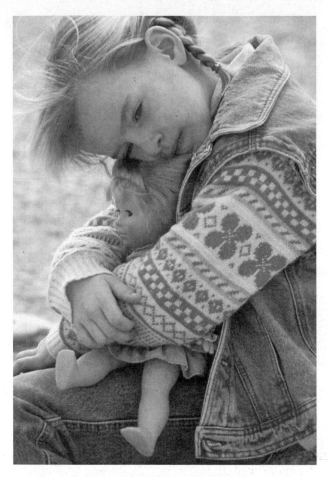

FIGURE 19.3. Abusive behavior can occur in any family and may continue for generations.

attitude is changing among professionals who work with children and other community members.

For many years states have had mandatory reporting laws. The first reporting law was passed in 1963 and required mandatory reporting of suspicious cases of child abuse, only by physicians. By 1966 all states had a reporting law. Over the years, numerous amendments have expanded the definition of child abuse and the persons required to report. Procedures for reporting categories of child abuse have also been clarified. Today professionals and the public are more aware of the problem, and there is an increase in reporting. Nonetheless, it is estimated that less than 10% of abused child cases are actually reported (Child Abuse Prevention Handbook, 1988). In 1974, the National Center for Child Abuse and Neglect was established as a result of the Child Abuse Prevention and Treatment Act. The center collects and analyzes information on child abuse and

neglect, serves as an information clearinghouse, publishes educational materials on the subject, offers technical assistance, and conducts research into the problem. Most professionals adopt the levels of prevention model to define child abuse and neglect prevention efforts:

Primary Level of Prevention

Establish community education to enhance the general well-being of children and their families. Provide educational services which are designed to enrich the lives of families and improve the skills of family functioning, and to prevent the stress and problems that might lead to dysfunction and abuse or neglect. Prevention should focus on parent preparation during the prenatal period, practices that encourage parent-child bonding during labor, delivery, the postpartum period, and early infancy, and provision of information regarding support services for families with newborns. Provide parents of children of all ages with information regarding child rearing and community resources.

Secondary Level of Prevention

Services are designed to identify and assist high risk families to prevent abuse or neglect. **High-risk families** are those families exhibiting the symptoms of potentially abusive or neglectful behavior or are under the types of stress associated with abuse or neglect.

Tertiary Level of Prevention

Intervention and treatment services to assist a family in which abuse or neglect has already occurred, to prevent further abuse or neglect. Intervention ranges from "early" intervention in the initial stages of abuse or neglect to "late stage" intervention in severe cases or after services have failed to stop the abusive or neglectful behavior (Child Abuse Prevention Handbook, 1988).

The community health nurse has a major role in primary prevention of child abuse. In addition, the nurse is in a unique position to detect early signs of neglect and abuse, establish rapport with abusing parents, family members, or others, and assist with appropriate interventions and referrals at the secondary and tertiary levels of prevention in an interdisciplinary manner with teachers, the department of social services, foster families, and other health care providers. See the cases below of reasons children come to foster care. The effectiveness of local programs depends, in large measure, on the willingness of community health professionals to increase their awareness and work as a team to detect, report, and develop interventions for abusers and abused children. Ongoing education of health care providers is recommended to increase their awareness of changing child abuse patterns, new reporting laws, and resources available to families.

Proper Oral Hygiene and Dental Care

Fluoridation of community water supplies is the most effective, safe, and low-cost means of protecting children's dental health. Fluoride makes teeth less susceptible to decay by increasing resistance to the bacteria-produced acid in the mouth. Public acceptance of community water fluoridation has been slow, despite 35 years of research demonstrating its unquestioned safety and effectiveness. As of 1987, 100 million people in the United States still were not served by fluoridated water supplies. For these people, supplemental fluorides, both systemic and topical, should be used (U.S. Public Health Service, 1990). However, there remains the need to have good dental health care. Professional dental health care has not changed dramatically in recent years, yet there are new products such as fluoride-releasing sealants, antibacterial rinses, plaque and tartar control dentifrices, and slow-release, intraoral drug delivery systems. However, none of these products or treatments take the place of personal oral health care supplemented with regular professional care.

CASE STUDY

REPORTS OF AN EMERGENCY FOSTER HOME

The following are examples of the various situations from which abused and neglected children come as reported by a couple who had an emergency foster home for the county department of social services. The examples represent a two year period in which 250 children were placed.

■ Two week old Jose was brought to their home because the parents (under the influence of drugs) were found swinging Jose upside down in circles in an infant carrier as they walked along a downtown street at 3 a.m. After being returned to his parents he returned to foster care one month later after being found abandoned in an infant carrier at the county fair.

■ Andre, Otis, and Selma ages 8, 5, and 4 were brought to the foster home when social services discovered they had been living with their father in an abandoned car for 2 years. They stayed for three weeks while the social worker found suitable housing for this family and counseling for the father.

■ Victoria, 5 years old, a loving and passive child, arrived wearing a diaper and appeared developmentally delayed. She had a history of being physically and sexually abused. Her family was very dysfunctional, and it took the social worker several weeks to sort out relatives and their intentions before placing Victoria in a long term foster home.

■ Ronald and Randall, 6 year-old twin boys who were forced to "sexually please their mother" for several years, came to the emergency foster home before being placed with relatives while their mother underwent psychiatric treatment. The boys began counseling during their stay in the emergency foster home.

■ Antoinette, aged 7, who had severe asthma and was very withdrawn, came to the emergency foster home because her mother (and boyfriend) refused to care for her. The child came with every photograph and momento of herself because the mother wanted no reminders of the child. The social worker was locating a grandmother who would be the child's guardian.

■ Thirteen year old Robert came home from school one day and found his mother and all their furniture gone. After a few weeks of living in the basement of the apartment building, someone alerted social services and Robert was placed in the emergency foster home for two months. His mother finally called social services after six weeks saying Robert was too difficult for her to handle, but she may want to see him again someday. Robert was eventually placed in a group home for boys.

■ YuFen, a 17 year-old Laotian girl, came into foster care after being referred by the school nurse because of wounds observed on her wrists and ankles. YuFen reported being strapped to a chair for 12 or more hours at a time by her father because she was not following the old ways and was shaming the family by being seen in public, unchaperoned, with a boy. Several meetings were held between the parents, a Southeast Asian community leader, and the social worker to resolve this situation so YuFen could go home safely.

There are barriers to care which are more prevelant among the poor and those who are institutionalized. Financial barriers and lack of education lead to poor dental health values, and adversely affect use of dentists and conscientious personal oral health care. Less than half the population have dental insurance, and use of oral health services has increased only modestly in recent years with 57% of people visiting a dentist during a 12 month period (National Institute of Dental Research, 1989). In addition to regular dental care, good nutrition, and proper oral hygiene, community health nurses can safely promote public water fluoridation as an important program for protecting children's dental health. In *Healthy People 2000* the recommendation is to expand the use of fluoridated water as the most effective and efficient preventive method in reducing oral diseases; it should be given the highest consideration (U.S. Public Health Service, 1990).

HEALTH PROMOTION PROGRAMS

Day Care and Preschool Programs

Early childhood development programs serve an increasingly important function for the escalating number of children enrolled in day-care centers and preschools. More than half of all children today have mothers who work, and that figure is rising. Economic pressures eat into family time together and often diminish the quality of children's physical and psychosocial nourishment. Childhood development programs, such as Head Start (federally funded preschool programs for 3–5 year old children from families in disadvantaged communities), provide physical, emotional, intellectual, and social stimulation during a critical period of children's growth when impressions are being made and patterns are formed that will influence what kind of adults these children will be in the future. Comprehensive preschool programs promote good physical health, proper nutrition, a positive self-concept, and cognitive and social skill development. Many such programs exist, but more are needed.

The president and the state governors have set six national education goals to be reached by the year 2000; the first is "By the year 2000, all children in America will start school ready to learn" (Department of Education, 1990). A physically and emotionally healthy child *will* be able to start school ready to learn. Where and how they achieve that health is the challenge to society. The stresses some parents feel are compounded when affordable and accessible licensed child care is not available; these stressed parents are more likely to abuse their children or place their children at risk of abuse, neglect, or exploitation.

"Availability and accessibility of affordable, quality licensed day care is recognized as a long-term solution for the prevention of child abuse" (Child Abuse Prevention Handbook, 1988, p. 21). The quality of day care and preschool programs varies considerably. Licensing laws can regulate only minimum safety and health standards. In addition, numerous child care operations are too small to require licensing, which leaves their quality open to individual discretion. Community health nurses can influence the quality of day care and preschool programs through active educational efforts, through monitoring of health and safety standards, and working to improve the state's role in passing stronger licensing laws.

Nutrition and Exercise Programs

Nutrition and weight control programs form another important set of health promotion services. Children need to learn sound dietary habits early in life to establish healthy lifelong patterns (Perry, et al., 1988). Overweight acquired during childhood or adolescence may persist into adulthood and increase the risk for some chronic diseases later in life (U.S. Public Health Service, 1990). Some preschool and school programs teach, as well as provide, good nutrition and encourage the kinds of eating patterns that prevent obesity. For overweight children and adolescents, there are a number of weight control programs available through schools, health departments, community health centers, health maintenance organizations, and private groups. Adolescents are particularly vulnerable to media and peer pressures for nonnutritious snacks, including diet sodas, based on a desire to be accepted and to look trim. Fad diets can also be harmful if they are not nutritionally balanced. Programs aimed at more nutritionally sound advertising are having a positive effect. Parents and children are becoming more aware of the need to cut down their consumption of saturated fat, salt, sugar, and overprocessed foods in order to feel better and look better. Acceptance of the U.S.D.A.'s Food Guide Pyramid as a guide to daily food choices is an approach to sensible eating that assists people in limiting consumption of the foods shown to affect health negatively. The nurse, through nutrition education and reinforcement of positive practices, plays a significant role in promoting the health of children. See the Levels of Prevention discussion on obesity below.

The value of exercise and physical fitness programs for young people has been recognized for some time. Organized groups, such as the YMCA, YWCA, Boy and Girl Scouts, and Campfire Girls, have offered sports and character development programs for many years. Good day care and preschool programs provide equipment and opportunities for large-muscle activity as well as fine motor development. Schools, parks, and recreation centers encourage exercise through use of playground equipment and organized sports activities. Despite these opportunities, many young people do not exercise often enough or vigorously enough. Members of minority groups, females, and inner-city residents exercise less than do white, suburban males (U.S. Public Health Service, 1990; Schlicker, et al., 1994). Even team sports keep players inactive much of the time and are not activities that young people continue in their adult lives. More comprehensive physical education programs that encourage and focus on vigorous individual exercise and self-discipline as lifetime habits would better serve the health needs of this population group. Community health nurses can promote such programs through the schools as well as encourage these activities in their contacts with students of all ages (see Fig. 19.4).

Education to Prevent Substance Abuse

The demonstrated hazards of cigarette smoking, alcohol, use of inhalants, and drug abuse have prompted the development of substance abuse programs particularly targeting children and adolescents. Health education efforts involving school nurses, teachers, and counselors have been a major source of influence encouraging students to make responsible decisions about smoking, drinking, and other behaviors affecting their health (Goldstein, 1994; Hass, 1993; Keenan, 1986).

Health departments, community health nursing agencies, and private groups such as the American Cancer Society and the National Lung Association also provide educational materials and promote anti-smoking and drug use prevention campaigns. The more successful programs emphasize how the human body works and how behaviors affect it. They also help young people resist social pressures to smoke and take drugs by pointing out that those who do are in the minority and by showing the deleterious effects of these practices. Using students themselves as health educators is a positive use of peer pressure and has proved to be a successful means of influencing attitudes (Goldstein, 1994). A media campaign that promotes the slogan, "Just say no!" was begun in the 1980's, and does express a valid goal. However, by itself it is too simplistic, and a set of skills has to be taught in order to make, "Just say no!" a reality (Ibid.).

Other groups, such as 4-H clubs, churches, the Catholic Youth Organization, and Scouts, use peer counseling to influence young people to assume responsibility for healthy life styles. Decision-making skills that lead to healthy life-style choices, enhanced in adolescence and remaining through adulthood, are the goals. The community health nurse participates in and supports existing programs in addition to counseling and referring young people who need help.

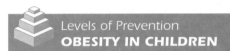

Levels of Prevention
OBESITY IN CHILDREN

PRIMARY PREVENTION

Foster good eating habits from infancy. Introduce foods according to health care provider's recommendations. Reserve empty calories for special occasions only. Reward good behavior with items/activites rather than food. Family dietary practices should model the recommendations in the Food Pyramid (see Chapter 1). Encourage an active life style with physical activity as much a part of childhood as TV and video games.

SECONDARY PREVENTION

Increase age appropriate physical activity. Have fruits and vegetables available for snacks. Limit purchasing empty calorie foods. Don't focus on the child dieting, the entire family should eat appropriately. A child should not necessarily lose weight, if the increased weight is mild to moderate, but weight should stabilize as child grows.

TERTIARY PREVENTION

Assist child and family to recognize the need to lose weight. Have a physical examination by a health care provider before dieting. Initiate other actions according to those listed in primary and secondary prevention. If child is morbidly obese, additional medical intervention may be necessary, including psychiatric intervention.

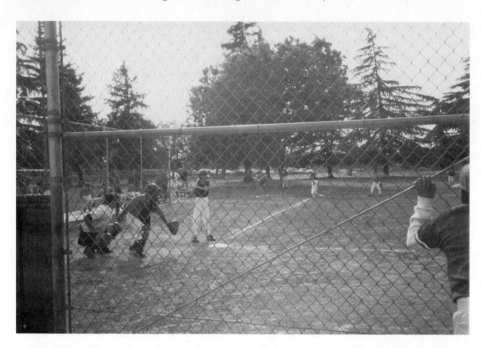

FIGURE 19.4. Vigorous exercise that promotes fitness and self-discipline is an important contributor to young people's health. Team sports further enhance the development of social skills and healthy relationships.

Counseling and Crisis Intervention

Stress control programs for children and adolescents do not exist in any great numbers, yet they are very much needed. Many of the health problems discussed in this chapter relate to the emotional health of young people. Reckless driving, suicide, homicide, unplanned pregnancy, smoking, alcoholism, illicit drug use, obesity, anorexia nervosa, and bulimia, as well as other problems—all signal the presence of stress and the absence of coping skills sufficient to handle it. Crisis intervention programs and services that treat a problem after it occurs are helpful and can prevent problems from worsening. More needed, however, for this population group are programs that build coping skills early, including self-help, peer counseling, peer intervention, and mutual support activities.

Programs offered in a group context, such as those mentioned earlier—4-H, Scouts, various character-building clubs, and organizations like Outward Bound (a team building and personally challenging outdoor experience lasting a day or several days)—have proven most effective. For the nurse, recognition of young people at risk (Hass, 1993; Mercer, 1990), counseling, and early referral to sources of help can prevent crisis situations. Reduction of stresses in the family and community environments can further enhance this group's health.

Role of the Community Health Nurse

Community health nurses face the challenge of continually assessing each population group's current health problems as well as determining available and needed services. Some gaps can be filled by nursing interventions. Others must be referred to various members of the community health team with whom the nurse may sometimes collaboratively develop services.

Community health nursing interventions with toddler, preschool, school-age, and adolescent populations are the same as those outlined in the basic conceptual model discussed in Chapter 4: education, engineering, and enforcement. The nurse uses educational interventions when teaching proper nutrition and exercise, family planning, physical and psychological effects of drug abuse, safety precautions, or weight control. Each of these involves providing information and encouraging client groups to participate in their own health care. Engineering interventions are those strategies in which the nurse uses a greater degree of persuasion or positive manipulation such as conducting voluntary immunization programs, encouraging safe sex and use of contraceptives, counseling for stress reduction, identifying and treating STD sexual contacts, or encouraging use of safety devices, such as stairway guards. Finally, the nurse uses enforcement interventions which are those in which the nurse must use coercion to make people comply with the law such as requiring certain immunizations, reporting illegal drug use, reporting suspected child abuse, or environmental health standards violations, such as sanitation issues.

SCHOOL NURSING PRACTICE

In community health practice, nursing service to a school-age population requires a shift in focus away from the individual schoolchild, or small groups of children, toward the needs of the school-age population as a whole.

School nursing is a speciality branch of professional nursing that serves the school-age population. "School nursing delivers services to students of all ages from birth through age 21 and serves students, families, and the school community in regular education, in special education, and in other educational arenas" (Hass, 1993, p.11). A **school nurse** is a registered nurse (frequently with additional educational preparation beyond the bachelor's degree in nursing) who has primary responsibility for the health care of school-age children and school personnel in an educational setting. There is a professional organization of school nurses that has been incorporated since 1979; the National Association of School Nurses (NASN). They have chapters in each state and meet locally to address the professional needs of school nurses. The NASN, using the American Nurses' Association, Standards of Clinical Nursing Practice, has developed, "Guidelines for a Model School Nursing Services Program" (Proctor, 1990).

The primary functions of the school nurse are to prevent illness and to promote and maintain the health of the school community. The community health nurse not only serves individuals, families, and groups within the context of school health, but also the school as an organization and its membership (students and staff) as aggregates.

School nursing practice incorporates three functions: health services, health education, and improvement of the school environment (Proctor, 1990). Health services include programs such as vision and hearing screening, scoliosis screening, health examinations, emergency care, and referrals. There are special corrective and training services for speech, hearing, or psychological problems. Student and family counseling are important services provided and programs to control communica-

ble diseases such as enforcing immunization requirements by law (see more about this in the Issues in Community Health Nursing display below). School health services also include health appraisal and services for school personnel.

The health education function of school nursing practice involves planned and incidental teaching of health concepts; curriculum development which includes classes in health science and healthful living; and use of educational media, library resources, and community facilities. These activities aim to integrate health information with students' daily living experiences, to build positive attitudes toward health, and to establish sound health practices.

The third function of school nursing practice is the promotion of healthful school living. Emphasis on a healthful physical environment includes proper selection, design, organization, operation, and maintenance of the physical plant. Consideration should be shown for areas such as adaptability to student needs; safety; visual, thermal, and acoustic factors; aesthetic values; sanitation; and safety of the school bus system and food services. Healthful school living also emphasizes planning a daily schedule that monitors healthful classroom experiences, extra class activities, school breakfasts and/or lunches, emotional climate, program of disci-

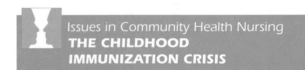

Issues in Community Health Nursing
THE CHILDHOOD IMMUNIZATION CRISIS

More than one-third of all 2 year olds in the United States have not received the recommended vaccinations. Some statistics show that complete immunization coverage in children is as low as 40 percent. The patchwork nature of the public and private systems responsible for financing immunizations adds to the problem. Half the families with private insurance do not have vaccines covered and a significant portion of families on Medicaid mistakenly believe it does not cover immunizations. Health care reform that has been long in coming will be longer in implementing uniformly nationwide. Reform that only pays for vaccines may have limited effects on increasing access unless vaccine administration and other preventative services are also covered (Lieu, et al, 1994).

pline, teaching methods, and reporting illegal drug use, suspected child abuse, or reporting violations of environmental health standards. It also seeks to promote the physical, mental, and emotional health of school personnel by being accessible as a resource to teachers and staff regarding their own health and safety.

A current problem today is the increase in violence and drugs in schools. Guns, knives, and other weapons brought to school by students create an unsafe learning environment for children and for the teaching and support staff of adults in many urban and suburban school districts. Drugs on school campuses create disruption in the classroom, interruption of the learning process for those under the influence, and is closely related to the increased violence. These issues create new challenges for the school nurse who is attempting to promote healthful school living.

LIAISON WITH THE INTERDISCIPLINARY SCHOOL HEALTH TEAM

School health, like all health programs in the community, requires an interdisciplinary team effort (Butcher et al., 1988; Kirby, 1990: Wold, 1981). Although the school nurse plays a central role, collaboration with many other individuals is important. The school principal influences all phases of the school health program by promoting good school health through actively supporting all the school's health services, participating in the setting of policies, and tapping community resources. The principal can reinforce positive efforts within the school ranging from health teaching to cleaning activities of the custodian. Because of the principal's influential position, it is absolutely essential for the nurse and principal to maintain a positive and cooperative working relationship.

Teachers, whether they are involved in regular instruction, physical education, or special education classes, play a major role in school health. Because they spend so much time with students, their observations, health teaching, and personal health habits have a profound effect on student health and the quality of school health services. The school nurse and teachers must collaborate constantly.

Other health team members, such as health educators, health coordinators, psychologists, audiologists, speech therapists, counselors, health care providers, dentists, dental hygienists, social workers, security personnel, or health aides, and volunteers may be present depending on the size and financial resources of the school. All team members, including students, parents, and the custodian, have a specialized role complementary to that of the school nurse. Consultation and referral between team members are crucial to implementing the school health program.

If the school system desires the services, a physician may work part-time, or be available on a consultation basis only. This role focuses largely on advising and consulting in policy and medical-legal matters. A community physician may serve on a school advisory panel and serve as a liaison with the community, other health agencies, and the school. The physician may be available to consult with those who plan and develop school health programs. In some communities, the physician may become involved in student health appraisal, rescreening, health problem intervention, sports physicals, or be in attendance at sporting events. See the "Standards of School Nursing Practice" listed in the display.

Special Training and Skills of the School Nurse

School nurses operate from one of two administrative bases, the school system or the health department. There is controversy over which system best serves the population's needs. In most localities, school nurses are hired through the public or private school system and maintain a specialized, school-based service. An advantage of this specialized school nurse's role is that the nurse can concentrate all the time and effort on the school health program and thus develop specialized skills in school health assessment and intervention. Today, with emphasis on delivering health care at community sites where clients spend most of their time (e.g. schools for children, the workplace for adults), the nurse specializing in school health care seems better prepared to meet the complex needs of the school-age population. In contrast, the more generalized role of the community health nurse who operates under the board of health's jurisdiction provides services to schools as one part of generalized services provided to the community. The community health nurse working through the health department devotes only a portion of the workday in the school and has other responsibilities such as clinic nursing and making home visits. Many argue that such generalized school nurses are at a disadvantage with not enough time spent on meeting school health needs. Although the advantage is this

NASN "STANDARDS OF SCHOOL NURSING PRACTICE"

The school nurse:

uses a distinct knowledge base for decision making in nursing practice.

uses a systematic approach to problem solving in nursing practice.

contributes to the education of the client with special health needs by assessing the client, planning and providing appropriate nursing care, and evaluating the identified outcomes of care.

uses effective written, verbal, and nonverbal communication skills.

establishes and maintains a comprehensive school health program.

collaborates with other school professionals, parents, and caregivers to meet the health, developmental, and educational needs of clients.

collaborates with members of the community in the delivery of health and social services, and utilizes knowledge of community health systems and resources to function as a school-community liaison.

assists students, families, and the school community to achieve optimal levels of wellness through appropriately designed and delivered health education.

contributes to nursing and school health through innovations in practice and participation in research or research-related activities.

identifies, deliniates, and clarifies the nursing role, promotes quality of care, pursues continued professional enhancement, and demonstrates professional conduct.

Source: Proctor, S.T. (1990). Guidelines for a model school nursing service program. Scarborough, ME: National Association of School Nurses.

tion or a master's degree in nursing) with experience in physical assessment, diagnosis, and treatment so that primary care can be provided to school-age children. Today many school districts see the advantage of having school nurse practitioners on staff rather than having the limited services of a physician. In the nurse practitioner role, assessments, diagnosis, treatment, and referral of injuries, communicable diseases, or other health problems can be managed more efficiently by a practitioner who is educationally prepared to work holisitcally with the school-age population and is part of the educational setting. If this is impractical, one school nurse practitioner available to the school nurses for consultation or employed on a part-time basis is a start to the development of more comprehensive school health services.

Some states are requiring even more specialized training for school nurses as the needs of school-age populations become increasingly complex. In California, school nurses are expected to hold a school health credential. This credential is obtained after having a bachelors degree in nursing. It involves a university program of study that includes coursework in audiology,

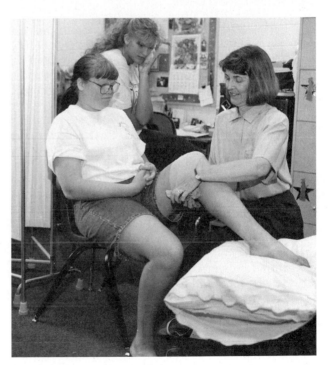

FIGURE 19.5. A school nurse assesses and treats an injured child. This is an essential component of a comprehensive school health program.

broader base allows contact with preschoolers and families, strengthened knowledge of the community and its resources, and integration of in-school and out-of-school care.

School nurse practitioners are registered nurses with advanced academic and clinical preparation (certifica-

guidance and counseling, exceptional children, school health principles and practice, a practicum in school nursing, child psychology, and health curriculum development in addition to other courses. There are many school nurses in California who feel that the future of health care delivery for children is at the school site, and so are preparing themselves for an expanded role in school nursing by combining the school health credential coursework with a nurse practitioner program. These school nurses are professionals who bring a multitude of skills to the school district. In California, a high percentage of school-age children are from migrant farm families; many are from ethnically diverse backgrounds where English is a second language; adolescent pregnancy rates in some counties are the highest in the nation; and the state has the nation's lowest rates of immunization coverage. The school nurse with additional educational preparation is able to work effectively with children and families in communities with increasingly complex health care needs. This nurse needs to be a specialist, in that she or he is in the school district as a full time health team member (see Fig. 19.5).

CASE STUDY

ELLEN RAMSEY, SCHOOL NURSE

Ellen Ramsey, a community health nurse for six years, recently took a job with the Washington County Board of Education to become a school nurse at Keeler Elementary School. The district will now have six school nurses to serve it's 8,000 students in five elementary schools, one middle school, and one high school. Ellen has been working with families and groups in the community and has taken coursework in school health at the local university, but she has not done school nursing before.

Mrs. Murray, the principal, shares her goals with Ellen, who is the first full-time nurse the school has ever had. She comments that she expects the children to be kept as healthy as possible and that Ellen will be the major consultant on health matters in the school. She prefers that Ellen carves out her own role in consultation with the school administration.

Built 20 years ago, Keeler has 926 students in grades kindergarten through sixth grade and is on the traditional academic schedule. With 31 teachers, its pupil-teacher ratio is approximately 30:1. Ellen reads materials Mrs. Murry has given her about the history of the school, acquaints herself with the teachers during the week before school starts, and attends meetings with the other school nurses and the pupil-personnel director of the school district. Since Ellen is familiar with the region and city resources, she uses this first week to focus on orientation to the school community as an aggregate within the larger community. Ellen also spends time looking through student records, confers with teachers, school psychologist and counselor to assess children at risk.

During the first weeks of school, Ellen arranges to go into each classroom and introduces herself to the children and explains what she will be doing regarding health appraisal and screening with each class. She also explains what the children can expect if they come into the nurse's office if they are ill or injured.

The school year is six weeks old and Ellen is overwhelmed by the numbers of identified health problems and the required follow up. She sends over 20 ill children home each day, seeks answers to teacher's questions about various students, visits families of some of the children with disabilities, and started a babysitters' safety class for interested sixth-graders. Yet there are so many children she has not assessed. Moreover, what about the teachers' needs? She knows that she is not really providing service to the whole school community as yet. She realizes that she must shift her focus. A meeting with the other school nurses has helped give her direction.

Changing her focus means Ellen now must adopt a broader set of goals for school nursing that involve the school organization and population levels, yet still include the individual, family, and group levels. Ellen bases her goals on the NASN "Standards of School Nursing Practice," (Proctor, 1990).

Ellen concentrates on selected individuals, selected families, or special groups needing nursing or other professional intervention. For example, she may seek to identify children with speech and language delays. Many of these clients will be referred to other community resources for assistance (Barnfather, 1991; Kirby, 1990). She plans to get to know personally each member of the school family and staff, including the secretaries and the custodian, in order to cultivate their good will and encourage their help. She will sharpen their observation skills regarding the students and she will assess their own health needs. A faculty or staff member who is not well physically or emotionally may significantly influence the health of the school community.

At the organizational level, Ellen aims to fulfill the following responsibilities spelled out in her job description:

1. Establish and revise school and district health philosophy, policies, and procedures pertaining to school health services.
2. Develop and maintain a system of emergency care.
3. Provide for school safety and a healthful school environment.

4. Facilitate comprehensive community health care planning and resources development to include the health needs of the preschool and school-age populations and their families.

This level requires more attention than Ellen has given to it in the past. She makes certain all staff are trained in administering first-aid and that the entire school community knows what to do and where to go in the event of an emergency such as a tornado, fire, or earthquake. Some school safety issues have been addressed, but now she needs to examine the overall safety of the building and check with administration about safety of the school buses. She looks into the effectiveness of fire drills and alternate routes for emptying the building. She oversees the handling of dangerous materials for science activities, among custodial supplies, and in the kitchen.

The school environment needs more careful assessment. Ellen starts checking the nutritional value of the school lunches and the ventilation of classrooms. She familiarizes herself with each teacher and classroom while observing students, and consults with teachers about her observations. The dingy halls of the old building soon take on a more cheerful appearance through the work of a volunteer paint crew from the PTA.

As an organization, Keeler Elementary School is functioning fairly well, Ellen decides. The pupil-teacher ratio is high by ideal standards, but classes of 30 students are being managed well by this group of experienced teachers at Keeler. To provide students with more individual attention, Ellen suggests adding more teacher aides and using some sixth graders to help the first graders with reading. Faculty on the whole get along well with each other and with Mrs. Murray. There is open communication and positive feedback. Working conditions are pleasant, and faculty requests are answered in a reasonable amount of time. There is also adequate space, equipment, personnel assistance, and support for the school health program.

To influence school health policy and resource planning, Ellen volunteers to serve on a district committee that meets once a month. Meeting other professionals concerned about school health broadens her understanding of school and community needs and also gives her ideas on intervention strategies and ways to tap community resources.

At the population group level, Ellen aims to achieve the following goals that are a part of her job description:

1. Assess the collective needs of preschool and school-age children and school personnel.
2. Identify existing and potential health problems in the school population (and in the larger community affecting it), determine those at greatest risk, develop a plan, and intervene to minimize or prevent problems.
3. Promote and maintain optimal health of the student body and the school personnel population.

4. Prevent and control communicable disease in the student population (in order to protect the well-being of students and the community).
5. Evaluate and upgrade the contribution of the school nurse role toward promoting the health of the school community.

During a conference with the pupil-personnel coordinator, Ellen reviews the goals and make plans for conducting a broader assessment of the school population's health. Journal articles and discussion with other school nurses at district school nurse and school nurse association meetings give her additional ideas. For example, one school nurse, instead of performing a routine physical examination on every child, developed a systematic method of classroom assessment. She evaluated an entire class of 25 to 30 children at one time through regular observation of their behavior and developmental status and through close consultation with teachers who alerted her about special student behaviors to observe. Ellen decides to try this method in combination with further data gathering on selected children through screening, interviews, and family visits. The vision and hearing screening done yearly on all children and scoliosis screening on the sixth grade students, offers another opportunity to observe them closely for signs of child abuse, malnutrition, or other physical or emotional problems that might be prevalent among this population group.

Ellen assesses preschool-age children who will be starting kindergarten next year by holding a Saturday afternoon preschool fair. Invitations are sent out to all the families in the community with four-year-old children. PTA volunteers help her organize games and refreshments and conduct school tours. Registered nurses from the Head Start Program and volunteers from the community assist in cursory physical exams that include vision and hearing screening and a review of immunizations. She notifies parents immediately if children need follow-up care.

While conducting this preschool assessment, Ellen keeps in mind that she wants a profile of this population of four-year-olds, not just each individual child's health picture. She looks for recurring problems that are common to the group, such as skin rashes, orthopedic defects, headaches, eating or respiratory difficulties, and signs of communicable diseases. Such population screening has sometimes uncovered widespread community health problems. For instance, in 1992 in a community in Fresno, California, recognition of a high incidence of cancers among students and staff in one elementary school that was situated beneath high tension wires led to an investigation and finally a relocation of portions of that school population. In 1980, a community in Memphis, Tennessee, whose incidence of miscarriages, cancer, and infant deaths had markedly increased, discovered that nearby chemicals buried many years previously were the cause. Identifying common problems among the preschool or school-age populations, including problems specific to each age group (Bocchino, 1991; Kirby, 1990), enables Ellen to take corrective action on a broader scale and thus to help many children at once as well as to take preventive action.

Ellen begins to collect data on the needs of the school personnel population by observing and talking informally with faculty and staff. She discovers that some of the teachers seem on the verge of burning out. They do not enjoy their teaching, feel tired most of the time, take piles of work home with them every night, do not sleep well, and often feel irritable toward the children. With school administration's approval, she plans a workshop to prevent teacher burnout. Expert consultants help the teachers learn to recognize symptoms and avoid burnout. During the workshop the teachers develop specific plans to help them cope with their present situations and design strategies for alleviating future stress.

The three sets of goals for school nursing have helped Ellen refocus her thinking and expand her service to include not only individual, family, and group levels of nursing intervention but school organization and school population group levels as well. Ellen is finding the role of school nurse challenging and rewarding as she sees positive changes in the health of all people in this community aggregate.

Summary

Children are an important population group to community health nurses because their physical and emotional health is vital to the future of society and because they are unable to help themselves without guidance and direction.

Mortality rates for children have decreased dramatically since the early 1900s but morbidity rates among children, remain high. Children are still vulnerable to many illnesses, injuries, and emotional problems often as a result of our complex and stressful environment.

Toddlers and preschoolers, are still at risk for accidents (falls, drownings, burns, and poisonings), acute illnesses, particularly respiratory illness, and nutritional, dental, and emotional ailments. Violence against children and deaths due to homicide have an alarming occurence in the U.S. Violent deaths, suicides, injuries and HIV/AIDS are the leading threats to life and health for adolescents. Other health problems include alcohol and drug abuse, unplanned pregnancies, STDs, and poor nutrition. All these problems create major challenges to the community health nurse who seeks to prevent illness and injury among children and promote their health.

Health services for children span three categories: preventive, health protecting, and health promoting. The community health nurse plays a vital role in each. Preventive services include quality child care, immunization programs, parental support services, family planning programs, services for those with STDs, and alcohol and drug abuse prevention programs. Health protection services include accident and injury control, programs to reduce environmental hazards, control of infectious diseases, services to protect children from child abuse, and fluoridation of community water supplies to protect children's dental health. Health promotion services include programs in early childhood development; nutrition and weight control; exercise and physical fitness; smoking, alcohol, and drug abuse education; and stress control.

The role of community health nurses includes three basic interventions while serving children's health needs. With educational interventions, such as nutrition teaching, nurses provide information and encourage clients to act responsibly on behalf of their own health. With engineering interventions, such as encouraging use of contraceptives, nurses employ persuasive tactics to move clients toward more positive health behaviors. With enforcement interventions, such as reporting and intervening in child abuse, nurses practice some form of coercion to protect children from threats to their health.

Nursing of the school-age population involves providing health services, health education and ensuring a healthful school environment. School nurses may provide these services as part of their role within a health department or be hired by the school district full time. The increasingly complex needs of the school-age population and the collective accessiblity to children in schools as a site to provide primary health care services is prompting schools to hire nurses with advanced preparation as nurse practioners and credentialed school nurses to expand the services to this aggregate.

Activities to Promote Critical Thinking

1. What is the major cause of death among school-age children? What community-wide interventions could be initiated to prevent these deaths? Select one intervention and describe how you and a group of community health professionals might develop this preventive measure.

2. Describe one health promotion program you, as a community health nurse, could initiate and carry out to improve the health of children in a day-care center or pre-school program.

3. How can environmental health protection programs affect the future health of infants? Why is control of environmental hazards important for children of any age? List three things a nurse can do to protect children from environmental hazards.

4. A 14-year-old girl from a middle-class family and a 14-year-old girl from a poor family both come to the office where you work as a school nurse. The girls have similar symptoms that possibly indicate gonorrhea. Would your assessment and interventions be the same or different for the two girls? What are your values and attitudes toward people with diseases that are sexually transmitted? Does social class, race, age, or sex make any difference in how you feel about them? What is one action the community health nurse can take to prevent such diseases in this population group?

REFERENCES

Aust, P.H. (1994). When the problem is not the problem: Understanding attention deficit disorder with and without hyperactivity. *Child Welfare, 73*(3), 215–227.

Barkley, R.A. (1990). *Attention deficit hyperactivity disorder: A handbook for diagnosis and treatment.* New York: The Guildford Press.

Barnfather, J.S. (1991). Restructuring the role of school nurse in health promotion. *Public Health Nursing, 8*(4), 234–238.

Bassoff, B.Z. & Willis, W.O. (1991). Requiring formal training in preventative health practices for child day care providers. *Public Health Reports, 106*(5), 523–529.

Belsky, J. (1990). Parental and nonparental child care and children's socioemotional development: A decade in review. *Journal of Marriage and the Family, 52,* 157–167.

Berger, D., Inkelas, M., Myhre, S., & Mishler, A. (1994). Developing health education materials for inner-city low literacy parents. *Public Health Reports, 109*(2), 168–172.

Bocchino, C. (1991). School-based clinics: Ensuring access to the health care for adolescent America. *Pediatric Nurse, 17*(4), 398, 418.

"Breaking down the barriers." (1994). *Maternal and Child Nursing, 19,* 80–81.

Browne, K.D. (1993). Violence in the family, and its links to child abuse. *Bailliere's Clinical Pediatrics, 1*(1), 149-164.

Browne, K. (1995). Preventing child maltreatment through community nursing. *Journal of Advanced Nursing, 21,* 57–63.

Butcher, A. H., et al. (1988). Heart smart, A school health program meeting the 1990 objectives for the nation. *Health Education Quarterly, 15*(1), 17–34.

Capitol Bulletin. (1992, September 16). *Minnesota Women's Consortium.* St. Paul, MN: Author.

Chernoff, R., Combs-Orme, T., Risley-Curtiss, C., & Heisler, A. (1994). Assessing the health status of children entering foster care. *Pediatrics, 93*(4), 594–601.

Crime Prevention Center. (1988). *Child Abuse Prevention Handbook.* Sacramento, CA: Office of the Attorney General.

Childrens Defense Fund. (1988). *What every American should be asking political leaders in 1988.* Washington, DC: Author.

Children's Defense Fund. (1991). *The state of America's children 1991.* Washington, DC: Author.

Clark-Stewart, A. (1989). Infant day care: Maligned or malignant? *American Psychologist, 44,* 266–273.

Community childhood hunger identification project. (1991). *A survey of childhood hunger in the United States.* Washington, DC: Food Research and Action Center.

Corby, R. (1992). Assessing child abuse in community health nursing. *Imprint, 39*(2), 77–78.

Cowan, C.P. & Cowan, P.A. (1992). *When partners become parents: The big life change for couples.* New York: Basic Books.

Department of Education. (1990). *America 2000: An education strategy sourcebook.* Washington, DC: Author

DeRienzo-DeVivio, S. (1992). Childhood lead poisoning. Shifting to primary prevention. *Pediatric Nursing, 18*(6), 565–567.

Falco, M. (1993). *The making of a drug-free America: Programs that work.* New York: Random House.

Goldstein, A. (1994). *Addiction: From biology to drug policy.* New York: W.H. Freeman.

Greenwood, M.R.C., Johnson, P.R., Karp, R.J., & Wolman, P.G. (1993). Obesity in disadvantaged children. In R.J. Karp (Ed.), *Malnourished children in the United States: Caught in the cycle of poverty.* (pp. 115–129). New York: Springer.

Hass, M.B. (Ed.). (1993). *The school nurse's source book of individualized healthcare plans* (Vol.1.). North Branch, MN: Sunrise River Press.

Henson, C. (1995, February, 9). Women getting hit hard by AIDS. (A1) *The Fresno Bee.*

Herbert, M. (1989). *Working with children and their families.* Chicago: Lyceum.

Hewlitt, S. (1991). *When the bough breaks: The cost of neglecting our children.* New York: Harper Collins.

Johansen, A., A. Leibowitz, A., & Waite, L. (1988). Child care and children's illness. *American Journal of Public Health, 78*(9), 1175–77.

Johnson-Russell, J. & Anema, M.G. (1989). Physical assessment skills: A new dimension to traditional school nursing. *School Nurse. 2,* 14,16–18, 20–21.

Karp, R.J. (Ed.). (1993). *Malnourished children in the United States: Caught in the cycle of poverty.* New York: Springer.

Keenan, R. (1986). School-based adolescent health care programs. *Pediatric Nursing, 12,* 365–69.

Kipke, M.D., Futterman, D., & Hein, K. (1990). HIV infection and AIDS during adolescence. *Medical Clinics of North America, 74*(5), 1149–1167.

Kirby, D. (1990). Comprehensive school health and the larger community: Issues and a possible scenario. *Journal of School Health, 60*(4), 170–177.

Lieu, T., Smith, M.D., Newacheck, P.N., Langthorn, N.D., Venkatesh, P., & Herradora, R. (1994). Health insurance and preventative care sources of children at public immunization clinics. *Pediatrics, 93*(3), 373–378.

Markowitz, D.L. (1993). Oral care for the disadvantaged child. In R.J. Karp (Ed.), Malnourished children in the United States: Caught in the cycle of poverty (pp. 168–173). New York: Springer.

McKay, M.M. (1994). The link between domestic violence and child abuse: Assessment and treatment considerations. *Child Welfare, 73*(1), 29–39.

Mercer, R.T. (1990). *Parents at risk.* New York: Springer Publishing Company.

National Institute of Dental Research. (1989). *Oral health of United States children. The national survey of dental caries in U.S. school children, 1986–1987.* DHHS Pub.No.(NIH) 89-2247. Bethesda, MD: U.S. Department of Health and Human Services.

National Safety Council. (1990). *Accident facts.* Chicago: Author.

Perry, C.L., et al. (1988). Parent involvement with children's health promotion: The Minnesota home team. *American Journal of Public Health, 78*(9), 1156–60.

Proctor, S.T. (1990). *Guidelines for a model school nursing services program.* Scarborough, ME: National Association of School Nurses.

Schlicker, S.A., Borra, S.T., & Regan, C. (1994). The weight and fitness status of United States children. *Nutrition Reviews, 52*(1), 11–16.

Shaywitz,S. & Shaywitz,B. (1991). Introduction to the special series on attention deficit disorder. *Journal of Learning Disabilities. 24*(2), 69.

Stark, E. & Flitcraft, A. (1988). Women and children at risk: A feminist perspective on child abuse. *International Journal of Health Services, 18*(1), 97–118.

Straus, M.A. & Gelles, R.J. (1990). *Physical violence in American families: Risk factors and adaptions to violence in 8,145 families.* New Brunswick, NJ: Transaction.

Tucker, V.L. & Cho, C.T. (1991). AIDS and adolescents. *Postgrauate Medicine, 89*(3), 49–53.

Urquiza, A.J., Wirtz, S.J., Peterson, M.S., & Singer, V.S. (1994). Screening and evaluating abused and neglected children entering protective custody. *Child Welfare, 73*(2), 155–171.

U.S. Bureau of Census. (1990). Money, income and poverty status in the United States: 1989. In *Current Population Reports* series P-60, No. 168, 59. Washington, DC: Author.

U.S. Department of Health and Human Services, Public Health Service, Centers for disease control. *HIV/AIDS Surveillance Report,* April, 1991, 12.

U.S. Public Health Service. (1995, January 6). Centers for Disease Control. Morbidity and Mortality Weekly Report, General Recommendations on Immunizations: Recommendations of the Advisory Committee on Immunization Practices (ACIP), American Academy of Pediatrics and American Academy of Family Physicians.January 06, 1995.

U.S. Public Health Service. (1990). *Healthy people 2000.* Washington, DC: Author.

U.S. Department of Commerce. (1993). *U.S. Statistical abstracts* (113th ed.). Washington, DC: Author.

Wagner, J. & Menke, E. (1991). No place to call home. *The Ohio State University College of Nursing Magazine, 1*(10), 11–13.

Wold, S. (1981). *School nursing: A framework for practice.* North Branch, MN: Sunrise River Press.

Zanga, J.R. & Oda, D.S. (1987). School health services. *Journal of School Health, 57*(10), 413–416.

SELECTED READINGS

American Nurses Association. (1991). *Standards of school nursing practice.* Kansas City, MO: Author.

Bagnato, S.J., Neisworth, J.T., & Munson, S.M. (1989). *Linking developmental assessment and early intervention: Curriculum-based prescriptions* (2nd ed.). Rockville, MD: Aspen.

Clayton, E.W., Hickson, G.B., & Miller, C.S. (1994). Parents' responses to vaccine information pamphlets. *Pediatrics, 93*(3), 369–372.

Cohen, F.L. & Nehring, W.M. (1994). Foster care of HIV-positive children in the United States. *Public Health Reports, 109*(1), 60–67.

Davidhizar, R. & Frank, B. (1992). Understanding the physical and psycholosocial stressors of the child who is homeless. *Pediatric Nursing, 18*(6), 559–562.

Drewnowski, A., Hopkins, S., & Kessler, R. (1988). The prevalence of bulimia nervosa in the U.S. college student population. *American Journal of Public Health, 78*(10), 1322–25.

Harold, R.D. & Harold, N.B. (1993). School-based clinics: A response to the physical and mental health needs of adolescents. *Health and Social Work, 18*, 65–74.

Kolbe, L.J. (1994). Our children's future. *Healthcare Trends and Transition, 6*(1), 14–17.

Kusserow, R.P. (1990). *Inspector general's report on crack babies.* (Report OEI-03-89-01540.). Washington DC: Department of Health and Human Services.

Logan, B.N. (1991). Adolescent asubstance abuse prevention: An overview of the literature. *Family Community Health, 13*, (4), 25–36.

Malloy, C. (1992). Children and poverty: America's future at risk. *Pediatric Nursing, 18*(6), 553–557.

Martin, D.A. (1992). Children in peril: A mandate for change in health care policies for low-income children. *Family Community Health, 15*(1), 75–90.

Must, A., Jacques, P.F., Dallal, G.E. Bajema, C.L. & Dietz, W.H. (1992). Long-term morbidity and mortality of overweight adolescents. *New England Journal of Medicine, 327,* 1350–1355.

National Center on Child Abuse and Neglect. (1992). [Working paper 1:1990 summary data component]. DHHS Pub. No. (AC) 92-30361.

Novello, A.C., Degraw, C., & Kleinman, D. V. (1992). Healthy children ready to learn: An essential collaboration between health and education. *Public Health Reports, 107*(1), 3–10.

Salsberry, P.J., Nickel, J.T., & Mitch, R. (1994). Immunization status of 2 year olds in middle/upper and lower income populations: A community survey. *Public Health Nursing, 11*(1), 17–23.

U.S. Department of Education. (1991). *Preparing young children for success: Guideposts for achieving our first national goal.* Washington, DC: Author.

Waller, A., Baker, S., & Szocka, A. (1989). Childhood injury deaths: National analysis and geographic variations. *American Journal of Public Health, 79*(3), 310–15.

Waszak, C. & Neidell, S. (1991). *School-based and school-linked clinics update.* Washington, DC: Center for Popuation Options.

workers between 1989 and 1991, and 10 deaths per 100,000 workers between 1986 and 1988 (U.S. Statistical Abstracts, 1994). See Levels of Prevention display below.

CHEMICAL FACTORS

Chemical factors are the chemical agents present in the work environment that may threaten worker health and safety. Numerous chemicals are found in the raw materials, production processes, and daily operations of industries and businesses such as dry cleaners, painters, food companies, photographers, automobile manufacturers, plastics factories, farms, pharmaceutical companies, and hospitals. In addition, the petroleum and chemical industries have introduced substances at the alarming rate of several hundred untested new compounds a year, subjecting workers to unknown hazards (Last, 1987; U.S. DHHS, 1991). Although chemicals are frequently associated with gases, they are also present in solvents, mists, vapors, dusts, and solids. Depending on their form and structure, chemicals can enter the human body through the lungs, gastrointestinal tract, and/or skin. Therefore, understanding the toxicology of chemicals is essential for identifying (1) the amount of chemical exposure that produces toxicity, (2) the routes by which chemicals enter the body, and (3) the appropriate personal protection for workers (Smisko, 1990). For example, lead enters the body through all three routes—lungs, gastrointestinal tract, and skin. Workers exposed to toxic levels of lead must wear protective clothing, maintain good hand-washing practices, avoid eating or smoking on the job to prevent ingestion, and employ appropriate respiratory protection to prevent inhalation.

Many toxic chemicals, such as insecticides, are taken for granted in daily use, and their toxicity is frequently ignored. But careless handling and needless exposure can cause serious burns, poisoning, asphyxia, tissue damage, or even cancer. For example, 4 workers in a factory of 500 in Kentucky experienced a rare type of liver cancer from intensive exposure to vinyl chloride monomer (Olsen, et al., 1991). This specific form of liver cancer occurs at a rate of 20 to 30 new cases per year in the entire U.S. population. Some inert, nontoxic industrial materials, such as resins and polymers, may decompose and form toxic byproducts when heated. Workers need to be warned of and protected from the hazards associated with the materials they use on the job. With proper handling and protection, toxicity can be prevented. Ideally, all toxic substances should be eliminated through substitution of nontoxic agents, when such chemicals exist.

BIOLOGICAL FACTORS

Biological factors are the organisms and potential contaminants found in the work environment. These include bacteria, viruses, rickettsiae, molds, fungi, parasites of various types, insects, animals, and even toxic

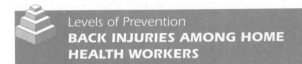

Levels of Prevention
BACK INJURIES AMONG HOME HEALTH WORKERS

GOAL

To prevent work-related back injuries among nurses, home health aides, and physical therapists employed in one home health agency.

PRIMARY PREVENTION

In-service training is required of all staff who provide direct client care that includes positioning, transferring, and lifting clients. On home visits, supervisors should observe appropriate safety techniques used with clients. They should also observe appropriate use of lifting devices, back supporters, and other appropriate working attire, such as wearing sturdy shoes.

SECONDARY PREVENTION

The injured employee should report the injury immediately and take appropriate actions, including rest, medical follow-up, drug therapy, exercise, heat, or hydrotherapy. On return to work, the employee should gradually work up to full potential and utilize all safety precautions mentioned above.

TERTIARY PREVENTION

For a long-term back injury, seek alternative treatment including transcutaneous electric nerve stimulation (TENS) units, acupressure, acupuncture, biofeedback, surgery, or other treatment modalities offered at reputable pain clinics. If those treatments provide no relief, consider a change of occupation, part-time work, or, as a last resort, disability and the consequences of living on a limited income.

plants. Potential hazards, such as infectious or parasitic diseases, may derive from exposure to contaminated water or to insects. Other vehicles include improper waste or sewage disposal, unsanitary work environments, improper food handling, and unsanitary personal practices.

Workers in every setting have a unique set of potential biological hazards (Levy and Wegman, 1988). Agricultural workers, for instance, are subject to a condition called "farmer's lung" that comes from inhaling fungi-contaminated grain dust. Staphylococcal, Hepatitis B, HIV, and other infectious agents threaten health care workers. Brucellosis (undulant fever) and Q fever from infected cattle are a threat to slaughterhouse workers. Outdoor workers, such as builders, forest rangers, or environmental specialists, face the hazards of insect and animal attack as well as exposure to toxic plants, such as poison oak and ivy.

ERGONOMIC FACTORS

Ergonomic factors include all the interactions between the worker, the demands of the job, the work setting, and the overall environment. **Ergonomics** (sometimes called human engineering) has become a field of study in occupational health concerned with "the design of workplaces, tools, and tasks to match the physiological, anatomical, and psychological characteristics and capabilities of the worker" (Pheasant, 1991; Ross, 1994).

For our purposes, ergonomic factors are the customs, laws, design, and expectations of the work itself. They include all the physiological and psychological demands on the job as well as other **workplace stressors** that can cause anxiety. These can include physical conditions in a work space (called engineering stressors) such as the design of necessary tools, equipment, lighting or ventilation, physical positions workers must assume, motions they must make to do the job, or bad habits associated with carrying out the work, such as improper lifting habits (see Fig. 20.1).

Mexican migrant field workers in some southwestern states as recently as 1984 were required to use short-handled hoes to speed production and maximize crop yield and were required to spend hours stooping over plants in this doubled-up position. This caused serious skeletal and internal injuries, some of which were permanent. Farm workers often suffer from a lack of toileting facilities or drinking water in the fields (The Network News, 1992). Stooping or squatting for hours can

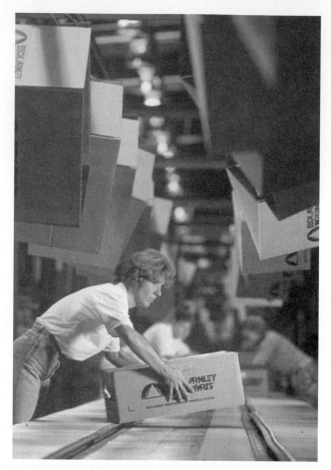

FIGURE 20.1. Repetitive lifting from this position is an ergonomic factor that places this worker at risk.

cause bladder and uterine problems in females. There can be organizational stressors in the company or industry itself involving the chain of command, policies, or procedures. Sometimes an employer's expectations or unrealistic job demands can provoke stress as well (Grant and Brisbin, 1992). In such situations the organization becomes the target of treatment, not the individual (Crawford, 1993). When these factors begin to have an impact on individuals' health, job stress results. Long periods of **job stress**, which is manifested in feelings of anxiety, frustration, and fatigue, can lead to job burnout. **Job burnout** can cause the worker to lose interest in the job; it can also undermine the morale of others and may even be unsafe. Some extreme cases of job burnout result in former employees using violence or sabotage against the company or its employees.

PSYCHOSOCIAL FACTORS

Psychosocial factors include the responses and behaviors that workers exhibit on the job. These behaviors come from the attitudes and values learned from their culture, life experiences, and work-site norms. They are the workers' responses to the work and the work milieu. Similar work conditions can evoke different responses. Within the same work setting some people may seem fatigued, tense, bored, angry, depressed, or agitated while others may seem enthusiastic and energized. Repetitive work may bore some people, while others may see it as an opportunity for reflection. Certain types of work may challenge some but threaten others.

The nature of the work as much as the working conditions can evoke certain responses. Work that is time sensitive or that conflicts with personal values may create tremendous stress for some employees (Gough et al., 1988). Ethical dilemmas, such as selling or promoting a product or service that might be injurious to the public, such as selling unreliable used cars, can cause emotional conflict for individuals. Peer pressure can also add stress, for instance when one employee is forced to agree with the majority, such as during strikes on labor disputes. Unrealistic personal expectations and unattainable aspirations can lead to chronic stress and fatigue and eventual burnout (Veninga and Spradley, 1981). Psychological stress can result from the personal problems such as a terminally ill spouse, a painful divorce or child custody battle, or other family difficulties or crises. These types of personal dilemmas influence the quality and quantity of work produced and in many professions can compromise worker safety if a worker is preoccupied and functioning inadequately.

Obviously, these five factors will vary in intensity and potential for threat to worker health, depending on the individual (see Fig. 20.1) and the work environment. They present a core of critical data for occupational health assessment and planning. Table 20.1 summarizes these five environmental factors.

Historical Perspectives

Over the years, working conditions have improved considerably. Modern occupational health is an outgrowth of the 19th century Industrial Revolution in England. Deplorable work conditions and worker exploitation created a growing public concern and spawned the development of many protective laws. This influence was felt in the United States, which was rapidly becoming an industrialized nation. Between 1890 and 1914, more than 16.5 million immigrants from all over the world poured into the United States. As industrial growth escalated, these new citizens worked in the plants, factories, railroads, and mines, creating a new market for manufactured goods (Parker-Conrad, 1988). Workers, children as well as adults, commonly worked 12- to 14-hour shifts, 7 days a week, under unspeakable conditions of grime, dust, physical hazards, smoke, heat, cold, and noxious fumes. People accepted work-related illnesses and injuries as part of the job and lived shorter lives, frequently dying in their 40s and 50s, with workers in some trades dying in their 30s (Lee, 1978).

No connection was made between work conditions and health. Employers attributed employees' poor health and early deaths to the workers' personal habits on the job or their living conditions at home. Physicians, uneducated in the relationship between work and health, blamed industrial-related diseases, such as silicosis, lead poisoning, and tuberculosis, on other causes.

It was not until the early 1900s that the Public Health Service conducted one of the first scientific studies on occupational hazards by investigating dust conditions in mining, cement manufacturing, and stone cutting. Other studies followed. Lead poisoning was as high as 22% among the pottery workers studied. A 1914 study of garment workers showed a high incidence of tuberculosis related to poor ventilation, overcrowding, and unsanitary work conditions. Other investigations revealed phosphorous poisoning among workers in the match industry (1912), radium poisoning among watchmakers (1920s), and mercury poisoning in those who manufactured felt hats (1930s) (Lee, 1978). The public was awakening to the effect of work conditions on people's health.

The birth of the labor movement increased the demand for healthful and safe working conditions. Workers' compensation laws provided for occupational injury and disease coverage, and other efforts were made to protect workers against the health hazards of the workplace. The health of American workers is better today than it has ever been, but health hazards still exist and new ones continue to develop as technology and environmental influences change. Occupational health must continue to protect and promote worker health and to improve the work environment.

TABLE 20.1. *Factors Influencing Health and Productivity in the Work Environment*

Variable	Physical	Chemical	Biological	Ergonomical	Psychosocial
Definition	Structural elements of workplace	Chemical agents present in work environment	Biological organisms and potential contaminants in work environment	Customs, rules, design, and expectations of the work itself	Workers' values, attitudes, and responses

Selected Types	Radiation
	Noise
	Vibration
	Light
	Temperature
	Space
	Color
	Pressure
	Construction
		Mists
		Vapors
		Gases
		Solids
		Liquids
		Dusts
		Solvents
			Viruses
			Insects
			Molds
			Fungi
			Bacteria
			Animals
			Plants
			Parasites
			Rickettsias
				Design of work space
				Design of job
				Work habits
				Required motions
				Design of tools
				Work standards
				Work flow
					Emotional:
					  Boredom
					  Anger
					  Depression
					Behavioral:
					  Fatigue
					  Tension
					Cultural:
					  Values
					  Norms

Illustrative Potential Hazards	Excessive noise Electromagnetic radiation Excessive ionizing radiation Temperature extremes Excessive vibration Pressure extremes Unsafe objects or structures	Excessive airborne concentrations Topical irritants Toxic absorption through skin Toxic ingestion	Contaminated water or food Improper waste or sewage disposal Unsanitary work environment Improper food handling Insect or animal attack Unsanitary personal practices	Improper lifting Poor motions or positions Improper tools Inadequate space to do work Interruptions Unrealistic work expectations Repetitive motion	Boring work Unchallenging work Time pressure Conflicts with worker values Group dissatisfaction Unrealistic personal expectations Peer pressure Unrealistic employer expectations Personal problems brought to the work environment

Pertinent Legislation

The preceding history shows that public awareness and understanding were necessary before changes could be made to improve working conditions. That understanding is based on continuing study and research.

In 1700, Bernardino Ramazzini, known as the "father of occupational medicine" (Lee, 1978), conducted the earliest systematic study of occupational disease. The Italian physician had the foresight, when attempting a diagnosis, to ask about his patient's occupation. Despite his influence, interest in and information concerning worker health evolved slowly. A few classic studies, such as those mentioned in the previous section, influenced the gradual development of protective legislation. Unfortunately, it took such disastrous events as the Triangle Shirtwaist Factory fire to create additional legislation. That notorious fire, which occurred in New York City in 1911, took the lives of 154 workers, most of whom were young women. Investigations after the incident revealed nonexistent fire escapes and locked exit doors. That tragic event resulted in establishment of the first serious safety laws to protect working people (Morris, 1976). Today a growing body of legislation exists to protect the health and safety of workers.

The following is a list of current laws that employers must follow to meet health and safety codes.

The **Workmen's Compensation Act of 1911** was initially enacted in New Jersey before it became national law in 1948. This law requires employers to carry employee insurance that provides compensation for lost wages and medical and rehabilitative costs associated with work-related disease and injury. Application of the law varies from state to state. All states, however, emphasize early intervention and rehabilitation.

The **Social Security Act of 1935** was enacted to provide financial resources to the "aged, blind, and disabled" as well as state and federal unemployment insurance programs. Amendments to the act in 1965 and 1972 created benefits for high-risk mothers and children and additional benefits for the elderly.

The **Federal Coal Mine Health and Safety Act of 1967** is the only federal program that deals with a specific occupational disease. The act originally established health standards in coal mines and provided medical examinations for actively employed underground coal miners. Through the Social Security Administration, it also provided benefits for black lung (pneumoconiosis) disease. Specifically, it required all exposed workers to have radiographic examinations and made available federal funds to compensate victims and their families. The subsequent Federal Mine Safety and Health Amendments Act of 1977 retains most of the original provisions.

The **Occupational Safety and Health Act of 1970** (Public Law, 91-596) generally provides workers with protection against personal injury and illness resulting from hazardous working conditions. More specifically, its purpose and functions are "to assure safe and healthful working conditions for working men and women by authorizing enforcement of the standards developed under the Act; by assisting and encouraging the States in their efforts to assure safe and healthful working conditions; by providing for research, information, education, and training in the field of occupational safety and health; and for other purposes" (Lee, 1978, p. 80).

The act created two federal agencies. The Occupational Safety and Health Administration (OSHA), housed in the Department of Labor, became its regulatory branch. The National Institute for Occupational Safety and Health (NIOSH), based in the Public Health Service (under the Department of Health and Human Services), is responsible for research.

OSHA's responsibilities include the following (Levy and Wegman, 1988):

Develop and update mandatory occupational safety and health standards.

Monitor and enforce regulations and standards.

Require employers to keep accurate records on work-related injuries, illnesses, and hazardous exposures.

Maintain an occupational safety and health statistics collection and analysis system (collaborating with NIOSH).

Supervise employer and worker education and training to identify and prevent unsafe or unhealthy working conditions (collaborating with NIOSH).

Provide grants to states to assist in compliance with the Act.

NIOSH responsibilities include the following (NIOSH, 1986):

Research on occupational safety and health problems.

Hazard evaluation.

Toxicity determinations.

Work-force development and training.

Industrywide studies of chronic or low-level exposures to hazardous substances.

Research on psychological, motivational, and behavioral factors as they relate to occupational safety and health.

Training of occupational safety and health professionals.

The **Privacy Act of 1974** ensures that only necessary information be collected on individuals by federal agencies. Furthermore, that information, including medical history, education, and financial and employment history, must be maintained to protect the individual's privacy (Lee, 1978).

The **Toxic Substances Control Act of 1976** serves to ensure that chemical substances do not present an "unreasonable risk of injury to health or the environment" (Lee, 1978, p. 83). The act requires that certain chemical substances and mixtures be tested and their use restricted. It is also concerned with the manufacture, processing, commercial distribution, and disposal of such substances (see Figure 20.2). The Environmental Protection Agency enforces the Act.

The **Hazard Communication Act of 1986**, known as the worker Right-to-Know legislation, ensures that workers are adequately educated regarding hazards in their places of work through a hazards communication program. This is especially important since all hazards and toxic substances cannot be removed from workplaces because of the nature of the product being developed or service provided by a company. Figure 20.2 depicts the conditions under which some workers are employed. This standard was extended in 1988 to

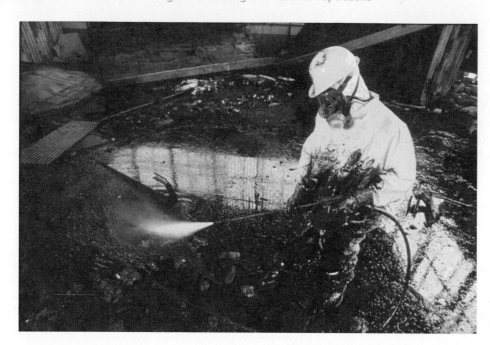

FIGURE 20.2. Disposal of toxic substances is mandated by the Toxic Substance Control Act of 1976.

all employers covered by OSHA. One of the most frequently cited OSHA violations has been noncompliance with this standard.

The **Americans with Disabilities Act (ADA)** was passed by Congress in 1990 as a civil rights law to prevent discrimination against qualified workers with disabilities. For employers with 25 or more employees, the law went into effect in 1992. For those employers with 15 to 24 employees, it went into effect in 1994 (McKenna, 1994). A **disabled person** is someone with a physical or mental impairment that substantially limits an aspect or aspects of daily living and work activity. Employees must identify themselves as disabled. The employer and employee then begin a process of defining the essential characteristics of the job and the accommodations that need to be made to allow the employee to work. This is usually done through a job description or a collective-bargaining contract.

The **OSHA Blood-borne Pathogens Standard** was enacted in 1992. Guidelines published since the early 1970s addressed infection-control compliance for the protection of health care workers against the transmission of blood-borne diseases. This new standard requires employers to do two things: offer the hepatitis B vaccine free of charge to all employees and practice general infection control, as recommended by the Centers for Disease Control and Prevention (CDC). The **uni-versal precautions** recommended by the CDC instruct health care workers to consider any direct contact with blood or body fluids as potentially infectious and provide guidelines on ways of handling such materials. This requires employers to provide such personal protective equipment as gloves, masks, gowns, and eye protectors, and to establish education, training, and some form of record keeping.

Annual compliance costs to employers have exceeded $800 million, and noncompliance with this new standard puts employers at risk of costly citations (Roup, 1993). However, the responsibility for adhering to universal precautions remains literally in the hands of the employees. With HIV infection—the most significant public health crisis of this century—compliance with standards for blood-borne pathogens becomes the responsibility of every health care employer and employee.

The **Family and Medical Leave Act of 1993** was enacted as a labor standards act. It requires employers of 50 or more people to provide unpaid leave of up to 12 weeks to their employees to care for family members with serious health conditions, their own serious medical condition, or newborn or newly adopted children. The employer must also continue providing medical benefits and ensure that the employee can return to the same or comparable job (McKenna, 1994).

Health Problems of the Working Population

As previously noted, the working population comprises adults whose health determines the productivity and well-being of each community as well as the nation as a whole. For all American adults, aged 25 to 64, the major causes of death are accidents, cancer, heart disease, suicide, and HIV (*U.S. Statistical Abstracts, 1994*). Table 20.2 shows the leading causes of death for adults in the United States.

Chronic disease poses a significant threat to the health of American adults (U.S. Bureau of the Census, 1993). Cancer is the major chronic illness in the U.S. It affects more people over the age of 15 than any other disease and remains the leading cause of death for these people. Major preventable risk factors that contribute to cancer include smoking, alcohol abuse, diet, exposure to radiation and sunlight, water and air pollution (U.S. DHHS, 1991). There is a proven link between exposure to cigarette smoke and lung cancer, and until legislation curtailed it, many workers were exposed to secondhand smoke in the workplace.

Chemicals and other potential cancer-causing materials are produced and used every year. In addition, known carcinogens, such as asbestos and vinyl chloride, continue to threaten the health of workers who, without adequate protection, develop malignancies not commonly found in the general population. In fact Mesothelioma, a lung cancer related to asbestos exposure, has been documented among people whose only known exposure was from the contaminants carried home on the shoes and clothing of a worker (Rosner and Markowitz, 1991). Because asbestos was once a common construction material, it is being removed from older buildings to protect people from asbestos exposure. Asbestos-removal experts are at risk of exposure and therefore must follow elaborate procedures to protect themselves. It has been estimated that up to 20% of all cancer deaths may result from occupational hazards (U.S. DHHS, 1991).

More than one-fourth of all deaths of adults aged 25 to 64 are due to cardiovascular diseases, primarily coronary artery disease and cerebral vascular accidents (CVAs). Heart disease has been the leading cause of death for men older than 40. Women, on the other hand, prior to menopause have only one-third the heart-disease rate of men. After menopause, however, the incidence among women increases. But men still have twice the incidence rate up to age 75. By age 85 the rates are nearly the same (U.S. Statistical Abstracts, 1994).

Heart disease is also the largest contributor to permanent disability claims for workers younger than 65 and accounts for more days of hospitalization than any other single disorder. It is the principal cause of limited activity for some 5 million to 6 million Americans under age 65 (U.S. Statistical Abstracts, 1994).

CVAs, in addition to being the fourth-leading cause of death among 25 to 64 year olds (3.5% of the total mortality rate for 25 to 64 year olds), leave many adults with paralysis as well as speech and memory impairments. Between 400,000 and 500,000 Americans suffer nonfatal strokes each year. African Americans between

TABLE 20.2. *Leading Causes of Death for American Adults Aged 15 to over 65 Years*

Age 15–24	25–44	45–64	65 and over
Accidents (Motor Vehicle)	Accidents (Motor Vehicle)	Cancer	Heart Disease
Homicide and Legal Intervention	Cancer	Heart Disease	Cancer
Suicide	HIV	CVA	CVA
Cancer	Heart Disease	Accidents	COPD
Heart Disease	Homicide and Legal Intervention	COPD	Pneumonia and Flu
HIV	Suicide	Chronic Liver Disease	Diabetes
		Diabetes	Accidents

Source: U.S. Bureau of the Census. (1994). *Statistical Abstract of the United States, 1994*. (114th ed.). Washington, D.C.: U.S. Government Printing Office.

the ages of 25 and 64 are almost twice as susceptible to stroke as whites, largely because of the high incidence of hypertension among the black population. In the southeastern United States (the "Stroke Belt") stroke death rates for both blacks and whites are higher than in any other part of the country (U.S. DHHS, 1991).

Risk factors contributing to coronary artery disease can be separated into three categories: personal, hereditary, and environmental. Personal risk factors include gender, age, race, cholesterol level (specifically low-density lipoprotein to high-density lipoprotein ratio), blood pressure, and cigarette smoking. The most preventable of these include cholesterol, high blood pressure, and cigarette smoking (Figure 20.3). Heredity obviously cannot be changed. The understanding of environmental risk factors, especially as they relate to occupational exposures, is currently quite limited (Levy and Wegman, 1988). The likelihood of heart disease or CVA multiplies with the increasing number of risk factors present.

Changes in society and changes that affect health and well-being are occurring in large enough numbers to be reflected in the mortality statistics. Violence is taking the lives of many people in the United States. Violence against children and spouses occurs in families. The increase of crimes that did not exist a decade ago, such as drive-by shootings and car jackings, puts everyone at risk. Sexually active teens and young adults who do not practice safe sex are exposing themselves and their unborn children to HIV and other sexually transmitted diseases. By 1994 the leading cause of death among *all* Americans between the ages of 25 and 44 was acquired immune deficiency syndrome (AIDS). (AIDS has been the leading cause of death for men between 25 and 44 since 1992.) The victims of HIV are getting younger each year, and the incidence of HIV among females is also increasing (CDC, 1995).

Three other problems that threaten the health of American adults, and thus that of the working population, are accidents, alcohol abuse, and mental illness. Each has taken a tremendous toll in lives lost and on health and productivity. The National Health Promotion and Disease Prevention Objectives, outlined in Healthy People 2000 states a compelling case for the preventability of these problems (U.S. DHHS, 1991).

Work-Related Health Problems

What are the health problems of the working population specifically? As previously mentioned, Americans are exposed to numerous safety and health hazards in the workplace. The following have been identified as the ten leading work-related health problems (Millar, 1988; NIOSH, 1989):

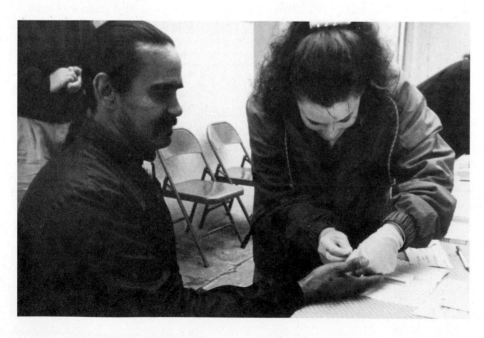

FIGURE 20.3. This man is participating in a cholesterol-screening program sponsored by community health nurses at a health fair. The information he will receive will assist him in planning for improving his own health care practices.

1. Occupational lung disease
2. Musculoskeletal injuries
3. Occupational cancer
4. Severe occupational traumatic injuries
5. Cardiovascular disease
6. Reproductive problems
7. Neurotoxic illness
8. Noise-induced hearing loss
9. Dermatological problems
10. Psychological disorders

It is estimated that 17 million work-related injuries or illnesses and 99,000 work-related deaths occur in the United States each year (U.S. Statistical Abstracts, 1994). Although the incidence of some of these injuries and diseases will diminish through preventive efforts, light on the nature, causes, and linkages of occupational diseases, contributing to a likely increase in their reporting.

Collecting data on occupational diseases has been difficult because the lag time is so great between exposure and onset of the disease and actual clinical evidence. Silicosis, for example, takes 15 years to develop. Some cases of mesothelioma have not become evident until 25 years after the worker was last exposed to asbestos (Rosner and Markowitz, 1991). The lag time for solid tumors is at least 10 to 20 years and possibly as long as 50 years (Levy and Wegman, 1988). Lung disease in workers occurs gradually over time. Most often exposures do not result in acute symptoms, and once the symptoms do occur, little can be done. It is for this reason that respiratory disease prevention is so important. Many workers who have changed jobs or retired are only now discovering disease that may be connected to previous employment. Documenting this connection poses problems.

Nonetheless, more sophisticated epidemiological methods and an improved database are enabling public health and industrial researchers to demonstrate linkages and make more accurate predictions. They have estimated, for instance, that of the 6000 current and past uranium workers, approximately 600 to 1100 will die of lung cancer in about 20 years because of radiation exposure (Ball, 1993). In two mines in Utah and Arizona at which the exposure to radon was the highest, 50% of the uranium miners died from lung cancer, as of 1981 (Ringholz, 1989). Until the 1960s, when safety regulations were enforced and many mines were closed, the coal miners in Appalachia worked in deep tunnels, constantly exposed to coal dust. If they survived the slag falls, the explosions, the fires, and the gases, the workers were often left crippled for life with black lung disease (or pneumoconiosis, an emphysema-like disease with progressive breathlessness and racking cough).

Over the years, black lung has killed and disabled an estimated 365,000 miners in the United States (Frazier and Brown, 1992). More than 12% of active coal miners have radiographic evidence of pneumoconiosis (Millar, 1988). Workers exposed to heavy metals, such as lead, mercury, and arsenic, will likely develop related diseases. Brown lung partially disables 15% to 25% of the active and retired cotton mill workers (Botsch, 1993).

Researchers have also demonstrated the relationship between cotton mill dust and byssinosis, a lung disease formerly thought not to exist in the United States. Epidemiologists are studying the connection between skin diseases and materials used on the job, a problem of considerable magnitude since dermatological problems are among the most common occupational diseases. It is estimated that 15 million workers are exposed to noise levels that can cause impaired hearing, and more than 8 million workers in the United States have some degree of noise-induced hearing loss (Harrison, 1989). As knowledge of occupational illnesses increases, nurses will be better equipped to design more effective protective and preventive measures.

A final set of health problems affecting workers encompasses all the ergonomic and psychological stresses that workers experience on the job or bring to the job from their personal lives. With increasing technology and changing work environments, new concerns over such things as lack of natural light and air, poor lighting, loud noise, isolation, and temperature extremes have surfaced (Pheasant, 1991). Also, an increasing amount of research is being devoted to the study of video display terminal exposure, which involves the visual problems associated with computer use and musculoskeletal problems from inappropriate positioning at workstations (Centers for Disease Control, 1988; Pheasant, 1991).

There is some evidence that up to 30% of absenteeism is due to emotional disturbances. Pressures at work to increase productivity, or a physically stressful work environment (for example, excessive noise, heat, or vibration) can send a worker home to take out his or her frustrations through domestic violence or alcohol and drug abuse. Personal problems, such as those dealing with finances or relationships, can, on the other hand, affect the worker's job performance. Either source of stress creates a vicious cycle perpetuating and escalating the problems in both settings with the potential for unsafe practices at work and harmful behavior at home.

A new concern that is all too frequently reported in the newspapers, is violence in the workplace stemming from "disgruntled employee syndrome," or from interpersonal relationship problems that escalate into violent acts against an employed spouse or significant other. Clearly workers' mental health influences their safety, their productivity, their levels of health, and the safety of others.

One societal change that is affecting the health and safety of adults is the violence in America that also affects the worker. Homicide is the second-leading cause of death at work. Workers in retail establishments, taxi drivers, and people working at night are the most vulnerable when robbery is the motive. The Labor department reported 6271 job-related deaths in 1993 (McClain, 1994). Twenty percent of those deaths were highway accidents (truck drivers, train engineers, etc.), however 17% were homicides.

Occupational Health Programs

Because the working population is primarily composed of healthy adults, the goal of occupational health is to maintain that healthy, productive work force by providing a safe and healthy work environment and promoting healthy personal health behavior. Thus, oc-

cupational health programs encompass the entire spectrum of the health care, including the practice of disease prevention, health protection, and health promotion (Maciag, 1993). Table 20.3 lists these priorities.

Occupational health programs have grown tremendously since World War II. Many manufacturing plants, service organizations, and commercial establishments, including department stores, have instituted some kind of health program for employees. Some programs still concentrate on providing emergency care, but most are beginning to recognize the importance of prevention and health promotion. For example, in 1981 the Adolph Coors Company opened the nation's first comprehensive wellness facility. Mesa Petroleum estimates an annual savings of $1.6 million in health care costs for its 650 employees as a result of its wellness program. Other major companies, such as General Electric Aircraft, Tenneco, AT&T Communications, and Johnson & Johnson have lowered absenteeism and health care costs by initiating health promotion programs (Upton, 1992).

In the mid-1980s, General Mills, Inc., instituted a health promotion program called the "TriHealthalon Program." This program incorporates a multidisciplinary approach to healthy lifestyles through education that emphasizes employee awareness and participation. After 2 years in the program participants improved their lifestyles: 5% stopped smoking, 37% began using seatbelts, and 23% exercised three times a week (Wood,

TABLE 20.3. *Practice Priorities in Occupational Health*

Goal and Function	Prevention	Protection	Promotion
Goal	Elimination of hazardous substance or condition	Avoidance of injury or illness of high-risk workers	Attainment of an optimal level of personal health
Function	Job analysis Preplacement exams Hazard communication Materials handling and training Industrial hygiene sampling Health surveillance Safety measures on equipment Safer work procedures Walk-through evaluations	Personal safety measures: Hard hats Ear muffs or plugs Safety glasses Respirators Foot protection Skin barrier creams Legislation and regulation: OSHA standards Employees right-to-know laws	Wellness: Physical fitness Smoking cesation Nutritional awareness Stress management Screening: Health risk appraisal Cancer detection Diabetes and hypertension screening Health policy formulation: Smoking Alcohol Cafeteria meal planning

Olmstead, and Craig, 1989). In 1991, after the program had been in practice for several years, General Mills built a 5300 square foot TriHealthalon Fitness Center at its corporate headquarters and several General Mills plants also have fitness centers.

The variety of work in the United States, as well as the number and type of workers employed, creates a wide range of potential hazards and the need for various on-site health programs. For example, construction and mine workers are a high-risk group for certain types of injuries and illnesses. These workers require an aggressive surveillance program that focuses on prevention and personal protection. In contrast, professionals, such as lawyers and accountants, are generally at low risk for encountering hazardous physical conditions at work, but may experience psychological stress and therefore may benefit from a health promotion program that emphasizes stress management and physical fitness.

In order to determine the priorities for intervention and the appropriate health goals and objectives for an aggregate of workers, it is essential that an environmental and workers' assessment be conducted. Knowledge of workers' job classifications, the types of materials they handle and are exposed to will provide clues to potential hazardous substances and working conditions. This information, together with data on the characteristics of the aggregate in terms of age, gender, race, and existing health conditions, should be compiled. In addition, workers' compensation claims and occupational safety and health reports should be examined to identify subpopulations at risk for occupational illness and injury (Ashford, et al., 1990; Kavianian and Wentz, 1990; Maciag, 1993).

DISEASE PREVENTION PROGRAMS

The practice of making prevention a priority holds primary importance in occupational health because work-related injuries and illnesses are frequently irreversible. Limb loss or mesothelioma from asbestos exposure are conditions for which there are no cures. Interventions, therefore, are aimed at eliminating the hazards by such methods as redesigning the equipment to provide safeguards and to substitute materials that are as effective but less toxic. The USDHHS publication, *Healthy People 2000*, in an effort to promote health and disease-prevention objectives in the area of occupational health and safety, points out that "the reduction of leading work-related injuries and illnesses and the prevention of new problems require that accrediting bodies of all scientific disciplines understand the role of their professions in recognizing or preventing occupational and environmental problems. Progress in this area also depends greatly on improvements in surveillance to identify high-risk groups and to assist in developing appropriate prevention strategies" (U.S. DHHS, 1991. p. 297).

Once occupational hazards are defined, they can be controlled. Safer materials can be substituted; manufacturing processes can be changed; hazardous materials can be isolated; exhaust methods and other engineering techniques can be used to control the source; special clothing and other protective devices can be used (Figure 20.2); and efforts must be made to educate and motivate employees and employers to comply with safety procedures that focus on prevention (Rossignol, 1991).

HEALTH PROTECTION PROGRAMS

Making protection a priority becomes essential when hazardous exposures cannot be eliminated. Construction workers, for example, wear hard hats and steel-toed safety shoes to protect themselves from falling objects. Health care workers who may be exposed to bodily fluids wear gloves, gowns, masks, and/or eye protectors. The protection of workers is frequently achieved through legislation and regulation. The Occupational Safety and Health Act of 1970 has provided the impetus for worker protection. More recently, employee right-to-know legislation has been passed, focusing on training of employees who are working with potentially hazardous agents, use of international symbols (electrical hazard is red on white background, biohazard is black on red background, radiation hazard is black on yellow background), Material Safety Data Sheets (MSDS), and OSHA's new standard regarding exposure to blood-borne pathogens has made health care delivery safer for employees. The enforcement of such regulations will continue to be the key intervention for ensuring that workers are adequately protected on their jobs.

Until 1982, 60% of the nation's work sites had no occupational health and safety staff or consultants (U.S. DHHS, 1991). Now, occupational safety programs are available in most industries, especially those employing larger numbers of workers. These programs include plant surveillance, safety-violation reporting, and worker safety education. All have the goal of protecting the employee. See Issues in Community Health Nursing display.

Issues in Community Health Nursing
THE AGING EMPLOYEE

The health care delivery system at work will need to change by early into the 21st century. Age 55 will be considered young in the workplace, and a new definition of middle age may emerge (Hart and Moore, 1992). The entire population is expected to grow 33% in the next 50 years. For those older than 55, however, the group is expected to grow by 113% (Miller, 1989). Occupational health nurses will need to deal with the age-related health problems of older adults in the work force, such as arthritis, hypertension, cardiovascular disease, hearing impairments, diabetes mellitus, and depression. The focus of care will be on reducing the decline in the worker's health status and consequently work productivity.

Another issue is the increasing responsibilities of many older workers in rearing grandchildren. Statistics indicate that more grandparents are assuming the parenting role for grandchildren because of their own children's inability to parent. That inability may be because they are teenagers themselves, they are single parents, both parents are working, they are substance abusers, they have mental health problems, or they have died as a result of AIDS.

That trend seems to span all ethnic, racial, and socioeconomic groups. This new role adds additional stress for the older employee. Health promotion programs will need to focus on stress management, early cancer detection, cholesterol screening, the benefits of exercise, and issues such as purpose in life, loss, co-dependency, coping techniques, and retirement planning (Campanelli, 1990).

support (Upton, 1992). Employee Assistance Programs are offered in federal and state governmental agencies and many private industries. These programs are cooperatively sponsored by employers and bargaining agencies. The intent is to promote the mental health of the employee by providing an outlet for employee concerns.

Of significance for community health is that health promotion activities in the workplace can involve long-term interventions that will permit the use of various educational and motivational strategies as well as a systematic plan for monitoring and evaluating the programs. The work environment itself can serve as a model for a healthy community. Such health policies as creating a smoke-free environment, offering low-fat meals in the company cafeteria, discouraging alcohol abuse, and encouraging seat-belt use will establish health norms for company personnel. Many of these healthy behaviors can also have a positive impact on employees' homes and families (Wood, Olmstead, and Craig, 1989).

Typical health promotion programs include exercise, weight loss, smoking cessation, and nutrition education. There is growing evidence that wellness efforts are effective. Some research indicates that, as a result of wellness promotion, employees have increased self-esteem, improved job performance and job satisfaction, decreased absenteeism, and used company health services less frequently (Christenson et al., 1988; Grant and Brisbin, 1992; Upton, 1992; Wood, Olmstead, and Craig, 1989). Health promotion programs in the workplace have the potential to provide a significant contribution to adult health as well as to research and development in this new arena of wellness. Cost and production incentives increase employers' acceptance of methods that enhance employee wellness. More research is needed to demonstrate the correlation between healthy employees and increased productivity on the job. Health promotion will continue to be a vital area of emphasis for the working community as the nation enters the 21st century.

HEALTH PROMOTION PROGRAMS

The practice of making health promotion a priority has appropriately received much attention and activity in the workplace over the past decade (Christenson et al., 1988; Upton, 1992; Wood, Olmstead, and Craig, 1989). The workplace is ideal for conducting health promotion efforts for two important reasons: (1) the majority of the healthy population can be reached at work and (2) employers view wellness programs as legitimate, worthwhile employee benefits to promote and

Nonoccupational Health Services

Although employers are not presently required to provide treatment for **nonoccupational injuries and illnesses**—that is, injury and illness not incurred at work—many companies do provide such services. One reason is that it is difficult to determine where such health problems as muscle strain, influenza, and minor rashes, are acquired. Therefore it is simpler to provide care for the problem regardless of its source. The on-site treatment of minor acute injury and illness as well as employee counseling depends on the philosophy of the company, the employment of an occupational health nurse (OHN), and the company's prior experience with offering these services as an employee benefit.

From the nurse's perspective, the advantages of offering nonoccupational health services are the following:

1. The OHN develops rapport with employees and can detect health problems early.
2. Loss of employee productivity is minimized when treatment is given on site.
3. The OHN, through triage, can decide which cases require medical attention and which can be managed by the nurse.
4. The OHN can provide needed, ongoing, personal health education and counseling in the context of a more holistic view of the worker.
5. On-site chronic disease management, such as hypertension monitoring, increases compliance, thereby saving costs of physician visits and complications associated with noncompliance.
6. The OHN provides employees with personal contact—a valued commodity in our high-technology work environments.

A number of OHNs have expressed concern that spending too much time on nonoccupational illnesses could keep them from pursuing an aggressive occupational health surveillance program. As OHNs learn more about environmental factors that threaten workers' health, they will likely spend less time with illness management and move more aggressively toward primary prevention, protection, and health promotion efforts. The direction of health care programs in the future is covered later in this chapter. See Research in Community Health Nursing display.

The Role of the Occupational Health Nurse

Community health nurses have a long history of involvement in occupational health. In 1895, the Vermont Marble Company hired the first industrial nurse in the United States to care for its employees and their fami-

Research in Community Health Nursing
TIPS FOR CONDUCTING SUCCESSFUL RESEARCH IN THE WORKPLACE

Lusk, S. L. and Kerr, M. J. (1994) Conducting work-site research: Methodological issues and suggested approaches. *AAOHN Journal*, 42(4): 177–181.

■ Labor relations play a large part in getting into the workplace.
■ If the topic being researched is useful to management, they may be more likely to be supportive of the researcher. Keep in mind that management generally does not like controversial topics.
■ If there is loss of productivity time, management will be less interested in participation.
■ Random sampling is nearly impossible to obtain in the workplace.
■ It's difficult for assembly line workers to participate in studies, however, white-collar workers are most easily recruited because they can be approached at their desks. Personal contact is important
■ Incentives of valuable prizes promotes participation.
■ Good explanations are needed in order to avoid reluctance in signing an informed-consent form because of unfamiliarity with the research process.
■ Data collectors need to become familiar with the safety practices used at a plant, including the use of protective equipment and the recognition of various warning sirens.
■ In order to deal with various reading levels of workers and questions about the research, multiple data collectors should be available to assist individual workers.
■ The time and money needed for incentives and multiple data collectors need to be considered when financing the research. Some grants do not cover the cost of incentives.

lies. At the time, it was an unusual demonstration of interest in employee welfare. The nursing service, which consisted mostly of home visiting and care of the sick, was free to employees and their families. Gradually that role changed. World War II showed a marked increase in employment of industrial public health nurses who practiced illness prevention and health education among employees at work.

In addition to emergency care and nursing of ill employees, the activities of many industrial nurses involved safety education, hygiene, nutrition, and improvement of working conditions. Yet a significantly high number of industrial injuries and sick employees kept many nurses too busy to do anything but care for the ill. They might see more than 75 patients a day in the plant dispensary, where they provided first aid and medications (Brown, 1988; Kalisch and Kalisch, 1978; Parker-Conrad, 1988). Employee health programs have improved as socioeconomic and political pressures have created improved safety and health standards for the work environment. Similarly, these developments have changed and expanded the nurse's role.

An occupational health nurse designed a hearing conservation training program for a company in which employees were exposed to excessive noise. Employee training and education was an essential part of the program that also included the use of hearing protectors. After 3 years, the hearing conservation program was examined for effectiveness. The goals of the program had been achieved: (1) noise-induced hearing loss was prevented, (2) speech interference complaints were minimized, (3) governmental noise regulations were complied with, and (4) the company workers' compensation costs were under control (Harrison, 1989). Hearing loss is usually gradual and takes years to occur; however, the short-term evaluation of this program was encouraging.

SPECIAL SKILLS AND DEMANDS

The nurse's role in occupational health, as previously mentioned, has traditionally focused on illness and injury care. That directly resulted from the knowledge and skills obtained in basic nursing education. During the last decade a number of nursing education programs (primarily on the graduate level) have developed a specialty focus in occupational health. In addition, many continuing-education programs provide OHNs with updated information and skill training for identifying and assisting in the management of the physical, chemical, biological, ergonomic, and psychosocial factors in the work environment that can affect worker health and safety. As a result, the OHN's role is not universal; it is dependent on the type and philosophy of the company, type and number of workers, the health professionals involved, exposures and potential hazards in the work environment, and the knowledge and skills of the nurse.

Nurses who select the field of occupational health and safety will encounter significantly different experiences than those found in an acute-care setting (Bey et al., 1988; Maciag, 1993). In order to make the adjustment, the nurse should be aware of the factors that make occupational health unique (American Association of Occupational Health Nurses, 1988; Rogers, 1994).

That setting, unlike hospitals or ambulatory care centers, is a nonhealth-care institution in which production or service (not health care) is the primary goal of the organization. The OHN participates in the organization's goals through activities that will contribute to a productive work force.

An OHN in the organization is in a **staff position**, taking on the role of a consultant, educator, or role model in the workplace, but one who has no supervisory responsibilities or power to hire or fire workers. The nurse is generally responsible for the management of the occupational health unit, serving the needs of **line position** employees (workers who supervise or are supervised by others and have a hierarchical relationship with those who have hiring and firing responsibilities) and as health consultant to line management personnel. Therefore, the power to effect change is not within the position of authority but in the OHN's expertise.

The OHN, especially in many smaller organizations, may be the only nurse in the company. As a result, such OHNs have no on-site consultation and direction that is needed for comfortable, competent, and independent decision making. Their isolation can also lead to job stress, which can be significant for many occupational health nurses. The types of job stress OHNs experience fall into five major categories (Crawford, 1993):

1. intrinsic job factors, such as role conflict, role ambiguity, work overload, and insufficient control;
2. organizational structure, such as red tape, politics, and rigid policies;
3. reward systems, such as inequitable rewards and faulty or infrequent feedback;
4. human resource systems that offer limited career opportunities and continuing education;
5. leadership that has the potential to create poor relationships and a lack of respect.

OHNs need to apply strategies to reduce job stress and potential job burnout by modeling health affirming choices, networking with other nurses and professional organizations in the community, and setting appropriate occupational health standards. "Because occupational health nurses promote stress reduction in worker populations, modeling these behaviors is important to enhance the credibility of those promoting such strategies" (Crawford, 1993).

The client base served in occupational health is a well population with whom long-term contact is possible. OHNs therefore have the chance to know their clients well and have opportunities to work with them through various stages of personal as well as health service–related incidents. Such continuity of health care can challenge OHNs to utilize all the community health nursing model interventions—education, engineering, and enforcement—described in Chapter 4.

Finally, the practice focus is oriented to the aggregate; the nurse serves a worker population. Environmental factors significantly influence the health and safety of workers. Therefore, OHNs need to constantly monitor the work environment and assess the health needs of the entire worker population in order to identify those at risk, such as workers in hazardous lines of work (Ross, 1994) or older workers (Hart and Moore, 1992), and develop prevention, promotion, and protection programs. Bachelor-degree educated nurses who have community health experience, an aggregate focus, excellent assessment skills, and strong managerial skills are the best prepared to meet the needs of this population. See World Watch display.

COMMUNITY-BASED OCCUPATIONAL HEALTH NURSING

Agencies external to business and industry also provide occupational health nursing services. Historically, public health nurses from visiting-nurse associations made home visits to sick employees and their families. In subsequent years, public health agencies provided part-time nursing services to small companies. These services included supervising the work environment, conducting health examinations, keeping records, teaching about and counseling on health issues, providing first aid, giving immunizations, and referring workers to community resources. More recently, community health nursing services have offered health screening and health promotion programs (American Association of Occupational Health Nurses, 1988). Furthermore, OHN consultants based in state departments of health provide consultation and continuing education programs to nurses employed in occupational health settings.

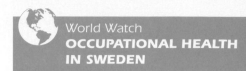

World Watch
OCCUPATIONAL HEALTH IN SWEDEN

Menckel, E. (1992). Occupational health nurses and accident prevention: An inventory of activities in one industrial sector in Sweden. *AAOHN Journal, 40*(10): 477–483.

Sweden has had nurses at major companies and other workplaces since the 1700s. As industrialization accelerated during the 20th century, increasing numbers of nurses were employed in industries. More than 2600 nurses work at approximately 900 occupational health service (OHS) units. More than 80% of the employees in Sweden are covered by OHS. After joining OHS, the nurses attend a training course for 10 weeks at the National Institute of Occupational Health where 200 occupational health nurses are trained each year. After analyses of the work of occupational health nurses in the 1950s and 1960s, the Swedish government concluded that the nurses' work should be preventative—that is, they should provide medical checks, work-place visits, and instruction and information on health matters. In 1991 a government bill placed even greater emphasis on primary prevention.

Each occupational health nurse in Sweden serves many companies. For example, one nurse serves 26 companies with five or more employees in a slaughterhouse and meatpacking OHS unit. The nurses report spending more time providing treatment after an accident than they did in primary prevention. As with occupational health nurses in the United States, Swedish nurses report they lack the time to focus on preventative work.

Hospital-based occupational health programs, large medical–industrial health clinics, and insurance companies also provide occupational health nursing services. These services may be in the form of direct care (rehabilitation of an injured worker) or indirect care (consultation on implementing regulations regarding record keeping or compiling health statistics).

A continuing unmet need is attending to the health of workers in smaller companies. These companies have more hazards because equipment and controls are often inadequate. They seldom, if ever, have a health professional on site, neither has the community provided health services that would meet their needs. Attempts have been made by some communities, but no sustained efforts exist. Community health nurses are in a position to accept this challenge and develop a system that will ensure ongoing service to this high-risk population.

FUTURE TRENDS

A broad goal for occupational health is to promote and maintain the highest level of physical, social, and emotional health for all workers (American Association of Occupational Health Nurses, 1988; Ross, 1994). In practice, this goal is only beginning to be realized in selected instances. Nevertheless, it is a worthy and, more important, an essential objective in the realization of an energized and productive working community. However, the rapid and fundamental changes in U.S. businesses in the 1990s have added three critical issues that affect the practice of occupational health nursing: (1) increasing worldwide competition that requires business to remain competitive by reducing costs; (2) increasing technological hazards that require sophisticated approaches as well as the knowledge of toxicology, epidemiology, ergonomics, and public health principles; and (3) the rising health care costs that are growing at faster rates than most company profits (12% increase per year) (Maciag, 1993).

In a study of 173 *Fortune* 500 companies (Lusk, 1990), corporate executives were asked to rank the most common current occupational health nursing activities and also identify those responsibilities that will be most needed in the future. The results indicated that current OHN practices would need to change to meet future needs with the focus moving away from one-on-one health services to a new OHN role involving broader business and research skills.

Current OHN activities:

1. Supervising care for emergencies and minor illnesses.
2. Counseling employees about health risks.
3. Following up with employees' workers' compensation claims.
4. Performing periodic health assessments.
5. Evaluating the health status of employees returning to work.

Future OHN activities:

1. Analyzing trends (health promotion, risk reduction, and health expenditures).
2. Developing programs suited to corporate needs.
3. Recommending more efficient and cost effective in-house health services.
4. Determining cost-effective alternatives to health programs and services.
5. Collaborating with others to identify problems and propose solutions.

For the remainder of the 1990s and into the 21st century, occupational health nurses and management will share a common purpose: developing a healthy, productive, and profitable company (Maciag, 1993). A healthy company consists of healthy and productive employees, and healthy employees mean lower health care costs. Lower costs result in an increased competitive edge and higher profits. Higher profits can make more resources available to support more programs and to improve employee health.

Members of the Multidisciplinary Occupational Health Team

Today the two professionals who generally provide on-site occupational health services are the occupational health nurse (OHN) and the safety engineer. Other members of the interdisciplinary team may include an industrial hygienist, epidemiologist, toxicologist, and occupational physician (U.S. DHHS, 1991). However, only large corporations usually employ these specialists or they provide only selected part-time services on a contractual basis. Therefore, the position of occupational health nurse in a large company or the community health nurse who serves smaller companies is the cornerstone of occupational health.

Collaboration may take time but will be worth the investment. The OHN must gain the respect and trust of management and establish open communication in order to influence company policies regarding the nature and scope of health programs.

Depending on the size of the company and its products or services, the OHN may also collaborate with any or all of the following people: insurance carriers, the union representatives, employee-assistance counselors, industrial hygienists, safety engineers, company and/or outside lawyers, toxicologists, and human resources personnel. Any comprehensive assessment of employee health and safety problems, as well as any health promotion program, requires cooperation and assistance from many individuals working in various departments within the organization.

Finally, the occupational health team is not complete without the workers themselves. Employees can help identify problems and needs and contribute to decision making about health programs. Their cooperation in implementing and evaluating programs is essential for an effective health protection and promotion effort.

The OHN will particularly need skills in effective communication, leadership, change management, research, business acumen, and assertiveness. These tools will be crucial for effectively interpreting the OHN's role and promoting ideas. The goal is to establish positive working relationships with the other team members, on whom success of programs depend.

Nurses involved in occupational health have a unique opportunity to help shape the health profile of the working population. The degree of that influence depends on how the nurse defines the OHN role. Also, the nurse must be able to overcome the many obstacles found in the occupational setting, including restrictive company policy, misunderstanding of the nurse's role, and lack of time for innovative program development. The nurse's role in occupational health, therefore, varies considerably. It ranges from only providing emergency care for on-the-job injuries or illness to establishing comprehensive policies and programs covering health promotion, accident and disease prevention, and innovative care for disease and disability (Maciag, 1993).

CASE STUDY

VICTOR RAMOS

Victor Ramos is a full-time OHN at Allied Electronics, a company that manufactures and sells electronic components and equipment. Allied's 750 employees are scattered throughout its sprawling 5-acre plant. At present, Allied's health program consists of several components. Health services, which Victor runs, provides emergency care for employees who are injured or become ill while at work. A private physician group in town provides standing orders for the nurse to use in emergencies and in caring for sick employees. The safety division's plant safety engineer regularly checks for existing or potential hazards at Allied.

Allied pays for a large percentage of employee health care through its health benefits program, which is precisely why Allied has hired Victor. Health insurance premiums per employee have skyrocketed, and managers are looking for alternative solutions to lower health provision costs. They would like Victor to develop an approach to employee health that would lower health care costs.

Victor's usual nursing activities include history taking, conducting partial and complete physical examinations, ordering laboratory diagnostics, and administering emergency care. He refers many employees for further treatment and follow-up care. Keeping health records is an expected part of his job, but it can be largely delegated to clerical help. He helps conduct health education and health counseling sessions for groups as well as for individual employees. Health assessment, screening, and monitoring are also important aspects of his job.

In order to keep a proper perspective on his goals and also to begin developing a more innovative approach to meeting employees' health needs (the reason he was hired),

he does some strategic planning. He reviews Allied's current expectations and long-range goals and develops specific objectives that fit the needs of Allied Electronics and its workers. Victor has also developed a time line for the activities to meet those objectives.

Meeting most of the individual and group needs of employees can be accomplished by scheduling health service hours, classes, and counseling sessions. Victor plans time to visit departments and to observe and interview selected personnel as part of his health assessment process.

He is aware of the relationship between the health of the employees (the population group) and the health of Allied Electronics (the organization). Consequently, he keeps a running log of observations on how the company functions and how that affects the employees. For example, he has noticed that some departments have a higher rate of stress-related health problems. These workers have a higher incidence of hypertension, headaches, gastrointestinal disturbances, and other somatic complaints. In response, he has begun to collect data on the working conditions in those departments. Is there high production pressure? Are there opportunities for relieving stress on the job? Do workers receive any positive feedback about their work? Are the symptoms caused or aggravated by some environmental factor, such as chemicals, gases, or noise?

Victor uses several approaches to assess the health needs of the total employee population and selected subgroups within the company. First, he uses the company's computer services to compile the results of individual health histories and physical examinations, and he then analyzes the findings. A picture emerges of dominant health problems among the employees and of the workers at greatest risk for other problems. As a result, Victor begins planning occupational health nursing activities needed now and those that will be most needed in the future (analysis and program development brought about by research).

It appears that hypertension, obesity, cigarette smoking, and inadequate exercise are the major problems common among Allied's employee population. Victor approaches these problems on several fronts. He starts a regular program to monitor blood pressure and upgrades the employee health education program with new videotapes and literature to make workers more health conscious and to show them ways of improving their health. Specifically, they learn ways to lose weight, manage stress, stop smoking, and maintain an exercise program. More importantly, however, is motivation. Victor convinces management that company inducements, similar to Coor's Wellness Center or Prudential's fitness program, are effective ways to stimulate employee participation. He tells them about the Dunlop Tire Company of Grand Island, New York, which provides employees with an on-site conditioning room and specific fitness programs to reduce musculoskeletal injuries, which accounted for 63% of its workers' compensation claims. Also, the Scoular Grain Company opened a fitness center for its 600 employees, and, as a result, the company's health care costs dropped by $1 million annually (Upton, 1992). Allied's management has agreed to give employees time for exercise breaks, to award quarterly bonuses to employees who stop smoking at work, and to begin planning a fitness center in an adjacent building not presently being used by the company.

Another approach that Victor is using to assess the health needs of the employee population is to conduct an environmental survey of health hazards. He uses data from the safety division's regular spot checking and collaborates with that division to systematically observe working conditions and interview workers. Victor serves on a multidisciplinary committee to analyze absenteeism, accidents, injuries, and illnesses. In addition, he posts suggestion boxes and gains management's approval to give any employee half a day off with pay for suggesting a safety or health improvement that is implemented.

Victor gains further ideas from other companies, such as stocking vending machines with nutritionally beneficial foods, like granola bars, yogurt, fruit drinks, fresh fruit, and nutritious sandwiches. He is also promoting regular exercise through the President's Council on Physical Fitness and Sports, which provides Presidential Sports Awards to employees who can earn the award in any of 58 sports/fitness categories. Moreover, Victor is forming a committee of employees to plan wellness activities. A "Live For Life" program at Johnson & Johnson lowered absenteeism and slowed the rise of health care expenses, resulting in saving $378 per employee yearly. Tenneco Corporation found that employees who used the company fitness center were less likely to leave the company, thus reducing expensive turnover rates (Upton, 1992).

Victor's analysis has also uncovered a rising incidence of back injuries among Allied's production workers. He learns that other companies have similar problems and that back problems are the leading cause of absenteeism and disability in the work environment. Low back pain afflicts about 75 million workers and annually accounts for $1 billion in lost output, plus $250 million in workers' compensation claims (Upton, 1992). With that information Victor, offers literature on backache prevention and presents classes on ways to strengthen back muscles and the proper body mechanics to use to prevent injuries.

Each set of data gathered through the various assessment approaches gives Victor information to guide his planning and development of health programs. An important dimension in this process is accurate record keeping. Exact figures on incidence and prevalence of health problems in the company helps him justify programs and provides data with which to compare the results as he evaluates program outcomes.

Occupational health nursing demands a great deal from the nurse. Individual needs in the workplace will always compete for the nurse's time and take attention away from aggregate needs, often to the detriment of the latter (Menckel, 1992). To maintain a proper focus on aggregate needs requires discipline and commitment—commitment based on a different mindset and the realization that the health and productivity of workers is interrelated with the health of the community.

Summary

The working population, composed of well adults, makes up the majority of the American people. The profile of this aggregate is changing from an industrialized labor force to one of a more white-collar workers and professionals. The environment of the workplace is changing as well.

Five types of environmental factors, common to all work settings, can influence worker health or safety. Physical or structural elements include such things as temperature and noise extremes. Chemical factors refer to the presence of potentially hazardous chemical agents. Biological organisms, such as viruses, bacteria, and fungi, may contaminate the work environment and cause disease. Ergonomic factors include the customs, design, and expectations of the job that influence the way people interact with their work environment. Psychosocial factors are the workers' feelings and behavior at work. Assessment of all of these is critical in determining appropriate occupational health interventions.

Historically, workers' health has been of little importance to the government. As a result, many have suffered unhealthy, dangerous working conditions and have contracted debilitating, often fatal, diseases and injuries. More recently, however, worker health has become a target for health intervention. The government has become more involved and passed major legislation to ensure workers' rights to a safe and healthy work environment. Three of the most significant pieces of legislation are the Occupational Safety and Health Act of 1970, the Hazard Communication Act of 1986, and the Americans with Disabilities Act of 1990.

Chronic diseases are prime threats to the health of the adult working population and the three leading causes of death in this population are cancer, heart disease, and accidents. Leading work-related health problems include occupational lung disease, injuries, and occupational cancers. New health concerns have arisen in this population that reflect our changing society, work patterns, and environment. They include job stress, job burnout, and ergonomic issues that relate to the computer age, violence, and HIV/AIDS.

Programs designed to serve the health needs of the working population vary with the work environment and should be based on an assessment of the unique needs of that setting. Occupational health services encompass the three public health practice priorities—prevention, protection, and health promotion. Preventive programs seek to eliminate potential hazards to worker health and safety. Protective services shield workers from remaining hazards. Health promotion or wellness programs seek to maintain and improve workers' health. Health services for workers may also cover nonoccupational illnesses.

Occupational health nursing applies the philosophy and skills of nursing and community health to protecting and promoting the health of people in their work environment. As business becomes more competitive, health care costs escalate at a frightening rate, and companies focus on controlling costs, the OHN's role will expand and change. That expanded role will include analyzing current trends, recommending more efficient and cost-effective in-house health services and innovative new programs, and collaborating with other members of the multidisciplinary occupational health team to work with management in developing appropriate programs. The focus will move from one-on-one health assessment and management and will instead focus on the health concerns of the entire working population. The nurse must view the client population as a whole, work with other professionals to assess worker health needs and the needs associated with the work environment, and then design, implement, and evaluate health services.

Activities to Promote Critical Thinking

1. Select an industry, agency, or corporation with which you are familiar, and identify employee health hazards that pertain to each factor: physical, biological, ergonomic, chemical, and psychosocial. Explain one method of control (protection or prevention) that you would suggest for each of the five health hazards identified.

2. You are asked to offer a weight-control program for a local milk-processing plant that has 100 employees. What steps would take to develop a successful program?

3. Explain how the role of OHN has been affected by the Americans with Disabilities Act of 1990 and OSHA's (1992) standards regarding exposure to blood-borne pathogens.

4. Compare the anticipated role of the OHN in the 21st century with the OHN in the 1990s. What areas will be different? Why?

REFERENCES

American Association of Occupational Health Nurses. (1988). The year 2000: Health objectives for the nation. *American Association of Occupational Health Nurses' Journal, 36*(6), 285–88.

Ashford, N. A., Spadafor, C. J., Hattis, D. B., & Caldart, C. C. (1990). *Monitoring the worker for exposure and disease.* Baltimore: The Johns Hopkins University Press.

Bailey, L. (1994). Confined space: Occupational health hazards. *AAOHN Journal, 42*(4), 182–188.

Ball, H. (1993). *Cancer factories: America's tragic quest for uranium self-sufficiency.* Westport, Connecticut: Greenwood Press.

Barlow, R. & Handelman, E. (1993). OSHA's final blood-borne pathogens standard. Part II. *AAOHN Journal, 41*(1), 8–15.

Bey, J. M., et al. (1988). How management and nurses perceive occupational health nursing. *American Association of Occupational Health Nurses' Journal, 36*(2), 61–69.

Botsch, R. E. (1993). *Organizing the breathless.* Lexington: The University of Kentucky Press.

Brown, M. L. (1988). An historical perspective: One hundred years of industrial or occupational health nursing in the United States. *AAOHN Journal, 36*(10), 433–436.

Campanelli, L. (1990). The aging work force: Implications for organizations. *Occupational medicine, 5*(4), 817–825.

Centers for Disease Control. (1988). NIOSH recommendations for occupational safety and health standards. *Mortality and Morbidity Weekly Report, 37*(S-7), 1–29.

Centers for Disease Control. (February 10, 1995). Update: AIDS among women. *Mortality and Morbidity Weekly Report.* U.S.D.H.H.S.

Christenson, G., et al. (1988). Highlights from the National Survey of Work Site Health Promotion Activities. *Health Values, 12*(2), 29–33.

Crawford, S. L. (1993). Job stress and occupational health nursing: Modeling health affirming choices. *AAOHN Journal, 41*(11), 522–528.

Frazier, C. A. & Brown, F. K. (1992). *Miners and medicine: West Virginia memories.* Norman: University of Oklahoma Press.

Girgis, A., Sanson-Fisher, R. W., & Watson, A. (1994). A workplace intervention for increasing outdoor workers' use of solar protection. *American Journal of Public Health, 84*(1), 77–81.

Gough, P., et al. (1988). Combating the pressure . . . occupational stress. *Nursing Times, 84*(2), 43–45.

Grant, C. B., & Brisbin, R. E. (1992). *Workplace wellness: The key to higher productivity and lower health costs.* New York: Van Nostrand Reinhold.

Harrison, K. (1989). Hearing conservation: Implementing and evaluating a program. *AAOHN Journal, 37*(4), 107–111.

Hart, B. G. & Moore, P. V. (1992). The aging work force: Challenges for the occupational health nurse. *AAOH Journal, 40*(1), 36–40.

Kalisch, P., & B. Kalisch. (1978). *The advance of American nursing.* Boston: Little, Brown.

Kavianian, H. R. & Wentz, C. A. (1990). *Occupational and environmental safety engineering and management.* New York: Van Nostrand Reinhold.

Last, J. (1987). *Public health and human ecology.* East Norwalk, CT: Appleton and Lange.

Lee, J. (1978). *The new nurse in industry: A guide for the newly employed occupational health nurse.* (DHEW [NIOSH] Pub. No. 78–143). Cincinnati: U.S. Government Printing Office.

Levy, B. S., & D. H. Wegman. (1988). *Occupational health: Recognizing and preventing work-related disease.* (2nd ed.) Boston: Little, Brown.

Lusk, S. L. (1990). Corporate expectations for occupational health nurses' activities. *AAOHN Journal, 38*(8), 368–374.

Maciag, M. E. (1993). Occupational health nursing in the 1990s: A different model of practice. *AAOHN Journal, 1*(1), 39–45.

McClain, J. D. (1994, June 30). Homicide second leading cause of death at work. *Fresno Bee.* p. C2.

McKenna, B. (1994, July/August). The Americans with Disabilities Act and the health care worker. *Healthwire.* Washington, DC: Federation of Nurses and Health Professionals.

Menckel, E. (1992). Occupational health nurses and accident prevention: An inventory of activities in one industrial sector in Sweden. *AAOHN Journal, 40*(10), 477–483.

Millar, J. D. (1988). Summary of proposed national strategies for the prevention of leading work-related diseases and injuries. Part I. *American Journal of Industrial Medicine, 13,* 223–240.

Miller, M. A. (1989). Social, economic, and political forces affecting the future of occupational health nursing. *AAOHN Journal, 37*(9), 361–366.

Morris, R. B. (Ed.). (1976). *The United States Department of Labor bicentennial history of the American worker.* Washington, DC: U.S. Government Printing Office.

National Institute for Occupational Safety and Health. (1986). *NIOSH recommendations for occupational safety and health standards.* Atlanta: Center for Disease Control, DHHS.

National Institute for Occupational Safety and Health. (1989). *National prevention strategies for the ten leading work-related diseases and injuries.* Atlanta: Center for Disease Control, DHHS.

Network news. (1992). *Farmworker women's health project.* Washington, DC: National Women's Health Network.

Olsen, J., Merletti, F., Snashall, D., & Vuylsteek, K. (1991). Searching for causes of work-related diseases: An introduction to epidemiology at the work site. Oxford: Oxford University Press.

Parker-Conrad, J. E. (1988). A century of practice: Occupational health nursing. *AAOHN Journal, 36*(4), 156–161.

Pheasant, S. (1991). *Ergonomics, work, and health.* Gaithersburg, MD: Aspen Publishers.

Ringholz, R. C. (1989). *Uranium frenzy: Boom or bust on the Colorado plateau.* New York: Norton.

Rogers, B. (1994). Advancing the profession of occupational health nursing. *AAOHN Journal, 42*(4), 158–163.

Rosner, D. and Markowitz, G. (1991). *Deadly dust: Silicosis and the politics of occupational disease in twentieth-century America.* Princeton: Princeton University Press.

Ross, P. (1994). Ergonomic hazards in the workplace: Assessment and prevention. *AAOHN Journal, 42*(4), 171–176.

Rossignol, M. (1991). Planning preventive occupational health services at the community level. *Canadian Journal of Public Health, 82*(2), 115–119.

Roup, B. J. (1993). OSHA's new standard: Exposure to blood-borne pathogens. *AAOHN Journal, 41*(3), 136–142.

Smisko, B. (1990). Hazardous material compliance training pays off. *Journal of Environmental Health, 53*(5), 37–38.

U.S. Statistical Abstracts of the United States (1994, September). 114th ed. Washington, DC: U.S. Government Printing Office.

U.S. Department of Health and Human Services. (1991). Healthy people 2000: National health promotion and disease prevention objectives. Public health service. Washington, D.C.: U.S. Government Printing Office.

Upton, D. E. (1992, May). When health is money. World traveler. Northwest Airlines.

Veninga, R., & J. Spradley. (1981). *The work-stress connection.* Boston: Little, Brown.

Wood, E.A., Olmstead, G.W., & Craig, J.L. (1989). An evaluation of lifestyle risk factors and absenteeism after two years in a worksite health promotion program. *American Journal of Health Promotion, 4*(2), 128–133.

SELECTED READINGS

Babbitz, M. A. (1992). Approaching the 21st century: Congressional agenda for health care and occupational health. *AAOHN Journal, 40*(1), 12–16.

Bacon, C. A. (1993). On the job conflict. *AAOHN Journal, 41*(11), 529–532.

Bamford, M. (1994). *Work and health: An introduction to occupational health care.* London: Chapman & Hall.

Bromberger, J. T. & Matthews, K. A. (1994). Employment status and depressive symptoms in middle-aged women. *American Journal of Public Health, 84,* 202–206.

Covey, L. S., Zang, E. A., & Wynder, E. L. (1992). Cigarette smoking and occupational status 1977–1990. *American Journal of Public Health, 82:* 1230–1234.

Cummings, P. H. (1991). Farm accidents and injuries among farm families and workers: A pilot study. AAOHN Journal. 39(9): 409–415.

Doebbeling, B. N., Li, N., & Wenzel, R. P. (1993). An outbreak of Hepatitis A among health care workers: Risk factors for transmission. *American Journal of Public Health, 83*(12), 1679–1684.

Durham, J. D., & Douard, J. (1993). The challenges of AIDS for health care workers. In F. L. Cohen & J. D. Durham (Eds.), *Women, children, and HIV/AIDS.* New York: Springer Publishing.

Freeman, S. H. (1991). *Injury and litigation prevention: Theory and practice.* New York: Van Nostrand Reinhold.

Howlett, M., & Archer, V. E. (1991). Worker involvement in occupational health and safety. In B. Spradley (Ed.), Readings in community health nursing. (4th ed.). Philadelphia: Lippincott.

Ivey, F. D. and Morris, M. W. (1993). *Liability issues for occupational health nurses: An overview. AAOHN Journal, 41*(1), 16–23.

Kimbrough, R., LeVois, M., & Webb, D. (1995). Survey of lead exposure around a closed lead smelter. *Pediatrics, 95*(4), 550–554

Komulainen, P. (1993). Occupational health nursing in Finland. *AAOHN Journal, 41*(3), 131–135.

Lusk, S. L. (1992). Selling health promotion programs: Recommendations for occupational health nurses. *AAOHN Journal, 40*(9), 414–418.

Lusk, S.L., Kerr, M.J., & Ronis, D.L. (1995). Health-promoting lifestyles of blue-collar, skilled trade, and white-collar workers. *Nursing Research, 44*(1), 20–24.

McCasland, L. J. (1992). *Development of an ergonomic program. AAOHN Journal, 40*(3), 138–142.

McNeely, E. (1991). Who's counting anyway; The problem with occupational health and safety statistics. *Journal of Occupational Medicine, 33*(10), 1071–1075.

McNeely. E. (1992). Tracking the future of OSHA: Regulatory policies into the '90s. *AAOHN Journal, 40*(1), 17–23.

Pickett, G., & Hanlon, J. (1994). *Public health: Administration and practice.* (10th ed.). St. Louis: Times Mirror/Mosby.

Robertson, B. (1993). *Alcohol disabilities primer.* Boca Raton, FL: CRC Press.

Robinson, J. C. (1991). *Toil and Toxics.* Berkeley: University of California Press.

Rogers, B., & Cox,. A. (1994). Advancing the profession of occupational health nursing: AAOHN's strategic planning process. *AAOHN Journal, 42*(4), 158–163.

Savitz, D.A., & Loomis, D.P. (1995). Magnetic field exposure in relation to leukemia and brain cancer mortality among electric utility workers. *Americal Journal of Epidemiology, 141*(2), 123–134.

Shortridge, L. A. (1990). Advances in the assessment of the effect of environmental and occupational toxins on reproduction. *Journal of Perinatal and Neonatal Nursing, 3*(4), 1–11.

Sluchak, T. J. (1992). Ergonomics: Origins, focus, and implementation considerations. *AAOHN Journal, 40*(3), 105–112.

U.S. Department of Labor/OSHA. (1992). *Occupational exposure to blood-borne pathogens.* Booklet #3127.

Wold, J. L. (1990) Workers' compensation law and the occupational health nurse. *AAOHN Journal, 38*(8), 385–387.

Yelin, E. H., Greenblatt, R. M., & Hollander, H. (1991). The impact of HIV-related illness on employment. *American Journal of Public Health, 81,* 79–84.

21

Promoting and Protecting the Health of the Older Adult Population

LEARNING OBJECTIVES

On completion of this chapter, readers should be able to do the following:

- Describe the health status of older adults in the United States today.
- List some of the major misconceptions held about the older adult population.
- Describe the major health needs of the older population.
- Discuss four primary criteria for effective programs for older adults.
- Describe various living arrangements and care options for older adults.
- Describe the future role of the community health nurse when working with older adults.

KEY TERMS

- Ageism
- Alzheimer's Disease
- Assisted living
- Board and care homes
- Capable elderly
- Case management
- Confidant
- Continuing care centers
- Custodial care
- Frail elderly
- Geriatrics
- Gerontics
- Gerontology
- Group home
- Hearty elderly
- Hospice care
- Intermediate care
- Long-term care
- Personal care homes
- Respite care
- Senility
- Skilled-nursing facility

Barbara Walton Spradley and Judith Ann Allender
COMMUNITY HEALTH NURSING: CONCEPTS AND PRACTICE, 4th ed.
© 1996 Barbara Walton Spradley and Judith Ann Allender

Introduction

Older Americans constitute a large and growing population group. In fact, people aged 65 and older make up the fastest-growing segment of the American population (National Institute on Aging, 1993). The most rapid increase is expected between the years 2010 and 2030 when the "baby boom" generation reaches 65 (American Association of Retired Persons, 1993). Older adults make up a group whose health needs are not fully understood, and the nation has yet to offer the full complement of services they require and deserve.

For community health nursing, this population group poses a special challenge. The increasing number of seniors in the community increases the need for health-promoting and preventive services. These services help maximize an older person's ability to remain an independent, contributing member of society and maintain a quality life. With this group's potential for longevity comes the myriad problems brought on by these extended numbers of years, including dwindling finances that may not be keeping up with inflation; increasing chronic disease and disability; diminishing functional capacity; dealing with ongoing and decreasing losses regarding work, home, family members and other loved ones. Significant economic, environmental, and social changes create a demand for greater protective and preventive services for older adults in addition to requiring adjustments in health care provision patterns. The challenge is clear. Nursing must study the needs of this group and respond with appropriate, effective, and cost-effective interventions.

The focus in this chapter is on population-based nursing for the elderly. There are four fundamental requirements for effective nursing of any population:

1. Know the characteristics of the population.
2. Set aside stereotypes based on misconceptions about the population.
3. Know the health needs of the population as a basis for nursing intervention.
4. View the population from an aggregate, public health perspective that emphasizes health protection, health promotion, and disease prevention.

This chapter first examines the characteristics of the aging population and looks at some misconceptions about the elderly. Next, the health needs of older adults are explored. Finally, population-based health services and nursing interventions applied to the health of the aging population are discussed in light of cost containment and comprehensive care.

Health Status of The Older Adult Population

Never before has the population of older adults been so large, and its numbers are on the increase. More than 32 million people in the United States (12.7% of the population) are older than 65 (American Association of Retired Persons, 1993), and by 2030 that number is expected to increase to 70 million (Figure 21.1). Women outnumber men in the older population because they live an average of 8 years longer. In fact, "older women outnumber older men in most countries, with older men tending to be married and older women, widowed" (National Institute on Aging, 1993, p. 11). More than half of the women older than 65 are widowed (Eliopolous, 1993).

People are living longer as a result of improved health care, eradication and control of many communicable diseases, use of antibiotics and other medicines, and accessibility to a better quality of life for residents of the United States. The average life expectancy has increased to 75.5 years (71.5 for men, 78.3 for women). The av-

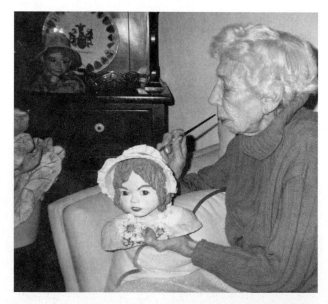

FIGURE 21.1. This widowed older adult, like other adults, benefits from satisfying activities and continues to express her interest and talents in art through painting.

erage life expectancy for white males and females is 75.6 years, compared with 69.2, which is the average for nonwhite males and females (U.S. Bureau of Census, 1990). Although life expectancies have been increasing, such factors as unhealthy lifestyles; societal problems, such as deaths caused by gun shots, drugs, and AIDS; and the rise of Alzheimer's disease among the elderly has caused those figures to level off in recent years.

But older people are healthier than ever before. Although statistics indicate people aged 65 years have 16.4 years of life remaining, it is estimated that 12 of those years will be healthy (National Center for Health Statistics, 1990). Increasing numbers of **capable elderly** older than 65 are living independently, and even **hearty elderly** older than 65 who maintain a high level of wellness and activity well above present expectations for that age are increasing in number. Not only can many people older than 65 maintain independent living but they can and do contribute to society and become involved in community programs and activities. Some have become valuable volunteers, helping others in such community activities as foster grandparents and literacy programs for adults, working in libraries and homeless shelters, or providing services such as Meals on Wheels.

The older population does, however, have a high percentage (80%) of chronic conditions, some of which may limit activities. These chronic illnesses include arthritis, heart disease, high blood pressure, diabetes, and visual and hearing impairments (Burke and Walsh, 1992).

Within the elderly population, the number of people living into "older" old age (75 years and older) is also increasing. Forty-one percent of elderly people in the United States are older than 75, more than 3.3 million are 85 or older, and more than 150,000 claim to be more than 100 years old. Until the year 2030, the 85-and-older age group (old-old age group) is projected to be the most rapidly growing segment of the entire U.S. population (U.S. Bureau of Census, 1992). As the number of old-old increases, so too will the need for assistance with activities of daily living. The **frail elderly** are those older than 85 who need assistance in attending to activities of daily living, such as dressing, eating, toileting, and bathing.

Other statistics on older adults are also useful for community health nurses to know in order to anticipate the needs of the older population. Most older men (76%) live out their years with their spouse and thus have someone for companionship, whereas more than half of older women are widowed, single, or divorced. In fact there are five times as many widows (8 million)

as widowers (1.5 million) in the U.S., and the incidence of widowhood increases with advancing age. Community health nurses should anticipate the needs of many older adults (particularly women) who will face the loss of a spouse, helpmate, and companion and may experience loneliness, social isolation, and depression.

Only about 5% of all older adults live in institutions. The majority of older people live in family settings. Only 30% live alone. Nearly three-quarters (73%) of older adults live with their children or live within 30 minutes of a child. Approximately 80% of older adults have seen one of their children within the previous week. These figures contradict the popular notion of abandoned elderly who have been "dumped" into nursing homes by their families (Staab and Lyles, 1990).

More than one-eighth (12.9%) of older Americans are poor, and many live in profound poverty. They are unable to afford clothing, recreation, transportation, or other items that people consider necessary for mental health, social status, and continued personal growth. It has been noted that among the elderly poor, 33% of African American elderly and 22% of Hispanic elderly live below the poverty level. In the total population almost twice as many women (16%) as men (9%) live below the poverty level (U.S. Bureau of Census, 1992).

The education level of the older population is increasing. Sixty percent of today's older population graduated from high school, and in 1992, 12% had bachelor's degrees (13.5% men and 8.5% women). These figures are predicted to change as the United States witnesses a trend toward a more educated senior population because of the significant numbers of people completing high school during and since the 1940s (Eliopoulos, 1993).

Misconceptions and Stereotypes of Older Adults

Stereotyping older adults and perpetuating false information and negative images and characteristics is called **ageism**. These misconceptions often arise from negative personal experience, myths shared throughout the ages, and a general lack of current information. Ageism can interfere with effective practice and prevent the kind of comprehensive and interdisciplinary service aging persons need and deserve. Community health nurses must guard against ageism in their practice by dispelling the common misconceptions that follow.

MISCONCEPTION: MOST OLDER ADULTS CANNOT LIVE INDEPENDENTLY

On the contrary, 95% of the elderly live in the community, outside formal facilities or institutions. Some live alone or with friends, and others may live in the homes of nonrelatives where room and board are provided. In some homes assistance in activities of daily living is provided. There are also alternative-housing arrangements; group living situations for older adults in which many types of housing arrangements and care possibilities are offered. This concept is not new, but these centers are being built now in greater numbers to meet the needs of a growing segment of the older adult population. These situations are well-suited to those who desire such comprehensive living choices and have the financial means for the housing and care arrangements provided.

Most elders, however, who are vigorous and functioning independently live in their own homes. Only 5% live in institutions, such as skilled-nursing facilities, extended care facilities, supervised living facilities, and Alzheimer's disease centers, and not all of these are permanent residents. Many are recovering from illnesses or rehabilitating from injuries and/or surgeries and will return to their living situation in the community within weeks.

MISCONCEPTION: CHRONOLOGICAL AGE DETERMINES OLDNESS

Older people are quite distinct from one another in the aging process, and they age at widely disparate rates (Bortz, 1991). Some people at age 75 still play golf, drive a car, and participate in social and community activities; others are frail and cannot move about well. Physical, social, and mental health parameters, life experiences, and genetic traits all combine to make aging an individualized process. (See Levels of Prevention display.)

MISCONCEPTION: MOST OLD PEOPLE HAVE DIMINISHED INTELLECTUAL CAPACITY OR ARE SENILE

Studies show that intelligence, learning ability, and other intellectual and cognitive skills do not decline with age. Cognitive deficits are caused by certain risk factors. Nutritional status has been singled out as a

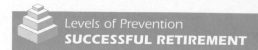

Levels of Prevention
SUCCESSFUL RETIREMENT

GOAL

Client will have a healthy transition into a satisfying retirement

PRIMARY PREVENTION

Early preparation emotionally, financial, avocation planning (pre-retirement workshops, support groups, financial planning)

SECONDARY PREVENTION

Celebration activity, reflect on contributions to the work force, organization of new free time; allow time for adaptation to this life transition

TERTIARY PREVENTION

Adaptation to changed roles with spouse and significant others, maintenance of health, participation in avocational activities, assess increasing dependency needs including alternative housing, modifications in transportation, and changing health care needs. Periodically review and update will, insurances, and other important documents as needed; keep beneficiaries or executors aware of changes in and location of documents and personal wishes regarding funeral arrangements and burial.

physical health variable that influences cognitive functioning, particularly memory performance, regardless of a person's age. Anticholinergic ingredients that are present in many medications can interfere with memory and cognitive functioning. In healthy, mentally stimulated, older adults, deficits are generally minimal and probably not even noticed. Speed of reaction tends to decrease with age, but basic intelligence does not. In fact, some abilities are viewed collectively as crystallized intelligence. Wisdom, judgment, vocabulary, creativity, common sense, coordination of facts and ideas, and breadth of knowledge and experience actually improve with age (Miller, 1995). Most older people are largely capable of making their own decisions; they want and need the freedom to make choices and to be as independent as their limitations will allow.

Senility, although not a legitimate medical diagnosis, is widely used by health professionals and laypeople alike to denote deteriorating mental faculties associated with old age. Yet fewer than 1% of people aged 65 years, and 20% of people older than 85 are affected by senility, cognitive impairment, dementia, or Alzheimer's disease, which are all physiological consequences of disease processes (Katzman, 1988). Alzheimer's disease as a growing community health problem is discussed in more detail later in this chapter. Although most cases of cognitive impairment are not treatable, 10% to 20% of them may be reversible. These include problems caused by drug toxicity, metabolic disorders, depression, or hyperthyroidism (National Institutes of Health, 1992).

Certainly Alzheimer's disease and arteriosclerosis cause memory loss and altered behavior in the elderly, but many older adults may have similar symptoms because of anxiety, losses, grief, or just from changes in their routine. These reactions need to be diagnosed and differentiated from disease processes by health care providers.

MISCONCEPTION: ALL OLDER PEOPLE ARE CONTENT AND SERENE

The tranquil picture of Grandma sitting in her rocker with her hands folded in her lap is misleading. It is true that many older people have learned to accept rather than fight the hardships and vicissitudes of life. Yet, for most people, advancing age brings increasing physical, social, and financial problems to harass and worry them. Depression, which may be a problem among the elderly, may sometimes be confused with dementia because of such symptoms as disorientation, failing memory, and eccentric behavior. However, one must not forget that in order to attain the status of senior citizen (meaning one who has survived 65 years or more of living) one has had a great deal of strength, tenacity, adaptation, and a sense of humor about many of the trials, tribulations, and absurdities in life. These people are survivors, and survivors do not always sit contentedly in a rocking chair on the sidelines of life.

MISCONCEPTION: OLDER ADULTS CANNOT BE PRODUCTIVE OR ACTIVE

More than two-thirds of the work force retire before age 65, and the median age of retirement is 60.6 years. Some reasons for early retirement include health, availability of private pension benefits, social expectations, and long-held plans to do something else with their time (Staab and Lyles, 1990). These additional years give older adults time for travel and hobbies. For some

people a third of their life is left to pursue these interests. Many older retired adults become volunteers, care for grandchildren or great-grandchildren, or even care for their very old surviving parent. One-fifth of women older than 65 have a living parent who may be 90 or older and need some degree of assistance. Most older adults are very active and productive.

More than 4 million Americans older than 65 work full or part time, and many others, not included in labor statistics, work but do not report their earnings because of Social Security restrictions. Healthy older people generally do not disengage or withdraw and isolate themselves from society, rather, they are active and involved. Remaining active, through a daily routine, organized purposeful behavior, and a positive view of life produces the best psychological climate for the elderly (Palmore, 1987).

MISCONCEPTION: ALL OLDER ADULTS ARE RESISTANT TO CHANGE

People at any age can learn new information and skills. Research indicates that older people can learn new skills and improve old ones, including how to use a computer (National Institute on Aging, 1993). The elderly have spent a lifetime adapting to change, with varying measures of success. The ability to change does not depend on age but rather on personality traits acquired throughout life or perhaps socioeconomic difficulties. For example, an elder may have financial concerns on a fixed income and be faced with inflationary costs. This may cause the property owner to vote against a school levy that would increase taxes, when he or she would support schools if finances were different.

Characteristics of Healthy Older Adults

No one knows conclusively all of the variables that influence healthy aging, but it is known that a lifetime of healthy habits and circumstances, a strong social support system, and a positive emotional outlook all significantly influence the resources people bring to their later years. Most people recognize a healthy older person when they meet one.

What is healthy old age? As we said earlier, the vast majority (95%) of the elderly, even those with chronic diseases and other disabilities, are living outside institutions and are relatively independent. Their ability to function is a key indicator of health and wellness and is an important factor in understanding healthy aging. Good health in the elderly means maintaining the maximum degree possible of physical, mental, and social vigor. It means being able to adapt, to continue to handle stress, and to be active and involved in life and living. In short, healthy aging means being able to function, even when disabled, with a minimum of ordinary help from others (Department of Health and Human Services, 1991; Speake, 1987).

Wellness among the older population varies considerably. It is influenced by many factors including personality traits, life experiences, current physical health, and current societal supports. Some elderly people demonstrate maximum adaptability, resourcefulness, optimism, and activity. See the case study that follows. Others, often those from whom we tend to draw our stereotypes, have disengaged and present a picture of dependence and resignation. Most of the elderly population fall somewhere in between those two extremes. Although the level of wellness varies among the elderly, that level can be raised. The challenge in community health nursing is to maximize the wellness potential of the elderly. Nurses must analyze and capitalize on an older person's strengths rather than to focus on the difficulties. The goal is to enable older people to thrive, not merely survive (Eliopoulos, 1993; Burke and Walsh, 1992).

Health Needs of The Older Adult

Effective nursing in any population requires familiarity with that group's health problems and needs. Aging in and of itself is not a health problem. Rather, aging is a normal, irreversible physiological process. Its pace, however, can sometimes be delayed, as researchers are discovering (Bortz, 1991), and many of the problems associated with aging can be prevented (Wold, 1993). The aging process is subtle, gradual, and lifelong. One can see remarkable differences among different individuals' rates of aging and even in a single individual. Various systems of the body age differently (Wold, 1993; Burke and Walsh, 1992; Bortz, 1991). Thus, chronological age cannot serve as an indicator of health needs, however, the proportion of people with health problems increases with age, and as a group, older adults are more likely than younger ones to suffer from multiple, chronic, and often disabling conditions.

The elderly, like any age group, have certain basic needs: physiological and safety needs as well as the need for love and belonging, self-esteem, and self-actualization. Their physical, emotional, and social needs are complex and interrelated.

CASE STUDY

PROFILE OF A HEALTHY OLDER ADULT

Minerva Blackstone, affectionately called Minnie by her friends, is a lively 87-year-old woman who enjoys life. Every day, except in bad weather, she walks a half mile to visit her granddaughter, Karen. There she is working on the quilt, which is stretched on a frame, that she is making for Karen. In addition, twice a week Minnie takes the city bus to the senior citizens' center to join her friends in an exercise class. Although her eyesight has somewhat diminished, Minnie enjoys reading in the evening or crocheting while she watches television. Mysteries and comedies are her favorite kinds of stories.

She is not content, however, unless she is up on the latest political developments. She always has opinions on current events and expresses them with vigorous shakes of her curly white hair at her monthly group meeting on women and politics. She has a good appetite and generally sleeps well. Minor arthritis does not hamper her activities, nor does the hypertension that she controls by taking her medication with conscientious regularity. Minnie is enjoying a healthy, successful old age.

NUTRITION AND EXERCISE NEEDS

People who have maintained sound dietary habits throughout life have little need to change in old age. Many have not established such habits but may wish to. It is generally felt that older people need to maintain their optimal weight by eating a diet that contains low fats, moderate carbohydrates, and high protein. However, John E. Morley (1994) of the division of geriatric medicine at St. Louis University states that as people age (70 and older) the need for calories increases. He states, "over age 70 there is no need to be on a diet except to eat anything you can. [In fact,] older fat women live longer than older thin women." Older adults should avoid habitual use of laxatives, adding instead more fiber and bulk to their diet.

Loss of teeth causes some to need foods that are easier to chew. However, since the 1960s water supplies and toothpastes have been fluoridated and regular dental care has become more accessible and acceptable to most people, all of which has helped prevent periodontal disease, a major component of tooth loss in adults. It is not normal for older adults to have lost their teeth. Oral health and hygiene needs do not decrease with age (Renn,1989). Eating, chewing, and swallowing should be an uncomplicated and natural process (National Institutes of Health, 1993). Frequently older adults are on medications that cause dry mouth, taste alterations, and loss of appetite that limit the desire for food. Eating should remain a pleasurable social experience, preferably taking place in the company of others.

Older people continue to need exercise (Figure 21.2). Aging does not and should not involve passivity; instead, physical activity and movement contribute to the quality of intellectual and physical performance in old age. Exercise, such as a daily walk, can keep muscles in good tone, enhance circulation, and promote mental health. Exercise may occur in connection with such activities as homemaking chores, gardening, hobbies, or recreation and sports. Often such physical outlets are done in the company of other people, which meets social and emotional needs as well.

PSYCHOSOCIAL NEEDS

Coping with Multiple Losses

Depression may be a difficult problem for older adults. Loss of employment, a spouse, and friends along with economic problems, physical disease and disability, loneliness, or drug side effects can make an older person feel that life holds no meaning (Cole, 1990). Social and emotional withdrawal can often occur, as can suicide. White men older than 65 have a suicide rate that is more than double that of adolescents (National Institutes of Health, 1993). Concern for the increased suicide rates among that group of white men has led to a key health objective in *Healthy People 2000*: By the year 2000, the goal is to reduce the suicide rate to 39.2 per 100,000 from 46.1, which was the rate in 1987 (U.S. Dept. of Health and Human Services,1990).

Mortality after bereavement is high (Kaprio et al., 1987, Gass and Chang, 1989) and can be prevented through nursing intervention. Loss and the mourning process has been studied by Pollock (1987), who found that crucial to successful aging is the ability to mourn prior states of one's self and the past. This, he finds, can be liberating and can give energy for current living, including "planning for the future" (Pollock, 1987, p.12).

In addition to preventing early deaths after the loss of a spouse, the greater goal for the nurse in promoting successful aging can be accomplished when the nurse

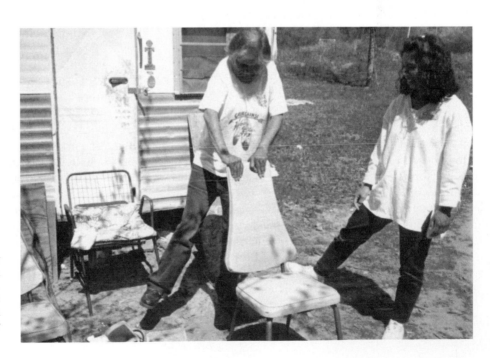

FIGURE 21.2. Community health nurses must be flexible in meeting the needs of each client. Here a nurse teaches a Native American elder range-of-motion exercises outside his rural trailer home.

recognizes the significance of accepting all the losses of aging. The loss of a spouse is much more frequent for women than for men (Ebersole and Hess, 1990; Wolinsky and Johnson, 1992). With this knowledge, a woman can age successfully by planning for the future through anticipatory guidance, with the help of a community health nurse. Women may survive their spouses by 20 years or more, and the nurse can help to make these years meaningful and as healthy as possible.

Economic Security Needs

Economic security is another major need for older adults. Worrying about finances is often one of the most debilitating factors in old age. Fearing the potential costs of major illness and not wanting to be a burden on family or friends, many older people will conserve their limited finances by eating cheaply, using health resources sparingly, taking medications in partial doses, and spending little on themselves. Too often, the fear, let alone the reality, of financial difficulties prevents older adults from leading full and active lives.

For older adults today, living many years past retirement and perhaps not planning for financial security for those later years, is a reality, not an unfounded fear. Putting older people in touch with appropriate community resources can do much to relieve the source of that stress and anxiety. The community health nurse can also help the younger, working adult plan for a physically and emotionally, as well as financially, vigorous old age.

Need for Independence

Older people need independence. As much as possible, the elderly need to make their own decisions and manage their own lives. Even those with activity limitations because of disability can still exercise decision-making options about many, if not most, aspects of their daily living. The need for autonomy—to be able to assert ourselves as separate individuals—is great for all of us. With life's restrictions ever increasing for the elderly person, this need is all the greater (Eliopoulos, 1993). Independence helps to meet the need for self-respect and dignity. The elderly need to have their ideas and suggestions heard and acted upon and to be addressed by their preferred names in a respectful tone of voice. Respect for the older adult is not a strong value in the American culture, but it is highly valued in Asians, Ital-

ians, Hispanics, and Native Americans. Older people represent a rich resource of wisdom, experience, and patience that is generally wasted in the United States.

Need for Social Interaction, Companionship and Purpose

Older people need companionship and social interaction, particularly when they live alone. The company of other people as well as the companionship of a household pet offers avenues for expression and response and adds meaning to life. Many studies of mortality patterns demonstrate that older adults living together have a greater survival rate and retain their independence longer than those who live alone (Hanlon and Pickett, 1984). The problem is of greatest significance for women, who outnumber men considerably in the later years and who live alone more frequently.

It is also important for older adults without companions to discover and develop a friendship with someone who can be considered a **confidant**, someone in whom the older adult can confide, can reflect on the past, and can trust. It could be a close friend, a sibling, a son or daughter, or an acquaintance. In particular, mothers and daughters form confidant bonds (Martin Matthews, 1991). This person may be someone who is seen daily or talked with on the telephone each month. In one study, women consider a sibling as a confidant, especially if that person lives close by; that is especially true for childless and single women (Connidis and Davies, 1992).

Meaningful activity is another need of the elderly that also adds purpose to life. Some kind of active role in community life is essential for mental health, satisfaction, and self-esteem. These activities can range from involvement in hobbies, such as gardening or crafts, to volunteer work or even full-time employment. One current example is the federally supported Foster Grandparents and Senior Companions programs that engage the help of more than 20,000 seniors. These older adults work part-time offering companionship and guidance to handicapped children, the terminally ill, and other people in need. Senior Partners is another program that keeps older adults involved. Volunteers earn service credits by providing support services so that persons aged 60 or older can remain independent and active in their own homes. Each hour of volunteer service earns one service credit. Credits may be "spent" in several ways. They can be used to obtain services, should the volunteer need them, or they can be donated to another person in need or donated back to Senior Partners to help others.

NEEDS OF OLDER ADULTS WITH CHRONIC HEALTH CONDITIONS

Although most of the elderly population is healthy, 80% have at least one chronic condition, causing nearly half of the elderly to experience some kind of limitations in activity (Burke and Walsh, 1992). A small portion suffer more disabling forms of disease, such as chronic obstructive pulmonary disease (COPD), cerebral vascular accidents (CVAs), or cancer or diabetes mellitus, both of which can require more extensive care. The most frequent health problems of older people in the community are arthritis, reduced vision, hearing loss, heart disease, peripheral vascular disease, and hypertension. In those older than 65, two in five persons have blood pressure recordings that are high enough to be considered hypertensive. "Hypertension increases with age, is twice as prevalent among blacks as whites, and generally affects men more than women. But older black women have the highest rates of hypertension of any group" (Older Women's League, 1987). Older adults do, however, need to have a blood pressure high enough to have sufficient cerebral circulation to avoid lightheadedness and dizziness. Hypotension leads to problems of safety, including being at a higher risk of falling. This point is mentioned to alert the community health nurse of the negative effects of a blood pressure that is too low. Both hypertension and hypotension can have significant detrimental effects on the health of older adults.

Drug Interactions and Side Effects

A significant safety issue for the older adult arises from adverse drug effects. Older people may need to take several medications to control the effects of chronic conditions, and their bodies may react differently than a younger person(on whom most new drugs are tested). Thus, multiple medications or complicated drug regimens for many older persons can lead to unexpected and dangerous drug interactions. The elderly need education about the drugs they take and their possible effects. They also need proper supervision of their overall medication intake. This is an area in which the community health nurse can intervene very effectively and with much success.

Alzheimer's Disease

Alzheimer's disease has been recognized in the medical literature since it was first described by Alzheimer (1907) as a "unique illness involving the cerebral cortex." Today approximately 4% of the population is diagnosed with Alzheimer's disease, and that is expected to rise to 12% of the population in the next 50 years. It is seen as the fourth leading cause of death among the very old in the United States (Margolin, 1994). This disease robs its victims of everything learned in life so they are unable to fall back on preserved intelligence. A simple way to describe the difference between the normal forgetfulness of aging and Alzheimer's disease is seen in the behavior described below.

With advancing age, or with increased stress, an individual may say, "Where are my keys? Where did I place them? I can't find them anywhere." After several stressful moments, the keys are usually found and the event is over. However, if a person with Alzheimer's disease is handed a set of keys, he or she looks at them blankly, handles them awkwardly, and has no idea *what they are for* or what to do with them.

Onset is gradual and verbal memory is often affected first. Alzheimer's patients lose judgment and reasoning, and safety becomes an issue early in the disease process. They neglect their health and are even unaware if they are experiencing major health problems. Probable causes of Alzheimer's disease include genetics, toxins, or possibly an infectious agent. Discovering the cause and preventing the disease will be a significant achievement that will hopefully be realized in this century. However, there are presently 16 agents under study as compared with 90 for cardiovascular disease. The medical community is not putting the amount of effort into research for Alzheimer's as it does for other diseases. That lack of research interest today affects what will be available for those in need tomorrow.

How does this disease affect the role of the community health nurse? Often until very late in the disease the person is cared for at home. The intense care-giving needs these clients require drain the reserve of their families. The client demonstrates depression, agitation, sleeplessness, and anxiety, which upsets the family's normal routine. In many situations the main caregiver is an aged spouse. The stress of care-giving puts the caregiver's health at risk as well. The intensity of care giving is aptly described in a book written for Alzheimer's disease family members, called *The 36 Hour Day* (Mace and Rabins, 1991). Medications may be prescribed but have limited effectiveness. At best, available medications may "turn back the clock by 6 months" and the disease worsens at a slower rate (Margolin, 1994).

The community health nurse is in a position to assess the level of stress on the family, provide them with methods and means to cope and adapt as needed, and make referrals when appropriate. Most communities have resources for clients and their families. They may provide family and caregiver support groups, respite care (see discussion about respite care later in this chapter), counseling, and/or legal and financial consultation. These services are available through local agencies, but there are also government-sponsored national resources that offer information, referral services, and educational materials, all of which can be accessed by the community health nurse and/or families in need. The nurse needs to know that resources are available in order to guide families to them. See Research in Community Health Nursing display.

THE NEED TO PREPARE FOR DEATH

A final need of the elderly, and one that is receiving increasing attention, is that of preparing for a dignified death. Elisabeth Kübler-Ross (1975) describes death as the final stage of growth and one that deserves the same measure of quality as other stages of life. Many older people fear death as an experience of pain, humiliation, discomfort, or financial concerns for their loved ones. Planning for a dignified death is an important issue for many older people. For most, this includes choosing, if possible, where and under what circumstances death will occur, being free of financial worries, knowing that their affairs and their family members are taken care of, having the opportunity to receive spiritual counseling, and dying in peaceful surroundings, preferably at home with the support of loved ones. Living wills, advance directives, and durable power of attorney give people legal power over some of these choices.

Community Health Perspective

THREE DISCIPLINES: GERIATRICS, GERONTOLOGY, AND GERONTICS

Another requirement for the nursing of older adults as a population group is to view them from a broad, community health perspective. In general, we can di-

Research in Community Health Nursing
OLDER ADULTS: PREVENTING DISABILITY AND FALLS

Wagner, E. H., LaCroix, A. Z., Grothaus, L., Leveille, S. G., Hecht, J. A., Artz, K., Odle, K., & Buchner,D.M. (1994). Preventing disability and falls in older adults in Los Angeles population-based randomized trial. *American Journal of Public Health, 84*, 1800–1806)

The purpose of this CDC grant–supported study was to test a multicomponent intervention program to prevent disability and falls in ambulatory older adults. Morbidity associated with advanced age can be delayed or compressed by interventions to prevent disability; this is a national priority.

More than 1550 ambulatory adults 65 years and older were randomly selected from health maintenance organization (HMO) enrollees. They were randomly placed in one of three groups: group one (N-635) received a nurse assessment visit and follow-up interventions targeting risk factors for disability and falls; group two (N-317) received a general health promotion nurse visit; and group three (N-607) received the usual care (the control group). The average age of the subjects was 73, 59% were female, 93% white, and 25% held college degrees. Data collection consisted of a baseline and two annual follow-up surveys.

The findings indicated that after 1 year, group one subjects reported a significantly lower incidence of declining functional status and a significantly lower incidence of falls than group three subjects. Group two subjects had intermediate levels of most outcomes. However after 2 years of follow-up, the differences narrowed.

The results of this study suggest that a modest, one-time prevention program appeared to confer short-term health benefits on ambulatory HMO clients, although the benefits diminished by the second year of follow-up if the intervention is not sustained over time. The recommendations are to intensify and sustain a disability and fall prevention/intervention without making costs prohibitively expensive for community health application.

vide nursing service to seniors into three approaches: geriatrics, gerontology, and gerontics.

Geriatrics is the medical specialty that deals with the physiology of aging and with the diagnosis and treatment of diseases affecting the aged. Geriatrics focuses on abnormal conditions and the treatment of those conditions, and geriatric nursing in the past has focused primarily on the sick aged.

Gerontology refers to the study of all aspects of the aging process, including economic, social, clinical, and psychological, and their affect on the older adult and society. Gerontology is a broad, multidisciplinary practice, and gerontological nursing concentrates on promoting the health and maximum functioning of older adults (Eliopoulus, 1993).

The name, **Gerontics**, or gerontic nursing, was coined in 1979 to define the nursing care and services provided to seniors. "The aim of gerontic nursing is to safeguard and increase health to the greatest extent possible, and to provide comfort and care to the extent necessary" (Wold, 1993). The newer view of gerontics aims to safeguard, extend, and enhance the health care and comfort of older adults. Although all three are important dimensions of nursing practice, a community health perspective emphasizes the gerontological or gerontic approach.

Community health nurses work with many older people. In one instance, the nurse may promote and maintain the health of a vigorous 80-year-old man who lives alone in his home. As another example, the nurse may give postsurgical care at home to a 69-year-old woman, teach her husband how to care for her, and help them contact community resources for shopping, meals, housekeeping, and transportation services. Perhaps such nursing intervention should focus on teaching nutrition and maintaining a healthful lifestyle in an extended family, including the 73-year-old grandmother who lives with them. The nurse may also lead a bereavement support group for senior citizens whose spouses have recently died.

The community health nurse's work with older adults is at the individual, family, and group levels. However, a community health perspective must also concern itself with the group of older adults as a whole. There are many instances of groups composed of seniors, for instance, those attending an adult day-care center, belonging to a retirement community, living in a nursing home, or using Meals on Wheels. Others include residents of a senior citizens' apartment building, retired business and professional women, older postcataract-

surgery patients at risk for glaucoma, the older poor, Alzheimer's disease sufferers, and the homeless elderly.

CASE MANAGEMENT AND NEEDS ASSESSMENT

The **case management** concept involves assessing needs, planning and organizing services, and monitoring responses to care throughout the length of the illness. This concept, which has been practiced by community health nurses for many years, focuses primarily on the health needs of clients. Social workers use case management to address their clients' social needs, including their financial problems. Some health maintenance organizations provide a coordinated system of services for their enrolled clients. Unfortunately, many communities provide no such advocate for their older residents. Therefore, a more comprehensive, communitywide system is needed to serve the entire older population. Such a system might be based on an agency specifically designed to serve as case manager, or "agent," to assess clients' needs and assemble existing agencies and services to meet those needs (Handy, 1990).

Various techniques are available to assess the needs of older adults. A comprehensive one, the Older Americans Resources and Services Information System (OARS), developed by Duke University, established baseline data on clients' well-being, available economic and social resources, physical and mental health status, and clients' capacity for self-care (Eliopoulos, 1993; Staab and Lyles, 1990). Clients' capacity for self-care is assessed by the Capacity for Self-Care Index, which ascertains clients' ability to go outdoors, climb stairs, move about their homes, bathe, dress, and cut their toenails (Shanas, 1980).

The Barthel Index assesses functional independence, and the Instrumental Activities of Daily Living Scale looks at an older adult's ability to perform such activities as using the telephone, shopping, doing laundry, and handling finances (Burke and Walsh, 1992). Other techniques, like the Ability to Perform Work-Related Activities survey (Kovar and LaCroix, 1987), determine an elderly person's physical, psychological, and social needs.

A frequently overlooked area of assessment is an elderly clients' spiritual needs. Religious dedication and spiritual concern often increase in later years. Limited ability or lack of transportation may prevent older people from attending religious services or engaging in spiritually enhancing activities. Self-health ratings, including clients' reporting on their spiritual needs, is another useful assessment technique.

Health Services for Older Adult Populations

How well are the needs of older adults being met? In order to answer this question, other questions must be raised. Do health programs for the elderly encompass the full range of needed services? Are programs both physically and financially accessible? Do they encourage elderly clients to function independently? Do they treat senior citizens with respect and preserve their dignity? Do they recognize older adults' needs for companionship, economic security, and social status (Fig. 21.3)? When appropriate, do they promote meaningful activities instead of overworked games or activities like bingo, shuffleboard, and ceramics? Games can be useful diversions but must be balanced with opportunities for creative outlets, continued learning, and community service through volunteerism.

CRITERIA FOR EFFECTIVE SERVICE

There are several criteria that help define the characteristics of effective community health service delivery system for the elderly. Four, in particular, deserve attention.

For a delivery system of a community health service to be effective, it should be *comprehensive*. Many com-munities provide some programs, such as limited health screening or selected activities but do not offer a full range of services to more adequately meet the needs of their senior citizens. Gaps and duplication in pro-grams most often result from poor or nonexistent com-munitywide planning. Furthermore, such planning should be based on thorough assessment of elderly peo-ple's needs in that community. A comprehensive set of services should provide the following (Ford, 1987; Timms, 1990):

Adequate financial support
Adult day care programs
Health care services (prevention, early diagnosis and treatment, rehabilitation)
Health education (including preparation for retire-ment)
In-home services
Recreation and activity programs
Specialized transportation services

A second criterion for a community service delivery system is *coordination*. Often older persons go from one agency to the next. After visiting one place for food stamps, they may go to another for answers to Medicaid questions, another for congregate dining, and still an-other for health screening. Such a potpourri of services reflects a system organized for the convenience of providers rather than consumers. It encourages misuse and discourages use. Instead, there should be coordi-

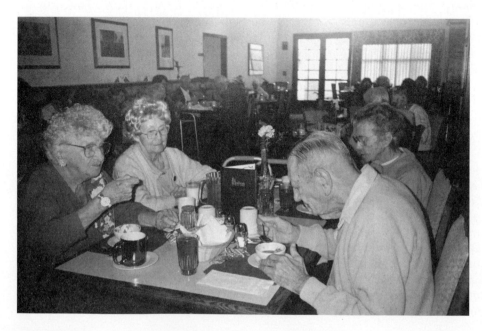

FIGURE 21.3. This group of older adults is enjoying compan-ionship while eating lunch in the dining room of their continuing-care center.

nated, communitywide assessment and planning. Communities must consider alternatives, such as multiservice agencies, that can meet many needs in one location.

A coordinated information and referral system provides another link. Most communities need this type of information network that contains a directory of all resources and services for the elderly and includes the name and telephone number of a contact person with each listing. Such a network is available in some communities and should be developed in those without one. A simplified information and referral system that includes one number, such as an (800) number, to call to find out what resources and services are available and how to get them is particularly helpful to older people.

A third criterion is *accessibility*. Too often, services for the elderly are not conveniently located or are prohibitively expensive. Some communities are considering multiservice community centers to bring programs and services for the elderly closer to home. More convenient and perhaps specialized transportation services and more in-home services, such as home health aides, homemakers, and Meals on Wheels, may further solve accessibility problems for many older adults. Federal, state, and private funding sources can be tapped to ease the burden on the economically pressured elderly population.

Finally, an effective community service system for older people should promote *quality* programs. This means services that truly address the needs and concerns of a community's senior citizens. Evaluation of the quality of a community's services for the elderly is closely tied to their assessed needs. What are the needs of this specific population group in terms of nutrition, exercise, economic security, independence, social interaction, meaningful activities, and preparation for death? Planning for quality community services depends on having adequate, accurate, and current data. Periodic needs assessment is a necessity to ensure updated information and to initiate and promote quality services.

Unfortunately, in most communities this is not done at all, or it is not done with any regularity or thoroughness. Many agencies in a given community do not coordinate services and deliver their own services to the elderly in a patchwork and uncoordinated fashion. Collaboration among those who provide services to seniors can provide vital information for planning and implementing needed programs which has been documented in a seven county area in California through the services of the San Joaquin Valley Health Consortium (Allender et al., 1993).

SERVICES FOR HEALTHY OLDER ADULTS

Maintaining functional independence should be the primary goal of services for the older population. Assessing needs and the ability to function and using techniques such as OARS, Instrumental Activities of Daily Living Scale, or other previously mentioned tools, form the basis for determining appropriate services. Although many of the well elderly can assess their own health status, some are reluctant to seek needed help. Thus, outreach programs serve an important function in many communities. They locate elderly persons in need of health or social assistance and refer them to appropriate resources.

Health screening is another important program for early detection and treatment of health problems among older adults. Conditions to watch for include hypertension, glaucoma, hearing disorders, cancers, diabetes, anemias, depression, and nutritional deficiencies (Eliopoulos, 1993). At the same time, assessment of elderly clients' socialization, housing, and economic needs, along with proper referrals, can prevent further problems from developing that would compromise their health status.

Health maintenance programs may be offered through a single agency, such as a health maintenance organization, or they may be coordinated by a case management agency with referrals to other providers. These programs should cover a wide range of services needed by the elderly, such as those given in Table 21.1.

LIVING ARRANGEMENTS AND CARE OPTIONS

Facilities Offering Nursing Care

While only 5% of the elderly population live in formal institutions, such organizations remain the most visible type of health service for older adults. **Long-term care facilities** make up the largest portion. These facilities provide skilled nursing care along with personal care that is considered nonskilled or **custodial care**, such as bathing, dressing, feeding, and assisting with mobility and recreation. In 1990, 1.6 million elderly persons were receiving institutional care.

Nursing home reform was enacted in 1987 with the Omnibus Budget Reconciliation Act (OBRA), which put increased demands on facilities to provide competent resident assessment, timely care plans, quality improve-

TABLE 21.1. *Health Maintenance Programs for Older Adults*

- Communication services (phones, emergency access to health care)
- Dental care services
- Dietary guidance and food services (such as Meals on Wheels, commodity programs, or group meal services)
- Escort and protective services
- Exercise and fitness programs
- Financial aid and counseling
- Friendly visiting and companions
- Health education
- Hearing tests and hearing-aid assistance
- Home health services (including skilled nursing and home health aide services)
- Home maintenance assistance (housekeeping, chores, and repairs)
- Legal aid and counseling
- Library services (including tapes and large-print books)
- Medical supplies or equipment
- Medication supervision
- Podiatry
- Recreational and educational programs (community centers, Elderhostel)
- Routine care from selected health care practitioners
- Safe, affordable, and ability-appropriate housing
- Senior citizens' discounts (food, drugs, transportation, banks, retail stores, and recreation)
- Social assistance services offered in conjunction with health maintenance
- Speech or physical therapy
- Spiritual ministries
- Transportation services
- Vision care (prescribing and providing eye glasses; the diagnosis and treatment of glaucoma and cataracts)
- Volunteer and employment opportunities

ment, and protection of resident rights. However, this increased complexity of services has caused costs in these facilities to rise. Staffing needs increase as care becomes more complex and the resident population grows. This requires licensed personnel to be knowledgeable decision makers, managers of unskilled staff, staff educators and role models, and efficient and effective administrators in an essentially autonomous practice setting.

In the past, nursing homes or long-term care facilities have had stigmas attached to them. Many people saw them as places that enforced dehumanizing and impersonal regulations, such as segregation of sexes, strict social policies, and sometimes overuse of tranquilizers or restraints. Media attention to such conditions as well as the current licensing regulations should make these

types of practices the rare exception. Gradually, the fear and despair associated with such facilities will begin to dissipate.

Even institutions in which the quality of care is acceptable to outstanding, costs are so high that family resources are soon depleted if not planned for long in advance of the need. Although Medicaid and other government sources pay a share of skilled nursing costs, patients and families pay more than half (Eliopoulos, 1993). Life savings that older parents had hoped to leave to their children may be quickly consumed, forcing them into indigence.

Institutions that offer only one level of care include **skilled nursing facilities** and provide a skilled level of nursing care that is reimbursable by Medicare, Medicaid, and other third-party payers such as private insurance companies. **Intermediate-care facilities** are less costly and still provide health care, but the amount and type of skilled care given is decreased. Frequently older adults need **assisted living**, which includes help with activities of daily living, reminders to take medications, and some meal preparation. This is a less-intense level of care than intermediate care units or facilities provide. Medicare (federal health insurance for those older than 65) generally only pays for skilled nursing facilities and services after hospitalization for a limited time. Medicaid (state subsidized health insurance for the medically indigent) pays for care in skilled as well as intermediate-care facilities.

Personal-care homes offer basic custodial care, such as bathing, grooming, and social support, but provide no skilled nursing services. Payment may also come from private funds, Title XIX or XX (Social Security Act) funds, or Supplemental Security Income (aid to the aged, disabled, or blind). Boarding homes, or **board-and-care homes**, house elderly persons who only need meals and housekeeping and can manage most of their own personal care. Government funds are not available to support these institutions. **Group homes** are an alternative for specific elderly populations, such as the mentally ill, alcoholics, or developmentally disabled, and are often subsidized by concerned community organizations.

The concept of the **continuing care center** (sometimes called total life centers), in which all levels of living, from total independence to the most dependent of skilled nursing care, provides the continuous living needs of older adults as they age (see Issues in Community Health Nursing display that follows). This choice is usually expensive; however, it is a very attractive alter-

Issues in Community Health Nursing
CONTINUING CARE CENTERS— THE WAVE OF THE FUTURE?

Otterbein Homes have five continuing care centers in Ohio. The Otterbein-Lebanon Center is a model continuing care center. With housing options for 760 residents on a 1500-acre campus in rural southeastern Ohio, older adults can choose housing options that include freestanding two-bedroom homes, one-bedroom cottages, or apartment-style studios or one- or two-bedroom units, as they live independently. Three hundred and fifty-six licensed beds include assisted-living options in private one- and two-bedroom apartments (with limited facilities for meal preparation) to semiprivate rooms in which nurses oversee medications, and staff is available to assist with personal care. But the residents are free to come and go as they wish. If assisted-living needs become greater, additional services are available. There is a freestanding 40-bed Alzheimer's living unit in which residents are cared for in wings of 12 to 14 beds.

Otterbein-Lebanon also provides home health care services, adult day care, a children's day care center on the campus, and the other usual services found in a community: a bank, a post office, an ice cream parlor, a hairdresser, a library, and a church (the choir has 70 members, a bell choir, and men's and women's clubs). Because of the popularity of this Otterbein-Lebanon location, there is a waiting list of 2 to 8 years for the independent living area.

Many of the health care beds are occupied by residents who moved into the independent living areas 10 to 15 years ago while they were in their 70s or 80s. Their ages now range from the late 80s to older than 100, and they need assisted or skilled care. In this type of setting, frail elderly persons do not have to leave their community to get the care they need, and longtime friends are nearby to care for them or to provide companionship. It is not unusual to see many of the independent seniors volunteering to help feed frail elderly in the skilled care units. In fact, they volunteer more than 80,000 hours a year to the Otterbein-Lebanon community. They know that when they need the care, a senior friend will be there for them (Otterbein-Lebanon Center, Lebanon, Ohio, 1994).

native to some segments of the aging population. Others may choose to remain in their own home because they do not desire the consolidated living arrangements in which only older adults reside or they may not be able to afford this comprehensive living arrangement. Nevertheless, demand is increasing for this type of housing option. For adults today nearing retirement, that concept is being looked into as a viable choice as they actively plan for a long old age.

Home Care and Day Care Services

Most older adults want to remain in their own homes for the remainder of their lives and be as independent and in control of their lives as possible. Some struggle to appear to be doing well in maintaining their independence. Often they fear that their children or others will make decisions for them that include leaving their homes. Home, whatever form it takes, is where these people feel they are the happiest. There is increased emphasis on providing needed services for elders at home. The trend started several years ago when it became evident that people improved more quickly and at lower costs when they were cared for as outpatients in their own homes.

Today's heightened emphasis on health care cost control gives added support for providing services at home. Given the increase in longevity, the potential for cost savings appears great if dependent older people can be maintained at home. This encourages functional independence as well as emotional well-being.

Home care provides services such as skilled nursing care, psychiatric nursing, physical and speech therapies, homemaker services, social work services, and dietetic counseling. Day care services offer a place where older adults can go during the day for social activities, nutrition, nursing care, and physical and speech therapies. Both services are useful for families caring for an elderly person when no one is at home or available during the day.

One disadvantage to those remaining at home is that services for the dependent elderly in the community are often fragmented, inadequate, and inaccessible, and at times they operate with little or no maintenance of standards or quality control.

Thus, the dependent elderly need someone in the community to assess their particular needs; assemble, coordinate, and monitor the appropriate resources and services; and serve as their advocate. Such case management roles are most appropriately filled by the community health nurse. This case management approach tailors services to the long-term needs of clients and enables them to function longer outside of institutions (ANA, 1988; Handy, 1990).

Hospice and Respite Care Services

Respite care is a service receiving increasing attention and is aimed primarily at caregivers' needs (Andreopoulos and Hogness, 1989). Many older persons at home are cared for by a spouse or other family member. The demands of such care can be exhausting unless the caregiver can get some relief, or respite—thus the name of this service. Respite care may be available through an agency that provides volunteers to relieve caregivers, giving them time off regularly or permitting a periodic vacation. Some skilled nursing facilities or board and care homes provide an extra room to give temporary institutional housing for the elderly while caregivers take a break. Elderly clients may also need a change from the constant interaction with their caregivers.

Hospice care may be offered through an institution such as a hospital, a home health agency, or be a free-standing facility existing solely as a hospice. Hospices and other agencies providing hospice care offer services that enable dying persons to stay at home with the support and services needed. The purpose of hospice care is to make the dying process as dignified, free from discomfort, and emotionally, spiritually, and socially supportive as possible. Some community health nursing agencies offer hospice programs staffed by their nurses. For the elderly, it is a service that has been well received, meets important needs, and is growing in use. Hospice and respite care are two services most needed and used by the families of Alzheimer's victims.

Future Goals and Roles

FOCUSING ON GOALS

The U.S. Department of Health and Human Services has identified three broad areas concerning those older than 65 as goals to reach by the year 2000—health status, risk reduction, and services and protection.

Health status objectives include reducing deaths from suicides (especially among white men); motor vehicle accidents; falls and fall-related injuries; and residential fires. They also include reducing hip fractures from falls, vision and hearing impairments, and pneumonia and influenza outbreaks. Additional goals include improving oral hygiene so that fewer people will lose their natural teeth and increasing the number of personal care activities people can do and the number of years of healthy living.

Risk reduction objectives include increasing the number of people engaged in leisure-time physical activity, receiving immunizations for pneumonia and influenza, and regular and periodic screening and other health promotion services.

Services and protection objectives include increasing home-delivered food services; increasing participation in at least one organized health promotion program a year; increasing oral health care during each year; increasing the following regularly scheduled medical tests: breast exams and mammograms; Pap smears, within the preceding 1 to 3 years; a fecal occult blood test, within the preceding 1 to 2 years; oral, skin, and digital rectal examinations during the year; regular evaluation for urinary incontinence and impairments of vision, hearing, cognition, and functional status from their primary care provider; and counseling about the benefits and risks of estrogen-replacement therapy (combined with progestin, when appropriate) for prevention of osteoporosis (U.S. Department of Health and Human Services, 1990).

FUTURE ROLES FOR THE COMMUNITY HEALTH NURSE

Community health nurses can make a significant contribution to the health of older adults. Because these nurses are in the community and already have contact with many seniors, they are in a prime position to begin needs assessments and mutual planning for the health of this group. Case management is often a critical aspect of the nurse's role since the community health nurse must know what resources are available and when and how to make referrals for these older clients.

The health care scene in terms of the availability of services for the elderly is changing dramatically. The numbers and types of home care services, for example, are mushrooming. Many entrepreneurs, including nurses, who are recognizing the potential of this growing market, have begun offering goods and services targeted for older adults. Community health nurses must keep abreast of new developments, programs, regulations, and social and economic forces and their potential impact on the provision of health services.

More importantly, community health nurses need to be proactive, designing interventions that maximize nursing's resources and provide the greatest benefit to elderly clients. For example, community health nurses might develop a case management program for older adults as a communitywide assessment, information, and referral service. Such a program might contract with existing agencies to serve as a clearing-house for the elderly and channel clients to appropriate services. Financing of such a program might be based on tax dollars (if a public agency), grants, or some innovative fee-for-service reimbursement system.

Many of the older population's health problems can be prevented and their health promoted. Changing to a healthier lifestyle is one of the most important preventive measures the nurse can emphasize. The following strategies for aging successfully are proposed (Bortz,1991):

1. Do at least 30 minutes of sustained, rhythmic, vigorous exercise four times a week.
2. Eat "like a bushman" (a healthy diet of fruits, whole grains, vegetables, and lean meat).
3. Get as much sleep and rest as needed.
4. Maintain a sense of humor and deflect anger.
5. Set goals and accept challenges that force you to be as alive and creative as possible.
6. Don't depend on anyone else for your well-being.
7. Be necessary and responsible: live outside yourself (give to others, become involved).
8. Don't slow down. Stick with the mainstream. Avoid the shadows. Stay together. Maintain energy flow in a purposeful direction; aging need not be characterized by losses.

The role of community health nurse as a teacher is an important one. Educating the elderly about their health conditions, safety, and use of their medications is another important way to prevent problems. Influenza and pneumonia can be prevented through regular health maintenance and immunizations. Other problems associated with environmental conditions and the aging process, such as arthritis, diabetes, and some cancers, can be diagnosed and treated early, thereby minimizing their effect on functional independence.

Many types of accidents that frequently happen to older adults are totally preventable. Community health nurses can make a difference through their work with individuals, families, and aggregates in teaching safety measures to avoid such accidents. Falls are a leading cause of injury and death and are caused by a combination of internal (diseases, effects of medicines) and external (lighting, scatter rugs) factors that are preventable or controllable (Perkins-Carpenter, 1989). Nurses can make a difference in the lives of older clients by using available materials and their own resources when teaching safety.

With a growing and aging elderly population, community health nurses face a serious challenge in addressing their needs. At the same time nursing can be on the forefront of developing innovative health services for that group and rising to meet the opportunity and the challenge.

Summary

The number of older adults (aged 65 and older) is increasing. That age group is also becoming a larger percentage of the overall population. Because women outlive men by about 20 years, women are a larger part of this older population. With improved medicines and medical technology, many people are now living into their 70s, 80s, and even 90s in relatively good health. They are able to enjoy these latter years and still make contributions to their families and society. This extended life expectancy is, of course, good news; however, it has also created a myriad of new health needs and concerns, not only for the older population, but also for health care facilities and professionals who deliver services to older adults.

Healthy longevity is the goal for the aging population. That means being able to function as independently as possible, to maintain as much physical, mental and social vigor as possible, and to adapt to life's changes and cope with the stresses and losses while still being able to engage in meaningful activity.

The most frequent health problems of older adults are chronic and often progressive conditions such as arthritis, vision and hearing loss, heart conditions, hypertension, and diabetes, all of which can become disabling conditions. Other major causes of death or disability are cancer, cerebral vascular accidents, Alzheimer's disease, and accidents and injuries from falls, fire, or automobile accidents. Older adults also often suffer adverse side effects from taking multiple medications prescribed for various chronic conditions. Many of these health problems associated with old age are preventable to some extent, such that early diagnosis and treatment of some conditions can minimize the condition's adverse effects. Many accidents and injuries that render older adults unable to live independently are preventable.

Many older adults also suffer from the emotional side effects of aging, such as feelings of distress and anxiety regarding their future, loneliness, and social isolation when loved ones or friends die, and even depression—feeling that life is over and they have no purpose or meaningful function in life. But older people can also enter this phase of life determined to keep physically and mentally healthy, interacting with others and making viable contributions to others and society.

In order to promote and maintain health and prevent illness, older people need to be educated about their own health care needs. In particular, they should understand potential hazards of drug interactions if they are taking multiple medications. They also need good nutrition and adequate exercise; they need to be as independent and self-reliant as possible; they need coping skills to face the possibility of financial insecurity and the loss of a spouse and other loved ones; they need social interaction, companionship, and meaningful activities; and they need to resolve anxieties regarding their own disability and death.

Many programs are available to older adults, both for those who are healthy, hearty, and active and for those who need some level of dependent or semi-dependent care. Programs for hearty older people include health maintenance programs that cover a wide range of health services, wellness programs, health screening, outreach programs, social assistance programs, and information about volunteering opportunities in the community. A variety of living arrangements and care options are available from which to choose according to the older person's desires and needs. These include the newest concepts of continuing-care centers that offer a full range of living arrangements from totally independent living to skilled nursing services, all within one community. There are also long-term care facilities that provide both skilled nursing and custodial care, home care or day-care services, respite care, and hospice care.

The community health perspective includes a case management approach that offers a centralized system for assessing the needs of older people and then matching those needs with the appropriate services. The community health nurse should also seek to serve the entire older population by assessing the needs of the population, examining the available services, and analyzing their effectiveness. The effectiveness of programs can be measured according to four important criteria—com-

Activities to Promote Critical Thinking

1. Picture an elderly person whom you know well or know a great deal about. Make a list of characteristics that describe this person. How many of these characteristics fit your picture of most senior citizens? What are your biases (ageisms) about the elderly?

2. If you were Minnie Blackstone's community health nurse, what interventions would you consider using to maintain and promote her health? Why?

3. As part of your regular community health nursing workload, you visit a senior day care center an afternoon a week. You take the blood pressures of several people who are on antihypertensive medications and do some nutrition counseling. The center accommodates 60 senior clients, and you would like to serve the health needs of the aggregate population. What are some potential health needs of this group? What actions might you consider taking at an aggregate level? With whom would you consult as you plan programs at the center?

4. Assume you have been asked by your local health department to determine the needs of the elderly population in your community. How would you begin conducting such a needs assessment? What data might you want to collect? How would you find out what services are already being offered and whether they are adequate?

5. Visit a continuing care center in your community. Assess the housing options, services, and health care provisions. Would you live here when you are older? Why or why not? What would you change?

prehensiveness, effective coordination, accessibility, and quality (targeted to the specific needs of the population).

The community health nurse can make significant contributions to the health of the older population as a whole by being aware of new developments and programs that are available, new regulations, and new social and economic forces and their impact on the provision of health services. But more importantly, the community health nurse can design interventions that maximize nursing resources and provide the greatest benefit to the older adult population.

REFERENCES

Allender, J., Fitzgerald, G., Guarnera, J., & Hewett, L. (1993). *Train the trainer: A program for elder care providers.* Fresno, CA: San Joaquin Valley Health Consortium.

Alzheimer, A. (1907). A unique illness involving the cerebral cortex. In D. A. Rottenberg & F. H. Hochberg (Eds.). (1977). *Neurological classics in modern translation.* New York: Hafner Press.

American Association of Retired Persons. (1993). *A profile of older Americans.* Washington, DC: AARP.

American Nurses Association. (1988). *Nursing case management.* Kansas City, MO: The Association.

Andreopoulos, S., & J. Hogness. (1989). *Health care for an aging society.* New York: Churchill Livingstone.

Bortz, W. M. (1991). *We live too short and die too long.* New York: Bantam Books.

Burke, M. M., & Walsh, M.B. (1992). *Gerontologic nursing: Care of the frail elderly.* St. Louis: Mosby Year Book.

Cole, M. G. (1990). The prognosis of depression in the elderly. *Canadian Medical Association Journal, 143*(7), 633–9.

Connidis, I. A., & Davies, L. (1992). Confidants and companions: Choices in later life. *The Journals of Gerontology, 47*(3), S115–122.

Department of Health and Human Services. (1991). *Healthy people 2000: National health promotion and disease prevention objectives.* DHHS Pub. No.(PHS) 91-50212. Washington, DC: U.S. Government Printing Office.

Eliopoulos, C. (1993). *Gerontological nursing.* (3rd ed.). Philadelphia: Lippincott.

Ebersole, P., & Hess. P. (1990). *Toward healthy aging: Human needs and nursing response.* (3rd ed.). St. Louis: Mosby.

Ford, A. B. (1987). Looking after the old folks. *American Journal of Public Health, 77*(12), 1499–1500.

Gass, K. A., & Chang, A. S. (1989). Appraisals of bereavement, coping, resources, and psychosocial health dysfunction in widows and widowers. *Nursing Research, 38,* 31–36.

Handy, J.(1990). Private case management. *Home Health Management Advisor, 3*(7), 1, 4.

Hanlon, J. J., & Pickett, G. E. (1984). *Public health: Administration and practice.* (8th ed.). St. Louis: Times Mirror/Mosby.

Kaprio, J., Koskenvuo, M., & Rita, H. (1987). Mortality after bereavement: A prospective study of 95,647 widowed persons. *American Journal of Public Health, 77*(3), 283–87.

Katzman, R. (1988). *Alzheimer's disease a an age-dependent disorder. Research and the aging population.* (CIBA Foundation Symposium 134). New York: Wiley (pp. 69–85).

Kovar, M. G., & LaCroix, A. Z. (1987). Aging in the eighties, ability to perform work-related activities. (Data from the supplement on aging). *National Health Interview Survey: United States.* (1984). National Center for Health Statistics Advance Data Number 136 (8, May), DHHS Pub. No. (PHS)87-1250. Hyattsville, MD: Public Health Service.

Kübler-Ross, E. (1975). *Death: The final stage of growth.* Englewood Cliffs, NJ: Prentice-Hall.

Mace, N. L., & Rabins, P. V., (1991). *The 36 hour-day.* (2nd ed.). Baltimore: Johns Hopkins University Press.

Margolin, D. I. (1994, March 19). *Alzheimer's disease: Update on diagnosis and treatment.* Address to the Seventh Annual Walter A. Rohlfing Medical Lectureship in Geriatrics and Long-Term Care, Fresno, CA.

Martin Matthews, A. (1991). *Widowhood in later life.* Toronto: Butterworths.

Miller, C. A. (1995). *Nursing care of older adults; Theory and practice.* (2nd ed.). Philadelphia: Lippincott.

Morley, J. E. (1994, March 19). *Malnutrition in the nursing home: A common life-threatening problem.* Address at the Seventh Annual Walter A. Rohlfing Medical Lectureship in Geriatrics and Long-Term Care, Fresno CA.

National Center for Health Statistics. (1990). *Health, United States, 1989 and Prevention Profile.* DHHS Pub. No. (PHS) 90-1232. Hyattsville, MD: U.S. Department of Health and Human Services.

National Institutes of Health. (1992). *Who? What? Where? Resources for Women's Health and Aging.* (NIH Publication No.91-323). Washington, DC: U.S. Government Printing Office.

National Institutes of Health. (1993). *Special Report on Aging, 1993.* (NIH Publication No.93-3409). Washington, DC: U.S. Government Printing Office.

National Institute on Aging. (1993, November). *Research Bulletin.* Bethesda, MD: Information Office.

Older Women's League. (1987). *The picture of health for midlife and older women in America: Mother's day report.* Washington, DC: OWL.

Otterbein-Lebanon Center. (1994, May 10). Lebanon, OH: (personal communication).

Palmore,E.B, (1987). Centenarians. In G. L. Maddox (Ed.). *The encyclopedia of aging.* (pp. 107–108). New York: Springer.

Perkins-Carpenter, B. (1989). *How to prevent falls: A comprehensive guide to better balance.* Rochester, New York: Senior Fitness Productions.

Pollock, G. (1987). The mourning-liberation process: Ideas on the inner life of the older adult. In J. Sadavoy and M. Leszcz (Eds.). *Treating the elderly with psychotherapy: The scope for change in later life.* (pp. 3–30). Madison, CT: International Universities Press.

Renn, N. (1989). Oral health and hygiene for the elderly; a shared learning experience. *Home Health Nurse, 7*(3), 37–39.

Shanas, E. (1980). Self-assessment of physical function: White and black elderly in the United States. In S. Haynes and M. Feinleib (eds.), *Epidemiology of aging.* (NIH Pub. No.

80-969). Washington, DC: U.S. Department of Health and Human Services.

Speake, D. L. (1987). Health promotion activity in the well elderly. *Health Values, 11*(6), 25–30.

Staab, A., & Lyles, M. (1990). *Manual of Geriatric Nursing.* Glenview, IL: Scott, Foresman.

Timms, J. (1990, Winter). Innovative community-based health care for the elderly: A university-community partnership. *Nursing Administration Quarterly, 14*(2), 75–78.

U.S. Bureau of Census. (1990). *Statistical Abstracts of the United States.* (110th ed.). Washington, DC: U.S. Government Printing Office.

U.S. Bureau of Census. (1992). *Statistical Abstracts of the United States.* (112th ed.). Washington, DC: U.S. Government Printing Office.

U.S.D.H.H.S. (1990). *Healthy People 2000.* (DHHS Publication No. [PHS] 91-50212). Washington, DC: U.S. Government Printing Office.

Wold, G. (1993). *Basic geriatric nursing.* St. Louis: Mosby Year Book.

Wolinsky, F. D., & Johnson, R. J. (1992). Widowhood, health status, and the use of health services among older adults: A cross-sectional and prospective approach. *Journal of Gerontology: Social Sciences, 47,* S8-16.

SELECTED READINGS

Anderson, G. (1995). *Caring for people with Alzheimer's disease.* Baltimore: Health Professions Press.

Boyle, J. S., et al. (1988). Toward healthy aging: A theory for community health nursing . . . in an Appalachian community. *Public Health Nursing, 5*(1), 45–51.

Brody, C. M., & Semel, V. G. (1992). *Strategies for therapy with the elderly: Living with hope and meaning.* New York: Springer.

Brody, E. M. (1990). *Women in the middle: Their parent-care years.* New York: Springer.

Chambre, S. M. (1993). Volunteerism by elders: Past trends and future prospects. *The Gerontologist, 33*(2), 221–228.

Cole, M. G. (1990). The prognosis of depression in the elderly. *Canadian Medical Association Journal, 143*(7), 633–639.

Crawford, G. (1987). Support networks and health-related change in the elderly: Theory-based nursing strategies. *Family and Community Health, 10*(2), 39–48.

Department of Health and Human Services (1991). *Physical frailty: A reducible barrier to independence for older Americans.* (NIH Publication no. 91-397.). Washington, DC: U.S. Government Printing Office.

Duffy, M. E. (1993). Determinants of health-promoting lifestyles in older persons. *Image: Journal of Nursing Scholarship, 25*(1), 23–28.

Eliopoulos, C. (Ed.). (1990). *Caring for the elderly in diverse care settings.* Philadelphia: Lippincott.

Fillenbaum, G. G., & Smyer, M. A. (1981). The development, validity, and reliability of the OARS multidimensional functional assessment questionnaire. *Journal of Gerontology, 36*(4), 428.

Fisher, P. P. (1995). *More than movement for fit to frail older adults.* Baltimore: Health Professions Press.

Grau, L. (1984). Case management and the nurse . . . long-term community care to the elderly. *Geriatric Nursing, 5*(8), 372–75.

Haber, D. (1994). *Health Promotion and Aging.* (2nd ed.). New York: Springer.

Hogstel, M. O. (1992). *Clinical manual of gerontological nursing.* St. Louis: Mosby Year Book.

Institute of Medicine. (1990). *The second fifty years: Promoting health and preventing disability.* Washington, DC: National Academy Press.

Kaprio, J., Koskenvuo, M., & Rita, H. (1987). Mortality after bereavement: A prospective study of 95,647 widowed persons. *American Journal of Public Health, 77*(3), 283-87.

Logan, J. R. and Spitze, G. (1994). Informal support and the use of formal services by older Americans. *Journal of Gerontology: Social Sciences, 49*(2), S25–S34.

Martx, S. (Ed.). (1991). *When I am an old woman I shall wear purple.* Watsonville, CA: Papier-Mâché Press.

McDaniel, S. A. (1988). Challenges to health promotion among older working women. *Canadian Journal of Public Health, 79*(1), Centre Appl. Health Research: S29–32.

Morley, J. E. (1991). Why do physicians fail to recognize and treat malnutrition in older persons? *Journal of the American Geriatric Society, 39,* 1139–1140.

Morley, J. E., & Miller, D. K. (1992). Total quality assurance: An important step in improving care for older individuals. *Journal of the American Geriatric Society, 40,* 974–975.

National Institute on Aging (October, 1991). *What's Your Aging I.Q.?* Washington, DC: U.S. Government Printing Office.

Older Women's League. (1988). *The road to poverty: A report on the economic status of midlife and older women. Mother's day report.* Washington, D.C.: OWL.

Pfeiffer, E. (Ed.) (1978). *Multidimensional functional assessment: The OARS Methodology.* (2nd ed.). Durham, NC: Duke University Center for Study of Aging and Human Development.

Shimon, D. A. (1991). *Coping with hearing loss and hearing aids.* San Diego: Singular Publishing Group.

Tout, K. (1993). Elderly care: A world perspective. London: Chapman & Hall.

Yale, R. (1995). *Developing support groups for individuals with early-stage Alzheimer's disease.* Baltimore: Health Professions Press.

CHAPTER

22

Promoting and Protecting the Health of the Home Care Population

LEARNING OBJECTIVES

By the end of this chapter the reader should be able to do the following:

- Define home health care.
- Describe the evolution of home care services to the present.
- Describe the range of services provided to clients by home health agencies.
- Compare and contrast community health nursing and home health care.
- Explain the future of the nurses' role in the home care movement including concepts of quality management, case management, and managed care.

KEY TERMS

- Home health care
- Homebound
- Homemakers
- Hospital-based home health agency

- Official home health agency
- Proprietary home health agency
- Voluntary home health agency

Barbara Walton Spradley and Judith Ann Allender
COMMUNITY HEALTH NURSING: CONCEPTS AND PRACTICE, 4th ed.
© 1996 Barbara Walton Spradley and Judith Ann Allender

Introduction

Home health care, broadly defined, refers to all the services and products provided to clients in their homes to maintain, restore, or promote their physical, mental, and emotional health. Its purpose is to maximize a client's level of independence and minimize the effects of existing disabilities through noninstitutional services; its primary goal is to use these supportive services to prevent institutionalization (Haddad and Kapp, 1991; Lindemann, 1992).

Aggregates of well, acutely ill, and chronically ill people of all ages have traditionally utilized home health services. However, today the health care needs among clients and families at home and the role of the nurse in home care is changing dramatically. Indeed, the entire picture of home health care is changing because of drastic shifts in financing, provider roles, and increasing client acuity (Rowland and Lyons, 1991; Woerner, Donnelly, and Edwards, 1993). Not only are the numbers of people needing home services growing rapidly, but the type of care is becoming increasingly complex. There are increasingly more dependent elderly and, correspondingly, a rise in the incidence of chronic illness. Early hospital discharges as a result of third-party payers' efforts toward cost containment have forced clients back into their homes and their communities to recuperate after surgeries or illnesses. These early discharges have resulted in the need for more home care and services. Moreover, these third-party payers require some procedures to be performed only on an outpatient basis, which also contributes to the need for increased at-home services.

Hospital stays for new mothers and their babies have been shortened to an average of 1 to 2 days, requiring home care to provide postpartum and infant care. Public awareness and demand for home services as an alternative to institutional care, broader third-party payment coverage for home care, and greater physician acceptance have all influenced the size and number of groups utilizing home health care. New technology and rising costs of hospital care have moved the care of acutely ill clients of all ages away from acute- and chronic-care facilities. Many clients also prefer to be cared for at home or in some other type of noninstitutional setting (Stricklin, 1993; Lepler, 1994). Such complex procedures as intravenous chemotherapy and pain management, parenteral nutrition, and mechanical ventilation, all of which were once only provided in hospitals or skilled-care facilities, are today routinely being provided and maintained at home.

Organizations Fostering Quality Home Health Care

Several prominent national organizations are involved with and particularly concerned about providing quality home health care. These include the Council of Home Health Agencies and Community Health Service, the National League for Nursing; the National Home Care Council; the National Association of Home Health Agencies; the Assembly of Outpatient and Home Care Institutions; and the American Hospital Association.

These organizations have agreed on the following goals and definitions of home health care: Home health service is that component of a continuum of comprehensive health care whereby services are provided to individuals and families in their home for the purpose of promoting, maintaining, or restoring health, or minimizing the effects of illness and disability. Services appropriate to the needs of the individual patient and family are planned, coordinated, and made available by an agency or institution that is organized for the delivery of health care through the use of employed staff, contractual arrangements, or a combination of administrative patterns (Dieckmann, 1988).

These goals could not have been easily set without the proactive groups whose members are concerned about the future of home care and hospice services. The National Association for Home Care (NAHC) is one such proactive group whose mission is to improve the quality of home health care (see Issues in Community Health Nursing display). Through a variety of publications and activities, the NAHC tries to inform and inspire home- and hospice-care providers in the community.

Historical Overview of Home Health Services

Early home health services in the United States were organized and administered by laypeople in the late 1800s. They provided nursing care and taught cleanli-

Issues in Community Health Nursing
THE MISSION OF THE NATIONAL ASSOCIATION OF HOME CARE

The purpose is to provide the following:

1. Serve as the unified voice for the home care and hospice community.
2. Provide directly needed services to the members.
3. Heighten the political visibility of home care and hospice interests.
4. Influence the legislative, judicial, and regulatory processes regarding issues of importance to hospice and home care.
5. Sponsor research and gather and disseminate home care and hospice data.
6. Promote home and hospice care as a viable component of the health care delivery system.
7. Foster, develop, and promote high standards of patient care at home and in hospice services.
8. Provide expert advice and assistance to members with respect to management, legal, or operational issues.
9. Disseminate information to the media and the general public to promote the acceptance of home care and hospice services and to support family/informal caregivers.
10. Expand private health insurance and other third-party sources for financing hospice and home care services.
11. Promote collaboration among national, state, and local organizations relating to home care and hospice services and issues.
12. Initiate, sponsor, and promote educational programs.
13. Represent the interests of caregivers (nurses, homemakers, home health aides, physicians, and therapists) who work in the home care field; and encourage individuals to choose a career in home care and hospice services.
14. Protect the legal rights of hospice and home care beneficiaries and those of the organizations and their employees who provide consumers with such services.
15. Promote independence to potential home care clients, thereby shattering the myth that dependence is a necessary state for the aged and disabled in America.

Reproduced by permission of the National Association of Home Care, from Homecare News. Not for further reproduction.

---

ness and home care techniques to the ill and their families. The Women's Branch of the New York City Mission in 1877 was first to employ a graduate nurse to deliver home care (Spiegel, 1983). Since then, nurses have played a primary role in home care. In 1900, home care was the dominant form of nursing in the United States; student nurses trained in hospitals, but they worked in the community. That trend persisted until the 1940s (Haddad and Kapp, 1991).

The Visiting Nurse Service of New York City, established in 1893 by Lillian Wald and Mary Brewster, was the first U.S.-organized home nursing service. The first government health department offering visiting-nurse care was the Los Angeles Health Department, established in 1898 (Spiegel, 1983). In 1909, through Lillian Wald's influence, the Metropolitan Life Insurance Company began a home nursing service for its New York City policyholders that, by the 1920s, became a model for other insurance companies.

Home care continued to be a part of nursing practice as the nursing profession developed. Twenty visiting nurse agencies serving the urban poor were operating by 1900, and in 1912, again through the influence of Lillian Wald, the Red Cross initiated a visiting nurse service for rural communities. Service was provided to the sick, to well babies, and to school children. County health departments, too, were soon providing home nursing care in rural areas, with service delivery enhanced by the development of the automobile.

Before World War II physicians were actively involved in home care. The war, however, created a physician shortage, and for the sake of efficiency, clients came to physicians. The cost-effectiveness of this pattern prompted its continuance, leaving a gap in home care that was filled by a growing number of visiting nurse associations. (See Chapter 4 for a more detailed history of community health nursing in the United States.)

The first hospital-based home care program was founded in 1947 by Dr. E. M. Bluestone at Montefiore Hospital in New York City. That program resulted from the many people who had lengthy hospitalizations because of chronic illnesses. A team approach, utilized for posthospital acute care, began the concept of convalescent care in the home. The program was also unique in that services were not limited to the poor or the elderly. The first paraprofessional home services—**homemakers**—were also instituted then, bringing people to the clients' home to cook, clean, run errands, and do simple personal care services. By 1958, that program had added physical therapy, nutrition, and X-ray and laboratory services to the initial team of physicians, nurses, and social workers. Housekeeping and chores were provided indirectly through other community resources (MacNamara, 1982).

The passage of Medicare and Medicaid legislation in 1965 drastically changed the home health care delivery system. Before the creation of Medicare, most home care was provided by voluntary visiting nurse associations (VNAs). The majority of home care clients were elderly persons, suffering from various chronic conditions, whose greatest need was for nursing care complemented by some home health aide and homemaker services. Typical home care, before Medicare, included bathing the client, reviewing basic self-care practices, and perhaps providing vitamin B12 or insulin injections, or changing dressings for chronic ulcers. Payment came either from welfare or from personal payment based on a sliding scale subsidized by charity or the agency providing service. In 1960, 250 official agencies provided nursing care to the sick on a regular basis. By 1968 (after Medicare laws came into effect, July 1, 1966), 1328 public health nursing agencies—half of all official agencies—provided that service (Harris, 1994).

With the advent of Medicare, the payment source as well as client eligibility, the provision of home care, and the purpose of that care all changed. For the more than 70 years before Medicare, since Lillian Wald's establishment of the first visiting nurse service, nurses had successfully provided home care on their own to the sick, the disabled, and children. Prior to a federal payment system, physicians did not direct home care. It was not expected or necessary. The need for some kind of gatekeeper to ensure provision of services to those who truly needed them as well as political pressures from medical groups concerned about the impact Medicare would have on medical practice led the federal government to appoint physicians to direct the traditionally nonmedically directed home services. Home care became more narrowly defined as a substitute for costly, extended hospitalization, and became a medical-based model of practice (Kaye, 1992).

Eligibility for Medicare reimbursement of home care costs is carefully defined and is based on patients' acute care conditions. Patients must be **homebound** (that is, someone has much difficulty and needs a great deal of assistance when leaving the house), need skilled care (medically directed service given by a nurse or other professional), and be under the treatment of a physician. Furthermore, the referring physician must plan, review, and certify as necessary the care to be given.

The medical model radically changed what had been historically the mission of home health care. Previously, home services sought to provide nursing care, assistance, and support. Community health problems, after Medicare's advent, were viewed as medical problems whose solution was disease eradication. Home care became medical care in the home. This view overlooked the need for preventive and health-promoting services and discounted the need homebound clients have for support services. Physicians and policymakers did not seem truly aware of the range of health needs clients had in the home (Neiman, et al. 1986). Somehow the assumption was made that if people could go home from the hospital, they had no need for supplemental assistance to manage meals, laundry, shopping, cleaning, and psychosocial support. Home services during those years still included health promotion, health teaching, and holistic family care. Medicare and Medicaid, however, did not cover these services; instead public health agencies provided the services without charge, or the services were delivered by **voluntary home health agencies**. Voluntary agencies have no mandates and can offer services of their own choosing. They do not receive government funding for many of the services provided. Services are offered on a set fee-for-service, sliding-scale, as a free service, or any combination thereof.

The passage of Medicare also influenced the structure of home care services. For the first time, home care agencies, in order to receive Medicare reimbursement, were required to provide one other service in addition to nursing. This service could be physical therapy, occupational therapy, speech therapy, social services, or home health aide services.

The total number of home care agencies actually declined shortly after the implementation of Medicare in the late 1960s. Many smaller **proprietary home health agencies** (freestanding for-profit agencies) went out of business because they could not develop the service scope and complexity required. This led to the growth of public home health agencies or **official agencies** (those supported by tax dollars and mandated to offer a particular group of services), and **hospital-based home health agencies** (operating units or departments of a hospital that provide home health care to discharged clients).

During the first decade after the passage of Medicare, those agencies that met the standards increased by 71%. The greatest growth was in hospital-based agencies. The number of proprietary agencies did not significantly increase until the early 1980s when it was assured that Medicare would pay for home care services. Even then, many functioned with limited budgets and failed as business ventures or consolidated with other more-profitable agencies. Table 22.1 depicts the differences among three main types of agencies: official, hospital-based, and proprietary.

It was evident by the early 1980s that the home health care movement provided a needed service to clients. Third-party payers, primarily Medicare, reimbursed agencies for selected services and home health care agencies were increasingly employing more nurses. That was a new role with new responsibilities for both hospital-based nurses and community health nurses who were making the change to home health care. The American Nurses Association (ANA), in their attempt to assist nurses to fulfill the profession's obligation to provide quality care to consumers, has established standards of practice for home health nursing. These are based on the Standards of Community Health Nursing Practice developed in 1973 (and revised in 1986) by the ANA's Division of Community Health Nursing Practice. The Standards of Home Health Nursing Practice (see Issues in Community Health Nursing display) represent agreed-on levels of practice and have been developed to characterize, to measure, and to provide guidance in achieving excellence in care (ANA, 1986).

From an historical perspective, the escalation in home health care would seem to suggest that health care is back where it started—in the home. Health care originated in the home and moved to the hospital with the advent of technology and improved diagnostic and treatment modalities. As the technologies became more expensive and the funding system to hospitals changed in the 1980s, hospitalized patients began leaving the hospital earlier. Such changes created a new emphasis on care in the home, primarily to control costs. However, opinion polls show an overwhelming consumer preference for home care over equivalent care provided in an institution (NAHC, 1991). Although home care is in the spotlight, its mission, services, financing, and providers have all changed.

The Current Home Care Population

The elderly are the largest portion of the U.S. population who use home care. Half of all home care recipients are older than 65 (Stulginsky, 1993). However, this

TABLE 22.1. *Agency Descriptions and Funding Sources*

Official Agency	Hospital Based Agency	Proprietary Agency
Mandated to offer a particular group of services and supported by tax dollars	Has no mandates, can offer services of their own choosing, no tax support to the agency and is an operating unit or department of a hospital	A free standing for-profit home care agency, services are provided based on third-party reimbursement schedules or by self pay
EXAMPLES		
City and county health departments e.g. Madera County Health Department, Madera, California, and the Health Services Agency of Fresno County.	St. Agnes Medical Center, Fresno, CA has: St. Agnes Home Health, Private Care Home Services, and San Joaquin Healthcare, Inc. (each provides a different set of home care services)	National chains/franchised agencies: Nurses Calling, Kimberly Care or locally/regionally and operated agencies: Best Care Home Health Care, in California and Interim Healthcare of Fresno, CA.

Any agency can provide home health care services. However, third-party payment (Medicare, Medicaid, or private insurance companies) depends on the mix of services available that is offered by a variety of licensed staff or contracted specialists.

Issues in Community Health Nursing
AMERICAN NURSES ASSOCIATION HOME HEALTH STANDARDS OF CARE

In the ANA publication, *Standards of Home Health Care,* each standard is followed by a rationale, structure criteria, process criteria, and outcome criteria (ANA, 1986).

Standard:

1. **Organization of home health services**—All home health services are planned, organized, and directed by a master's-prepared professional nurse with experience in community health and administration.
2. **Theory**—The nurse applies theoretical concepts as a basis for decisions in practice.
3. **Data collection**—The nurse continuously collects and records data that are comprehensive, accurate, and systematic.
4. **Diagnosis**—The nurse uses health assessment data to determine nursing diagnoses.
5. **Planning**—The nurse develops care plans that establish goals. The care plan is based on nursing diagnoses and incorporates therapeutic, preventive, and rehabilitative nursing actions.
6. **Intervention**—The nurse, guided by the care plan, intervenes to provide comfort; to restore, improve, and promote health; to prevent complications and sequelae of illness; and to effect rehabilitation.
7. **Evaluation**—The nurse continually evaluates the client's and family's responses to interven-

tions in order to determine progress toward goal attainment and to revise the data base, nursing diagnoses, and plan of care.

8. **Continuity of care**—The nurse is responsible for the client's appropriate and uninterrupted care along the health care continuum, and therefore uses discharge planning, case management, and coordination of community resources.
9. **Interdisciplinary collaboration**—The nurse initiates and maintains a liaison relationship with all appropriate health care providers to assure that all efforts effectively complement one another.
10. **Professional development**—The nurse assumes responsibility for professional development and contributes to the professional growth of others.
11. **Research**—The nurse participates in research activities that contribute to the profession's continuing development of knowledge of home health care.
12. **Ethics**—The nurse uses the code for nurses established by the American Nurses' Association as a guide for ethical decision making in practice.

Reprinted with permission from American Nurses Association. (1986). *Standards of Home Health Nursing Practice.* Washington, DC.

group receives 78% of the home visits, averaging 22.3 home health visits a year (Keating and Kelman, 1988). In a report (NAHC, 1991) of home care statistics, the number of institutionalized and noninstitutionalized persons with health problems severe enough to require assistance with such activities of daily living (ADLs) as eating, toileting, dressing and bathing, is estimated between 9 million and 11 million. Only a few are in institutions (16% or 1.7 million). The vast majority live in the community (84% or 8.9 million). These people are of all ages. However, the need for assistance rises sharply with age. Between the ages of 65 and 74, about one in ten need help, but half of those 85 and older

need help. Two-thirds of all home care clients are women, and approximately one-third of all home care patients live alone. These elderly can avoid institutionalization by receiving help with their personal care.

Along with the elderly and the chronically ill, recently hospitalized acute-care patients also need home care. Although there are no exact figures on the size of this group, it is increasing rapidly. Rising hospital costs and prospective payment incentives motivate an early hospital discharge. In addition, technological advances have made it possible to administer complicated procedures in the home. Such advances contribute to a growing population of home care recipients (Davis, et al., 1993; Stulginsky, 1993: Twardon and Gartner, 1992).

Many of these are elderly persons who have been hospitalized with an acute illness or disability and need convalescent home care. Others who need home care include babies and children with disabilities or adults sent home needing various involved therapies (Figure 22.1). An increasing number of AIDS clients, of all ages, also need home care. Due to a better understanding of these clients' needs and advances in medications and treatments to prolong life, more AIDS clients receive intermittent home care services for extended periods of time (Stanhope and Knollmueller, 1992).

Another subpopulation receiving home services are residents in continuing care centers or retirement communities who have "wellness nurses" available to them.

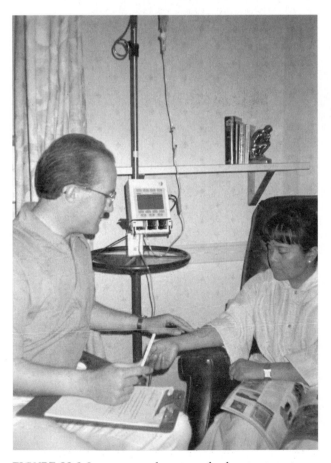

FIGURE 22.1 Intravenous therapy and other treatments are routinely administered in the home, serving the needs of a home care population that spans all ages.

A wellness nurse is employed by the continuing care center and makes home visits to residents. The goal of the service is to maintain the health of the residents by providing continuity of care, encouraging participation in educational programs, and monitoring their health status (Petit, 1994).

Specific services that are available within each setting are defined by the philosophy of each retirement community. However, the wellness nurse has a unique opportunity to practice autonomous case-management with healthy older adults. In this role the nurse functions as consultant, adviser, teacher, triage nurse, and friend. It is the nurse who regularly sees the residents and manages the care of each client in coordination with other disciplines. Such healthy individuals do not need medical care primarily, but have concerns about their health and well-being. They are receptive to health-promotion and illness-prevention strategies and use services such as diagnostic testing and screening (blood-pressure monitoring, for instance); educational counseling in such areas as nutrition information; support for daily living, including home maintenance and housekeeping; and illness prevention that might include information on exercise, stress management, and adapting to the trauma of relocation.

The concept of continuing care centers is not new. There are about 800 in the United States, housing more than 250,000 residents (see Chapter 21). That number is expected to double by the year 2000 (Garland, 1992), with new opportunities for the home care nurse and the community health nurse.

Other groups also benefit from this wellness approach, such as parents of infants and young children (see Chapter 18); children and teens (see Chapter 19); and the adult working population (see Chapter 20). Actually the entire population of a community can benefit from some form of wellness education. The hospitalized client, and frequently family members, are given explicit discharge instructions about medications, treatments, or dressings in order to continue the recovery process.

For the hospitalized client, wellness is part of the client's discharge plan when the client leaves the acute care setting. Ideally, discharge planning should start before admission and focus on continuing the care at the level needed as the client makes the transition to home. That should be a smooth transition with no gaps in services and with all involved (client, family, and/or other care givers) adequately prepared for managing the recovery process at home. (See Discharge Planning Matrix).

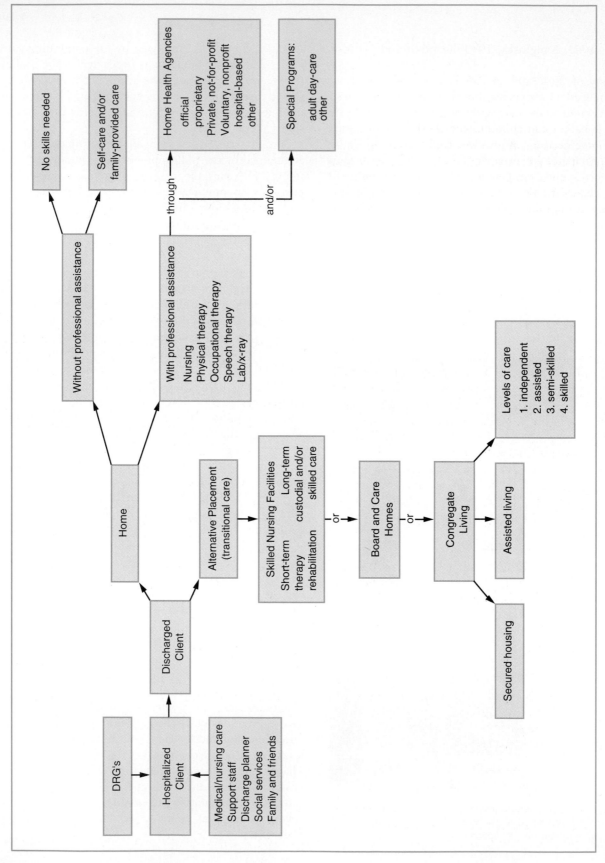

Discharge Planning Matrix.

Needs of the Home Health Care Population

The major subgroup of home health service recipients are older than age 65. Their home health needs fall into five categories: chronic illness and disability care, social support and interaction, alternative housing options, personal services and day care needs, and financial support or reimbursement.

CHRONIC ILLNESS AND DISABILITY CARE

The most common diagnoses of elderly home care clients are cancer, diabetes, cardiovascular disease, and chronic obstructive pulmonary disease (COPD). Each is chronic, degenerative, and disabling. Each can lead to progressive pathology and deterioration with the increased possibility of complications and growing dependency needs. The majority (80%) of older adults older than age 65 live with at least one chronic illness, and many with a combination of several acute and chronic illnesses and disabilities. Older adults, for example, may have arthritis and hypertension in addition to cancer or diabetes. The complexity of their conditions leads to a greater variety of home care service needs.

SOCIAL SUPPORT AND INTERACTION

Meaningful contact with people is a basic human need, especially of the homebound elderly, many of whom live alone. Social supports are a vital component of home care. Research demonstrates that when such support is present, people are less prone to depression and live longer (Burke and Walsh, 1992; Miller, 1995)—a fact that should make a comprehensive social assessment part of home care providers' overall needs assessments(Stanhope and Knollmueller, 1992). Additionally, there is the need for an informal network of help from friends and family members. This network, which is vital for many older adults, helps them remain independent.

ALTERNATIVE HOUSING OPTIONS

Because families are scattered geographically and unable to care for their elderly relatives and because people are living longer, group or congregate living for the mostly independent older adult fills an important need. Minor supervision or assistance with activities of daily living are available in a variety of housing options. (See Chapter 21 for detailed discussions of these options for older people.) Residents can assist one another with tasks, meals may be taken in the company of others, recreation and other activities are planned, transportation is provided, and a nurse is often available or on call. Such family-type housing enables older people to live independently for a longer period of time. In continuing-care retirement centers, as the resident ages and becomes more dependent, semi-skilled and skilled nursing care options are available within the housing community.

PERSONAL SERVICES AND DAY CARE NEEDS

A large number of elderly persons need assistance with personal care or instrumental activities of daily living (IADL). These include preparing meals, doing laundry, shopping, bathing, house cleaning, and being transported to health and personal care services, such as to a physician, dentist, or hairdresser. Many elders in institutions would be living at home if their personal care needs could be met there. Home is where the older adult wants to be, and when the appropriate home care services are provided they will be the happiest at home.

Home care also serves to keep families together and to save the government billions of dollars (Halamandaris, 1988). Sometimes home care needs are met voluntarily by relatives, a spouse, or friends. This is not without sacrifices, however. For millions of families, home care is a heavy burden. Frequently family members give up jobs and sacrifice the quality of their own home life to provide the care-giving needs of a dependent family member. Most often the care giver is a middle-aged daughter who is in the "sandwich generation" (caught between the demands of her children and the demands of her aged parents). That can leave the family exhausted, resentful, and unable to give further care (Pollack, 1993). Support for these families is much needed.

In 1989 almost three-quarters of severely disabled elders receiving home care services relied solely on family members or other unpaid help (NAHC, 1993). And as recently as 1992 two-thirds of Americans who needed long-term care in their homes did not get professional help, according to a Families USA study (Pollack, 1993). Adult day care services for elders who are cared for at home rather than in an institution helps families with frail elders at home.

The day care alternative provides respite for family members who need a break from the stress of care giving or for those who fear for the safety of an elder left alone. In addition, with adult day care, family members can continue to work and still keep an older family member within the family unit. Day care centers for older adults provide supervision, social activities, meals and snacks, and rest periods. At some centers, outings, educational sessions, and interaction with children in day care are options for elders who can tolerate or desire more stimulation. These centers are ideal for the frail elderly or older adult with Alzheimer's disease who may not be safe at home alone during the day while the family is away. Day care may be the deciding factor between living at home and being institutionalized. Frequently home care providers can deliver their services to clients while they are in these centers; especially the services provided by nurses, physical therapists, and speech therapists. See Issues in Community Health Nursing display.

FINANCIAL SUPPORT OR REIMBURSEMENT

Insurance programs servicing elders frequently do not pay for medications, eyeglasses, preventive podiatry, and dentistry. Because these services are not paid for, elderly persons with limited resources often do not seek out such care. Lack of proper glasses, medications, or other necessary care can compromise the safety of older adults and can even cause new and possibly life-threatening health problems or can exacerbate chronic illnesses, all of which can lead to institutionalization.

Home Health Care Services

Home health services vary depending on the recipient's age and health conditions. Both chronic and acute care conditions require assistance that can be divided into three categories: (1) professional services, (2) support services, and (3) supplies and equipment.

A professional interdisciplinary team of nurses, physicians, aides, and physical, respiratory, speech, and occupational therapists are needed to meet the home-

Issues in Community Health Nursing
REIMBURSEMENT PARAMETERS DETERMINE SERVICE

Because many home care services are still not reimbursable by third-party payers, the quality of care is much less than it should be. Rather than offering quality family- and community-centered care, it has become a business in which care is determined by reimbursable services. As a result, services are narrowly focused on short-term skilled care that follows reimbursement policies. Frequently nurses contracted to work in home health agencies do not have the public health background to respond to the variety of problems presented by most clients, especially the elderly. "Long-term health maintenance, chronic illness management, preventative health care, and the focus on the family have been abandoned." (Benson and McDevitt, 1994)

Because older adults are most in need of the broad array of home health care services, they are most at risk for being denied needed services. Health care professionals are not making decisions about nursing care. Decisions that should be made by nurses are being made by insurance actuaries and other for-profit motivated business-people.

Nurses have an opportunity to rekindle their skills of client advocacy and to develop skills of negotiator and arbitrator of services rather than merely being gatekeepers of the present system. Political activism at local, regional, state, and national levels is needed from individual nurses and all nurses as a group so their voices are heard by the policy makers and holders of the purse-strings.

bound's first category of needs and are a major component of home health care. These needs include health teaching, psychosocial support, and prevention or reduction of disability.

Support personnel (such as social workers, ministers, and family members) and services (such as pharmaceutical, transportation, homemaker and nutritional services) fill other vital areas of need. Important additional services may include data and claims processing, legal, and home protection and safety services.

Home care clients also frequently need supplies and equipment. An increasing number of new products, generated by new technologies, are available to maintain ill or disabled people at home (Davis, et al, 1993; Ferrell, et al., 1993; Lindemann, 1992). They include oxygen and respiratory services and durable medical equipment, such as wheelchairs, lifts, and walkers. Rehabilitation equipment can include an exercise "horse" or hand grips. Nursing care supplies, such as dressings, decubiti cushions and treatments, or catheters, are frequently used along with such supplies as disposable syringes and equipment needed for intravenous therapy, inhalation and aerosol devices, oxygen concentrators, or needleless insulin injectors. Nutritional supplies for oral and total parenteral nutrition, phototherapy units for infants with elevated bilirubin levels, and home peritoneal dialysis equipment are needed for a growing segment of the home health care population.

Well clients have a different set of needs. Home nursing care focuses on health-promoting and illness-preventing activities including diagnostic screening, educational counseling and information, daily living support services, and illness-prevention services (such as exercise guidance and weight and stress control). This requires supplies and equipment such as products for self-diagnosis and screening and for self-treatment, vitamin and nutritional supplements, exercise equipment, products that assist in the activities of daily living, and communications and security devices.

Designing Relevant Home Health Services

Assessing clients' home health needs is essential for appropriate program development. A growing body of research data is shedding light on this area, and nurses should be aware of this information. Further research and community needs assessment should be conducted to ensure home care services are appropriately focused.

Home health care, when efficiently organized with good backup services and based on standards of care, is a highly cost-effective way of caring for people in the community. The following are examples and studies that have demonstrated the cost savings of special home

care programs that all third-party payers still do not accept as standard practice.

■ The Maryland Medicaid program reported a 76% reduction in the health care costs of a 2 year old Maryland boy with AIDS who was able to receive home care in place of hospital care. The cost was only $531 a day at home (for 24 hours of nursing to administer oxygen, IV's, and 37 medications) compared to $2,263 a day in the hospital (Goldstein, 1993).

■ In a study of respiratory technology-dependent children cared for at home rather than in an institution, the findings revealed an average annual savings per patient of $79,074 (Fields, et al., 1991).

■ In a study by Olds (1992), a home-visitation program for low-income women and children pays for itself by the time the children are 4 years old. The program includes home visitation by a nurse during pregnancy, during the child's first 2 years of life, and free transportation for regular prenatal and well-child visits. The program costs about $3,200 for 2 years of home visitation. During the 4 years after the delivery of their first child, low-income women who participated in the program used $3,300 less in government services than those not in the program.

■ Lewin/ICF (1991) studied differences between the cost and effectiveness of inpatient care plus home care and a shorter inpatient stay and more home care for patients hospitalized with a hip fracture, COPD, or ALS with pneumonia. Findings indicate that for all three diagnoses, substituting inpatient days with more home care days reduced costs by $2,300 for hip fracture clients, $520 for COPD clients, and $300 for ALS clients.

Many critically needed services are not reimbursable by third-party payers. These include home safety assessment, extensive family medications review, care adapted to the home setting, and coordination of care with medical and other community resources. Such deficiencies continue to exist in the reimbursement system for home health services. Hopefully, a restructured health care delivery system will alleviate these deficiencies and allow third-party reimbursement for special home care services.

A quantitative formula for analyzing community needs for home care services is helpful in program development. This formula enables the home service planner to estimate the number of potential clients in a given service area by examining the elderly population, acute care discharged patients, and those inappropriately placed in skilled or intermediate care nursing facilities. Use of a formula becomes more complex, however, as one agency competes with other agencies to provide care in the same service area to a given number of potential clients.

Planning for effective home health services must recognize that the majority of clients have chronic conditions compounded by periodic acute episodes. A diversified service system must meet this range of needs. However, reimbursement rules and other regulations affect home care planning and delivery (Woerner, et al., 1993). For example, a typical home health agency may include two service divisions—home health care and private care with each division offering similar services but each being financed differently. Home health care includes: intermittent nursing services, extended 24-hour on-call services, client education, medical social services, homemaker and home health aides, nutritional consultation, durable medical equipment, and rehabilitative services such as physical therapy. Private services include all home health care services, but might also provide 24-hour nursing, home health aide, or homemaker services. Ideally the family has a third-party payer that will cover the majority of the costs; however, that is rare and most frequently the client or family pays for these extended services out of their own pockets.

In order to compete with other agencies, a home health agency may provide the following additional special services:

- *Hospice care* includes emotional support and instituting resources for clients in the final stage of life and for their families. Hospice benefits cover such things as continuous care, respite care, and bereavement counseling.
- *Long-term care* typically includes meals delivered to the home, family care, and primary home care (personal care, housekeeping, meal preparation, and other home chores).
- *Mental health care* may involve intermittent home visits by psychiatric nurses, group supportive services (for clients and/or families), transportation services, and other assistance needed to maintain psychiatric clients in the community (Hellwig, 1993).

Third-party payers usually do not pay for social workers or nutritionists (Woerner et al,. 1993). An agency needs to be financially sound and managed efficiently in order to provide these services.

Cost containment, as a motivating factor in all areas of the health care delivery system, enables home health agencies to partner with the community and develop innovative services. Health care providers in decision-making positions need to be committed to finding alternatives to institutionalization. Clients can be better served by packaging diverse services that meet a much broad range of needs. As a result, billions of dollars spent on inpatient care can be saved. Unfortunately, the traditional medically oriented, single-purpose skilled services offered by home care agencies under Medicare is not meeting all the home care client's needs.

Ideally, home health services are centrally coordinated by health professionals and operated by a case management system based on assessed clients' needs. A case manager may or may not provide direct care and serves as the designated person to see that clients receive needed home care and supportive services (NAHC, 1993). Providing continuity of care between an institution, such as the hospital, nursing home, or long-term care facility, and the home, is part of this case management approach, as is assigning appropriate services and resources through formal and informal supports and activities (Kaye, 1992). (See World Watch display that follows.)

Current Status of Home Health Services

Home health services are on the cutting edge of change in health care provision. Spurred by multiple forces, home care is growing rapidly. Depending on the source quoted, home health services are expanding 12% to 15% a year (FIND/SVP, 1992; Health Care Reform Update, 1993). That growth is expected to continue well into the 21st century, as baby boomers reach old age. One major force is cost-containment pressures by government and third-party payers and employers who appreciate home care's lower costs. Research continues to be needed to substantiate these cost-cutting claims. Several previously mentioned studies have already demonstrated that costs are cut when home care is used to shorten hospitalizations.

Another force for change is the growth of an aging population with increasing dependency needs. In addi-

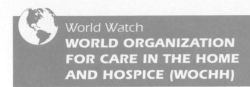

The first meeting of the World Organization for Care in the Home and Hospice (WOCHH) met in Bermuda in June 1993. Twelve countries sent delegates—Australia, Belgium, Bermuda, Canada, Egypt, France, Japan, the Netherlands, Saudi Arabia, Sweden, the United Kingdom, and the United States. The representatives from these countries acted as a steering committee for WOCHH, making all policy decisions including involvement and participation of other countries. The major purposes of WOCHH were identified and include data gathering and information sharing; influencing public policy, education, training, and quality assurance; and increasing public awareness.

The creation of WOCHH is in recognition that the world is becoming a smaller place—not of national markets, but global one in which the concerns of one nation become the concerns of the world. The steering committee is developing plans for the first World Assembly on Home Care in 1997 and will present them in concert with the World Health Organization (NAHC Annual Report, 1993).

tion, hospitals and nursing homes will eventually be unable to manage the load created by the rising number of elderly people needing medical attention. Fewer family caregivers are available since more women work outside the home (Callahan, 1988). Also, consumers are better educated and concerned about health care. As a result, clients are demanding greater satisfaction and a better quality of life, and care in the home needs to respond to these desires. A final force of growing significance in home health care is the impact of medical and computer technology. Advanced equipment design, electronics, and communication systems have the potential for enabling the ill and disabled to live near-normal lives outside institutions with home services as the sustaining intermediary.

The increased demand for home health care has also increased the number and variety of agencies providing services. No longer is home care the sole province of public health nursing agencies and visiting nurse associations (VNAs). According to the National Association for Home Care's inventory of home care agencies (1993), as of August 1993, 6902 home health agencies were certified by Medicare in the United States, which is an all-time high. However, 6231 noncertified home health agencies, home care aide organizations, and hospices remain outside Medicare for a variety of reasons. Some do not provide the services that Medicare covers. Other noncertified agencies are potentially eligible to participate in Medicare but choose to limit their services to private-paying patients (NAHC, 1993).

Hospital-based and proprietary agencies have grown faster than any other type of certified agency and now comprise more than a third of all certified agencies. That differs markedly from the industry composition in the early 1980s, when public health agencies dominated, and only one-fourth of the total were hospital-based or proprietary agencies (NAHC, 1993). By 1993, approximately 14,000 home care or hospice providers were operating in the United States. Medicare added hospice benefits in 1983, 10 years after the first hospice started in the United States. The number of Medicare certified hospices has grown from 31 in 1984 to 1288 in 1993 (NAHC, 1993).

Hospital expansion into home care is viewed as a logical extension of hospital services. One reason is that continuity of care can be maintained for clients. Another is that hospital staff are better trained to handle the demands of highly technical and skilled care now required in many home care situations. Finally, as hospitals retool their services to remain competitive, expanding into the home care market is an economic necessity. Escalating costs and a declining census are forcing many hospitals to explore alternative revenue sources, with home care being one of them.

Proprietary, for-profit agencies form the other fastest-growing group moving into home care. More than 2400 home health agencies were privately owned in 1993 (NAHC, 1993). Some are locally owned and operated and serve one area. Others, however, are large organizations with franchises or extensions in communities throughout the nation, such as Upjohn, Kimberly, and VIVRA. The proprietary companies have created businesses that supply the majority of home care personnel throughout the nation. Pharmaceutical companies, insurance companies, temporary staffing agencies, nursing homes, and many others have entered the competitive and mushrooming field of home care. Even some durable medical equipment and supply companies have expanded into providing skilled nursing and other comprehensive services in the home.

Home care services in the past were generally provided by non-profit agencies while the for-profit sector sold home care equipment and supplies. These patterns have changed. The traditional equipment and supply companies see an opportunity for financial profit in offering services, and the non-profit providers find the supply and service market, which offers even higher profit margins, financially attractive. Hospitals are important customers of supply companies. To avoid direct competition, many supply companies are attempting joint ventures with hospitals.

Home health care has become synonymous with both acute care and intensive at-home care (Weinstein, 1993). Advanced-practice nurses are needed to address the increasing complexity and acuity found in the home setting (dela Cruz, et al., 1991; Twardon and Gartner, 1992). Examples of the complexity and acuity follow.

Total parenteral nutrition (TPN) is performed in the home and until the 1990s was the fastest-growing home care service. Home TPN was introduced about 15 years ago as a technique to facilitate hospital discharge of those patients whose primary reason for hospitalization was parenteral nutrition support. TPN uses intravenous feeding to sustain people who have intestinal obstructions and digestive disorders and is occasionally used for those who need this form of feeding during the postoperative period.

In the 1990s clients with AIDS have become a new and growing group needing home care services. In 1993 more than 250,000 cases of AIDS were reported to the Centers for Disease Control and Prevention (Centers for Disease Control and Prevention, 1993). That number is projected to grow through the year 2010. People living with AIDS (PLWA) prefer the home care alternative, which also reduces acute care use and cost (Ungvarski, et al., 1994). In addition to a thorough HIV/AIDS home care assessment (Ungvarski and Nokes, 1992), AIDS clients need antibiotics for life-time suppressive therapy that necessitates medication-therapy compliance as well as medication instruction. Polypharmacy, or multiple drug therapy, used for organ/system-specific problems and the inherent drug interaction potential require the home care nurse to be alert to medication information, supervision, and administration. Home care nurses also must be knowledgeable in the areas of nutrition, rehabilitation therapy, specific treatments ordered, use of the necessary equipment and supplies, family support, the need for legal assistance, housing needs, spiritual needs,

and palliative and hospice care during the terminal stage of AIDS. This is a broad range of services, and as the number of AIDS cases increases, home care nurses will be challenged with planning the nursing care for this population.

People chronically ill with cancer make up another aggregate needing home health care services. Home intravenous cancer chemotherapy services allow clients to remain in the comfort of their homes while receiving care. Billions of health care dollars can be saved by home care for clients with cancer. This involves the use of home intravenous chemotherapy as well as home hospice services.

There are issues yet to be approached in providing home care services. While cost savings have been clearly demonstrated in studies of home care, additional questions need to be addressed. For example, care of a severely disabled person in the home may appear less costly than in a nursing home, but one must consider the total impact—physically, emotionally, and financially—on family members and the community (Kemper, 1992; Wallace, 1990). When all things are considered, nursing home care in some instances may be less costly than maintaining people at home.

Another concern in home care is the issue of quality. The number of new agencies entering the field, many of which are choosing not to be certified by Medicare, has opened up the potential for reduced quality of services that are not subject to any standards of care. There is an increasing emphasis in the field on assuring quality home care services (ANA, 1986; Lalonde, 1988; Stricklin, 1993; Taylor et al., 1991; Twardon and Gartner, 1991), including recognition of homebound clients' rights (see Issues in Community Health display that follows). Closely tied to the quality issue is the problem of fragmented and overlapping services, which emphasizes the need for coordination and case management.

Future Needs of Home Health Care Clients

The home care recipient of the future will be sicker and older. In 1989, 31 million people in the United States were older than age 65, and the Census Bureau projects that number to double by the year 2050 with those older than 85 making up 25% of the aged population (NAHC, 1991). As stated earlier, half of those older

Issues in Community Health Nursing
A HOME HEALTH CARE CLIENT'S BILL OF RIGHTS

Licensed and accredited home health care agencies must provide written statements of clients' rights similar to the one that follows. Clients are given information about whom to call if they have questions or comments.

As a patient receiving services from Personal Care Health Services, you are entitled to be informed of your rights, which are summarized below:

■ You have the right to expect fully qualified and experienced personnel to meet your individual home health needs.

■ You have the right to be informed of the information contained in your medical record unless medically contraindicated by your physician, as well as to be involved in the plan of treatment devised to meet your individual needs.

■ You have the right to be respected as an individual and to have major responsibility for making decisions on your own personal health care.

■ You and your family have the right to be instructed in your health care needs so that health management can continue at an optimal level when services are discontinued.

■ You have the right to refuse service, or accept or reject health teachings or treatments, but you must be informed of the medical consequence should you choose to reject the health care.

■ You have the right to privacy concerning your own medical care as well as confidentiality in all communications and records relating to your care, exclusive to designated authorized personnel.

■ You have the right to complete access to your own health care record on request.

■ You have the right to be informed of the procedures regarding complaints and to be assured of confidentiality when registering them.

■ You have the right to be fully informed of the services that are available, including the fees for service, and the party who has the final responsibility for payment of services rendered.

It is the policy to provide a grievance process for prompt and equitable resolution of complaints including complaints based on discrimination due to race, color, creed, religion, sex, age, national origin, or handicap. If you feel that any of your rights have been denied or you have any questions, please call.

(Adapted from Personal Care Health Services Corp., Laguna Hills, Calif., Patient Rights and Responsibilities, 1994.)

---

than 85 need some assistance to live independently. Some project the number of disabled elderly will increase from 14 million to 24 million by 2060 (NAHC, 1991). That would greatly increase the demand for personnel to provide care at home, requiring the number of full-time homemakers or home health aides to increase from just under 200,000 in 1985 to about 484,000 in 2040 (NAHC, 1991). It is also estimated that by the year 2000, national home care spending will quadruple to between $30 billion and $35 billion to meet the service needs of this increasingly older population (NAHC, 1992a). These are, however, projected costs based on the percentages of older adults that use formal services now. If more services become accepted as reimbursable by third-party payers, these projections may be vastly underestimated.

The second major change in the future home care population is that clients will continue to require increasingly technical services in the home. Surgeries will be more frequently performed in freestanding surgery centers or out-patient settings in which clients will do all of their recovering at home. During that recovery period the client may need professional monitoring, treatment, or care. The numbers of chronically ill clients dependent on ventilators, dialysis, IVs, and inhalation and/or aerosol therapies, massive and/or continuous complex dressing changes, and central-line medication or nutrition will also increase by the year 2000. As a result, the need for registered nurses will increase by 39%, primarily in the home care industry (Halamandaris, 1991). Home care and long-term care settings will be feeling the greatest impact from the demand for these services. The health care delivery system in the United States, undergoing recent scrutiny and proposed changes, can no longer support the model of care that was typical during the 1960s through mid-1980s. The only certainty about the future of the health care delivery system is that change is inevitable, and the changes will include more technical health care being delivered at home.

Community Health Nursing and Home Care

The changing picture in home health services has significantly affected community health nursing. Community health nursing agencies were once the sole provider of home health care. Now hospitals are serving these clients. Medicare and other reimbursements for home care have generated a sizable portion of community health nursing agencies' budgets, but decreased referrals have diminished those revenues. When a client's Medicare benefits or third-party coverage is exhausted, clients are often referred to tax-supported public agencies rather than home health agencies so that they can still receive follow-up care.

The changing financial structure of home health services poses a dilemma for community health nursing agencies faced with a conflict in values between the competition and basic public health values. Although hospital-based agencies and other technologically skilled home care providers can offer important and necessary services to clients at home, their personnel are not as prepared to give holistic, family-focused, preventive, and health-promoting care that is essential for the health of this client population. Also, most home care providers are unable to offer this broader range of services because of their added expense and limited reimbursement schedule from Medicare and/or Medicaid (Benson and McDevitt, 1994).

Community health nurses demonstrate the value of assessment of client health status by using a functional level as a predictor of need rather than gauging need only by diagnostic category (Duffy and MacDonald, 1990; Stanhope and Knollmueller, 1992). Both the Visiting Nurse Service of Omaha and the Ramsey County Nursing Service of St. Paul have been using a function code system for determining client health status and ability to manage the activities of daily living. Providers and legislators have been debating for some time about the appropriateness of applying a classification system like Medicare's diagnosis-related groupings (DRGs) to community health clients (Phillips, et al., 1989). Research in home care client assessment is an area for greater community health nursing involvement (see Research in Community Health Nursing display).

HOME CARE ACCOUNTABILITY AND QUALITY IMPROVEMENT

Program evaluation of a home care agency is part of the cycle of program development and is critical to agency survival (Harris, 1994). Evaluation is an important phase of the nursing process as well. Evaluations involve conducting research within an agency to acquire information that can be compiled and analyzed to enhance the agency's functioning and client care outcomes based on outcome criteria. Nurses in home care agencies are asked to contribute to the evaluation process by assisting with its formulation or adhering to agency philosophy, developing client-outcome criteria, collecting client data, maintaining thorough records, serving on audit or quality assurance committees, conducting peer evaluations, and generally participating in the components of evaluation that give the agency feedback about the care clients receive. After discharge from the agency's service, clients complete questionnaires regarding their perception of care and their personal outcome. This completes the evaluation cycle. All of the information gathered by agency self-evaluation contributes to accountability and continuous quality improvement and is essential to agency existence, growth, and development. An agency, through its governing body, is accountable to the community that it serves. An effective program evaluation can establish accountability and assure quality care (Joint Commission on Accreditation of Healthcare Organizations, 1991; Sherman and Malkmus, 1994).

A continuous quality improvement program was established between the Visiting Nurse Association (VNAC) of Chicago and the University of Chicago Hospitals. The VNAC relied on the university hospitals as their main referral source. To assure that the discharged clients were getting quality care, the two agencies set up a joint quality improvement program (Leimnetzer et al., 1993). When hospitals and home health agencies work together using a continuous quality improvement partnership plan, they can meet accreditation criteria for both organizations by creating an interdisciplinary quality-improvement system. This promotes collaboration and successful client outcomes.

Research in Community Health Nursing
USING THE ALBRECHT NURSING MODEL IN HOME HEALTH

The Albrecht model proposes that the combined effects of three categories of elements in a home visit have direct and indirect effects on client outcomes. The elements are structural, modifying, and process in nature. In the study described, structural elements were client and family. The modifying element was client classification, and the process element was type of care. The model suggests that with the right combination of structure and process elements, clients have positive outcomes. Using this model helps predict the elements that contribute to the outcome of home visits.

A quantitative study consisted of 154 subjects with arthritis. A correlational and explanatory design with secondary analysis of data from a national study of the effectiveness of the Arthritis Foundation's "Bone up on Arthritis" program was used. The outcome of interaction among the three elements described in the Albrecht Model was measured on a seven-point scale by the subjects responding to the question, "How satisfied are you with your life as a whole these days?" A three-step multiple regression model was developed from nine structure, modifying, and process elements.

Findings showed that the subjects were predominately white women who were married and had at least a high school education, the diagnosis of arthritis was made within a mean of 11 years, and they were highly satisfied with the home study intervention. Each category of the Albrecht Model for home healthcare explained an additional significant portion of the variance in the client satisfaction. Gender and age were noted to be most significant.

Outcomes of this study demonstrate that nurses in home health care should provide leadership in developing cost-effective and satisfying self-care interventions for clients at home. Clients are becoming more involved in their own care, and home care nurses must search for various ways to provide innovative approaches that are both satisfying and meaningful to maintain clients at home.

(Albrecht, M., Goeppinger, J., Anderson, M. K., Boutaugh, M. Macnee, C., & Stewart, K. (1994). The Albrecht nursing model for home health care. *Journal of Nursing Administration, 23*(1), 51–54.)

THE COMMUNITY HEALTH NURSE AS CASE MANAGER

Community health nurses face new challenges and new roles in home care. The home care client population still has the same basic needs, but the changing health care delivery structure requires that nurses develop creative new ways of meeting them. One role that community health nurses are particularly well-suited for is case management (Cohen, 1991; Lamb and Stempel, 1994; Lepler, 1994). Many nurses with community health backgrounds are becoming certified case managers and working for case management companies. Professional Dynamics Inc., in Washington State and California, has case managers who do field work. "They go on-site to see people in a variety of settings—in the hospital, at home, or at work—rather than assessing and coordinating care solely by the telephone or working internally for a hospital or other facility as many of their colleagues do" (Lepler, 1994, p. 1, 21). This "bonding with patients" helps the patient feel more connected and less anxious. Coordination of needed services and resources and provision of continuity of care are critical elements of the case manager's role and essential to an effective home health program (Bower, 1992; Lyon, 1993).

With health care cost containment a national priority, the role of case manager will become increasingly important. As the shift to outpatient care continues, clients will be more frequently managed in homes, hospices, and other community settings, which makes coordinating care more difficult than when they were inpatients. Care can become fragmented and gaps or overlapping services can compromise the quality of care as well as the cost. A nurse needs a unique combination of skills to succeed in the role of case manager (Fig. 22.2). Most nurses agree that the case manager must combine clinical and psychosocial nursing skills with management, business, and financial acumen and excellent interpersonal skills to work with all those involved in a case (Lepler, 1994).

MANAGED CARE AND THE HOME CARE AGENCY

A final consideration for nursing is where the nurse fits into the concept of managed care. The managed care concept was initially thought of as a panacea for escalating costs, and doubts persist about its effectiveness (Anderson, 1993; NAHC, 1992b). The home care market is going to expand beyond that of which most people can imagine. Along with this growth will come increasing financial incentives for agencies to divert patients to low-cost providers through the use of case managers, gatekeepers, and care coordinators. However, the promised savings have not materialized, and the administrative costs of managed care programs are high.

A managed care environment in which all angles, including the physician, the hospital, and the home environment, are examined by insurance companies, forces

patients back home faster than in the past. Posthospital facilities and services are not expanding rapidly enough, and appropriate follow-up care is not always prescribed or paid for. Nurses who work as case managers for private companies (as mentioned in the previous section) as a part of the broad managed care scheme may be forced to provide care that is "managed" to reduce costs, yet the additional cost of having the nurse to manage the care only increases costs to the agency and jeopardizes the stability of that role.

It may be a no-win situation for the nurse in this new role if the benefits of a nurse within the managed care arena is not translated into savings for the provider who employs the nurse. The ethical dilemma of quality of care versus cost of care, and the question of whether both can exist together, will be an ongoing challenge for the nurse within the managed care environment of the future.

If managed care is to survive and indeed be cost effective, changes will have to occur. Large groups of physicians will probably band together to guarantee referrals and build a market share in proprietary agencies as well as in hospital-based agencies. People speculate about other changes, however, a change in the health care delivery system in the United States is inevitable. More people are eligible for services, which increases volume for hospitals at a time when downsizing has

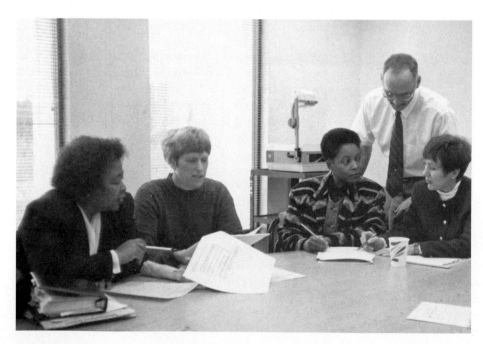

FIGURE 22.2 The case management role of the home health nurse involves working with health care team members to provide continuity of care.

been the focus. That increase will increase the number of clients into the home care system that is already growing at an alarming rate. This time of rapid change in the entire system of health care delivery provides new opportunities for nurses, demands that nurses be knowledgeable about the effects of these changes on client care, and that they must proactively determine their professional role in the system.

Summary

Many forces are influencing the current and future status of home health services. These forces include an increasing elderly population, a growing HIV/AIDS client population, advanced technology that allows more sophisticated care at home, rising costs of health care, and demands for consumer satisfaction. As the need for more home health care expands, so does the competition for services and products. Community health nursing programs, once the sole provider of home health care, are now one of many types of agencies that provide home health care. The fastest growing of these are hospital-based programs and proprietary for-profit home care programs.

The major target aggregates for home health services are the elderly, the disabled (those needing noninstitutionalized long-term care), patients recently discharged from acute care settings, and those interested in wellness and self-care. Home care programs provide a variety of services, including a multidisciplinary group of professionals, support personnel, and the variety of increasingly sophisticated equipment and supplies that are needed to maintain the care given at home.

A relevant system for home health services requires a proper needs assessment, and providers should plan diversified services to accommodate the complex and wide-ranging needs of this population. A full range of services includes home health, hospice, respite, and day care. Case management is a crucial factor for coordinating continuity of care.

Community health nursing faces a critical time of challenge and opportunity. Competing home health agencies are greatly influencing the number and type of clients that community health nurses normally serve. Changing financial structures and costs require that community health nursing develop new partnerships and innovative service delivery patterns. Case management techniques and managed care are critical services that allow agencies to improve continuity of care and to curtail spiraling costs. Also, the community health nurse's challenging role will include program evaluation and accountability, including conducting research and developing more effective ways to measure home care client needs, health status, and outcomes of care, for adequately meeting the needs of clients today and in the future.

Activities to Promote Critical Thinking

1. Assume you have been assigned to provide home care to a 75-year old woman with arthritis, hypertension, and chronic leukemia who lives alone. What are some general areas of information you will need to gather before beginning to plan her care? Contrast what her care will involve now with what it might have been 40 years ago.

2. As part of the planning team of your community health nursing agency, you are concerned about developing a comprehensive home health services system. What elements should you consider including? How would you determine the exact programs to include?

3. From the home care client population's point of view, quality of care is probably the most important criterion for home health services today. What are the needs of the homebound elderly and what actions might you take to ensure that these needs are met? Design a hypothetical home care program for an agency's elderly population.

REFERENCES

ANA. (1986). Standards of home health nursing practice. Washington, DC: American Nurses Publishing.

Anderson, P. A. (1993). Consider this . . . Making it in the managed care environment. *Journal of Nursing Administration, 23*(12), 7.

Benson, E. R., & McDevitt, J. Q. (1994). When third-party payment determines service: The elderly at risk. *Holistic Nursing Practice, 8*(2), 28–35.

Bower, K. Case Management by Nurses. (1992). Washington, DC: American Nurses Publishing.

Burke, M. M., & Walsh, M. B. (1992). *Gerontologic nursing: Care of the frail elderly.* St. Louis: Mosby Year Book.

Callahan, D. (1988). Families as caregivers: The limits of morality. *Archives of Physical Medicine and Rehabilitation, 69*(5), 323–28.

Centers for Disease Control and Prevention. (1993). *HIV/AIDS surveillance* (Report Vol. 5, No., pp. 1–22). Atlanta: Centers for Disease Control and Prevention.

Cohen, E. (1991). Nurse case management: Does it pay? *Journal of Nursing Administration, 20,* 20–25.

Davis, J. H., Berry, R. K., Lettow, J., & Foltin, J. J. (1993). An innovative preceptor program for intravenous home care nursing. *Journal of Intravenous Nursing. 16*(5), 287–292.

dela Cruz, F., Jacobs, A., & McCown, D. (1992). Home health care nursing: A clinical specialty in need of graduate education. *Home Healthcare Nurse, 10*(2), 44–50.

Dieckmann, J. (1988). Home health administration: An overview. In M. D. Harris (Ed.). *Home Health Administration.* Owings Mills, MD: National Health Publishing.

Duffy, M. E., and MacDonald, E. (1990). Determinants of functional health of older persons. *Gerontologist, 30,* 503.

Ferrell, B. R., Taylor, E. J., Grant, M., Fowler, M., & Corbisiero, R. M. (1993). Pain management at home: Struggle, comfort, and mission. *Cancer nursing, 16*(3), 169–178.

Fields, A. L., Rosenblatt, A., Pollack, M. M., & Kaufman, J. (1991). Home care cost-effectiveness for respiratory technology–dependent children. *American Journal of Disabled Children, 145,* 729–733.

FIND/SVP (1992). *The market for home care services.* New York: FIND/SVP.

Garland, S. (4 May, 1992). Homes with nursing that aren't nursing homes. *Business Week,* 182.

Goldstein, A. (1993). A tragedy in red tape—family wins 5 month battle to let gravely ill child die at home. Washington, DC: Washington Post, A1, A6.

Haddad, A. M. & Kapp, M. B. (1991). *Ethical and legal issues in home health care.* Norwalk, CN: Appleton & Lange.

Halamandaris, V. J. (1991). *Basic statistics about home care—1991.* Washington, DC: National Association for Home Care.

Halamandaris, V. J. (1988). The future of home care. In M. D. Harris (Ed.), *Home Health Administration.* Owings Mills: National Health Publishing.

Harris, A. D. (1994). Handbook of home health care administration. Gaithersburg: Aspen Publishers Inc.

Health Care Reform Update. (14 May, 1993). Home care industry to experience continued rapid growth, NAHC presi-

dent tells Wisconsin association. 1(9). *National Association for Home Care, 1,* 2.

Hellwig, K. (1993). Psychiatric home care nursing: Managing patients in the community setting. *Journal of Psychosocial Nursing, 31*(12), 21–24.

Joint Commission on Accreditation of Healthcare Organizations. (1991). *An introduction to quality improvement in health care.* Chicago: JCAHO.

Kaye, L. W. (1992). *Home health care.* Newbury Park: Sage Publications.

Keating, B. & Kelman, G. B. (1988). *Home health care nursing: Concepts and practice.* Philadelphia: Lippincott.

Kemper, P. (1992). The use of formal and informal home care by the disabled elderly. *Health Services Research, 27*(4), 421–51.

Lalonde, B. (1988). Assuring the quality of home care via the assessment of client outcomes. *Caring, 7*(1), 20–24.

Lamb, G. S. & Stempel, J. E. (1994). Nurse case management from the client's view: Growing as insider-expert. *Nursing Outlook, 42,* 7–13.

Leimnetzer, M. J., Ryan, D. A., & Neimann, V. G. (1993). The hospital-visiting nurse association *partnership. Journal of Nursing Administration, 23*(11), 20–23.

Lepler, M. (1994). In the field, case managers provide patient advocacy and streamlined care. *Nurseweek, 7*(16), 1,21.

Lewin/ICF. (1991). Economic analysis of home medical equipment services. Washington, DC: May 29, 1991.

Lindemann, C. (1992). Nursing and technology, moving into the 21st century. *Caring, 11*(9), 5–10.

Lyon, J. C. (1993). Models of nursing care delivery and case management: Clarification of terms. *Nursing Economics, 11,* 163–169.

MacNamara, E. (1982). Home care: Hospitals rediscover comprehensive home care. *Hospitals, 16*(21), 60–66.

Miller, C. A. (1995). *Nursing care of older adults: Theory and practice.* (2nd ed.). Philadelphia: Lippincott.

National Association for Home Care. (1991). *Basic statistics about home care—1991.* Washington, DC: National Association for Home Care.

National Association for Home Care. (1992a). *National home care spending to see record growth.* (Report No. 488, pp. 3–4).

National Association for Home Care. (1992b). *NAHC requests readers' advice on managed care.* (Report No. 480, p. 2).

National Association for Home Care. (1993, April 9). NAHC's Mission. *Homecare News,* 2.

National Association for Home Care. (1993, October). Home care: The people's choice. *Annual Report,* 22–24.

Neiman, E., et al. (1986). Bridging the gap: Hospital to home in a changing health care environment. *Emphasis on Nursing, 2*(1), 12–17.

Olds, D. L. (1992). Home visitation for pregnant women and parents of young children. *American Journal of Disabled Children, 146,* 704–708.

Petit, J. M. (1994). Continuing care retirement communities and the role of the wellness nurse. *Geriatric Nursing, 15,* 28–31.

Phillips, E. K., et al. (1989). DRG ripple and the shifting burden of care to home health. *Nursing and Health Care, 10*(6): 325–27.

Pollack, R. (1993). Long-term care at home: A heavy burden for millions of American families. Families USA Foundation (Press Release).

Rowland, D. & Lyons, B. (1991). Financing home care. Baltimore: Johns Hopkins University Press.

Sherman, J. J., & Malkmus, M. A. (1994). Integrating quality assurance and total quality management/quality improvement. *JONA, 24*(3): 37–41.

Speigel, A. D. (1983). *Home health care: Home birthing to hospice care.* Owings Mills, MD: National Health Publishing.

Stanhope, M. and Knollmueller, R. N. (1992). *Handbook of community and home health nursing.* St. Louis: Mosby Year Book.

Stricklin, M. V. (1993). Home care consumers speak out on Quality. *Home Healthcare Nurse, 11*(6), 10–17.

Stulginsky, M. M. (1993). Nurses' home health experience. Part I: The practice setting. *Nursing & health care, 14*(8), 402–407.

Taylor, A., Hudson, K., & Keeling, A. (1991). Quality nursing care: The consumer's perspective revisited. *Journal of Nursing Quality Assurance, 5*(2), 23–31.

Twardon, C., & Gartner, M. (1991). Empowering nurses: Patient satisfaction with primary nursing in home health. *Journal of Nursing Administration, 21*(11), 39–43.

Twardon, C., & Gartner, M. (1992). A strategy for growth in home care: The clinical nurse specialist. *Journal of Nursing Administration, 22*(10), 49–53.

Ungvarski, P. J., Schmidt, J., & Neville, S. (1994). Planning home care services for people living with AIDS. *Home Healthcare Nurse, 12*(2), 17–22.

Ungvarski, P., & Nokes, K. (1992). Community-based and long-term care. In J. H. Flaskerud, and P. J. Ungvarski (Eds.), HIV/AIDS: A guide to nursing care. (2nd ed., pp. 225–313). Philadelphia: Saunders.

Wallace, S. P. (1990). The no care zone: Availability, accessibility, and acceptability in community-based long-term care. *The Gerontologist, 30*, 254–261.

Weinstein, S. (1993). A coordinated approach to home infusion care. *Home Healthcare Nurse, 11*(1), 15–20.

Woerner, L., Donnelly, P., & Edwards, P. (1993). Challenges facing the home health care industry. *Nursing Dynamics, 2*(3), 5–8.

SELECTED READINGS

Bedrosian, C. A. (1988). *Home health nursing: Nursing diagnoses and care plans.* East Norwalk, CN: Appleton and Lange.

Bergen, A. (1991). Nurses caring for the terminally ill in the community: A review of the literature. *International Journal of Nursing Studies, 28*(1), 89–101.

Biegal, D. E., Sales, F., and Schulz, R. (1991). *Family caregiving in chronic illness.* Newbury Park: Sage Publications.

Brent, N. J. (1994). Healthcare reform: Implications for home healthcare nursing and agencies. *Home Healthcare Nurse, 12*(1), 10–11.

Buck, J. N. (1991). Planning for successful home health care. *Home Healthcare Nurse, 9*(1), 24–29.

Bull, M. J. (1994). Use of formal community services by elders and their family caregivers 2 weeks following hospital discharge. *Journal of Advanced Nursing, 19*(3), 503–508.

Chromiak, D. M. (1992). Referral sources in home healthcare. *Journal of Nursing Administration, 22*(12), 39–45.

Chubon, S. J. (1991). An ethnographic study of job satisfaction among home care workers. *Caring, 10*(4), 52–56.

Cline, B. A. (1990). Case management organizational models and administrative models. *Caring, 9*(7), 14–18.

Cloonan, P. A and Belyea, M. J. (1993). Limits of using patient characteristics in predicting home health care coordination. *Western Journal of Nursing Research, 15*(6), 742–751.

Cloonan, P. A., & Brodie, B. M. (1993). Home health care agencies: What constitutes success? *Nursing Economics, 11*(1), 29–33.

Coughlin, T., McBride, T., Perozek, M., & Liu, K. (1992). Home care for the disabled elderly: Predictors and expected costs. *Health Services Research, 27*(4), 453–479.

de Savorgnani, A. A., Haring, R. C., & Davis, H. (1992). A survey of home care aides: A personal and professional profile. *Caring, 11*(4), 28–32.

de Savorgnani, A. A., Haring, R. C., & Galloway, S. (1992). Caught in the middle: A profile of licensed practical nurses in home care. *Caring., 11*(9), 8–11.

de Savorgnani, A. A., Haring, R. C., & Galloway, S. (1993). Recruiting and retaining registered nurses in home healthcare. *Journal of Nursing Administration, 23*(6), 42–46.

Feldman, J., et al. (1988). *Patients and purse strings: The productivity, effectiveness, and efficiency of home care programs for the elderly.* (Vol. 2, Publication No. 201-2191, pp. 367–87). New York: National League for Nursing.

Gabe, M., & Gill-Forney, B. (1993). Reaching for the ideal in home care. *Home Healthcare Nurse, 11*(6), 30–34.

Glasheen, L. K. (1994). Homeward bound. *AARP Bulletin, 35*(8), 7, 11.

Goodwin, D. R. (1992). Critical pathways in home healthcare. *Journal of Nursing Administration, 22*(2), 35–40.

Helberg, J. L. (1993). Factors influencing home care nursing problems and nursing care. *Research in Nursing & Health 16*, 363–370.

Hood, J. N., & Smith, H. L. (1994). Quality of work life in home care: The contribution of leaders' personal concern for staff. *Journal of Nursing Administration, 24*(1), 40–47.

Jaffe, M. S., & Skidmore-Roth, L. (1993). *Home health nursing care plans.* (2nd ed.). St. Louis: Mosby.

Kaufman, J. (1991). An overview of public sector financing for pediatric home care: Part 1 *Pediatric Nursing, 17*(2), 280–281.

Kirkis, E. J. (1993). Home health/public health/visiting nurse returning to our past: A comparison of public health nursing at the turn of the century. *Home Healthcare Nurse, 11*(5), 9–13

Maraldo, P. J. (1989). Home health care should be the heart of a nursing-sponsored national health plan. *Nursing and Health Care 10*(6): 300–304.

Marrelli, T. M. (1993). *Handbook of home health standards and documentation guidelines for reimbursement.* St. Louis: Mosby.

Martin, K. S., Scheet, N. J., & Stegman, M. R. (1993). Home health clients: Characteristics, outcomes of care, and nursing interventions. *American Journal of Public Health, 83*(12), 1730–1734.

Mason, S. G. (1992). When a ventilator patient is going home. *RN, 55*(10): 60–64.

Montgomery, P. (1993). Starting a hospital-based home health agency: Part III: marketing. *Nursing Management, 24*(10), 29–32.

Nadwairski, J. A. (1992). Inner-city safety for home care providers. *Journal of Nursing Administration, 22*(9), 42–47

National homecare and hospice directory. (1993). Washington, DC: Author.

Peters, D. A. (1992). A new look for quality in home care. *Journal of Nursing Administration, 22*(11), 21–26.

Polick, C., Parker, M., Hottinger, M., & Chase, D. (1993). *Managing healthcare for the elderly.* New York: Wiley.

Rice, R. (1992). *Home health nursing practice: Concepts and application.* St. Louis: Mosby.

Stephany, T. M. (1993). Health hazard concerns of home care nurses: A staff nurse perspective. *Journal of Nursing Administration. 23*(12), 12–13.

Sullivan, G. H. (1994). Home care: More autonomy, more legal risks. *RN, 57*(5), 63–69.

Trojan, L. & Yonge, O. (1993). Developing trusting, caring relationships: Home care nurses and elderly clients. *Journal of Advanced Nursing, 18,* 1903–1910.

Zuckerman, C., Neveloff, N., & Collopy, B. (Eds.). (1990). *Home health care options.* New York: Plenum Press.

23 Protecting Community Health Through Control of Communicable Diseases

LEARNING OBJECTIVES

Upon completion of this chapter, readers should be able to:

- Explain the significance and use of surveillance methods in communicable disease control.
- List sources of food and water-borne diseases.
- Describe control strategies for vector-borne diseases.
- Discuss specific ways to prevent sexually transmitted diseases, including HIV/AIDS.
- Differentiate between HIV infection and AIDS.
- Explain the significance of immunization as a communicable disease control measure.
- Describe the nurse's role in contact investigation.
- Discuss ethical issues affecting communicable disease and infection control.

KEY TERMS

- Acquired immunodeficiency syndrome (AIDS)
- Active immunity
- Communicable disease
- Direct transmission
- Endemic
- Epidemic
- Herd immunity
- Human immunodeficiency virus (HIV)
- Immunization
- Incubation period
- Indirect transmission
- Infection
- Infections
- Isolation
- Pandemic
- Passive immunity
- Quarantine
- Reservoir
- Screening
- Surveillance
- Vaccine
- Vector

Barbara Walton Spradley and Judith Ann Allender
COMMUNITY HEALTH NURSING: CONCEPTS AND PRACTICE, 4th ed.
© 1996 Barbara Walton Spradley and Judith Ann Allender

Communicable diseases pose a major threat to public health and are of significant concern to community health nurses. A **communicable disease** is one that can be transmitted from one person to another and is caused by an infectious (capable of producing infection) agent that is transmitted from a source or reservoir to a susceptible host. The host may be a person, animal, or insect on which the infectious agent survives or multiplies. The source or **reservoir** can be a person, animal, insect, or inanimate material in which the infectious agent lives and multiplies and which is a source of infection to others. Transmission of a communicable, also called infectious, disease can occur by direct or indirect methods. **Direct transmission** can occur by direct contact with the source, such as occurs in sexually transmitted diseases. **Indirect transmission** occurs when the infectious agent is transported by some contaminated inanimate materials such as air, water, or food or through a **vector**, which is a non-human carrier such as an animal or insect. Common vectors include fleas, ticks, lice, bats, raccoons, or skunks. During vector-borne transmission the infectious agent may be transported mechanically without multiplication or change in the infectious agent or the infectious agent may develop biologically prior to passage to a susceptible host. The host-agent-environment model is described in detail in Chapter 12.

Communicable diseases have challenged health care providers for centuries. They have led to the development of countless nursing and medical preventive measures, from simple procedures such as hand washing, sanitation, and proper ventilation, to the research and development of vaccines and antibiotics. Because these preventive measures have greatly reduced the spread of communicable diseases, many people consider communicable diseases to be a threat of the past. Yet this is not so. Communicable diseases, particularly those of epidemic and pandemic proportions such as Acquired Immunodeficiency Syndrome (AIDS), continue to cost millions of lives and billions of dollars to the global human society every year. **Epidemic** refers to disease occurrence that clearly exceeds normal or expected frequency in a community or region. **Pandemic** means an epidemic that is worldwide in distribution.

Knowledge of communicable diseases is fundamental to the practice of community health nursing because they are diseases and conditions that spread through communities of people. Understanding the basic concepts of communicable and infectious disease control, as well as the numerous issues arising in this area, will help a community health nurse work effectively to prevent and control communicable disease in populations and groups. It will help nurses teach important and effective preventive measures to community members, advocate for those affected, and protect the well being of uninfected persons (including the nurse).

Several issues and circumstances have emerged during the past 20 years which are important areas of concern to community health nurses. They are listed below:

- *AIDS*, as a result of *HIV* infection, has become the leading cause of death in the United States for men aged 25–44 years and was the fourth leading cause of death in women of the same age in 1993 (CDC, 1995b). It is also increasingly affecting infants and children and draining a large portion of scarce health care dollars away from other important health initiatives.
- *Tuberculosis*, now frequently related to HIV infection, has re-emerged in virulent, drug-resistant forms, presenting a significant threat not only to clients but to their caregivers.
- Despite significant declines in mortality, communicable diseases are responsible for persistently high morbidity among various age and population groups.
- Rates of some communicable diseases, especially tuberculosis and *sexually transmitted diseases* remain disproportionately (in some cases, shockingly) high in selected population groups, a fact often masked when statistics are aggregated.
- *Immunization* rates of coverage have declined in some areas, with subsequent increases in immunizable, preventable diseases such as measles.
- The development of *multidrug resistant strains* of bacteria and viruses, pose significant occupational health as well as practice issues for health workers.
- Recent outbreaks of *cholera* worldwide and in the United States provide evidence that everyone remains vulnerable to the communicable diseases that continue to ravage the developing world.
- Lastly, current research reveals that infectious agents may be responsible for a number of the *chronic diseases*, including some forms of cancer, that have occupied the interest of health care providers in the last few decades.

This chapter provides community health nurses with information to assess the communicable disease burden in a community. It describes ways to plan appropriate prevention interventions including immunization of children and adults, environmental interventions, community education, screening programs, and case-finding and contact investigation. Ethical issues of communicable disease control are discussed. A list of communicable disease information sources useful to the nurse are given in Appendix A at the back of this book.

Assessing the Communicable Disease Status of Communities— Surveillance Measures

The term **surveillance** in the context of communicable disease control is a methodology used to detect and monitor all aspects of communicable disease occurrence. It involves three steps: (1) systematic collection of data pertaining to the occurrence of specific diseases, (2) analysis and interpretation of data, and (3) dissemination of aggregated and processed information for the purposes of program interventions (Evans, 1989). Although surveillance methods enable one to demonstrate the success of effective control strategies, the reporting methods are often controversial. There are issues such as conflicts between individual privacy versus what information is in the public domain. Some even argue that surveillance methods can be manipulated to place blame or focus on certain population groups. These criticisms have prompted trends toward developing national health data systems that statistically summarize health status and outcomes of interventions across populations and eliminate inaccurate or unreliable data. There is a growing need for improved data from a more scientific and mathematical model which uses computer-supported techniques to predict infectious disease trends in populations (Anderson & May, 1992).

Surveillance methods have been used at least since the 14th century, when individuals were appointed to monitor ships for plague-affected passengers (Evans, 1989). Modern surveillance of communicable disease in the United States is controlled centrally by the Centers for Disease Control and Prevention (CDC), a branch of the United States Public Health Service (USPHS) based in Atlanta, Georgia. Among its many functions the CDC is responsible for monitoring communicable diseases, conducting research, and developing and disseminating information including publishing a list of approximately 40 diseases that must be reported. In addition, individual states may enact legislation requiring the reporting

of various conditions including HIV infection. A list of notifiable diseases for the year 1994 is displayed in Table 23.1. Surveillance measures provide an essential means for estimating disease incidence (all new cases of a disease appearing at a given time) and prevalence (the number of people with a given disease at a given time) in populations and communities over time.

Several important limitations affect current surveillance methods. Numerous health organizations have an interest in accumulating reliable and valid statistical measures of various conditions, yet there is no uniform consensus on the means for accumulating and disseminating such data. Differences in methods of collecting and reporting statistics from agency to agency can lead to misleading or inaccurate statistics. Most surveillance data depends on voluntary reporting by individual clinicians. Cases of some types of diseases may be vastly underreported, particularly if they do not require medical intervention, which causes the infected person to make contact with a health professional, or if providers or clients are reticent or frightened to report some controversial disease such as AIDS or other sexually transmitted diseases. Sometimes health providers may even be ignorant or unmotivated about their obligations to report certain illnesses.

Another aspect of unreliability in surveillance data stems from developments in diagnostic technology. Newer detection methods may result in improved reporting of a disease suggesting an increase in its occurrence when its presence was simply underreported in the past.

The difference between active surveillance and passive surveillance can further slant the statistics. Active surveillance occurs when public health officials contact providers to specifically inquire whether cases have been detected and passive surveillance relies solely on clinicians' initiative to report. Characteristically, active surveillance results in increased cases reported. Passive surveillance may also reflect an upward swing if a certain disease is a current news topic or the focus of well-funded research. For all these reasons it may be difficult to compare disease statistics over time when such changes may have occurred.

Despite the potential limitations discussed above, surveillance data can be very useful for community health nurses because they provide a well-accepted basis for planning community interventions, as well as measuring change as a result of those interventions. Surveillance data may also be extremely useful for identifying population groups at highest risk, based on fac-

TABLE 23.1. *Summary of Cases of Specified Notifiable Diseases, United States,*
Cumulative, Week Ending December 24, 1994 (51st Week)

	Cum. 1994		Cum. 1994
AIDS*	72,888	Measles	
Anthrax	—	Imported	186
Botulism		Indigenous	696
Foodborne	58	Plague	14
Infant	74	Poliomyelitis, Paralytic§	1
Other	7	Psittacosis	40
Brucellosis	93	Rabies, human	2
Cholera	31	Syphilis, primary and secondary	19,783
Congenital rubella syndrome	6	Syphilis, congenital, age < 1 year¶	1,123
Diphtheria	1	Tetanus	36
Encephalitis, post-infectious	107	Toxic shock syndrome	180
Gonorrhea	388,234	Trichinosis	35
Haemophilus influenzae (invasive disease)†	1,113	Tuberculosis	21,694
Hansen Disease	111	Tularemia	85
Leptospirosis	34	Typhoid fever	405
Lyme Disease	11,144	Typhus fever, tickborne (RMSF)	437

* Updated monthly to the Division of HIV/AIDS, National Center for Infectious Diseases; last update November 29, 1994.
† Of 1047 cases of known age, 301 (29%) were reported among children less than 5 years of age.
§ This case was vaccine-associated. The remaining 6 suspected cases with onset in 1994 have not yet been confirmed.
¶ Total reported to the Division of Sexually Transmitted Diseases and HIV Prevention, National Center for Prevention Services, through second quarter 1994.
From CDC (1995) Morbidity and Mortality Weekly Report 43(Nos. 51 & 52):962.

tors such as age, behavioral and cultural characteristics, socioeconomic status, occupation, geographical location, and other characteristics. Surveillance data for community health nurses is most valuable when the data are both current and local. CDC has developed software for personal computers that can enhance the capability of local community-based health services to monitor disease rates (as well as other measures of health status).

FOOD AND WATER-BORNE DISEASES

Communicable diseases result from interplay between the disease-causing or infectious agent, the susceptible host, and the environment in which the two interact. A discussion of food and water-borne diseases demonstrates how people may be affected by certain communicable diseases merely through carrying on the normal activities of eating food and drinking beverages. Chapter 6 describes both government's role and the nurse's role in helping to prevent food and water contamination by infectious agents.

Food-borne illnesses frequently reported to CDC in the last few years include salmonellosis, a bacterial agent; hepatitis A, a viral agent; and shigellosis, a bacterial agent. The most commonly reported water-borne illness is due to *Giardia lamblia,* an infection-causing protozoan, which also occurs as a food contaminant as do hepatitis A and *Escherichia coli*. Most of the disease-causing agents typically found in foods also survive in water to cause disease, though water may provide a less nutritive environment and result in lower concentrations of the agent. Most commonly, exposure to infectious food or water results in symptoms relating to gastrointestinal function, including diarrhea, nausea, vomiting, stomach cramps and jaundice. Onset of symptoms may occur within a few hours of exposure or not until days and even weeks later, depending upon the organism. This time interval between exposure and onset of symptoms is called the **incubation period**. Interestingly, however, water-borne diseases are not exclusively those that affect the gastrointestinal tract. CDC compiles reports as well on skin infections associated with recreational water use.

Bacterial contamination of food resulting in human illness occurs as a result of infection or intoxication. Infection occurs through ingesting food contaminated with adequate doses of *salmonella*, *shigella*, or *E. coli*. The cycle begins when the infectious agent multiplies and grows in the food medium. The agent subsequently invades the host upon ingestion of the food. **Infection** then occurs, which is the entry and development or multiplication of an infectious agent in the body usually accompanied by an immune response, such as the production of antibodies with or without clinical manifestation. The infectious organism produces illness by direct irritation of the normal gastrointestinal mucosa. Intoxication refers to the production of toxins as a by-product of normal bacterial life-cycle, such as *Staphylococcus aureus* or *Clostridium perfringens*. It is the toxin that is illness-producing upon ingestion.

The distinction between infection and intoxication is relevant for a number of reasons. Toxins may be difficult to isolate and identify, particularly in the absence of the bacteria; thus some suspected food-borne illnesses go unidentified. While the bacteria itself may be killed upon heating of foodstuffs before consumption, some bacteria-produced toxins are stable in normal cooking temperatures, and thus the food cannot be rendered safe. A bacteria that establishes itself in the human gastro-intestinal system may require medical treatment in order to be eradicated. A person suffering from food intoxication may require essentially supportive care while in the process of ridding him or herself of the toxin.

The most important aspects of food and water-borne diseases for nurses in community health may be in recognizing that outbreaks of illness affecting large numbers of people continue to occur fairly regularly. This is true despite well-recognized standards for decontamination of water supplies and safe commercial food preparation. Secondly, such outbreaks may not be detectable by usual surveillance means because of individuals' mobility. For example, an outbreak of illness in Minnesota in 1990 was associated with food served on an international airline. Had a large group of the affected travellers not communicated among themselves and to providers, the outbreak may never have been identified. Thirdly, such outbreaks can serve to remind all community health practitioners that there continues to be a need to teach and observe the most basic methods for preventing food and water contamination. Table 23.2 summarizes correct methods for preserving the safety and cleanliness of food.

TABLE 23.2. *Correct Methods for Preserving the Safety and Cleanliness of Food*

BEFORE HANDLING FOOD

- Wash hands and all food preparation surfaces and utensils thoroughly with soap and water.

WHEN PREPARING FOOD

- Wash foods that are to be eaten raw and uncooked thoroughly in clean water. This includes foods that are to be peeled that grow on the ground or come in contact with soil.
- Cook all meat products thoroughly.
- Do not allow cooked meats to come in contact with dishes, utensils, or containers utilized when the foods were raw and uncooked.

WHEN STORING LEFT-OVER FOODS

- Cool cooked foods quickly; store under refrigeration in clean covered containers.

WHEN REHEATING LEFT-OVER FOODS

- Heat foods thoroughly. Bacteria contaminating food grow and multiply in a temperature range between 39 and 140 degrees Fahrenheit.

VECTOR-BORNE DISEASES

As described in Chapter 6, a vector is a non-human organism that transports an infectious agent from a reservoir or source to a susceptible host. Vector-borne illnesses, those transmitted by vectors, prove challenging in communicable disease control because individuals who become infected need not have direct personal contact with other infected persons. The disease is transmitted or carried by a "third-party" (the vector), usually a biting insect such as a mosquito, tick, flea, or louse. Human history has been significantly impacted by vector-borne diseases, as louse-borne typhus and flea-borne plague together were responsible for a majority of devastating disease epidemics occurring in the last six centuries. Vector-borne illnesses have received renewed attention in recent years with accumulating information about tick-borne Lyme disease, a viral disease tranmitted to humans by a tick vector, resulting in symptoms of varying severity including rash, joint pain, and progressive weakness, vision changes, and other neuromuscular dysfunction. Mosquito-borne malaria and snail-borne schistosomiasis alone currently cause major human suffering to hundreds of millions of people in tropical settings every year. The fact that most of these diseases are **endemic** (habitually present within a geographic area) to certain areas suggests the need for tight controls for prevention and intervention.

Control strategies directed to vector-borne diseases typically involve complex environmental measures to hinder the vector from reaching the host (see Chapter 6) as well as community education. Such strategies include:

- reducing the population of insect vectors, for example by spraying insecticides to kill mosquitoes;
- treating the natural habitat of the vector in order to reduce the population density;
- reducing the population of other animal hosts that harbor the vector, as when rats are exterminated to reduce the risk of plague;
- erecting barriers between the susceptible human and the vector, such as use of mosquito nets or screened windows to control malaria or protective clothing and sprays against tick-borne diseases;
- educating the public about preventive and protective measures including actions to take when attacked by the vector to prevent disease from developing.

In the United States in the 1990's, vector-borne diseases receiving the most attention are Lyme disease and tick-borne fevers, such as Rocky Mountain Spotted fever, relapsing fever, or rabies (rabies vector usually is a domestic animal, bat, skunk, or raccoon). Occasionally imported vector-borne tropical diseases, including malaria and dengue fever, are reported. The return of military personnel from Southeast Asia through the 1960s and 1970s had a significant effect on the numbers of imported cases of malaria reported in the United States.

SEXUALLY TRANSMITTED DISEASES

Sexually transmitted diseases (STDs) are those infections spread by transfer of organisms from person to person during sexual contact. STDs are of critical importance in any discussion of communicable disease control because, as a single class of disease, they account for almost 12 million case-events each year in the the United States, 86% of them occurring in people aged 15 through 29 years (CDC, 1992a). The total cost to society of treating STDs exceeds $3.5 billion annually, with the cost of pelvic-inflammatory disease (PID) and PID-associated ectopic pregnancy and infertility alone exceeding $2.6 billion (USPHS, 1991). The sexually transmitted diseases discussed in this section include syphilis, gonorrhea, chlamydia, and genital herpes and genital warts. Acquired immunodeficiency

syndrome (AIDS), of course, is a sexually-transmitted disease, as is hepatitis B, although transmission of these diseases can also occur through intravenous drug use, transfusion of blood products prior to 1986, or accidental or intentional needle-stick injury. These diseases are discussed later.

Of further concern to community health nurses is the fact that women and children suffer an inordinate amount of the sexually transmitted disease burden. Leaving aside for the moment the risk of acquired immunodeficiency disease and subsequent death, the most serious complications of STDs are pelvic inflammatory disease, sterility, ectopic pregnancy, blindness, cancer associated with human papillomavirus, fetal and infant death, birth defects, and mental retardation. The medically underserved, particularly the poor, ethnic and racial minorities, shoulder a disproportionate share of this problem, experiencing higher rates of disability and death than the population as a whole (USPHS, 1991).

Syphilis

Syphilis is the first STD for which control measures were developed and tested. Although syphilis incidence has decreased in recent years (from more than 50,000 cases in 1990 to 20,000 cases in 1994), it continues to be a serious health threat (Webster, et al., 1991; CDC, 1995a). (See Fig. 23.1.) For minority populations in the United States, this dramatic overall increase tells only a portion of the story. In the period 1985 through 1990,

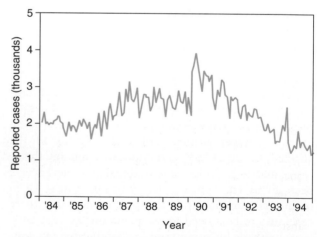

FIGURE 23.1. Syphilis cases, by 4-week period of report—United States, 1984–1994 (From CDC (1995). *Morbidity and Mortality Weekly Report* 44(3), 57).

primary and secondary syphilis rates rose from 69 to 156 per 100,000—an increase of 126%. The rate for black women, however, rose from 35 to 116 per 100,000—an increase of 231% (CDC, 1991f). Concern over these increases is intensified by the fact that genital ulcer diseases, including syphilis, have been epidemiologically linked with HIV infection and transmission.

Syphilis presents in several forms during the life cycle of the disease. Approximately three weeks following exposure, a primary lesion called a chancre characteristically appears as a painless ulcer at the site of initial invasion of the causative organism, *Treponema pallidum*, a spirochete. After four to six weeks, the chancre will heal without treatment, to be replaced by the development of more generalised secondary skin eruption, classically appearing on the soles of the feet and palms of the hands, often accompanied by constitutional symptoms. Secondary manifestations resolve spontaneously, followed by a latent period which may last from weeks to years. Unpredictably, severe, systemic involvement with disability or even death may occur (Benenson, 1990).

Treatment of early primary, secondary, and early latent syphilis is generally accomplished through antibiotic therapy. Clients should be reexamined at three and six months post-treatment to ensure cure (Ibid.).

Gonorrhea

Gonorrhea is the most frequently reported communicable disease in the United States; its causative agent is the gonocossus bacteria *Neisseria gonorrhoeae*. The incidence of gonorrhea has declined somewhat in the past decade but it continues to be a major public health problem (See Fig. 23.2). High risk groups include blacks, adolescents, and women of child-bearing age (USPHS, 1991). A major concern in working to reduce the incidence of gonorrhea is the increase in antibiotic resistant strains of the bacteria. The proportion of all gonorrhea cases attributed to antibiotic-resistant strains increased dramatically from 0.8% in 1985 to 7.0% in 1989 (Whittington & Knapp, 1989).

The cost-benefit ratio of gonorrhea screening and outreach efforts is estimated to be more than 2:1 (CDC, 1994a). There is no uniform reporting system to track the number of gonorrhea cases that are repeat infections, however, there is some evidence indicating that a substantial proportion of gonorrhea infections occur in individuals who previously received treatment (USPHS, 1991; McEvoy & Le Furgy, 1988). Successful interventions with these individuals could prove to be the most

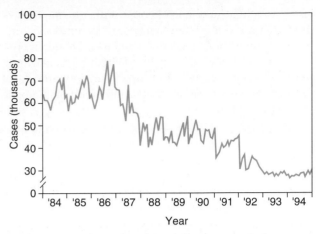

FIGURE 23.2. Gonorrhea cases, by 4-week period of report—United States, 1984–1994 (From CDC (1995). *Morbidity and Mortality Weekly Report 44*(33), 57).

cost-effective. Helping individuals avoid repeat infections will most likely begin with a thorough personal history, including partner characteristics and willingness to also be treated. It will also require a more comprehensive multiagency approach focusing on some of the other social, economic, and environmental issues that demand attention for successful, lasting behavior change (USPHS, 1991).

Gonorrhea commonly presents in men as a purulent drainage from the penis accompanied by painful urination within two to seven days after an infecting exposure. In females, symptoms may be so mild as to go unnoticed. Progression of untreated gonorrhea may lead to serious reproductive system involvement and subsequent infertility (Benenson, 1990). The recommended treatment regimen for gonorrhea has been Ceftriaxone in a single intramuscular injection plus doxycycline twice daily by mouth for seven days. Because treatment failure with the combined ceftriaxone/doxycycline regimen is rare, a follow-up test of cure is not considered essential. Clients treated with any other drug regimen, however, should receive a follow-up culture four to seven days following completion of therapy.

Chlamydia

Chlamydia is the most common sexually transmitted bacterial infection in the United States, causing an estimated 4 million acute infections annually. Yet, until recently, chlamydia was probably the least recognized of the STDs and is not presently part of the national disease surveillance system. People with uncomplicated infection are quite often symptom-free until late and serious complications occur. Women and children typically are the most adversely affected, particularly in terms of sequelae, including pelvic inflammatory disease (PID), infant conjunctivitis, and infant pneumonia (USPHS, 1991).

Control of chlamydial infections of the cervix is considered key to effective reduction in the rates of pelvic inflammatory disease, particularly among teenage women. Although chlamydia can be successfully treated with relatively inexpensive therapy, efforts to identify infected asymptomatic people has been hindered by the lack of a widely-available, inexpensive, easy to perform diagnostic test (a problem shared by a number of the communicable diseases, including tuberculosis). In addition, lack of compliance with the required seven day treatment regimen is a major barrier to effective control (USPHS, 1991). The current recommended treatment regimen for uncomplicated chlamydia infection is doxycycline twice daily for seven days or tetracycline four times a day for seven days. Because no antibiotic resistant strains of chlamydia have been detected, CDC does not presently recommend any follow up to ensure cure (CDC, 1993).

Genital Herpes and Genital Warts

The estimated annual incidence of symptomatic genital herpes in the United States is 200,000 cases, with total prevalence estimates of genital herpes infection as high as 30 million cases. By their late teens, about 4% of whites and 17% of blacks have been infected with herpes type 2 virus (Johnson, et al., 1989).

Control efforts for genital herpes are currently hampered because as many as three-fourths of genital herpes infections are transmitted by people who are unaware of their own infection and because no cure for the condition exists (Mertz, et al., 1988). Symptomatic management is usually accomplished by treatment of the first clinical episode of genital herpes with acyclovir orally five times daily for seven to ten days or until clinical resolution occurs. Subsequent recurrent episodes may be relieved to some extent with short-term courses of acyclovir, though this has proven to be ineffective for many people. Alternatively, a long-term course of daily suppressive therapy may reduce the frequency of recurrences (CDC, 1993).

Genital warts are caused by human papillomavirus (HPV), which has been strongly associated with cervi-

cal dysplasia and genital cancers. Genital warts are a common STD and account for approximately 5% of all STD clinic visits (USPHS, 1991). Genital HPV infection can be transmitted to newborns during passage through the birth canal.

Many individuals infected with HPV are asymptomatic and transmit the infection unknowingly. Genital HPV infections are difficult to treat and commonly reoccur. No culture method is available to diagnose HPV, so diagnosis is commonly made on clinical presentation. Current recommendations are to treat visualized warts with a topical solution of podophyllin or by cryotherapy or electrocautery. The goal of therapy is removal of the warts and relief of symptoms (CDC, 1993).

Prevention of STDs

The United States Public Health Service document, *Healthy People 2000,* identifies the availability and quality of public services for sexually transmitted disease as key factors in reducing the spread of STDs and preventing complications (1991). Effective health promotion approaches in the community must include STD prevention in the curricula of middle and secondary schools. Focus on the adolescent population is mandated by data demonstrating that youth are not risk averse *and* tend to be sexually active. While the proportion of youth sexually active between the ages of 15 and 19 years has been over 50%, less than half of these sexually active young people used a condom in their last sexual intercourse (CDC, 1991e). The initiation of sexual activity early in life results in an increased number of sexual partners over a person's lifetime and thus establishes the behavioral link to higher levels of STDs.

In addition to the need for more innovative and effective sexual health promotion approaches in school settings, a number of recommendations have been made for improvements in current delivery systems (CDC, 1992a; USPHS, 1991). The number of clinics offering STD screening, diagnosis, treatment, counseling and referral services should increase substantially to improve access to comprehensive services. Certainly consideration, planning, and the allocation of resources should be directed to the quality of life issues that operate in young adults' lives and contribute to inappropriately early initiation of unprotected sexual activity. Case management by providers often does not conform to CDC recommendations in the nature of medical treatment, follow-up strategies to confirm cure, or notification and treatment of sexual partners. This in turn may contribute to inadequate treatment, continued transmission, higher risk of complications, and the increase in drug-resistant strains of gonorrhea and other diseases. *Healthy People 2000* (USPHS, 1991) strongly recommends expansion of contact tracing efforts. Treating individuals who present with symptoms is only half the job. The partner or partners of infected persons must be notified and also require treatment for effective and lasting "cure" of the case.

In 1992, the CDC published data about the prevalence of sexual intercourse, contraceptive use, condom use, and STDs among U.S. high school students (CDC, 1992a). The data came from the national school-based Youth Risk Behavior Survey, using a sample of over 13,000 youths. Of all students in grades 9–12, 60.8% of males and 48.0% of females reported having had sexual intercourse. Black students were significantly more likely to have had sexual intercourse than white or Hispanic students (72.3%, 51.6%, and 53.4%, respectively). Among sexually active students, only 49.4% of males and 40.0% of females reported they or their partner used a condom during the last sexual intercourse. Four percent of all students reported having had an STD (black, 8.4%; white, 3.4%, and Hispanic, 3.5%).

Adolescent and young adult females and males who have multiple sex partners over a specified period (e.g., several months), are at increased risk for gonorrhea, syphilis, chlamydia, and chancroid (See Fig. 23.3). Increased numbers of sex partners over a lifetime is associated with a greater cumulative risk for acquiring viral infections such as hepatitis B, genital herpes, HPV, and HIV. National health objectives for the year 2000 include efforts to reduce the proportion of sexually active adolescents to no more than 15% by age 15, and no more than 40% by age 17 (USPHS, 1991). Other objectives are to increase the use of condoms during last intercourse to 60%–70% among sexually active unmarried persons aged 15–19 years.

These changes in behavior will require diverse and multidisciplinary interventions over an extended period of time. Such interventions must integrate the efforts of parents, families, schools, religious organizations, health departments, community agencies, and the media. The goals of educational programs should be to provide adolescents with the knowledge and skills they need to refrain from sexual intercourse, and to increase the use of condoms as well as other contraceptive measures among those unwilling to postpone onset of sexual activity (Ibid.). Studies have suggested that parent-child conversations about sexual matters have

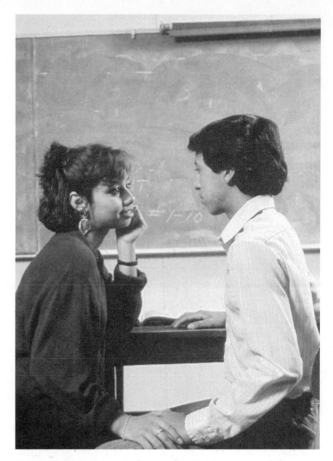

FIGURE 23.3. Increased sexual activity among adolescents makes them vulnerable to contracting STDs.

been associated with delays in initiation of sexual activity and with the increased use of contraceptives by adolescents who engaged in sexual intercourse. Additional recommendations to promote sexual health in adolescent populations included (1) innovations for early detection and treatment of STDs among teenagers, (2) specialized training for clinicians providing health services for adolescents, (3) school education combined with accessible clinical services, and (4) behavioral interventions to prevent exposure to and acquisition of STDs (CDC, 1991e).

HIV INFECTION AND AIDS

Human immunodeficiency virus (HIV) is a retrovirus that attacks the body's immune system. It is "transmitted from person to person through sexual contact, sharing HIV-contaminated intravenous needles and syringes, and through transfusion of infected blood or its components" (Benenson, 1990, p.3). **Acquired immunodeficiency syndrome (AIDS)** is a severe, life-threatening condition representing the late clinical stage of infection with HIV in which there is progressive damage to the immune and other organ systems, particularly the central nervous system. HIV-infected persons may be asymptomatic for months or years and onset of the illness is usually gradual with such non-specific symptoms as anorexia, fever, chronic diarrhea, weight loss, lymphadenopathy, and fatigue. Presence of these non-specific symptoms in an HIV-infected individual (when evidence was insufficient for a diagnosis of AIDS) was formerly called AIDS-related complex (ARC) or "symptomatic HIV infection" but this diagnosis is no longer used by CDC. Eventually the vast majority of those infected with HIV develop AIDS and, although newer therapies may be prolonging their lives, most cases (80% to 90%) are fatal within approximately five years after diagnosis (Benenson, 1990).

Incidence and Prevalence of HIV/AIDS

Current estimates based on various studies are that 1 million people in the United States are infected with HIV (Anderson & May, 1992; CDC, 1994d; CDC, 1995b), and the majority of these individuals are unaware they harbor the infection. The number of AIDS cases reported in the United States each year continues to climb. (See Fig. 23.4). On a global scale, 8–10 million adults and 1 million children are infected *each year* with HIV. By the year 2000, 26 million people may be infected with HIV with more than 85% of these residing

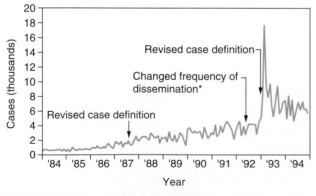

FIGURE 23.4. Acquired immunodeficiency syndrome cases, by 4-week period of report—United States, 1984–1994 (From CDC (1995). *Morbidity and Mortality Weekly Report 44*(3), 56).

in developing countries, furthermore, an annual death toll of 2 million is predicted (UNICEF, 1995). Without treatment, within 10 years of infection with HIV, about 50% of HIV-infected people develop AIDS and another 40% or more develop other clinical illnesses, including many types of infections and cancers, associated with HIV infection (Hessol, et al., 1988). Annual costs of AIDS care in the United States have been in the billions of dollars. With a growing emphasis on the benefits of early drug therapy, such as zidovudine (ZDV) treatment for HIV infection (CDC, 1994e), more people will be drawn into the health care system at an earlier point for intervention of long duration. Consequently it is expected that AIDS-related care costs will continue to grow.

Populations-at-risk for AIDS

AIDS was first recognized as a distinct syndrome in 1981 and during the early years was seen as a disease of male homosexuals, intravenous drug abusers, and/or people with a history of multiple blood transfusions. The at-risk population for AIDS includes people with large numbers of sexual partners, adolescents, injecting drug users and their sexual partners, homosexual men and their male or female partners, people who exchange sex for drugs or money, and people already infected with HIV (USPHS, 1991). Sexual transmission of HIV is closely associated with other STDs, particularly those that have an ulcerative phase, including syphilis. With belated but growing awareness of the AIDS epidemic on a global scale, it is becoming recognized as a universal threat to health and well-being—of individuals and of populations. Worldwide, the AIDS epidemic affects men and women in equal proportions and in Africa women account for 55% of all new cases of HIV (UNICEF, 1995). A tragically high incidence of neonatal AIDS now occurs due to maternal-fetal transmission of the virus. An estimated 20% to 40% of the infants of infected mothers develop HIV infection (Ginzberg, et al., 1990). AIDS is now seen in the United States as a potential health threat to all sexually active people and their offspring (Anderson & May, 1992). Heterosexually acquired AIDS has increased significantly in the 1990s (CDC, 1994d). AIDS was the fourth leading cause of death among women aged 25–44 years in 1993 (CDC, 1995b).

Adolescents and young adults are considered to be at particular risk for HIV infection because many of them engage in high-risk behavior, believing themselves to be invulnerable to infection. In addition to the considerable risks posed by potential HIV infection, other adverse outcomes related to early initiation of sexual activity include higher levels of all STDs (CDC, 1991e). Most persons (90%) who contract AIDS are between 20 and 49 years of age (Benenson, 1990).

HIV Prevention and Intervention

National HIV prevention and intervention efforts depend on two important factors: (1) self-perception of risk and (2) adoption of risk-reducing behaviors in response to awareness of the risk. Consequently education about HIV/AIDS, including safe sex and injecting drug use, has become the key to prevention. See the Research in Community Health Nursing display. Public health workers seek to identify and intervene with the at-risk population, providing counseling and prevention education as well as testing services. The primary purposes of counseling are to prevent further spread of HIV infection and, where possible, to slow progression of HIV infection to AIDs. HIV counseling can help uninfected people initiate and sustain behaviors to reduce their risk of infection; help infected people adopt behaviors to reduce the risk of transmission to others; encourage spouses and partners of infected people to adopt safe behaviors; and help infected people take better care of themselves. Proper use of condoms, reducing the number of sexual partners, and abstinence from injecting drug use decrease, but do not eliminate, risk of HIV infection (USPHS, 1991).

Care for the HIV-infected Population in the Community

HIV infection and AIDS are important topics of concern to community health nurses for a number of reasons. They present an intriguing service delivery problem requiring complex and sophisticated multidisciplinary interventions. Sexual behaviors, illegitimate drug use, end-of-life issues, and other psychosocial aspects provide very human dimensions to a problem also demanding of nursing, medical, social, epidemiological, political, and economic resources.

Care of persons with HIV infection presents a special opportunity for community health nurses to meet an important and visible challenge in modern society. Individuals with HIV/AIDS are living longer, requiring nursing care that is widely integrated with other community services. This population requires knowl-

Research in Community Health Nursing
KNOWLEDGE OF AIDS

DiIorio, C., Parsons, M., Lehr, S., Adame, D., & Carlone, J. (1993). Knowledge of AIDS and safer sex practices among college freshmen. *Public Health Nursing, 10*(3), 159–165.

A critical primary prevention measure against AIDS is education. Programs to inform people about HIV/AIDS and the measures they can take to protect themselves have been aggressively developed throughout the world. While providing information is an important step toward promoting behavior change, it is also important to determine what at-risk populations do, in fact, know that will enhance risk-reducing sexual practices.

This study assessed the AIDS-related knowledge of single college freshmen at three private colleges in the South. Students were asked to complete an AIDS information survey, a questionnaire regarding their knowledge of safe sex practices, and a demographic form. Of the 689 respondents, 51% were men, 63.4% were black, 30.9% were white, 5.7% of other ethnic groups, and 71% were sexually active.

Results of the study showed that the students had a high level of knowledge about the cause, transmission, and seriousness of AIDS Nearly all knew about protection during sexual intercourse but their knowledge about specific protection was lower. Some did not know that latex condoms are more effective than nonlatex condoms in preventing spread of HIV or that using a spermicide containing nonoxynol-9 was considered a safer sexual practice.

The researchers concluded that misperceptions still exist and that students know least about the medical aspects of AIDS and the specifics of safer sex practices. Educational implications included the need to counteract misperceptions about AIDS transmission, be aware of who is at risk (increasingly it is the heterosexual population), reinforce which contraceptive methods protect against HIV infection, and make educational messages culturally sensitive.

edgeable, skilled, often aggressive therapeutic and preventive nursing services for acute as well as chronic illness, supported by an interdisciplinary network of providers. Three major goals of care with this population are: (1) promoting general health and resilience, (2) preventing infections of all sorts, and (3) delaying the onset of clinical symptoms with antiviral therapy. To meet these goals, the community health nurse's role involves getting HIV positive clients engaged in wellness programs such as promoting nutritional health, exercise, drug management, and preventing opportunistic infections. Stress reduction is essential for these clients; the nurse can facilitate relaxation activities, client and family counseling, and support groups to assist clients' coping abilities. An important part of nursing care with these clients is use of "universal precautions" which refers to CDC recommendations to prevent infections that are transmitted by direct or indirect contact with infected blood or body fluids (bloody body secretions, semen, vaginal secretions, tissue, CSF, and synovial, pleural, peritoneal, pericardial, and amniotic fluids). These are covered in a later section entitled, "health care provider precautions". Nurses can also make important contributions to the evolution of HIV/AIDS care and services by participating in the debates that occur and will likely continue over the ethical dimensions of the AIDS crisis, including HIV screening, contact investigation, and AIDS-related discrimination which are discussed later in this chapter.

The therapeutic management of HIV infection and AIDS is evolving and in fact largely experimental. Attempts at vaccine development are ongoing, and include experimentation with vaccines for those already infected, to increase resistance to multiplication of the viral agent and development of clinical symptoms. Nurses wishing timely updates on clinical and medical aspects of AIDS case management are urged to refer to recent issues of CDC's *Morbidity and Mortality Weekly Report*, as well as professional journals devoted to disseminating information to practitioners working with AIDS patients.

TUBERCULOSIS

Tuberculosis, once nearly eradicated, now poses a major threat to the public's health. There is evidence of recent alarming increases in overall rates, sharply disparate rates of tuberculosis among minority populations, a fatal association of tuberculosis with HIV infection and AIDS, increasing rates of tuberculosis among children, and a proliferation of multidrug-resistant strains.

Roughly 20% of the world's population is infected with *Mycobacterium tuberculosis*. Thus, one billion people in the world have the potential for developing active tuberculosis at some point in time (Glittenberg, 1990; Snider, 1989). Tuberculosis kills about three million people worldwide every year, more than any other single infectious disease (USPHS, 1991), and this despite the fact that effective anti-tuberculosis treatment has been known since the 1940's.

Exposure to tuberculosis does not lead to actual disease in all cases. A long latent period may persist for many years (even for a lifetime) before the infected person develops disease and becomes infectious. The probability of becoming infected depends primarily on exposure to air contaminated with *M. tuberculosis*. Approximately 75% of individuals exposed to infectious cases do not become infected. Of those who become infected, about 10% develop clinically apparent infectious disease at some point in life (Snider, 1989). The remaining 90% harbor the organism though they are not **infectious** (capable of spreading infection to others) and represent a persistent pool of potential cases in a population. The likelihood of being among the 10% who develop clinical infectious disease is variable, depending on the initial dose of infection and certain other risk factors. Groups at increased risk include men, young and old persons, those infected within the past two years, and individuals with impaired cell-mediated immunity (Glittenberg, 1990). Unlike some other infectious diseases that spread rapidly in a susceptible community, immunizing or killing large numbers of people, tuberculosis can be maintained at endemic levels in populations for generations (Rieder, 1989). Endemic levels are those at which the disease or infectious agent is habitually present in a geographic area but disease outbreaks are contained to a minimum.

Tuberculosis Surveillance

Uniform national surveillance for tuberculosis was initiated in 1953 (Snider, et al., 1989). Until 1951, reported data included both active and inactive cases. Starting in 1952, only active cases were reported. In 1953, 84,304 cases were reported nationally, declining by 1987 to 22,517 cases (Ibid.). This decrease of over 73% is attributed largely to widespread use of anti-tuberculosis medications, primarily isoniazid. The decrease in cases with the disease is seen as contributing to the medical and political complacency that has resulted in lax control efforts and now to the resurgence of tuberculosis.

In 1988 the number of tuberculosis cases began to rise, and continued to accelerate through the early 1990s, with an increasing proportion of cases occurring among members of racial and ethnic minorities in the United States, increases in cases among children, and increases among foreign-born persons living in the United States. The incidence of tuberculosis has remained high over the past decade and continues to be a major public health problem (CDC, 1994b). (See Fig. 23.5).

Populations at Risk for Tuberculosis

Minority populations tend to be at greater risk for tuberculosis. The proportion of tuberculous cases among nonwhites compared to whites climbed from 24% of all cases in 1953 to 65% of cases in 1988 (Dowling, 1991). In 1987, the overall case rate for whites was 5.7 per 100,000 while among non-whites it was 29.3 per 100,000. Among minorities, the age group of peak incidence was 30–34 years, while among non-Hispanic whites, peak age group was 70–74 years (Snider, et al., 1989). Blacks are as resistant as whites to progression from infection to active disease, but appear to be more susceptible to infection than whites (Stead, et al., 1990). Although reasons for this difference are not clear, susceptibility may relate to socioeconomic factors. Other groups at risk for higher rates of tuberculosis in the United States include foreign born persons, prison and jail inmate populations, and individuals

infected with HIV. Tuberculosis rates are high among refugees and immigrants and noncompliance is a major factor in continued transmission of the disease.

Immune suppressed individuals such as those with AIDS can develop fulminant active tuberculosis within weeks of exposure to the mycobacterium, and the disease progresses much faster than in those with normal competent immune systems. Consequently, a suspected case of tuberculosis in a person with AIDS is usually treated immediately without waiting for sputum test or chest x-ray results. As the incidence of HIV infection has shifted from a predominantly homosexual, white, middle-class male population to a more impoverished, heterosexual, inner-city minority population with a high prevalence of *M. tuberculosis* infection, the incidence of HIV-related TB mortality can be expected to rise (Dowling, 1991).

The risk of HIV-infected groups for tuberculous infection is further complicated by inaccuracy of the tuberculin skin test due to the HIV-infected client's impaired immunity. Specific recommendations for testing the HIV-infected person have been promulgated by CDC in response to these problems. The basic approach involves testing for tuberculin reactivity in combination with at least one other skin-test antigen (mumps, tetanus toxoid, Candida) to which most healthy persons in the U.S. population can be assumed sensitized. A positive response to the other antigen, but not to PPD tuberculin, is considered evidence of absence of infection with *M. tuberculosis*. Absence of response to both warrants further investigation.

Increasing numbers of tuberculous cases among children are especially worrisome because they point to escalated transmission in the United States. Cases in children most often result from recent infection which is in contrast to cases among older adults that may develop as a result of infection occurring many years previously. Tuberculosis among children suggests rising case rates among persons of reproductive age, who have contact with and transmit infection to susceptible children. This underscores the need to investigate the household and community contacts of the child for untreated disease. Likewise, when adult active tuberculous cases are identified, it is essential to evaluate child contacts of the case.

Among children with active tuberculosis, minority groups account for more than 80% of the cases (Dowling, 1991). Girls have a much higher incidence during elementary and high school years than do boys of the same age. Susceptibility in children and adoles-

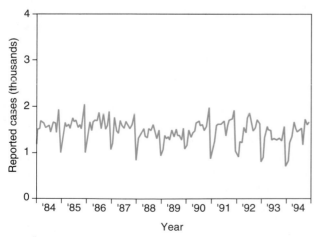

FIGURE 23.5. Tuberculosis cases, by 4-week period of report—United States, 1984–1994 (From CDC (1995). *Morbidity and Mortality Weekly Report 44*(3), 56).

cence peaks during infancy and again in puberty. Infants show decreased ability to localize infection, and have limited stores of acquired antibodies. It is unclear whether the increased susceptibility in adolescents is the result of increased contacts with infected persons, rapid hormonal changes, suboptimal diets, or a combination of all of these (Richardson, et al., 1991).

Problems with Drug-Resistant Tuberculosis

Epidemiologists and communicable disease specialists cite a number of factors contributing to the development and spread of tuberculous strains resistant to one or more of the standard arsenal of tuberculosis drugs. Strains now exist that are resistant to as many as 9 of 11 standard anti-tuberculous drugs. Chief among the factors contributing to drug-resistance seems to be the political and social response to declining rates of tuberculosis over past decades, resulting in cuts in funding for surveillance, treatment, and research, and a premature sense that tuberculosis was beaten. Federal surveillance of drug-resistant tuberculosis strains was discontinued in 1986 due to budgetary constraints. On an individual case basis, non-compliance with therapy for the full recommended period has been significant in the development of drug-resistant strains. Public health services with limited resources have been unable to provide the intensive follow-up necessary to assure that persons essentially feeling well remain on medication (that may produce unpleasant though usually mild and manageable side effects) for the 6–18 months considered necessary to achieve cure. Public health officials face a challenge to network effectively to provide continuous case management for highly mobile and often disenfranchised infected minority populations (Jereb, et al., 1990).

The reality of drug-resistant strains of tuberculosis significantly complicates the crisis of AIDS. Thus, when candidates for drug therapy are identified, it is essential to provide program support to ensure that the maximum number of individuals comply with their medication regimen for the full duration of therapy. Isoniazid therapy for individuals infected with tuberculosis, but without evidence of active disease, has been shown to be highly effective in preventing progression to infectiousness and clinical symptoms. Isoniazid is also a key component of treatment for active disease. Adverse effects of isoniazid therapy are often overestimated, leading to inappropriate withdrawal of therapy.

Commitment and flexibility on the part of health providers and services can substantially enhance medication compliance. Significant improvement in compliance has been demonstrated with programs designed to provide directly observed therapy, using community-based health workers who meet with clients in residences, at job sites, and other local venues. In many cases, the community health workers are former program participants, trained and supervised by professional health workers (Snider, et al., 1989). In addition, new variations on the standard treatment regimens are being researched. Approaches include allowing individuals to take larger medication doses on a twice-weekly schedule, or providing an observed medication program for a limited period, followed by a course of self-administered medication with periodic revaluation by health care providers (Glittenberg, 1990).

Prevention and Control of Tuberculosis

Tuberculin testing, the standard method for evaluating tuberculous infection, is a simple skin test which measures by visible reaction whether the body has had immunologic experience with *M. tuberculosis*. From there evaluation procedures differentiate between classification status of the disease, ranging from 0 to 5. The two most used terms would be infected, classification 2, and with the disease, classification 3 (See Table 23.3).Thus, the skin test is not diagnostic of disease. There are two widely available skin test products. The tine test delivers a premeasured dose of purified protein derivative (PPD) under the skin by puncture. The Mantoux test delivers 0.1 ml of PPD by intradermal injection. The Mantoux (the dose is measured at time of injection) is generally considered the more reliable test,

TABLE 23.3. *Tuberculosis Classification Status*

Classification	Hx of Exposure	PPD	Sputum and X-ray
0	−	−	−
1	+	−	−
2	+	+	−
3	+	+	+

(Classification 2 means the person is infected, classification 3 means the person has the disease, classifications 4 & 5 [not shown] refer to stages of being treated or post-treatment.)

as the dose of the tine test and the technique of inoculation may be highly variable.

Interpretation of the tuberculin test is critical to subsequent evaluation of clients' status. The interpretation of this screening method must be as sensitive as possible while maintaining specificity for exposure (these terms are further explained later in this chapter in the section on screening). Table 23.4 presents interpretation criteria for various groups based on measured reaction to skin testing.

The Committee on Infectious Disease of the American Academy of Pediatrics in 1988 developed guidelines based on cost-effectiveness for routine periodic skin testing only in high-risk populations. Such populations include children of American Indians, native Alaskans, children in neighborhoods where case rates are higher than the national average, children of immigrants from Asia, Africa, the Middle East, Latin America or the Caribbean, and children from households with one or more cases of active tuberculosis. Routine periodic screening was recommended for all children at 12 to 16 months of age, 4 to 6 years of age, and 14 to 16 years of age (Richardson, et al., 1991). Adults should be tested periodically once negative status has been determined. Frequency of testing depends on risks of exposure and symptoms, if any. Once an individual is known to be a positive reactor to a skin test, the tuberculin test is not a valid means of assessing tuberculous infection, and subsequent evaluation calls for a chest x-ray to identify tuberculous lesions.

Community health nurses working with ethnically diverse populations may meet clients who, upon relating vaccination and/or tuberculosis histories, may have records of or recall receiving Bacille Calmette-Guerin (BCG) vaccination. BCG is an antituberculous vaccination first developed in 1906, which has been widely used on a global scale since 1921 in all countries except the Netherlands and the United States It is not used in the United States as it destroys this country's one control measure of a positive PPD to identify classification 3 individuals who should receive treatment. BCG is one of the oldest vaccine products still in use today. After receiving BCG all recipients are positive for up to 10 years although protection may wane after 5 years. Another reason BCG has never been used in this country is that it has never been cloned, and vaccine products made in different locations may vary widely in effectiveness, providing from 0%–80% effectiveness protection for inoculated individuals (Glittenberg, 1990).

BCG vaccine is an attenuated substrain of M. bovis and will usually induce a positive skin tuberculosis test, although skin test reactivity tends to diminish with time. By 10 years post vaccination, most recipients do not have measurable reactions (Richardson, et al., 1991). Table 23.5 provides guidelines for interpretation of tuberculin test reactions for a person with previous history of BCG vaccination.

In 1987, the Secretary of the Department of Health and Human Services established the Advisory Committee for Elimination of Tuberculosis. This committee was charged with developing a strategy for eliminating tuberculosis from the United States by the year 2010. As a part of this effort, CDC published guidelines for the elimination of tuberculosis (CDC, 1989) and guidelines for preventing tuberculosis transmission in health care facilities (CDC, 1994c). To accomplish this goal, spe-

TABLE 23.4. *Cutoff Points for Significant PPD Test*

REACTION ≥ 5 MM

Persons with HIV infection
Household or close contact of a patient with infectious
    tuberculosis
Persons with chest x-rays consistent with old healed
    tuberculosis

REACTION ≥ 10 MM

Foreign-born persons from countries with high
    tuberculosis prevalence
Medically underserved, low-income populations,
    including high-risk minorities; especially blacks,
    Hispanics and Native Americans
Intravenous drug users
Other populations that have been identified locally
Persons with other medical factors known to increase
    the risk of tuberculosis
        Silicosis
        Diabetes
        Immunosuppressive or steroid therapy
        Hematologic and reticuloendothelial disease
        End-stage renal disease
        Intestinal bypass
        Postgastrectomy
        Carcinomas of the oropharynx and upper gastro-
            intestinal tract
        Persons 10 percent or more below ideal body weight

REACTION ≥ 15 MM

All other persons

PPD = purified protein derivative; HIV = human immunodeficiency virus.
{From CDC (1990) Morbidity and Mortality Weekly Report 39:462.}

TABLE 23.5. **Interpretation of PPD**
Following BCG Vaccination

The probability that a skin test reaction results from exposure to *M. tuberculosis* increases in the following situations:

1. As the size of the reaction increases
2. When the patient is a known contact of a person with tuberculosis
3. When there is a family history of tuberculosis or when the patient's country of origin has a high tuberculosis prevalence
4. As the length of time between vaccination and tuberculin testing increases

PPD = purified protein derivative; BCG = bacille Calmette-Guérin.
{From CDC (1988) Morbidity and Mortality Weekly Report 37:664.}

cific populations must be protected against the potential of exposure to individuals with latent infection (Jereb, et al., 1990). Public education and outreach are needed to develop positive working relationships with the target communities, involving them in successful program planning and implementation. Successful interventions will also require tuberculosis control programs to focus resources on high-risk persons, including contacts of persons recently diagnosed as having tuberculosis. Techniques for contact investigation are discussed later in this chapter. Also targeted for prevention efforts are members of racial and ethnic minorities, and persons born in countries where tuberculosis prevalence is high. Persons with tuberculous infection who have conditions placing them at increased risk of active tuberculosis, such as HIV infections, also require special attention.

IMMUNIZABLE DISEASES

Immunizable diseases, such as measles, polio, diptheria, and pertussis are diseases that can be prevented through immunization. **Immunization** is the process of introducing some form of disease-causing organism into a person's system causing the development of antibodies that will resist that disease and making the person immune (able to resist a specific infectious disease-causing agent) to that particular infectious disease. As discussed in Chapter 12, immunity may be either passive or active. **Passive immunity** is short term resistance to a specific disease-causing organism that may be acquired naturally (as with newborns through maternal antibody transfer) or artificially through innoc-

ulation with a vaccine that gives temporary resistance. Such immunizations must be repeated periodically to sustain immunity levels as with influenza vaccinations. **Active immunity** is long term (sometimes life long) resistance to a specific disease-causing organism and is also acquired either naturally or artificially. Naturally acquired active immunity occurs when a person contracts a disease, developing long-lasting antibodies that provide immunity against future exposure. Artificially acquired active immunity occurs through innoculation with a vaccine, such as the diphtheria, pertussis, tetanus vaccination series given to children. A **vaccine** is a preparation made either from killed, living attenuated, or living fully virulent organisms and is administered to produce or artificially increase immunity to a particular disease.

Because of the success of immunization strategies, few practicing nurses today have treated clients with tetanus or diptheria (although some have cared for clients with residual polio disabilities). However, immunizable diseases still exist in force in the developing world today, and outbreaks occur in the United States in groups of unimmunized or susceptible populations, for example certain groups are constitutionally exempt from immunization for religious reasons and certain refugee populations can also be vulnerable.

Prevention Approaches

IMMUNIZATION: PRIMARY PREVENTION

Control of acute communicable diseases through immunization has been a common practice since the 19th century in the United States (Grad, 1990). The fact that immunization requirements are acceptable in American society today is evidenced by high levels of immunization in schoolchildren and the fact that aggressive enforcement of school immunization requirements, starting in the late 1970's, has not met with widespread opposition (Hinman, 1991).

The statutes that exist to ensure adequate immunization levels by school entry, place the school in the role of controlling agency while public health departments and private health care providers are authorized to administer the required vaccines. An emerging drawback of this mechanism is the fact that many parents may delay immunizations until the fifth year (Pickett &

Hanlon, 1990). Preschool-aged children represent a major proportion of all cases of immunizable diseases and are the group at highest risk of infection (Hutchins, et al., 1989; CDC, 1991d). A child appropriately vaccinated at 3 months of age is 3.1 times more likely to be appropriately vaccinated at 2 years of age (CDC, 1992b; CDC, 1992c). The national objective, stated in *Healthy People 2000,* is for 90% of American children to be vaccinated by their second birthday with four doses of DPT, three doses of oral polio, and one dose of the combined measles, mumps, and rubella vaccine (USPHS, 1991). In addition, infants are now to receive three doses of hepatitis B vaccine and four doses of *H. influenzae* type b before their second birthday, as recomended by the Advisory Committee on Immunization Practices (ACIP) and the Committee on Infectious Diseases of the American Academy of Pediatrics (AAP) (CDC, 1995a).

Half of all children in the United States receive vaccination services in the public sector, while the other half are served by private medical providers (Hinman, 1991). Unvaccinated children are more likely to be recipients of health care in the public sector (Hutchins, et al., 1989). Children who are not vaccinated on time are more likely to have single mothers and parents who are unknowledgeable about existing vaccines. They are more likely to be members of racial and ethnic minorities and to be socioeconomically disadvantaged (USPHS, 1991). Thus, it is critical to discover the social and cultural characteristics affecting health status, attitudes about preventive measures, behaviors in seeking services, acceptability of intervention, and perceptions of health care providers that, in turn, determine parental action in having a child immunized in a regular and timely fashion. This is a unique area of health care delivery, where nurses must rely on parental initiative to obtain a form of care for the well child that may be perceived as producing pain and temporary illness, for no observable benefit.

Schedule of Recommended Immunizations

A schedule for the administration of childhood vaccinations recommended by the Centers for Disease Control effective January 1995 is shown in Table 23.6. CDC also provides schedules for children not receiving their first immunization at two months of age according to the standard schedule. Current recommendations call for a child to receive nine different vaccines or toxoids (many in combination form and all requiring more than one dose) in five to six visits to a provider, between birth and school entry (CDC, 1995a).

Factors influencing the recommended age at which vaccines are administered include the age-specific risks of disease, age-specific risks of complications, ability of persons of a given age to produce adequate and lasting immune response, and potential for interference with the immune response by passively transferred maternal antibodies. In general, vaccines are recommended for the youngest age group at risk whose members are known to develop an acceptable antibody response to vaccination (ACIP, 1994). Recommendations for vaccine administration may be revised in light of specific circumstances. For example, in response to a rising incidence of hepatitis B among sexually active individuals, it is now recommended that infants receive hepatitis B vaccine in doses varying depending on whether their mothers have positive or negative responses to the hepatitis B surface antigen (CDC, 1995a).

Assessing Immunization Status of the Community

Determining the immunization status of children in a community can be a time-consuming but worthwhile task. Community health nurses may consider assessing groups of children with some common characteristics such as children served by WIC, by private medical providers, or attending public schools in various neighborhoods. Because all children attending school in the United States must show proof of immunization upon school entry, review of immunization records at school can provide a means of retrospectively determining the proportion of these children whose immunizations were up to date at age 3 months or age 2 years. CDC strongly promotes the retrospective school vaccination record survey as a means of estimating current levels and monitoring trends over time in immunization status (CDC, 1992b). If no unusual immunization events occur in the intervening period, this retrospective record review gives a reasonable estimate of current immunization status of those age groups in the community. In addition, such a record review targeting children who were not up to date on their immunizations prior to school entry helps identify younger siblings who may also not be up to date.

With increasing numbers of children entering day care services in the preschool years, more states now require immunization for preschool children, often including immunization against influenza, which is not

TABLE 23.6. *Recommended Childhood Immunization Schedule*—*United States, January 1995*

Vaccine	Birth	2 Months	4 Months	6 Months	12[†] Months	15 Months	18 Months	4–6 Years	11–12 Years	14–16 Years
Hepatitis B[§]	HB-1	HB-2		HB-3						
Diphtheria, Tetanus, Pertussis[¶]		DTP	DTP	DTP		DTP or DTaP at ≥15 months		DTP or DTaP	Td	
H. influenzae type b[**]		Hib	Hib	Hib		Hib				
Poliovirus		OPV	OPV	OPV				OPV		
Measles, Mumps, Rubella[††]						MMR		MMR [or] MMR		

* Recommended vaccines are listed under the routinely recommended ages. Shaded bars indicate range of acceptable ages for vaccination.

[†] Vaccines recommended in the second year of life (i.e., 12–15 months of age) may be given at either one or two visits.

[§] Infants born to hepatitis B surface antigen (HBsAg)-negative mothers should receive the second dose of hepatitis B vaccine between 1 and 4 months of age, provided at least 1 month has elapsed since receipt of the first dose. The third dose is recommended between 6 and 18 months of age. Infants born to HBsAg-positive mothers should receive immunoprophylaxis for hepatitis B with 0.5 ml Hepatitis B Immune Globulin (HBIG) within 12 hours of birth, and 0.5 ml of either Merck Sharpe & Dohme (West Point, Pennsylvania) vaccine (Recombivax HB®) or of SmithKline Beecham (Philadelphia) vaccine (Engerix-B®) at a separate site. In these infants, the second dose of vaccine is recommended at 1 month of age and the third dose at 6 months of age. All pregnant women should be screened for HBsAg during an early prenatal visit.

[¶] The fourth dose of diphtheria and tetanus toxoids and pertussis vaccine (DTP) may be administered as early as 12 months of age, provided at least 6 months have elapsed since the third dose of DTP. Combined DTP-Hib products may be used when these two vaccines are administered simultaneously. Diphtheria and tetanus toxoids and acellular pertussis vaccine (DTaP) is licensed for use for the fourth and/or fifth dose of DTP in children aged ≥15 months and may be preferred for these doses in children in this age group.

[**] Three *H. influenzae* type b conjugate vaccines are available for use in infants: 1) oligosaccharide conjugate Hib vaccine (HbOC) (HibTITER®, manufactured by Praxis Biologics, Inc. [West Henrietta, New York], and distributed by Lederle-Praxis Biologicals, [Wayne, New Jersey]); 2) polyribosylribitol phosphate-tetanus toxoid conjugate (PRP-T) (ActHIBN™, manufactured by Pasteur Mérieux Sérums & Vaccins, S.A. (Lyon, France), and distributed by Connaught Laboratories, Inc. [Swiftwater, Pennsylvania], and OmniHIB™, manufactured by Pasteur Mérieux Sérums & Vaccins, S.A., and distributed by SmithKline Beecham); and 3) *Haemophilus* b conjugate vaccine (Meningococcal Protein Conjugate) (PRP-OMP) (PedvaxHIB®, manufactured by Merck Sharp & Dohme). Children who have received PRP-OMP at 2 and 4 months of age do not require a dose at 6 months of age. After the primary infant Hib conjugate vaccine series is completed, any licensed Hib conjugate vaccine may be used as a booster dose at age 12–15 months.

[††] The second dose of measles-mumps-rubella vaccine should be administered EITHER at 4–6 years of age OR at 11–12 years of age.

Source: Advisory Committee on Immunization Practices, American Academy of Pediatrics, and American Academy of Family Physicians. {From CDC (1995) Morbidity and Mortality Weekly Report, 43 (Nos. 51 & 52):960.}

presently required for older age groups. Preschool or day care operators therefore now obtain information about immunization status of this younger cohort, a group that has until now often escaped surveillance and immunization initiative.

Other community settings where community health nurses may identify underimmunized children include homeless shelters and other public service settings used by families and children including local churches. A family with one underimmunized child may have other underimmunized children of other ages, as well as any number of other unmet preventive health care needs which the community health nurse might help address.

Understanding disease rates and immunization status by race or ethnicity requires population data accurately showing the multicultural composition of the community. Such data can be obtained from census figures, augmented by refugee or immigration records. Noting the racial or ethnic heritage of the underimmunized child may lead to valuable insights about unique barriers for the group that must be addressed in order to reduce disease rates and increase healthy resilience.

Herd Immunity

Herd immunity is central to understanding immunization as a means of protecting community health. **Herd immunity** (as described in Chapter 12) is the immunity level present in a particular population of people (Benenson, 1990). Low herd immunity occurs when there are few immune persons within a community and the spread of disease is more likely . . . When more individuals in a community are vaccinated so that a high proportion of the individuals have acquired resistance to the infectious agent, this contributes to high herd immunity. High herd immunity reduces the probability that the few unimmunized persons will come in contact with one another, making spread of the disease unlikely. Outbreaks may occur when immunization falls below 85% (Pickett & Hanlon, 1990), or if nonimmunized susceptible persons are grouped together rather than dispersed throughout the immunized community. An example of lack of herd immunity is presented below in World Watch display.

Barriers to Immunization Coverage

Improving immunization coverage requires examination of reasons children are not immunized. Many barriers exist. They include religious, financial, social and cultural factors, and provider limitations that form barriers to adequate immunization.

Religious Barriers. The right to religious freedom gives some groups of individuals in the United States the constitutional right to exemption from immunization when they object to vaccination on religious grounds (Grad, 1990). Children from these families are identified at school entry. Such exemptions must be specifically enacted by law, and although it is not necessary to belong to a specific denomination, courts have required those seeking exemption to demonstrate that such belief against immunization is sincere, and that no clear danger exists due to the particular disease. Problems arise when members of exempted groups are found together in school or community settings, raising the risk of disease spread (Ibid.).

Financial Barriers. Finances may be significant in accounting for immunization delays in families with limited incomes. Such families may have more immediate priorities than vaccinations for an otherwise well child. Hinman (1991) calculated that the total cost of a complete childhood series of vaccinations in the private sector was $303.55, often paid by third-party payers or health plans. In the public sector the total cost was $92.53, usually paid by public funds supplemented by donations. Financial barriers also limit agencies' ability to deliver services. Funding for vaccination services by the Centers for Disease Control accounts for approximately half of the vaccines administered in the public

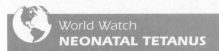

World Watch
NEONATAL TETANUS

Throughout the world, a newborn dies every minute from tetanus infection and a new mother dies from the same disease every 10 minutes (UNICEF, 1994). The tetanus vaccine has been available for 30 years and goals to eradicate tetanus from every country by 1995 should have been realized. Yet the deadly problem persists.

Estimates state that 50,000 maternal deaths and close to 600,000 neonatal deaths each year from tetanus could be prevented through two approaches; (1) tetanus vaccination and (2) hygienic birth practices. Two doses of tetanus toxoid during pregnancy will protect both mother and baby until the infant can be immunized, starting at two months. In many countries childbirth is practiced under unhygienic conditions bringing tetanus spores in contact with the unhealed umbilical cord as well as the birth canal. The World Health Organization states that of all deliveries only half are "clean" and only half have a trained person in attendance (Ibid.).

Some countries are changing. The Peoples Republic of China developed the "three cleans"—clean hands, a clean delivery surface, and clean cutting and care of the cord—and in addition to practicing these has instituted mass tetanus vaccination of women in 300 counties. Zimbabwe now has three out of five pregnant women fully immunized against tetanus and all women who perform deliveries are trained in the three cleans. In Thailand one quarter of neonatal mortality was caused by tetanus but now the country is close to eradicating the disease. By 1992 they had raised the level of women immunized with tetanus toxoid to 72%, improved disease reporting, conducted mass educational campaigns to promote vaccination, taught safe birth practices, gave tetanus shots and boosters to nine out of ten schoolchildren, and delivered safe delivery kits to high-risk areas. Within three years, two of the Thai provinces showing the highest neonatal tetanus rates had cut those rates in half. There is hope that other countries will follow these examples.

sector, about one-quarter of the national total. The level of grant funding increased from $5 million in 1976 to $185 million in l991 (Ibid.). Although at face value this increase seems phenomenal, the portion of funding allowed for program operations, including surveillance, assessment, education, and evaluation increased very little. The overall increase was largely a function of rising costs of existing vaccines and new vaccines (Hinman, 1991). CDC funding does not cover the administrative costs of delivering immunization services. These costs must be provided for through some other public fund source, at a time when there is fierce competition for these dollars.

Social Barriers. Low educational levels, transportation problems, and access to and overcrowding of facilities pose further barriers to adequate immunization coverage (Terris, 1990). Formidable quantities of paperwork involved in obtaining informed consent of parents may be intellectually intimidating as well as time consuming. Single working parents may find it difficult, if not impossible, to reach an immunization clinic with their child during working hours. Requirements for appointments versus walk-in clinics, or for physical exam prior to vaccination may present additional deterrents.

Cultural Barriers. Meeting the immunization needs of minority groups may involve cultural barriers related to differing concepts of health care and preventive measures between cultures. Language barriers may intervene to make parents feel confused, overwhelmed, and unable to access services. Depending on how long a family may have resided in the United States and the level of active sponsorship, expectations of the health care system for parental action on behalf of the well child may be very unfamiliar.

Provider Limitations. Another barrier to immunization coverage are provider limitations. Health care providers may have contact with an eligible child yet fail to offer the vaccination (Hinman, 1991). This occurs when providers see children for different reasons and do not review their immunization records, missing the opportunity to provide vaccination services at what may be a very convenient time for parents. Sometimes children come for immunization services and receive some vaccines but not others, even though the safety and efficacy of administering multiple vaccines on the same occasion (different sites) is well-established and recommended by CDC (ACIP, 1994). Providers may erroneously defer administration of a vaccine based on a condition (e.g. symptom of illness) that is not a true contraindication to immunization (Hutchins, et al., 1989). To address this particular issue, CDC has developed guidelines for providers showing misconceptions concerning contraindications to vaccination (ACIP, 1994). (See Table 23.7). Another provider limitation or

---

TABLE 23.7. *Misconceptions Concerning Contraindications to Vaccination*

Some health-care providers inappropriately consider certain conditions or circumstances contraindications to vaccination. Conditions most often *inappropriately* regarded as routine contraindications include the following:

1. Reaction to a previous dose of DTP vaccine that involved only soreness, redness, or swelling in the immediate vicinity of the vaccination site or temperature of <105 F (40.5 C).
2. Mild acute illness with low-grade fever or mild diarrheal illness in an otherwise well child.
3. Current antimicrobial therapy or the convalescent phase of illnesses.
4. Prematurity. The appropriate age for initiating immunizations in the prematurely born infant is the usual chronologic age. Vaccine doses should not be reduced for preterm infants.
5. Pregnancy of mother or other household contact.
6. Recent exposure to an infectious disease.
7. Breastfeeding. The only vaccine virus that has been isolated from breast milk is rubella vaccine virus. There is no good evidence that breast milk from women immunized against rubella is harmful to infants.
8. A history of nonspecific allergies or relatives with allergies.
9. Allergies to penicillin or any other antibiotic, except anaphylactic reactions to neomycin (e.g., MMR-containing vaccines) or streptomycin (e.g., OPV). None of the vaccines licensed in the United States contain penicillin.
10. Allergies to duck meat or duck feathers. No vaccine available in the United States is produced in substrates containing duck antigens.
11. Family history of convulsions in persons considered for pertussis or measles vaccination.
12. Family history of sudden infant death syndrome in children considered for DTP vaccination.
13. Family history of an adverse event, unrelated to immunosuppression, following vaccination.

[From: Advisory Committee on Immunization Practices. (1989). General recommendations on immunizations. *Morbidity and Mortality Weekly Report*, 38(13), 224.]

barrier to timely immunization coverage is that few providers have the initiative and resources to establish a uniform system for recall and notification when the next immunization is due (Hinman, 1991). In the United States, clients of private providers are not often encouraged or assisted to maintain their own copies of personal written medical records.

Planning and Implementing Immunization Programs

Immunization programs targeting specific subgroups can be effective when they include the following: (1) community assessment parameters by race or other cultural groupings in the planning phase, (2) assessment of specific characteristics of the groups such as language, child care practices, preventive health behaviors, extreme poverty or high illiteracy, and (3) make appropriate planning decisions to deal with these potential barriers. Successful outreach efforts are motivated by the desire to reach the target population, even though specific or unusual accommodations must be made. Clinics are scheduled and held at times and places specifically intended to make the service more accessible and convenient to the target group. Materials are designed and presented with the needs and abilities of target parents in mind. Interpreters are present as needed. Table 23.8 outlines the necessary steps and considerations for administering immunization clinics in community settings.

Adult Immunization

Many people erroneously assume that vaccinations are for children only. Well advertised influenza vaccination campaigns in recent years have helped somewhat to correct this notion. However, media coverage about adverse effects of such vaccination has done little to increase either community or provider enthusiasm about adult vaccination in general.

Adults may require vaccination for a variety of reasons. Occupational exposure to blood, blood products, or other potentially contaminated body fluids provides the basis for Occupational and Safety Health Administration (OSHA) requirements for hepatitis B vaccine. All persons should receive tetanus vaccine every 10 years unless they have experienced major and/or contaminated wounds. If this is the case, individuals should receive a single booster of a tetanus toxoid on the day of the injury if more than 5 years have elapsed since their last tetanus toxoid dose. Beside influenza vaccination already mentioned, adult immunizations may also include pneumonia vaccine and adult diphtheria/tetanus (DT). Other reasons for adult vaccination include international travel or suspected failure of earlier vaccines to produce lasting immunity.

A substantial portion of vaccine-preventable diseases still occur among adults despite the effectiveness and availability of safe and effective vaccines. At least six reasons contribute to low vaccination levels among adults (CDC, 1991g).

1. No comprehensive vaccine delivery systems are available in the public and private sectors.
2. Although statutory requirements exist for vaccination of children, no such requirements exist for all adults.
3. Vaccination schedules are complicated because of the detailed recommendations that may vary by age, occupation, lifestyle, or health condition.
4. Health care providers frequently miss opportunities to vaccinate adults during contacts in offices, outpatient clinics, and hospitals.
5. Vaccination programs have not been established in other settings where adults congregate (e.g. the workplace).
6. Clients and providers may fear adverse effects following vaccination.

COMMUNITY EDUCATION: PRIMARY PREVENTION

Although the use of vaccines is one form of controlling some communicable diseases, there are other strategies which are as important including health education, helping at-risk individuals understand their risk status, and promoting behaviors that decrease exposure or susceptibility. The community health nurse must use all these strategies.

Chapter 14 deals more extensively with the concepts of learning theory and the variety of health education approaches and materials available to community health nurses today. In the context of communicable disease control, two particular themes are included here: (1) using the mass media to combat AIDS and other communicable diseases and (2) successfully targeting meaningful health messages to aggregates.

*TABLE 23.8. **Administrative Aspects of Immunization Programs***

STUDY THE TARGET COMMUNITY

Assess disease incidence and level of immunization coverage.
Identify the target group.
Assess conditions in the community: is the target group scattered or localized?
Assess level of community involvement and awareness of the problem.
Identify means of communicating with target group: through the media or through leaders or other.
Consider political and social structure of the community. Identify important leaders.
Identify sites for immunization clinics that are appropriate, accessible, and available.

PLAN THE IMMUNIZATION PROGRAM

Review budget for immunization services.
Determine goals for clinic performance or outcome measures.
Communicate with target group to notify them of need and promote involvement and participation.
Estimate needs for vaccines and supplies and obtain them.
Plan care of vaccines before, during, and after clinic.
Develop team coordination among staff.
Plan clinic logistics: available supply of needed materials; medical waste disposal; anaphylaxis supplies; records and means of clinic registration; staffing; floor plan for traffic control and efficient management of crowds.
Prepare staff with information regarding objectives for clinic; criteria for who shall not be immunized; mechanisms for referral of clients with other health needs.

PUBLICITY

Inform target group of date, location, and times of immunization clinic.
Provide information on reasons for and benefits of (and contraindications to) immunization.
Encourage parents to bring existing immunization records to clinic.
Provide contact information for those with questions or inquiries.

IMMUNIZATION CLINIC

Registration system and records (for parent and clinic) ready.
Registrar or assistant(s) ready to assist parents not familiar with language of paperwork.
Parent education: informed consent; reporting of adverse reactions; date next vaccine due.
System for call-back, follow-up.
System for dealing with other health issues and/or adverse events.

EVALUATION OF PROGRAM

Assess numbers of immunizations given in relation to goals.
Assess suitability of approach in identification of target group, selection of sites, means of communication with group, availability of resources, etc.
Invite parental as well as community and staff feedback.
Evaluate results in relation to expenditures.

Use of Mass Media for Health Education

As the earlier discussion of communicable diseases demonstrates, many hard-to-reach groups, such as low-income and racially and ethnically diverse sections of society, are most at risk for communicable diseases. One way to reach them is through the media.

In order to disseminate public health information to large numbers of people, Flora and Cassady (1990) find four major roles of the media.

1. Use the media as a primary change agent; community education programs can successfully increase knowledge about communicable diseases and preventive measures.

2. As a complement to other disease prevention efforts, the media can effectively model preventive behaviors, such as condom use and drug abstinence (Shilling & McAlister, 1990).

3. As a promoter of communicable disease control programs, the media can help to increase participation of community members in immunization and STD services.

4. Disease prevention messages can contribute to creation of a social environment that promotes health, for example increasing acceptance of regular condom use in the prevention of sexually transmitted disease.

The body of literature on mass communication and marketing theory for promoting health and preventing disease through the voluntary adoption of healthy behaviors, is growing rapidly (Atkin & Wallack, 1990; Fontana, 1991).

The urgency to combat AIDs, as well as other life-threatening diseases, provides a strong rationale and impetus for developing effective disease prevention and control messages for dissemination through the media. (See Fig. 23.6). Messages need to be tailored to the specific characteristics of target audiences and the media channels to which the audiences are exposed. Studies show that low-income and ethnic-racial minority families (often those at highest risk) watch and listen to more television and radio than do more affluent, majority culture families. Blacks and Hispanics rely on the broadcast media as a source of information more than do socioeconomically similar persons of the majority culture (Shilling & McAlister, 1990). CDC studies show that the behavior changes essential to control the spread of AIDS depend on successful communication between community health providers and target audiences. Participation in media and education efforts depends on groups, such as injection drug users, being aware of these programs and how to access them. Carefully and thoughtfully designed disease prevention messages disseminated through the media have proven to be a reliable and effective way of reaching this hard-to-reach population (CDC, 1991c).

Targeting Meaningful Health Messages to Aggregates

To effectively deliver a communicable disease prevention message, the message must reach the target (at-risk) population. This requires correctly identifying the

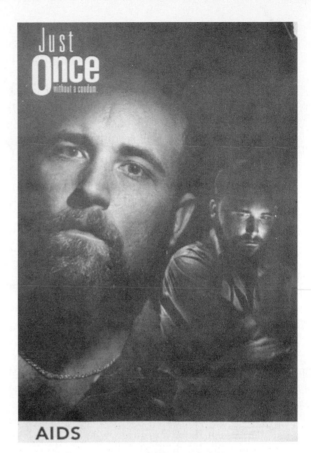

FIGURE 23.6. This poster conveys a powerful message about AIDS.

characteristics of the target audience, in terms of educational level, salience of the issue, involvement of the target audience with the issue, and access of the target audience to the media channels used (Flay & Burton, 1990). Cultural issues affect people's interpretation of messages and must be considered in the presentation of a disease prevention message to ethnic and racial minority groups (Shilling & McAlister, 1990; Nolde and Smillie, 1987). Rice and Valdivia (1991) present "operating principles" for adapting health messages to specific population subgroups:

1. Develop educational materials from the community perspective, reflecting respect for community values and traditions, relevance to community needs and interests, and participation of the community in the preparation and use of the materials.

2. Ensure that materials are an integral part of a health education program, supported by other components of intervention, not standing alone as the educational program in itself.
3. Materials must be related to the delivery of health services that are available, accessible, and acceptable to the target population.
4. All materials must be pretested and have demonstrated attractiveness, comprehension, acceptability, ownership, and persuasiveness.
5. Materials must be distributed with instructions for their use, that is how, when, and with whom they are to be used.

SCREENING FOR DISEASE: SECONDARY PREVENTION

The term **screening** is used in community health and disease prevention to describe programs that deliver a testing mechanism to detect disease in groups of asymptomatic, apparently healthy individuals. Familiar examples include the rapid plasma reagin (RPR) test for syphilis, the tine or Mantoux tuberculin test for tuberculosis, or the ELISA and Western Blot tests for HIV infection. Screening is a secondary prevention method because it discovers those who may have already become infected in order to initiate prompt early treatment.

It is important to remember that the screening itself is not diagnostic but rather seeks to identify those persons with positive or suspicious findings who require further medical evaluation and/or treatment. Any community health nurse working with clients in a screening setting must be prepared to clearly and correctly explain to individuals that screening tests are not definitive and positive findings require subsequent investigation before diagnostic conclusions can be drawn.

Criteria for Screening Tests

There are some important criteria for deciding whether to carry out a screening intervention in a community.

Validity and Reliability. The screening test must be valid and reliable. Validity refers to the test's ability to accurately identify those with the disease. Reliability refers to the test's ability to give consistent results when administered on different occasions by different technicians.

Test Predictive Value and Yield. The predictive value of a screening test is important for determining whether the screening intervention is justified. Yield refers to the number of positive results found per number tested. The predictive value and the yield of screening tests become important in planning screening programs for communicable disease detection and prevention because they can help planners locate screening efforts in areas or within population groups that are known to be at high-risk for the disease. The predictive value of screening tests increases as the prevalence of the disease increases. For example, a screening test for syphilis targeted at the population included in crack-houses in a particular city, would have greater predictive value and yield than a screening test for syphilis given to the city population-at-large.

Epidemiologic criteria for screening interventions for the detection of health problems are as follows (Mausner & Kramer, 1985):

1. Is the disease an important public health problem?
2. Is there a valid and reliable test?
3. Is there an effective and tolerable treatment that favorably influences the early stages of the disease?
4. Are facilities for diagnosis and treatment following positive screening results available and accessible?
5. Is there a recognizable early asymptomatic or latent stage in the disease?
6. Do clear guidelines for referral and treatment exist?
7. Is the total cost of the screening justifiable compared to the costs of treating the disease if left undiscovered?
8. Is the screening test itself acceptable?
9. Will screening be ongoing?

The ethics or values represented by these statements include a commitment to ensuring that resources are allocated to areas where they will have the most benefit in preventing disease and premature death. They speak to respect for the individual receiving the screening service, that the person should only take on the burden of diagnosis if access to acceptable further intervention exists. Woolhandler and Himmelstein (1988) pointed out that socioeconomically disadvantaged persons are often the most at-risk for disease yet the least likely to receive screening services, due to financial barriers including lack of health insurance coverage for preventive care.

CONTACT INVESTIGATION AND CASE-FINDING: SECONDARY PREVENTION

Another secondary approach is contact investigation and case-finding in which the community health nurse seeks to discover and notify those who have had contact with a person diagnosed with a communicable disease. The objective in contact tracing and partner notification is specifically to reach contacts of the index case (diagnosed person) before the contacts in turn become infectious (CDC, 1991a). Thus, the rapidity with which contact investigation can be accomplished is a concern.

Healthy People 2000 further differentiates between two types of partner notification. Patient referral describes those clients who voluntarily advise their partners of the risk of disease and the need for contact with a health provider. Provider referral describes the community health workers who contact the individuals exposed to the index case and encourage them to receive appropriate medical care. In both types of notification, clients need information and encouragement as well as assurance of confidentiality.

It is a fact that not all individuals with disease can accurately identify the persons with whom they have had close or intimate contact. This is particularly the case with sexually transmitted diseases associated with drug abuse and the selling of sex for drugs. It is also true in situations involving highly mobile or transient people whose lifestyles preclude establishing relationships that can be traced or followed. These problems lead to the need for alternative approaches in case-finding, including the provision of screening activities in locations where people with similar risky lifestyle behaviors are likely to congregate. It further points to the critical need for tests that provide reliable results very rapidly, as it may not be possible to relocate the person 24 hours or 2 weeks later for follow-up.

Contact investigation is most commonly practiced today in sexually transmitted disease and tuberculosis control programs. It is also used with some types of food-borne illness outbreak control efforts. Rapidly evolving diseases and those which produce acute identifiable symptoms are not of concern in contact investigation so much as finding the cases of disease with incipient onset and long periods of infectiousness. The latter allow infected persons to reside and interact extensively in the community in an infectious state without being aware of their illness. An example of a community health nurse-initiated model for contact investigation is found in the case study below.

CASE STUDY

CONTACT INVESTIGATION

A community health nurse-initiated contact investigation concerning tuberculosis (TB) provides a useful model (Kellogg, et al., 1987). In planning the contact investigation, the nurses initially contacted and gained the support of a person with authority at the workplace, then learned about the work environment of the index case. From this information, they were able to distinguish those potentially exposed persons as having low, moderate, or high exposure to the case, based on proximity of work areas and frequency of association. First the nurses targeted the highest exposure group, and administered the Mantoux tuberculin test at the workplace. Guided by Los Angeles County Health Department Tuberculosis Control criteria, the nurses were aware from the start that a positive reaction rate of 30% or greater among high exposure contacts would warrant testing of the moderate exposure group.

Evaluation of the project showed: (1) High-risk contacts of the index case had been quickly identified; this timing was critical for promoting compliance with the contact investigation process. (2) The nurses gained support and involvement from a key contact person at the workplace. This provided important coordination of activities and a communication channel between nurses and employees. (3) The nursing process was utilized to assess the workplace environment and plan the intervention, first targeting the most highly exposed. This strategy proved to be an efficient way to organize the use of resources. (4) Education materials emphasizing implications of the disease and preventive measures were distributed to all those exposed to the source case; the goal was to promote compliance with the intervention. (5) Compliance was enhanced by organizing the contact investigation services and making them conveniently available in the workplace to contacts of the index case. (6) The nurses worked closely with administration at the workplace to make followup services for positive Mantoux reactors conveniently accessible without disrupting the work environment. (7) Nurses and contacts interacted frequently over a period of time, allowing the nurses opportunity to address concerns and reinforce information given. A limitation of the project was that it focused only on the workplace contacts of a person diagnosed with active TB, thus effectively omitting similar contact investigation activities needed in the residential or non-work environment. However, The authors provide a helpful framework for use by other health professionals.

Confidentiality and Ethics in Contact Investigation

The issue of confidentiality has always been a major concern in contact investigation. It continues to be a source of debate in balancing the values of protection of the individual with protection of the public's health. Not only must the identity of the individual be protected to the maximum extent possible, but any breaches of confidentiality must be clearly justified based on a threat to the safety of any individual. That is, failure to provide essential information must jeopardize the well-being of the exposed person or contact. It is important to ensure that accessible services exist for the exposed partner or contact in the event that as a result of screening intervention they are burdened with the emotional, physical, and financial consequences of diagnosis.

HEALTH CARE PROVIDER PRECAUTIONS: TERTIARY PREVENTION

Isolation and Quarantine

Communicable disease control includes two methods for keeping infected persons and noninfected persons apart so as to prevent spread of the disease. **Isolation** refers to separation of the infected persons (or animals) for the period of communicability from others in order to limit the transmission of the infectious agent to susceptible persons. **Quarantine** refers to restrictions placed on healthy contacts of an infectious case for the duration of the incubation period to prevent disease transmission if infection should develop (Benenson, 1990).

Safe Handling of Contaminated Infectious Waste

Also important to control of infection in community health is the proper disposition of contaminated wastes (Hayden, 1990). CDC has developed universal precautions in which it encourages health workers to think of all blood and body fluids, and materials that have come in contact with same, as potentially infectious (Benenson, 1990). The universal precautions include:

- Basic handwashing after contact with infected persons or contaminated articles and before care of other clients.
- Appropriate discarding or bagging and labeling of articles contaminated with infectious material before being sent for decontamination and reprocessing.

- Isolation of infected person if hygiene is poor.
- Wearing of protective gowns and gloves by health workers when coming in contact with blood or body fluids.

The Environmental Protection Agency (EPA) defines infectious waste as "waste capable of producing an infectious disease". The agency notes that for waste to be infectious, "it must contain pathogens with sufficient virulence and quantity so that exposure to the waste by a susceptible host could result in an infectious disease" (Fay, et al., 1990, p. 1496). EPA requirements for medical waste disposal are for waste to be segregated into categories of (1) sharps, (2) toxic, hazardous, regulated, or infectious fluids of greater than 20 ml, and (3) other materials. Although incineration has long been recognized as an efficient method of disposing safely of sharps and other contaminated medical waste, fewer incinerators are available now with increasing regulation of emissions, particularly those related to burning chemical wastes.

Four key elements of an infectious waste management program are applicable to community practice (Fay, et al., 1990). (1) Health professionals must be able to correctly distinguish waste that poses a significant infection hazard from other biomedical waste that poses no greater risk than general municipal waste; and such infectious waste must be clearly defined. (2) The waste management program must have administrative support and authority in order to institute practice guidelines and provide the containers and other resources needed for safe disposal of infectious wastes. (3) Handling of the infectious wastes must be minimized. Containers should be rigid, leak resistant, impervious to moisture, have sufficient strength to prevent rupture or tearing under normal conditions, and be sealed to prevent leakage. For sharps, containers must also be puncture-resistant. (4) There must be an enforcement or evaluation mechanism in place to ensure meeting the goal of reducing potential for exposure to infectious waste in the community.

Transmission by Health Care Workers

The problem of multidrug resistant organisms has been increasing since the 1960s, when the first strains of methicillin-resistant *Staphylococcus aureus* were identified in England. The problem is not limited to hospitals, as clients who are colonized or infected with multiresistant strains are discharged into and admitted from the community. Colonization refers to multiplication of an organism on a body surface, such as the skin, without evoking a tissue or immune response. Over the past 10 years, methicillin-resistant and other resistant strains of aureous have become one of the most common agents of hospital and community-acquired infections (Shovein & Young, 1992). This is a special concern for nurses because not only is there potential for the nurse to carry the infectious agent from client to client, but also because there is considerable uncertainty about the implications for practice of the nurse who becomes colonized with drug-resistant bacteria in the course of caring for individuals. Although there is no definitive evidence that colonized health workers are implicated in outbreaks of drug-resistant infections, some agencies furlough colonized workers or limit their practice to infected patients. Studies have shown that effective decolonization may take from 3 weeks to a year. Employee health care programs must include infection control policies that address this problem and provide recommendations to the nurse for the prevention not only of infection but colonization, and provide agency policies regarding care of the infected or colonized nurse.

Communicable Disease Control with High Risk Populations

Some groups and populations are clearly more at risk than others for communicable diseases. This section will examine some groups that are particularly vulnerable to communicable diseases, populations that include pregnant women and infants, children in day care, the homeless, the mentally ill and disabled, international travelers and refugees, persons with home care, and community health nurses themselves.

PREGNANT WOMEN AND INFANTS

Special communicable disease control needs accompany pregnancy. Earlier sections dealing with sexually transmitted diseases and HIV infection discussed the threat of these diseases on the health and reproductive lives of affected mothers as well as on their babies. Women and children are at increasing risk for AIDS throughout the world (UNICEF, 1995). (See Fig. 23.7). Other types of maternal infections, such as rubella, are known to be of great risk to the unborn child, even though the clinical experience of the mother may be quite mild or even unnoticed. Low herd immunity for tetanus among pregnant women in developing countries place them and their newborns at serious risk for contracting tetanus (Ibid.).

Various types of maternal infections place infants at risk for congenital anomalies as well as fulminant infections (Sharts-Engel, 1991). The most prevalent organisms with the potential to cause congenital malformations are the rubella and herpes viruses including *Cytomegalyvirus* (CMV). Congenital manifestations occur in approximately 255 of infants born to mothers who acquired rubella during the first trimester of pregnancy; the incidence drops to 10% by the 16th week, and is rare in infections acquired after the 20th week (Williamson, et al., 1988). Up to 25% of young adults in

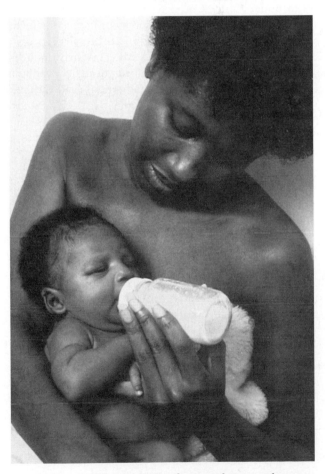

FIGURE 23.7. Maternal HIV infection places newborns at great risk for developing AIDS.

the United States show negative rubella antibody titers and are therefore vulnerable to infection.

DAY CARE CHILDREN

Children in day care are at risk for certain communicable diseases. Currently more than half of all women with children under the age of six years are in the work force. The majority of their children are cared for outside their homes, in small family day care settings, or larger group day care (Johansen, et al., 1988). This daily interaction with groups of young children has been closely associated with the spread of infectious disease, mainly *Haemophilus influenzae*, and enteric diseases including diarrhea, giardia, and hepatitis A (USPHS, 1991; Johansen, et al., 1988; Wenger, et al., 1990). The highest incidence of acute and recurrent otitis media occurs in day care children (Wald, et al., 1988). Children under the age of two and one-half years are at greater risk than older preschoolers for infection, due to a less developed immune system, lack of toilet training, and habit of putting shared toys in their mouths (Johansen, et al., 1988). Pediculosis (head lice) shows a higher incidence in preschool and school-aged children over all other groups.

HOMELESS POPULATION

Homeless people are difficult to quantify in terms of health care needs and characteristics due to the very nature of a transient and often disenfranchised existence. However, as public health services have developed to meet the needs of this growing population, more information is becoming available that is relevant to issues of communicable disease control.

The homeless population of the 1990s is young (averaging 35 to 40 years old), non-white (50%), often female (25%), and highschool educated (30%–35%). The evolution from the alcoholic, older, white male homeless population of past generations has been attributed to a decline in low-income inner-city housing, high unemployment rates, a breakdown in family systems, social service cutbacks, and deinstitutionalization of the chronically mentally ill. Health assessment surveys have shown members of the homeless population to neglect routine health care and ignore health problems, and often to be unable to navigate a complex system of health care (Bowdler, 1989).

A study of homeless black men in Florida identified a high prevalence of substance abuse and at-risk sexual behaviors, both of which are closely associated with a high incidence of sexually transmitted diseases, including AIDS (CDC, 1991b). Failure to thrive syndrome, delayed immunizations, and iron-deficiency anemia are all overrepresented in the homeless-child population (Bowdler, 1989) placing them at greater risk for contracting additional diseases. Other studies show a high risk for tuberculosis among the homeless due to several factors. There is a higher prevalence of active and latent tuberculosis among the homeless population. Shelters are overcrowded and have insufficient ventilation. The prevalence of other conditions, such as HIV infection, poor nutrition, alcoholism and drug use, and psychological stress, may increase susceptibility to active tuberculosis if infection occurs. Transience among this population results in very high rates of noncompliance with or incomplete therapy, further increasing the risks of relapse, drug resistant strains, and transmission (CDC, 1991h). Strategies for control of tuberculosis in this population are similar to those already discussed in the section on tuberculosis. CDC strongly promotes directly observed therapy for individuals receiving treatment or preventive therapy. CDC also recommends HIV-infection status for appropriate identification and management of those requiring intervention for tuberculosis. Other important prevention regimes include proper ventilation and environmental controls in shelters, routine monitoring of tuberculin reactivity of shelter staff members, and close cooperation between shelter staff and local health departments to develop and monitor effective tuberculosis control programs.

CHRONICALLY MENTALLY ILL AND DISABLED POPULATION

The chronically mentally ill and mentally disabled are another population at risk for communicable disease. Many of these individuals were previously institutionalized and released to less restrictive community settings with government-sponsored initiatives of the late 1960s and 1970s. These people are vulnerable to infectious agents because they often lack or do not exercise self-care skill, such as proper hygiene and good nutrition. Their mental instability makes them further vulnerable to drug abuse and contact with persons infected with HIV, hepatitis B, or other communicable diseases.

INTERNATIONAL TRAVELERS AND REFUGEES

As Americans interact more and more with their neighbors in other parts of the world, the incidence of Americans with tropical or imported diseases also rises. Information necessary for a potential traveler to go to new and exotic places, remain healthy, and return healthy, is available from a number of sources. At the very minimum all international travelers must take steps to be adequately immunized as required by international health practices. These include being immunized with immunoglobulin to prevent hepatitis A, having the necessary chemical prophylaxis on hand (and taking it regularly as instructed) if the traveler is to be in a malarious area, and being knowledgeable about food and water hygiene precautions as well as basic first aid for the care of simple injuries. Yet every year, 5000 hepatitis A infections and 20% to 60% of all malaria cases are due to poorly prepared and careless international travelers. In many major cities of the United States one finds tropical medicine or travelers' medicine specialists who can assist in being adequately prepared for travel. CDC offers a travelers' hotline with up to date recommendations regarding malaria prophylaxis. Health departments and large libraries usually offer materials on international travel, including those listed in Appendix A.

Refugees or international travelers who arrive in the United States are often unfamiliar with its health systems, health precautions, and practices. Refugees and immigrants must follow prescribed guidelines for their acculturation including extensive health screening mandated by U.S. immigration laws. More than ever before, community health nurses have professional contact with these new Americans, whether close to time of their arrival or later, in schools and immunization clinics or other locations. Visitors from other countries may also require the assistance of community health professionals. For this reason community health nurses are encouraged to develop and maintain a global perspective on communicable diseases.

HOME CARE POPULATION

While infection control procedures have been recognized as part of institutionalized in-patient care for many years, only more recently have home health and community settings been recognized as locations for patients with infectious or potentially infectious conditions. An increasing incidence of surgical wound and other types of infections are cared for at home, including those attributed to drug-resistant organisms. Family members and other caregivers, as well as the occasional waste handler, are all at risk (Hayden, 1990). In a review of infection control practices in nursing, Larson noted that while nosocomial infections occurred in 5%–10% of hospitalized patients, rates were much higher in extended care facilities, day care centers, and home care settings (Larson, 1989).

A number of problems confront community health nurses working to control transmission of infection in the home care environment. Infection control problems for home care nurses include:

1. Poor communication between hospitals discharging patients with nosocomial or surgical wound infections and the nurse receiving the referral in the community.
2. An increased number of patients in home settings with indwelling medical devices including urinary and intravenous or central line catheters.
3. Safe disposal of needles and clinical waste with minimal handling by the nurse, patient, or other caregivers.
4. Proper use of protective clothing and antiseptic products to avoid carrying infection from one setting to another.

COMMUNITY HEALTH NURSES

Community health nurses require information and administrative support to maintain their health and freedom from occupationally-related communicable diseases. Nurses in a variety of community settings may be exposed to hepatitis B, tuberculosis, HIV, herpes simplex type II viruses (including CMV), and rubella, as well as other immunizable diseases (Williamson, et al., 1988). Employee health programs for community health workers should include: (1) identification of infection hazards in the work environment; (2) education on the responsibilities of the employee in infection control that emphasizes maintenance of sound personal hygiene habits including rigorous handwashing between clients and before and after handling supplies and equipment, and safe disposal of infectious waste; (3) the provision of care for work-related injuries and exposures; (4) institution of protective practices to prevent transmission of disease to employees (Williamson, et al., 1988). Important in this last step is the review of employee immunization status with encouragement to update immunizations as needed (Hayden, 1990), including hepatitis B vaccination for health care workers which is recommended by CDC.

Ethical Issues in Communicable Disease and Infection Control

While working to effectively control communicable diseases in communities and population groups, it is important to ensure that the activities undertaken are ethically sound and justified. See the Issues in Community Health Nursing discussion of ethics. It is important in communicable disease control to consider the ethical aspects of access to disease prevention and treatment services; enforced compliance with preventive measures; screening programs; privacy, confidentiality, and discrimination; and issues involving the health worker employee who is infected with or is a carrier of an infectious agent.

HEALTH CARE ACCESS IN COMMUNICABLE DISEASE CONTROL

Access to health care means that persons needing services find them available, acceptable, and appropriate, unrestricted by barriers to use. Such access has been advocated as an essential public health value by Priester (1992). It would be misleading to say that rates of communicable diseases in population subgroups provide reliable indicators of health care access. The issue is significantly confounded when health care providers miss opportunities to vaccinate and when parents, who have the means, fail to seek out services to ensure immunizations are up to date (Hinman, 1991). It is clear that in the absence of access to health care services, opportunities for people to receive the information and the services necessary to prevent transmission and progression of infectious diseases are sharply curtailed.

ENFORCED COMPLIANCE

Legally, the responsibilities of public health officials in communicable disease control include the police power to enforce compliance with treatment or restrict the activity of infectious individuals in order to protect the welfare of others (Grad, 1990). In disease preven-

Issues in Community Health Nursing
ETHICS OF MASS IMMUNIZATIONS

In critically examining existing or potential regulations pertaining to communicable disease control, it is also interesting to examine how the benefits and burdens are distributed in the population. As an example, recent recommendations for universal immunization of infants against hepatitis B (CDC, 1995a) in the United States are controversial. The purpose of the recommendation is to create an immune cohort in order to reduce the peak incidence of hepatitis B that occurs at the onset of young adulthood, closely associated with sexual behaviors and illicit drug use. CDC has determined that the at-risk population is difficult to reach at or immediately prior to this period of peak incidence, so the proposed alternative approach involves immunizing all individuals at a time in life when, unless the mother is infected, there is very little risk of becoming infected. Still unproven in this matter is the duration of immunity which is provided by infant hepatitis B immunization: Is this intervention in fact an effective one? Have all means to promote voluntary immunization among those truly at-risk for disease, and able to give voluntary consent, been exhausted? Have other health promotion strategies to alter the behavioral and environmental factors been exhausted? Who is to bear the economic burden, and the economic benefits of this strategy?

tion, completely voluntary measures to encourage healthier lifestyles tend to be ineffective.

Regulations that enforce compliance with disease prevention strategies are a justifiable restriction if the measures proposed are demonstrably effective and grounded in ethical principles (Pelligrino, 1981). Coercion must be of the mildest sort compatible with achieving the goals of the regulation. Information must be provided to allow consumers to see the consequences of deleterious habits and the value choices that must be made. Inducements should be favored over disincentives. Remediable conditions that make choice less than free should be ameliorated (through education, by restraints on misleading advertisement, reducing peer or group pressure, and treating emotional problems). Regulation should be confined to actions with direct public impact and be limited severely in matters that are personal and private.

SCREENING FOR COMMUNICABLE DISEASES

As discussed earlier in this chapter, screening programs for communicable diseases are conducted to detect existing or potential public health problems. One can argue that they are morally and ethically justified if they protect and serve both infected individuals as well as those who might be at risk for exposure. However, other issues arise that must be addressed. Are screening resources allocated to areas where they will have the most benefit in preventing disease and premature death? Should individuals receiving the screening service take on the burden of diagnosis if treatment is unavailable because of cost or access? Are screening costs justified in light of scarce health care dollars?

Levine and Bayer (1989) suggest that there is no ethical justification for HIV screening programs. There is at present no known intervention that renders the infected person with HIV non-infectious. Treatment protocols remain largely experimental. Prevention of transmission of the virus continues to require voluntary changes in behavior of infected persons. If screening was to be carried out, identification of the estimated 1 million or more HIV-infected persons in the United States would exceed the capacity of the health care system to provide services.

CONFIDENTIALITY, PRIVACY, AND DISCRIMINATION

To carry out communicable disease interventions, client needs for confidentiality and privacy must be ensured. Screening and other interventions must take place in a physical setting that does not allow overt differentiation between those clients with positive and negative results. As agency and national data systems and programs continue to evolve, it is essential to make confidentiality and data protection measures clear priorities. Studies have reported between 60 and 100 individuals having access to an average hospital record. Bayer (1991) points out that anonymity is frankly incompati-

ble with early intervention. Two areas of current practice that may benefit from closer ethical scrutiny in regard to protection of privacy are contact investigation in sexually transmitted disease programs (Ibid.) and school-based screening for pediculosis (Donnelly, et al., 1991).

Human society has had a long standing aversion to infectious diseases that is still true today. Ostracism in the past of persons with leprosy and other contagious conditions has shifted to discrimination against persons with tuberculosis, AIDS, head lice, and other current forms of communicable disease. Such discrimination should be of as much concern to those in public health as in the legal sector (Carroll & Maher, 1989; Bayer, 1991).

Passage of the Americans with Disabilities Act in 1990 hopefully will result in legal protections for individuals diagnosed with communicable diseases who suffer discrimination regardless of status of infectiousness. The objectives of *Healthy People 2000* encourage community-based agencies to expand communicable disease services, among other strategies, by offering expanding contact follow-up services. Such expansion should occur only with careful planning for the ethical standards which will spell out the protections due each individual client while still effectively advancing the cause of disease prevention.

INFECTED HEALTH WORKERS

Health workers have historically been at high risk caring for clients with communicable diseases, be it plague, typhus, or tuberculosis. Advances in treatment strategies for these clients, however, have consistently resulted in a safer working environment for their caregivers and those exposed to body fluids and various contaminated fomites. Trends in increasing community-based rather than inpatient care for communicable diseases have further contributed to equalizing the risk faced by health workers and the general population.

Yet the pendulum swings. HIV infection, multidrug resistant tuberculosis, and nosocomial infections, particularly with methicillin-resistant *Staphylococcus aureous* (MRSA), now threaten caregivers in significant ways, and the ethical implications of these issues are considerable and evolving. Legislation is proliferating requiring health care workers who are known HIV positive to report to their local and state health authorities. MRSA is a growing problem in many facilities where health care workers are undergoing screening for colonization by the organisms, patients with MRSA are being refused admittance, and the work activities of colonized workers are curtailed (Shovein & Young, 1992). Strategies for health care workers' protection and prevention need to be mandated and enforced in much greater measure.

Summary

Communicable diseases pose a major threat to the public's health. Such diseases can be transmitted through direct contact from one person to another or indirectly through contaminated objects (air, water, food) or a vector (animal or insect). Communicable diseases affect large groups of people and have world wide significance.

Assessment of a community's communicable disease status is accomplished through surveillance measures that collect data regarding disease occurrence, analyze and interpret data, and disseminate information to be used for intervention. These activities are coordinated through the Centers for Disease Control and Prevention, a branch of the United States Public Health Service, which has developed standardized methods for communicable disease reporting and national data systems.

Some communicable diseases occur as a result of ingesting food or water contaminated with disease-causing organisms. Outbreaks of such illnesses occur fairly often and can affect large groups of people. Such disease occurrences need identification and the public educated on preventive measures.

Communicable diseases transmitted by vectors pose different problems for control. Strong environmental meaures must be taken to hinder the vector from reaching the host with the disease-causing agent. Preventive and protective actions include community education.

Sexually transmitted diseases (STDs) threaten the health and lives of millions of citizens. At risk are the sexually active, particularly adolescents and young adults, as well as minorities, women of childbearing age, and children. Control of STDs can be accomplished through effective screening, treatment, contact investigation, and aggressive public education.

Human immunodeficiency virus (HIV) infection, which can lead to acquired immunodeficiency syndrome (AIDS) (the late clinical stage of HIV infection), has become a pandemic and is a major threat to world health. HIV is transmitted primarily through sexual contact and injecting drug use making adolescents and young adults at particularly high risk. It threatens men and women in equal proportions and infants and children are increasingly affected. Prevention and intervention efforts include aggessive education about HIV/AIDS, contact investigation, counseling, support and tertiary prevention with the HIV infected population, and stringent infection control.

Tuberculosis has returned as a major public health threat, particularly for the immune-suppressed population, minorities, and children. The disease-causing organism is transmitted through the air. Problems in treatment include drug-resistant tuberculosis strains along with client compliance with medication regimens. Tuberculosis control includes early detection of tuberculosis through skin testing or chest x-rays, promoting compliance with medication regimens, and preventive education.

Certain communicable diseases, such as common childhood diseases, are preventable through immunization (introducing a form of the disease-causing organism into a person's system to make them immune). Immunity is accomplished through adminstration of a vaccine which is a preparation made from the disease-causing organism. The success of preventing immunizable diseases depends on maintaining a high level of immunity in a population. Recommended pre-school and certain adult immunizations are aimed at this goal.

Additional preventive approaches in communicable disease control include use of mass media and education to inform the public regarding infectious disease prevention and intervention, screening programs for early detection of disease, contact investigation to find and notify those who have had contact with infected persons, and appropriate handling of infectious wastes and infection control.

High-risk groups who are vulnerable to communicable disease include pregnant women and infants, day-care children, homeless persons, chornically mentally ill and disabled, international travellers and refugees, the home care population, and health workers.

Ethical issues in communicable disease and infection control include access to health care, enforced compliance, the justifiability of screening, preservation of confidentiality and privacy, avoidance of discrimination against infected persons, and problems posed by infected health workers.

Community health nurses play an important role with regard to all populations at risk for communicable diseases. Nurses concerned with communicable disease control must recognize who is at risk, where the potential reservoirs and sources of infectious disease agents are located, what environmental factors promote their spread, and what comprises the characteristics of vulnerability of community members and groups—particularly those subject to intervention. Community health nurses must work collaboratively with other public health professionals to establish immunization and education programs, to improve community infection control policies, and to develop a broad range of services to populations at risk.

Activities to Promote Critical Thinking

1. Interview a professional in your local or state health department who works in communicable disease control. Determine: (a) how they conduct communicable disease surveillance, (b) what diseases must be reported in your state, and (c) which communicable diseases are posing the greatest threat to the health of your states' citizens?

2. Compare a recent issue of *Mortality and Morbidity Weekly Report* with the same issue published a year earlier in terms of cases of specific notifiable diseases in the United States. Which diseases appear to be increasing? Decreasing? Select one disease and read at least one recent publication on this subject to determine the reasons for its rise or decline.

3. Determine through your local health department what percent of pre-school children are immunized in your city or county. Is this a safe level of herd immunity? Propose some recommendations for preserving or raising this level.

4. Select one high-risk population discussed in this chapter and list the factors that make this group vulnerable to communicable disease. Use at least one other published source to enhance your understanding. Now propose one nursing intervention (such as a specific screening or educational program) and outline how it might be accomplished.

5. Interview a professional who works in STDs services and/or with the HIV-infected population. Determine what methods they use for contact investigation. How do they preserve privacy and confidentiality? What measures have proven most effective in reaching contacts? What is your evaluation of their success?

REFERENCES

Advisory Committee on Immunization Practices. (1994). General recommendations on immunization. *Mortality and Morbidity Weekly Report, 43*(No. RR-1), 1–38.

Anderson, R.M. & May, R.M. (1992). Understanding the AIDS pandemic. *Scientific American,* May, 58–66.

Atkin, C. & Wallack, L. (Eds.) (1990). *Mass communication and public health: Complexities and conflicts.* Newbury Park, CA: Sage Publications.

Bayer, R. (1991). AIDS: the politics of prevention and neglect. *Health Affairs, 10*(2), 87–97.

Benenson, A., (Ed.). (1990). *Control of communicable diseases in man* (15th ed.). Washington, DC: American Public Health Association.

Bowdler, J. (1989). Health problems of the homeless in America. *Nurse Practitioner, 14*(7), 44,47,50–51.

Carroll, R. & Maher, V. (1989). Legal aspects of contagious infectious disease. *Advancing Clinical Care, 4*(4), 6.

Centers for Disease Control. (1989). A strategic plan for the elimination of tuberculosis in the United States. *Morbidity and Mortality Weekly Report, 38*(S-3), 1–25.

Centers for Disease Control. (1991a). Alternative case-finding methods in a crack-related syphilis epidemic—Philadelphia. *Morbidity and Mortality Weekly Report, 40*(5), 77–80.

Centers for Disease Control. (1991b). Characteristics and risk behaviors of homeless black men seeking services from the Community Homeless Assistance Plan—Dade County, Florida, August 1991. *Morbidity and Mortality Weekly Report, 40*(50), 865–868.

Centers for Disease Control. (1991c). HIV infection prevention messages for injecting drug users: sources of information and use of mass media—Baltimore, *1989. Morbidity and Mortality Weekly Report 40*(28), 465–469.

Centers for Disease Control. (1991d). Measles—United States, 1990. *Morbidity and Mortality Weekly Report, 40*(22):369–372.

Centers for Disease Control. (1991e). Premarital sexual experience among adolescent women—United States, 1970–

1988. *Morbidity and Mortality Weekly Report, 39*(51 & 52), 929–932.

Centers for Disease Control. (1991f). Primary and secondary syphilis—United States, 1981–1990. *Morbidity and Mortality Weekly Report, 40*(19), 314–323.

Centers for Disease Control. (1991g). Successful strategies in adult immunization. *Morbidity and Mortality Weekly Report, 40*(41), 700–703,709.

Centers for Disease Control. (1991h). Tuberculosis among residents of shelters for the homeless—Ohio, 1990. *Morbidity and Mortality Weekly Report, 40*(50), 869–871, 877.

Centers for Disease Control. (1992a). Early childhood vaccination levels among urban children—Connecticut, 1990 and 1991. *Mobidity Mortality Weekly Report, 40*(51 & 52), 888–891.

Centers for Disease Control. (1992b). Retrospective assessment of vaccination coverage among school-aged children—Selected U.S. cities, 1991. *Morbidity and Mortality Weekly Report, 41*(6), 103–107.

Centers for Disease Control. (1992c). Sexual behavior among high school students—United States, 1990. *Morbidity and Mortality Weekly Report, 40*(51&52), 885–888.

Centers for Disease Control. (1993). Special Focus: Surveillance for STDs. *Morbidity and Mortality Weekly Report, 42*(No.SS-3).

Centers for Disease Control. (1994a). Division of STD/HIV Prevention Annual Report, 1994. Atlanta, GA: U.S. Department of Health and Human Services.

Centers for Disease Control. (1994b). Expanded tuberculosis surveillance and tuberculosis morbidity—United States, 1993. *Morbidity and Mortality Weekly Report, 43*(20), 361–366.

Centers for Disease Control. (1994c). Guidelines for preventing the transmission of *Mycobacterium tuberculosis* in health care facilities, 1994. *Morbidity and Mortality Weekly Reports, 43*(No. RR-13).

Centers for Disease Control. (1994d). Heterosexually acquired AIDS—United States, 1993. *Morbidity and Mortality Weekly Report, 43*(9), 155–160.

Centers for Disease Control. (1994e). Recommendations of the USPHS task force on the use of Zidovudine to reduce perinatal transmission of HIV. *Morbidity and Mortality Weekly Report, 43*(No. RR-11).

Centers for Disease Control. (1994f). Sexually transmitted diseases treatment guidelines. *Morbidity and Mortality Weekly Report, 43*(RR-S).

Centers for Disease Control. (1995a). Summary—Cases of specified notifiable diseases, United States, cumulative, week ending December 24, 1994 (51st week). *Morbidity and Mortality Weekly Report, 43*(Nos. 51 & 52), 962.

Centers for Disease Control. (1995b). Update: AIDS among women—United States, 1994. *Morbidity and Mortality Weekly Report, 44*(5): 81–84.

Dilorio, C., Parsons, M., Lehr, S., Adame, D., & Carlone, J. (1993). Knowledge of AIDS and safer sex practices among college freshmen. *Public Health Nursing, 10*(3), 159–165.

Donnelly, E., Lipkin, J., Clore, E.R., & Altschuler, D.Z. (1991). Pediculosis prevention and control strategies of community health and school nurses: A descriptive study. *Journal of Community Health Nursing, 8*(2), 85–95.

Dowling, P. (1991). Return of tuberculosis: Screening and preventive therapy. *American Family Physician, 43*(2), 457–467.

Evans, A.S. (1989). *Epidemiological Concepts and Methods* (3rd ed.). New York: Plenum Medical Book Co.

Fay, M., Beck, W., Fay, J. & Kessinger, M.K. (1990). Medical waste: The growing issues of management and disposal. AORN Journal, *51*(6), 1493–1508.

Flay, R.R. & Burton, D. (1990). Effective mass communication strategies for health campaigns. In Atkin, C. & L. Wallack (Eds.) *Mass communication and public health: Complexities and conflicts.* (Chapter 10) Newbury Park, CA: Sage.

Flora, J. & Cassady, D. (1990). Roles of media in community-based health promotion. In N. Bracht (Ed.), *Health promotion at the community level.* Newbury Park, CA: Sage.

Fontana, S. (1991). Applying marketing concepts to promote health in vulnerable groups. *Public Health Nursing, 8*(2), 140–143.

Ginzberg, H.M., Trainor, J., & Reis, E. (1990). A review of epidemiologic trends in HIV infection of women and children. *Pediatric AIDS and HIV Infection: Fetus to Adolescent, 1*(1), 11–15.

Glittenberg, J. (1990). Problems of global control of tuberculosis. *Journal of Professional Nursing, 6*(2), 73, 129.

Grad, F. (1990). *The Public Health Law Manual* (2nd. ed.). Washington, DC: American Public Health Association.

Hayden, D. (1990). Infection control in public health: A new perspective. *American Journal of Infection Control, 18*(1), 47–9.

Hinman, A.R. (1991). What Will It Take to Fully Protect All American Children With Vaccines? *American Journal of Diseases of Children, 145*(5), 559–562.

Hutchins, S.S., Escolan, J., Markowitz, L.E., Hawkins, C., Kimbler, A., Morgan, P.A., Preblud, S.R. & Orenstein, W.A. (1989). Measles outbreak among unvaccinated preschool-aged children: Opportunities missed by health care providers to administer vaccine. *Pediatrics, 83*(3), 369–374.

Jereb, J., Kelly, G., Dooley, S., Cauthen, G., Snider, D. Tuberculosis morbidity in the United States: Final data, (1990). *Morbidity and Mortality Weekly Report, 40*(SS-3), 23–27.

Johansen, A., Leibowitz, A., & Waite, L. (1988). Child care and children's illness. *American Journal of Public Health, 78*(9), 1175–1177.

Johnson, R.E., Nahmias, AJ., Magder, L.S., Lee, F.K., Brooks, C.A. & Snowden, C.B. (1989). Distribution of genital herpes (HSV-2) in the United States: A seroepidemiologial national survey using a new type-specific antibody assay. *New England Journal of Medicine, 321*(1), 7–12.

Kellogg, B., Dye, C., Cox, K., & Rosenow, G. (1987). Public health nursing model for contact follow-up of patients with pulmonary tuberculosis. *Public Health Nursing, 4*(2), 99–104.

Larson, E. (1989). Infection control. *Annual Review of Nursing Research, 7,* 95–113.

Levine, C. & Bayer, R. (1989). The ethics of screening for early intervention in HIV disease. *American Journal of Public Health, 79*(12), 1661–1667.

Mausner, J. & Kramer, J. (1985). *Mausner and Bahn—epidemiology: An introductory text.* Philadelphia: Saunders.

McEvoy, B.F., & Le Furgy, W.G. (1988). A 13-year longitudinal analysis of risk factors and clinic visitation patterns of patients with repeated gonorrhea. *Sexually Transmitted Diseases, 15*(1), 40–44.

Mertz, G., Coombs, R., Ashley, R., Jourden, J., Remington, M., Winter, C., Ducey, H., Corey, L. (1988). Transmission of genital herpes in couples with one symptomatic and one asymptomatic partner: A prospective study. *Journal of Infectious Diseases, 157*(9), 1169–1175.

Nolde, T. & Smillie, C. (1987). Planning and evaluation of cross-cultural health education activities. *Journal of Advanced Nursing, 12*(2), 159–165.

Pelligrino, W. (1981). Health promotion as public policy: The need for moral groundings. *Preventive Medicine, 10*(3), 371–378.

Priester, R. (1992). A values framework for health system reform. *Health Affairs, 11*(1), 84–107.

Pickett G. & Hanlon, J.H. (1990). *Public health: Administration and practice* (9th ed.). St. Louis: Times Mirror/Mosby.

Priester, R. (1992). A values framework for health system reform. *Health Affairs, 11*(1), 84–107.

Rice, M. & Valdivia, L. (1991). A simple guide for design, use, and evaluation of educational materials. *Health Education Quarterly, 18*(1), 79–85.

Rieder, H.A. (1989). Tuberculosis among American Indians of the contiguous United States. *Public Health Reports, 104*(6), 653–657.

Richardson, V., Zickler, C., & Wheat, L.J. (1991). Tuberculosis screening and treatment in children. *Journal of Pediatric Health Care, 5*(1), 11–17.

Sharts-Engel, N. (1991). An overview of maternal-child infectious diseases (1976–1990). *Maternal Child Nursing*, 16, 58.

Shilling, R.F. & McAlister, A.L. (1990). Preventing drug use in adolescents through media interventions. *Journal of Consulting and Clinical Psychology, 58*(4), 416–424.

Shovein, J. & Young, M. (1992). MRSA: Pandora's Box for hospitals. *American Journal of Nursing, 92*(1), 49–52.

Snider, D. (1989). Introduction: Research towards global control and prevention of tuberculosis with an emphasis on vaccine development. The Fogarty International Center Workshop. *Review of Infectious Diseases, 11*(suppl 2), S336–338.

Snider, D.E., Salinas, L., & Kelly, G.D. (1989). Tuberculosis: An increasing problem among minorities in the United States. *Public Health Reports, 104*(6), 653–657.

Stead, W.W., Senner, J.W., Reddick, W.T., & Lofgren, J.P. (1990). Racial differences in susceptibility to infection by *Mycobacterium tuberculosis*. *New England Journal of Medicine*, 322, 422–7.

Terris, M. (1990). Public Health Policy for the 1990's. *Journal of Public Health Policy*, Autumn, 281–295.

UNICEF. (1994). *The state of the world's children, 1994.* New York: Oxford.

UNICEF. (1995). *The state of the world's children, 1995.* New York: Oxford.

U.S. Department of Health and Human Services. (1991). *Healthy People 2000: National Health Promotion and Disease Prevention Objectives.* DHHS Publication No. (PHS) 91-50212, Washington, DC:Author.

Wald, E., Dashefsky, B., Byers, C., Guerra, N., & Taylor, F. (1988). Frequency and severity of infections in day care. *Journal of Pediatrics, 112*(4), 540–545.

Webster, L.A., Rolfs, R.T., Nakashima, A.K., & Greenspan, J.R. (1991). Regional and temporal trends in the surveillance of syphilis, United States, 1986–1990. *Morbidity and Mortality Weekly Report, 40*(SS-3), 29–33.

Wenger, J., Harrison, L., Hightower, A., & Broome, C. (1990). Day care characteristics associated with *Haemophilus influenzae* disease. *American Journal of Public Health, 80*(12), 1455–1458.

Whittington, W.L. & Knapp, J.S. (1989). Trends in resistance of Neisseria gonorrhoea to antimicrobial agents in the United States. *Sexually Transmitted Diseases, 15*(3), 202–210.

Williamson, K., Selleck, C., Turner, J., Brown, K., Newman, K., & Sirles, A. (1988). Occupational health hazards for nurses, infection. *IMAGE, 20*(1), 48–53.

Woolhandler, S. & Himmelstein, D. (1988). Reverse targeting of preventive care due to lack of health insurance. *Journal of the American Medical Association, 259*(19), 2872–4.

SELECTED READINGS

Alter, M., Hadler, S., Margolis, H., et al. (1990). The changing epidemiology of hepatitis B in the United States. Need for alternative vaccination strategies. *Journal of American Medical Association* 263, 1218–22.

Anderson, C. (1995). Childhood sexually transmitted diseases: one consequence of sexual abuse. *Public Health Nursing, 12*(1), 41–46.

Aral, S. & Holmes, K. (1991). Sexually transmitted diseases in the AIDS era. *Scientific American* 264, 62–9.

Bayer, R., N. Dubler, N., & Landesman, S. (1993). The dual epidemics of tuberculosis and AIDS: Ethical and policy issues in screening and treatment. *American Journal of Public Health, 83*(5), 649–54.

Brunham, R. & Plummer, F. (1990). A general model of sexually transmitted disease epidemiology and its implications for control. *Medical Clinics of North America*, 74, 1339–52.

Centers for Disease Control. (1994). Addressing emerging infectious disease threats: A prevention strategy for the United States. *Morbidity and Mortality Weekly Report, 43*(RR-5).

Centers for Disease Control. (1994). Human plague—India, 1994. *Morbidity and Mortality Weekly Report, 43*(38), 689–91.

Centers for Disease Control. (1995). Physician vaccination referral practices and vaccines for children—New York, 1994. *Morbidity and Mortality Weekly Report, 44*(1), 3–6.

Centers for Disease Control. (1994). Summary of notifiable diseases, United States, 1994. *Morbidity and Mortality Weekly Report, 43*(53).

Centers for Disease Control. (1990). Tuberculosis among foreign-born persons entering the United States. Morbidity and Mortality Weekly Report 39, 1–21.

Coward, D.D. (1994). Meaning and purpose in the lives of persons with AIDS. *Public Health Nursing, 11*(5), 331–336.

Fillit, H. (1991). Acquired immunodeficiency in the elderly: Normal, reversible, and irreversible causes. *AIDS Medical Report*, 4, 20–24.

Ghendon, Y. (1990). WHO strategy for the global elimination of new cases of hepatitis B. *Vaccine*, 8 (suppl), S129–132.

Grimes, D. (1991). *Infectious diseases*. St. Louis: Mosby Year-book.

Joseph, S. (1993). Editorial: Tuberculosis, Again. *American Journal of Public Health, 83*(5), 647–8.

Kuehnert, P.L. (1991). Community health nursing and the AIDS pandemic: case report of one community's response. *Journal of Community Health Nursing, 8*(3), 137–46.

Lilienfeld, D. E. & Stolley, P. (1994). *Foundations of epidemiology* (3rd ed.). New York: Oxford.

Nokes, K., Wheeler, K., & Kendrew, J. (1994). Development of an HIV assessment tool. *IMAGE, 26*(2), 133–38.

Reichman, L. B. (1993). Fear, embarrassment, and relief: The tuberculosis epidemic and public health. [Editorial] *American Journal of Public Health, 83*(5), 639–41.

Sellers, D.E., McGraw, S.A., & McKinlay, J.B. (1994). Does the promotion and distribution of condoms increase teen sexual activity? Evidence from an HIV prevention program for Latino youth. *American Journal of Public Health, 84*(12), 1952–1959.

Salsberry, P.J., Nickel, J.T., & Mitch, R. (1994). Immunization status of 2-year-olds in middle/upper- and lower-income populations: A community survey. *Public Health Nursing, 11*(1), 17–23.

Stein, Z. (1993). HIV prevention: An udate on the status of methods women can use. *American Journal of Public Health, 83*(10), 1379–82.

Strunin, L. (1991). Adolescents' perceptions of risk for HIV infection: Implications for future research. *Social Science and Medicine, 32,* 221–28.

Wuorenma, J, et al. (1994). Implementing a mass influenza vaccination program . . . 15-site health maintenance organization. *Nursing Management, 25*(5), 81–2, 84–5, 88.

24

Promoting and Protecting the Health of At-Risk Populations

LEARNING OBJECTIVES

Upon completion of this chapter readers should be able to:

- Explain the concept of vulnerability and why some groups of people are at greater risk for health problems.
- Analyze each of the four causal domains contributing to vulnerability.
- Describe the etiology of the three types of homelessness.
- Discuss the health-related needs of the homeless population.
- Identify the factors from the four causal domains contributing to the problems of the mentally impaired population.
- Explain the causal factors and health-related problems of the substance abusing population.
- Discuss the community health nurse's role with at-risk populations.

KEY TERMS

- At-risk population
- Chemical addiction
- Chemical dependence
- Chronically homeless
- Depressants
- Episodically homeless
- Genetic predisposition
- Hallucinogens
- Homelessness
- Inhalants
- Marijuana
- Mentally impaired
- Narcotics
- Risk factors
- Steroids
- Stimulants
- Substance abuse
- Temporarily homeless
- Vulnerability

Barbara Walton Spradley and Judith Ann Allender
COMMUNITY HEALTH NURSING: CONCEPTS AND PRACTICE, 4th ed.
© 1996 Barbara Walton Spradley and Judith Ann Allender

For all the decades that nurses have served community clients, certain populations have stood out as needing special assistance. Throughout the history of public health and public health nursing, these populations consistently appear as primary targets for intervention. Who are these people? Why do they need a more concentrated focus in the planning and delivery of health services? As one examines community health needs today, even when reading the daily paper or listening to the news, the answer becomes clear. There are certain groups of people who are particularly vulnerable to problems affecting their health and well being. They are the homeless wandering the streets without adequate provision for their basic needs, such as food, shelter, and employment. They are children, women, and elders who have been victims of abuse and neglect. They are the discharged mentally ill without the emotional and economic resources to cope in a confusing and stressful world. They are people of all ages who have become dependent on alcohol or drugs. They are minorities or immigrants who experience disadvantaged circumstances. They are migrant farmworker families and other economically disadvantaged people eking out a marginal existence. The list could go on. What do these groups have in common? They are populations who are vulnerable or at risk. Persons at risk are those whose chance of experiencing some kind of harm is much greater than the rest of the population. The document, *Healthy People 2000: National Health Promotion and Disease Prevention Objectives*, describes an **at-risk population** as a group with a greater probability of acquiring certain diseases or unhealthy states than the population as a whole (U.S. Department of Health and Human Services, 1991). Low birthweight infants are a population at risk because their chance of experiencing health problems greatly exceeds those of normal weight infants. Studies show children born to parents who were abused are more at risk of abuse than children of parents who were not abused. Residents living near a toxic chemical spill are at risk of diseases, such as cancer, caused by these toxins. Pregnant teenage girls and frail elderly persons are other groups that have conditions that place them at risk. This chapter explores the meaning of vulnerability, factors contributing to vulnerability, and issues surrounding vulnerability. It examines the unique needs of specific vulnerable populations and discusses community health nursing's role in serving them.

Causes of Vulnerability (Risk Factors)

Populations at risk are vulnerable. The concept of **vulnerability** refers to a state of defenselessness, fragility, or susceptibility to harm. The condition of vulnerability stems from many possible variables or **risk factors** which are factors that increase the probability of developing a disease or health problem (Green & Kreuter, 1991). Dever calls them "preconditions" or factors which, if present singly or in combination, contribute to being vulnerable (Dever, 1991, p.14). They derive from four general causal domains: biological, behavioral, sociocultural, and environmental. Within each domain are variables that influence people being at risk (see Fig. 24.1).

BIOLOGICAL DOMAIN

In the biological domain five variables have a significant impact on people's vulnerability. They are genetic predisposition, age, gender, race or ethnicity, and physical or mental impairment. Since these variables, for the most part, cannot be changed, one could easily overlook their importance for intervention. Community health nurses need to remember the crucial role they play among the multiple determinants of vulnerability.

Genetic Predisposition

Genetic predisposition refers to an inherited disease or condition that increases the risk of developing certain diseases or health problems for some people. Persons with a family history of a disease or condition, such as heart disease or renal problems, are more likely to be at risk for developing similar problems. Other diseases that have hereditary links include diabetes mellitus, hemophilia, cycstic fibrosis, and muscular dystrophy. The rapid growth of genetic research in recent years enhances understanding of human development and facilitates better diagnosis and manipulation of genetic-related problems. Genetic engineering also creates risks, such as the unknown long-range consequences of altering gene structures in the hope of making a person more resistant to a health problem, and raises serious ethical dilemmas.

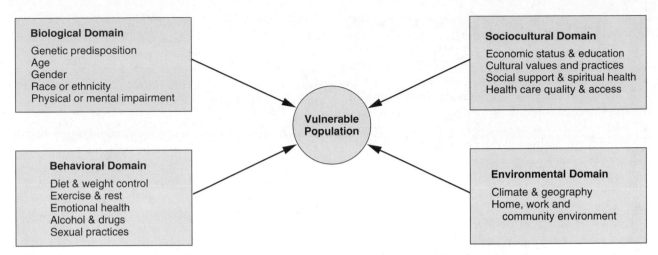

FIGURE 24.1. Model of causal domains influencing vulnerability.

Nursing Actions. Community health nurses can help reduce the incidence of genetically-related problems by first determining who is at risk by history-taking and examination of records. Families can then be referred to appropriate genetic counselling resources or to other community agencies that provide services to cope with such disabling conditions. Nursing interventions also include educating and counseling at-risk groups. Primary prevention occurs when families at risk choose to adopt children instead of having their own biological children whose chances of disability are very high. Secondary prevention occurs when the severity and impact of the genetically predisposed condition is reduced through early and consistent health measures, such as diet and exercise for diabetes.

Age

Age becomes a risk factor under certain conditions. Prematurely born infants, for instance, are at-risk for disease and other health problems because their immune systems and other physiological functions have not had the opportunity to fully develop. Adolescent girls who become pregnant are at risk because pregnancy places an undue strain, physically and emotionally, at a time when normal growth and development already make heavy demands. Children and frail elderly persons can both be at risk for abuse and neglect because of the powerlessness and limitations associated with their ages. Advancing age also places older persons

at risk for other health problems, such as fractures from brittle bones or arteriosclerotic or neurologic changes leading to memory loss and senility.

Nursing Actions. Assessing clients' potential risk for age-related health hazards is a major community health nursing responsibility. Here nurses can have considerable impact on reducing vulnerability. We can prevent many premature births by ensuring access to and use of quality prenatal services. We can reduce adolescent pregnancy through improved education, counseling and support services to teenagers. Child abuse or elder neglect can be prevented through assessing at-risk individuals, vigilant monitoring and reporting, and provision of services to abusers as well as the abused. Other age-related risk factors leading to health problems can be prevented through education and early adoption of healthy life-style behaviors. For example, osteoporosis (decreased bone mass and density with accompanying fragility) in older women, can be prevented through adequate calcium in the diet and weight-bearing exercise during the early and middle years of life.

Gender

Gender influences vulnerability when a person's sex predisposes that person to harm. Throughout history women have been at greater risk because of pregnancy and child birth complications, economic and social exploitation, and physical and emotional abuse. See the World Watch display about women at risk for violence.

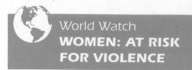

World Watch
WOMEN: AT RISK FOR VIOLENCE

An appalling global problem, mostly hidden, is the violence inflicted on women by their male partners. An estimated 25% of the world's women are violently abused in their own homes with surveys showing higher figures in Thailand (50%), Papua New Guinea and the Repubic of Korea (60%), and Pakistan and Chile (80%) (UNICEF, 1995). Domestic violence in the United States is the largest single cause of injury to women leading to more hospital admissions than muggings, rapes, and road accidents combined (Ibid.).

It is not an easy problem to measure or solve. In many countries, including subcultures within developed nations, women are conditioned from birth to see themselves as inferior and existing for the sole purpose of serving and satisfying others. These women tend to respond to abusive situations by blaming themselves, feeling ashamed, and hiding their injuries—not believing that they deserve any better. The children of these families are at risk as well for physical and emotional problems. Many countries are attempting to address the problem by bringing it to public awareness, providing help for the victims, and exposing the causes. For example, Latin America alone has over 400 private organizations dealing with violence against women (Ibid.).

Recent studies suggest an additional concern. As women become more equal with men, such as closing the literacy gap, the risk of domestic violence increases when male partners find their traditional superiority and control is threatened (Carrillo, 1992; Heise, et al., 1994). Interventions to protect women at risk of violence must also take these factors into account.

For many decades women have been vulnerable to greater health risks and currently are at greater risk than men for AIDS (UNICEF, 1995). Most early research focused on men in the study of growth and development, of common health problems, and of working conditions. Only recently has the emphasis shifted to include a concerted effort to study issues affecting women's health. The Women's Health Equity Act, providing for the establishment in 1990 of the Office for Research on Women's Health at the National Institutes for Health, demonstrates this concern. Because of their gender, women still remain at considerable risk for illness and harm at home, in the workplace, and in the community-at-large.

Men, too, experience certain gender-related health risks. Because men tend to be physically stronger, society's expectations for them to perform strenuous tasks and jobs often places them under greater physical and mental strain. Social role prescriptions for men to be strong and withstand social and economic pressure to provide for their families creates additional stress with concomitant risks.

Nursing Actions. Community health nurses can intervene in several ways to reduce risk factors associated with gender. Rigorous assessment of client populations will reveal the groups most at risk and these groups bear careful monitoring. Community health nurses are often the key professionals for detecting signs of potential harm if they train themselves to be vigilant in watching for early warning signs. A family history or subtle evidence of physical or emotional abuse, for example, will alert the observant nurse to follow up and design interventions. Furthermore, the nurse can help develop programs targeted at enhancing self-esteem and providing support, thus preventing further abuse for many individuals. Pregnancy and childbirth complications can be eliminated or ameliorated through promotion and use of appropriate services. Nursing intervention with political, civic, and employer groups can influence safer communities and working conditions for women and men.

Race or Ethnicity

Race or ethnicity becomes a risk factor when racial origin or ethnic ties predispose people to certain health problems. Studies show minorities are statistically more vulnerable to certain diseases, such as sickle cell anemia among African Americans and alcoholism among some Native American groups. In 1992 death rates from HIV infection, kidney disease, diabetes, and heart disease were all higher for blacks than for whites (CDC, 1994). South East Asian refugees have been at risk for diseases related to their culturally prescribed diet or practices or to communicable diseases, such as measles, from which they had no acquired immunity. Life expectancy remains lower for blacks, especially black males. (See Fig. 24.2.) In some instances, however, whites are at greater

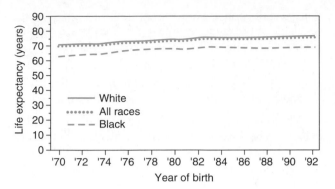

FIGURE 24.2. Life expectancy at birth, by year of birth and race*—United States, 1970–1992.

risk for conditions, such as Down's Syndrome, which occurs mainly in whites, uncorrelated with socioeconomic level or sex.

Nursing Actions. It is important for community health nurses to know the health problems associated with race or ethnicity to which their community clients may be most vulnerable. Such knowledge can then lead to preventive interventions. Promoting appropriate immunizations and other health programs among vulnerable immigrant groups is one example. Assessment of migrant workers' health needs and development of improved services to address them is another. Native Americans' vulnerability to alcoholism can be addressed with a variety of programs targeting improved self-esteem and coping with stress related to cultural adaptation.

Physical or Mental Disability

Physical or mental disability can place individuals at risk. Whether caused by a birth defect, illness, or injury at any stage of life, the disability can render people vulnerable to many types of health problems. Children with Down's Syndrome, for example, are at risk for upper respiratory infections and acute lymphocytic anemia (Pillitteri, 1991). Quadriplegics are vulnerable to problems associated with their limited activity, such as infections or contractures. Mentally-retarded individuals may more likely experience accidents and injuries because of impaired judgement. Nerve-deaf children who have not learned sign language or developed the ability to communicate are at risk for emotional and behavioral problems (Spradley & Spradley, 1985).

Nursing Actions. Although the disabilities themselves may not be changed, community health nurses can intervene to reduce the severity of the disability's

impact on affected individuals' quality of life and well-being. Secondary problems, such as infections, contractures, or injuries, can be prevented with appropriate measures. Support services and training programs for the deaf, sheltered workshops for the mentally retarded, or programs providing employment opportunities for the physically disadvantaged are all examples of interventions that can be promoted by community health nurses.

BEHAVIORAL DOMAIN

The behavioral domain encompasses life style choices. These are variables that can, in combination with each other or with those from other domains, place people at risk of health problems. They include diet and weight control, exercise and rest, emotional health and stress management, alcohol and drug use, and sexual practices. Unlike the biological domain, the majority of these variables can be influenced through intervention.

Diet and Weight Control

Diet and weight control influence vulnerability in several ways. Most people know that a well balanced diet with low fat and low cholesterol is important for good health. Despite general knowledge about diet and weight control, many people are poorly nourished. Reasons for this may vary from simple convenience of fast foods to complex psychological or economic problems causing under consumption or over indulgence. Over concern about weight may lead to fad dieting or even eating disorders, such as anorexia and bulimia. Malnourished people are more vulnerable to developing a variety of health problems, such as heart or liver disease, gastrointestinal problems, and osteoporosis. Obesity, too, causes physical and emotional health problems, such as diabetes, and heart disease. Both weight extremes place people at risk.

Nursing Actions. Populations at risk because of poor diet or weight control problems can be helped. Community health nurses intervene through careful assessment of causal factors and through development of educational and service programs to promote healthier eating habits. Specific vulnerable groups, such as obese children or teenagers who are anorexic or bulimic, often benefit from group counselling and support programs as well as referral to medical services.

Exercise and Rest

Moderate exercise and adequate rest are important for health and well-being. In fact, balance and moderation in all areas of one's life promotes health. People at risk tend to be those who go to life style extremes. Those who choose mostly sedentary patterns, often with accompanying weight problems, can be vulnerable to heart disease, stroke, cancer, and diabetes. Those who exercise excessively and sleep little may be at risk for problems affecting their musculoskeletal and neurological systems.

Nursing Actions. Educational programs that emphasize exercise and rest, particularly targeting children, can help individuals establish healthy habits for life. Community health nurses can work through schools, community recreation programs, and parent groups to encourage exercise and rest as ways to feel better and improve performance in sports and at work.

Emotional Health

Emotions play a major role in determining whether or not people will be at risk. The level of people's emotional health influences the way they work, play, interact with others, and view their world. Poor emotional health prevents people from coping effectively with stress. They may be at risk for developing unhealthy behaviors, such as excessive consumption of alcohol, tobacco, or drugs which lead to additional health problems. Many types of stress, including divorce, unemployment, or overwork add to the risk for poor emotional health. Low self-esteem and depression contribute significantly to vulnerability for destructive behavior. Depressed adolescents and elderly persons are particularly vulnerable to suicide. Violence, now acknowledged as a serious public health problem (Rosenberg, et al., 1992), is attributable in most instances to emotional disturbance. Shootings, reckless behavior resulting in unintentional injuries or death, and physical and mental abuse are all forms of violence resulting from poor emotional health. The primary population at risk affected by violence is the victims'. However, both perpetrators and victims need intervention.

Nursing Actions. Community health nurses can work with existing mental health services or help to develop new programs to address the needs of groups at risk for emotional problems. Nurses working with any given community should collaborate with other health professionals to assess the mental health needs of vulnerable populations in that community, such as the homeless, discharged mentally ill, or teenagers at risk for suicide, and ensure that appropriate services are available. A broad range of programs may be needed, including food and shelter, employment, support groups, counseling, and nursing and medical services.

Alcohol and Drugs

When abused, alcohol and drugs become serious risk factors. The association between alcohol abuse and motor vehicle accidents, homicides, suicides, and family violence has been well established (U. S. Department of Health and Human Services, 1991; Archer, et al., 1995). Use of alcohol causes depression. Alcohol abuse also contributes to other health problems, such as cirrhosis of the liver and cancer. Misuse of over-the-counter and prescription drugs creates additional risk factors. Stimulants, sedatives, tranquilizers, and other drugs are used to excess by many people to combat neuroses and escape from stress. Many individuals engaged in competitive sports have abused the use of steroids and other drugs leading to serious health consequences. A further concern for community health nurses is the heavy trafficking in illicit drugs, particularly among youth and young adults. Use of marijuana and cocaine has risen sharply for all ages (U. S. Department of Health and Human Services, 1991). Misuse of and injecting of drugs leads to placing people at risk for many health problems, including heart disease, strokes, injuries, suicide, homicide, and HIV infection.

Nursing Actions. A number of programs, such as Alcoholics Anonymous or drug rehabilitation centers, exist to work with these vulnerable groups. Community health nurses should be aware of available services so that appropriate referrals can be made. Often the nurse can serve as case finder in determining individuals who need help and also as case manager in coordinating services. Community health nurses can promote more studies of the factors contributing to these health risk behaviors and can assist in the development of more preventive programs in the community.

Sexual Practices

Sexual practices, under certain conditions, place people at risk. In an era when freedom of sexual expression is encouraged and advertising and films promote sexual activity, adolescents and young adults are particularly vulnerable. Incidence of sexually transmitted diseases is rising, 86% of them occurring in individuals 15 to 29 years of age (CDC, 1992). Approximately a million individuals in the United States are infected with the Human Immunodeficiency Virus (HIV), many of them unaware

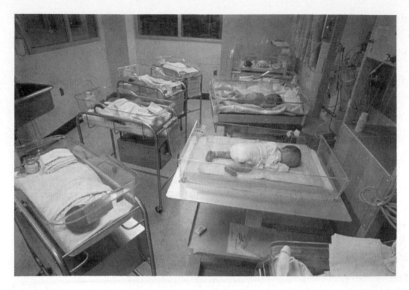

FIGURE 24.3. Increasing numbers of HIV-positive infants are directly related to rising numbers of infected women.

that they carry the infection. Without treatment, nearly 50% of these people can expect to develop Acquired Immunodeficiency Syndrome (AIDS) and 40% more will likely develop other clinical illnesses associated with HIV infection (Hessol, et al, 1988). Although intravenous transfusions may be one cause, sexual contact is the primary means for contracting HIV infection and AIDS, diseases that have reached epidemic proportions in the United States and world-wide. The victims of these diseases, initially mostly homosexual men in urban areas, now include heterosexuals and people of all ages. Throughout the world, women have been exposed and are now becoming infected with HIV, the virus that causes AIDS, as often as men. By the year 2000 the World Health Organization (WHO) predicts that most new infections will be in women. And the rising infection rates for women have been accompanied by a corresponding rise in the number of children born to them infected with HIV (UNICEF, 1995). (See Fig. 24.3.) Many of these infants may escape infection but are at risk for becoming orphans of mothers who die of AIDS (Merson, 1992).

Women and children are at serious risk for additional health problems related to sexual practices. Among the complications of sexually transmitted diseases are pelvic inflammatory disease, sterility, ectopic pregnancy, blindness, cancer associated with human papillomavirus, fetal and infant death, birth defects, and mental retardation. Within this group, the poor and ethnic and racial minorities experience the highest rates of disability and death (U. S. Department of Health and Human Services, 1991).

Nursing Actions. Health teaching and counseling are important weapons for community health nurses to use in fighting this risk variable. Young people, a particularly vulnerable group, can be reached through school, community, and church programs that teach the dangers of unhealthy sexual practices and that promote self-esteem and safe sex. Single adults comprise another at-risk group needing similar encouragement. Services exist through health departments and other agencies in many communities to provide education, examinations, and even free condoms. The nurse can refer clients to these services or help to ensure their development in communities where the services do not exist.

SOCIOCULTURAL DOMAIN

A third causal domain presents several additional variables influencing people's vulnerability. These include economic status and education, cultural values and practices, social support systems including spiritual health, and health care quality and access. Once again, some of these variables can be changed. Their impact on vulnerability and the important role they play in designing community health nursing interventions must not be underestimated.

Economic Status and Education

Economic status and education may influence people's degree of vulnerability to health problems. Research has established that low income groups tend to experience higher rates of mortality and morbidity. Economic deprivation is often associated with poor nutrition and living conditions, less than optimal life-style behaviors, as well as limited use of and access to health services. Low income groups constitute the greatest number of uninsured and underinsured for health services in the United States (Goodman, 1992). They are generally less educated and consequently less well informed about health and health care. Minimal education also limits people's ability to obtain meaningful work and the needed income to improve their standard of living. For all these reasons the poor tend to be an at-risk population.

Many middle income people are also vulnerable. Self-employed individuals, for example, find they cannot afford the extraordinary costs of paying for their own health insurance and preventive health services when not available to them at discounted group rates. Ten to fifteen percent of the population lacks adequate health insurance and the number of middle income people in this group is increasing (Rice, 1992). Many others covered by employer-based insurance have experienced erosion of their benefits because of rising costs. Although this socioeconomic group is generally better educated, increased living costs and other stressors may interfere with use of health services offsetting what their education has taught them about healthy living.

Nursing Actions. Although economic status itself may be an unchangeable variable, community health nurses can intervene in several ways to reduce the vulnerability of these populations. With low income groups health education and efforts to ensure improved quality and access to health care are important nursing actions. In addition, influencing policy development and legislation will be critical to providing adequate health insurance coverage to all vulnerable groups. Community health nurses can play an active role in this process by informing legislators of the needs of these groups and testifying at legislative hearings.

Cultural Values and Practices

Cultural values and practices play an important role in determining whether or not a population is at risk. In Chapter 7 culture is defined as a learned set of beliefs that govern people's perceptions and actions. For each cultural group these beliefs provide a set of standards for individual members' behavior and for interpreting the behavior of others. Most often these beliefs and standards derive from a process of adaptation to the group's environment over a long period of time. When that environment changes and members of a cultural group are transplanted to a new setting or must adapt to a different dominant culture, as is the case with immigrants, refugees, and many Native Americans, some of their traditional beliefs and practices may no longer be useful. Inappropriate adaptation to the new environment can lead to unhealthy practices, such as use of certain folk medicine remedies, placing the group at risk for illness.

Nursing Actions. To reduce the vulnerability of these populations, community health nurses must assess the cultural practices that could potentially cause harm and then apply the cultural intervention principles described in Chapter 7. They include the following:

■ Recognize and appreciate the differences between your clients' culture and your own.
■ Understand the cultural basis for your clients' behaviors.
■ Listen and learn before suggesting any changes.
■ Empathize with and show respect for clients and their culture.
■ Be patient. It takes time to build trust and effect cultural change.

Services exist in many communities for groups who may be at risk because of differing cultural values and practices such as South East Asian refugee programs, migrant worker services, and Latino centers. Community health nurses can refer clients to these services or, if none exist, work collaboratively with the community to develop those that are needed.

Social Support Systems and Spiritual Health

Inadequate social and spiritual supports may place people at risk for health problems. A time-honored support system, the family, has been eroded in recent years through divorce and mobility. Family members who are scattered geographically or those who experience conflict within their families often do not find needed support to cope with the stresses of raising children, the demands of single parenting, or other strains imposed when both parents work. Improved day care programs, after school activities, and other social services all help. But the fact remains that many individuals in the community receive inadequate support—emotionally, socially, financially, and spiritually. Low income single parents are one particularly vulnerable group. Another is the unemployed. People living alone, such as widowed elderly persons, constitute an additional group at risk. Others, such as the homeless or discharged mentally ill, are more vulnerable when the community fails to provide needed support and rehabilitation.

In many settings, community agencies, businesses, and churches work together to provide relief. Food shelves, donated clothing and toys, emotional and financial counseling services, housing and employment programs are available in increasing numbers. (See Fig. 24.4.) Support groups, too, have been developed in many communitites to addresss the concerns of such people as single parents, the unemployed, recently divorced or widowed, or individuals coping with cancer, AIDS, and other diseases or disabling conditions. Churches, synagogues, and other community groups offer spiritual support and encouragement in faith. But none of these services help if vulnerable groups do not know about them or do not have the emotional, physical, or financial resources to use them. The isolated elderly, for example, may lack transportation, single parents may feel they don't have the time, or unemployed persons may feel too depressed to use existing supports. Other community settings may offer limited or no support services.

Nursing Actions. Community health nurses can play an important role in preventing health problems and reducing the impact of these risk factors. The challenge lies in determining which are the vulnerable groups in a given community that lack support systems, what supports exist that these people might be assisted to use, what support services need to be developed, and what strategies will ensure that the at-risk groups receive needed support. Collaborative efforts with other community members will provide the answers and promote improved use of needed support for these vulnerable groups.

Health Care Quality and Access

The quality of and access to health services also influence the degree to which people are at risk for health problems. As technology has improved, health care costs have risen, and health regulations have tightened, certain groups have become vulnerable to receiving inadequate health services with resulting health risks. The poor and those with inadequate insurance are at greater risk of developing health problems because they have limited access to health care services and quality of care is often inadequate.

Geographic placement of services also affects quality of health care. Urban settings provide a greater concentration of resources for health education and other preventive efforts as well as available diagnostic equipment, treatment facilities, and research capabilities. Consequently, rural communities can rarely attract the

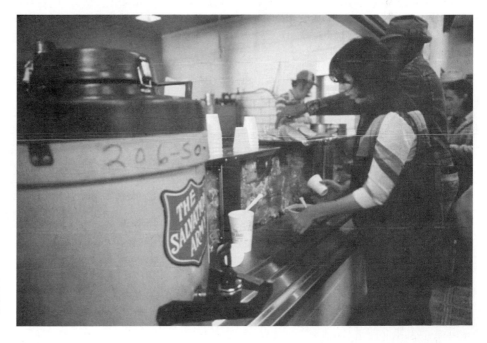

FIGURE 24.4. This food shelf, run by the Salvation Army, provides meals for vulnerable groups.

same quality of health services. Rural residents must often travel great distances to receive care, a factor that influences the degree to which they use services.

Lack of physical access to health care creates another risk factor. Many individuals lack transportation and if elderly or disabled cannot manage public transportation. Others must take time off work with a loss in pay to attend health programs or receive health services not offered at convenient times. The poor and the elderly are often the most vulnerable populations to risk factors associated with health care quality and access.

Nursing Actions. Intervention to reduce the impact of these risk variables is essential. Community health nurses face a clear challenge to change the system to one that is more consumer friendly. Efforts to influence policy, legislation, and planning for health services at all levels, from local to international, will be critical to ensure success in reducing the vulnerability of these groups. A useful reference for community health nurses is the 1992 publication, *Improving Access to Health Care: What Can the States Do?*, edited by John Goddeeris and Andrew Hogan. Various authors describe ways to address the access problem, propose insurance solutions, and analyze issues in policy implementation. Examples include lobbying for program funding and taking services to outlying areas through mobile units.

ENVIRONMENTAL DOMAIN

A fourth and final causal domain influencing vulnerability is the environmental domain. Once again, certain variables, this time associated with the environment, may place people at risk for health problems. The variables are climate, geography, and the home, work and community environment.

Climate and Geography

Climate and geography may generate several kinds of risk factors. Climate extremes in areas that are excessively cold or hot, wet or dry; where there is too much sun exposure or too little, often put people at risk for health problems. Even in more moderate climates, severe winters or hot and humid summers take their toll on certain vulnerable individuals, particularly the elderly and those with cardiac or respiratory conditions. Some people are vulnerable to the dusts and pollens that promote a higher incidence of allergies and asthma in certain areas. In climates that have long rainy seasons and many overcast days people can be more prone to depression. Studies have shown that depression and anxiety for some people are directly associated with seasonal changes leading to a condition called seasonal affective disorder (Allen, et al., 1993). Depending on where people live, many may be at risk for natural geographic or climatic occurences such as hurricanes, tornados, earthquakes, floods, and volcanic eruptions. Indiginous plants and animals can pose additional risks. Examples are poisonous plants, venomous snakes and scorpions, and disease-carrying insects or animals such as rodents, ticks, and fleas.

Nursing Actions. Community health nurses working in a given area should be aware of the potential health risks imposed by the climate and geography of that region. You can learn about the resources available or work with other community professionals to develop needed screening services, educational efforts, disaster preparedness and relief programs. Records from health departments, insurance companies, relief agencies, and other sources can tell the nurse which people have been most vulnerable in the past to the risks unique to that area and, knowing which groups are most vulnerable, interventions can be designed. Chapter 6 provides the reader with more in-depth discussion on this topic.

Home, Work, and Community Environment

The environment of the home, worksite, and community may offer potential risk factors affecting people's health. Safety issues generate a large area for concern. Accidents are one of the leading causes of death in the United States and many are preventable, particularly for young children and the older population. Most common accidental injuries result from motor vehicle accidents, firearms, falls, drownings, and fires. In the home there are many substances and conditions which place people at more risk to accidents. Unsafe situations for children include unsafe toys which can cause choking, toxic cleaning agents, firearms, asbestos insulation, lead-based paint, unguarded stairways and electrical outlets. Loose scatter rugs can cause falls and fires can be caused by poor wiring, overloaded electrical outlets, improperly used heaters, and careless smoking. Improper use of tools and other dangerous equipment can also cause injuries.

The work environment, too, may present risk factors affecting people's health. Since the passage of the Occupational Safety and Health Act in 1970, employee working conditions in the United States have improved considerably and exposure to hazardous substances and unsafe equipment and procedures has been greatly reduced. Nonetheless, injuries and illnesses occur in the workplace when standards are not met and proper procedures are not followed. Some workers are at risk for specific types of health problems because of the physical demands of their job or substances with which they come in contact such as workers who do heavy lifting and are at risk for muscle and back strain, furniture refinishers are at risk for leukemia, miners are at risk for lung cancer, firefighters are at risk for carbon monoxide poisoning and burns, and computer programmers are at risk for carpal tunnel syndrome and headaches. (See Fig. 24.5). Other physical conditions of the work environment, such as lighting, ventilation, odors, temperature, and space may have adverse health effects. Psychosocial environment factors add another layer of possible risk factors. Unsatisfying work, the stress of overwork, or difficult interpersonal relationships on the job can place individuals at greater risk for heart disease and other illnesses. In addition, some workers are more vulnerable to illness or injury at work when their life style outside of work or general physical and emotional health are not good. Chapter 20 provides a more detailed discussion of factors affecting health and safety in the workplace.

In the community other conditions may create potential health risks. Outbreaks of communicable disease, such as tuberculosis, influenza, or HIV become real threats to the health of unaffected but vulnerable groups. Urban settings may develop such things as an unsafe water supply, contamination from a nuclear power plant, toxic wastes, airport noise, high crime, drug trafficking, or highway congestion that can contribute to safety and health problems. Rural communities may face different potential threats to health, such as leaking septic tanks, pesticide poisoning, and unsafe farm equipment.

Nursing Actions. It is important for community health nurses to remember that while each home, workplace, and community environment may have some common features, all have certain aspects that are unique to each setting. Nursing actions must begin with careful environmental assessment focused on answering two important questions. First, what are the factors in this particular environment that are potentially threatening to health and safety? Second, who are the people most vulnerable to health problems associated with these environmental factors? In gathering assessment data the nurse will draw from several sources including the nurse's own observations, interviewing consumers, examination of health department and other records, and collaborative review with professional colleagues. Once the nurse knows the potential environmental threats and which groups of people are most vulnerable, then she or he can work with consumers and other

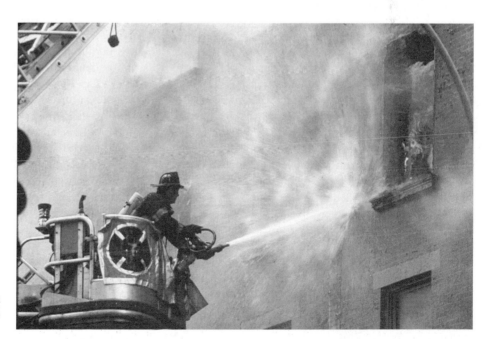

FIGURE 24.5. Smoke inhalation and burns are an occupational risk of firefighting.

community health workers to design preventive interventions, such as distributing information on how to child proof one's home. Educational programs can be started in the workplace to promote proper lifting techniques, exercise, diet and other healthy life style behaviors. In the community, the nurse can promote such things as safe playground equipment, bicycle paths, and escorts for elderly pedestrians. In sum, community health nurses have a three part role. One, they need to assess for environmental risk factors. Two, they inform consumers and agencies about the impact of the environment. And three, they advocate for a healthier environment.

Specific At-Risk Populations

The preceeding discussion of causal domains graphically portrays the many variables, singly or in combination, that place certain groups of people at risk for health problems. Throughout the discussion, three populations emerge as particularly vulnerable to health problems: they are the homeless, the mentally ill and disabled, and substance abusers. These people lack the needed ability or resources to avoid the obstacles leading to health problems. The following discussions focus on these selected at-risk populations to examine their unique vulnerabilities and explore how community health nurses can promote and protect their health.

THE HOMELESS POPULATION

Homelessness has become an increasingly urgent social and public health concern. **Homelessness** refers to the condition of lacking resources and community ties necessary to provide for one's own adquate shelter (Committee on Community Health Services, 1988). Homeless persons may fall into one or more of three categories. The **temporarily homeless** are those who are forced to find temporary shelter because of a sudden disaster, such as as a fire or flood, which leaves them without a home. A second group are **episodically homeless** individuals who "frequently go in and out of homelessness" (Institute of Medicine, 1988, p.23), such as runaway young persons, migrant workers, and families experiencing financial difficulties who seek periodic housing with family members or friends. These people without their own home but sharing the home of friends or family go uncounted in homeless statistics

and are often called the "hidden homeless" population. The third category are the **chronically homeless** or those persons who have no permanent residences for a year or more (Ibid.). Many of the deinstitutionalized mentally ill as well others mentioned above fall into this category. Most experience some form of financial exigency and are unable to obtain affordable housing of their own.

Homelessness exists today throughout the world in both developed and underdeveloped countries. In increasing numbers, political refugees, war and disaster victims, the poor and others sleep in temporary and inadequate housing in such countries as Hungary, Austria, Belgium, the Sudan, Britian, Denmark, Mexico, India, and the Philippines (Berne,et al., 1990). The United Nations reported in 1985 that 100 million people were without shelter and it named 1987 the International Year of Shelter for the Homeless (Ramachandran, 1988).

Like other developed nations, the United States has seen an increase in homelessness with close to four million persons estimated to be homeless. There has also been a dramatic change in the demographics of the homeless. No longer is this population comprised solely of older white men; 31% of the homeless in the United States are women, of whom 25% are single and have children (Ugarriza & Fallon, 1994). Mothers with young children constitute the fastest growing segment of the homeless population. See the Research in Community Health Nursing discussion on homeless children. The majority of the homeless population is still male, but the average age male is younger, in his thirties (Winkleby, et al., 1992). Many of the female homeless are young also. "Nearly 50% of the homeless parents seeking shelter during 1985 in Boston were between the ages of 17 and 25 years . . . 20% of the families admitted to a San Antonio shelter were headed by teen parents" (U.S. House, 1987, p.4). Overall the homeless population is younger and better educated than in the past. One study showed that "two thirds of the homeless were betweeen the ages of 25 and 44 years (mean age = 36 years); virtually none were 65 or older . . . 68% of the homeless had completed at least high school and 30% had attended college" (Winkleby, et al, 1992, p. 1395). The homeless population includes an increasing number of women, children, and ethnic and racial minorities, particularly African Americans. Even though fewer of the homeless are the stereotypical alcoholic, many (an estimated 30% to 40%) are mentally ill (Wright & Weber, 1988; Ugarriza & Fallon, 1994). Substance abuse and psychiatric disorders are high

Research in Community Health Nursing
HOMELESS CHILDREN

Riemer, J. G., Van Cleve, L., & Galbraith, M. (1995). Barriers to well child care for homeless children under age 13. *Public Health Nursing, 12*(1), 61–66.

With increasing numbers of children among the homeless, they have become a new population-at-risk. The investigators in this study sought to determine what homeless families perceived as barriers to preventive health care and whether there was a relationship between these barriers and the families' duration of homelessness.

Fifty-three families (with 120 children) at three shelter sites in three California counties were surveyed using a questionnaire at the shelters during evening hours. The four barriers affecting the children's care that were cited most frequently were (1) difficulties in selecting a provider; (2) waiting to obtain a well child appointment; (3) waiting during well child appointments; and (4) high cost of transportation and/or parking.

This study did not show a relationship between duration of homelessness and the perceived barriers. However, the barriers identified in this study confirm findings from previous studies about potential barriers to preventive services. The investigators concluded that innovative services to reduce these barriers need to be developed, such as shelter-site clinics, mobile units, and use of a nurse liaison between shelters and hospital-based clinics.

among the homeless but research has yet to demonstrate whether these conditions precede homelessness or are the consequences of homelessness (Winkleby, et al., 1992). It has been demonstrated that the stresses of poverty and homelessness coincide with an increase in mental health problems, particularly for homeless mothers and children (Berne, et al., 1990).

Etiology of Homelessness

The factors contributing to homelessness derive from all four of the causal domains. In the biological domain, genetic predisposition to chemical addiction or mental illness may place some individuals at higher risk of homelessness. Any type of physical or emotional illness

or impairment, including war-stressed veterans, may limit an individual's ability to find employment or cope with the demands of living. Those without resources of their own or those lacking outside assistance are particularly vulnerable. Age, gender, and race or ethnicity are additional biological variables influencing the vulnerability of this population as evidenced by the statistics demonstrating increased numbers of minorities, single women and children, who are homeless. A rising number of the homeless are battered women who, in desperation, leave their husbands or boyfriends to find safety in shelters for themselves and their children (Newman, 1993).

Behavioral factors may contribute to being at risk for homelessness. Poor physical and emotional health practices, such as alcohol and drug abuse, inadequate nutritional intake, or poor stress management, may lead to an inability to earn a living or function adequately. When some individuals fall on hard times or experience tragedy or disappointment, and have no family or support systems upon which to temporarily depend for help, they may be unable to cope. Unhealthy behavior patterns or being the recipients of abuse often contribute to this inadequate coping. A recent study of adult homeless individuals showed that "excessive alcohol use as an adult and physical abuse during childhood were the factors most strongly related to length of time homeless" (Winkleby, et al, 1992, p.1394).

Social and economic factors play the largest role in causing homelessness. Poverty, unemployment, and lack of affordable housing, in particular, have combined forces to create homelessness. Poverty is the largest single common denominator among the homeless (Francis, 1991). James O'Connell, director of the Homeless Families Program, states, "Homelessness will never be 'solved' until persistent poverty has been eradicated in our society" (O'Connell, 1994, p. 3). Poverty is highest among female-headed and minority families (Waxman & Reyes, 1989). Many of these women lack job skills and cannot earn an adequate living. Some of the homeless are employed but do not earn enough to afford the costs of housing. Others have lost their jobs and are unable to find employment. While some go to subsidized hotels and shelters, others live in public parks, sleep in tents or their cars and use public facilities, double up with family or friends or sleep in subways. (See Fig. 24.6.) For these reasons it is difficult to accurately count the number of homeless or to design programs and develop policies that address their needs.

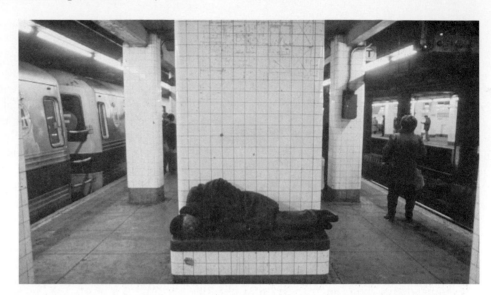

FIGURE 24.6. A homeless city dweller takes refuge in a subway station.

A serious lack of affordable low income housing contributes greatly to the problem of homelessness. The cost of housing for low income people can be prohibitive, some paying as much as 75% of their monthly income on rent (Waxman & Reyes, 1989). While inflation has driven up the cost of housing, the proportion of people living below federal poverty levels has risen sharply. The Chairman of the Select Committee on Children, Youth, and Families stated:

"Limited affordable housing and insufficient AFDC grants contribute to family homelessness . . . families . . . are displaced from their homes every year as a result of eviction, revitalization projects, economic development plans and spiraling rent inflation. One-half million low rent dwellings continue to be lost each year as a result of condominium conversions, abandonment, arson and demolition (U.S. House, 1987, p.4).

Thus the poor are often unable to pay for even the most squalid living quarters. Furthermore, because there is only a limited number of shelters and community resources, many homeless remain on the street with no place to turn for help.

Deinstitutionalization of the mentally ill has added to the problem of homelessness. Since 1963 with the passage of the Community Mental Health Centers Act, many inpatient facilities for the seriously mentally ill have discharged patients into the community in the hope of providing less restrictive care and promoting their gradual reintegration into society (Riesdorph-Ostrow, 1989). However, many of these individuals have not received adequate support from their families or the community. They find it difficult to follow prescribed medication regimens, to assume self-care responsibilities, and to function stably enough to maintain employment. Large numbers have relapsed into a marginal or non-functional existence resulting in their homeless and disenfranchised state. Among homeless women 33% are mentally impaired (Ugarriza & Fallon, 1994).

A related set of variables in this domain exacerbates the vulnerability of the homeless. A serious lack of adequate social and health care services leaves the homeless without the needed resources to cope with daily living and to regain some measure of independent living. Existing shelters are overcrowded, social service agencies' resources stretched to the limit, and health facilities unable to cope with the many needs of this population.

Finally, environmental factors can contribute to the vulnerability of the homeless. Some geographic locations lend themselves only to seasonal employment, such as the harvesting of fruit and vegetable crops, leaving many individuals without work and without sufficient income to provide for their needs for the remainder of the year. Insect and rodent vectors, numerous in many settings, add to the vulnerability of the homeless. Scabies and infestation of lice are common problems (Lindsey, 1989). Other disease-carrying vectors further erode the health and promote the problem of homelessness. Harsh climates, too, make survival for the poor more difficult. Rain, snow, and cold temperatures leave those without the means for adequate food and shelter vulnerable to numerous illnesses and threaten their very survival. Figure 24.7 summarizes the causal

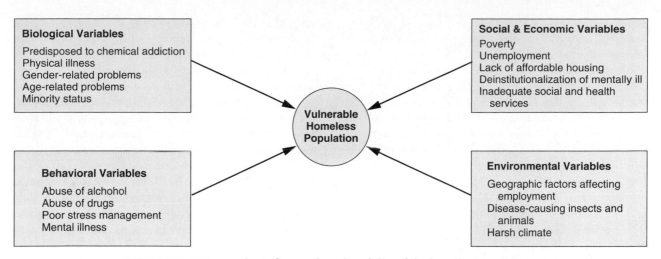

FIGURE 24.7. Factors that influence the vulnerability of the homeless population.

variables influencing the vulnerability of the homeless population.

Problems of the Homeless

The homeless encounter numerous problems affecting their health and well-being. They face all the needs associated with poverty only compounded by the condition of homelessness. How, for example, do the homeless care for simple ailments that require nourishing food and a day of rest in bed when they have neither the money to buy the food, a place to prepare it in, or a bed on which to rest? Simple acts of hygiene that the majority of the population takes for granted, like a daily shower and brushing one's teeth, are denied the homeless. Instead, homeless individuals live from one day to the next not knowing where they will sleep, what they will eat, or how they will protect themselves from exposure to the elements and the dangers of street-living. Because of their marginal existence, the homeless are vulnerable to many more health threats than the rest of society. In fact, it has been said that "the homeless may well harbor the largest pool of untreated disease left in American society today" (Wright & Weber, 1988, p. 88). The needs of the homeless can be grouped into three categories: physical problems, emotional problems, and social problems.

The physical problems of homeless people encompass a wide range of diseases and conditions. Chronic diseases abound in this population with diabetes, hypertension, alcoholism, and drug addiction among the most frequently reported in some studies (Lindsey, 1989, Brickner, et al, 1985). The homeless are at serious risk for many communicable diseases, particularly tuberculosis, AIDS, scabies, lice, and respiratory infections. Some develop peripheral vascular problems and many are at risk for malnutrition, dental problems, hypothermia in winter, or assault and other traumatic injuries (Ugarriza & Fallon, 1994).

Homeless children are especially vulnerable to abuse and neglect as well as a host of other physical health problems. They include scabies, skin problems, lice, dental problems, anemia, asthma and bronchitis, neurological disorders, chronic cardiovascular problems, and inadequate immunization status (Institute of Medicine, 1988).

The emotional problems of homeless people are numerous. Severe addictive and psychiatric disorders are clearly present in many homeless individuals; although the degree of psychopathology in this population may have been exaggerated, more of the homeless appear to have depression, phobias, and anxiety (Ugarriza & Fallon, 1994). It is still unclear if the existence of these disorders leads to homelessness or whether homelessness causes or contributes to the development of these disorders. One study showed that adverse childhood events, namely removal from parents and placement in foster care, physical abuse, and sexual abuse, had some association with homelessness. Although this study showed 20% of the men and 41% of the women entered homelessness with a history of adverse childhood events (placement in foster care or sexual or physical abuse), it was concluded that overall the homeless population is less deviant, in terms of social, addictive, and psychiatric behavior, than previously reported (Winkleby, et al., 1992).

It appears that a great number of emotional health problems arise while people are homeless. While a large number of the homeless (30% to 40%) are mentally ill, the remaining group needs to be distinguished as being no more mentally ill than the general population. Yet the stresses of poverty compounded by homelessness make this population at greater risk for developing emotional health problems (Berne, et al., 1990). Many of the homeless experience poor self-esteem and a sense of shame and stigmatization because of their low social status and dependence on society. Unrelieved stress leads to feelings of anxiety, hopelessness, and despair along with a sense of demoralization and powerlessness in the face of being unable to live independently. In many instances, poor emotional health then promotes exacerbation of physical violence, and alcohol and drug dependence.

Homeless children are vulnerable for other emotional health problems. Without the stability and support of home and family life, many homeless children do not thrive developmentally. Instead, they exhibit anxiety, depression, acting out, and other behavioral problems. School attendance tends to be poor among homeless children who feel stigmatized and unwelcome.

The third category of needs experienced by the homeless are social problems. First and foremost is the problem of poverty. With little or no income, the homeless are deprived of most of the basic necessities of life including food, shelter, and decent clothing, not to mention the luxuries, like entertainment and recreation, that the majority of people take for granted. Unemployment further deprives the homeless of self-esteem and pride in accomplishment. The homeless are socially isolated, cut off from the connections with family, friends, and community that provide support and promote well-being. Other social problems include inadequate drug and alcohol treatment and rehabilitation programs, little or no available health insurance, limited access to health services, and, in some settings, no access for children to the educational system. The latter has been addressed by the McKinney Homeless Assistance Act of 1987 that provides grants to participating states to give homeless children the same services in the schools as received by non-homeless children (Francis, 1991). The health-related problems of the homeless population are listed in Table 24.1.

NURSING ACTIONS FOR PREVENTION AND INTERVENTION WITH THE HOMELESS POPULATION

Health care services for the homeless have varied in the success with which they have been able to address their problems. A major barrier has been access (Institute of Medicine, 1988). There are probably several reasons for access problems but one stands out in importance—the lack of adequate numbers, types, and distribution of services available to serve the needs of the homeless. Despite increased national concern about homelessness and a growing number of services in most states, many homeless still lack access to any care but that available in emergency rooms. This precludes early

TABLE 24.1. *Health-Related Problems of the Homeless Population*

Physical Problems	Emotional Problems	Social Problems
Chronic diseases (diabetes, hypertension, heart disease, chronic lung disease, peripheral vascular disease)	Psychotic disorders	Poverty
Communicable diseases (TB, AIDS, respiratory infections)	Anxiety	Unemployment
Scabies, lice	Behavioral disorders	Lack of affordable housing
Malnutrition	Low self-esteem	Social isolation
Anemia	Shame	Stigmatization
Skin problems	Depression	Educational problems
Dental problems	Despair/hopelessness	Inadequate drug/alcohol programs
Traumatic injuries	Powerlessness	Limited health services
Hypothermia	Demoralization	Limited social services
	Low motivation	
	Non-compliance	

screening, early intervention, or prenatal care. Clinics and on-site services for the homeless, both traditional approaches, have often not proven effective (Berne, et al, 1990). Reasons for this include the mobility of many of the homeless, lack of continuity of care, understaffing, stigmatization of homelessness, anxiety, and low motivation leading to "non-compliance" by homeless individuals. Some comprehensive outreach programs have been more effective in assisting the homeless. A New York project took services to the homeless in their "hotels" and nurses were able to do intake, casefinding, referral, and health teaching successfully (Berne, et al., 1990). Various organizations exist to serve the homeless. One such organization is The Homeless Families Program, based in Princeton, New Jersey, and initiated through the Robert Wood Johnson Foundation and the U.S. Department of Housing and Urban Development. This program provides homeless families with health and social services as well as permanent housing (O'Connell, 1994).

It is important for community health nurses to remember that effective services for the homeless must take into consideration a broad spectrum of needs—physical, emotional, and social—since all are intricately related. Even when a program targets only one area, such as a drug rehabilitation service, homeless persons will be best served if nursing assessments determine what other needs remain unmet (whether physical, emotional, or social) and what referrals or interventions are indicated. Homeless people need and deserve to be treated with respect and dignity. They need and deserve to have food, shelter, health care, and other necessities such as basic human rights. They need and deserve human caring and supportive relationships. It is in these areas that community health nurses can play a major role. These emphases can be built into the services offered to the homeless through careful planning and team effort.

Services for the homeless tend to be mostly secondary and tertiary prevention. To engage in primary prevention of homelessness, Berne, et al. (1990) advocate working to change social policies. Among other things they suggest that housing needs to become more affordable for low income persons who also need education and job training. The homeless need to be provided with meaningful work and adequate compensation, better public assistance programs, child care, and access to health services. These are areas in which community health nurses can influence policy development through political advocacy. Chapter 28 provides many practical suggestions for community health nurses' involvement in the political arena.

THE MENTALLY IMPAIRED POPULATION

Another vulnerable group in the community is the **mentally impaired** who are people with limited ability to function due to significant behavioral or psychological disorders. These are individuals with a range of mental disorders from severe psychoses and neuroses to behavior disorders and inadequate adjustment. To define mental disorders or epidemiologically measure their incidence and prevalence has not been easy. Mental illness has not been a reportable condition by law, thus in the past only those individuals housed in mental hospitals or asylums could be accurately counted. Yet, an even larger number of persons, either receiving treatment through mental health centers and in private practice or untreated and living in the community, were unknown to public health policy makers and program planners. It was not until 1952 that the American Psychiatric Association first published it's *Diagnostic and Statistical Manual of Mental Disorders* (Pickett & Hanlon, 1990).

The Diagnostic and Statistical Manual lists the following 17 categories of mental disorders:

- Disorders usually first evident in infancy, childhood, or adolescence;
- Dissociative disorders;
- Sexual disorders;
- Organic mental syndromes and disorders;
- Psychoactive substance use disorders;
- Schizophrenia;
- Delusional disorders;
- Psychotic disorders not elsewhere classified;
- Mood disorders;
- Anxiety disorders;
- Somatoform disorders;
- Sleep disorders;
- Factitious disorders;
- Impulse control disorders not elsewhere classified;
- Adjustment disorders;
- Psychological factors affecting physical condition;
- Personality disorders;
- Conditions not attributable to a mental disorder that are a focus of attention or treatment (DSM, 1987).

For epidemiological purposes, this list has made it possible to more accurately define disorders and estimate their occurrence in the community. The latter has been enhanced through a program sponsored by the National Institute of Mental Health which has targeted three goals: (1) to determine reliable estimates of the incidence and prevalence of mental disorders, (2) to explore possible causes, and (3) to assist with planning and development of mental health services (Eaton, et al., 1981; USPHS, 1991).

Despite these advancements, the size of the mentally ill and disabled population can only be roughly estimated. There were close to half a million, or 468,831, mentally ill and impaired patients being treated as inpatients or in residential treatment centers in 1969. By 1983, that number had decreased by approximately one half to 224,169 (Manderscheid & Barrett, 1987). But these figures do not tell the whole story. With deinstitutionalization of the mentally ill, one would expect a decline in inpatient census. Many of those formerly treated as inpatients now receive care in various outpatient and ambulatory settings. The numbers admitted to these services has increased dramatically in recent years. Furthermore, some estimate that as many as 300,000 have been transferred to nursing homes (Kiesler & Sibulkin, 1987) while numerous others remain untreated in the community, many of whom are the homeless.

Etiology of Mental Impairment

To describe the etiology of mental disorders in any detail is beyond the scope or purpose of this chapter. However, as one considers the vulnerability model, it is important to be aware of the major causative factors contributing to the at-risk status of this population. Certain biological factors can place people at risk for mental disorders. Since the physical and psychological are interrelated, mental disorders often have their origin in a physiological disturbance. Genetic factors predispose some individuals toward mental disorders particularly when there is a history of mental illness or disability in the family. Birth defects and injuries sustained at birth can also cause mental disorders. Some individuals later acquire mental impairment from traumatic brain injuries or illnesses that cause tissue damage or anoxia (lack of oxygen). Age is another biological factor influencing vulnerability for mental disorders, particularly for infants and children. "Most mental illnesses have their origins in early childhood but do not become manifest until the developmental or productive years of life" (Pickett & Hanlon, 1990, p.461). At the other end of the age continuum, as the size of the el-

derly population increases, there is a growing incidence of senile dementia, Alzheimers disease, and other forms of mental disability among the elderly.

Behavioral factors also influence the vulnerability of this population. Psychologic stress from a variety of sources, such as being an unwanted child, or experiencing job burnout, can be a major contributer to mental disorders when individuals affected have not developed healthy coping responses (Lindgren, 1990). Neglect and abuse during childhood appear to be associated with various psychoses, neuroses, and behavior disorders, including schizophrenia, depression, withdrawal, or violent behavior (Cook & Fontaine, 1991). Low self-esteem tends to accompany and often influences mental functioning. Depending on the severity of their poor self-esteem, people so afflicted may be unable to hold jobs, withdraw into depressive states, or exhibit other neurotic behaviors. Finally, alcohol and/or drug abuse can lead to chemical dependence, physiological damage, and mental impairment.

Sociocultural factors can also influence the vulnerability of the mentally impaired. Economic stress affects the mental health of numerous individuals. Anxiety over such things as inadequate income, financial pressures, unemployment and inability to provide for family may create emotional stress with which some people cannot cope. People from all socioeconomic levels may experience this although the poor are most vulnerable because they have relatively few, if any, resources to provide for even the basics of food, shelter, clothing, and health services. The lack of adequate mental health services in the community, lack of adequate community support systems, and little emphasis on prevention are major sociocultural factors increasing vulnerability. See the Issues in Community Health Nursing display. Many mentally impaired individuals who would have formerly been institutionalized in a secure and ordered residential setting are left to wander the streets, unable to sustain employment or function adequately in a stressful and confusing world. Their feelings of abandonment, loneliness, and fear only exacerbate their mental disability. Stigmatization further jeopardizes the health of this population. Misperceptions and fears of the general public cause the mentally ill to become even more socially isolated and cut off from needed support. Data on racial or ethnic distribution among the mentally ill and disabled is limited and inconclusive. Among the impoverished mentally ill in the community a higher proportion of minorities appear, while figures on inpatient psychiatric services show 80% to be white, 18%

Issues in Community Health Nursing
MAKING MENTAL HEALTH A PRIORITY

The problems associated with mental impairment present a tremendous challenge to public health. Certainly there are access, adequacy, and cost of treatment issues, that must be addressed. Many of the mentally impaired are among the homeless, substance abusers and other populations with multiple problems and service needs. There is a clear association between mental illness and much of the dysfunctional behavior, family violence, crimes, and substance abuse that health and social services are inadequately equipped to address. Many of the children growing up in dysfunctional and abusive environments are almost certain to become part of the next generation of substance abusers and criminals. And the cost to the taxpayer for treatment or incarceration of these mentally impaired adults is double the amount of money needed to provide preventive services at an early age. Isn't it time to start emphasizing preventive mental health?

To make mental health a priority will require some radical paradigm shifts for policy makers and providers. Documentation of the cost-effectiveness and community benefits needs to be accomplished through clinical practice and research. Community health nursing is strategically positioned to influence these changes by accepting the challenge to develop innovative preventive services with this at-risk population. It will require collaborative work with other community providers to target at-risk children, in particular, and develop sports programs, esteem building activities, employable skills, and other programs whose effectiveness can be documented and the results disseminated to influence policy decisions.

African American, and the remainder Native American, Asian American, and Hispanic in origin (Pickett & Hanlon, 1990).

Environmental factors appear to play a lesser role in affecting the vulnerability of the mentally ill and disabled. Nonetheless, one must not overlook the impact of climate and geography on some individuals' mental state. Living with the fear of eminent earthquakes, tornados or hurricanes and then living through them, for example, can create severe stress for certain people. Some may become depressed by excessively wet and gloomy weather, long winters, or severely cold temperatures. Many of the conditions in urban areas are stressful; transportation problems, excessive noise, crowded streets, and impersonal sevices may cause anger, anxiety, or frustration.

Lead poisoning continues to be a serious public health problem contributing to impaired intelligence. Its source may be from exhaust fumes, drinking water channelled through lead pipes in older homes, from ceramic mugs or bowls whose glaze has been unsafely fired, or from crystal glassware whose lead has "leaked" through repeated dishwasher use. Finally, a number of ergonomic factors in the workplace, such as poor lighting, crowded space, noise, and irregular shifts, can contribute to mental health problems as well. (See Chapter 20 for details). Figure 24.8 summarizes the factors influencing the vulnerability of the mentally impaired population.

Problems of the Mentally Impaired

In assessing the needs of the mentally ill and disabled, one finds a variety of health-related problems, some of which are preventable. The nature of these problems as well as the degree to which they are preventable, varies of course with the type and severity of the mental disorder, whether or not the affected individuals are receiving and complying with needed treatment, and the degree of independence with which they can function in the community. Although the mentally ill and disabled population is disparate in terms of its wide range of diagnoses and conditions, there are nonetheless many problems shared in common by the members of this group. Furthermore, interventions designed to address specific needs can often provide wide-reaching benefits to the whole mentally impaired population. The problems of this group, as with the homeless, fall into three categories, (1) physical problems, (2) emotional problems, and (3) social problems.

The physical problems of the mentally impaired are numerous. Since many people in this population take medications for a prolonged period of time, a major problem for them is dealing with serious medication side effects. Prolonged tranquilizer use, for example, can cause tardive dyskinesia, an irreversible condition in which damage to the cerebral cortex from the drug

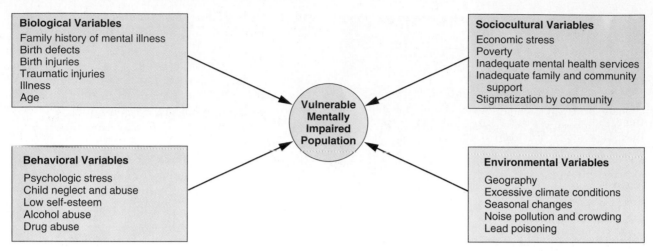

FIGURE 24.8. Factors that influence the vulnerability of the mentally impaired population.

leads to tremors and loss of motor control. Clients on psychotropic drugs tend to have increased problems with constipation and regular elimination. They frequently have sleep distrubances that lead to sleep deprivation and make them vulnerable to other physical health problems.

Poor compliance in taking prescribed medications is an additional problem for this population. Many forget to take their medications or do not value their importance and others lose track in moving from one group home or living situation to the next. Generally, the medications are needed to enable the mentally impaired to function and live independently. When treatment protocols are not followed consistently, many are at risk for exacerbation of symptoms and need more supervised living accomodations.

Poor nutrition is another major problem with the mentally ill and disabled, particularly those living on their own. Low income and limited mental abilities combine to promote poor choices in food selection with many people in this group consuming a high fat, high carbohydrate, "junk food" diet. The consequences are considerable obesity in this population as well as being at greater risk for coronary artery disease, diabetes, and dental problems. Because of their high dependency, particularly among males, on alcohol, drugs, and cigarette smoking, the mentally ill are also vulnerable to liver disease, cardiac disease, and cancer. The mentally impaired, depending on the extent of mental dysfunction, face problems associated with limited motor coordination and self care ability. As a population, the mentally impaired are also vulnerable to a number of communicable diseases, including sexually transmitted diseases, AIDS, and tuberculosis.

The emotional problems of the mentally ill and disabled vary depending on the etiology and severity of their condition. The stresses of coping with daily living, compounded by the complexities of city life for most, create such responses as confusion, depression, frustration, and anger. Psychological isolation, loneliness, and poor self-esteem are interrelated problems for people with mental disorders. People with these conditions are often unable to establish supportive relationships and feel the stigma that society places on mental disabilities. In addition, few have adequate, if any, family or friendship supports. The developmentally disabled, such as people with spina bifida, cerebral palsy, or mental retardation, experience similar emotional problems although this group, due to better funded programs, generally receives better services overall.

Many of the social problems experienced by the mentally ill and disabled are related to system inadequacies. Income for these individuals is limited. Finding employment and sustaining it is difficult given their disabilites. If they have worked they are eligible in the United States for Social Security Disability income and if they have never worked they can receive supplemental income under the Social Security Act. But in both cases it allows only a subsistence level of living. Another problem is that people with mental disorders are generally isolated physically with little sense of support or acceptance in the community. Those who live in group homes must move every two years because of regulatory time restrictions on how long an individual can stay in one residence. Thus, for many in this population unstable housing creates mobility with additional problems. Although the intent of deinstitutionalization of the mentally ill has been to promote independence, the system per se with its regulations and restrictions frequently does just the opposite. Needed services for this population are often fragmented. Collaboration between the many providers should be required so that services, such as public health nursing, social work, recreational therapy, occupational therapy, nutrition, and drug rehabilitation, could be coordinated to better meet this population's needs. Table 24.2 summarizes the problems of the mentally impaired population.

Nursing Actions with the Mentally Impaired Population

Many services exist in the community to address the needs of the mentally ill and disabled. Beside possible referral to inpatient facilities in state psychiatric hospitals and private hospitals, there are a variety of public and private programs. Counseling services, medical and dental care, public health nursing services, drug rehabilitation, occupational therapy, recreational therapy, nutritional counseling, group homes, sheltered workshops, housing and income assistance are among those on the list.

As the community health nurse works with this population, it is important to understand the community support system concept that underlies the development of quality mental health services (Stroul, 1986). In the past, services for the mentally ill and disabled were poorly organized and inadequately funded. This led to development, by the National Institute for Mental Health in 1977, of a model for community mental health centers. The model, called a community support system, demonstrated that services alone were not enough and recommended a combination of elements to enhance community support to the mentally ill and disabled. It included the following:

- Client location and outreach to ensure that services are received.
- Helping to meet basic needs by coordinating with social service providers to ensure adequate food, shelter, and clothing.
- Mental health treatment including assessment, intervention, and evaluation.
- A 24-hour crisis service using such measures as a hot line and emergency and stabilization centers.
- Social and vocational counseling and rehabilitation to assist with development of skills for daily living and employment.
- Affordable housing suited to clients' level of independence.
- Income assistance including identification of sources and help with application.
- Peer support through structured groups, day programs, recreational activities.
- Family and community support through education and involvement in mental health programs.

TABLE 24.2. *Health-Related Problems of the Mentally Impaired*

Physical Problems	Emotional Problems	Sociocultural Problems
Medication side effects	Depression	Low income
Loss of motor control	Confusion	Unemployment
Constipation	Anger/frustration	Physical isolation
Sleep disturbances	Lack of motivation for compliance with treatment	Unstable housing
Poor nutrition	Anxiety	System does not foster independence
Dental problems	Loneliness	Disjointed and inconsistent mental health services
Obesity	Low self-esteem	
Chronic diseases (coronary artery disease, diabetes, heart disease, liver disease, cancer)	Unable to establish relationships	
Limited self-care ability	Feelings of stigmatization	
Communicable diseases (STDs, AIDS, Tbc)	Psychological isolation	
	Neuroses	
	Psychoses	

■ Advocacy and protection of client rights including informing them of their rights and helping them to find the most suitable treatment and resources.

■ Health and dental services including location and payment for services.

■ Case management to coordinate efforts and ensure that all needs of clients are met.

Community health nurses can play an important role in implementing the community support system concept in their clients' communities. The above elements could be used as a check list or standard for ensuring comprehensive services to the mentally ill and disabled. Within this role, community health nurses function in a variety of ways as case managers, educators, advocates, counselors, and collaborators in the planning, implementation and evaluation of services.

While a large share of community health nursing's role with the mentally ill and disabled is to assist with treatment and management of their care and the problems associated with their resulting dependency, one must not lose sight of the importance of and possibilities for prevention. Many of the risk factors, outlined earlier in the etiology section, can be eliminated or ameliorated. Depression, for example, can be prevented or minimized when interventions focus on early recognition and treatment of those at-risk women, minorities and the elderly (in whom depression occurs more frequently), those with a family history of depression, people experiencing bereavement and loss, and other stressful life events, such as unemployment or retirement (Cook & Fontaine, 1991). Education, establishment of support groups, referral to counseling, and connecting with resources, are all appropriate nursing actions to accomplish primary or secondary prevention. Other problems of the mentally ill and disabled can be minimized through tertiary preventive nursing actions, such as combatting low self-esteem through provision of rehabilitation and skill training programs.

THE SUBSTANCE ABUSING POPULATION

Substance abuse refers to excessive and prolonged use of some chemical (alcohol, drugs, tobacco) that leads to serious physical, emotional, and social problems. The people who make up the substance abusing population are those who abuse the use of chemicals in three areas—alcohol, drugs (both legal and illegal) and tobacco. A portion of this group may become dependent on alcohol, drugs, or tobacco but may not be addicted. **Chemical dependence** refers to a strong, overwhelming preoccupation with and desire to have the drug, experienced as a craving. Only a portion of substance abusers (7%–15%) experience **chemical addiction** which means a compulsion to use a chemical in a way that is beyond a person's self control (Peele, 1985). People who become addicted first develop a tolerance so that it takes increasing amounts of the drug to achieve the desired effect. Withdrawal occurs when drug dependent individuals go without the drug (either intentionally or because they cannot obtain it) and is accompanied by distressing physical and psychological symptoms unless the drug is taken in increasingly smaller doses.

Substance abuse leading to chemical dependence and addiction is a serious public health problem. The substance abusing population spans all ages and socioeconomic and cultural groups. Thus, it is difficult to know the size of this population since the definitions for alcoholics, drug abusers, and smokers vary considerably depending on whether one is counting light users, moderate users, heavy users, or all three. The prevalence of alcohol abusers and/or dependents over the age of 21 years in the United States was more than 13 million in 1988 (Grant, et al., 1991). Studies show that nearly one quarter of the United States population drinks moderately which is defined as not more than two drinks per day for healthy men and not more than one drink per day for healthy, nonpregnant women (Archer, et al., 1995). Statistically men tend to drink more than women, although the number of women and youth who drink heavily appears to be increasing and is cause for concern. Among the elderly, the proportion of those who drink heavily tends to increase with age (Atkinson, 1984). Overall, drinking rates have declined slightly in the past decade but alcohol abuse remains a major problem.

Drug abusers fall into four groups. The first group consists of individuals, primarily adolescents and young adults, who try drugs on an experimental basis, often because of peer pressure. Repeated use in many cases leads to addiction. Second, are those relatively well-adjusted persons who become addicted as a result of overprescription of medications for treating insomnia, pain, obesity or other medical reasons. The third group is composed of people with neurotic tendencies who use drugs to excess to cope with personal problems. Finally, there are individuals with psychopathic tendencies who become addicted as they repeatedly seek escape or release through illicit drug use. Characteristics commonly noted among drug dependent persons include "under-achievement, loneliness, mistrust and fear of closeness, identity problems, social conflicts, and self-destructive tendencies" (Pickett & Hanlon, 1990, p.483).

Commonly Abused Drugs

A wide variety of drugs are used by substance abusers. Currently, some of the commonly abused drugs include alcohol, marijuana, cocaine, crack, caffeine, and tobacco. Mood altering or psychoactive drugs include those that are legal as well as illegal. They fall into seven categories—cannabis, depressants, hallucinogens, inhalants, narcotics, steroids, and stimulants.

1. Cannabis, more commonly known as marijuana, is an illegal substance made from the hemp plant, Cannabis sativa, when smoked or consumed, makes users feel mildly euphoric and relaxed with more intense sensory perception. Today's drug is more powerful than the 1960's version, called "pot." Hashish or hashish oil come from the same plant and has similar effects as marijuana. Adverse reactions and abuse can cause hallucinations, anxiety, and paranoia. Users may develop tolerance and physical dependence. Among illicit drugs in the United States, it is the most commonly used (Doweiko, 1990) but, because of its illegal status, the quality of the drug is not controlled nor is it legally permitted to be used for medicinal purposes. The psychoactive ingredient in marijuana, tetrahydrocannabinol (THC), was used widely as a safe therapeutic agent, particularly as an antinauseant for cancer patients receiving chemotherapy.

2. Depressants are drugs that slow down the central nervous system, relax muscles and reduce coordination, decrease pulse and respirations, calm nerves, and generally lower energy level, producing sleep. If taken in high enough doses they can cause coma and death. Depressants are made up of sedative-hypnotic and tranquilizer drugs. They are addictive and users develop a tolerance for them so that increasingly larger doses must be taken to achieve the same effect. Alcohol, a depressant, is the most abused drug; alcoholism ranks third, after coronary disease and cancer, as a leading cause of death in the United States. Mortality in alcoholics is two and a half times greater than in non-alcoholics (Kinney & Leaton, 1991). By the year 2000, the World Health Organization predicts that alcoholism will become the world's leading health problem (Spickard, 1986). Tranquilizers, such as Valium and Librium, constitute the second most abused category of drugs after alcohol. It is now recognized that they have been prescribed to excess in the treatment of both chronic and acute mental disorders. Other depressants include barbiturates, chloral hydrate, and well known brands such as Doriden, Quaalude, Equanil, and Miltown.

3. Hallucinogens, called psychedelic drugs, stimulate the central nervous system and are mind-altering, producing hallucinations that affect perception, feelings, thinking, and self-awareness. Two categories include indole hallucingens and phenylethylamines. Of the first group, lysergic acid diethylamide (LSD) is the best known and an extremely potent drug. Ingested in minute amounts orally, it ideally produces a "high" with heightened awareness, distorted perceptions, and psychedelic sounds and images. A bad "trip" causes a negative physical (hypertension) and psychological reaction leading to panic and possible psychosis. A "flashback," or recurrence of the "trip," may occur weeks later without taking the drug. In the second group of hallucinogens, peyote and mescaline are known to have been used by Native Americans for centuries. Phencyclidine (PCP), a powerful psychedelic drug, stands alone as a third type and is the only hallucinogen that can cause addiction.

4. Inhalants include gases and solvents inhaled through the nose which initially act as stimulants and then slow body functions, causing depression. Their effects tend to be rapid in onset but of short duration. This group of drugs are easily obtainable as household or industrial products, and are used most often by children and adolescents. Cleaning solvents, aerosol sprays, paint thinner, and airplane glue are examples. They can be extremely dangerous because of the high concentration of chemicals per dose.

5. Narcotics include opiates, derived from the Asian poppy seed, and synthetic drugs that produce the effects of opiates by initially stimulating the higher centers of the brain but then depressing the central nervous system. They are used to relieve pain and induce sleep. The better known narcotics include heroin, codeine, morphine, opium and others known by brand names such as Percodan, Darvon, and Lomotil. Some, like heroin, may be diluted and injected. Others are ingested orally or inhaled. Narcotics are extremely addictive. Addiction to heroin in the United States has been estimated as high as several hundred thousand individuals (Pickett & Hanlon, 1990). Users develop a tolerance to narcotics so that increasingly larger doses must be taken to achieve the same effect.

6. Steroids, chemically related to the male hormone testosterone, increase muscular strength and body weight. They appeal particularly to athletes and young adults because of their function in accelerating physical

development and athletic prowess. They are called anabolic-androgenic because anabolic means to build up muscle and body tissue and androgenic means development of male sex characteristics. Steroids may be taken orally or injected directly into the muscle. Their use and abuse can lead to a variety of problems including hypertension, liver and kidney damage, heart disease, risk of injury to tendons and ligaments, and sterility in men.

7. Stimulants are chemicals that increase alertness and activity by stimulating the central nervous system. Caffeine, a mild stimulant found in coffee, tea, chocolate, and soft drinks, is the most widely used psychoactive drug in the world. The effect of stimulants is to cause nerve fibers to release noradrenaline and other stimulating neurotransmitters, which allow the body to expend more of its own energy sooner. Thus harmful effects can be avoided by allowing the body time to replenish itself. Abusers repeat the dose to avoid the "down" time and become dependent. The most well known stimulants include caffeine, cocaine, crack (a smokeable form of cocaine), methamphetamines, and nicotine. Cocaine, a euphoria-producing drug used more by the rich, is largely taken intranasally, some by inhalation, and a small percent intravenously (Higgins, 1989). Crack, a cheaper form of smokeable cocaine, is more frequently used by lower income African Americans. Amphetamines tend to give an intense "high" that can last, with use, for days followed by a "crash" and prolonged deep sleep. Benzedrine, Dexedrine, and Methedrine are better known amphetamines. Nicotine, a chemical stimulant derived from the tobacco plant, is mostly smoked in cigarettes, pipes, and cigars but is also available in chewing tobacco and snuff. Studies show recent declines in smoking prevalence for women and men but adolescents, particularly white males, remain a high risk group (Nelson, et al., 1995). Both active and passive smoking cause health problems including cardiovasular and pulmonary disease, cancer, and health effects on newborns from smoking during pregnancy. Table 24.3 summarizes all these drug types, their "street" names, signs of use/abuse, and their associated health risks.

Etiology of Substance Abuse

There is no general consensus about the causes of alcohol and drug abuse. Research approaches to studying the population of substance abusers have pointed to a variety of possible causal factors, some physiological, some social, and some psychological. There is evidence, for example, that certain individuals using alcohol seem to "need" more, even at the onset of their drinking, suggesting a chemical predisposition leading to addiction. Other evidence points to psychological factors, like low self-esteem, or behavioral patterns, such as drug experimentation, promoting use and abuse. Social factors, too, such as overprescription and drug advertising influence use and abuse. And the environmental milieu surrounding certain individuals, such as peer pressure, dysfunctional families, as well as societal attitudes about drugs—both "good" and "bad" drugs—can promote use and eventual dependence. There seem to be few, if any, single causes but rather an interaction of multiple factors operating to influence substance abuse.

Biological causative factors include a family history of alcoholism or drug abuse. Although there is little conclusive evidence that genetic predisposition is an actual cause, there is reason to believe that in some cases, individuals who begin use of alcohol or certain drugs are more readily susceptible to addiction. The physiological makeup of these people, related perhaps to body chemistry, may prompt the cravings that lead to abuse. Regardless, the belief that alcohol or drug dependence and addiction are a disease has basis in fact when one considers their effect on the health of substance abusers.

The behavioral/psychological causative factors are varied. For children and adolescents, trying new and risky things is part of normal developmental behavior and this often includes experimentation with drugs, alcohol, and tobacco. Peer pressure for adolescents is a major influence and combined with drug experimentation can lead to dependence. Even people who are relatively well adjusted emotionally turn to alcohol or drugs as a way to relieve stress from such things as divorce, death of a loved one, chronic pain, job loss, work pressures, family conflict, or simply a too fast-paced life. Drug choices may range from excessive coffee consumption and smoking, self medication with over-the-counter drugs, overuse of prescribed medications such as tranquilizers, all the way to use of illicit drugs. Social activities incorporating alcohol consumption are commonplace and even illicit drugs, such as marijuana or cocaine, are encouraged in some social groups. When these patterns persist, tolerance and dependence can result. People with low self-esteem are at greater risk for substance abuse as are those with personality disorders or other psychological disturbances who may be seeking thrills or defying authority through drug use. Their mental impairment contributes to maladaptive coping patterns prompting some in society to unfairly label substance abuse as a "moral failing."

(text continues on page 568)

TABLE 24.3. Drugs Involved in Substance Abuse

Drug Type	The Facts	Possible Signs of Use/Abuse	Possible Health Risks of Use/Abuse
CANNABIS			
Hashish (Hash, herb, kif) Hashish oil (Hash oil, honey) Marijuana (Grass, weed, dope, ganja, reefer, pot, Acapulco gold, Thai sticks)	Cannabis is made from the hemp plant, Cannabis sativa. When smoked or ingested produces mild euphoria, relaxation, and intense sensory perception. Users may develop tolerance and physical dependence. Sinsemilla is a highly potent form of marijuana.	Relaxation and euphoria. Altered perceptions of time & space Hallucinations or anxiety attacks with Sinsemilla use	Damage to heart and lungs Damage to brain nerve cells Memory disorders Temporary loss of fertility Psychological dependence
DEPRESSANTS			
Alcohol (Brew, Juice, Liquor) Barbiturates (Downers, Barbs) Benzodiazepines (Valium, Librium, Tranquilizers) Chloral Hydrate (Knock Out, Mickey Finn) Glutethimide (Doriden) Methaqualone (Quaalude, Ludes) Other Depressants (Equanil, Miltown, Noludar, Placidylm, Valmid)	Depressants depress or slow down the central nervous system by relaxing muscles, calming nerves and producing sleep. Alcohol is a depressant. Depressants are composed of sedative-hypnotic and tranquilizer drugs. Depressants are addictive. Users of depressants develop a tolerance to the drugs, meaning larger doses must be taken each time to produce the same effect.	Relaxation and drowsiness; lack of concentration; disorientation; loss of inhibitions; lack of coordination; dilated pupils; slurred speech; weak and rapid pulse; distorted vision; low blood pressure; shallow breathing; staggering; clammy skin; fever, sweating; stomach cramps; hallucinations; tremors; and delirium.	Liver damage; convulsions; addiction with severe withdrawal symptoms; coma; death due to overdose. For pregnant women: the newborn may be dependent and experience withdrawal or suffer from birth defects and behavioral problems.
HALLUCINOGENS			
Lysergic Acid Diethylamide (LSD) Phencyclidine (PCP, Angel Dust) Mescaline and Peyote (Mexc., Buttons, Cactus) Psilocybin (Mushrooms) Amphetamine Variants (MDMA/ Ectasy, MDA/Love Drug, TMA, DOM, DOB, PMA, STP, 2.5-DMA) Phencyclidine Analogues (PCE, PCPy, TCP) Other Hallucinogens (Bufotenine, Ibogaine, DMT, DET, Psilocybin	Hallucinogens are psychedelic, mind-altering drugs that affect a person's perception, feelings, thinking, self-awareness, and emotions. A "bad trip" may result in the user experiencing panic, confusion, paranoia, anxiety, unpleasant sensory images, feelings of helplessness, and loss of control. A "flash-back" is a reoccurrence of the original drug experience without taking the drug again.	Dilated pupils; increased body temperature, heart rate, and blood pressure; sweating; loss of appetite; sleeplessness; dry mouth; tremors; hallucinations; disorientation; confusion; paranoia; violence; euphoria; anxiety; and panic.	Agitation; extreme hyperactivity; psychosis; convulsions; mental or emotional problems; death.

(continued)

TABLE 24.3. *Drugs Involved in Substance Abuse* (Continued)

Drug Type	The Facts	Possible Signs of Use/Abuse	Possible Health Risks of Use/Abuse
INHALANTS			
Amyl Nitrite (Poppers, Snappers) Butyl Nitrite (Rush, Bolt Bullet) Chlorohydrocarbons (Aerosal Sprays, Cleaning Fluids) Hydrocarbons (Solvents, Airplane Glue, Gasoline, Paint Thinner) Nitrous Oxide (Laughing Gas, Whippets)	Inhalants are substances which are breathed or inhaled through the nose. Inhalants are depressants and depress or slow down the body's functions. Inhalants are normally not thought of as drugs because they are often common household or industrial products. However, inhalants are often the most dangerous drugs per dose.	Euphoria and lightheadedness; excitability; loss of appetite; forgetfulness; weight loss; sneezing; coughing; nausea and vomiting; lack of coordination; bad breath; red eyes; sores on nose and mouth; delayed reflexes; decreased blood pressure; flushing (skin appears to be reddish); headache; dizziness; and violence.	Depression; damage to the nervous system and body tissues; damage to liver and brain; heart failure; respiratory arrest; suffocation; unconsciousness; seizures; heart failure; sudden sniffing death.
NARCOTICS			
Codeine (School Boy) Heroin (H. Harry, Junk, Brown Sugar, Smack) Hydromorphone (Lords) Meperdine (Doctors) Methadone (Dollies, Methadose) Morphine (Morpho, Miss Emma) Opium (Dovers Powder) Other Narcotics (Percodan, Talwin, Lomotil, Darvon, Numorphan, Percocet, Tylox, Tussionex, Fentanyl)	Narcotics are composed of opiates and synthetic drugs. Opiates are derived from the seed pod of the Asian poppy. Synthetic drugs called opioids are chemically developed to produce the effects of opiates. Initially, narcotics stimulate the higher centers of the brain, but then slow down the activity of the central nervous system. Narcotics relieve pain and induce sleep. Narcotics, such as Heroin, are often diluted with other substances (i.e. water, sugar) and injected. Other narcotics are taken orally or inhaled. Narcotics are extremely addictive. Users of narcotics develop a tolerance to the drugs, meaning larger doses must be taken each time to produce the same effect.	Euphoria; restlessness and lack of motivation; drowsiness; lethargy; decreased pulse rate; constricted pupils; flushing (skin appears to be reddish); constipation; nausea and vomiting; needle marks on extremities; skin abscesses at injection sites; shallow breathing; watery eyes; and itching.	Pulmonary edema; respiratory arrest; convulsions; addiction; coma; death due to overdose. For users who share or use unsterile needles to inject narcotics: tetanus, hepatitis, AIDS. For pregnant women: premature births, stillbirth, and acute infections among newborns.

STEROIDS

Anabolic-Androgenic (roids, juice, d-ball)	Steroids may contribute to increases in body weight and muscular strength. The acceleration of physical development is what makes steroids appealing to athletes and young adults. Anabolic-Androgenic steroids are chemically related to the male sex hormone testosterone. Anabolic means to build up the muscles and other tissues of the body. Androgenic refers to the development of male sex characteristics. Steroids are injected directly into the muscle or taken orally	Sudden increase in muscle and weight; increase in aggression and combativeness; violence ("roid rage"); hallucinations; jaundice; purple or red spots on body, inside mouth, or nose; swelling of feet or lower legs (edema); tremors; and bad breath. For women: breast reduction, enlarged clitoris, facial hair and baldness, deepened voice. For men: enlarged nipples and breasts, testicle reduction, enlarged prostate, baldness.	Acne; high blood pressure; liver and kidney damage; heart disease; increased risk of injury to ligaments and tendons; bowel and urinary problems; gallstones and kidney stones; liver cancer. For men: impotence and sterility. For women: menstrual problems. For users who share or use unsterile needles to inject steroids: hepatitis, tetanus, AIDS.

STIMULANTS

Amphetamines (Uppers, Pep Pills) Cocaine (Coke, Flake, Snow) Crack (Rock) Methamphetamines (Ice, Crank, Crystal) Methylphenidate (Ritalin) Phenmetrazine (Preludin, Preludes) Other Stimulants (Adipex, Cylert, Didrex, Ionamin, Melfiat, Plegine, Sanorex, Tenuate, Tepanil, Prelu-2)	Stimulants stimulate the central nervous system, increasing alertness and activity. Users of stimulants develop a tolerance, meaning large doses must be taken to get the same effect. Stimulants are psychologically addictive.	Increased alertness; excessive activity; agitation; euphoria; excitability; increased pulse rate, blood pressure, and body temperature; insomnia; loss of appetite; sweating; dry mouth and lips; bad breath; disorientation; apathy; hallucinations; irritability; and nervousness.	Headaches; depression; malnutrition; hypertension; psychosis; cardiac arrest; damage to the brain and lungs; convulsions; coma; death.

Sociocultural factors form another set of variables influencing substance abuse. Substance abusers include all ages, sexes, race, and economic levels but the poor and minorities are often more vulnerable because they lack the education and resources to cope with life stresses and find needed assistance. Many individuals do not realize the dangers inherent in certain drugs or know how to use other drugs safely, such as the dangers of drinking alcohol when taking tranquilizers which can be lethal. Misleading information is another factor. Over-the-counter drugs are often not considered drugs and their ready access plus heavy advertising promotion leads to abuse. Examples are the excessive use of diet pills, cold remedies, and nonprescription pain killers. Overprescription of medications, such as morphine for pain or valium for depression, can also lead to addiction. The quality of illegal drugs cannot be controlled so that many drugs, such as heroin and cocaine, may be poorly mixed and have unpredictable dosages. Social values that promote competition, productivity, and involvement in too many activities further contribute to stress that can lead to alcohol and drug abuse. Drug laws labelling users as criminals often prevent these individuals from seeking appropriate help that might prevent addiction or treat dependency. Some cultural groups promote moderate substance use or even abstention but generally in the United States these influencing variables are not present.

Environmental factors related to the physical and social milieu can influence substance abuse. Dysfunctional families and abusive relationships both contribute to alcohol or drug use leading to dependence. Peer pressure with a desire for social acceptance among adolescents and young adults especially is a strong contributing factor. Availability of legal and illegal drugs, particularly in highly populated urban settings, further promotes use. Widespread public misconceptions about which drugs are dangerous to one's health can influence abuse, many people feel that alcohol, tobacco, over-the-counter and prescription drugs are all right because they are legal. A summary of these influencing factors is listed in Figure 24.9.

Problems of the Substance Abusing Population

Many health-related problems result from the abuse of alcohol and other drugs. Each drug has its own particular side effects and possible consequences. These are listed more specifically in Table 21.7. But, as we consider the overall health needs of this at-risk population, we can group those needs into three categories, physical, emotional, and social.

Serious physical health problems can arise from substance abuse. Damage to organs and other body parts is common from most drugs and includes damage to the liver, brain, central nervous system, heart, kidneys, skin, ligaments and tendons, bowel, and lungs. Disease resulting from substance abuse includes cirrhosis of the liver with alcohol abuse, heart disease and liver cancer with abuse of steroids, AIDS and hepatitis from needle sharing with narcotics, and lung cancer with tobacco and marijuana abuse. Infants whose mothers abused depressants, narcotics, or marijuana during pregnancy

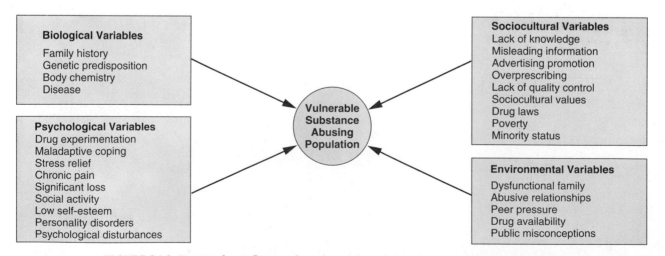

FIGURE 24.9. Factors that influence the vulnerability of the substance abusing population.

may experience one or more of the following: addiction and withdrawal, birth defects, low birth weight, premature birth, stillbirth, and acute infections. Abuse of steroids can cause impotence and sterility in men and menstrual problems for women while marijuana abuse can lead to infertility in both women and men. Other physical problems include headaches, malnutrition, severe withdrawal symptoms from addiction, memory disorders with marijuana, pulmonary edema with narcotics, convulsions, respiratory arrest, heart failure, suffocation, unconsciousness, and, with overdose, coma and death. Polysubstance use and abuse can also lead to serious results from multiple drug interactions.

Two major psychological health problems occurring with substance abuse are addiction and psychological dependence. Addiction occurs with the abuse of depressants, narcotics, and the hallucinogen, PCP. Psychological dependence occurs with the abuse of other drugs, such as marijuana, caffeine, and nicotine. Other problems experienced by substance abusers include anxiety and depression with inhalants, agitation, hyperactivity, and hallucinations with hallucinogens, plus neuroses, psychoses, violence, and suicide.

Social problems resulting from substance abuse cover a broad area affecting individual abusers, their families, and the community. Monetary and social costs to the individual of maintaining a drug habit can lead to poverty, unemployment, social stigma, and punishment for crime. Alcohol and drug abuse creates family disruption, family neglect and abuse, and depletes family financial and emotional resources. For the community, problems include an increased incidence of violence, traffic accidents and deaths, homicides, and crime related to obtaining money or possession of illicit drugs. Further problems for the community come from added costs of law enforcement, welfare programs, drug abuse surveillance, and drug treatment and rehabilitation services. Table 24.4 summarizes these problems.

Nursing Actions with the Substance Abusing Population

Addressing the needs of the substance abusing population is a challenging task. Public health interventions include two major emphases, prevention and treatment, and community health nurses can play an important

TABLE 24.4. *Health-Related Problems of the Substance-Abusing Population*

Physical Problems	Psychological Problems	Social Problems
Physical damage (liver, brain, heart, central nervous system, kidneys, skin, ligaments and tendons, bowel, lungs)	Psychological dependence	Poverty
	Anxiety	Unemployment
Disease (heart, lung cancer, AIDS, cirrhosis of liver, hepatitis)	Depression	Stigma
	Agitation	Punishment for crimes committed to support habits
Exposed newborns (low birth weight, birth defects, addiction, stillbirth, premature birth, infections)	Hyperactivity	Family disruption
	Hallucinations	Family neglect/abuse
Polysubstance interactions	Neuroses	Depleted family resources
Sterility	Psychoses	Increased violence in community
Headaches	Violence	Homicide
Malnutrition	Suicide	Crime
Addiction and withdrawal		High cost of drug treatment and rehabilitation
Memory disorders		
Pulmonary edema		
Convulsions		
Respiratory arrest		
Cardiac arrest		
Suffocation		
Unconsciousness		
Coma and death		

role in both. Prevention of substance abuse should be a major goal in serving this vulnerable population. Community health nurses have opportunities to intervene at all three levels of prevention: primary, secondary, and tertiary.

Primary prevention efforts aim at preventing abuse from occurring at all. First, and perhaps the most important intervention, is educating people about drugs, their use and abuse, and the potential dangers of these practices. People need to be aware that so-called "good" drugs, like caffeine, alcohol, cold medications, or diet drugs, can produce harmful effects as can "bad" or illegal drugs. Many people have become dependent on caffeine in coffee or soft drinks without even realizing it. Individuals taking medications need to be helped to assume responsibility for learning their actions and side effects and the potential dangers of multiple drug interactions. The nurse can assist in providing and clarifying this information. People need to learn other ways to enjoy social activities than with drinking alcohol or taking drugs. They need to develop alternative methods for coping with stress, including planned physical activity and recreational outlets. When adults model these behaviors then children and adolescents will more likely develop healthier practices too. Drug education programs, in which the community health nurse can play an important part, should address all of these issues, emphasizing stress management, assertiveness skills, and drug information. Nurses can develop such programs, assist with existing ones, and serve as consultants to school systems and organizations in the community.

Secondary prevention measures aim at halting and reversing drug use patterns. To develop effective interventions, the community health nurse needs information about these people. Who are they, where are they located, what drugs are they using, and what are their problems? Some surveillance systems, such as the Drug Abuse Warning Network (DAWN), determine abuse patterns in the community or the presence of contaminated drugs. DAWN's information comes from daily selected hospital emergency room reports, compiled nationally, and is available to those providing treatment (Pickett & Hanlon, 1990). Other surveillance and needs assessment information can come through community professionals, such as school nurses, health department nurses, drug treatment providers, and law enforcement officers. Interviewing students in the schools and clients in drug treatment programs provides further information to gain understanding about drug users (or potential users) and to assist in planning and carrying out programs. Two other important secondary prevention measures are drug testing, to screen for individuals who are using drugs, and employee assistance programs, to identify and assist with health problems including drug use.

Tertiary prevention aims at treating problems and preventing them from getting any worse. Treatment for drug abuse must be concerned with the harm to abusers as well as the problems abuse creates for the abusers' families and the community. Alcohol and drug treatment and rehabiltation programs exist in most large communities, but unless the treatment addresses multiple variables, it is often not long lasting as evidenced by the high recidivism rate among substance abuse clients. Community health nurses must use the nursing process in a framework of collaboration with other professionals to mount a comprehensive approach that examines the many factors influencing drug abuse patterns and design services to meet abusers' needs as well as their families and the community. Needs assessment is a first step, then community health nurses can assist in the design, implementation, and evaluation of a variety of services targeted for this vulnerable population. They include detoxification centers, drug treatment programs, half way houses, counseling services, support groups like Alcoholics Anonymous, smoking cessation programs, and church and synagogue outreach.

Meeting the holistic needs of these individuals is an essential goal. Treating the drug problem only without addressing needs for income and employment, housing, supportive relationships, or improved stress-coping patterns contributes to the recidivism mentioned earlier. The community health nurse needs to know what resources and programs are available or need developing and then can assist abusers and their families to find and use these services. The nurse can also help to initiate and implement new efforts such as support groups or smoking cessation programs, in addition to providing counseling and coordination of services.

Summary

Certain groups of people have always been more vulnerable or at risk of health problems, harm, or injury than the rest of the general population. Community health nurses need to know which groups are at risk, what constitutes their needs, and how to serve them. A variety of risk factors contribute to the condition of vulnerability and can be grouped into four causal domains: biological, behavioral, sociocultural, and environmental. Biological factors include genetic predisposition, age, gender, race or ethnicity, and physical or mental impairment. Behavioral factors include risk factors related to diet and weight control, exercise and rest, emotional health, alcohol and drugs, and sexual practices. Sociocultural factors include economic status and education, cultural values and practices, social and spiritual support, and health care quality and access. Environmental factors include those related to climate and geography, and the home, work, and community environment.

Specific vulnerable populations examined in this chapter include the homeless population, the mentally impaired, and the substance abusing population. The homeless population, still mostly males, is increasingly younger and made up more and more of women and children, many of whom leave their homes to seek shelter from domestic violence and abuse. Poverty, stress, lack of job skills, and lack of adequate health and social services all add to this population's vulnerability. Health needs of the homeless include such problems as chronic diseases, communicable diseases, malnutrition, anemia, hypothermia, psychotic disorders, anxiety, stress, low self-esteem, depression, social isolation, and stigmatization. Community health nursing interventions with the homeless include assessment, intervention, and referrals to address their needs for food, shelter, and health and social services. The nurse's role also involves collaborative planning and advocacy to improve health policy and services for this at-risk population.

The mentally impaired population experiences a broad spectrum of disabling conditions from severe psychoses and mental disorders to mild neuroses and distress or depression. Many in this population formerly received mental health services as inpatients but, since the deinstitutionalization of the mentally ill, now live and receive treatment in the community. Risk factors for this population include genetic predisposition for some mental disorders (such as schizophrenia and Alzheimer's disease), economic and psychological stress, child neglect and abuse, stigmatization and feelings of abandonment, loneliness, or low self-esteem, urban crowding, and noise pollution, climates of long

and gloomy rainy seasons or threats of earthquakes or hurricanes. The health needs of the mentally impaired include a variety of problems, such as poor nutrition, chronic diseases like diabetes and coronary artery disease, communicable diseases such as sexually transmitted diseases and tuberculosis, lack of supportive relationships, low income, unemployment, isolation, and inadequate mental health services. Nursing actions with this population focus on assisting and improving existing services to manage their care and foster independence. It also includes efforts to promote mental health in the community and prevent or minimize the problems encountered by the mentally impaired.

Substance abusers are persons who use alcohol, drugs, or tobacco to excess for a prolonged period of time resulting in serious health and social consequences. Some in this population become dependent on the chemical, and an even smaller portion (7%–15%) become addicted. Substance abuse is a serious public health problem affecting all ages and socioeconomic levels. Drugs used by substance abusers fall into several categories: depressants (such as alcohol) slow down the central nervous system, hallucinogens (such as LSD) stimulate the central nervous system, inhalants (such as paint thinner) provide stimulation then cause depression, narcotics (such as heroin) depress the central nervous system relieving pain and inducing sleep, steroids build muscle and body tissue, stimulants (such as caffeine or cocaine) stimulate the central nervous system, and marijuana promotes euphoria and sensory perception.

Various factors may contribute to substance abuse. Among them are a family history of drug or alcohol abuse, drug experimentation, stress relief, chronic pain, psychological disturbances, advertising promotion of substance use, poverty and minority status, abusive relationships, and peer pressure. The substance abusing population experiences many health and social problems. Among them are various organ (heart, lung, liver) diseases and cancer, addiction, depression, psychoses, poverty, unemployment, family disruption, stigma, violence and crime, Community health nursing actions aim at primary, secondary, and tertiary prevention. They accomplish this through educational programs, assessing the needs of drug users, assisting them to find healthier ways to cope, and working collaboratively with other professionals to improve existing and develop needed services.

Activities to Promote Critical Thinking

1. Identify a population-at-risk in your community. From the literature and community health data, determine what specific risk factors are present that make this group vulnerable? Group these risk factors into the four causal domains described in this chapter.

2. Visit a shelter for the homeless or for battered women and children. Talk with people at the shelter (clients and providers) and learn what they perceive as their greatest needs. Are providers' and clients' stated needs the same? Analyze the similarities and/or differences.

3. Interview a public health professional who works with the mentally impaired. Determine what service approaches have been most effective and propose three community health nursing interventions, one for each of the three levels of prevention, to assist the mentally impaired population.

4. Attend an Alcoholics Anonymous meeting. What purpose do these meetings serve and are they effective? Why?

5. Review a recent article in the literature on substance abuse. Describe the author's purpose and conclusions in writing this report. Identify the implications of what you learned from this article for community health nursing action with the substance abusing population.

REFERENCES

Allen, J.M., Lam, R. W., Remick, R.A., &. Sadovnick, A.D. (1993). Depressive symptoms and family history in seasonal and nonseasonal mood disorders. *American Journal of Psychiatry, 150*(3), 443–448.

American Psychiatric Association. (1987) Diagnostic and Statistical Manual of Mental Disorders (3rd ed.). Washington, DC: Author.

Atkinson, R.M. (1984). *Alcohol and drug abuse in old age.* Washington, DC: American Psychiatric Press, Inc.

Archer, L., Grant, B.F., & Dawson, D.A. (1995). What if Americans drank less? The potential effect on the prevalence of alcohol abuse and dependence. *American Journal of Public Health, 85*(1), 61–66.

Berne, A.S., Dato, C., Mason, D.J., Rafferty, M. (1990). A Nursing model for addressing the health needs of homeless families. *Image: Journal of Nursing Scholarship, 22*(1), Spring, 8–13.

Brickner, P.W., et al., (Eds.). (1985). *Health care of homeless people.* New York: Springer.

Carrillo, R. (1992). *Battered dreams: Violence against women as an obstacle to development.* New York: United Nations Development Fund for Women.

Centers for Disease Control (1994). Mortality patterns—United States, 1992. *Morbidity and Mortality Weekly Report, 43*(49), 916–919.

Centers for Disease Control (1992). Sexual behavior among high school students—United States 1990. *Morbidity and Mortality Weekly Report 40*(51,52), 885–888.

Committee on Community Health Services, American Academy of Pediatrics (1988). Health needs of homeless children. *Pediatrics, 82*(6), 938.

Cook, J. S. & Fontaine, K.L. (1991). *Essentials of mental health nursing* (2nd edition). Redwood City, CA: Addison-Wesley.

Dever, G.E.A. (1991). *Community health diagnosis: Global awareness at the local level* (2nd ed.). Gaithersburg, MD: Aspen.

Doweiko, H.E. (1990). *Concepts of chemical dependency.* Pacific Grove, CA: Brooks/Cole Publishing.

Eaton, W., et al. (1981). The epidemiological catchment area program of the National Institute of Mental Health. *Public Health Reports, 96,* July–Aug. 319.

Francis, M.B. (1991). Homeless families: Rebuilding connections. *Public Health Nursing, 8*(2), 90–96.

Goddeeris, J. & Hogan, A., (Eds.). (1992). *Improving access to health care: What can the states do?* Kalamazoo, MI: W.E. Upjohn Institute for Employment Research.

Goodman, J.C. (1992). The uninsured: Special report—Health care in America: Is there a cure? *Current Issues in Health Care,* June, 25.

Grant, B. F., Harford, T., Chou, P., et al. (1991). Prevalence of SDM-III-R alcohol abuse and dependence: United States, 1988. *Alcohol Health Research World, 15,* 91–96.

Green, L.W. & Kreuter, M.W. (1991). *Health Promotion Planning: An Educational and Environmental Approach* (2nd ed.). Mountain View, CA: Mayfield.

Heise, L., Pitanguy, J., & Germain, A. (1994). *Violence against women: The hidden health burden* (discussion paper). Washington, DC: World Bank, Population, Health, and Nutrition Department.

Hessol, N.A., Rutherford, G.W., Lifson, A.R., et al., (1988). The natual history of HIV infection in a cohort of homosexual and bisexual men: A decade of follow up. Abstract 4096. *Proceedings of the IV International Conference on AIDS*: Stockholm, Sweden. Higgins, R. (1989). Cocaine abuse: What every emergency nurse should know. *Journal of Emergency Nursing, 15*(4), 318.

Institute of Medicine. (1988). *Homelessness, health and human needs*. Washington, DC: National Academy Press.

Kiesler, C.A. & Sibulkin, A.E. (1987). *Mental hospitalization: myths and facts about a national crisis*. Newbury Park, CA: Sage.

Kinney, J. & Leaton, G. (1991). *Loosening the grip*. St. Louis: Mosby-Year Book.

Lindgren, C. L. (1990). Burnout and social support in family caregivers. *Western Journal of Nursing Research, 12*, 469–87.

Lindsey, A.M. (1989). Health care for the homeless. *Nursing Outlook, 37*(2), 78.

Manderscheid, R.W., & Barrett, S.A., (Eds.). (1987). *Mental health, U.S., 1987*. Rockville, MD: U.S. Department of Health and Human Services.

Merson, M. (1992). World Health Organization address at the International Conference on AIDs. Amsterdam, Netherlands.

Nelson, D. E., et al. (1995). Trends in cigarette smoking among U.S. adolescents, 1974 through 1991. *American Journal of Public Health, 85*(1), 34–40.

Newman, K. (1993). Giving up: shelter experiences of battered women. *Public Health Nursing, 10*(2), 108–113.

O'Connell, J. J. (1994). Yetta Adams' legacy is a call to action. *Home Again: Newsletter of the Homeless Families Program, 1*(2), 3.

Peele, S. (1985). *The meaning of addiction: Compulsive experience and its interpretation*. Lexington, MA: Heath.

Pickett, G. & Hanlon, J. (1990). *Public health: Administration and practice* (9th ed.). St. Louis: Times Mirror/Mosby.

Pilliteri, A. (1991). *Maternal and child health nursing. Care of the growing family*. Philadelphia: Lippincott.

Ramachandreon, A. (1988). International year of shelter for the homeless. *Cities 5*, 144–162.

Rice, J. (1992). What's right and wrong with United States health care. Special report—Health care in America: Is there a cure? *Current Issues in Health Care*, June, 22–29.

Riemer, J. G., Van Cleve, L. & Galbraith, M. (1995). Barriers to well child care for homeless children under age 13. *Public Health Nursing, 12*(1), 61–66.

Riesdorph-Ostrow, W. (1989). Deinstitutionalization: A public policy perspective. *Journal of Psychosocial Nursing and Mental Health Services, 27*(6), 4

Rosenberg, M, O'Carroll, P., & Powell, K. (1992). Let's be clear: Violence is a public health problem. *Journal of the American Medical Association, 267*(22), 3071–2.

Spickard, A. Jr. (1986). Alcoholism: The missed diagnosis. *Southern Medical Journal, 79*, 1489.

Spradley, T. S. & Spradley, J.P. (1985). *Deaf like me*. Washington, DC: Gallaudet College Press.

Stroul, B.A. (1986). *Models of community support services: Approaches to helping persons with long-term mental illness*. Boston: Sargent College of Allied Health Professions.

Ugarriza, D. N. & Fallon, T. (1994). Nurse's attitudes toward homeless women: A barrier to change. *Nursing Outlook, 42*(1), 26–29.

UNICEF (1995). *The state of the world's children 1995*. New York: Oxford.

U.S. House Select Committee on Children, Youth, & Families (1987). *The crisis in homelessness: Effects on children and families hearing*. Feb. 24, (Serial no. 72-237). Washington, DC: U.S. Government Printing Office.

U.S. Department of Healthe and Human Services (1991). *Healthy People 2000: National Health Promotion and Disease Prevention Objectives*, Pub. No. (PHS) 91-50212, Washington, D.C.: Department of Health and Human Services.

Waxman, L.D., and Reyes, L.M. (1989). *A status report on hunger and homelessness in America's cities: 1988*. Washington, DC: U.S Conference of Mayors.

Winkleby, M.A., Rockhill, B., Jatulis, D., & Fortmann, S.P. (1992). The medical origins of homelessness. *American Journal of Public Health, 82*(10), 1394–97.

Wright, J.D. & Weber, E. (1988). *Homelessness and health*. New York: McGraw-Hill.

SELECTED READINGS

Alexander, M.A., J. Sherman, J., & Clark, L. (1991). Obesity in Mexican-American preschool children—A population group at risk. *Public Health Nursing, 8*(1), 53–58.

Borgford-Parnell, D., et al. (1994). A homeless teen pregnancy project: an intensive team case management model. *American Journal of Public Health 84*(6), 1029–30.

Carskadon, M.A. & Acebo, C. (1993). Parental reports of seasonal mood and behavior changes in children. *Journal of the American Academy of Child and Adolescent Psychiatry, 32*(2), 264–269.

Centers for Disease Control (1994). Preventing tobacco use among young people. A report of the Surgeon General. *Morbidity and Mortality Weekly Report, 43* (No.RR-4), 1–10.

Centers for Disease Control (1994). Programs for the prevention of suicide among adolescents and young adults. *Morbidity and Mortality Weekly Report, 43* (No.RR-6), 3–7.

Centers for Disease Control (1994). Surveillance for selected tobacco-use behaviors—United States, 1900–1994. *Morbidity and Mortality Weekly Report, 43* (No.SS-3), 1–43.

Chen, K. & Kandel, D.B. (1995). The natural history of drug use from adolescence to the mid-thirties in a general population sample. *American Journal of Public Health, 85*(1), 11–17.

Fontana, S. A. (1991). Applying marketing concepts to promote health in vulnerable groups. *Public Health Nursing, 8*(2), 140–143.

Kane, C., DiMartino, E., & Jimenez, M. (1990). A comparison of short-term psychoeducational and support groups for relatives coping with chronic schizophrenia. *Archives of Psychiatric Nursing, 4*, 343–353.

Leavitt, F. (1995). *Drugs and behavior* (3rd ed.). Thousand Oaks, CA: Sage.

Link, B. G., Susser, E., Stueve, A., et al. (1994). Lifetime and five-year prevalence of homelessness in the United States. *American Journal of Public Health, 84*(12), 1907–1912.

Lipton, R. I. (1994). The effect of moderate alocohol use on the relationship between stress and depression. *American Journal of Public Health, 84*(12), 1913–1917.

North, C. R., (1994). Access to psychiatric services for homeless mentally ill people. *British Journal of Nursing, 3*(9), 446–449.

Peled, E., Jaffe, P.G., & Edelson, J.L., (Eds.). (1994). *Ending the cycle of violence: Community responses to children of battered women.* Thousand Oaks, CA: Sage.

Reilly, F. E., et al. (1992). Living arrangements, visit patterns, and health problems in a nurse-managed clinic for the homeless. *Journal of Community Health Nursing, 9*(2), 111–121.

Stroul, B.A. (1989). Introduction to the special issue: The community support systems concept. *Journal of Psychosocial Rehabilitation, 12*(3), 5.

Taft, L. & Barkin, R. (1990). Drug abuse? Use and misuse of psychotropic drugs in Alzheimer's care. *Journal of Gerontological Nursing, 16,* 4–10.

Talashek, M. L., et al. (1994). The substance abuse pandemic: determinants to guide interventions. *Public Health Nursing, 11*(2), 131–139.

Wagner, J. D., et al (1992). Case management of homeless families. *Clinical Nurse Specialist, 6*(2), 65–71.

Watkins, E., Larson, K., Harlan, C., & Young, S. (1990). A model program for providing health services for migrant farmworker mothers and children. *Public Health Reports, 105*(6), 567–575.

Weisner, C., T. Greenfield, T., & Room, R. (1995). Trends in the treatment of alcohol problems in the U. S. general population, 1979–1990. *American Journal of Public Health, 85*(1), 55–60.

UNIT

V

Expanding the Community Health Nurse's Influence

CHAPTER

25

Leadership, Power, and Effecting Change in Community Health Nursing

LEARNING OBJECTIVES

Upon completion of this chapter readers should be able to:

- Describe three characteristics of leadership.
- Summarize six leadership theories.
- Explain the difference between transformational and transactional leadership.
- Describe five leadership functions.
- Differentiate between four power bases and four power sources.
- Discuss the concept of empowerment and its significance for community health nursing.
- Explain the three stages of change.
- Discuss the eight steps in planned change.
- Identify three planned change strategies.
- Summarize six principles for effecting change in community health.

KEY TERMS

- Autocratic leadership style
- Autonomous leadership style
- Change
- Empirical-rational change strategy
- Empowerment
- Evolutionary change
- Force field analysis
- Leadership
- Normative-reeducative change strategy
- Participative leadership style
- Planned change
- Power
- Power bases
- Power-coercive change strategy
- Power sources
- Revolutionary change
- Stages of change
- Transactional leadership
- Transformational leadership

Barbara Walton Spradley and Judith Ann Allender
COMMUNITY HEALTH NURSING: CONCEPTS AND PRACTICE, 4th ed.
© 1996 Barbara Walton Spradley and Judith Ann Allender

Influencing people to change to healthier beliefs and practices lies at the heart of all community health nursing. With clients at every level, from families and groups to large aggregates, the ability to influence change requires knowledge and skill in the practice of leadership, the acquisition and use of power, and the management of change.

How do nurses carry out their roles as both leaders and change agents at the aggregate level? With rapidly expanding opportunities, one can find many examples. A community health nurse becomes a member of the Governor's Commission on the Handicapped. In addition to understanding the entire state as a community and the handicapped as a special population, the nurse assists the commission to formulate new policies for meeting the needs of the handicapped. Another nurse, as a member of a metropolitan health planning board, works to improve health care for a group of Hmong immigrants from Southeast Asia. In a rural community of farms and small towns, the county nurse organizes a grass-roots task force concerned about the rising number of farm machinery injuries. The task force decides to survey farm families to determine the causes and develop preventive measures. All three of these nurses are involved in leadership and change at the aggregate level. They are working to change people's beliefs regarding health and health activities and to involve them in creating organized responses to community problems. (See Fig. 25.1.)

Community health nurses also lead people to change at the organizational level. For example a staff nurse in a public health nursing agency who feels overburdened by paperwork, is burned out, and seems to lack clear goals for daily tasks, observes that other staff members seem to be feeling the same. At a staff meeting, the nurse brings up the problem of job stress and suggests that everyone read an article on the subject to discuss at the next staff meeting. The first discussion is successful and a regular staff development meeting evolves with rotating leadership. Over a few months' time the staff begins to feel a new sense of direction and more competent to cope with job stress, and morale improves. This is an example of how a nurse can lead informally, to bring about organizational change. The result not only left individuals feeling better able to cope with their jobs, but also improved the health of the organization and the quality of its services.

Many nurses do not see themselves as leaders, nor do they wish to become leaders. All too often, leadership for some nurses means assuming a formal position with heavy responsibilities but leadership also takes place informally in nursing practice. Nurses are often called upon to assume leadership roles and they should realize that professional accountability includes this leadership role (Krichbaum, 1993).

Many advocate that all nurses should exercise leadership and accept responsibility for continually revitalizing professional nursing practice, broadening nursing's sphere of influence, and improving health services (Clifford, 1991; Krichbaum, 1993; Moloney, 1979). Moloney declares: "Accountability for professional

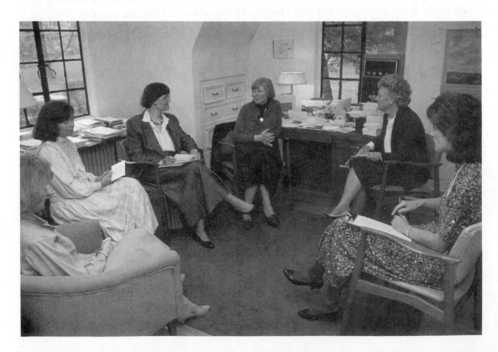

FIGURE 25.1. A community health nurse functions as both leader and change agent in discussions with college faculty about the increase in eating disorders among students.

practice implies that nurses are functioning as leaders in health care. If nurses are to become accountable for practice, they must broaden their view of what responsible leadership entails" (p. 3).

Nurses have many opportunities to exercise leadership. In acute care, they may lead in the improvement of health services. As nurse managers, they may facilitate improved professional practice. Nurse faculty may promote the quality of educational programs and influence the preparation of students for leadership roles (Chait, 1988; Flynn, et al., 1987; Krichbaum, 1993). For community health nurses the opportunities for leadership are staggering in number. Among them are the need to influence health reform, promote healthy public policies, and design more effective health services. A number of authors emphasize that community health nurses prepare themselves to move into leadership positions (Josten, 1989; Salmon, 1993).

Becoming an effective leader and change agent requires specialized knowledge and skills. This chapter examines the theoretical and applied aspects of leadership, power, and change. It describes how leadership, empowerment, and effecting change are inextricably linked, and how community health nurses incorporate them into practice.

What is Leadership?

Leadership is an interpersonal process in which one person influences the activities of another person or group of persons toward accomplishment of a goal (Robbins, 1993). In its simplest terms, leadership involves creating a vision and guiding and directing people's beliefs and behavior toward fulfilling that vision. It is accomplishing goals with and through people (Hersey & Blanchard, 1988). To lead requires interacting with other people to influence them to achieve a goal.

Three major characteristics of leadership are implied in the definition above. It involves a purpose or goal; it is interactive with people; and it influences people.

LEADERSHIP IS PURPOSEFUL

Leadership is purposeful and always has a goal (Adams, 1986; Robbins, 1993). No act of leadership exists without a reason. A mayor seeks low-cost housing for the poor; a community nurse wants to see teen parents develop parenting skills; a minister desires transportation that is accessible to all the physically handicapped. In each instance, the leader has a purpose and seeks to involve others in accomplishing that purpose.

A leader will work to achieve goals by making them clear, attainable, specific, and agreeable to the follower constituency.

LEADERSHIP IS INTERPERSONAL

Leadership is interpersonal and always involves a social exchange, a relationship between the two parties of leader and followers (Nicoll, 1986). These parties mutually agree upon roles and share information in a variety of patterns. A community agency director of nursing sets policy and standards for client services; a nurse chairing a community task force makes informal suggestions to members. In both cases, however, the leader and followers must maintain a relationship that fosters ongoing communication and facilitates the movement-toward-a-goal process.

LEADERSHIP IS INFLUENTIAL

Leadership is influential by helping to motivate others to change behaviors and achieve some goal (Fritz, 1986). For example, in a suburb of a larger city, a nurse received reports that several children had encountered rats while playing and two children had been bitten. A casual survey revealed alleys with piles of garbage and trash that attracted rats. The nurse, as a leader, wanted to influence or motivate members of the community to eliminate this public health problem. In order to mobilize the local citizens to achieve this goal, the nurse needed to influence them. The nurse began by inviting the parents of children who had encountered rats to call their neighbors together. At that meeting, the nurse facilitated the discussion and offered suggestions; the group decided to form a task force and hold a clean-up day with proper disposal of refuse and adequate containers. As a leader, this nurse offered guidance and direction, thus influencing the ideas and activities of this group of followers. Leadership, then, in community health means to influence people toward development of an optimally healthy life-style and environment. Any purposeful effort to influence behavior is an example of leadership; thus, every community health nurse can act as a leader (Krichbaum, 1993).

Leadership Theory

Some nurses effectively influence change in community health. Others do not. What explains the difference? What accounts for effective leadership? Six theoretical approaches provide insight into the nature of leadership: trait theory, behavioral theory, contingency theory, leadership style theories, attribution theory, and charismatic theory.

TRAIT THEORY

Trait theory began to emerge as early as the 1870s in which researchers theorized that certain individuals exhibited specific personality qualities or traits that made them leaders. Qualities such as intelligence, enthusiasm, self-confidence, charisma, and decisiveness appeared to be common to many leaders. They sought to identify leaders' personal traits, at first concluding that leaders were born with these characteristics but later determining that for some these traits were acquired. However, trait theorists were unable to identify specific qualities possessed by all leaders. For example, Geier reviewed 20 different research investigations that had isolated 80 different traits but only five traits were common to four or more of the studies (Geier, 1967). Research did establish that six traits distinguished leaders from nonleaders: (1) desire to lead; (2) ambition and energy; (3) intelligence; (4) self-confidence; (5) honesty and integrity; and (6) job-relevant knowledge (Kirkpatrick & Locke, 1991). Nevertheless, trait theories were unsuccessful in establishing any one group of traits that would predict selection of leaders or leadership effectiveness (Moloney, 1979). The trait approach did not examine the needs of followers. It did not clarify the relative importance of various traits. It did not reveal whether traits are present before or acquired as a result of leadership. And it failed to consider the influence of situational factors (Robbins, 1993).

BEHAVIORAL THEORY

Dissatisfied with the limitations of the trait approach, researchers began in the 1940s to focus on the behavior of leaders during interaction with followers. Behavioral theory proposed that leaders' behavior, rather than leaders' personality traits, were the chief determinants of who would become leaders and how effective they would be. This approach held out the hope that leadership ability could be developed.

As stated earlier leadership involves accomplishing goals with and through people. Consequently, behavioral theorists determined that leaders must be concerned with production in order to achieve goals and with relationships to show concern for people. These two dimensions, concern for people and concern for

productivity or tasks, became the focus of many studies (Blake & Mouton, 1964; Hersey & Blanchard, 1988; Robbins, 1993). Research showed that leaders who exhibited high concern for tasks while neglecting concern for people tended to be less effective. Similarly, leaders demonstrating high concern for people with little emphasis on tasks did not yield desired results. Figure 25.2 describes this two-dimensional behavioral approach. Research revealed that leaders who showed high concern for people as well as high concern for production (upper right quadrant) were the most effective. The behavioral research findings, however, could not demonstrate a leadership style that was effective in all situations.

CONTINGENCY THEORY

Contingency theory described leadership in terms of the leader's ability to adapt to the situation. It became the focus of research starting about the mid 1960s when researchers recognized that predicting leadership success was more complex than had been envisioned previously. One type of leadership used in one organization was not always successful in another organization. It appeared that leadership success was contingent upon the situation and researchers began to examine situational factors that influenced leadership effectivness.

Several contingency models emerged to explain leadership effectiveness. Researchers studying contingency

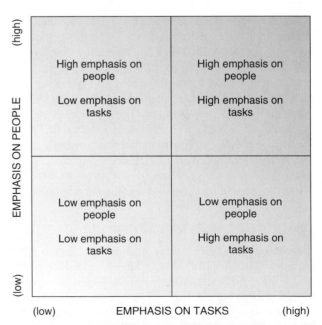

FIGURE 25.2. Leadership behavior grid. Adapted from Blake and Morton, 1964 and Hersey and Blanchard, 1988.

theory concluded that the situation dictated which style of leadership should be used. Because every situation was unique, leadership became a dynamic process of adapting one's style to the demands of the situation. Hersey and Blanchard (1988) referred to this process as "adaptive leader behavior" and said leadership style should be adapted to followers' level of maturity or their ability and willingness to assume responsibility. Figure 25.3 illustrates this approach. Its implications for community health nursing can be summarized: the more nurses adapt their style of leadership behavior to meet the particular situation and the needs of clients or followers, the more effective they will be in reaching health-related goals (Bernhard & Walsh, 1981; Reed, 1992).

LEADERSHIP STYLE THEORIES

Early research identified three general styles of leadership: (1) autocratic, (2) participative, and (3) autonomous (formerly called laissez-faire) (Hersey & Blanchard, 1988).

Autocratic Leadership Style

Autocratic leadership style is an authoritarian style in which leaders use their power (usually the power of their position) to influence their followers. The autocratic leader gives orders and expects others to obey without question. This style is generally evident in the military. Suggestions from followers are not, as a rule, invited or accepted. The leader is dominant and followers have little power or freedom of choice. In times of extreme crisis, an autocratic style can enhance results and even survival. Sometimes a nurse finds that members of a group will expect to be led in an autocratic style. They may see the nurse as the qualified expert among them. Autocratic leadership must be used with caution, and many current organizational structures do not lend themselves to its practice (Robbins, 1993).

Participative Leadership Style

Participative leadership style is a democratic style in which leaders involve followers in the decision-making process (Kinsman, 1986). This form of leadership has been increasingly popular in recent years as it tends to promote followers' self-esteem and to increase motivation and productivity. Leaders using this style encourage all members of the group to have a voice and participate in decisions which are made by group con-

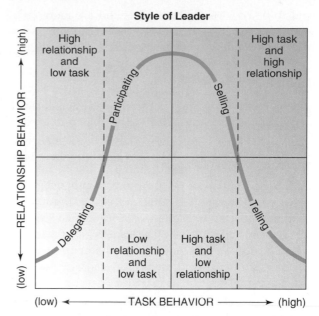

FIGURE 25.3. Leadership adapts to the situation and followers' readiness. Adapted from Hersey and Blanchard, 1988.

census. Some participative leaders encourage followers to exercise more freedom and power than others. Generally, however, this leadership style allows followers considerable freedom to make choices (Nicoll, 1986; Terry, 1993).

Autonomous Leadership Style

Autonomous leadership style is facilitative and encourages group members to select and carry out their own activities, and function independently. The leader's role is to set general parameters and to facilitate followers' progress. This style is used in certain industries, for example, where creative design of new products such as computer applications or medical technologies, is being encouraged. It is effective in a group whose members have both the motivation and competence to achieve the goals (Kinsman, 1986). Although someone is formally the leader, this style uses little or no direct influence; rather, the leader exercises indirect influence by establishing an overall purpose and encouraging follower creativity and innovation.

Building on these leadership styles, Hersey and Blanchard (1988) developed a continuum of leader behavior, illustrated in Figure 25.4, that describes style in relation to concern for people versus concern for production. Research has shown that autocratic leaders tend to be concerned about goals and are more task-oriented, whereas participative leaders tend to be more concerned about people and emphasize relationships.

ATTRIBUTION THEORY

Attribution theory says that leadership is made up of a set of characteristics ascribed or attributed to leaders by other people. For example, Mother Theresa is considered an exceptionally inspiring and humane leader, characteristics which are attributed to her because of people's perceptions of her style and accomplishments This theoretical approach combines aspects of trait, behavioral, and contingency theories to explain leadership-style and effectiveness. The leader's performance is judged by people's perceptions as to whether the leader's behavior is internally caused, meaning whether it is under personal control, or externally caused, meaning does the situation dictate the leadership behavior (Robbins, 1993).

CHARISMATIC THEORY

Charismatic theory says that leadership occurs because of a magnetic and inspirational personality and behavior. Charismatic theory is similar to attribution theory in that followers attribute extraordinary leadership ability to someone who exhibits exceptional appeal and persuasive ability. An example is Martin Luther King Jr. Conger and Kanungo (1988) describe charismatic leaders as:

1. Having an exceptionally clear vision and goal;
2. Being strongly committed to their vision;
3. Skilled at communicating their vision to others;
4. Perceived by others as unconventional;
5. Self-confident and assertive;
6. Seen as radical agents of change;
7. Able to realistically assess the environment.

Research shows a high correlation between charismatic leadership and followers' high performance and satisfaction. Furthermore, additional research has demonstrated that individuals can learn "charismatic" behaviors (Robbins, 1993) thus not limiting this type of leadership to only those who are born with these qualities.

Transformational vs. Transactional Leadership

Transactional leadership refers to the exchange relationship between leader and followers which emphasizes clarification of required roles and tasks and fo-

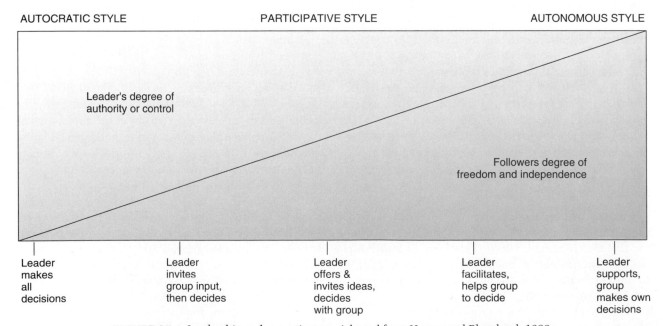

FIGURE 25.4. Leadership styles continuum. Adapted from Hersey and Blanchard, 1988.

cuses on goal accomplishment. Leader and followers engage in a reciprocal transaction. Most of the early leadership theories involved transactional leadership. However, the literature shows an increasing emphasis on transformational leadership which is more charismatic in nature (Burns, 1978; Bass, 1990; Terry, 1993). **Transformational leadership** is leadership that inspires followers to high levels of commitment and effort in order to achieve group goals (Robbins, 1993). Transformational leaders gain the respect and trust of their followers, instill in them a sense of pride and mission, communicate high expectations, promote intelligent, rational problem-solving, and give followers individualized consideration (Bass, 1990). Nurses are being challenged to engage in transformational leadership (Beecroft, 1993; Porter-O'Grady, 1992).

Closely related to transformational leadership is the reflective leadership view, an ethical perspective proposed by Robert Terry (1993), director of the Hubert H. Humphrey Institute of Public Affairs Education for Reflective Leadership Program at the University of Minnesota. He emphasizes that true leadership must be transformative rather than transactional to effect positive change. He states that a leader is an ethically motivated person who sees the possibilities for improvement in a situation and works in concert with followers to effect the change.

Community health nurses will need to determine their most appropriate leadership style by assessing the unique qualities of each situation, their followers' needs and degree of independence, and their own personalities and abilities (Guidera et al., 1988).

Leadership Functions

What are the functions of leadership in community health nursing? Kouzes and Posner (1987) describe leaders as challenging the process, inspiring a shared vision, enabling others to act, modeling the way, and encouraging the heart. Leaders know how to ask the right questions, how to develop problem-solving networks to find solutions to these questions, and how to marshall human energy and commitment to create the solutions. More specifically, five essential functions are required for effective leadership at any level: (1) the creative function, (2) the initiating function, (3) the risk taking function, (4) the integrative function, and (5) the instrumental function. These functions do not occur in any particular order; rather, they operate simultaneously throughout the leadership process.

CREATIVE FUNCTION

Leaders must be creative and able to envision new and better ways to solve problems. This first step involves creative thinking about problems that includes developing methods and activities for carrying out their solutions. This function requires ingenuity, innovation, vision, and a future orientation (Fritz, 1986). For instance, a nurse in a rural agency recognized that the home health aides or homemakers could potentially meet more client needs, find their jobs more fulfilling, and better serve the agency through an expanded role. She revised their job descriptions and instituted an expanded role-training program (Hennes, 1979). The creative leadership function is one that includes generating ideas and developing designs for action. It also involves empowering others to use their own creativity to accomplish goals (Harman, 1986; Hagberg, 1994).

INITIATING FUNCTION

A leader introduces change and sets its process in motion. For a nurse, the initiating function includes convincing clients or followers of the need for change, starting the problem-solving process, and launching the activities needed to carry out the plan. Like all the other leadership functions, it requires decision-making skills. For example, after seeing an increased number of pregnancies, a nurse who works in a high school convinces the girls to start a sex education and prenatal counseling group and initiates a series of teen parenting seminars. The initiating function begins the process toward goal accomplishment. It is the stimulus or "push" that starts clients or followers on their course of action (Fritz, 1986).

RISK-TAKING FUNCTION

Every leader is faced with uncertainty, and to proceed under uncertain conditions is to take risks (Lee, 1987). Leaders cannot guarantee outcomes. Most nurses, working with a family or group in the community, encounter a number of unpredictable variables during the process of planning with clients for health goals. Examples are new government policies that may alter programs and funding, or whether a proposed program will be well received by clients and actually bring about the needed change. The leadership process requires careful planning based on all available data and the creation of scenarios in order to predict all possible obstacles and outcomes. It even requires preparation of alternative courses of action, should earlier plans fail. Nevertheless, some variables cannot be predicted beyond a certain point, and leaders must be willing to take risks and expose themselves to possible failure and embarrassment. Taking risks also means they may expose clients or followers to potential negative outcomes. Effective leaders, however, take calculated risks (Kouzes & Posner, 1987); they weigh the potential consequences, pro and con, of each action before proceeding. Their concern is to minimize harmful consequences and maximize positive outcomes for followers.

INTEGRATIVE FUNCTION

The integrative aspect of the leadership role focuses on strengthening collective ties and uniting clients or followers through a strong sense of purpose. The leader reminds the followers of their goals, encourages pride in their group identity, stabilizes intragroup relations, and mediates interpersonal conflict (Kouzes & Posner, 1987). Community health nurses working with families, groups, and aggregates frequently find members at odds or cross-purposes with one another. Individuals in any group setting tend to have their own hidden agendas and separate needs. One of the nurse leader's jobs is to keep the client group on target by clarifying and reinforcing the goals they have mutually identified. The integrative function requires good interpersonal skills for establishing positive relationships with, as well as between, followers. This function supports the aim of promoting member commitment and cooperation.

INSTRUMENTAL FUNCTION

Leaders must also keep followers moving in the right direction; this is the purpose of the instrumental or facilitative function. Inspired by vision and goals, the leader serves as enabler to move followers to act (Hersey & Blanchard, 1988; Kouzes & Posner, 1987). For nurse leaders, this function involves good communication. They must keep in constant touch with clients or followers to make certain that goals and activities are understood and agreed upon, and to encourage both negative and positive feedback. Leaders further stimulate followers to progress toward achievement of goals

by reinforcing desired behaviors and by setting the pace themselves. The latter is particularly important for gaining followers' respect and sustained commitment. To set the pace means nurse leaders must demonstrate competence, practice what they preach, and show followers that they believe in them and in what they are asking followers to accomplish.

Community Health Nurses' Leadership Roles

Community health nurses exercise the functions of leadership in ever-widening spheres of influence, as is shown in Figure 25.5. The central aim of this leadership role is to positively influence community health. The first area of focus is to improve the immediate environment, which includes physical, psychological, social, and spiritual factors, by influencing consumer health-related behavior. Community health nurses exercise leadership when they influence the quality of nursing practice of their co-workers through, for instance, peer consultation and review. They may also influence the service provision vehicle, the agency or organization through which care is offered, by accepting a formal leadership position or by serving on committees and taking an active part in quality control. For example, listed below are some areas of influence associated with various positions in a large community health nursing agency:

Director	Influences organizational policy and decision making
Associate director	Influences management of specific aspects of the organization
Supervisor	Influences structure and process of providing services
Case manager	Influences coordination of assessment and referral activities
Team leader	Influences day-to-day quality of nursing practice
Staff nurse	Influences client health, behavior, and environment

In other settings for community health nursing practice, such as rural or occupational environments, there may be only one nurse present to provide leadership

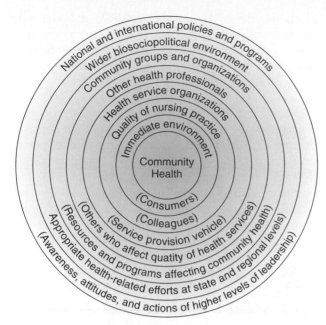

FIGURE 25.5. Areas of potential leadership influence within community health nursing practice.

that encompasses many, if not all, of these activities. Beyond the agency itself, the leadership role of each nurse extends to influencing those community attitudes, programs, and environmental factors that affect community health. Each nurse must assess the situation and determine the kind and extent of leadership needed.

Community health nurses may influence other professionals involved in the health system through ongoing communication to promote awareness of health needs and facilitate development of appropriate services. Nurses may influence groups and organizations, such as clubs, churches, or the legislature, by keeping them informed about health problems and suggesting ways they can improve community health levels. Extending their leadership influence even wider, community health nurses may focus on the wider biosociopolitical environment of the city, county, state, or region (Williams, 1981; Salmon, 1993). For example, a nurse may support anti-smoking programs or may campaign for proper disposal of nuclear waste. Finally, community health nursing leadership may extend to influencing national and international policies and programs that affect health, such as those of the World Health Organization. Participating in citizens' lobbies, serving on national committees, or contacting senators and representatives at the national and international levels are

some of the many possible actions nurses could take. The number of spheres in which the community health nurse exercises a leadership role varies, depending on health needs, the work situation, the nurse's abilities, and available time.

CONDITIONS FOR EFFECTIVE NURSING LEADERSHIP

The ultimate test of nurse leadership is in the outcomes. Are goals met? What did the leader accomplish? Reaching a successful outcome involves certain factors. Adherence to these factors will contribute to positive results, but violation of one or more of them will create negative results. They form the conditions necessary for leadership to be effective.

1. Followers must understand the suggestion, advice, or directive in order to make compliance possible (Henry et al., 1987).
2. Followers must be able to carry out the suggestion. They must have or be supplied with the needed resources or abilities (Lee, 1987).
3. The required action must be consistent with the followers' personal values and interests (Fritz, 1986).
4. The required action must be consistent with the followers' collective purposes, values, and norms; that is, followers must be in tune with group or organizational goals (Guidera, et al., 1987)

Central and most important to effective leadership is a relationship of trust, respect, and mutual exchange between leader and followers. It is through this transformational relationship that community health nurses can satisfy the conditions for effective leadership and accomplish positive health outcomes. See the Issues in Community Health Nursing display.

Power and Leadership

Power is the ability to influence or control other people's behavior to accomplish a specific purpose. Leadership and power are closely related as leaders use power in the process of achieving goals. The concept of power has both positive and negative connotations. Positive synonyms for power are strength, energy, force, and might. Although the power to influence people for good

Issues in Community Health Nursing
LEADERSHIP DEPENDS ON EFFECTIVENESS OF FOLLOWERS

A great deal of attention has been focused on leadership. Yet for every leader there must be followers. There is evidence that the success of leadership depends on the effectiveness of followers (Hollander & Offermann, 1990). Simple observation demonstrates that some followers do a good job of supporting leader goals while others may be indifferent or incompetent. What role do followers play in successful leadership outcomes? It is becoming evident that ineffective followers may be more of a handicap to accomplishing goals than ineffective leaders (Robbins, 1993).

Four qualities are characteristic of effective followers:

1. **Commitment**—They are committed to the vision, goals, and purpose of the leadership effort, in addition to concern for their own goals. They are physically and psychologically dedicated to their work.
2. **Self-management**—Effective followers manage their own lives well, working independently, and not needing close supervision. They are disciplined and can think and solve problems for themselves.
3. **Integrity**—Effective followers are honest and trustworthy. Their ideas, judgement, and ability to follow through can be trusted. They have high moral and ethical standards, acknowledge their mistakes, and give credit where it is appropriate.
4. **Competence**—Effective followers learn to master the skills necessary for accomplishing leadership goals. They seek to expand their competence and have higher standards for their own performance than the job requires. (Kelley, 1988)

of mutual dependency (Robbins, 1993). A leader only has as much power over her or his followers as the followers grant to the leader. The leader is dependent on the followers. At the same time, the greater the followers' dependency on the leader, the greater the power the leader has over the followers.

When a college student is financially dependent on her parents, the parents have a certain amount of power over the student. But the amount of the parents' power over their daughter depends on how much she allows them to control her behavior. People make choices. Followers can choose the degree of dependency they wish to have on the leader as well as the amount of power they wish to exercise for themselves. Leaders can also choose the amount of power they exert and the degree of their dependency on their followers. Thus the amount of power one has over others is determined by two things: (1) the amount one chooses to take and (2) the amount others are willing to give.

POWER BASES AND POWER SOURCES

Where does power come from? What is it that actually gives people the ability to influence others? In 1959, French and Raven identified five bases of power: (1) coercive power that used force to gain compliance, (2) reward power that provided something of value in exchange for compliance, (3) expert power that exerted influence by means of special knowledge or skills, (4) legitimate power derived from the person's position or title, and (5) referent power that came from other people's admiration and emulation of the powerholder. These five categories proved useful but did not clearly distinguish between bases of power and sources of power (Bacharach & Lawler, 1980).

Power Bases

Power bases refer to knowledge or skills the powerholder possesses that enable him or her to exert influence over others. As a powerholder, one's power bases are those things that one controls. Power bases come from four types of power: information power, persuasive power, reward power, and coercive power.

Information Power. Information power refers to a person's access to or possession of valued information. It has often been said that knowledge is power. When an individual controls unique information needed for such things as decision making they are in a position of power.

is a goal in community health, power may also be abused. Authority, control, domination, coercion, and manipulation are negative terms often associated with power.

Although power is often viewed as being exercised by the leader, many now see power as a social relationship

Persuasive Power. Persuasive power is the ability to influence people to adopt changed beliefs and actions through convincing discussion. The discussion may take such forms as argumentation, entreaty, or expostulation. A political leader who arouses a crowd to rally around a certain cause and a clergyman passionately raising money for the poor are both using persuasive power.

Reward Power. Reward power is the ability to influence people by granting rewards that they view as valuable. People comply with a request if they believe that a positive benefit will result from their compliance. They are thus voluntarily granting power to the person giving the reward. When a child is offered candy for good behavior or an employee a raise in salary if performance improves, the individuals offering the benefits have reward power.

Coercive Power. Coercive power refers to forced compliance based on fear. People will comply with orders if they believe that to not do so would result in some penalty, pain, or even death. A mother insisting that her children complete their homework before play has coercive power. A robber holding a gun to the head of a jewelry store owner has coercive power.

Power Sources

Power sources refer to qualities or situations from which the powerholder gains a power base (Robbins, 1993). Although individuals may hold one or more of the types of power just described in their power base, the question still remains, "where did that power come from?" Robbins describes four sources of power; they come from one's position, personal qualities, expertise, and opportunities.

Position Power. Position power means the ability to influence or control people as a result of one's formal position. Being in a formal position of authority, such as a corporation CEO, a classroom teacher, or head of a nursing department, gives one power over those who are lower in the structural hierarchy. Position power enables one to use various power bases. For example, a college professor exercises persuasive and reward power, a police officer uses coercive power, and a secretary applies information power.

Personal Power. Personal power is the ability to influence people because of one's personality. Trait theory and charismatic theory demonstrate that personal characteristics are a source of power. An individual who is charming, articulate, or physically dominating is usually able to influence others through personal power.

Expert Power. Expert power refers to the ability to influence people based on specialized knowledge or skills. Expertise in some specialized area enables one to use one or more of the power bases. For example, a computer expert's knowledge is the source for his or her information power as well as persuasive power in making computer-related decisions. Nurses, physicians, environmentalists, epidemiologists, tax accountants, and many more have expert power.

Opportunity Power. Opportunity power is the ability to influence people by taking advantage of a special or timely situation. Martin Luther King, Jr. seized an opportune moment in history to create awareness and change concerning civil rights. Often in a crisis, for example a car accident scene, someone who does not necessarily have any position power will emerge to take charge and tell people what to do. They are using opportunity power. Being in the right place at the right time and using that opportunity to influence people is drawing on opportunity power.

EMPOWERMENT FOR CHANGE IN COMMUNITY HEALTH

Community health nurses need to develop their sources of power. Nurses can move into positions of influence in the health system as professional practitioners, managers, teachers, researchers, and consultants. They can use these positions to exercise information power, persuasion power, reward power, or coercive power to effect change. Nurses can also capitalize on their personal characteristics as a power source. Self knowledge becomes critical in cultivating this power source. Nurses need to know their own strengths, limitations, and proclivities in order to find and sharpen the traits that will serve to enhance the ability to influence people. Developing expertise is another source of nurse empowerment. In community health, nurses who expand their knowledge and competence in such areas as group dynamics, health policy and politics, computer technology, epidemiologic research, occupational health, school health, environmental health, health planning, or community assessment, can use this expertise to build their power base of knowledge, persuasion, reward, and coercion. Nurses also need to take better advantage of opportunities. Sometimes nurses shy away from chances to serve on influential committees in the community, testify before the legislature on important health issues, attend community meetings where issues are being aired, or provide input for planning decisions. These are only a few of the opportunities where community health nurses can gain power and influence change. Nursing's input into health reform discussions is a prime example of gaining nursing power and influence.

Empowerment is a process of developing knowledge and skills that increase one's mastery over the decisions that affect one's life (Kreisberg, 1992). To empower means to enable. As community health nurses learn to empower themselves, they can then empower others. To empower people in the community requires helping them to develop competence to take charge of their lives and find ways to meet their own needs (Zerwekh, 1992). See the Research in Community Health Nursing display. It means helping them to develop knowledge and skills so that they can participate in their social and political worlds (Krichbaum, 1993). Nurses can assist community clients to develop the four power sources for themselves—use of position, capitalizing on personal characteristics, developing expertise, and taking advantage of opportunities. The elderly population, for example, could be encouraged to take advantage of a local election (opportunity power) to lobby for crime prevention. Adolescents could participate in school educational projects to gain knowledge (expert power) about family values and sexuality. Such programs have, in fact, proven effective in preventing teen pregnancy (American Hospital Association, 1994).

Vulnerable groups in the community, such as the homeless or abused women and children, often perceive themselves to be powerless. To promote client choice and self-determination requires empowering strategies that foster clients' self-esteem. To promote client self-esteem, nurses can provide consistent affirmations, set clear expectations, encourage increasing responsibility, model empowering behavior, facilitate client choices, and promote a sense of meaning and hope (Zerwekh, 1992). When people are unable to act in a positively autonomous manner, for example abusive parents or the mentally ill, the nurse may need to use persuasive or coercive power bases to protect them and the people their actions affect.

Empowerment of self and others is germaine to effective leadership for community health nurses (Eng, et al., 1992). The use of power can and should be a positive force for protecting and promoting aggregate health.

Research in Community Health Nursing
EMPOWERMENT AND COERCION

Zerwekh, J. V. (1992). The practice of empowerment and coercion by expert public health nurses. *Image: Journal of Nursing Scholarship, 24*(2), 101–105.

Public health nurses seek to empower families in self care. At the same time nurses must exercise coercion when family members need protection from neglect and violence. This qualitative study examined expert public health nurses' home visit anecdotes (N-95) to learn how these apparently contradictory activities were handled.

In the study, empowerment was defined "as enabling a parent to develop personal capacity and authority to take charge of everyday family life" (p. 102). The nurses used four strategies to promote client power in making their own choices. First was *believing* in clients' ability and encouraging choice making. Second was *listening* to family concerns and starting with their preferences. Third was *expanding* family vision of what was possible. Fourth was candid *feeding back* of reality and unhealthy choices. "The expert public health nurse has learned to do a figurative dance, stepping forward with nurse assertion and then backing off to await client initiative" (p. 102).

For the nurses in the study coercion, which is "the use of force by social authority" (p.103), was exercised through three levels of persuasion: reasoning, confronting, and requiring. When family members were at risk the nurses used *reasoning* by persuading through logical argument, giving evidence that would help convince clients of the need to change. They used persuasion through *confronting* by directly opposing unhealthy action or inaction. And finally, they exercised authority, *requiring* accountability and change. Exercising authority included the nurse detecting risk, judging whether to take authoritative action, representing authority, and choosing between divided loyalties. The study showed that expert public health nurses were able to successfully incorporate both advocacy and coercion into their practice.

The Nature of Change

To be a leader is to effect change in people's behaviors (McPherson, 1991; Moloney, 1979). When nurses suggest that families adopt healthier communication patterns, they are asking them to change. Teaching parenting skills to teenagers is introducing a change. Promoting a community's self-determination in choosing a safer environment again, requires that the individuals involved must change. Since community health nursing's responsibility is to accomplish health goals and thus promote change, nurses cannot lead without introducing change into people's lives. Therefore, it becomes imperative for community health nurses to understand the nature of change, how people respond to it, and how to effect change for improved community health.

DEFINITION AND TYPES OF CHANGE

Change is "any planned or unplanned alteration of the status quo in an organism, situation, or process" (Lippitt, 1973, p. 37). This definition explains that change may occur either by design or by default (Rantz, et al., 1987). Over the years various theorists have contributed to understanding the nature of change. From a systems perspective, change means that things are out of balance or the system's equilibrium is upset (Spradley, 1980; Bennis, et al., 1985). For instance, when a community is devastated by a flood, that community's normal functioning is thrown off balance. Adjustments are required; new patterns of behavior become necessary. Other theorists explain change as the process of adopting an innovation (Spradley & McCurdy, 1994). Something different, such as an organization-wide smoke-free policy, is introduced; change occurs when the innovation is accepted, tried, and integrated into daily practice. Some have explained change in terms of its effect on behavior—that change requires adjustment in thinking and behavior and that people's responses to change vary according to their perceptions of it. Change threatens the security that people feel when following established and familiar patterns (Nordstrom et al., 1987). It generally requires the adoption of new roles. Change is disruptive.

The way people respond to change depends, in part, on the type of change it is. One can describe the change process as sudden or drastic (revolutionary) or gradual change over time (evolutionary) (Gerlach & Hine, 1973).

Evolutionary change is change that is gradual and requires adjustment on an incremental basis. It modifies rather than replaces a current way of operating. Some examples of evolutionary change include becoming parents, gradually cutting back on the number of cigarettes smoked each day, and losing weight by eliminating desserts and snacks. (See Fig. 25.6.) Since it is gradual, this kind of change does not require radical shifts in goals or values; in fact, it may enhance current goals or values (Nordstrom et al., 1987). This type of change may sometimes be viewed as reform.

Revolutionary change, in contrast, is a more rapid, drastic, and threatening type of change that may completely upset the balance of a system. It involves different goals and perhaps radically new patterns of behavior (Ibid.). Sudden unemployment, stopping smoking overnight, losing the town's football team in a plane accident, or suddenly removing children from abusive parents are examples of revolutionary changes. In each instance, the people affected have little or no advance warning and no time to prepare. High levels of emotional, mental, and sometimes physical energy and rapid behavior change are required to adapt to revolutionary change. If the demands are too great, some may experience defense mechanisms such as incapacitation, resistance, or denial of the new situation. See Chapter 15 for detailed discussion of coping with stress and defense mechanisms.

The impact of a proposed change on a system will clearly depend on the degree of the change's evolutionary or revolutionary qualities, a factor to be considered in planning for change. Some situations lend themselves better to one kind of change than the other. A community in need of improved facilities for the handicapped, such as ramps and wider doors, can introduce this change on an evolutionary, incremental basis; whereas a community involved in an unsafe, intolerable, or life-threatening situation, such as a flood or serious influenza epidemic, may require revolutionary change.

STAGES OF CHANGE

The phrase **stages of change** refers to the three sequential steps leading to change that include unfreezing (when desire for change develops), changing (when people accept and try out new ideas), and refreezing (when the change is integrated and stabilized in

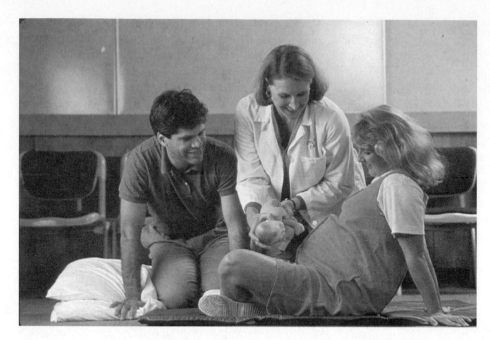

FIGURE 25.6. Becoming parents is an evolutionary change that occurs over time.

practice). These stages were first described by Kurt Lewin and have become a cornerstone for understanding the change process (cited in Lippitt, et al., 1958; Noone, 1987).

Unfreezing

The first stage, unfreezing, occurs when a need for change develops causing disequilibrium in the system. A system in disequilibrium is more vulnerable to change. People are motivated to change either intrinsically or by some external force (Ryan, 1987). People have a sense of dissatisfaction; they feel a void that they would like to fill. The unfreezing stage involves initiating the change.

Unfreezing may occur spontaneously. A family requests help in solving a problem with alcoholism; a group seeks assistance in adjusting to retirement; a community desires a solution to noise pollution. However, the nurse as change agent may need to initiate the unfreezing stage by attempting to motivate clients, through education or other strategies, to see the need for change (Ibid.).

Changing

The second stage of the change process, changing, occurs when people examine, accept, and actually try the innovation. For instance, this is the period when

participants in a prenatal class are learning exercises or when the elderly in a senior citizens' center are discussing and trying ways to make their apartments safe from accidents. During the changing stage, people experience a series of attitude transformations ranging from early questioning of the innovation's worth to full acceptance and commitment to accomplishing the change. The change agent's role during this stage is to help clients see the value of the change, encourage them to try it out, and assist them in adopting it for use (Cobb-McMahon et al., 1984).

Refreezing

The third and final stage in the change process, refreezing, occurs when change is established as an accepted and permanent part of the system. The rest of the system has adapted to it. Since it is no longer viewed as disruptive, threatening, or even new, people no longer feel resistant to it. As the change is integrated, the system becomes refrozen and stabilized. It is evident that refreezing has occurred when weight loss clients, for example, are routinely following their diets and losing weight, or when senior citizens are using grab bars in their bathrooms and have removed scatter rugs from their homes, or when a community has erected stop signs and established crosswalks at dangerous intersections.

Refreezing involves integrating or internalizing the change into the system and then maintaining it. Simply because a change has been accepted and tried does not guarantee that it will last (Spradley, 1980). Often there is a tendency for old patterns and habits to return; consequently, the change agent must take special measures to assure maintenance of the new behavior. A later section discusses ways to stabilize change.

Planned Change

Planned change is a purposeful, designed effort to effect improvement in a system with the assistance of a change agent (Ibid.). Planned change is crucial to the development of successful community health nursing programs. The following characteristics of planned change are key to its success:

The change is purposeful and intentional; there are specific reasons or goals prompting the change. These goals give the change effort a unifying focus and a specific target. Unplanned change occurs haphazardly, and its outcomes are unpredictable.

The change is by design, not by default. Thorough, systematic planning provides structure for the change process, and a map to follow toward a planned destination.

Planned change in community health aims at improvement. That is, it seeks to better the present situation, to promote a higher level of efficiency, safety, or health enhancement. Planned change however, aims to facilitate growth and positive improvements. Plans to provide shelter and health care for a homeless population, for example, are designed to improve this group's well being.

Planned change is accomplished by means of an influencing agent. The change agent serves as a catalyst in developing and carrying out the design; the change agent's role is a leadership role.

PLANNED CHANGE PROCESS

The planned change process involves a systematic sequence of activities that uses the nursing process. Following its eight basic steps leads to the successful management of change: (1) recognize symptoms, (2) diagnose need, (3) analyze alternative solutions, (4) select a change, (5) plan the change, (6) implement the change, (7) evaluate the change, and (8) stabilize the change (Spradley, 1980). Figure 25.7 shows how forces acting on a system create a need for change.

Step 1: Assess Symptoms

The first step in managing change is to recognize and assess the symptoms that indicate a need for change. In this step, one should gather and examine the presenting evidence, not diagnose or jump ahead to treatment. For instance, assume that a group of clients show interest in receiving help with parenting skills. The nurse cannot assume that these clients feel inadequate in the parent role, neither can she assume that they lack information about parenting or are having difficulty with their children. The nurse must assess the specific needs to discover that some of the parents have trouble talking to their teenagers, others wonder if their children's behavior is normal, a few question how strictly they should set limits, and still others are not certain about how to handle punishment. These symptoms are pieces of evidence that will assist diagnosis in the next step. This first step is an assessment phase. Before moving on, however, change agents need to ask themselves what their motives are for pursuing this change. Inappropriate motives of the change agent, such as wanting to feel needed, can cloud judgment and interfere with effective management of change.

Step 2: Diagnose Need

Diagnosis means to analyze the symptoms and reach a conclusion about what, if anything, needs changing. First, describe the situation as it is now (the real) and compare it to the way it should be (the ideal). For example, loud arguing and conflict may be quite normal and functional behavior for an adolescent support group. There is no discrepancy between the real and the ideal and therefore no need for change within the group. If, however, there is a discrepancy between the real and the ideal, then a need exists and a change effort is justified (Hersey & Blanchard, 1988). For example, the community health nurse in talking with a group of parents, hears the following comment: "I'm not sure how much freedom to allow Karen. She came in late twice last week and I'm not sure how to punish her." Clearly the nurse notices a discrepancy between this family's present and ideal situations; hence, there is a need.

The next step is to determine the exact nature and cause of the need. Gathering data by means such as questioning clients, checking the literature, or seeking consultation is important for making a more accurate diagnosis (Porter, 1987). The parents should be questioned in more detail about the difficulties they are having with their children. Asking questions such as: How

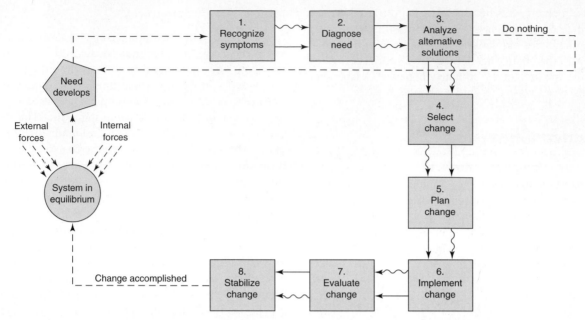

FIGURE 25.7. Planned change model. The planned change process begins when one recognizes a need. When the change agent fails to respond to a need for change, the need continues and may escalate. Client system (those involved and affected by the change) and change agent must work together throughout the entire planned change process. Their respective roles vary depending on the situation and the players' abilities, but no planned change is truly effective without utilization of this collaborative relationship. The client system (wavy arrow), which may be an entire community, will fluctuate in its involvement with the change process. The change agent (straight arrow), as a good leader, analyzes the situation thoroughly, plans carefully, and sets a steady course for effecting the change.

do they feel about being parents? What are the most difficult aspects of parenting for them? Have they read any books or used any other resources to help them in their parenting activities? To whom do they talk (if anyone) about parenting problems? When they have a problem handling the raising of their children, how do they usually solve it? Secondary data should be obtained by checking the literature to determine the most effective approaches to solving parenting problems or consulting an expert on family life to get ideas about what this group of parents might need. The parents should also be asked directly what information they desire or need. Conclusions should be drawn about what specific changes are needed for these parents. Unless the diagnosis is made accurately, the entire change effort may be addressing its attention to the wrong problem. Also, when possible, the client system should help diagnose. Ask the parents exactly what it is that they want and need.

The findings should be formulated into a single diagnostic statement that also includes the cause. After data collection, the nurse discovers the parents are insecure

in their parenting roles partially because of lack of knowledge about how to carry out parental responsibilities but primarily because they lack a supportive reference group. Most of them live some distance from relatives or no longer maintain close ties with relatives. The diagnosis for these parents is insecurity in the parenting role due to lack of support and some lack of knowledge.

Step 3: Analyze Alternative Solutions

Once the diagnosis and its cause are determined, it is time to identify solutions or various alternative directions to follow. Brainstorming is helpful here and the client system should be involved as much as possible in the process. A review of the literature is helpful at this point to suggest solutions tried by others. Make a list of all the reasonable broad alternatives, and then analyze them thoroughly to determine the advantages, disadvantages, possible consequences, and risks involved in each. For the parents, one might consider general alternatives such as family counseling, a support group, or education in family life. Each of these alternatives has some advantages and disadvantages toward meeting the parents' need for confidence in their roles.

Next, each alternative should be analyzed. For example, the counseling solution could provide insight and awareness into family behavior. It would give family members opportunities to express feelings and gain understanding of how other members feel. However, it would not provide a frame of reference that they could use to compare their own parenting behaviors with other acceptable ones, nor would it provide adult peer support for the parents. The consequences of this alternative would most likely be to promote parents' self-understanding and better family communication. Risks would include the possibility that children, especially teenagers, might not be willing to participate and that parents might not gain self-confidence in their roles. Each alternative should be examined to determine its usefulness and feasibility again using literature and other resources, such as consultants, to learn the best ways to meet the parents' need for change.

Step 4: Select Change

After having carefully analyzed all the alternatives, one must select the best solution. The parents support the idea that the best solution seems to be a parenting support group. The risks involved in the change choice should be reexamined such as whether this action might be too costly in time, money, or potential for failure. Ways to reduce these risks might be explored.

It is important to know what the change is aiming to accomplish by formulating a clearly stated goal. For this parenting group, the mutually agreed-upon goal is to provide a supportive, reinforcing climate while increasing members' parenting skills.

Step 5: Plan the Change

This step is at the heart of planned change because it is at this stage that change agent and client system together prepare the design, the blueprint that guides the change action. In steps 1 through 4, data are gathered, a diagnosis made, resources assessed, and a goal established, all preparatory actions for planning the change. The plan tells the change agent and client system how to meet that goal. Preferably they develop the plan together.

Talk with the parents about ways to meet their goal, considering such possibilities as weekly discussion groups on selected topics, monthly meetings with an informed speaker, or reading books and articles on parenting with regular sessions to discuss their application. After analysis and discussion, the group decides to meet one evening a month, rotating the location between members' homes. Group sessions will include a variety of approaches: a speaker will be invited every three months; a book or article discussion will be held quarterly; and the remaining meetings will be spent on topics of the group's choice. All sessions will provide opportunities for parents to discuss their concerns or problems. You and the group design this plan around a set of objectives.

The most important activity in planning is to have clear, specific objectives. These should be measurable and, preferably, stated as outcomes. For example, the following objective is measurable and describes an outcome. "By the end of the second session, each parent in the group will have participated in the discussion at least once." It is helpful to prepare a list of activities to help accomplish each objective, and develop a time plan. It is also important to assess the potential costs in terms of time, money, and number of people and materials needed, and to determine the resources available. Design the evaluation plan, and start a list of ways to stabilize (refreeze) the change.

During planning, it is useful to perform a **force field analysis** (Hersey and Blanchard, 1988), a technique developed by Kurt Lewin (1947) for examining all the positive (driving) forces and negative (restraining) forces influencing a change situation. Force field theory says there are driving forces that favor change and restraining forces which decrease or discourage change. Examples of driving forces include clients' desire to be healthier, more productive, or have a safe environment. Examples of restraining forces include apathy, fear of something new, low self-esteem, or hostility. When the strength of the driving forces is equal to the strength of the restraining forces, equilibrium exists. To introduce a change and move the client system to a higher level of health, that balance must be altered. To do so, the change agent either increases the driving forces, decreases the restraining forces, or both. The change agent uses force field analysis to study both sets of forces and to develop strategies to influence the forces in favor of the change (see Fig. 25.8).

The procedure for conducting a force field analysis follows a few simple steps. The change agent may perform the analysis alone but preferably will consult with clients and a change-planning resource group, such as

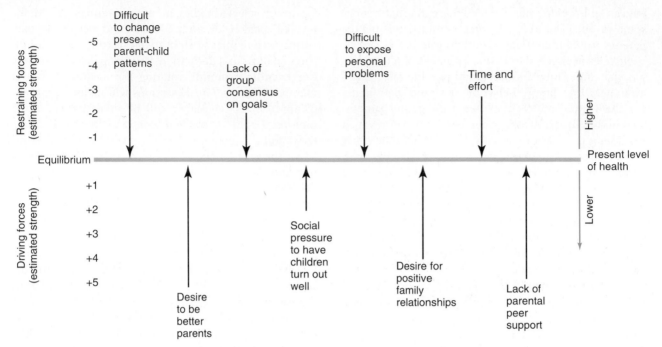

FIGURE 25.8. Analysis of restraining and driving forces.

community health colleagues. The following are steps for force field analysis:

1. Brainstorm to produce a list of all driving and restraining forces. (For the parenting group, one driving force is the parents' desire to be more successful parents; a restraining force might be lack of group agreement on discussion topics.)
2. Estimate the strength of each force.
3. Plot the forces on a chart such as the one shown in Figure 25.7.
4. Note the most important forces; then research and analyze them.
5. List and document possible responses or action steps that might strengthen each important driving force or weaken each important restraining force.

Finally, as a consideration in planning the change and in analyzing the driving and restraining forces, study the social network and interaction of the system involved in the change. The change agent needs to be aware of formal and informal leaders, cliques within larger groups, influential persons, and all the other possible social network influences on the change process. For instance, one nurse attempting to improve the in-

fant-feeding practices of a group of young Southeast Asian mothers failed to consider the strong cultural influence of the infants' grandmothers living near by. The older women had strong opinions based on long-held cultural traditions about what infants were to eat and how they were to be fed. To ignore their influence could cause the proposed change to fail; involving the grandmothers could be a way of turning their influence into a driving force for the change.

Step 6: Implement Change

The implementation step involves enacting the change plan. Because the objectives and activities have been clearly defined in previous steps, change agent and client system know exactly what needs to be done and begin the process. For example, the parenting group and their nurse-change agent begin group discussions meeting every Tuesday evening at a local school.

At the start of implementation, it is important to make certain that *all* persons concerned clearly understand and are prepared for the change. When working with an aggregate, for example, the nurse may do most of the planning with a few key members. The nurse must make certain each member who will be affected by the proposed change knows what to expect and that they understand the meaning of the change and what will be required of them in adapting to it. An unprepared client system, especially in a large group or organization, may bring disaster (Kanter, 1985). No matter how well a change effort is planned, people who are unprepared for it may resist it strongly and render it useless.

When implementing change that will affect a large group of people, such as introduction of a mass screening or immunization program, it is helpful to do a pilot study. The pilot study is done to test the change on a small scale in order to iron out problems and revise the change before implementing it into the larger system. One advantage of a pilot study is that it demonstrates the change to the client system on a small scale that is less threatening so that clients are more receptive. It gives people time to adjust their thinking and to discover that the change will not disrupt their lives too much or require drastic adaptations.

Step 7: Evaluate Change

The success of this step also depends on how well the change is planned. Well-written objectives with specific criteria for their measurement will make the evaluation step much simpler. However, evaluation does not end with saying whether or not the objectives were met. Each objective requires analysis: (1) Was it met? (2) What evidence (documentation) shows that it was met? (3) Was it accomplished using the best means possible, or would some other method have been better? The objective for the parenting group stated that each member should enter into the discussion by the end of the second session. Although this objective could be easily evaluated by the nurse leader, the objective could have been improved by more specific description of how this participation would occur. A better method to achieve this objective would have been to suggest that more active group members could solicit ideas from those who had not had an opportunity to speak. This would facilitate more group participation rather than the nurse leader calling on nontalkers to speak. Finally, considering the evaluation, the change agent makes needed modifications in the change before stabilization.

Step 8: Stabilize Change

The final step in the planned change process requires taking measures to reinforce and maintain the change (see Fig. 25.8). A well-developed change plan includes a design for stabilization. The change agent actively encourages continued use of the innovation by establishing two-way communication; thus any future resistance can be overcome, and the client's full commitment to the change can be maintained (Noone, 1987). Stabilization occurs by soliciting reactions from the client system. Do the clients perceive any potential problems? Do they have doubts? Reinforcing the desired behavior and following up on the change as long as necessary will help assure its permanence. Alcoholics Anonymous, for example, stabilizes the change to nondrinking by providing a regular support group that reinforces the nondrinking pattern. The group rewards compliance with praise and replaces drinking with other satisfying experiences, such as social acceptance, to keep the alcoholic from returning to the old behavior. In the example of the parenting group, the nurse stabilizes changed behaviors by focusing on the group's increased confidence in their parenting roles and emphasizing the greater number of successes they are having in coping with their children. The group decides to reward successes by giving a "Parent of the Month" plaque to the member who demonstrates the most growth in parenting skills and agree to nominate one member as "Parent of the Year" in the community newspaper contest. When stabilization occurs and the system achieves a new equilibrium (see Figure 25.7), the change agent-client system relationship can be terminated for this specific change effort.

APPLYING PLANNED CHANGE TO LARGER AGGREGATES

This section has viewed the planned change process primarily in the context of introducing change to smaller aggregates. Community health nurses also utilize these eight steps when managing change at the organization, population group, community, and larger aggregate levels. For example, a nurse may suspect that there is a widespread lack of confidence among young parents. This hypothesis could be tested through a survey using a mailed questionnaire to determine parenting needs among the entire community's population of young parents. If symptoms are present (step 1), the nurse, in collaboration with health department personnel or other appropriate professionals, could analyze the symptoms and reach a diagnosis (step 2), perhaps that a large percentage of young parents in the community are lacking in confidence and knowledge of parenting skills. Several approaches to meeting this need could be considered, such as instituting a parenting center in the community with satellite clinics; organizing churches, clubs, or both, to sponsor parenting support groups; or working through the community college system to hold workshops and classes on parenting skills (step 3). The most feasible and useful alternative could be selected (step 4), and a parenting program for the community planned (step 5) and implemented (step 6). The nurse, with parents and the other professionals involved, would then evaluate the outcomes (step 7) and make any necessary adjustments in the parenting program before finally stabilizing it (step 8), making certain that this change, undertaken to meet a population group need, remained an established and effectively functioning service. See the World Watch discussion.

PLANNED CHANGE STRATEGIES

The literature describes three general change strategies (Bennis, et al., 1985; Haffer, 1986). In any given situation, the change agent may use one or a combination of these strategies to effect a change (Haffer, 1986; Lundeen, 1992). They are (1) empirical-rational, (2) normative-reeducative, and (3) power-coercive.

Empirical-Rational Strategies

Empirical-rational strategies are strategies used to effect change based on the assumption that people are rational and when presented with empirical information will adopt new practices which appear to be in their best interest. To use this approach, which is common in community health, one simply offers or makes new information available to people. For instance, most family planning programs use empirical-rational strategies. Clients are given basic information on reproductive anatomy and physiology, and they are told about the benefits of contraception with an explanation of a variety of family planning methods. Health workers hope that once clients have this information, they will adopt some method of family planning. Some clients respond well to this approach, while others do not. The difference lies in client ability and interest in self-help. The nurse-change agent uses empirical-rational strategies with clients who can assume a relatively high degree of responsibility for their own health. In some respects, this set of strategies parallels the participative leadership style, described in Figure 25.4, that fosters maximum client autonomy.

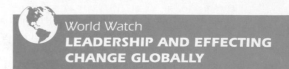

World Watch
LEADERSHIP AND EFFECTING CHANGE GLOBALLY

We live in a global community. The problems and affairs of one country can no longer be viewed in isolation; rather, they influence trade, economic conditions, health, and welfare on an international level. Wars, famine, floods, earthquakes, population overcrowding, limited food supply, economic disasters, and epidemics of communicable diseases are among the many events that have a global impact.

World population growth, for example, continues to escalate, increasing close to 90 million per year. The distribution of this growth is predominantly in developing countries where the rate of increase is at least 12 times that of developed countries and mortality is approximately four times greater in developing countries than in developed countries. Of persons under 25 years of age, 80% live in developing countries and this figure is rising each year. In addition, the global population of elderly (aged 65 years and over) is increasing by 800,000 *a month*, adding to the need for health services to address chronic disabilities (WHO, 1994). Environmental health problems and disease distribution follow similar global patterns. AIDS is a disease of world-wide concern with as many as eight to ten million adults and one million children infected each year with HIV. Projections state that by the year 2000, 26 million people could be infected with HIV with more than 85% of these from developing countries, and an annual death toll of 2 million is predicted (UNICEF, 1995). Public health leadership is needed to address these problems and it must be leadership that is population- and prevention-focused.

Community health nurses face an unparalled opportunity to provide leadership and influence change internationally. Many nurses already serve in influential positions with the World Health Organization, the Pan American Health Organization, the Peace Corps, and numerous other national and international organizations assisting developing countries. However many more community health nurse leaders are needed to effect improvement in global health.

Normative-Reeducative Strategies

Normative-reeducative strategies are strategies used to influence change that not only present new information but directly influence people's attitudes and behaviors through persuasion (Ryan, 1987; Flynn, 1992). It is a sociocultural reeducation. This approach assumes that people's attitudes and practices are determined by sociocultural norms and that they need more than presentation of information to change behavior (Chin & Benne, 1985). This approach attempts to strengthen client self-understanding, self-control, and commitment to new patterns through direct urging and influence. For example, a health-teaching program that aims to increase safety practices in an industrial setting not only provides safety information such as posters and warning signs but also uses persuasive tactics such as individual rewards for safe practices, division recognition for minimum number of accidents, or discipline for noncompliance. Nurses use normative-reeducative strategies with clients who have a measure of self-care skill but, at the same time, need external assistance to effect lasting behavioral change. This type of client is found in teaching, counseling, and therapy situations.

Power-Coercive Strategies

Power-coercive change strategies use coercion based on fear to effect change. Change agents may derive power from the law (such as health regulations or administrative policies), from position (such as political, social, or managerial positions), from a group (such as a social, work, or professional group), or from personal power (such as personal charisma, competence, or respect of followers) (Gorman et al., 1986). They use this power to coerce change; the result is more or less forced compliance on the part of the client system. Some situations, particularly those that are life-threatening, may require power-coercive strategies. In community health practice, power-coercive strategies may be used with people who cannot help themselves or in situations that threaten individuals' safety or the public's health. An example is the stringent enforcement of infection control policies regarding the treatment of contaminated objects, such as needles used by HIV infected individuals, and the safe disposal of infectious wastes. In another example, if officials find a restaurant in violation of health codes they will most likely either force compliance with the code or close down the restaurant. Occasionally clients cannot exercise responsibility because of tempo-

rary or permanent physical or psychological incapacitation, such as the mentally ill, abusive parents, or developmentally disabled persons. In such cases, the nurse may need to use the power of the law, for example with abusive parents, to effect changes that are in clients' best interests. Although power-coercive strategies are appropriate in some situations, they should be used with caution because they can rob people of opportunities to grow in autonomy and capacity for self-care.

Planned change strategies may be combined; for instance, a normative-reeducative approach might have a power-coercive backup. This combination is evident in programs that, for example, educate and persuade groups of people to be immunized against an impending epidemic or to keep their garbage contained to avoid insect and rodent infestation. Behind this normative-reeducative strategy is an implied coercive threat of official disapproval, or worse, for noncompliance.

The effectiveness of a change strategy, then, varies with each situation and particularly with the degree of client capacity for self-care. As in the approach to leadership styles and use of power discussed earlier in the chapter, the nurse-change agent adapts strategies to fit each change situation.

PRINCIPLES FOR EFFECTING POSITIVE CHANGE

Community health nurses introduce change every day that they practice. Every effort to solve a problem, prevent another from occurring, meet a potential community need, or promote people's optimal health requires changes. To make these changes truly successful so that desired outcomes are reached, they must be managed well. The following six principles provide guidelines for effecting positive change: (1) principle of participation, (2) principle of resistance to change, (3) principle of proper timing, (4) principle of interdependence, (5) principle of flexibility, and (6) principle of self-understanding.

Principle of Participation

Persons affected by a proposed change should participate as much as possible in every step of the planned change process (Nicoll, 1986). This involvement is important for several reasons. Collaboration with those who have a vested interest in the change can produce a wealth of ideas and insights that can greatly improve the change plan. Furthermore, such participation can help remove obstacles and reduce resistance. Participation ensures a greater likelihood that the change will be accepted and maintained (Kanter, 1985; Flynn, 1992). (See Fig. 25.9.) One nurse, for instance, when planning with a school's parent-teacher association for a drug education program, involved students as well as teachers and parents. As a result, she secured all their support and cooperation, gained many helpful suggestions that she herself had not considered, and discovered that students were more responsive to the program because the change plan was specifically tailored to their needs.

Principle of Resistance to Change

Because all systems instinctively preserve the status quo, the change agent can expect people to resist change (Fritz, 1986). The homeostatic mechanism operating in any system seeks to maintain equilibrium; change poses a threat to that stability and security. Furthermore, all systems experience inertia; that is, they resist beginning movement. People do not undertake a change until they are convinced of its worth. Resistance may also come from a conflict over goals and methods or from misunderstanding about what the change will mean and require. Involving people in the planned change process, discussed in the previous section, is one way to overcome resistance. Another way is establishing and maintaining open lines of communication in order to make ideas clearly understood and to resolve disagreements quickly (Lundeen, 1992). Prepare people thoroughly for the change, provide support and patience during the change process, and encourage response and expression of feelings.

Principle of Proper Timing

Sometimes a change, even a well-designed and much needed one, should be postponed because the present is not the right time to introduce it. For example, perhaps the client system is experiencing too many other changes to handle the stress of another change. Other projects or activities in which the client system is currently engaged may compete for energy and other resources, depleting the energy and resources needed to make the proposed change successful. For example, in November some middle-aged women, eager to start a book club that focused on discussion of preparing for menopause, had to postpone the project because Christmas was approaching. Shopping, entertaining, and vacations made it impossible to give the kind of time and energy needed to make the book club effective.

Proper timing is as important to a planned change as well-timed seed planting is to a good harvest. The change idea must be appropriate, the change recipient

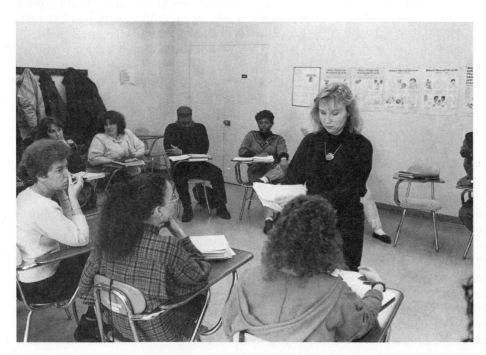

FIGURE 25.9. Collaborating with community residents in planning a change increases their receptivity.

prepared, the climate right, and the resources available before the change can be fostered to grow into full maturity and usefulness (Cobb-McMahon et al., 1984; Flynn, 1992).

Principle of Interdependence

Every system has many subsystems that are intricately related to and interdependent upon one another. A change in one part of a system affects its other parts, and a change in one system may affect other systems (Chin, 1980). A county community nursing agency made a change in its use of home health aides. Because many homebound clients needed more care than the agency staff could provide, the agency contracted with a private home-care service for extra home health aides. These paraprofessionals worked in the homes of agency clients, supplementing the care given by agency staff. The private company preferred to supervise its own aides, whereas the county agency had a policy of using community health nurses to supervise aides. The county agency was legally responsible and professionally accountable for the quality of care given to clients. The private company wanted to retain control of its workers. The matter was resolved by contracting with another private service. The change, however, had affected the roles of nurses and aides within the system as well as the relationships between the two systems.

This principle of interdependence reminds the nurse that change does not take place in a vacuum. When workers learn new health and safety practices associated with their jobs, their relationships with each other and with their bosses, their overall productivity in the organization may easily be affected. One must anticipate and prepare for the impact of the proposed change on the clients involved, other persons, departments, organizations, or even geographic areas.

Principle of Flexibility

Unexpected events can occur in every situation. This fifth principle emphasizes two points; first, the nurse needs to be able to adapt to unexpected events and make the most of them. Perseverance and flexibility are the marks of a good change manager. One community health nurse had tried unsuccessfully to contact a young mother who was reportedly abusing her two-year-old son. After several phone calls and visits to an empty house, she finally found the mother and son at home with a neighbor who insisted on staying for the entire visit. At first the nurse was irritated by the neighbor's presence and viewed it as interfering with her goal of getting to know the mother and child. Then she realized that this situation offered an opportunity to learn more about the situation through the neighbor's input and viewed it as an opportunity to influence another client as well. She asked if the neighbor had children and began to include them both in the discussion and explained what she had to offer in terms of health teaching and support. This nurse was flexible in her approach to this situation.

The second point to remember about flexibility is that a good change planner anticipates possible blocks or problems by preparing strategies and alternate plans. During step 3 of the planned change process, it is helpful to rank the alternative solutions considered. Then, if the first choice does not work out for some reason, an alternative is ready to be put into action. Flexibility involves a willingness to consider a variety of options and suggestions from many sources (Haffer, 1986).

Principle of Self-Understanding

Self-understanding is essential for an effective change agent (Hersey & Blanchard, 1988). A leader and change agent should be able to clearly define their role and learn how others define it. It is important to understand one's values and motives in relation to each change that one might ask people to make. Nurses as well should understand their personality traits and typical leadership styles to capitalize on or alter these in order to be more effective leaders and change agents. Understanding oneself is crucial to learning to make use of one's best qualities and skills to effect change.

Summary

Community health nurses, at every level of practice, must be leaders and change agents in order to influence people to adopt healthier behaviors. Formally or informally, they act as leaders to change people's health beliefs and practices and promote organized responses to community health problems. For example, they may provide leadership in initiating programs to meet the needs of at-risk populations, such as the homeless, or may lead groups, such as the elderly, toward self-empowerment.

Leadership includes three important characteristics: it is purposeful, it is interpersonal—involving interaction with others, and it is influential in that the change agent influences others toward accomplishing a goal. Several theories assist in understanding leadership. Their differing emphases include personality traits, leader behaviors, adapting leadership to the situation, differing leadership styles, attributed qualities, and charisma. Some leadership is transactional, focused more on roles, tasks, and accomplishing goals. Other leadership is transformational, emphasizing inspiring motivation and commitment in followers.

Effective leadership incorporates the functions of creative problem-solving, initiating ideas and events, taking risks, uniting people around a purpose, and facilitating movement toward the goal. Community health nurses use these leadership functions in the context of ever-widening spheres of potential influence. They inspire and motivate people to believe in themselves, develop high self-esteem, and empower themselves to solve problems and effect change.

Leadership influence depends on use of power. This power is based on ability to use information, ability to be persuasive, ability to grant rewards, and ability to enforce compliance. The sources of these abilities or power bases come from the leader's position of authority or influence, the leader's personality, the leader's ex-pertise, and effective use of opportunities. Nurses need to empower themselves and others to effect change in community health.

The purpose of leadership is to effect change which alters the equilibrium in a system and may occur gradually with time for people involved to adjust or it may occur in a drastic fashion, such as in a crisis or natural disaster. Change occurs in three stages: unfreezing when the system is ready for change, changing when the innovation is implemented, and refreezing when the change is stabilized.

Planned change is a purposeful, designed effort to effect improvement in a system with the help of a change agent. It involves a process of eight steps, similar to the nursing process, that nurses can use to create change. These steps include: assessing symptoms, diagnosing need, analyzing alternative solutions, selecting a change, planning the change, implementing the change, evaluating the change, and stabilizing the change. During planned change, the nurse can use one or a combination of three major strategies: a rational approach of providing information to influence people to change, an educative approach of combining new information with persuasion to effect change, and a coercive approach of enforcing compliance. Several important principles

Activities to Promote Critical Thinking

As a staff community health nurse, you have been asked to chair an ad hoc committee in your health department made up of interdisciplinary colleagues and community members. The committee's task is to plan a health fair for the local community.

1. As chairperson of the committee, discuss how you would exercise each of the five leadership functions as you chaired the planning committee.

2. Identify and analyze your own sources of power and bases of power. Which of these power bases and sources would you use to influence committee members and community citizens?

3. Describe your leadership style and determine whether it is appropriate for this situation and group.

4. Outline the specific planned change steps your committee would need to take to ensure a successful health fair with outcomes that promoted improved levels of community health.

5. Select one specific objective of your health fair (e.g. cholesterol screening of an at-risk aggregate with reduced cholesterol levels in a year). Does the proposed objective require an evolutionary or revolutionary change in citizens' health-related behaviors? Justify your choice of the type of change.

6. Explain the strategies you would use to effect the change.

7. Six principles for effecting positive change were presented in this chapter. Briefly discuss how you would use each one as you and your committee developed the health fair.

serve as guidelines for community health nurses to effect change. They include involving all persons affected by the change, introducing change in a timely fashion, considering the impact of the change on other systems, being flexible, and understanding oneself and one's own qualities that can be groomed to provide the most effective leadership.

REFERENCES

Adams, J. D. (Ed.). (1986). *Transforming leadership: From vision to results*. Alexandria, VA: Miles River Press.

American Hospital Association (1994). Fostering a culture of innovation. *American Hospital Association News,* Sept. 5, 6.

Bacharach, S.B. & Lawler, E.J. (1980). *Power and politics in organizations*. San Francisco: Jossey-Bass.

Bass, B. M. (1990). Transformational leadership: Beyond initiation and consideration. *Journal of Management,* December: 693–703.

Beecroft, P.C. (1993). Where are the transformational leaders? *Clinical Nurse Specialist.* 7(4), 163.

Bennis, W. G., Benne, K.D., & Chin, R. (1985). *The planning of change* (4th ed.). New York: Holt.

Bernhard, L. & Walsh, M. (1981). *Leadership—The key to the professionalization of nursing*. New York: McGraw-Hill.

Blake, R. R. & Mouton, J.S. (1964). *The Managerial Grid*. Houston: Gulf.

Burns, J. M. (1978). *Leadership*. New York: Harper.

Chait, R. (1988). What makes a leader in higher education? *Journal of Professional Nursing,* 4(3), 223–29.

Chin, R. (1980). The utility of system models and developmental models for practitioners. In J. Riehl and S. Roy (Eds.), *Conceptual models for nursing practice* (2nd ed.). New York: Appleton-Century-Crofts.

Chin, R. & Benne, D. (1985). *General strategies for effecting changes in human systems*. In W. G. Bennis, K.D. Benne, & R. Chin (Eds.), *The planning of change* (4th ed.). New York: Holt.

Clifford, J. C. (1991). The practicing nurse as leader. *American Journal of Maternal Child Nursing,* 16(1), 18–20.

Cobb-McMahon, B., Williams, D., & Davis, J. (1984). Changing health behavior of community health clients. *Journal of Community Health Nursing,* 1(1), 27–31.

Conger, J. A. & Kanungo, R.N. (1988). *Charismatic leadership*. San Francisco: Jossey-Bass.

Eng, E., et al. (1992). Community empowerment: The critical base for primary health care (review). *Family and Community Health,* April, 15(1), 1–12.

Flynn, B.C. (1992). Healthy cities: A model of community change. *Family and Community Health,* 15(1), 13–23.

Flynn, B., et al. (1987). Preparation of community health nursing leaders for social action. International Journal of *Nursing Studies,* 24(3), 239–48.

French, J., Jr. & Raven, B. (1959). The bases of social power. In D. Cartwright (Ed.), *Studies in Social Power.* Ann Arbor: University of Michigan, Institute for Social Research.

Fritz, R. (1986). The leader as creator. In J. D. Adams (Ed.), *Transforming leadership*. Alexandria, VA: Miles River Press.

Geier, J. G. (1967). A trait approach to the study of leadership in small groups. *Journal of Communication,* Dec., 316–323.

Gerlach, L. & Hine, V. (1973). *Lifeway leap: The dynamics of change in America*. Minneapolis: University of Minnesota Press.

Gorman, S., et al. (1986). Power and effective nursing practice. *Nursing Outlook,* 34(3), 129–34.

Guidera, M., et al. (1988). Working with people: In defense of followership. *American Journal of Nursing,* 88(7), 1017.

Haffer, A. (1986). Facilitating change: Choosing the appropriate strategy. *Journal of Nursing Administration,* 16(4), 18–22.

Hagberg, J. O. (1994). *Real Power*. Salem, WI: Sheffield Publications.

Harman, W. (1986). Transformed leadership: Two contrasting concepts. In J.D. Adams (Ed.), *Transforming leadership*. Alexandria, VA: Miles River Press.

Hennes, K., Sr. (1979). *Expansion of the aide's role in home care*. Unpublished manuscript. University of Minnesota, Minneapolis.

Henry, B. & Le Clair, H. (1987). Language, leadership, and power: Research-based theories of language in organizations. *Journal of Nursing Administration,* 17(1), 19–25.

Hersey, P. & Blanchard, K. (1988). *Management of organizational behavior: Utilizing human resources* (5th ed.). Englewood Cliffs, NJ: Prentice-Hall.

Hollander, E. P. & Offermann, L.R. (1990). Power and leadership in organizations. *American Psychologist,* Feb., 179–189.

Josten, L. E. (1989). Wanted: Leaders for public health. *Nursing Outlook,* 37(5), 230–232.

Kanter, R. M. (1985). *The change masters*. New York: Simon and Schuster.

Kelley, R. E. (1988). In praise of followers. *Harvard Business Review,* Nov–Dec, 142–148.

Kinsman, F. (1986). Leadership from alongside. In J. D. Adams (Ed.), *Transforming leadership*. Alexandria, VA: Miles River Press.

Kirkpatrick, S. A. & Locke, E.A. (1991). Leadership: Do traits matter? *Academy of Management Executive,* May, 48–60.

Kouzes, J. & Posner, B. (1987). *The leadership challenge: How to get extraordinary things done in organizations*. San Francisco: Jossey-Bass

Kreisberg, S. (1992). *Transforming power, domination, empowerment and education*. New York: State University of New York Press.

Krichbaum, K. (1993). Empowering nursing students for leadership. *University of Minnesota Health Sciences Learning Resources Journal,* April, 11–14.

Lee, J. L. (1987). Leadership in practice. *Imprint* 34(6), 57–58, 61.

Lewin, K. (1947). Frontiers in group dynamics: Concept, method, and reality in social science; social equilibria and social change. *Human Relations,* 1, 5.

Lippitt, G. L. (1973). *Visualizing change: Model building and the change process*. La Jolla, CA: University Associates.

Lippitt, R., Watson, J., & Westley, B. (1958). *The dynamics of planned change*. New York: Harcourt.

Lundeen, S. P. (1992). Leadership strategies for organizational change: Applications in community nursing centers. *Nursing Administration Quarterly,* 17(1), 60–68.

McPherson, W. (1991). Leadership is about change. *Nursing Standard,* 5(36), 51.

Moloney, M. (1979). *Leadership in nursing: Theory, strategies, action*. St. Louis: C. V. Mosby.

Nicoll, D. (1986). Leadership and followership. In J. D. Adams (Ed.), *Transforming leadership*. Alexandria, VA: Miles River Press.

Noone, J. (1987). Planned change: Putting theory into practice . . . Utilizing Lippitt's theory. *Clinical Nurse Specialist 1*(1), 25–29.

Nordstrom, R., et al. (1987). Cultural change versus behavioral change. *Health Care Management Review, 12*(2), 43–49.

Porter, E. J. (1987). Administrative diagnosis—Implications for the public's health. *Public Health Nursing, 4*(4), 247–56.

Porter-O'Grady, T. (1992). Transformational leadership in an age of chaos. *Nursing Administration Quarterly, 17*(1), 17–24.

Rantz, M., et al. (1987). Change theory: A framework for implementing nursing diagnoses in a long-term-care setting. *Nursing Clinics of North America, 22*(4), 887–97.

Reed, J. F. (1992). Situational leadership. *Nursing Management,* (Long term care edition) 23(1), 63–64.

Robbins, S. P. (1993). *Organizational Behavior* (6th ed.). Englewood Cliffs, NJ: Prentice-Hall.

Ryan, P. (1987). Strategies for motivating life-style change. *Journal of Cardiovascular Nursing, 1*(4), 54–66.

Salmon, M. (1993). An open letter to public health nurses (editorial). *Public Health Nursing, 10*(4), 211–212.

Spradley, B. (1980). Managing change creatively. *Journal of Nursing Administration, 10*(5), 32–37.

Spradley, J. & McCurdy, D. (1994). *Conformity and conflict: Readings in cultural anthropology* (8th ed.). New York: Harper Collins.

Tannenbaum, R. & Schmidt, W.H. (1973). How to choose a leadership pattern. *Harvard Business Review,* May/June.

Terry, R. (1993). *Authentic leadership: Courage in Action*. San Francisco: Jossey-Bass.

UNICEF (1995). *The state of the world's children, 1995*. New York: Oxford.

Williams, C. A. (1981). Nursing leadership in community health: A neglected issue. In J. McCloskey & H. Grace (Eds.), *Current issues in nursing*. Boston: Blackwell Scientific Publications.

World Health Organization (1994). Population and health. *World Health, 47*(3), 3–31.

Zerwekh, J. V. (1992). The practice of empowerment and coercion by expert public health nurses. *Image: Journal of Nursing Scholarship, Summer,* 24(2), 101–105.

SELECTED READINGS

Andrews, M. (1993). Importance of nursing leadership in implementing change *British Journal of Nursing, 2*(8), 437–439.

Archer, S. E., Kelly, C.D., & Bisch, S.A. (1984). *Implementing change in communities: A collaborative process*. St. Louis, C. V. Mosby.

Barker, A. (1992). *Transformational nursing leadership: A vision for the future*. New York: National League for Nursing.

Bass, B. M. & Stogdill, R.M. (1990). *Bass and Stogdill's Handbook of leadership: Theory, research, and managerial applications* (3rd. ed.). New York: Free Press.

Bobo, K.A., Kendall, J., & Max, S. (1991). *Organizing for social change*. Cabin John, MD: Seven Locks.

Brown, B.J. (1990). Leadership and followership. *Florida Nurse, 38*(10), 11.

Eng, E. and R. Young. (1992). Lay health advisors as community change agents. *Family and Community Health, 15*(1), 24–40.

Farley, S. (1993). The community as partner in primary health care. *Nursing and Health Care, 14*(5), 244–249.

Flynn, B., et al. (1987). Preparation of community health nursing leaders for social action. *International Journal of Nursing Studies, 24*(3), 239–48.

Gibson, C.H. (1991). A concept analysis of empowerment. *Journal of Advanced Nursing, 16*(3), 354–61.

Hempstead, N. (1992). Nurse management and leadership today. *Nursing Standard, 6*(33), 37–39.

Horsley, J. A. (1986). Factors associated with innovation in nursing practice. *Family and Community Health, 9*(1), 1–11.

Jenkins, H. M. (1989). Ethical dimensions of leadership in community health nursing. *Journal of Community Health Nursing, 6*(2), 103–112.

Jones, M.E. & Clark, D.W. (1990). Nurse practitioners develop leadership in community problem solving. *Journal of the Academy of Nurse Practitioners, 2*(4), 160–163.

Krackhardt, D. (1990). Assessing the political landscape: Structure, cognition, and power in organizations. *Administrative Science Quarterly,* June, 342–369.

Manfredi, C. & Valiga, T. (1990). How are we preparing nurse leaders? *Journal of Nursing Education, 29*(1), 4–9.

Marriner-Tomey, A. (1992). *Transformational leadership in nursing*. St. Louis: Mosby Year Book.

Mechanic, D. (1990). Nursing leadership: Global strategies. *Improving health status through health policy: An agenda for nursing leaders*. (National League for Nursing Publication, #41-2349), 181–188.

Milio, N. (1989). Developing nursing leadership in health policy. *Journal of Professional Nursing, 5*(6), 315–321.

Milio, N. (1991). Information technology and community health—invitation to innovation. *Journal of Professional Nursing, 7*(3), 146.

Morgan, M. (1988). Nursing leaders: adapting to change. *World Health,* April, 24–26.

Nazarey, P. (1993). The spirit of nurse empowerment: a leader's responsibility. *Emphasis: Nursing, 4*(2), 7–12.

Olson, J. K., et al. (1988). Learning planned change: A practicum for RN students. *Journal of Nursing Education, 27*(4), 178–80.

Ryan, S. A. (1990). A new decade of leadership: From vision to reality. *Nursing Clinics of North America, 25*(3), 597–604.

Siler, P. (1993). The leadership of change: a kaleidoscope of opportunity. *Emphasis: Nursing* 4(2), 1–2.

Smith, G. R. (1989). Using the public agenda to shape public health nursing practice. *Nursing Outlook, 37*(2), 72–75.

Spickerman, S., et al. (1988). Use of learning modules to teach nursing leadership concepts. *Journal of Nursing Education, 27*(2), 78–82.

Stevens, P. & Hall, J. (1992). Applying critical theories to nursing in communities. *Public Health Nursing, 9*(1), 2–9.

West, M. (1989). Innovation in health visiting. *Health Visitor, 62,* 46–48.

26

Research In Community Health Nursing

LEARNING OBJECTIVES

Upon completion of this chapter readers should be able to:

- Explain the difference between quantitative research and qualitative research.
- Describe the eight steps of the research process.
- Differentiate between experimental and nonexperimental research design.
- Analyze the potential impact of research on community health nursing practice.
- Identify the community health nurse's role in conducting research and using research findings.

KEY TERMS

- Conceptual model
- Control group
- Descriptive statistics
- Experimental design
- Experimental group
- Generalizability
- Inferential statistics
- Instrument

- Nonexperimental design
- Randomization
- Qualitative research
- Quantitative research
- Reliability
- Research
- Validity

Barbara Walton Spradley and Judith Ann Allender
COMMUNITY HEALTH NURSING: CONCEPTS AND PRACTICE, 4th ed.
© 1996 Barbara Walton Spradley and Judith Ann Allender

Research is the systematic collection and analysis of data related to a particular problem or phenomenon. If research is properly conducted and analyzed, it has the potential to yield valuable information that can affect the health of large groups of people and often serves as the basis for changing health care policies and programs.

The potential for **generalizability**, the ability to apply the research results to other similar populations, has great value to health profesionals. It allows researchers to test their hypotheses on smaller groups before instituting widespread changes in methods, programs, and even national health policies. In the current national atmosphere of economic crisis and spiralling health care costs, the importance of valuable research which can accurately predict how health care dollars can best be spent to benefit the greatest number of people cannot be overemphasized.

This chapter examines research as it relates to community health and nursing. It discusses the differences between quantitative and qualitative research and then describes the eight steps in the research process. Specific research in community health nursing is examined and the nurse's role with respect to research in community health is discussed.

Quantitative and Qualitative Research

Scientific inquiry through research is generally pursued by means of two different approaches: quantitative research and qualitative research. **Quantitative research** collects data on things that can be quantified or measured objectively. An example is a study that measured fecal contamination in a child day care center by taking a series of microbial samples from the play/sleep area, the diaper changing area, and from caregivers and childrens' hands (Holaday, et al., 1995). The investigators compared the influence of using cloth diapers versus paper diapers on the amount of fecal contamination and found no significant differences in type of diaper used but did learn useful information for preventing contamination. Quantitative studies tend to examine isolated parts of problems or phenomena and thus do not generally pay attention to the larger context or overall health of individuals. This research approach involves a reductionistic tendency (focusing on the parts rather

than the whole) and if used exclusively can limit nursing knowlege since many of the important aspects of client services such as quality of life, grieving, and spirituality cannot be measured objectively. (See Fig. 26.1).

A more subjective or qualitative approach is also needed in order to study areas that need a broader focus or that do not lend themselves to objective measurement. **Qualitative research** emphasizes subjectivity and the meaning of experiences to individuals. An example of this type of research is a study that surveyed 53 homeless families' in three shelters to determine what they perceived as barriers to receiving well child care (Riemer, et al., 1995). The four barriers identified by the homeless families were problems with selecting providers, waiting to get appointments, waiting during appointments, and high transportation and parking costs. Qualitative research involves a more holistic approach to understanding a problem or phenomenon and studies the context of events enabling investigators to examine people's experiences and perceptions (Brockopp & Hastings-Tolsma, 1994).

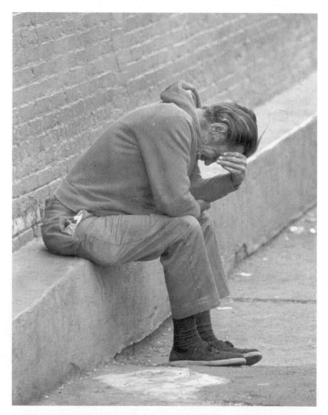

FIGURE 26.1. It is rarely possible to objectively measure the impact of factors, such as grief, on overall health.

Qualitative research methods can be as rigorous and systematic as quantitative research methods, although the design and purpose of the approaches differ. The choice of one approach over the other is largely determined by the nature of the phenomenon to be examined.

Steps in the Research Process

All effective research follows a series of pre-determined, highly specific steps. Each step builds on the next and provides the foundation for the eventual discussion of findings. Alone or in collaboration with others, investigators use the following eight steps to complete a research project: identify an area of interest, formulate a research question/statement, review the literature, select a conceptual model, choose a research design, collect and analyze data, interpret results, and communicate findings. While the process remains the same for any nurse conducting research, the area of interest may vary depending on specialty.

IDENTIFY AN AREA OF INTEREST

Identifying the specific problem or area of interest is frequently one of the most difficult tasks in the research process. When identifying a problem or interest area the nurse must be certain that the problem or interest is not too broad, that one has the resources and opportunity to study it, and that the area has relevance to community health nursing practice.

The problem needs to be specific enough to direct the formulation of a research question (specificity). For example, concern about quality of services for the mentally ill is too broad a problem, instead, one might focus on availability of health services for the homeless mentally ill.

Whether or not the area of interest can be examined given available resources should be addressed (feasibility). For example a state-wide study of the needs of pregnant adolescents might not be practical if time or funding is limited, but to study the same group in a given school district could be feasible.

The meaning of the project and its relevance to nursing must also be considered, such as exploring the implications for nursing practice in the pregnant adolescents study. Areas for study often evolve from personal interests, clinical experience, or philosophical beliefs. The nurse's specialty influences the selection of a problem for study and also the particular perspective used. The community health nurse functions within a context that emphasizes disease prevention, wellness, and the active involvement of clients in the service they receive. Clients' physical and social environments, as well as their biopsychosocial and spiritual domains, are of major concern. Community health nurses think in terms of the broader community and therefore their research efforts are developed with the needs of the community or specific populations in mind.

Problems recently identified and studied within community health nursing include the high incidence of drug abuse among children (Hahn, 1995), nurses' negative attitudes toward individuals diagnosed with the human immunodeficiency virus (HIV) (Tessaro & Highriter, 1994), the increasing number of women diagnosed with breast cancer (Wruble, et al., 1994), and the stress associated with providing care for an elderly family member (Theis, et al., 1994). Each of these problem areas provide direction for the formulation of related research questions. See the discussion on Research Priorities.

FORMULATE A RESEARCH QUESTION/STATEMENT

The research question or statement reflects the kind of information desired and provides a foundation for the remainder of the project. How the question or statement is phrased suggests the research design for the project. For example, the question, "What are nurses' attitudes toward patients diagnosed with HIV?" determines that the design will be a simple, non-experimental, exploratory one. Whereas, the question, "What is the effect of an educational program on nurses' attitudes toward individuals diagnosed with HIV?" suggests an experiment that will evaluate an intervention designed to influence nurses' attitudes.

Well formulated research questions identify (1) the population of interest, (2) the variable or variables to be measured and, (3) the interventions (if being used). It is extremely important when formulating research questions that specific terms are used to clearly represent the variables being studied. For example, if stress is identified as the variable measured in the research question, the investigator must focus only on the "stress" experienced by clients and must be careful not to measure

Issues in Community Health Nursing
RESEARCH PRIORITIES

Although topics abound that need to be studied through research, it is important for community health nurses to consider which topics are of highest priority. Meisner, Watkins, and Ossege (1994) addressed this issue by determining what practicing public health nurses perceived as important research questions and priorities, and also assessed whether the respondents believed that the profession should provide leadership in addressing these questions. The study was conducted using a two-round modified Delphi survey. In the first round public health nurses were asked an open-ended question—to identify research priorities. Respondents (290) identified 657 priorities which were reviewed by an expert panel, narrowed to categorical clusters, and condensed to 78 items. Respondents (347) prioritized these items in round two.

Results showed 76 ranked research priorities that fell into three categories: outcomes in maternal-child and family planning, outcomes in home health services, and public health nurse recruitment, retention, job satisfaction, and image. These results were consistent with the health objectives for the nation for the year 2000.

other related variables such as anxiety or depression. Consistency of terms used is crucial to the success of a project, so investigators must formulate the research question carefully. Good examples of research questions addressed recently by community health nurses include:

- "What is the scope of education (variable) provided for secondary school teachers (population of interest) regarding HIV?" (Gingess & Basen-Engquist, 1994);
- "What health care services (variables) are provided to children and adolescents in schools (population of interest)?" (Hacker, et al., 1994);
- "Will education about the advantages of prenatal care (intervention) influence community leaders (population of interest) to gain understanding and positive attitudes (variables) about promoting prenatal care for low income women?" (Kozlowski & Zotti, 1994); and

- "What are the dietary preferences (variables) of students in grades 5, 8 and 11 (population of interest)?" (Murphy et al., 1994).

REVIEW THE LITERATURE

There are two phases to a review of the literature. The first phase consists of a cursory examination of available publications related to the area of interest. While there are several nursing research journals that publish studies reflecting all areas of nursing practice, most specialty areas have journals dedicated to specific interests. *Public Health Nursing*, *Family and Community Health*, *Journal of Community Health Nursing*, and *Journal of School Health* are some of the journals that carry publications of interest to community health nurses. In this phase the investigator develops a somewhat superficial but sufficient knowledge about the area of interest to make a decision about the value of pursuing a given topic. If considerable research has been conducted in the area, the investigator may decide to ask a different question or to pursue another area of interest.

The second phase of the literature review involves an in-depth, critically evaluated search of all publications relevant to the topic of interest. Journal articles describing research conducted on the topic of interest provide the most important kind of information followed by clinical opinion articles (information on the topic described by experts in the field) and books. Journal articles provide more updated information than books and systematic investigations provide a foundation for another study.

Criteria for compiling a good review of the literature include: (1) articles that closely relate to the topic of interest (relevancy); (2) current articles which provide updated and recent information (usually within the past five years). Those written prior to the five year period are included based on their importance to the area of interest; and (3) inclusion of primary and secondary sources. A primary source is a publication which appears in its original form. A secondary source is an article in which one author writes about another author's work. Primary sources are preferred over secondary sources because the information can be reviewed in its original form and it provides the investigator with a more accurate and first-hand account of the study. For example, Anderson (1995) describes childhood sexually transmitted diseases (STDs) as the result of sexual abuse, citing many other studies including one by Strader and Beaman (1992) on STD counselors promotion of condom use. The Anderson article is important and useful for understanding childhood STDs but it becomes a secondary source for knowing about the results of the condom study. Direct reading of the Strader and Beaman report would provide a primary source for information gained from that research (see Fig. 26.2).

A major component of a review of literature is the investigator's critical evaluation of information collected. The conceptual base and research methods of studies must be critically assessed regarding the appropriateness of the methods used and the conclusions drawn, as well as how carefully the research was conducted. Examining the primary literature source assists this process. For nurses unskilled in this type of assessment, consultation with an experienced researcher can be helpful.

Following a careful and comprehensive review of the literature, the investigator writes a clear description of the information related to the area of interest. Conflict-

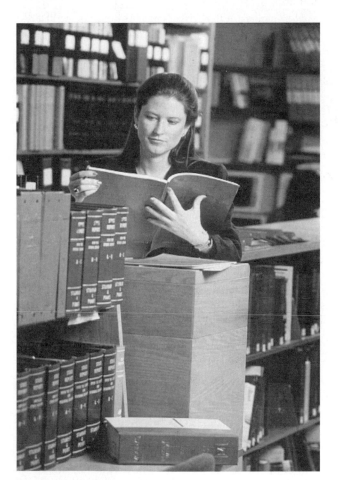

FIGURE 26.2. Primary sources are preferred for literature review prior to formulating a research proposal.

ing findings are included and each study/article is referenced. This review provides the basis for the proposed study.

SELECT A CONCEPTUAL MODEL

In relation to research, a **conceptual model** is a framework made up of ideas for explaining and studying a phenomenon of interest. A conceptual model conveys a particular perception of the world; it organizes one's thinking and provides structure and direction for research activities.

All fields of study, whether they be nursing, psychology, sociology, or physics, specify the major concerns and boundaries for their activities. Nursing is concerned with the interaction between humans and the environment in relation to health (Meleis, 1991). Nursing conceptual models such as Orem's (1985) self-care model or King's (1989) open systems model reflect the boundaries and major concerns of nursing as a profession. While nurse investigators frequently and successfully use conceptual models developed within other fields, the advantage of using nursing models is that they provide an understanding of the world in terms of nursing's major concerns.

The investigator can become familiar with various conceptual models by reviewing the literature in their area of interest as well as by reading any of the many texts available on conceptual models. A thorough understanding of the major concepts of a potential model and their relationships is necessary before attempting to use a model as a framework for a study. For example, Quinn and Strelkauskas (1993) studied the effects of therapeutic touch on the immune system of recently bereaved individuals using Rogers' theory of unitary human beings (1990). Rogers' theory supports the notion that an energy transfer is possible between practitioner and recipient and thus provides a foundation for an examination of therapeutic touch. Another group of investigators could study therapeutic touch from a caring perspective and use a model of caring to provide a foundation for a study.

CHOOSE A RESEARCH DESIGN

The design of a research project represents the overall plan for carrying out the study. This overall plan guides the conduct of the study and, depending on its effectiveness, can influence investigators' confidence in their results. A major consideration in selecting a particular design is to try to control as much as possible those factors that are not included in the study but can influence the results. For example, Yu (1995) studied 350 elderly persons living at home to determine their level of functioning for independent living (FIL). As a part of this study design it was important to thoroughly train the interviewers so that data collection would be done in a consistent and reliable manner. Although the interviewers were not a part of the study, a failure to control the quality of their interviewing would have skewed the results.

Complete descriptions of various research designs, specific methodologies, and sample selection are available in basic nursing research texts. For the purposes of this chapter, a few important considerations underlying design selection are described. It is important to understand that there are two major categories of research design within quantitative approaches to research: experimental and non-experimental, or descriptive. **Experimental design** requires that the investigators institute an intervention or change and then measure the consequences of the intervention. Investigators hypothesize that a change will occur based on their intervention and then they attempt to test whether or not their hypothesis was accurate. Experimental design also requires investigators to randomly assign subjects to an **experimental group** (those receiving the intervention) and a **control group** (those not receiving the intervention). This process of random assignment of subjects to a study group is called **randomization** which is the systematic selection of research subjects so that each one has an equal probability of selection. For example, Kendrick, et al., (1995) conducted a demonstration project to promote smoking cessation among pregnant women receiving prenatal services in public clinics in three different states. Selection of subjects was done through clinics being randomly assigned to intervention or control status. Interventions were integrated into routine prenatal care and included providing information on the effects of smoking on the fetus, the benefits of quitting, techniques for quitting, developing support, and preventing relapse. Intervention (experimental) clinics showed a higher quitting rate than control clinics. Less stringent research designs do not require randomization in either sample selection or assignment.

Another important distinction exists within the experimental category of research. There are true experiments and quasi-experiments. The true experiment is characterized by instituting an intervention or change, assigning subjects to groups in a specific manner (ran-

domization), and by comparing one group of subjects who experience the manipulation to another group that does not (control group). The quasi-experimental design lacks either the randomization of subjects or the formation of a control group. An example is the quasi-experimental study conducted by Kozlowski and Zotti (1994) to educate and influence community leaders to promote prenatal care for low income women. The community leaders were the experimental group under study and since there was no control group, the effect of the educational intervention was measured with a pre- and post-test. Study results showed a signficant increase in community leaders' knowledge, positive beliefs, and stated intents to promote prenatal care for low income women. Community health nurses conduct quasi-experiments more often than true experiments because it is often difficult (sometimes impossible) to provide a treatment for only one-half of a group and/or to randomize subjects.

Non-experimental (descriptive) designs are used in research to describe and explain phenomena or examine relationships among phenomena. Examples of this approach could include examining the relationship between sex and smoking behaviors among adolescents, describing the emotional needs of families of clients with AIDS, or determining the attitudes of parents in a given community toward sex education in the schools. In each of these instances the focus of the research would be on the relationships observed or the description of what exists.

These non-experimental designs are often the precursors of experiments. For example, Sorensen (1994) compared the daily stressors and coping responses of 21 rural children and 23 suburban children by having them keep semistructured diaries over a period of six weeks. The children reported stress coming from external sources such as home or school demands and interruptions affecting their choices and control over their lives. They reported internal stressors such as personal fears or disappointments or lack of achievement. Interpersonal stressors focused on relationships with family and friends. Coping resources included enjoying favorite school subjects (art, music, math, science), release from chores/demands, freedom to choose activities, organized group activities, sports, pets, new purchases, and support from family and friends. (See Fig. 26.3). There were many individual variations among the children suggesting the need for individual appraisal and futher study of stress-coping phenomena. Other investigators could use these findings to devise

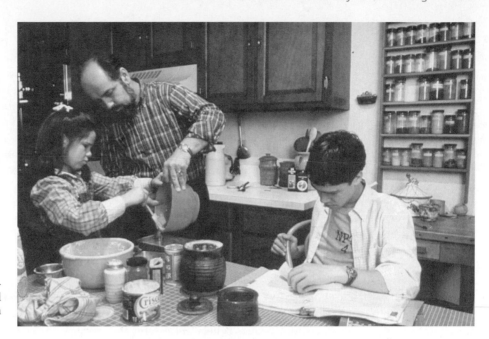

FIGURE 26.3. Shared family activities and interest in school subjects help children cope with stressors.

interventions (and test them using an experiment or a quasi-experiment) that would promote childrens' effective coping with stress into adulthood.

The choice of research design influences the generalizability of the results and the attention given to the details of the study affects the value of the knowledge derived.

COLLECT AND ANALYZE DATA

The value of the data collected in any research project largely depends on the care taken when measuring the concepts of concern or variables. The specific tool, often a questionnaire or interview guide, used to measure the variables in a study is called an **instrument**. The accuracy of the instrument used and the appropriateness of the choice of instruments can clearly influence the results.

To evaluate instrument accuracy, two tests are used: validity and reliability. **Validity** is the assurance that an instrument measures the variables it is supposed to measure. If a written questionnaire is the instrument being used in the study, questions included on the questionnaire would be evaluated to make certain they are appropriate to that subject (content validity) and whether the variable of interest is actually being measured (construct validity). For example, Yu, in studying

elderly persons' level of functioning for independent living (FIL), developed a questionnaire which was a modification of a previously published assessment scale. This instrument was tested for validity by an extensive literature review, the researcher's own previous experiences, and the opinions of five nursing and medical experts in geratrics, rehabilitation, gerontology, and community health who reviewed the instrument. Questions in this instrument explored personal factors (such as sex, age, religion, marital status, health insurance), physical health status (such as self-rated health, physical activity, chronic disease), and family and social factors (such as socioeconomic status, family type, caregiver present) to provide an overall FIL score for each subject. An example of an appropriate question was, "Would you rate your physical activity as 'relatively good,' 'fairly good,' 'fairly poor' (relatively immobile), or 'relatively poor' (bedridden)?" (1995) Without the addition of the clarifying descriptors placed in parentheses in the last two choices, respondents might have misinterpreted the meaning of 'fairly poor' and 'relatively poor' thus providing inaccurate data.

Reliability is how consistently an instrument measures a given research variable within a particular population. Test-retest reliability insures that similar results are obtained by the same instrument in the same population on two separate testings. If similar results are obtained on two separate occasions, the test can be considered reliable. A questionnaire is internally consistent to the extent that all of its subparts measure the same characteristic. In Yu's study, test-retest reliability was done by administering the questionnaire twice (with a four-week interval between testings) to 20 elderly persons living at home who were not study subjects. Their responses were similar enough each time to indicate a high internal consistency in the wording of the questionnaire. Statistical tests and measurements are often used to analyze subjects' responses to questionnaires in order to evaluate internal consistency.

Unfortunately, within the area of community health nursing research, instruments appropriate to the measurement of nursing concepts are often not available. Dawkins, et al. (1988) examined health orientations, beliefs, and use of health services among minority, high-risk, expectant mothers. They developed their own instruments and pretested them in a pilot study. DeVon and Powers (1984) examined the health beliefs and psychosocial adjustment to illness among clients with hypertension. They used questionnaires to measure compliance and psychosocial adjustment to illness that had been designed and tested by other investigators. Both approaches to measuring the variables of interest are acceptable; however, using available instruments of known reliability and validity saves considerable time.

A variety of methods can be used to collect data. They include *self-report* (subjects report their own experience verbally or in written form), *observation* (investigators observe subjects and document their observations), *physiological assessment* (measures of physical evidence such as blood pressure, impaired mobility, etc.), and *document analyses* (review and analysis of written materials such as health records). For example, using the four methods mentioned above, investigators examining the stress level of the caregiver when a family member chooses to die at home might: (1) design or use an existing written questionnaire or interview schedule (self-report); (2) outline a schema (such as a list of potential stress-induced behaviors) for observing caregivers as they function in the home (observation); (3) measure various physiological indicators of stress such as hypertension, insomnia, poor diet (physiological assessment); or (4) ask caregivers to keep a diary of their activities and feelings for two weeks then analyze the diaries for evidence of stress (document analysis). In most instances the nature of the data to be collected

dictates the best method of collection. One or more methods may be appropriate, given the topic of concern. In the example above, a combination of the first three would probably be appropriate or substitute the diary keeping for the questionnaire. In Yu's study, the elderly living at home were assessed using the first two methods, self-report and observation.

Once collected, data must be analyzed so that a meaningful interpretation can be made. Statistical procedures simply reduce great amounts of information to smaller chunks that can be easily interpreted. When deciding on an appropriate statistical procedure, it is helpful to consider the two major categories of statistical analysis: descriptive and inferential statistics.

Descriptive statistics describe in quantitative or mathematical terms the data collected. Commonly used descriptive statistics include calculating the average number or mean of a particular set of occurrences or calculating standard deviations (how much each score on the average deviates from the mean) and percentages. For example, an investigator analyzing data collected from 50 chronic pain clients might find their mean pain score to be 4.6 (scale used 0 = no pain, 10 = worst pain) with a standard deviation of 0.1. These descriptive statistics suggest that clients are grouped around the middle of the pain scale and differ very little in the amount of pain they experience. The investigator may also report that 40% of the female clients experience pain between 5 and 6 on the 10-point pain scale. These descriptive statistics can be reported graphically (using graphs or charts) or in written form.

Inferential statistics are statistical procedures which enable one to determine the extent to which changes or differences between sets of data are attributable to chance fluctuations and to estimate the confidence with which one can make generalizations about the data (Brockopp & Hastings-Tolsma, 1994). There are many inferential statistical techniques that vary considerably in their complexity; however, the goal of each technique is the same. Using inferential statistics enables one to determine as precisely as possible the probability of an occurrence. Investigators analyze their data to establish the likelihood that differences in the groups under study are the result of chance as opposed to the manipulation of variables. Because errors occur whenever one attempts to infer characteristics from a small group to the larger population, there is always some likelihood that the differences between groups could be the result of chance.

It is often appropriate to use both descriptive and inferential statistics to analyze the data from a study. For example, in a study designed to examine the effects of prenatal education on the health status of pregnant women, investigators might, using inferential statistics, find a significant difference in health status between the group who experienced the educational program (experimental group) and the group who did not (control group). The investigators might also use descriptive statistics to report the percent of women from the experimental group who attended all classes and the means and standard deviations for the women's health status scores. See the discussion on research in developing countries below.

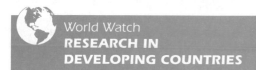

World Watch
RESEARCH IN DEVELOPING COUNTRIES

Community health nursing research at the international level is needed on numerous topics. As nurses are involved in establishing health programs in developing countries, research is needed to document their effectivness, enabling others to learn from this information and replicate similar programs in other areas. Research is needed to identify preventive dietary interventions in undernourished populations and to institute nutritional education programs. Women and children are particularly vulnerable in developing countries due to abuse and violence, low status, poor nutrition, and limited access to health care (UNICEF, 1995). Research is needed to address their needs and improve their health status (Carty, 1991). Communicable diseases, including AIDS, tuberculosis, and typhoid, are rampant in developing countries and challenge nurses to join forces with other public health professionals to study their spread and develop interventions.

Opportunities for community health nurses to serve in developing countries abound. Organizations such as Project Hope and the Peace Corps plus many others provide a means for nurses to make a contribution to the developing world. The challenge lies in capitalizing on these opportunities to also conduct research that will expand knowledge and improve practice.

INTERPRET RESULTS

The explanation of the findings of a study flows from the previously formulated research plan. Findings need to make sense in relation to the identified conceptual framework, research question, literature review, and methodology. When findings support the directions developed in the research plan, their interpretation is relatively straightforward. For example, a group of community health nurse investigators might design a study to determine the effect of parenting classes on the self-esteem of single welfare mothers between the ages of 21 and 35. They could use Coopersmith's (1967) ideas on self-esteem as their conceptual model, hypothesize that self-esteem will improve as a result of the classes, and design an experiment to test their idea. If self-esteem does in fact increase, their finding flows logically from their framework.

If the findings do not support the hypothesis of the study, investigators question various aspects of the research in order to develop an explanation. In this instance a number of questions could be posed. Coopersmith related feelings of success in an endeavor to assess self-esteem. Can that position be inaccurate? Could the parenting classes have been ineffective? Perhaps they did not enhance feelings of success. Were there problems with the methodology used—perhaps too few subjects, or intervening occurrences that affected the results? All of these questions and more could be considered in an attempt to explain the results.

If the study is descriptive in nature, i.e., one that was designed to describe particular characteristics of a population, the direction of the findings is not a concern. A detailed, accurate report of the results and their implications is appropriate. Given either an experimental or descriptive design, the importance of accuracy cannot be overemphasized. Leaps of faith when reporting the results of a study are not desirable unless labeled as such. One could not conclude, for example, from the study on the parenting classes that these classes develop expert parenting skills, given that parenting skills were not assessed.

A valuable contribution can be made to the advancement of nursing knowledge when investigators use their results to make suggestions for future research. The investigators' knowledge of a particular area and their experience in conducting a specific study give them an excellent background for identifying future research possibilities.

COMMUNICATE FINDINGS

The findings of nursing research projects need to be shared with other nurses regardless of the study's outcome. Findings contrary to the researcher's expectation are a valuable contribution to other researchers and consumers of research. Negative as well as positive findings can make a valuable contribution to nursing knowledge and influence nursing practice.

The research report itself should include the key elements of the research process. The research problem, methodology used, results of the study, and the investigators' conclusions and recommendations are presented. Whether investigators are presenting their findings verbally or writing for publication, they need to discuss the implications of their findings for nursing practice.

Impact of Research on Community Health and Nursing Practice

Research has the potential to have a significant impact on community health nursing in three ways: (1) on public policy and the community's health, (2) on the effectiveness of community health nursing practice, and (3) on the status and influence of nursing as a profession. Community health nurses have been involved in research addressing all three of these dimensions.

PUBLIC POLICY AND COMMUNITY HEALTH

Research with policy implications for addressing the health needs of aggregates has been conducted on numerous topics. See one example below. Many studies done by nurses and others examine issues related to prevention, lifestyle change, quality of life, and health needs of specific at-risk populations. (BABESworld, 1990; Theis, et al., 1994; Sorensen, 1994; Wruble, Alkobi-Kedushim & Musgrave, 1994). The results of these studies can influence public policy, the quality of services, and, in turn, the public's health. For example, Yu's study examined elderly persons' ability to function independently in the community. Analysis of interviews with 350 elderly people living at home revealed that five variables were significant in preserving their ability to

Research in Community Health Nursing
PORNOGRAPHY AND ABUSE OF WOMEN

Cramer, E. & McFarlane, J. (1994). Pornography and abuse of women. *Public Health Nursing, 11*(4), 268–272.

The investigators in this study were concerned that there might be an association between male pornographic use and the physical abuse of women. To address this question, they did a review of the literature learning that abuse of women was widespread and that recent research showed a relationship between male use of pornography and battering of women. They designed a nonexperimental study in which a sample of 87 battered women who were filing charges against their male partners were surveyed. The battered women were interviewed in a private location using a 24-item questionnaire developed by the investigator. An example of a question was: "Does your partner use magazines or films or videos that contain sexual violence such as naked women being beaten or girls being raped?" (p. 270). Study results showed that 40% of the subjects' male partners used one or more pornographic materials and that there was a significantly high association between male use of such materials and women being physically abused including being forced to participate in violent sexual acts. This research has strong policy implications. By disseminating these research findings and recommendations, policy makers and society at large can be made aware of the degrading view of women and children and promotion of violence that pornography perpetuates. Such awareness can lead to tighter restrictions and legal bans against violence-promoting materials. Futhermore, the investigators proposed specific nursing actions to take, such as routine assessment of all women for abuse including questions about pornography use, providing information about pornography in high school health classes, developing public awareness, and promoting actions against its use as a societal threat.

live independently: physical activity, chronic diseases, health care needs, age, and family care provider. The findings from this research support the fact that greater physical activity, appropriate health care, and family support are needed to promote elderly person's independence in the community. Clearly there are implications for health policy and nursing practice. Since the number and proportion of the elderly in all countries is expected to increase, the significance, both in terms of quality of life for the elderly as well as cost-savings in health services, of promoting elders' independence cannot be overemphasized. Actions to be taken should include early and regular assessment of elderly persons to prevent or institute early treatment of chronic and disabling conditions, improved access of health services, promotion of elders' physical and social activities, and support programs for family caregivers.

COMMUNITY HEALTH NURSING PRACTICE

A primary purpose for conducting community health research is to gain new knowledge that will improve health services and promote the public's health. Consequently most nursing research has implications for nursing practice. Many studies focus on a specific health need or population at-risk and then suggest nursing actions to be taken based on study findings (Anderson, 1995; Riemer, et al., 1995; Schmitz & Reif, 1994; Seiderman, et al., 1994). An example is Duffy's (1993) study of the unmet needs of divorced women with children. Using mailed questionnaires and telephone interviews with 148 recently divorced women, the investigator learned that within two years after their divorce the women experienced a significant decrease in the size of their social network and social supports outside of their families. The most frequently cited unmet needs (in descending order) were: emotional support, financial assistance, need for a significant other, time for herself, and child care. The results from this study provide useful information for nurses in targeting the unmet needs of this population.

Some nursing research specifically targets the improvement of nursing practice. For example, Tessaro and Highriter (1994) studied the intentions and willingness of public health nurses to work with HIV-infected clients by having 311 public health nurses complete an anonymous questionnaire. Nurses with more favorable attitudes about the disease, who perceived that family or

friends supported this kind of work, who had stronger profesional ties to public health, and who had less years of experience in public health had stronger intentions to work with HIV-infected clients. Implications for nursing practice include improved continuing education for nurses about HIV and promotion of programs that target changing nurses' normative orientations toward working with HIV-infected clients.

NURSING'S PROFESSIONAL STATUS AND INFLUENCE

The third way in which research has a significant impact on community health nursing is its potential to enhance nursing's status and influence. As community health nursing research sheds light on critical health needs of at-risk populations, exposes deficiencies in the health care system, demonstrates more efficient and cost-effective methods for delivering services, and documents the effectiveness of nursing interventions the profession will gain a stronger voice and have a greater impact on health policy and programs. In a review of the literature covering considerable research, Deal (1994) underscores these points and describes the effectiveness of services provided by community health nurses. In addition to home-based interventions, community health nurses have been effective in developing community partnerships in maternal and child health; in developing cost-effective, community-based follow-up preventive services; in promoting health in day care centers; in developing programs for vulnerable populations; in promoting multidisciplinary approaches to working with high risk youth; and assisting in development of effective health policies. Deal's review provides strong documentation for the effectiveness of community health nursing interventions. This kind of information along with other research findings must be made visible and used to influence legislators, planners, administrators, and other decision makers in health care. As this occurs, nursing's status and influence will increase.

The Community Health Nurse's Role in Research

Community health nurses have two important responsibilities with respect to research in community health: (1) to apply research findings and (2) to conduct nursing research. First, since research results provide essential information for improving health policy and the delivery of health services, community health nurses need to be knowledgeable consumers or users of research. That is, they need to be able to critically examine research reports and apply study findings to improve the public's health. An example is the work done by Anderson (1995) who through extensive review of existing research demonstrates that the problem of sexually transmitted diseases (STDs) among children is a very real problem of greater prevalence than society wishes to believe. Anderson reinforces the need for nurses and other health care providers to assess children for a history of child sexual abuse, describes several STDs found in children, and suggests appropriate interventions.

Community health nurses have many opportunities to apply the results of other investigators' research but a necessary prerequisite is to be informed about research findings. As an essential part of their role, community health nurses must read the journals in public health and community health nursing. Subscribing to some of these journals enables nurses to make regular review of research an ongoing part of their professional practice. Nursing agencies and employment sites in community health can encourage nurses becoming more knowledgeable about research findings by subscribing to journals and circulating them among staff, by holding seminars to discuss recent research results, and by promoting nurses' application of research findings in their practice.

Second, although the amount and quality of community health nursing research is expanding, many more community health nurses need to conduct research themselves. An increasing number of nurses have developed skill in research through advanced preparation and conduct investigations related to aggregate health needs. Many examples of community health nursing research have already been discussed in this chapter. Other community health nurses work collaboratively with trained investigators on a variety of research projects affecting community health. Whether these projects are initiated by the nurse or whether the nurse is involved as a team member, it is an opportunity to influence the types of research questions that are addressed and the way in which the research is carried out, ultimately affecting the community's health.

Summary

Involvement in community health nursing research can be an exciting opportunity to contribute to the body of nursing knowledge and influence changes in nursing practice and in community health programs and policies. Research findings also enable community health nurses to promote health and prevent illness among at-risk populations.

The community health nurse needs to understand the basic research process including the eight steps: (1) identify an area of interest, (2) specify a research question or statement, (3) review the literature, (4) select a conceptual framework, (5) choose a research design,

Activities to Promote Critical Thinking

1. As a community health nurse working in a large city, you notice a group of small children playing in a vacant, unfenced lot bordered by a busy street. List three research questions you might consider using to study the situation.

2. You want to determine whether a group of sexually active teenagers who are at risk of AIDS would be receptive to an educational program on AIDS. Formulate a research question and describe a conceptual framework you might use in your study and defend your choice.

3. Select a community health nursing research article from the references and readings listed in this chapter (or choose one of your own) and analyze its potential impact on health policy and on community health nursing practice.

4. You have just completed a study on the effectiveness of a series of birth control classes in three high schools and the results show a reduction in the number of pregnancies over last year. Describe three ways in which you could disseminate this information to your nursing colleagues and other community health professionals.

(6) collect and analyze data, (7) interpret the results, and (8) communicate the findings. While the process is the same regardless of nursing specialty, community health nurses have a unique opportunity to expand nursing knowledge in relation to community health issues and the health needs of aggregates.

Research has a significant impact on community health and nursing practice in three ways. It provides new knowledge that helps to shape health policy, improve service delivery, and promote the public's health. It contributes to nursing knowledge and the improvement of nursing practice. Research also offers the potential to enhance nursing's status and influence through documentation of the effectiveness of nursing interventions and broader recognition of nursing's contributions to health services.

The community health nurse's role in research is two-fold. The nurse must become a responsible user of research, keeping abreast of new knowledge and applying it in practice. More community health nurses must also engage in conducting research studies of their own or in collaboration with other community health professionals. It is this commitment to the use and conduct of research that will move the nursing profession forward and enhance its influence on the health of populations at-risk.

REFERENCES

Anderson, C. (1995). Childhood sexually transmitted diseases: one consequence of sexual abuse. *Public Health Nursing, 12*(1), 41–46.

BABESWorld. (1990). *Lower Elementary Basic BABES Teaching Guide.* (Available from the National Council on Alcoholism, Greater Detroit Area, 17330 Northland Park Court, Southfield, Michigan 48075, 1-800-542-2237).

Brockopp, D. and M. Hastings-Tolsma (1994). *Fundamentals of Nursing Research.* Boston: Jones and Bartlett.

Carty, L. (1991). The promotion and measurement of healthy coping. *Health Care Women International, 12*(2), 211–222.

Coopersmith, S. (1967). *The antecedents of self-esteem.* San Francisco. Freeman & Company

Cramer, E. & McFarlane, J. (1994). Pornography and abuse of women. *Public Health Nursing, 11*(4), 268–272.

Dawkins, C., Ervin, N., Weissfield, L., & Yan, A. (1988). Health orientation, beliefs, and use of health services among minority, high-risk expectant mothers. *Public Health Nursing, 5*(1), 7–11.

Deal, L. W. (1994). The effectiveness of community health nursing interventions: a literature review. *Public Health Nursing, 11*(5), 315–323.

DeVon, H.A., & Powers, M.J. (1984). Health beliefs, adjustment to illness, and control of hypertension. *Research in Nursing and Health, 7*(1), 10–16.

Duffy, M.E. (1993). Social networks and social support of recently divorced women. *Public Health Nursing, 10*(1), 19–24.

Gingess, P.L., & Basen-Engquist, K. (1994). HIV education practices and training needs of middle school and high school teachers. *Journal of School Health, 64*(7), 290–295.

Hacker, K., Fried, L., Bablorezian, L., & Roeber, J. (1994). A nationwide survey of school health services delivery in urban schools. *Journal of School Health, 64*(7), 279–283.

Hahn, E. (in press). Predicting head start parent involvement in an alcohol and other drug prevention program. *Nursing Research.*

Holaday, B., Waugh, G., Moukaddem, V., West, J., & Harshman, S. (1995). Fecal contamination in child day care centers: Cloth vs paper diapers. *American Journal of Public Health, 85*(1), 30–33.

Kendrick, J., Zahniser, S.C., Miller, N., et al. (1995). Integrating smoking cessation into routine public prenatal care: the smoking cessation in pregnancy project. *American Journal of Public Health, 85*(2), 217–222.

King, I.M. (1989). King's general systems framework. In J. Riehl-Sisca (Ed.), *Conceptual models for nursing practice* (3rd ed.). (pp. 149–158). Norwalk, CT: Appleton & Lange.

Kozlowski, L.A. & Zotti, M.E. (1994). Influencing community leaders toward the promotion of prenatal care at the community level. *Public Health Nursing, 11*(5), 343–351.

Meisner, T.R., Watkins, J.G., & Ossege, J. (1994). Public health nursing research priorities: A collaborative delphi study. *Public Health Nursing, 11*(2), 66–74.

Meleis, A. (1991). *Theoretical nursing: Development and progress* (2nd ed.). Philadelphia: Lippincott.

Murphy, A., Youatt, J., Hoerr, S., Sawyer, C., & Andrews, S. (1994). Nutrition education needs and learning preferences of Michigan students in grades 5, 8, and 11. *Journal of School Health, 64*(7), 273–278.

Orem, D.E. (1985). *Nursing: Concepts of practice* (3rd ed.). New York: McGraw Hill.

Quinn, J., & Strelkauskas, A. (1993). Psychoimmunologic effects of therapeutic touch on practitioners and recently bereaved recipients: A pilot study. *Advances in Nursing, 15*(4), 13–26.

Riemer, J.G., Van Cleve, L., & Galbraith, M. (1995). Barriers to well child care for homeless children under age 13. *Public Health Nursing, 12*(1), 61–66.

Rogers, M. (1990). Nursing: Science of unitary, irreducible, human beings: Update 1990. In E.A.M. Barrett (Ed.), *Visions of Rogers' science-based nursing.* New York: National League for Nursing.

Schmitz, K. & Reif, L. (1994). Reducing prenatal risk and improving birth outcomes: The public health nursing role. *Public Health Nursing, 11*(3), 174–180.

Seiderman, R.Y., Williams, R., Burns, P., Jacobson, S., Weatherby, F., & Primeaux, M. (1994). Culture sensitivity in assessing urban Native American parenting. *Public Health Nursing, 11*(2), 98–103.

Sorensen, E. S. (1994). Daily stressors and coping responses: A comparison of rural and suburban children. *Public Health Nursing, 11*(1), 24–31.

Strader, M. & Beaman, M. (1992). Theoretical components of STD counselors' messages to promote clients' use of condoms. *Public Health Nursing, 9*(2), 109–117.

Tessaro, I., & Highriter, M. (1994). HIV and the work intentions of public health nurses. *Public Health Nursing, 11*(4), 273–280.

Theis, S., Moss, J., & Pearson, M. (1994). Respite for caregivers: An evaluation study. *Journal of Community Health Nursing, 11*(1), 31–44.

UNICEF (1995). *The state of the world's children 1995.* New York: Oxford.

Wruble, A., Alkobi-Kedushim, Y., & Musgrave, C. (1994). Breast cancer prevention education at a shopping center in Israel: A student nurse community health project, *Journal of Community Health Nursing, 11*(3), 149–154.

Yu, S. (1995). A study on functioning for independent living among the elderly in the community. *Public Health Nursing, 12*(1), 31–40.

SELECTED READINGS

American Academy of Nursing Expert Panel on Violence (1993). Violence as a nursing priority: policy implications. *Nursing Outlook, 41*(2), 83–92.

Chen, S.C., Telleen, S., & H. Chen, E.H. (1995). Adequacy of prenatal care of urban high school students. *Public Health Nursing, 12*(1), 47–52.

Cobb, B. K. (1990). What areas of community health nusing would benefit from clinical investigation? *Florida Nurse, 38*(6),20.

Conn, V.S. &. Armer, J.M. (1994). A public health nurse's guide to reading meta-analysis research reports. *Public Health Nursing, 11*(3), 163–167.

Connelly, L., Keele, B., Kleinbeck, S., Schneider, J., & Cobb, A. (1993). A place to be yourself: empowerment from the client's perspective. *IMAGE, 25*(4), 297–303.

Ellickson, P., Bell, R., & McGuigan, K. (1993). Preventing adolescent drug use: Long-term results of a junior high program. *American Journal of Public Health, 83*(6), 856–861.

Leininger, M.M. (Ed.). (1985). *Qualitative research methods in nursing.* Orlando, FL: Grune & Stratton.

Martin, K., Scheet, N., & Stegman, M. (1993). Home health clients: Characteristics, outcomes of care, and nursing interventions. *American Journal of Public Health, 83*(12), 1730–1734.

Munhall, P.L., & Oiler, C.J. (1986). *Nursing research: A qualitative perspective.* Norwalk, CT: Appleton-Century-Crofts.

Robins, L. & Mills, J. (Eds). (1993). Effects of in-utero exposure to street drugs. *American Journal of Public Health, Supplement, 83*(12), 1–32.

Shortell, S.M. & Reinhardt, U.E. (Eds). (1992). *Improving health policy and management: Nine critical research issues for the 1990s.* Ann Arbor: Health Administration Press.

Zima, B., Wells, K., Freeman, H. (1994). Emotional and behavioral problems and severe academic delays among sheltered homeless children in Los Angeles county. *American Journal of Public Health, 84*(2), 260–264.

Zurlindern, J. K., et al. (1991). Community-based research offers new hope and therapy. *Journal of Home Health Care Practice, 3*(2), 77–79.

CHAPTER

27

Quality Management in Community Health Nursing

LEARNING OBJECTIVES

By the end of this chapter the reader should be able to do the following:

- Define quality care.
- Discuss the historical development of quality care attainment in the delivery of community health care.
- Compare and contrast the four models of quality management in community health care.
- Identify the three primary areas of focus in a quality management program.
- Identify the six characteristics of quality community health programs.
- Describe how quality care is assessed and measured.
- Discuss the role of the nurse in a quality management program in a community health care setting.

KEY TERMS

- Audit
- Concurrent review
- Peer review
- Quality assurance
- Quality care
- Quality circles
- Quality control
- Quality indicators
- Retrospective review
- Standards of care
- Total quality management

Barbara Walton Spradley and Judith Ann Allender
COMMUNITY HEALTH NURSING: CONCEPTS AND PRACTICE, 4th ed.
© 1996 Barbara Walton Spradley and Judith Ann Allender

Introduction

Quality is a relative term that defines something with high merit or excellence. Excellence compared with what? Quality must be measured according to some standard or norm. In business or industry, products and services are measured against a predetermined standard of quality established by using field testing to determine consumer response and then fashioning the product to meet consumer expectations.

Managers institute measures of **quality control** to ensure that all products and services conform to predetermined levels of quality and certain standards or norms that satisfy customers. Companies constantly monitor and control the purchase of supplies and production and presentation methods to make sure that standards are met and customers are satisfied.

In health care, it is more difficult to determine standards by which health care can be judged because of the variety of health care situations and services. But during the past 40 years, serious efforts have been made to set standards for measuring and monitoring health care services to ensure that quality care is provided. **Quality care** means that the services provided match the needs of the population, are technically correct, and achieve beneficial results. The escalating costs of health care have caused consumers and third-party payers to demand quality care at more reasonable costs. The rising costs and the impending changes in the health care delivery system are largely beyond a nurse's direct control, as are particular client outcomes.

But nurses do have control over the delivery and measurement of quality care, and they can evaluate the quality of their own nursing process and the outcomes of that care. They can use these measurements and evaluations to determine whether clients are receiving the best care possible and how limited resources can best be spent to bring about the most needed improvements and programs.

This chapter discusses how quality care in the community is measured and the role of the community health nurse in managing quality care.

Historical Perspectives

Nursing has evolved over the last 140 years as a self-regulating profession from three perspectives: (1) clinical competence of nurses, (2) organizational competence, and (3) nursing care review processes.

The move to quality assurance in health care has its roots in the medical and nursing professions. Both physicians and nurses as young professional groups in the mid-1800s assumed responsibility for maintaining standards in the services that each provided. That began by requiring minimum levels of education, which Florence Nightingale recommended as early as the mid-1800s. Later, in the 1900s, clinical competence was further determined by licensure and clinical certification in all states.

Nursing education began with a few intuitive, service-minded people who applied practical knowledge in the care of the ill. Today it includes standardized basic and advanced education. Various accrediting organizations were established in the early 1900s to oversee and stimulate nursing schools to keep up with changes in health care. Two of the most influential organizations are the American Nurses Association (ANA), which began in the 1890s, and the National League for Nursing (NLN), which was formed in 1952 from seven organizations established in the early 1900s. The NLN offers voluntary accreditation for nursing programs and works closely with schools to maintain standards of educational programs. The ANA has resources available to nurses including standards of practice in 10 nursing specialties. In 1986, the ANA developed **standards of care**, which are desired goals that can help plan and evaluate care in community and home health nursing (ANA,1986; 1986a & b).

The American Nurses Credentialing Center (ANCC), a subsidiary of the ANA, provides clinical certification for nurses in 25 clinical specialties. Certification exams and ongoing CEUs (continuing-education units) provide additional means for achieving and maintaining a high level of nursing skills. In addition, associations of nurses in specific disciplines influence the standards of care provided while providing a forum of support for nurses through regularly scheduled meetings and periodic conferences focusing on advances in that specific discipline (ANA, 1982).

By 1952 all states, the District of Columbia, and United States' territories had enacted nurse practice acts (Mitchell and Grippando, 1993) to ensure that minimum standards of education, practice, and expertise are maintained. In addition, today most states require CEUs as part of their qualifications for nursing license renewal. Professional organizations also offer in-services, workshops, and conferences in which nurses can update their clinical skills and keep current in nursing while earning needed CEUs.

As health care organizations have developed and diversified, many methods for managing large staffs, multiple departments, and missions have emerged. Organizational structures and methods were designed to promote effective operations of hospitals and other health care organizations. The many responsibilities that health care agencies have to their clients, staffs, boards of directors, and funders complicate their functioning and sometimes compromise care.

Institutional attention to quality-of-care issues first appeared in the 1940s and 1950s. At that time it became clear that organizations delivering health care services needed to monitor those services in order to meet the goals of the organization and its consumers, and to survive in a competitive environment (Bohnet, et al., 1993). External certification and accreditation processes began about the same time. These processes verified an organization's ability to provide adequate service. Voluntary accreditation boards, such as the Joint Commission on Accreditation of Health-care Organizations, examine all types of health care organizations to help them attend to all facets of their operations, and thus establish appropriate priorities (Joint Commission on Accreditation of Health-care Organizations, 1992).

Throughout the 1970s and 1980s, the Joint Commission (as it is commonly called) and a precursor to the Utilization and Quality Control Peer Review Organization (PRO) certified all organizations receiving Medicare and/or Medicaid dollars. Both organizations made the impact of organizational functioning on quality of care their primary emphasis. They began to consider how quality is affected by such factors as staff recruitment, organizational structure, management effectiveness, billing practices, and planning. Both bodies continue to require evidence of effective quality assurance programs in all agencies that they certify.

Formal quality management activities in the health care field began in earnest in the early 1970s. Nursing's efforts in **quality assurance** generally predated those of other health care fields and include methods of assuring that quality care is being delivered by using the following three-phase process: (1) comparing a health care situation with preestablished criteria believed to represent quality care; (2) identifying care strengths, deficiencies, and opportunities for improvement; and (3) introducing changes in the health care system. Additional quality assurance efforts developed and used during the 1950s and 1960s include initial setting of standards, formal auditing, and **peer reviews,** in which peer professionals use an organized system to assess the quality of care being delivered (Phaneuf, 1976).

Record keeping was incorporated into the evaluation when the problem-oriented medical record was implemented across the country in the 1970s, thus standardizing evaluative documentation in nursing records. That was significant in assuring quality because it made the nurses' internal problem-solving process available to outsiders for evaluation. Thus the quality assurance tools that began to be developed for nursing during the 1950s could be used to assess nurses' decision-making activities.

In its 1988 Peer Review Guidelines, the American Nurses Association proposed that nurses bear primary responsibility and accountability for the quality of nursing care their clients receive (ANA, 1988). Each nurse is responsible for interpreting and implementing the standards of nursing practice and must participate with other nurses in the decision-making process for evaluating nursing care.

Accrediting bodies focused most of their attention on hospitals in the 1970s. In the 1980s the attention shifted to include ambulatory or out-patient care, long-term care, and home health care. That shift occurred for many reasons, but the high costs of care and competition for health care dollars were the leading reasons why those agencies sought accreditation (Ellis and Hartley, 1995). The Community Health Accreditation Program, Inc. (CHAP), a subsidiary of the National League for Nursing, is setting a standard of excellence through its accreditation services and publications geared to home health care, hospice care, and community health care organizations (CHAP, 1993). Through their efforts they are attempting to determine levels of excellence (quality) in home care services through the "In Search for Excellence" project (See Issues in Community Health Nursing display). This project, funded by the W. K. Kellogg Foundation, is designed to strengthen the quality of care delivered at home by (1) defining quality outcomes using consumer feedback; (2) developing a system to assess quality using these outcomes; and (3) incorporating the process into CHAP's process of accreditation (CHAP, 1993; Peters, 1992). Project leaders work together with as many people as possible through advisory groups, expert consultants, and consumers to define the important values in home care. The project has combined various beliefs about quality to develop the following definition of quality: "The degree to which consumers progress toward desired outcomes, which they have established with the guidance and support of health care providers. These providers are part of an administratively and financially sound organization that monitors competent staff and an environment encouraging personal excellence." (Peters, 1992, p. 24.)

Over the past 35 years nursing has developed increasingly more formalized nursing care review models and
implemented them throughout the profession. The
American Nurses Association has contributed to formal
quality improvement evaluative processes through development of models, quality of care and peer review
guidelines, and nursing care standards, including those
for community health nursing and home health nursing.
In addition, nursing case management and managed
care concepts are incorporated in publications produced
by the ANA since 1982. Nursing has adapted and applied these models, guidelines, standards, and concepts
in many inpatient, ambulatory care, and community
nursing settings (ANA, 1986c and 1991).

Models for Quality Management

THE DONABEDIAN MODEL

Donabedian (1966, 1985) proposed a model for the
structure, process, and outcome of quality that is widely
used as the framework for more elaborate models. "The
structure of the care environment, the processes responsible to improve or stabilize the patient's health sta-

tus, and the resultant outcomes need to be causally
linked indicators of quality in order to have an organization-wide appreciation of quality . . ." (Sainfort, et al.,
1994, p. 75). The Donabedian paradigm is recognized
as a method of measuring quality as structure, process,
and outcome and can be depicted in the following linear model:

Structure $\longrightarrow$	Process $\longrightarrow$	Outcomes
Facility	Standards,	Client
resources,	attitudes,	health care
personnel	nursing	goals met,
mix and skills,	care plans,	efficiency
philosophy,	effectiveness,	and effec-
policies,	client satis-	tiveness
client mix	faction	of services

THE ANA MODEL

The American Nurses Association provides a quality
improvement model that is based on standards of care
and quality indicators within the Donabedian framework of structure, process, and outcomes (Dienemann,
1992). Nursing and its disciplines can use Donabedian's
concepts to construct models appropriate to its purposes. This ANA model has changed over time as more
information is gathered through research and as the profession of nursing grows. This circular model has a core
that includes the agency's philosophy or mission statement. The core identifies the values of the agency and
reflects its views of clients, nursing, the community, and
health. This is the first step in improving quality and
defining the beliefs of the agency. The three components
of structure, process, and outcomes are depicted as pie-
shaped wedges around the central core. Specific nursing
actions are added to more closely interrelate each section
and make the transition to the next section smoother.

Although each component is important, positive
client outcomes are the key indicators of success within
an agency and are focused on today. Successful outcomes are the purpose of the agency's existence and the
key to evaluation by accrediting bodies. Moreover, continued reimbursement by third-party payers, such as
private insurance companies, Medicare, and Medicaid,
depends on successful outcomes.

THE UPWARDLY SPIRALING FEEDBACK LOOP MODEL

This model takes the ANA model one step further. It
adds a feedback loop that makes the process dynamic
and subject to change in response to ongoing feedback,

which is used to assess and then implement revisions in care or plans. The model in Figure 27.1 illustrates this idea graphically. The right pole of the model represents the continuum of a client's health needs and personal health behaviors from a client's current status to optimal health and coping. The left pole depicts the contact between clients and the health care system. The spirals' movement from pole to pole demonstrates the quality assessment activities that nurses use to assess their clients, revise nursing care or plans, and implement changes. Any changes are assessed again at a future date as part of the ongoing review process.

This ongoing and repetitive process should result in improvements in the quality of care and the clients' health. The model makes two basic assumptions: first, that specific nursing activities are known to maintain and promote health, and second, that positive results are brought about by positive interventions.

This model shows the distance between the two poles of client needs and behaviors and contacts with the health care delivery system. It demonstrates that nurses should step back from the everyday demands of direct client care and assess that care and the desired outcomes. More specifically, stepping back from the process prompts nurses to do the following:

1. Identify and prioritize the health problems and needs of the populations served.

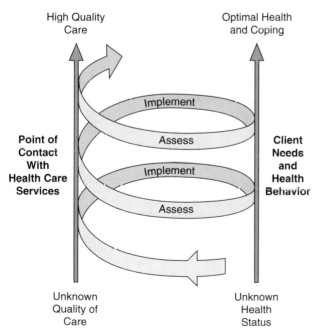

FIGURE 27.1. Upwardly spiraling quality assurance feedback loop.

2. Determine the systems, nursing actions, or outcomes in terms of client behaviors that are facilitated by the nurse.
3. Examine the success or failure of nursing efforts with a specific group.
4. Adjust nursing care, systems, or client goals as needed.
5. Plan for future quality assessments.

THE HOESING AND KIRK QUALITY MANAGEMENT MODEL

A final model focuses on the "big picture" and provides the clarity needed to manage quality and to monitor and evaluate the results (Hoesing and Kirk, 1990). The model is designed for supervisory and administrative personnel as well as for the individual professional nurse (Figure 27.2). The model begins with defining the major nursing responsibilities within the agency. "If nurses know what is desired and expected of them, they will also have direction and a knowledge of what it is they are working toward in achieving goals, as well as objective measures to monitor and evaluate results" (Hoesing and Kirk, 1990, p. 11).

The key to this quality management model is identifying measurable and verifiable indicators and being able to easily access timely and accurate information about them. Hoesing and Kirk use concepts of standards of care, practice, and finance (Kirk and Hoesing, 1991). Information gathered from monitoring the major responsibility areas is collected, organized, and analyzed. From that data can be determined whether the indicator is being met or exceeded and the appropriate action to take. The next step in the process is to communicate feedback, information, then praise, and then to go on to develop even higher targets to promote a higher level of improved quality. For example, within a community health agency, a practitioner performance indicator might be that nurses complete client assessments during the first home visit 95% of the time. If that 95% goal or indicator is met, feedback in the form of praise is shared with the staff and a higher target can then be implemented (97.5%). Agencies might use that model to determine whether it would ever be practical to expect 100% compliance with an indicator. For instance, would it ever be possible to expect 100% of the assessments completed on the first home visit? There may be circumstances beyond the nurse's control, such as a crisis may occur in the home at the time of the visit or the client may be aphasic and the caretaker may be unavailable at the time.

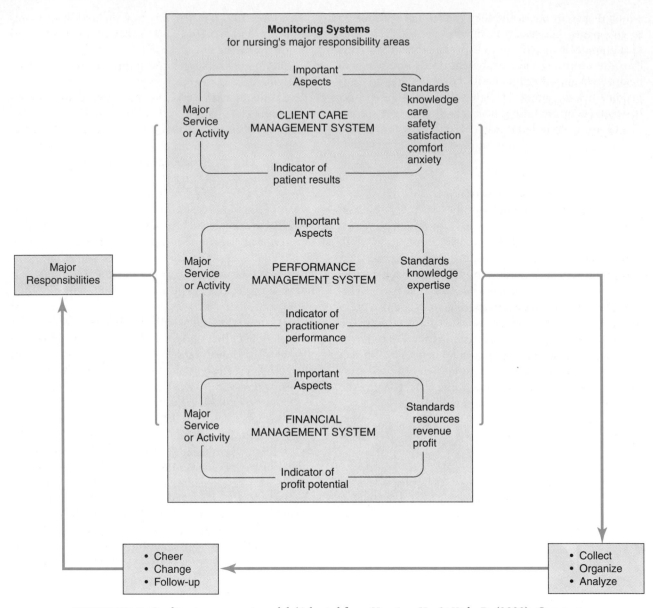

FIGURE 27.2. Quality management model (Adapted from Hoesing, H., & Kirk, R. (1990). Common-sense quality management. *Journal of Nursing Administration, 20*(10), 11).

An example of a client results indicator might be that on a scale of 1 to 10, client satisfaction should be at least 8. If that is not met because the results are 7.2, then these data are shared, some praise may be in order, especially if previous surveys indicated that client satisfaction had been 6. However, discussion may lead to changes in any or all parts of the program to achieve a higher level of client satisfaction. The more that successes, problems, and information are shared with agency staff, the greater the potential for quality improvement.

Principles of Quality Management

QUALITY ASSURANCE

"Quality is not an event, it's a way of life, a way to conduct business, an ongoing quest for excellence," (Kirk and Hoesing, 1990 p. 93). That quotation embodies the main principle of quality management. Programs that promote quality should consider quality to be an ongoing process and a standard rather than an afterthought of a specific event. The many terms used for describing various aspects of quality management may seem confusing, if not overwhelming. In order to evaluate a quality business, which any health care agency can and should be, several principles regarding the evaluation process need to be mentioned.

Measurable Goals and Objectives

Planned programs should have specific goals to help identify who the program is supposed to serve, what services are provided, the length of time in which the services are provided, and the resources that are needed. Then, measurable objectives are developed that describe the expected outcomes. Using selected verbs indicates the expected level of achievement, such as the client will be able to *demonstrate* safe administration of insulin. This is done when developing an educational program (see Chapter 14) or an entire health program or service. These statements of measurable goals are then examined during the program evaluation. Without such statements, accurate evaluations cannot be conducted.

Quality indicators or quality-focused objectives as markers are used to determine whether a goal has been achieved and to measure client outcomes or process outcomes, such as all clients are visited within 24 hours of receiving the referral. Quality indicators assure that quality issues are dealt with routinely within all organizational program evaluations. **Total quality management (TQM)** is a comprehensive term referring to the systems and activities used to achieve all aspects of quality care within a given agency. Quality indicators are a part of this broader concept.

In evaluating programs and care, outcomes must be measured against certain standards. Standards are generic guidelines of expected functioning and can focus on the client, the caregiver, or the organization (finances). All care and services must also be measured against these guidelines. The core standards of care, practice, and finance must be integrated and compatible if they are to ensure quality care.

Outcomes

The outcomes or results of care include the satisfaction of the clients involved and success of the care delivered. Client satisfaction is measured by how closely a client's expectations of nursing care are to the perception of the nursing care actually received (Megivern, Halm, and Jones, 1992). Client satisfaction can be determined by a telephone survey or a mailed questionnaire.

When responses indicate a program is meeting its goals, maintaining set standards, and having positive client outcomes and satisfied clients, that means the program is providing quality care. However, the accuracy of using outcomes as a primary measure of quality care is limited because some clients may have unsatisfactory outcomes despite receiving good care. Factors other than specific health interventions influence outcomes, such as a client's compliance or the client's ability to respond to care as a result of such situations as a compromised immune system. Nursing staff needs to keep all that in mind when evaluating care (Donabedian, 1969).

ASSESSING QUALITY CARE IN THE COMMUNITY

Assessing the quality of care delivered in the community is of paramount importance to the success of the services provided. Standards of care, practice, and finance as components of a total quality management process need to be reviewed regularly, as defined by each agency's philosophy or mission. The quality assessment process within community health nursing agencies may take a number of forms, depending on the values of the organization's leadership, the time available, and the staff's experience in research and quality assessment. Agency personnel need to initiate, coordinate, and implement assessment processes, with each employee having a role in the process. Formal controls that are found in the acute care setting may be lacking in the home and community settings. Monitoring of specific aspects of care is often done in response to funders' (Medicare, Medicaid or private insurers) requirements for periodic progress reports rather than as part of a program of quality management. If monitoring is done only for reimbursement purposes, the total quality of the program is not the agency goal, as it should be. A program of quality has specific pulse points (check points) and outcomes that are determined by the agency's mission statement and are measurable (Peters, 1992). The "In Search of Excellence" project, funded by the W. K. Kellogg Foundation to strengthen the home care industry, has identified 11 pulse points for quality. These pulse points are divided into three categories (Peters, 1992):

1. Consumer Outcome
   a. consumer empowerment
   b. caregiver relationship

c. knowledge and information needs
d. family support
e. consumer expectations.
2. Clinical Outcomes
  a. functional ability
  b. physiological functioning.
3. Organizational Outcomes
  a. team building
  b. commitment to quality
  c. coordination of care
  d. financial viability.

Ideally, a comprehensive community health nursing program will address in some fashion all of the agency services, the processes and resources utilized to accomplish the services, and client expectations and outcomes. This is done to improve quality and efficiency and are parts of an organized assessment process.

Audit Tools

A variety of audit tools can help achieve the best and most comprehensive data. These tools are: record reviews, checklists, questionnaires, and surveys and provide the audit committee with quantitative data with which to make decisions about future care as it relates to the agreed on standards. Involving the entire staff in the process is essential to increasing incentives for adhering to the standards (Robinson and Fitzgerald, 1990; Toms, 1992). The information gathered can also support plans for revising and perhaps modifying the standards as client needs change. In some instances the audit committee is empowered to implement those changes. Otherwise, the committee should receive follow-up reports on their recommendation from those who have taken the actions. In either case, the results of recommended actions should be reevaluated at a specified future date by the same group (ANA, 1988; JCAHO, 1988). The **audit** becomes an organized effort practicing professionals can use to monitor, assess, and judge the quality and appropriateness of nursing care provided by peers as measured against professional standards of practice.

Retrospective Review System. The most commonly known audit process is the **retrospective review** of client charts. This review is a quality assessment process that examines patterns of care over a specified period of time and includes closed-record audits and a statistical review of trends in services provided. Specific components of a home visit or care provided are reviewed, such as documented teaching, wound size in millimeters or centimeters, the nurse's signature, or dates of

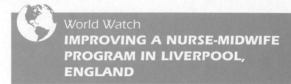

World Watch
IMPROVING A NURSE-MIDWIFE PROGRAM IN LIVERPOOL, ENGLAND

Source: Sgouros, J., & Moore, L. (1992). Improving community services. *Nursing Times, 88*(38), 28–30.

In 1989 a study of the services provided by 38 nurse-midwives serving Liverpool, England was conducted. They routinely deliver 4000 babies a year, and the majority of their time is spent on postnatal visits (more than 76,000 a year) and on prenatal home and clinic visits (more than 6500 a year). As busy as that schedule may appear, the midwives participated in an activity analysis to make sure their time was being spent wisely. Seventy-one percent of the midwives participated in 2 weeks of data collection. Results confirmed that the midwives were indeed very busy, but not necessarily doing midwifery. Fifteen percent of their time was spent on administration, which included doing paperwork; they spent 20% of the time traveling, and 13% using the telephone. Only 38% of their time was spent in direct client contact.

As a result of the study, the nurses met to clarify their aims and objectives, but mainly to increase direct client care to 62%. Changes were made in daily paperwork that focused on eliminating duplication, reorganizing midwife work groups, rescheduling visits around the city, and making more efficient use of midwives when they work with physicians in clinics. In the fall of 1990, a year after instituting these changes, the activity analysis was repeated. Direct client contact had increased to 57%, an increase of almost 20% from the previous year. Time spent on telephone and administrative work decreased, and travel time actually increased slightly. An unexpected bonus of the project was that it brought all the midwives together in a common goal, which provided them with an increased sense of teamwork and the knowledge that they could contribute to and improve the system.

care. However, the assumption that there is a relationship between the quality of documentation and the quality of nursing care is questionable(Edwards, et al., 1991; Griffin, 1988; Stewart and Craig, 1987). That type of audit should be viewed as a continuous process of reflective exploration (Morgan, 1983) rather than an attempt to determine the quality of care. Morgan advocates the need for exploratory tools as well as evaluative tools. One tool does not give an agency the holistic picture of care provided. An agency that relies only on one tool can get a distorted and incomplete view of the care delivered.

Concurrent Review System. The Public Health Nursing Services of Baltimore County, Maryland, instituted a **concurrent review** system that uses the chart audit, clients' opinions, and observations of the health center environment (Zlotnick, 1992). This approach combines a retrospective review with assessment of current clients' opinions and observations, while the care is still occurring. The Baltimore system tabulates and consolidates the combined data into a report that is shared with the staff. In order to understand this audit system, the staff members attend work sessions in which they review one client record using the combined monitoring tools. As a result, staff members gain insight and become invested in the system (Jenko, et al, 1990; Zlotnick, 1992).

Quality Circles. Nursing staff in the community can use quality circles to improve the quality of care provided to clients. **Quality circles** are a participative management approach in which employees and managers share the responsibility for decision making and problem solving in client care. The concept of quality circles is based on several well-established motivational and management theories (Maslow, 1954; Herzberg, Mauser, and Snyderman, 1968). The quality circles approach of workers and management sharing responsibility for decision making has been used in Japan since the 1950s and 1960s. Kaoru Ishikawa (1985) is recognized as the founder of that movement. More recently, quality circles have been used in American industry as a participative management tool based on W.G. Ouchi's Theory Z (Ouchi, 1981). Quality circles are subsequently being used as effective tools in the health care arena. Although this management technique was at first only used in the acute-care setting, it is now being identified as an excellent tool for those providing care in the home and community. The use of quality circles help home care agencies achieve program goals and multidisciplinary and interdisciplinary collaboration (Schmele, et al., 1991).

For a quality circle to be an effective problem-solving group, it must incorporate the following:

■ nurses are involved in identifying and solving problems that are encountered by utilizing the energies of nurses working in groups

■ contributions made by individuals and groups are recognized

■ continuous mechanisms are in place for further learning, decision making, and nursing research

■ processes are instituted for advocacy and negotiation, power from knowledge, networking through consultation, communication, collaboration, and coordination (O'Brien and McHugh, 1994).

Central to achieving the above purposes is the expectation that the formation of a quality circle ensures unity and a common sense of purpose. Employees are more satisfied in environments that are open and supportive of opportunities for self-determination and creative expression and in which their ideas are valued (Schmele, et al., 1991). The quality circle approach promotes such environments (O'Brien and McHugh, 1994). Staff members share their expertise, experiences, and ideas and critique the handling of past situations. This profoundly useful quality management tool uses sharing and quality practices to go beyond routine auditing of key nursing activities (Figure 27.3). The emphasis on group processes facilitates increased understanding among a staff who must consider the quality of care delivered by the department or agency and must work together across a range of skills, management levels, and job assignments to solve problems related to the nursing goals.

Measuring Client Outcomes. Quality indicators of client outcomes are the quantitative measures of a client's response to care. Defining and quantifying client outcomes from these indicators are worthwhile processes that enable the nursing staff to evaluate the results of the care they provide. The goal of care in the community is successful client outcomes. By starting with measurable indicators, successful outcomes can be demonstrated in quantifiable terms. When client care meets the standards set, client satisfaction—another quality indicator—is greater.

Quantifying the indicators can be accomplished through a rate or ratio of events for a defined population and time frame. These indicators can be tailored to express almost any patient outcome (Williams, 1991):

$$\frac{\text{outcome}}{\text{indicators}} = \frac{\text{number of patient care events}}{\substack{\text{total number of clients or total} \\ \text{number of times at risk for event} \\ \text{during a given period of time}}}$$

For example:

$$\begin{array}{l}\text{occurrence of} \\ \text{UTI's in} \\ \text{clients with} \\ \text{indwelling} \\ \text{urinary} \\ \text{catheters}\end{array} = \dfrac{\begin{array}{c}\text{number of clients experiencing} \\ \text{urinary tract infections (UTI) re-} \\ \text{lated to long term use of indwelling} \\ \text{urinary catheters} \\ \text{from 1/1 to 3/1, 1996}\end{array}}{\begin{array}{c}\text{number of clients with long term} \\ \text{indwelling urinary catheters} \\ \text{from 1/1 to 3/1, 1996.}\end{array}}$$

The nursing staff sets a standard for the number of UTIs the agency will tolerate in clients with indwelling urinary catheters (perhaps 5% to 7%, depending on client age, diagnosis, family support, and home environment). This is a quality outcome indicator. It is necessary to have indicators when setting standards in order to measure the success and quality of programs at home or in the community. The same types of indicators are used in acute care settings, using the focus appropriate to that population. If the standards are being met, but client outcomes are unacceptable, Nadzam (1991) suggests that the process indicators, such as the catheter care protocol an agency uses, and possible areas of weakness may need further study to identify the cause of the infections.

Measuring Client Satisfaction. The health care practices that consumers value have been receiving more attention in recent years. The client's perception of quality care has become very important, as health care agencies or programs compete for clients. However, client satisfaction is difficult to define. Many studies using reliable and valid measurement tools indicate that clients identify quality care by such attributes as kindness, pleasantness, the ability to listen and care, flexibility, and proficiency. In addition, the quality of the nurse–client interaction in providing holistic care is frequently mentioned when clients are asked about the quality of care received (Megivern, et al., 1992; Reeder and Chen, 1990; Taylor, et al., 1991).

The final step of the nursing process—the evaluation—is often the weakest yet one of the most crucial components. Failure to thoroughly evaluate services and care can result in delivering mediocre nursing care. If the delivery and outcome of care is not evaluated, then care may continue at an unsafe or below minimum standard. No longer will consumers tolerate mediocre care, nor can agencies afford to provide such care. Today's health care consumer demands a high level of quality care from beginning to end. That may begin by the pleasantness and timeliness of the first telephone call and continue with a proficiency and flexibility of services, to the follow-up survey 2 weeks after the termination of service. Questionnaires or telephone surveys can be used to collect feedback from clients. If clients are not

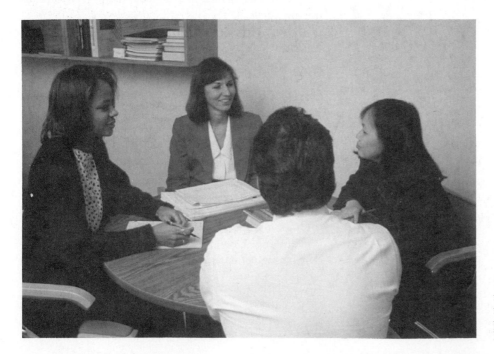

FIGURE 27.3. This group of nurses form a quality circle that is being used as a quality improvement tool in a community health care agency.

satisfied they may select a different agency, or they may be unreceptive to services by refusing to come to the door or to be at home, which often occurs in public agencies. Lack of follow-up and noncompliance with mutually set goals can often be traced to dissatisfaction with certain aspects of the care received.

In public agencies, many clients do not solicit the care they receive. As a result, noncompliance with instructions or goals, such as teaching parenting skills to substance abusers, educating pregnant teens, and instructing older adults about their medication, becomes an even more important and challenging issue. Issues of noncompliance also make it difficult to use questionnaires or surveys to gather information on client satisfaction. Measuring satisfaction, however, may be achieved through qualitative measures, such as statements from clients and family members. Quantitative measures may include such indicators as the number of times clients make themselves available for visits and comply with care-giving measures. Another factor affecting clients' perceptions of the care they receive is the nurse-to-client ratio. In many public programs, because one-on-one nursing care is not cost effective, more care is delivered to the aggregate. Using such aggregate approaches as group classes may affect the client's perception of quality care. In addition, only the most motivated and receptive clients may attend group sessions, which means the reticent or disinterested clients do not contribute to an evaluation process.

Quality Management in Community Health Nursing

Do the people in the health care field know what their customers want, need, and like? Can satisfied consumers of health care services be identified? Often the answers to these questions are no, leaving health care agencies with little knowledge about how to target their services.

Faced with limited resources available and escalating costs of care, health care agencies must be able to identify services and programs that best serve the needs of the community. Studying the impact of intervention and instituting tighter controls on the delivery of specific community health nursing services may not automatically result in satisfied clients or healthier clients; however, such methods can enhance the quality of care

delivered by the home care organization (Bohnet, et al., 1993). When various nursing interventions within a given group are proven to be highly satisfactory and cost efficient, these interventions should be consistently chosen over those that fail such tests.

The unique population-focused role of community health carries with it the challenge of sorting out top-priority health care needs from the many competing client needs. There are many areas of community health in which the current system of services does not meet the needs of large segments of the population. Frequently seen are preventable injuries, illnesses, and deaths caused by accidents, chemical abuse, sexually transmitted diseases, domestic violence, violent deaths, and suicide. Deficiencies in health services are also evident in the way care is given to those with existing problems, such as adolescent parents, handicapped children, frail elderly, and people entrenched in cycles of poverty and illness.

New and innovative public health programs arise from the realization by public health practitioners that time-honored methods have become ineffective in addressing the problems of those at risk. New strategies need to be found. Such realizations come from scrutinizing public health services. This careful examination requires objective data on services and self-reflection on health care delivered (Figure 27.4). The process of continually improving and assuring quality provides a framework for collecting and evaluating this data on an ongoing basis (Harvey, 1991; Jenko, et al, 1990; Peterson, 1991; Zlotnick, 1992).

CHARACTERISTICS OF QUALITY HEALTH CARE

An agency operates from an agreed-on definition of quality. That definition is incorporated into an agency's mission statement or philosophy and is the basis on which a quality health care program can be built. In other words, a quality health care program is built on the concepts that the agency and its staff value. Such a program must consider everything that has an impact on the agency and the clients it serves. The following is a list of six characteristics considered essential in the development and maintenance of quality community health programs.

A quality program includes the following:

1. It is comprehensive and addresses the interrelated health needs of the entire person or community.

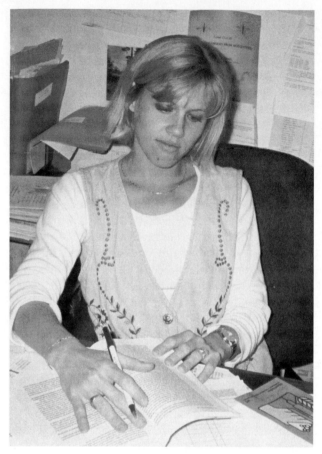

FIGURE 27.4. Quality management efforts begin with self-reflection on health care service delivery. This community health nurse spends time during the care planning phase to contemplate the care her clients need.

2. It demonstrates organizational competency and operates from within an expertly managed and financially sound organizational system.
3. It demonstrates professional competency and a commitment to an environment that encourages personal excellence among a competent staff.
4. It is accessible and demonstrates that its services are readily available to its clients in a timely manner, despite the financial, cultural, emotional, or geographic barriers that may exist.
5. It is efficient and demonstrates that it consistently makes the best use of available and, at times, limited resources.
6. It is effective and demonstrates its consideration of client priorities and concern with the positive effects of the health status of clients as measured

by client outcomes, client satisfaction ratings, and the client's ability to return to the same program when needed.

These six characteristics provide a framework for evaluating the quality of health care delivery. Consider how these six characteristics might be used to assess a program or services for adolescent mothers: (1) Are we looking at all the health care needs of our typical teen mothers? (2) and (3) Is the care being provided and delivered by competent staff who provide excellent care, from an agency that is well managed? (4) Are these young mothers actually functioning at a higher level as a result of our care, and do we connect with these women during their first trimester and find ways to effectively interact with them to meet their needs throughout their pregnancy and postpartum period? (5) Are the services provided consistent with the mother's specific needs, or are they too generalized to make efficient use of available funds? (6) Are the women satisfied with their care and do they return to our agency for continued services after this pregnancy? Such questions provide the basis for studying each dimension of quality. Each question refers to one of the key dimensions within the agency's mission statement or philosophy (Figure 27.5).

ROLE OF THE NURSE IN QUALITY MANAGEMENT IN THE COMMUNITY

Although nurses who deliver care directly to clients are not managers as such, improving or assuring quality is largely a "management" activity. And although com-

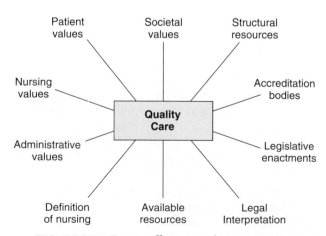

FIGURE 27.5. Factors affecting quality nursing care.

munity health nurses may not be responsible for a staff or agency budget and functioning, they are responsible for managing a caseload of clients with needs of varying degrees of urgency. Using the resources available, they must provide priority services that will promote the highest level possible of personal and group functioning and health. Thus, any activities the community health nurse engages in to realize these goals contribute to the quality management program.

Some quality management activities for community health nurses include daily prioritizing care needs for a caseload of clients, seeking supervision or skills development for a difficult case, systematizing charting so that needed documentation is efficiently completed (e.g., using flow sheets to chart maternal-child health visits), proposing better ways to organize care of chronically ill clients, or establishing new agency procedures. All these actions demonstrate that nurses are evaluating their work and looking for ways to improve care. Staff meetings, quality circle meetings, and case conferences are common settings for nurses to bring the lessons of their practices to the larger group for examination and potential adoption.

It is the role of nursing administration to develop a formalized quality management program that includes a three-pronged focus, based on a classic approach to quality management: (1) review organizational structure, personnel, and environment; (2) focus on standards of nursing care, methods of delivering nursing care (process); and (3)focus on the outcomes of that care (Donabedian, 1985). These formal evaluations include peer review audits (documented care delivered by peers), client satisfaction assessments, review of agency policies and procedures, analysis of demographic information, and the like (Berman, 1988).

Nurses who are new to formal quality management activities in the work setting need to see the value of these efforts and their part in assuring that quality care is being delivered. Direct service providers are the best judges of care problems and their potential solutions. It is critical, then, that quality assurance reviews and other quality improvement activities focus on issues relevant to staff and client concerns and be structured so that they can be accomplished quickly and with minimal effort. When these activities are clear, concise, and well integrated into daily routines, they become less time-consuming. Additionally, staff will clearly see the positive client outcomes as rewards of their contributions to the process. Moreover, when health care providers have

the opportunity to systematically examine the care they provide, and will generate useful ideas for improving that care and identify care issues sooner.

Agencies, whether small or large, are complex organizations with interrelated components. The nursing staff has input into or some control over the quality of care delivered to clients who use the services of the agency. The following is a review the nurse's role in each of the three areas of structure, process, and outcomes.

Structure. The organizational structure and financial stability of the agency should allow the mission statement or philosophy to be realized. The agency should be client focused with sufficient resources to maintain present services and introduce additional services as needed. Public agencies need to operate within budget and also have a well-developed system of acquiring additional funding for new services through grants and contract expansion. Private agencies should operate efficiently enough to realize a profit that encourages the owners and boards of directors to continue to support the services and look for additional ways to solicit clients in addition to employing highly motivated and qualified staff.

Process. The agency should maintain standards set by the professional staff that comply with or surpass those recommended by a variety of accrediting bodies mentioned earlier. The staff is encouraged to contribute to evaluation of the standards and revise them as needed. Staff members need to keep themselves current by attending in-services and acquiring additional education appropriate to their job requirements. The staff works collaboratively with others across disciplines to improve the quality of care given in the community by using a variety of participative management tools (audit instruments, quality circles). The agency is supportive of its staff and the needs of individuals. Staff turnover is minimal because employee values are compatible with the goals of the agency. Administration and staff have a compatible working relationship. A system of quality review is in place and each staff member contributes to this process as a member of a peer review committee or quality improvement or assurance committee. Staff also listens to clients and provides an outlet to evaluate the care received either by questionnaires, surveys, or interviews, and the agency acts on client suggestions and comments.

Outcomes. Standards of care are met or surpassed. Client outcomes are consistent with agency goals and quality care. They are measured against set standards.

Client satisfaction is monitored and a system of improving client satisfaction is part of the agency's agenda.

All services an agency provides should be reviewed periodically to determine whether standards are meeting the present needs of the population and whether the nursing staff is implementing these standards. The nursing services used most frequently, such as well-child care, self-care education with chronically ill adults, or various screening programs, are excellent places to begin the review. Generally these services involve the entire nursing staff and consume a significant amount of nursing care time.

Focusing on commonly served high-risk groups presents an opportunity to optimize care delivery as well as to benefit high-risk clients. Children living in neighborhoods that are known to have high lead toxicity rates from leaded paint in older homes stand to benefit tremendously by a consistently implemented lead screening, treatment, and advocacy program. Without review, such a program may not achieve its goals of decreasing toxic levels of lead in area children.

Incidents of poor client outcome are important areas for further study. Clinics or community health nurses who make home visits can routinely review records of deceased or hospitalized clients to assess whether any aspect of the clinic's care or home visit activities might have prevented these occurrences. For instance, a case of a child with repeated high serum lead levels who requires hospitalization for chelation might stimulate a clinic's examination of the adequacy of parent education on environmental sources of lead. The clinic could also explore the effectiveness of its advocacy with the area's lead-abatement staff to assure needed repairs in leaded homes and the removal of families to safe housing while repairs are being made. It is generally accepted that a sample of 20 randomly selected cases will provide useful information. If the population to be sampled numbers more than 200, some sources recommend that the sample include more than 20 cases.

A nurse who frequently visits older adults who take multiple medications reviews the charts of hospitalized clients to ascertain whether teaching or compliance issues regarding medication contributed to the hospitalization. This may prompt a change in home visit teaching techniques, an increase in the frequency of visits, or a change in vital-sign parameters for notifying a physician. If problems and deficiencies persist, that could be a clue that the nurse needs additional education in this area or that the nurse's caseload is too heavy and therefore exceeds the ability of the nurse to provide minimally expected care. Once the cause is determined, implementation of appropriate changes can commence,

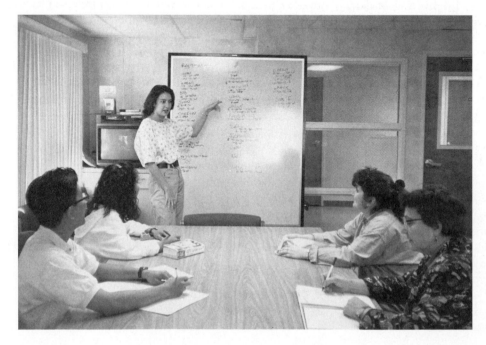

FIGURE 27.6. Quality care is more likely to occur when staff have been thoroughly trained and oriented to the setting and to clients' needs. Here an inservice program is being conducted with community health nursing staff.

after allowing adequate time for the staff to address critical issues. Should additional education be needed, it is the responsibility of the coordinating or in-service nurse to provide or arrange for the needed education (Figure 27.6). Frequently new pieces of equipment, such as beds used for infant phototherapy at home, are manufactured by companies that provide in-services on their products at no cost to the agency.

Given adequate resources, including sufficient time, information, and support, good care is the norm. Occasionally quality-of-care problems result from an individual provider's performance. Recommendations are made for counseling or other type of intervention by that person's supervisor, and appropriate corrective action should be taken to resolve the problem and preserve the employee's job.

Summary

Quality management for community health nursing is vital. It seeks to assure that sufficient health care services are provided in a timely manner and that the services being provided are very likely to produce positive effects on the health and perception of health of those being served. The changing health care climate necessitates that standards come from within the profession of nursing; otherwise, they will be imposed from forces outside of nursing, namely insurers and other purchasers of health care.

Over time, quality management tools have changed, becoming more inclusive and using participative management systems. Standards of practice and client care have been refined and new methodologies have been validated. The models or frameworks on which quality management systems are based include a classic way of looking at programs through organizational structure, process and outcomes, and the interrelatedness of each component. The current use of quality circles is having an impact on the health care arena. These circles provide new ways to involve staff in participative management opportunities.

All services an agency provides should be reviewed periodically to determine whether the current standards are being met. Increasing focus has been placed on quality care indicators, such as client outcomes and client satisfaction, because of the increasing competition among health care providers. Nurses need to define and quantify client outcomes and client satisfaction in order to assess the quality of care being delivered. The goal of care in the community is successful client outcomes. When client care meets the standards set there is greater potential for client satisfaction. Whether quality management techniques are formally or informally practiced, any time nurses monitor, assess, and judge the quality and appropriateness of care as measured against professional standards, the interests of clients are being served.

Activities to Promote Critical Thinking

1. Refer to an existing community health nursing program (home health agency, public health nursing service, or an adult health clinic) in your community and evaluate its quality based on the characteristics of a quality community health program.

2. Using one of the four models for quality management discussed in this chapter, create a quality management program in a community family planning agency. Select another model and create a quality management program in a prenatal clinic.

3. Select a community program with which you are familiar. Identify one topic for study and develop one or more standards and criteria you can use to measure the actual service provided.

4. Using the organizational tools (philosophy, mission, procedures, and protocols) of a community agency, participate in a quality circle with peers to improve an identified area of care an agency provides.

REFERENCES

American Nurses Association. (1986). *Standards: Maternal-child health nursing practice*. Kansas City, MO: Author.

American Nurses Association. (1982). *Credentialing in nursing: Contemporary developments and trends*. Kansas City, MO: Author.

American Nurses Association. (1986a). *Standards of community health nursing practice*. Kansas City, MO: Author.

American Nurses Association. (1986b). *Standards of home health nursing practice*. Kansas City, MO: Author.

American Nurses Association. (1986c). *Community-based nursing services: Innovative models*. Kansas City, MO: Author.

American Nurses Association. (1988). *Peer review guidelines*. Kansas City, MO: Author.

American Nurses Association. (1991). *Nursing's agenda for health care reform*. Kansas City, MO: Author.

Dienemann, J., (Eds.). (1992). *Continuous quality improvement in nursing*. Kansas City, MO: American Nurses Association.

Berman, S. (1988). Quality assurance in ambulatory health care. *Quality Review Bulletin, 13*(1), 18–21.

Bohnet, N. L., Ilcyn, J., Milanovich, P. S., Ream, M. A., & Wright, K. (1993). Continuous quality improvement: Improving quality in your home care organization. *Journal of Nursing Administration 23*(2), 42–48.

Community Health Accreditation Program, Inc. (CHAP). (1993). *Standards of excellence for community health organizations*. New York: author.

Dienemann, J., (Ed.) (1992). Continuous quality improvement in nursing. Kansas City, MO: American Nurses Association.

Donabedian, A. (1966). Evaluating the quality of medical care. *Milbank memorial fund quarterly 44*, 166–206.

Donabedian, A. (1969). Medical care appraisal: Quality and utilization. In *Guide to medical care administration*. New York: American Public Health Association.

Donabedian, A. (1985). *Explorations in quality assessment and monitoring* (Vol. 3). Ann Arbor: Health Administration Press.

Edwards, N., Pickard, L., & Van Berkel, C. (1991). Community health nursing audit: Issues encountered during the selection and application of an audit instrument. *Public Health Nursing, 8*(1), 3–9.

Ellis, J. R., & Hartley, C. L. (1995). *Nursing in today's world: Challenges, issues, and trends*. (5th ed.). Philadelphia: Lippincott.

Griffin, M. (1988). Assumptions for success. *Nursing Management, 19*(1), 32U–32X.

Harvey, G. (1991). An evaluation of approaches to assessing the quality of nursing care using (predetermined) quality assurance tools. *Journal of Advanced Nursing, 16*(3), 277–286.

Herzberg, F., Mauser, B., & Snyderman, B. (1968). *The motivation to work*. New York: John Wiley.

Hoesing, H. & Kirk, R., (1990). Common sense quality management. *Journal of Nursing Administration, 20*(10), 10–15.

Ishikawa, K. (1985). *What is total quality control?* Englewood Cliffs, NJ: Prentice-Hall.

Jenko, M., Gillette, B., & Gonzalez, L. (1990). The development of an evaluation tool for unit-based quality assurance. *Journal of Nursing Quality Assurance, 4*(2), 63–70.

Joint Commission on Accreditation of Health Care Organizations.(1992). *Ambulatory health care standards manual*. Chicago: Author.

Kirk, R. & Hoesing, H. (1991). *The nurses' guide to common sense quality management*. West Dundee, IL: S-N Publications.

Maslow, A. (1954). *Motivation and personality*. New York: Harper & Row.

Megivern, K, Halm, M. A., & Jones, G.(1992). Measuring patient satisfaction as an outcome of nursing care. *Journal of Nursing Care Quality, 6*(4), 9–24.

Mitchell, P. R. & Grippando, G. M. (1993). *Nursing perspectives and issues* (5th ed.). Albany: Delmar Publishers.

Morgan, G. (1983). *Beyond method: Strategies for social research*. Beverly Hills: Sage.

Nadzam, D. (1991). The agenda for change: Update on indicator development and possible implications for the nursing profession. *Journal of Nursing Quality Assurance, 5*(2), 18–22.

O'Brien, B.& McHugh, M. (1994). Quality circles: One organization's experience. *Journal of Nursing Care Quality, 8*(4), 20–24.

Ouchi, W. G. (1981). *Theory Z*. Reading, MA: Addison-Wesley.

Peters, D. A. (1992). A new look for quality in home care. *Journal of Nursing Administration, 22*(11), 21–26.

Peterson, G. (1991). Computer-assisted quality assurance. *ANNA Journal, 16*(3), 288–290.

Phaneuf, M. C. (1976). *The nursing audit and self-regulation in nursing practice*. New York: Appleton-Century-Crofts.

Reeder, P. J. & Chen, S. C. (1990). A client satisfaction survey in home health care. *Journal of Nursing Quality Assurance, 5*(1), 16–24.

Robinson, K. & Fitzgerald, M. (1990). A staff-centered approach. *Nursing Times, 86*(14), 42–43.

Sainfort, F., Ramsey, J. D., Ferreira, P. L., & Mezghani, L.(1994). A first step in total quality management of nursing facility care: Development of an empirical causal model of structure, process and outcome dimensions. *American Journal of Medical Quality, 9*(2), 74–86.

Schmele, J. A., Allen, M. E., Butler, S., & Gresham, D. (1991). Quality circles in the public health sector: Implementation and effect. *Public Health Nursing, 8*(3), 190–195.

Stewart, M. J. & Craig, D. (1987). Adaptation of the nursing audit to community health nursing. Nursing Forum. 23(4), 134–144.

Taylor, A. G., Hudson, K., & Keeling, A. (1991). Quality nursing care: The consumers' perspective revisited. *Journal of Nursing Quality Assurance, 5*(2), 23–31.

Toms, E. C. (1992). Evaluating the quality of patient care in district nursing. *Journal of Advanced Nursing. 17*, 1489–1495.

Vance, M. (1991, October 30) *Management by Values Seminar.* National Association of Home Care. Tenth Annual Meeting. Boston, MA.

Williams, A. D. (1991). Development and application of clinical indicators for nursing. *Journal Of Nursing Care Quality, 6*(1), 1–5.

Zlotnick, C. (1992). A public health quality assurance system. *Public Health Nursing, 9*(2), 133–137.

SELECTED READINGS

Al-Assaf. A. F. & Schmele, J. A. (Eds.). (1993). *The textbook of total quality in healthcare*. New York: National League for Nursing.

Ammentrop, W., Gossett, K., & Poe, N. (1992). *Quality assurance for long-term care providers*. Newbury Park, CA: Sage Publications.

Barry, T. L. (1994). Computer support for continuous quality improvement. *Journal For Healthcare Quality, 16*(2), 16–17, 40.

Bower, D., L. Linc, & D. Denega. (1988). *Evaluation instruments in nursing*. (Pub. No. 15-2178). New York: National League for Nursing.

Bower, K. A. (1992). *Case management by nurses*. Kansas City, Mo.: American Nurses Association.

Bull, M. (1994). Patients' and professionals' perceptions of quality in discharge planning. *Journal of Nursing Care Quality, 8*(2), 47–61.

Davis, E. R. (1994). *Total quality management for home care*. Gaithersburg, MD.: Aspen Publishers, Inc.

Enthoven, A. C.(1993). Why managed care has failed to contain health costs. *Health Affairs. 12*(3), 27–43.

Farren, E. (1991). Effects of early discharge planning on length of hospital stay. *Nursing Economics, 9*(1), 25–30.

Frost, M. H. (1992). Quality: A concept of importance to nursing. *Journal of Nursing Care Quality, 7*(1), 64–69.

Grossman, D. & Neubauer, J. (1992) Basic statistical concepts in quality improvement. *Journal of Nursing Care Quality, 6*(4), 1–8.

Hicks, L. L., Stallmeyer, J. M., & Coleman, J. R. (1993). *Role of the nurse in managed care*. Kansas City, MO: American Nurses Association.

Holmes, C. A. (1989) Health care and the quality of life: A review. *Journal of Advanced Nursing, 14*(10), 833–839.

Hough, B. L., & Schmele, J. A. (1987). The Slater scale: A viable method for monitoring nursing care quality in home health. *Journal of Nursing Quality Assurance, 1*(3), 28–38.

Joint Commission for Accreditation of Healthcare Organizations. (1992). *Accreditation manual for hospitals*. Chicago: Author.

Jones, D. J., & Ziegenfuss, J. T. (1993) The administrative and clinical rationale for the total organization approach to continuous improvement. *Quality Assurance Utilization Review, 8*, 112.

Joy, L. (1993). On the road to quality: A view of the journey. *Journal of Nursing Care Quality, 7*(4), 32–38.

Kelly, M. P., Bacon, G. T., & Mitchell, J. A. (1994). Glossary of managed care terms. *Journal of Ambulatory Care Management, 17*(1), 70–76.

Kemp, N. & Richardson, E. (1994) *The nursing process and quality care*. San Diego: Singular Publishing Group.

Kenyon, V., Smith, E., Vig Hefty, L., Bell, M. L., McNeil, J., & Martaus, T. (1990). Clinical competencies for community health nursing. *Public Health Nursing. 7*(1), 33–39.

Lang, N. M. & Marek, K. D. (1991) The policy and politics of patient outcomes. *Journal of Nursing Quality Assurance 5*(2), 7–12.

Lopresti, J. & Whetstone, W. R. (1993). Total quality management: Doing things right. *Nursing Management, 24*, 34–36.

McGuffin, B. (1990). Clinical nursing standards: Toward a synthesis. *Journal of Nursing Quality Assurance, 4*(3), 35–45.

Peters, D. A. (1991). Measuring quality: Inspection or opportunity? *Holistic Nursing Practice, 5*(3), 1–7.

Peters, D. A., & Eigsti, D. M. (1991). In search of excellence: The personnel issue of the future. *Caring, 10*(4), 12–15.

Peters, D. A., & Eigsti, D. M. (1991) Utilizing outcomes in home care. *Caring, 10*(10), 44–45.

Phillips, C. (1991). Developing a method of assessing quality of care in nursing homes, using key indicators and population norms. *Journal of Aging Health, 3*, 407–422.

Rinke, L. T., & Wilson A. A. (Eds.). (1987). *Outcome measures in home care: Research and Service* (Vols. 1 & 2). New York: National League for Nursing.

Roberts, J. & Schyve, P. (1990, May). QA to QI: The views and role of the Joint Commission. *Quality Letter,* 9–12.

Smith-Marker, C. G. (1988). Practical tools for quality assurance: Criteria development sheet and data retrieval form. *Journal of Nursing Quality Assurance, 2*(2), 43–54.

Ulrich, B. (1992). *Leadership and management according to Florence Nightingale*. Norwalk, CN: Appleton & Lange.

Warren, B. H. (1994). An outcomes analysis approach to utilization management: Quality assessment of appropriateness of specialty referrals. *American College of Medical Quality. 9*(1), 34–38.

Zinn, J. S., Aaronson, W. E., & Rosko, M. D. (1993). The use of standardized indicators as quality improvement tools: an application in Pennsylvania nursing homes. *American Journal of Medical Quality. 8*:72–78.

CHAPTER

28

Health Policy, Politics, and Community Health Advocacy

LEARNING OBJECTIVES

Upon completion of this chapter readers should be able to:

- Define health policy and explain how it is established.
- Analyze the influence of health policy on community health and nursing practice.
- Explain the role of special interest groups in health care reform and policy making.
- Identify the four stages in the policy process and briefly explain what each entails.
- Define political empowerment and describe ways in which community health nurses can become politically empowered.
- Explain the role of community health nurses in determining a community's health policy needs.
- Identify the ten steps in mobilizing a community for political action.
- Describe the steps involved in how a bill becomes law.
- Explain several methods of communicating with legislators on policy issues.
- List at least four political strategies for community health nursing.

KEY TERMS

- Community health advocacy
- Distributive health policy
- Health policy
- Health policy outcomes
- Lobbying
- Polarization
- Policy
- Policy analysis

- Policy system
- Political action
- Political action committee (PAC)
- Political empowerment
- Politics
- Public policy
- Regulatory health policy
- Special interest group

Barbara Walton Spradley and Judith Ann Allender
COMMUNITY HEALTH NURSING: CONCEPTS AND PRACTICE, 4th ed.
© 1996 Barbara Walton Spradley and Judith Ann Allender

Many community health nurses have a vision of health care that is more accessible, equitable, cost effective, and quality oriented than the present system. However, nurses must recognize that vision alone is not enough. For a myriad of reasons nurses have had a difficult time just making policy makers recognize the value of nursing's input, not to mention their vital role in providing essential health care services. Although most nurses recognize their role as essential providers of health care, many still do not understand the importance of health policy and politics in relation to their practice or to community health.

Behind all legislation and health care regulation there are power struggles. The outcomes of these struggles determine the availability and quality of all social services. Only the naive think that others will be persuaded by the facts alone. There are social and political factions at work, special interest groups, and business and industry—each bringing their power into play in these struggles and decision making. Clearly, nurses need to develop an operational knowledge of health policy and political process in order to protect individuals, families, communities, and their nursing practice.

Fortunately, nursing's interest and representation in public affairs is growing. Nurses are competing successfully for fellowships in public policy such as the Robert Wood Johnson Health Policy Fellows Program and the Kellog National Fellowship Program. In 1992, Eddie Bernie Johnson, RN (Texas) became the first nurse to be elected to the US House of Representatives. She was one of nine nurses who ran for the 103rd Congress (Mason, et al., 1993).

This chapter examines health policy, the political process involved in determining health policy, and community health nursing's role in the process. The underlying bias is that community health nurses should not only provide input to policy circles, but should be leaders who sit at the decision-making tables. The purpose is to emphasize the need for community health nurses to understand their role and power in providing an essential influence and unique perspective in health care.

What is Policy?

Policy is an authoritatively stated course of action that guides decision making. It is how an institution, organization, agency, or government exercises its authority; it is based on that group's goals, and it exists to provide guidelines for operation (Stimpson & Hanley, 1991). Policy can (and should) be written, formally, but many policies are unwritten, unclear, or "hidden" to prevent public or legal review. Government policy, whether the government is local, state, or federal, that makes decisions affecting the public is **public policy** (Dye, 1992).

Policies attempt to express the collective interests and beliefs of the social system or institution that generates them. Public policy usually comes about because policy makers perceive that something is not functioning as it should or the political pressure is so great that a change is mandated. The something needing change can be as large and complex as the health care system or as small and simple as a local agency's title. It should be noted, however, that the latter will not be perceived as small and simple by those with a vested interest in the title. Regardless, a policy is made because the perceived benefits outweigh the perceived costs, at least to the decision makers (Harrington & Estes, 1994).

Policies are enforced by the agency or organization for whom they were created. For example, noncompliance with employment policies in a health care agency may mean termination of services; violation of a government policy, such as illegally selling drugs, may mean paying a fine or imprisonment. Public policy is backed by law.

All public policy is inextricably linked to economics. Harrington and Estes (1994) state, "The growth of the medical-industrial complex (our health care system) . . . is driven by economic conditions and profit motives as well as a political climate that promotes competition" (p.xii). Policy problems come about because a policy, to a great extent, determines who gets what in a society or institution.

In other words, policy problems occur because resources are being redistributed resulting in some receiving a greater share and others receiving less.

Health Policy

Health policy is about health care choices (Mason, et al., 1993), and should reflect a community's values. However, the power to make policy decisions for any community is spread among a number of stakeholders (anyone with a vested interest) who may not live in the community. Because there are so many people with vested interests in the health care system, it is unlikely that anyone can know the real and full impact of a health policy on any one community until after its implementation.

Health policy is any policy that constitutes the governing framework (structure, process, outcomes) for providing health services on a local, state, national, or even international level. Structure is the number and types of agencies, programs and services, as well as providers and targeted clients. Process is how the agencies, programs and services are going to be provided, managed and funded, and how clients are to receive services. **Health policy outcomes** are the actual consequences of a health policy being implemented and are described in terms of effectiveness, efficiency, equity, innovativeness, and empowerment. Figure 28.1 outlines health policy from this perspective.

The passage of health care legislation at the federal and state levels ultimately leads to the formulation and implementation of health policy at a local level. For example, the Omnibus Budget Reconciliation Act (OBRA) of 1993 recognized the Vaccines for Children (VFC) program as a critical need. As a result, the President's Childhood Immunization Initiative (CII), a nationwide effort to vaccinate all children in the United States, was implemented in October 1994. This federal health policy provides guidelines and resources by combining the efforts of both public and private health care providers at a local level to vaccinate children, regardless of ability to pay.

Theoretically, health policy should empower the community for which it is intended. But often conflict can arise over empowerment when one community's empowerment threatens the values of another. For example, there is much conflict and argument over the controversial policies regarding the government funding of abortions for low income women. Some community groups oppose this policy, arguing that it violates the greater policy of preserving life, while other groups support it saying that it protects and promotes the overall health of the community. Such conflict dilutes the empowering ability of a given health policy.

Health policy also empowers the health care provider by deeming the provider's services as essential, subsidizing the provider's education, and directly reimbursing the provider. Because health policy affects a community's health status and determines who will be reimbursed for what by whom, politics are involved at every step of its development, implementation, and evaluation. When health policy fails to provide a workable framework at the community level, the health care needs of communities are not met in a cost effective manner. The Medicare Catastrophic Coverage Act of 1988, which was repealed in 1989, is a reminder that the intent of a policy may not be its outcome. The policy intent reflected by this bill was to provide significant

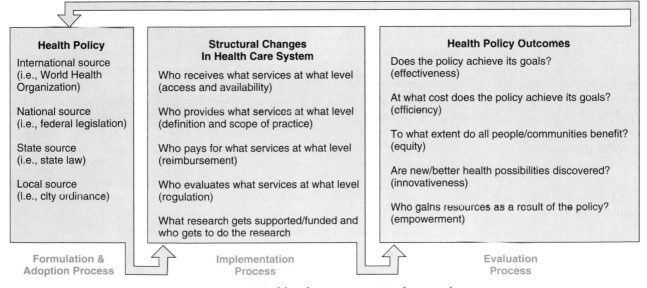

FIGURE 28.1. Health policy as a governing framework.

expansion of Medicare benefits, including coverage of outpatient prescription drug costs and home health benefits, but its repeal defeated the assistance this bill would have provided to the Medicare population.

Health policies can be distributive or regulatory. **Distributive health policy** promotes nongovernmental activities thought to be beneficial to society as a whole. An example of a distributive policy is the Nurse Training Act, Title VIII of the Public Health Service Act established in 1965, which provided federal subsidy for nursing education to address the need for a greater supply of nurses. Redistributive health policy changes the allocation of resources from one group to usually a broader or different group. Medicare is an example of redistributive policy in that provisions under Medicare expanded to provide a broader range of benefits and coverage to needy groups.

Regulatory health policy is policy that attempts to control the allocation of resources by directing those agencies or persons who offer resources or provide public services. For example, there are government regulations that set standards for licensure of health care organizations, such as hospitals, and health care providers, such as nurses. Public health often uses regulatory policy to protect the health of the community (McLeroy, et al, 1988).

Regulatory policy can be further categorized as either competitive or protective. Competitive regulation limits, or structures, the provision of health services by designating who can deliver them. Protective regulation sets conditions under which various private activities can be undertaken. Although professional licensure is most commonly identified by professions as primarily protecting the public, such policy is competitive regulation in terms of its social impact. Protective regulation is more clearly evident in utilization review organizations (regulatory bodies that critically examine health agency utilization patterns) or certificates of need (the legal requirement for a potential provider agency to demonstrate the need for its services before a license to practice is granted).

Health Policy Debate and Interest Groups

Health policy debate revolves around central issues such as overall cost of health care reform, the amount of control the federal government will exercise over the entire health care system, and the extent to which vari-

ous individuals and groups, including nurses, will be harmed by reform or perceive they will be harmed by reform. Any policy involving the redistribution of income will be opposed most vigorously by those affected most negatively. If a group perceives they will have to pay more for health care coverage they will attempt to block passage (Elwood, 1993/1994).

The most significant obstacles to the passage of effective health care legislation today are special interest groups and partisan politics. A **special interest group** is any group of people sharing a common goal which is politically active in attempting to influence policy formation to be in support of their goal. Policy solutions are, more often than not, eliminated by the outcry of politically motivated special interest groups. These interest groups come in many forms whether business groups, labor groups, neighborhood groups, minority groups, religious groups, environmental groups or even nursing specialty groups. The American Medical Association (AMA), the tobacco industry and the National Rifle Association (NRA) constitute three of the most powerful forces in the United States today influencing policy decisions. The impact of these three organizations on health services delivery, on continuing the ill effects of smoking and tobacco use, and on control of gun ownership contributing to high death and injury statistics is immeasureable. Interest groups employ many tactics to influence policy decisions, including public hearings, campaigns, litigation, protest, public relations, and especially lobbying (Christensen, 1995). **Lobbying** is the process by which an individual or group acts on the behalf of others to influence specific decisions of policy makers, such as legislators. Many special interest groups and organizations employ one or more full-time lobbyists to represent their interests. These individuals work behind the scenes to influence policy makers through informal sessions and written communication in addition to attending hearings and giving public testimony.

The four most powerful interest groups in health care have been physicians, hospitals, insurance companies, and the drug industry (Lee & Estes, 1994). Physicians recognized the implications and consequences of health policy in relation to their profession decades ago and have become increasingly empowered through most of this century. Medicine's strong social and political influence is the result of many factors, among them a strong professional organization (the AMA), active political lobbying for their interests, and formation of strategic coalitions with respected individuals and scientific groups.

POLICY, POLITICS, AND COMMUNITY HEALTH NURSING

Nursing has become a much stronger political voice in recent years and is learning to build strategic alliances and power bases. Health policy provides the conditions for empowering or disempowering certain groups in a variety of ways. (See the World Watch discussion that follows.) Community health nurses must understand that power is an essential and primary concept inherent to all political and policy systems. A power base can be created through collaboration, cooperation, and communication (Vance, 1993). Nurses have to negotiate and compromise with other interest groups to be politically effective. By forming strong health care coalitions, nurses gain a stronger voice in policy decisions affecting them and their clients.

Politics is inherent in any system where resources are absolutely or relatively scarce and where there are competing interests for those resources. **Politics** is an interactive process of influencing others to make decisions that favor (or at least do not threaten) a person's or group's chosen position and the allocation of scarce resources to support that position. (Mason, et al., 1993). For example, nursing's increasing influence on federal research development and funding policies is demonstrated by the National Center for Nursing Research (NCNR) being funded for $63,531,000 in 1994, compared to Allied Health's $3,467,000 (Elwood, 1993/1994).

The health care system is governed through complex interactions among different government representatives, health professionals, consumers, third party payers, and employers who may not agree upon each other's roles and jurisdiction in health care. These groups use politics to survive, as well as to pursue their respective health care goals. "There is no single source of governance or health policy, nor is there a single set of shared values or goals among these groups; the health care system is an amalgamation of many different agendas" (The Pew Health Professions Commission, 1991, p. 55). The significance of politics in the government is demonstrated by the fact that literally thousands of legislative bills are drafted each year yet only a few are ever signed into law. Although the political system within a local community may be less formalized, it has a profound influence on the collective health and well-being of its residents.

In the past, public policy primarily has restricted nurses in three related ways—scope of practice limitations, exclusionary definitions, and limits on eligibility for reimbursement. Although most community health nursing services constitute primary care by being first contact, continuous, comprehensive, and coordinated (Selker, 1994), most health policy definitions of primary care exclude community health nurses as providers of primary care. As a result community health nurses are not paid directly for their services, require physician supervision and have responsibilities that exceed their legal authority.

It is a major problem when health policy does not recognize nurses as providing reimbursable health care services or primary care services in any community context (Griffith, 1993). The exclusion of nurses, other than nurse practitioners, in primary care legislation and

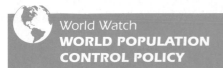

World Watch
WORLD POPULATION CONTROL POLICY

Population growth world-wide is increasing at an alarming rate. Currently world population is 5.6 billion people and is projected to rise to 10 billion (with some projections reaching 12.5 billion) by the year 2050 (UNICEF, 1995). What contributes to this growth and how can it be slowed?

The International Conference on Population and Development which met in Cairo, Egypt, in 1994, debated these questions. Drawing on research from the past 20 years, the Cairo Conference concluded that the solution to population growth lies in women having greater control of their own lives and their fertility. Dr. Nafis Sadik, Executive Director of the the United Nations Population Fund stated, "Empowerment of individual women, opening a wider range of choice for both women and men, . . . may be the key to social development, including the resolution of population problems, in the rest of the century and beyond" (Ibid., p. 15).

Global public health policy must target reduced levels of abortion and maternal mortality, universal availability of family planning services in all countries, progress in child health and survival, raised levels of women's education, and greater progress toward gender equality. Such a comprehensive approach could slow population growth, meet women's basic rights and needs, and begin to promote a sustainable future.

health policy statements, practically eliminates the possibility of community health nurses receiving direct fees for services or even practicing unless under the "direct" supervision of a physician. Community health nurses should be one of the major sources of influence (Courtney, 1987; Stimpson & Hanley, 1991), even though many strong and well-organized forces resist nursing's direct involvement in the politics and policy making of health care.

In spite of health policy restrictions on reimbursement and scope of practice, the demand for community health services is stronger than ever. Community health nursing has grown in part because many areas were abandoned or delegated by physicians, such as home- and community-based ambulatory care, and primary care. Finally, the importance and impact of quality community health care is receiving the national and political focus it deserves. In its conclusions the Pew Health Professions Commission 1993 report lists 17 competencies for future health care practitioners such as the need to care for the community's health, emphasize primary care, expand access to effective care, practice prevention, involve clients and families in the decision-making process, promote healthy lifestyles, understand the role of the physical environment, accommodate expanded accountability, and participate in a racially and culturally diverse society. Clearly, these are competencies that have long been expected of community health nurses.

Changes in federal health policy may present an opportunity to revisit the wisdom of giving community health nurses authority consistent with their actual practice. Commonly stated goals of health care reform are to provide more services to more people at a lesser cost. Community health nurses are well-positioned to provide these services.

No practicing nurse can escape politics whether it be in the workplace or in the context of local, state, and federal government. However, there are still many social and professional barriers in place that hinder nurses from becoming a unified, powerful political force. Fragmented communication patterns isolate individual nurses and prevent them from interacting around issues of health policy beyond their immediate work environment. Also, tight resources limit opportunities and strain nurse relationships in the work environment. Finally, prevailing methods of evaluation and reward in the work place often undermine attempts to create an environment more conducive to political involvement of nurses beyond their workplace issues. The extent to which political thinking and behavior is valued, supported and fostered within one's nursing practice arena is critical to the profession's future.

Community health nurses need to learn to effectively manage their immediate work environment and be able to participate in the context of a larger political system to support quality health care. They must work to create a supportive health care culture that encourages frequent interaction among the various constituencies. Political involvement is an important means to achieve this goal. They must understand that community health nurses, like all people, may hold significantly different or conflicting opinions about theory, methods, and the direction of health care. These differences should be aired and debated to promote dialogue and creative solutions to health care problems. Community health nurses face an unparalleled opportunity to influence health policy through political involvement (Vance, 1993).

THE NEED FOR HEALTH CARE REFORM

Although the United States' health care system has been remarkably successful with advances in practice, education, technology, and facilities over the past 50 years, today there is great demand and need for change in the health care system at the federal policy level. All the advances and new technology have come at a very high price. Furthermore, inflation has compounded the problem, so the United States is spending an extraordinary and disproportinate amount of its national income on health care.

"Far and away, the most troubling issue in health care is the growing aggregate cost and the seemingly disproportionate share of income that we pay for care when compared to other nations" (Pew, 1991, p.5). "By virtually all measures, U.S. health spending is the highest in the world" (Harrington & Estes, 1994, p. 36). Today, annual health care expenses are approaching one trillion dollars ($1,000,000,000,000).

There are also problems with accessibility of health care to certain segments of the population. Despite the enormous cost, 15% of the U.S. population (36 million) have no health insurance at all. Another 60 million are under-insured, although most are employed. One in four pregnant women receives no pre-natal care, and 43% of toddlers go without recommended vaccinations. These figures suggest why the United States ranks 21st in the world in infant mortality, and 16th in the world in life expectancy (Pelka, 1993).

President Clinton re-energized the health care debate by making health care reform a major theme of his 1992 presidential campaign and a primary goal of his administration. The proposed Clinton plan (the Health Security Act of 1993) was supposed to provide quality health care to everyone, regardless of ability to pay, while curbing the disastrous rise in medical costs. This legislation stirred national debate and controversy and ultimately was defeated in 1994. Its defeat demonstrates the complexities of health care reform at the federal level and the influence of partisan politics and special interests of business and labor, the insurance industry, government and education, health care providers and consumers. Although Starr (1982) stated that health care reform will be elusive, "As long as opposing interests remain sufficiently strong to block almost any coherent course of action, conservative or progressive" (p. 411); the fiscal need for health care reform may be the driving force that will eventually overcome whatever resistance exists.

One group with an enormous stake in health care reform is the disability community. People with disabilities are a population with great health care needs and most likely to be uninsured or under-insured (Watson, 1993). The current U.S. system spends enormous sums on nursing homes and hospitals, and very little on outpatient, home health, preventive care or on personal assistance services (Pelka, 1993). It is the latter services that the disability community needs most.

The challenge for United States health care reform into the next century is to reduce costs and increase accessibility. Figure 28.2 shows the uninsured who will help drive health care reform. What is needed is change from the present uncoordinated system to a consolidated health services delivery system that is accountable for costs, quality, and outcomes (Foster, 1994). Strategically, enhancing quality health care and reducing health care costs are the primary yardsticks for any health policy. Community health professionals must work to convince the political players that the health of the community is directly tied to quality health services, accessibility, and reasonable costs.

POLITICAL EMPOWERMENT AND PROFESSIONAL ORGANIZATIONS

Because politics is an inherent part of any professional organization's operations, it is through participation in organizations that many nurses develop and refine their political skills. A strong professional organization offers a more collective diversity and realistic

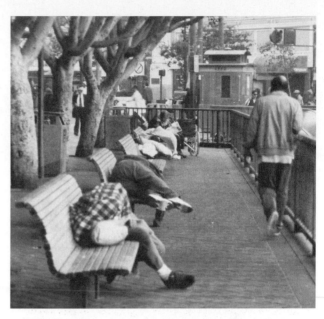

FIGURE 28.2. Increasing numbers of homeless people contribute to the alarming numbers of medically uninsured in the United States.

forum for political issues and debate and for enhancing a nurse's visibility. Leaders of professional organizations sit on decision-making boards, influence public policy, and define priorities for their communities. Professional organizations become seats of political empowerment. **Political empowerment** is a conscious state in which an individual, group, or organization becomes recognizably influential in determining policy. The nurse who is visible and influential in professional organizations can raise community awareness and mobilize community support (Decker & Sullivan, 1992).

Professional organizations come under fire by people outside their membership. Some feel professional organizations are nothing more than efforts to carve out turf or claim dominion at the expense of others. Morrison claims, "professional associations . . . have sought to control professional accreditation programs, to establish and maintain rigid scopes of practice that preserve professional monopolies, and to restrict the use of professionals in the work place through control of facility licensure and accreditation schemes"(p. 8, 1993).

Regardless of criticisms, professional organizations provide a critical mechanism for nurses to be collectively empowered. One nurse's opinions may not be recognized nor would one nurse have the resources to promote a cause, but several thousand nurses together could. Effective nursing organizations monitor governmental regulations and lobby public officials on a regular basis. They also work together to influence how the public views nursing, to set standards for nursing practice, and to participate in interdisciplinary efforts to shape public policy (Decker & Sullivan, 1992). An example is *Nursing's Agenda for Health Care Reform* (ANA, 1994) which has been endorsed by over 40 professional nursing organizations. This document, presented to legislators and many others, has raised national consciousness and given nursing a strong voice in shaping health reform.

Personal politics, as much as any other factor, sharpens conflict among individual nurses and makes communication difficult. The pursuit of personal agendas over the common good results in a piecemeal approach to problems and promotes polarization. **Polarization** is the process by which a group is seriously split into two or more factions over a political issue. Polarization can be so intense that people perceive each other as good or wicked depending upon their ideological opinion. One of the primary goals of a professional nursing association is to build a collective voice for nurses. A strong professional association limits polarization by developing the political skills of its members and insuring that its structure and processes equitably meet the needs of its constituencies.

Policy Systems and Policy Analysis

A **policy system** is an entity that receives input from external sources and has legal authority to generate or revise policies governing or managing the constituents it represents. Policy systems, such as city and county governments, are interrelated, complex, and highly political and receive input from many sources such as voters, lobbyists, special interest groups, and the media. Policy systems produce an output by generating policy that in turn determines feedback for subsequent policy decisions. Their boundaries are defined by their legal authority to make only certain types of policy decisions at a particular level. Ideally, policy systems revise or make policy (output) based on comprehensive, accurate information (input) from a variety of sources, including feedback from all constituencies being affected by the policy.

Community health nurses need a simple policy analysis framework to be effective in any practice arena. Nurses use the framework for determining the intentions and possible capacity of policy systems governing their practice, as well as her community. This framework allows nurses to protect themselves and, most important, to protect clients, whether families or groups.

Policy analysis is the systematic identification of causes or consequences of policy and the factors that influence it (Litman & Robins, 1991). Often nurses confuse policy advocacy with policy analysis. This mistake can be detrimental in community health nursing. Policy advocacy is subjective; policy analysis should be objective. What is most important is that policy analysis should come before policy advocacy.

Nurses can take several approaches when analyzing a policy, such as mandatory preschool immunizations, that affects the health of a community or target population. They can look at the reasons for policy formulation, the groups of people affected by the policy, or the policy's possible long-range consequences. When analyzing policy, nurses need to answer two general questions: (1) Who benefits from this policy? and (2) Who loses from this policy? Whether or not the policy should be advocated by the community as a whole depends upon the degree to which the policy benefits the community without being detrimental to individuals or the country.

Figure 28.3 provides a simple model for studying health policy. If nurses know something about the forces shaping health policy and the policy process, then they are in a better position to influence policy outcomes. The model identifies four major stages in the policy process: formulation, adoption, implementation, and evaluation. Policy formulation involves identifying goals, problems, and potential solutions. Policy adoption involves the authorized selection and specification of means to achieve goals, resolve problems, or both. Implementation follows adoption and occurs when the policy is put to use. Policy evaluation means comparing policy outcomes or effects with the intended or desired effects.

STAGE 1 AND 2: POLICY FORMULATION AND ADOPTION

Health policy formulation is the stage at which a policy is conceptualized and ultimately defined. It is approached in at least two ways. Most commonly, a health problem is identified, such as the increased infant mor-

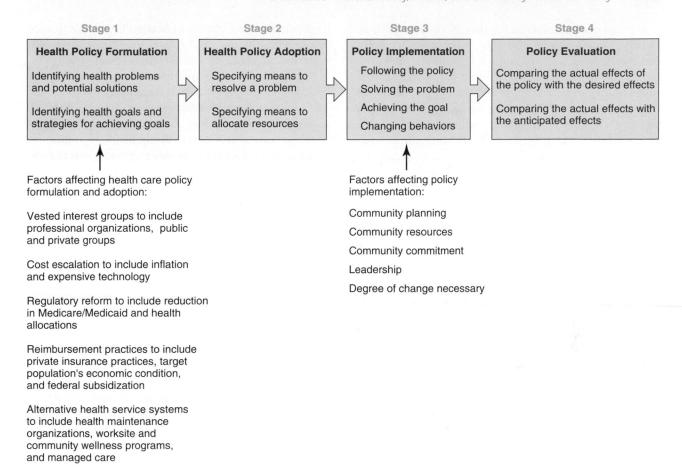

FIGURE 28.3. Policy analysis model. Policy analysis examines the entire process to determine (1) who benefits from the policy and (2) who loses from the policy.

tality rate associated with teenage pregnancy. Health policy is developed to correct the particular health problem. Another approach to policy formulation emphasizes health planning more than corrective actions, at least initially. This is a goal-oriented approach. Health goals and strategies for achieving the goals are identified. In this more proactive approach, resources may be created as well as allocated for health services. Whereas both approaches to policy formulation may lead to the solution of a health problem, the goal-oriented approach is less reactive in that it does not require problem identification before the making of health policy.

The social and political conditions that affect policy formulation are limitless, but public need and public demand should be the strongest influences (Hancock, et al., 1985). Health care providers can stimulate a community to identify its health needs and demand health policies to fulfill its needs. During this process the com-

munity health nurse should recognize that each community is unique, with its own mix of health services and public expectations.

STAGE 3: POLICY IMPLEMENTATION

Implementation of health policy occurs when an individual, group, or community puts the policy into use. It involves overt behavior changes as the policy is put into nursing practice. The degree and extent of compliance with a policy is the most direct measure of the policy's implementation (Harrington & Estes, 1994). Noncompliance refers to conscious or unconscious refusal to follow the policy directives. Community health nurses have always been health policy implementers and, recently, evaluators, regardless of whether these roles were consciously chosen.

Implementation of health policy is an essential part of effective, comprehensive client care for many documentable reasons. It should now be apparent that policies come in many forms and may have statutory or nonstatutory origins. Nurses are most cognizant of the latter in the form of procedure manuals and institutional guidelines. Communities are most aware of policies that limit or restructure their activities and growth, such as curfews and zoning regulations.

Once a health policy is written and adopted, its successful implementation depends heavily upon the manipulation of many variables. For example, the implementation of day-care standards depends, in part, on how they are interpreted and what resources are available to enforce them. The community health nurse as an implementer assesses the capacity of the community to formulate and define strategies that will enhance the community's compliance with the policy. This phase of policy analysis does not focus on the merits or shortcomings of the policy as is done in policy formulation, adoption, and evaluation.

STAGE 4: POLICY EVALUATION

Comparing what a policy does with what it is supposed to do is evaluation. Evaluation of a policy should result in continuance of the policy in its original form, revision or modification of the policy, or termination of the policy. Laws and policies are created to express the collective and powerful interests of the political system that generated them (Litman & Robins, 1991). The need for a particular health policy may be temporary, but a policy is difficult to change once adopted and implemented. Once a policy system is in operation, vested interests evolve as a result and become political influences. These vested interests under the guise of jobs, positions, titles, and wealth are perceptibly jeopardized by any change in the health policy that helped create them. Hence, tradition in the form of old policies tends to prevail.

One form of policy evaluation examines the health outcomes believed to be attributable to the health policy. Indicators such as mortality and morbidity statistics are used. Yet how the outcomes are defined and measured is highly political and more subjective than many recognize. For example, mortality statistics are often treated as objective data yet how statistics are collected can often render them more subjective. For example, if driving under the influence of alcohol or drugs data are not included in deaths from motor vehicle accidents, or

if smoking data is left out in deaths from lung cancers, this information is inadequate and policy decisions based on such data may be seriously misdirected.

Perhaps the major premise that should underlie policy evaluation is that the goal of health policy is to design a system whereby health services are equitably distributed and appropriate care is given to the right people at a reasonable cost (Donley, 1982; Stimpson & Hanley, 1991). This premise leads to the following basic criteria for evaluation:

1. Are the health services appropriate?
2. Are the health services accessible?
3. Are the health services comprehensive?
4. Is there continuity of care?
5. Is the quality of the services adequate?
6. Is the efficiency of the services adequate?
7. Is there an ongoing evaluation of the services?
8. Is appropriate action taken based on the findings of the evaluation?

Regardless of the factors that affect policy evaluation, continual comparison between what a community believes about and wants in health care with what it is getting is necessary. Nurses have a responsibility to increase community awareness of health issues. They help the community make sure that its health needs are met through productive, desirable health policies.

Community Health Advocacy

The health of a nation stems from the health of its communities, and nurses have a solid tradition in serving the community's needs (Pew Commission, 1993; Shoultz, et al., 1992). Nurses improve the quality of health services through community health advocacy. Advocacy, as defined in Chapter 5, refers to the community health nurse's role of pleading the cause of or working on behalf of others. **Community health advocacy** refers to efforts aimed at creating awareness of and generating support for meeting the community's health needs. Both nurses and communities have a common goal, and that is the best possible health services for all. The community health nurse helps communities achieve this goal by being politically active, as well as providing effective health programs. As an advocate the nurse works directly with community constituencies to support vulnerable groups such as low-income families, children, and the elderly. For example, community health advocacy might mean creating public awareness of the needs of battered women and exerting pressure on policy makers to provide protective legislation or it might mean demonstrating the effectiveness of early intervention. See the Research in Community Health Nursing discussion below.

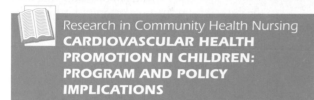

Research in Community Health Nursing
CARDIOVASCULAR HEALTH PROMOTION IN CHILDREN: PROGRAM AND POLICY IMPLICATIONS

Harrell, J.S. & Frauman, A.C. (1994). Cardiovascular health promotion in children: program and policy implications. *Public Health Nursing, 11*(4), 236–241.

Community health nurses need information about health conditions in order to promote sound public health policy. For this reason, ongoing research is needed to provide the essential knowledge for program and policy decisions (Raudonis & Griffith, 1991).

This study examined cardiovascular disease (CVD) risk factors in children. Since CVD is the leading cause of death in the United States and has contributed significantly to rising health care costs, to determine the presence of risk factors in childhood could provide information for early intervention at a time of forming life-long habits. The investigators conducted a state-wide study in North Carolina of 2209 children ages 8 to 11 years enrolled in 21 urban and rural schools. They studied the presence of risk factors such as obesity (rural children were at greater risk), poverty (poor children were at greater risk due to less access to and use of health services), eating habits (poor children had less adequate diets), smoking (more black children had smoked and had parents that smoked than white children), and exercise tolerance (children in coastal regions were at greater risk suggesting need for better exercise programs in those schools). The investigators concluded that prevention of heart disease can and should start with children and suggested a number of recommendations for program and policy development.

This recognition of a community's rights in determining its health policies inherently involves conflict. Nurses as community advocates are under pressure to define specific goals, delegate or implement actions to achieve these goals, and to establish controls to see that a community moves toward these goals. Sometimes specific health goals prove elusive or they have no validity save that they are agreed upon. One thing is certain, the goals, constraints, and consequences of actions are seldom known precisely at a community level.

Community health advocacy causes change to occur at the community level. The change can be through legislation at local level (traffic laws), state level (revision of nurse practice act), or federal (expansion of Medicaid coverage for a target population). The change can also be regulatory (higher reimbursement for home health care services) or budgetary (federal financing of training for nursing students). To be effective, community health nurses must be an impetus for change at the community level by increasing the community's awareness and supporting the community's decisions regarding health policies (Courtney, 1987).

DETERMINING A COMMUNITY'S HEALTH POLICY NEEDS

Data about a community's problems and needs are often incomplete. This results in ineffective policy decisions and usually occurs because people within a community allow others to determine policy for them instead of with them. When consultation with important policy implementers such as community health nurses is not considered, ineffective health policy is likely to be enacted. A notable effort to prevent these types of omissions in relation to health care policy has been the formulation of *Healthy People 2000: National Health Promotion and Disease Prevention Objectives* (U.S. Department of Health and Human Services, 1991). This document was developed with input from numerous groups and individuals among whom nursing was well represented. It proposed a national strategy for improving the health of the United States over the decade of the 1990s.

It is essential that the community health nurse take an active role in determining a community's health policy needs. The nurse serves as a facilitator in assessing the community's unique health care needs in relation to its existing health care policies. Legislation and policy must be reviewed from the community's viewpoint, as opposed to an individual's viewpoint (Williams, 1983).

Both public health efforts and community health systems are confronted with conflicting interests when individual rights interfere with aggregate rights. However, the community health nurse's primary mission is to promote and preserve the health of populations or aggregates for the benefit of the entire community.

To identify the health policy needs of a community requires an ongoing comprehensive assessment of the community, or what some policy analysts call a "community diagnosis." Chapter 9 identified the dimensions or variables of a community that are important in making a community assessment. Public opinion polls sometimes provide data for policy formulation but should be examined carefully to avoid biased research design. Bias by the tobacco interests resulted in flawed design and results of two polls on smoking, one in Michigan and the other in Los Angeles (Perlstadt & Holmes, 1987).

COMMUNITY ORGANIZATION FOR POLITICAL ACTION

Political action refers to actions taken by an individual or group to influence the political decisions of others toward issues or policies beneficial to the welfare of the individual or group. Organizing a particular community for political action involves taking the following steps:

1. In your role as the community health nurse, identify yourself as a potential community organizer. In this beginning step, nurses must perform a self-assessment in terms of what they have to offer the community.
2. Identify problems, concerns, and issues. This information should come from the community's perspective, not merely that of individuals. Such information may be obtained directly by conducting a survey in the community and indirectly by looking at vital statistics, voting practices, and the life-style of the community.
3. Assess the physical community. Physical environment can have a significant influence on a community. Characteristics of the location in which a population lives set the stage for particular health problems and practices. Information about the physical environment can be obtained from a variety of resources (see Chapter 6).
4. Assess community strengths, resources, and interests. This information is an important indica-

tor of the community's health potential and ability to organize for political action. In this step, the nurse identifies community skills, as well as assesses community strengths and limitations.
5. Assess political influences in the community. Each community has its own power base and political structure. Gaining knowledge of community political systems enables the nurse to identify key people and operations that are essential to the successful implementation of health goals. The community health perspective has a political advantage in terms of votes if the community is clearly defined and can be unified on a particular health issue.
6. Evaluate alternative courses of action. Community decision making is facilitated when the community is well informed. The nurse can play an important role in the decision-making process by helping to identify possible outcomes and alternative courses of action to meet health goals. Each community, as well as each individual, is different in its perspective of a situation. Decision making will be influenced by the impact the decision can have on the social systems of the community.
7. Redefine objectives, priorities, and the community health nurse's goals. After a careful assessment of the community's needs, the community health nurse must compare the relationship between existing programs and policies as they relate to the defined needs and goals. If an incongruent relationship does exist, plans must be made to redefine and reshape existing and future policy directions.
8. Develop a plan of action. Planning for an entire community requires the nurse to collaborate with other professionals and representatives of the community's social systems. Each member of the planning team is considered an equal resource, and each member's input is vital to the successful implementation of the plan. Target audiences include federal policy officials, state and local policy officials, community groups, the business community, professional groups, major institutions such as hospitals or universities, research organizations, advocacy groups, and the general public.
9. Implement the plan. Implementing the plan first and foremost requires effectively communicating it to those who have a vested interest in such a

way they will support it or at least not block it. One must figure out a way of reconciling differences that exist among those who: (1) favor taking major action, but in different ways; (2) favor taking action, but in incremental steps; (3) only see the necessity of correcting problem areas such as allowing workers to transfer the same health insurance coverage when they change jobs. Implementation of a plan requires several important considerations: involvement by representatives of the population to be affected, proper timing, and preparedness.

When implementing a community action plan it is critical that the nurse is prepared and understands the common ground that racial and ethnic groups share without losing sight of their differences. Understanding the community's cultural values and media behavior is the first step to bridging cultural gaps. The second step is to choose the right messages. When the Centers for Disease Control and Prevention tested public-service announcements about AIDS through focus groups, it found that single-race panels and multicultural panels reacted quite differently. In other words, a multicultural panel's perspective is not complete in itself (Rabin, 1994).

Rabin states, "Messages may or may not be controversial in themselves, but the chance of controversy increases greatly if you don't get permission to relay a message to a particular group. It is critical to win the support, respect, and invitation of community leaders before they can open an effective line of communication with their members" (p. 57, 1994).

10. Evaluate the outcome of the planned action. Evaluation of a plan or program requires analyzing the observed outcomes based on the specific goals, objectives, and criteria that were adopted. Evaluation should be a continuous process that guides decision making for the future.

The Legislative Process and Influencing Legislation

Theoretically, at the local level, health policies are guidelines for the implementation of health laws. A community's policy system exerts its control in distributing its health resources through its health policies. Sometimes nurses and clients come to think of policies as statutes and therefore as difficult to change as law. In reality, community health policies are often an interpretation of health laws and at best serve as a strategy for implementing health laws, whether they be state or federal.

The nurse's role as an indirect care provider includes active involvement in the community's political arena (Bagwell & Clements, 1985). Nurses particularly have a responsibility to generate new ways of providing health care and to modify or improve existing health care (Stimpson & Hanley, 1991). In order to influence and initiate changes in the health care system, the nurse needs to know about the legislative process and be directly involved in setting the health policy agenda for a community. The nurse also needs to know how to influence the passage of legislation or modify existing legislation (Williams, 1983; Wakefield, 1990). (See Fig. 28.4.) These skills are essential for all professional nurses because they are major ways that nurses can provide leadership in the improvement of health care.

HOW A BILL BECOMES LAW

All state governments and the three branches of the federal government make decisions that affect health care. All nurses have opportunities to provide input on the initiation, formulation, and revision of legislation at the local, state, and federal levels. Proposed drafts of bills originate from many places because the sources of legislative ideas are relatively unlimited. An idea may be forwarded to a legislator by individuals, groups, government agencies, or other interested parties. The process can be initiated when a concerned citizen or group writes or talks to a legislator.

The legislative process is well defined and guided by rules at all levels of government (U.S. House of Representatives, 1981). The process is similar at the state and federal levels, with the exception of some minor peculiarities. Public libraries have copies of a state's legislative process, or the nurse may write to the state's printing office for information.

There is a requirement that certain types of federal bills be started in the House of Representatives, as opposed to the Senate. This may not be true at the state level, depending upon the particular state's constitution. Once a senator or representative is found who is willing to author a bill, discussion takes place about

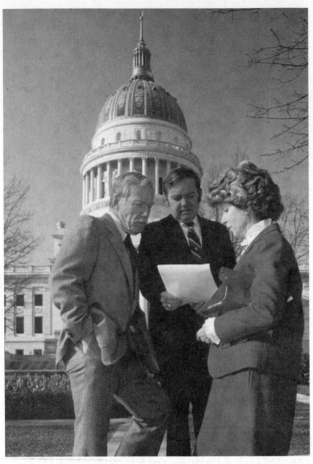

FIGURE 28.4. Nurses are an invaluable source of health care information for legislators.

what current law needs changing or what needs to be added to existing laws. When authoring a bill, a senator or representative consults with a legislative council. This council consists of legal specialists who assist legislators with the drafting of bills. The drafted bill is returned to its originator in the form of an "author copy." Content is carefully reviewed to ascertain that the bill does in fact state what it was intended to state.

A bill can be introduced at any time while the House is in session as long as the sponsoring representative has endorsed the bill and placed the proposal in the House's hopper. The procedure is more formal for the Senate, and any senator can postpone a bill by raising objections to it. All sponsored bills are assigned a legislative number and referred to committee. Currently there are 16 standing committees of the Senate, 22 standing committees of the House of Representatives, and five

joint committees. Most standing committees have two or more subcommittees.

Formal statements and details pertaining to each bill are published in the Congressional Record and printed for distribution. At the federal level, a bill may be considered at any time during the two-year life of that Congress.

The chairperson of the committee to which a bill has been referred must submit the bill to the appropriate subcommittee assigned to work on it within a specified time period, usually two weeks. The exception occurs when the majority of the committee members of the majority party vote to have the bill considered by full committee. Traditionally, many committees and subcommittees have had a policy that any member who insists on a committee hearing on a particular bill should have it. Standing committees must have regular meetings at least once per month, and the chairperson may call additional meetings.

The legislators appointed to a committee conduct the hearing on a bill. At the federal level a bill may have no hearings or several hearings at one time in different committees. At the federal level, the author of a bill is seldom a member of the committee hearing the bill, while at the state level, the bill's author may have connections not available to other legislators or the audience.

The committee chairperson selects individuals to present the first testimony at hearings. Individuals or representatives of groups who have requested to speak about the bill may or may not be called for testimony. It is a frustrating political reality that one may go to committee hearings planning to speak or expecting to hear witnesses, only to find that the voting action was determined before the meeting. Astute individuals and groups not only monitor legislation but also tactfully lobby legislators before committee and subcommittee hearings.

After studying a bill and possibly hearing testimony, there are three types of recommendations the committee can make. (1) The committee approves the bill and is ready to forward it (due pass). (2) The committee revises the bill (due pass with amendments). (3) The committee may refer the bill to another committee. If the bill is set aside by any committee it will eventually die; in so doing, committees can actually veto bills. Bills are usually revised and then forwarded or set aside. If a committee votes to pass a bill, a committee report is written that includes the bill's purpose, scope, and the reasons for the committee's approval. Containing a section-by-section analysis of the bill, the committee's report is one of the most valuable sources of information regarding policy formulation and adoption.

Amendments to state bills and federal bills are handled differently. At the state level, the original bill retains its assigned number throughout the legislative process regardless of amendments. At the federal level, amending occurs in "mark-up" sessions. A new bill is printed and reintroduced with a new number following each mark-up session. Obviously, it is more difficult to follow a bill through the federal process. Also, it should be noted that thousands of bills and joint resolutions are introduced each year yet fewer than 10% of these are enacted as laws.

Following committee action, the bill goes on the calendar and awaits being read before the originating house. The house considers the bill, and at this point its author states reasons why the bill is needed and responds to questions. Only legislators of the house may speak at the floor vote. The house may pass the bill or defeat the bill at this third reading. If the author knows in advance that there are not enough votes for the bill's passage, he or she will take action to delay the vote. At this point considerable compromise, negotiating, trade-offs and other strategies come into play. Success greatly depends upon the author's power base and political maneuvering.

If a bill passes the first house, it is forwarded to the second house. For example, if a bill passes the Senate, it then goes to the House of Representatives. It enters as a new bill with an introduction and first reading. In the second house the bill will again be assigned to committee. The committee will recommend due pass, due pass as amended, or amend and rerefer. Following this committee's actions, the bill has a second reading on the floor of the second house. The third reading results in a floor vote. If there are any changes in the bill by the second house, it is returned to the originating house for concurrence. When significant differences prevent concurrence, the bill is referred to a conference committee consisting of members from both houses.

The conference committee action is a very important step to which the public has no access. This committee determines which version of the bill, or whether a compromise from both versions, will go forward in the conference report. This is a point where a great deal of political trading goes on and major deals are cut. After adoption by both houses, the bill is enrolled and goes to the president.

The president has three options; to sign, hold, or veto the bill. Signing the bill causes it to become law. Holding the bill without signing it may be done for timing or political reasons but, even without signing, the bill becomes law after a delay of ten days if Congress is still in session. Vetoing the bill sends it back to Congress with the president's objections attached. Congress can override this veto by a two-thirds majority vote in both houses, and if the veto is overridden, the bill becomes law despite the president's objections.

Figure 28.5 outlines the process by which a bill becomes law. The fact remains that statutory law is only the beginning. The legislature enacts statutory law that enables a government agency to administer that law by means of regulation. Law is measured only in court. There are few laws other than criminal law by which one may be cited for noncompliance without going through a report mechanism. The executive branch, as represented by a government agency, administers the law through regulation. In the case of registered nurses, it is the Board of Registered Nursing that administers laws relating to nursing education, licensure, and practice, most often called the Nurse Practice Act. That is also the group accountable for disciplining registered nurses who do not meet the law.

A POLITICAL STRATEGY FOR NURSING

Community health nursing must be clearly defined as having a necessary and integral role with clear-cut responsibilities in the health care system. The role must be understood and appreciated by the public and legislators. The "selling" or marketing of the role can begin at the community or grass-roots level but must also occur at the state and national levels. Ideas of opposition groups or interest groups with conflicting goals must be met with constructive criticism and compromise. During this process of defining and marketing nursing, nurses should present a positive and unified image to the public, the legislators, and opposition groups (Mason, et al., 1993).

Nursing, like all other professions, has internal struggles and disagreements, but these internal disagreements need to be down played in the political arena. Nursing needs to present a unified, professional influence. Nursing holds a great deal of power, but that power remains unexerted (Gorman & Clark, 1986). A change in image is overdue. Nurses outnumber all other health care providers and are as well educated as most. They have enhanced the health care system throughout all its struggles. Nurses need to improve their individual and collective self-concept and learn to be personally

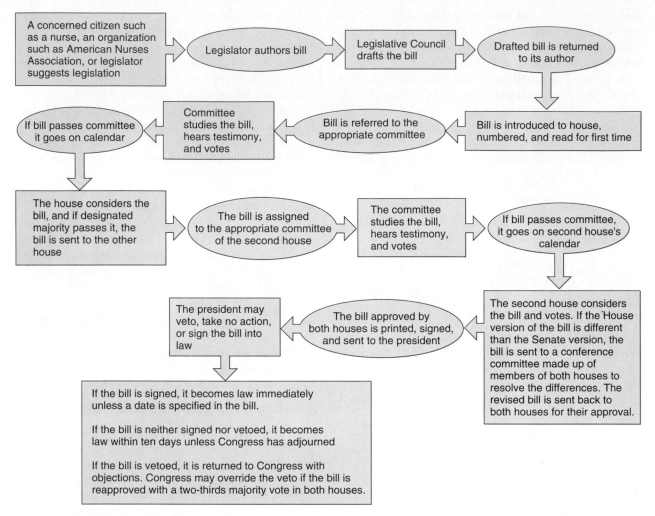

FIGURE 28.5. This flow chart diagrams the legislative process through which a bill becomes a federal law.

and politically assertive (Mason, et al., 1993). They must assist each other in achieving the highest possible levels of maturity, education, public service, and professionalism (Goldwater & Zusy, 1990). Again, the focus should be on construction and growth.

Nurses must give each other credit for their accomplishments and learn to support and assist each other. Community health as a movement was created by nurses, yet there are many other groups ready to take the credit. Many leaders in nursing have received little recognition from their peers. Nurses need their colleagues' respect and recognition.

Policy research has shown that economic resources continue to be the major determinant of public policy, although the attitudes of political leaders appear to be increasingly important (Litman & Robins, 1991). The fact that the bulk of federal law presently originates in the executive branch of the government supports this conclusion. A great deal of emphasis has been placed on pluralistic political variables such as voter participation, party competition, and majority party control.

A greater financial base for promoting nursing will have to be established. As with any investment, nurses must first invest money in their professional organizations, in supporting the work of nurse lobbyists, and in promoting research and dissemination of information about nursing's contributions, before expecting any returns. Also, it must be recognized there is an inherent risk to be taken by being politically involved before any short-term or, more importantly, long-term gains can be expected. That is, gains for clients and for the profession as a whole have been minimized because, until

Salutation   My dear Mr. or Ms. Doe:
                  Yours very truly,

U.S. Secretary of Health and Human Services

Name   The Honorable Donna E. Shalala
Address   200 Independence Ave, SW
                  Washington, DC 20201
Salutation   My dear Ms. Shalala:
                  Yours very truly,

Governor

Name   The Governor
Address   State Capitol
                  City, State, Zip
Salutation   Dear Governor Doe:
                  Respectfully yours,

Mayor or City Council Member

Name   Mayor (or) Council Member
Address   City Hall
                  City, State, Zip
Salutation   Dear Mayor or Council member:
                  Yours very truly,

2. When a bill is in committee, correspond with *all* members of the committee. The content of the letter may be the same, but each letter should be individually typed or handwritten.
3. Plan the wording of your letter to make points concisely and succinctly. Letters are scanned before they are read. The following is a content outline of what is appropriate to include in the correspondence:
   a. One sentence that clearly states the issue
   b. One sentence that clearly states your individual or group position
   c. A statement that delineates the status of the proposed legislation (for example, where it is in the legislative process and what appears to be its disposition)
   d. A list of the reasons to support or oppose the pending legislation
      (1) Financial
      (2) Groups adversely affected
      (3) Weaknesses of opposing view
      (4) Specific benefits that override weaknesses of your view, benefits of the opposing view, or both
   e. Specific data that support these reasons
      (1) Dollar amounts
      (2) Number of groups affected and their names

       (3) Numbers within those groups
       (4) Delineation of processes, systems, equipment, and loopholes that have adverse or positive effects
  f. A clear, concise statement of the action that you want the legislator to take on the piece of legislation such as to: vote for or against the legislation; meet with you or your organization; ask for additional information; convey contents of letter to interested, influential persons; provide you with those persons' names and titles so that you can contact them, or other similar action.

Personal Visits

An amazing number of bills are enacted with no input from constituents. Lobbyists exert great influence, as do other legislative colleagues and persons who use the physical proximity of sitting close to a legislator or the persuasive tactic of trading favors to sway legislators' decisions.

Personal visits by nurses to their legislators can have a profound impact. Many legislators welcome additional expert information and respect the professional commitment involved in making the visit. Because legislators are very busy, with as little as three to five minutes for an interview, the nurse will make the visit more profitable by sending a briefing sheet or letter prior to the meeting. Discussion with a legislator's staff members can also be worthwhile and may be the only route open to you. These individuals do the legislator's background research and help to develop the positions and language contained in the bills. Staff members are the gatekeepers and are often more knowledgeable than the legislator about the issues and have more time to discuss them.

Community health nurses, as advocates for a health issue, must know the opposition's arguments and be prepared to counter them. The prepared nurse will communicate far more effectively with the legislator and his or her staff.

Attending Hearings and Providing Testimony

Community health nurses attending a legislative hearing can have considerable impact on a pending bill or proposed regulation (Bagwell & Clements, 1985). Singly or as an organized group, the nurses' physical presence communicates to legislators that they are concerned, informed, and ready to take action. Again, nurses need to be prepared in advance of the hearing. Resources, such as a government relations committee or the state nurses' association, can provide useful information on the issues surrounding the bill. Other existing communication networks, such as nurses involved in political action committees, can provide additional information.

Once a community health nurse is versed in the particular topic of a bill, he or she may want to provide testimony (see Fig. 28.6). Testimony may be given verbally at the time of a hearing, or it may be written in advance. What should be included in one's testimony differs little from what should be included in a letter, with the exception of supportive materials, such as actual research or survey data.

Party politics has significant impact on the conduct of legislative business. Whether legislators belong to either the Democratic, Republican, or another party, they will often vote in favor of their party's view. The numbers of any given party in each house can make a considerable difference in passing bills. At times votes may reflect party allegiance and platforms rather than the individual legislator's response to the information provided at the hearing or through constituents' letters. Organized lobbying groups can exert more pressure on legislators to override party decisions.

If you as a community health nurse support a bill and wish to testify, contact the author of the bill. If you are opposed to a bill and wish to testify, notify the bill's author and the chairperson of the committee in which the bill is being heard. Organized groups with registered lobbyists are most familiar with the process and may provide the best entree to the committee hearings as a participant. Remember, votes are counted by the author before a committee meets, and if the number is not sufficient for a due pass, there are many ways to postpone an official vote.

Resources for Political Action and Studying Policy

Nurses must focus their reading and depend upon professional and political organizations and current literature for guidance in studying policy and becoming politically active. Many organizations are politically significant to community health nurses; a listing of some at the national level can be found in Appendix B at the end of this book. The chief objective is to provide directions in which political contacts and knowledge can be developed by the community health nurse.

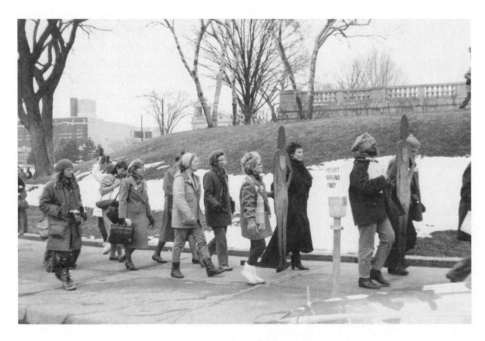

FIGURE 28.6. A group of community health nurses on their way to testify at a health-related hearing in the state capitol.

Summary

The need for health care reform has become critical as the costs of health care continue to escalate. The United States spends a disproportionate percentage of the national budget on health care and yet there are still major segments of the population which do not have adequate access to quality health services. Because of these economic concerns, health care reform and policy making have become politically charged issues involving many groups and factions including not only health care providers and health care professionals but government, third-party payers, insurance companies, and others with vested interests.

Many are concerned that health care is being viewed as a business, and that business interests and efforts to curb escalating costs may divert public services away from community health issues, such as preventive and primary care. Community health nurses know community needs and the value of such services and therefore need to be a major force in this political arena where health policy decisions are being made. Community health nurses need to become politically aware and active in order to assure quality health services—working as community health advocates. They must collaborate with community constituents and with nurses and other professionals to assure the safety and well-being of groups and populations at risk.

Although nurses' influence has been limited in the past, nurses must learn how to empower their own profession, themselves, and the communities they work with by becoming politically active and aware. If they are to fulfill their mission of promoting, protecting, and preserving the health of aggregates, they must become policy makers as well as policy implementers. They

Activities to Promote Critical Thinking

1. Investigate a major health policy system in your community or state; discover how it works and determine whether community health nurses are represented in this system. Areas to investigate include the boundaries of the system; the authority by which the system generates health policy; how the system receives input (formally and informally); resources the policy system uses and allocates to others; and the system's output over the past few years.

2. Describe a legislative bill related to community health at either the state or federal level and the issues involved in it. Identify who is sponsoring the bill, who is opposing it, and why. Determine who will be affected by the bill, if passed, and in what ways they will be affected. Discuss what you, as a community health nurse, could do to be involved in this bill and then develop a political action plan to support or oppose the bill. Write a letter to your legislator regarding your position.

3. Carefully review your own health care plan and determine whether you feel it is an adequate and equitable plan. Describe the plan and the issues involved in it. Include what health services are covered and who is authorized to provide services and receive direct reimbursement. Also determine who qualifies for the plan and who is excluded and what conditions can disqualify a person or a family once they have the plan. Compare the cost of this plan to one other plan.

4. Attend a meeting of a professional organization, board of directors, government agency or council when a health policy or health care issue is on the agenda. Analyze the positions of the major interest groups involved and describe to what extent economics comes into the discussion. Describe who controls the discussion and how this is done.

5. Interview a health care administrator in your local area and determine this person's position on health care reform including the rationale for the position. Determine at what level(s) this administrator is politically active and involved in influencing policy.

must learn to use policy systems and the political process so that their voice is heard and they have influence in policy decision making. They must learn to formulate, implement, and evaluate health policies. They must understand the legislative process and how to influence that process. The politically involved nurse should aim to accomplish three primary goals of (1) generating suppport for his or her views, by communicating ideas effectively and getting to know and influence representatives at local, state, and national levels; (2) creating professional legitimacy such as keeping abreast of current issues in health care and nursing and becoming involved in professional nursing organizations, community boards, and/or committees or running for office; and (3) resolving conflict and being able to effectively negotiate and compromise.

Many resources and opportunities exist to help community health nurses study policy issues and make political contacts. Community health nurses must recognize societal changes and their potential impact on community health. They must also be able to analyze policy and become active in the political process to influence policy decisions that are in the community's best interests.

REFERENCES

American Nurses' Association. (1994). *Nursing's agenda for health care reform*. Washington, DC: ANA publications.

Archer, S. E., & Goehner, P.A. (1982). *Nurses: A political force*. Monterey, CA: Wadsworth

Bagwell, M. & Clements, D. (1985). *A political handbook for health professionals*. Boston: Little, Brown.

Christensen, T. (1995). *Local politics*. Belmont, CA: Wadsworth.

Courtney, R. (1987). Community practice: Nursing influence on policy formulation. *Nursing Outlook, 35*(4), 170–73.

Decker, P.J., & Sullivan, E.J. (1992). *Nursing administration: A micro/macro approach for effective nurse managers*. East Norwalk, CT: Appleton & Lange.

Donley, R. (1982). Nursing and the politics of health. In N. L. Chaska (Ed.), *The nursing profession: A time to speak* (pp. 844–57). New York: McGraw-Hill.

Dye, T. R. (1992). *Understanding public policy*. Englewood Cliffs, NJ: Prentice-Hall.

Elwood, T. (Ed) (Dec 1993/Jan 94). Clinton health reform bill dropped into congressional hoppers. *Trends: Association of Schools of Allied Health Professions Newsletter*, p. 2.

Foster, J. (1994). Keynote address to national workshop, *The Role of Allied Health in the Delivery of Primary Care*, at Thomas Jefferson University, Philadelphia, PA, March 13, 1994.

Goldwater, M. & Zusy, M.J. (1990). *Prescription for nurses: Effective political action*. St. Louis: Mosby.

Gorman, S., & Clark, N. (1986). Power and effective nursing practice. *Nursing Outlook, 34*(1), 129.

Griffith, H.M. (1993). Needed—A strong nursing position on preventive service. *Image: Journal of Nursing Scholarship, 25*(4), p. 272).

Hancock, T., et al. (1985). Beyond health care: Proceedings of a conference on healthy public policy. *Canadian Journal of Public Health, 76*(3)(Suppl. 1), 99–104.

Harrell, J. S. & Frauman, A.C. (1994). Cardiovascular health promotion in children: Program and policy implications. *Public Health Nursing, 11*(4), 236–241.

Harrington, C., & C.L. Estes. (1994). *Health policy and nursing: Crisis and reform in the U.S. health care delivery system*. Boston: Jones and Bartlett.

Lee, P. R., & Estes, C.L. (Eds.) (1994). *The nation's health* (4th ed.). Boston: Jones and Bartlett.

Litman, T. J., & Robins, L.S. (1991). *Health politics and policy*. New York: Wiley.

Mason, D.J., Talbott, S.W., & Leavitt, J.K. (Eds.) (1993). *Policy and politics for nurses: Action and change in the workplace, government, organizations and community*. Philadelphia: Saunders.

McLeroy, K.R., Bibeau, D., Steckler, A., & Glanz, K. (1988). An ecological perspective on health promotion programs. *Health Education Quarterly, 15*(4), pp. 351–377.

Morrison, R. D. (1993). *Creating an agenda for change in Virginia: Virginia health care workforce*. A presentation to the twenty-sixth annual meeting, Association of Schools of Allied Health Professions, Galveston, TX, October 28, 1993.

Pelka, F. (1993). Trauma time: Disability issues must be a litmus test for evaluating the validity of any proposal for health care reform. *Mainstream, 17*(6), pp.35–41.

Perlstadt, H., & Holmes, R. (1987). The role of public opinion polling in health legislation. *American Journal of Public Health, 77*(5), 612–14.

Pew Health Professions Commission. (1991). *Healthy America: Practitioners for 2005. A report of the Pew Health Professions Commission*. Durham, NC: Duke University Medical Center.

Pew Health Professions Commission (1993). *Health professions for the future: Schools in service to the nation. A report of the Pew Health Professions Commission*. San Francisco: UCSF Center for the Health Professions.

Rabin, S. (1994). How to sell across cultures. *American Demographics, 16*(3), 56–57.

Raudonis, B.M. & Griffith, H. (1991). Model for integrating health services research and health care policy formation. *Nursing & Health Care, 12*(1), 32–36.

Selker, L.G. (1994). Descriptions of the current and future roles of allied health workers in the direct provision and support of primary care. White paper presentation at Thomas Jefferson University workshop. *The role of allied health in the delivery of primary care*. March 12–13, 1994.

Sharp, N., Biggs, S., & Wakefield, M. (1991). Public policy: New opportunities for nurses. *Nursing and Health Care, 12*(1), pp. 16–22.

Shoultz, J., Hatcher, P.A. & Hurrell, M. (1992). Growing edges of a new paradigm: The future of nursing in the health of the nation. *Nursing Outlook, 40*(2), 57–61.

Starr, P. (1982). *The social transformation of American medicine*. New York: Basic Books.

Stimpson, M., & Hanley, B. (1991). Nurse policy analyst: advanced practice role. *Nursing and Health Care, 12*(1), pp. 10–15.

UNICEF. (1995). *The state of the world's children 1995*. New York: Oxford.

U.S. Department of Health and Human Services (1991). *Healthy People 2000: National health promotion and disease prevention objectives* (S/N 017-001-00474-0). Washington, DC: U.S. Government Printing Office.

U.S. House of Representatives. (1981). *Our American government: What is it? How does it function? 150 questions and answers* (House Document No. 96-351). Washington, DC: U.S. Government Printing Office.

Vance, C. (1993). Politics: A humanistic process. In D.J. Mason, S.W. Talbott, & J.K. Leavitt. (1993). *Policy and politics for nurses: Action and change in the workplace, government, organizations and community*. Philadelphia: Saunders.

Wakefield, M. K. (1990). Perspectives on health policy: influencing the legislative process. *Nursing Economics, 8*(3), 188–190.

Watson, S. D. (1993). An alliance at risk: The disability movement and health care reform. *The American Prospect,* (winter).

Williams, C. A. (1983). Making things happen: Community health nursing and the policy arena. *Nursing Outlook, 31,* pp. 225–28.

SELECTED READINGS

Aday, L.A., Begley, C.E., Lairson, D.R., & Slater, C.H. (1993). *Evaluating the medical care system*. Ann Arbor, MI: Health Administration Press.

Allen, C. (1990). *Political campaigning: A new decade*. Washington, DC: National Women's Political Caucus.

American Nurses' Association. (1990). *Political and legislative handbook*. Washington, DC: Author.

Aroskar, M. A. (1993). Ethical issues: Politics, power, and policy. In D.J. Mason, S.W. Talbott, and J. K. Leavitt (Eds), *Policy and politics for nurses*. Philadelphia: Saunders.

Barry, C. T. (1990). Profiles of nurses professionally involved in public policy. *Nursing Economics, 8*(3), 174–176, 187.

Chin, P. L. (1993). What can just one nurse do? *Nursing Outlook, 11*(2), 54–55.

Ciglar, A.J. & Loomis, B.A. (1991). Interest group politics. *Congressional Quarterly*. Washington, DC: US Government Printing Office.

Congressional Quarterly. (1991). *How Congress works*. Washington, DC: Author.

Coss, C. (1993). Lillian D. Wald: progressive activist. *Public Health Nursing, 10*(2), 134–37.

deVreis, C. M. and M. W. Vanderbilt (1993). *The grassroots lobbying handbook*. Washington, DC: American Nurses Publishing, ANA Pub.No. GR-4.

Dionne, E.J. (1991). *Why Americans hate politics*. New York: Simon and Schuster.

Faherty, B. (1993). Now is the time to advocate. *Nursing Outlook, 41*(6), 248–49.

Feldstein, P. J. (1994). *Health policy issues: an economic perspective on health reform*. Ann Arbor, MI: Health Administration Press.

Gott, M. (1990). Policy framework for health promotion. *Nursing Standard, 5*(10, 30–32.

Hall-Long, B.A. (1995). Nursing's past, present, and future political experiences. *Nursing & Health Care, 16*(1), 24–28.

Heineman, R.A., Bluhm, W.T., Peterson, S.A., & Kearny, E.N. (1990). *The world of the policy analyst: Rationality, values, & politics*. Chatham, NJ: Chatham House.

Hrebenar, R.J. & Scott, R.K. (1990). *Interest group politics in America*. Englewood Cliffs, NJ: Prentice Hall.

Immerwahr, J. et al. (1992). *Faulty diagnosis*. New York: Public Agenda Foundation.

Ketter, J. (1994). Is there a cure for our ailing public health system? *The American Nurse, 26*(4), pp. 18, 20.

Kettl, D.F. (1992). *Deficit politics: Public budgeting in its institutional and historical context*. New York: MacMillan.

Kuehnert, P. L. (1991) The public health policy advocate: fostering the health of communities. *Clinical Nurse Specialist, 5*(1), 5–10.

Longest, B. B.(1994). *Health policymaking in the United States*. Ann Arbor, MI: Health Administration Press.

Mitchell, P.H., Krueger, J.C., & Moody, L.E. (1990). The crisis of the health care nonsystem. *Nursing Outlook, 36*(5), 214–217.

Pender, N. J. (1993). Health care reform: one view of the future. *Nursing Outlook, 41*(2), 56–57.

Schieber, G., Poullier, J., & Greenwald, L. (Fall, 1991). Health care systems in twenty-four countries. *Health Affairs, 1,* 22–38.

Sprayberry, L. D. (1993). Nursing's dual role in health care policy. *Nursing & Health Care, 14*(5), 250–254.

Thomas, P.A. & Shelton, C.R. (1994). Teaching students to become active in public policy. *Public Health Nursing, 11*(2), 75–79.

U.S. Office of Management and Budget, Executive Office of the President (199-). *Budget of the U.S. government, fiscal year, 199-*. Washington, DC: U.S. Government Printing Office.

Williams, D.M. (1991). Policy at the grassroots: community-based participation in health care policy. *Journal of Professional Nursing, 7*(5), 271–276.

Williams-Crowe, S. & Aultman, T. (1994). State health agencies and the legislative policy process. *Public Health Reports, 109*(3), 361–367.

Woodworth, J.R., & Gump, W.R. (1994). *Camelot: A role playing simulation for political decision making*. Belmont, CA: Wadsworth.

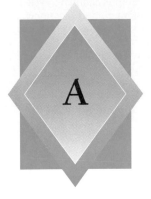

Communicable Disease Information Sources

COMMUNICABLE DISEASES (GENERAL REFERENCE)

■ Benenson, A.S., ed. (1990). Control of Communicable Diseases in Man (15th ed.) American Public Health Association: Washington, D.C.

An extremely useful and well-respected small reference book, updated every 5 years. A valuable library addition for any health professional needing reliable, accurate, updated information in the field of communicable disease control. Available from the American Public Health Association, 1015 Fifteenth St. NW, Washington, D.C. 20005.

■ Centers for Disease Control. The Division of Immunization, Center for Preventive Services, CDC, Atlanta GA, 30333, telephone 404-639-3311; offers technical advice on vaccine recommendations, disease outbreak control, and sources of immunobiologics.

■ Centers for Disease Control. HIV/AIDS Surveillance Report. Published quarterly in January, April, July, and October.

■ Centers for Disease Control. National AIDS Clearinghouse, P.O. Box 6003, Rockville, MD 20849-6003; telephone 1-800-458-5231.

■ National AIDS Hotline: 1-800-342-2437; 1-800-344-7432 (Spanish access) and; 1-800-243-7889 (TTY, deaf access).

NATIONAL SURVEILLANCE DATA AND CONTROL RECOMMENDATIONS

■ Centers for Disease Control. Summary of notifiable diseases, United States, 1995. Morbidity and Mortality Weekly Report 1995; 44(53).

This statistical summary of notifiable diseases in the United States is published to accompany each volume of the Morbidity and Mortality Weekly Report by the Centers for Disease Control, Atlanta, Georgia. Monthly summaries of notifiable diseases are also carried in the MMWR throughout the year, in addition to a plethora of other topics pertinent to communicable disease control.

Subscriptions are available through Superintendent of Documents, U.S. Government Printing Office, Washington, D.C. 20402; and through MMS Publications, C.S.P.O. Box 9120, Waltham, MA 02254.

IMMUNIZATION RECOMMENDATIONS

■ ACIP (Advisory Committee for Immunization Practices) General recommendations on immunization. Published by the Centers for Disease Control periodically in Morbidity and Mortality Weekly Report.

Gives immunization practices recommended by the U.S. Department of Health and Human services. It includes a summary of available vaccine products in the United States and recommendations for administration, including guidelines for scheduling serial immunizations, immunizations for HIV-infected children, appropriate and inappropriate contraindications to vaccination. In addition to this summary, updated recommendations for individual vaccines can be located through the MMWR index to specific issues.

■ "The Red Book." Committee on Infectious Diseases of the American Academy of Pediatrics. 1991. Report of the Committee on Infectious Diseases (Red Book) 22nd ed. American Academy of Pediatrics: Elk Grove, IL.

Used by many physicians, this text is updated every 2–3 years and contains recommendations on all licensed vaccines compiled by the American Academy of Pediatrics. Policy changes for individual recommendations for immunization practices are published as needed by the American Academy of

Pediatrics in the journal *Pediatrics*. They are available from the American Academy of Pediatrics, Publications Division, 141 Northwest Point Blvd. P.O. Box 927, Elk Grove Village, IL 60009-0927.

■ Guide for Adult Immunizations

Produced by the American College of Physicians for providers caring for adults, this guide covers immunization recommendations for healthy adults as well as those with specific health problems. Available from the American College of Physicians, Division of Scientific Activities, Health and Public Policy, 4200 Pine Street, Philadelphia, PA 19104.

■ Health Information for International Travel

Internationally accepted reference for international traveller immunization and prophylaxis requirement and recommendations. Helpfully broken down into regions as well as national entities to enhance traveler safety.

Available from the Superintendent of Documents, U.S. Government Printing Office, Washington, DC 20402.

■ World Health Organization, (1991). International Travel and Health: Vaccination Requirements and Health Advice. WHO: Geneva, Switzerland.

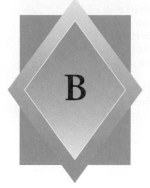

Resources for Political Action and Studying Policy

PUBLICATIONS REGARDING LAWS AND REGULATIONS

- *Federal Register*
  Lists (5 times/week) regulations of government agencies, notices, executive orders, and presidential proclamations. Responsible for publication of laws, presidential documents, and the United States Government Organization Manual.

- *United States Statutes at Large*
  Compilation of Congressional acts and public laws accumulated for each congressional session.

- *Code of Federal Regulations*
  Annual publication of all government regulations currently in effect.

- *Weekly Compilation of Presidential Documents*
  Includes presidential materials such as speeches and messages.

- *Congressional Record*
  Bimonthly publication containing a complete record of everything said on the floor of both House and Senate, printed by the U.S. Government Printing Office, Washington, D.C. 20402.

PUBLICATIONS RELATED TO HEALTH AND HEALTH POLICY

- *Monthly Vital Statistics Report*
  From National Center for Health Statistics, Hyattsville, Maryland 20872.

- *Public Policy*
  Offers detailed, theory-based case studies.

- *Journal of Policy Analysis and Management*

- *Policy Sciences*

- *Policy Studies Journal*

- *Policy Studies Review*

- *Policy Analysis*

- *From the Washington Office*
  Gives overviews of federal policy and laws, voting records of legislators, and action needed for nursing at the national level. Published by the American Nurses Association, Government Relations Division, 1030 15th St. NW, Washington, DC 20005.

PROFESSIONAL ASSOCIATIONS, POLITICAL ORGANIZATIONS, AND GOVERNMENT BODIES

- *The Encyclopedia of Associations*
  Published annually, available on-line, provides detailed information concerning nonprofit U.S. organizations, includes some for-profit groups which are voluntary or not primarily for profit, and citizen action groups. Includes addresses, phone and fax numbers, information about membership, staff, budget, and purpose of organization. Available in libraries and through Gale Research Company in Detroit, Michigan.

ORGANIZATIONS THAT DEAL WITH GOVERNMENT RELATIONS AND COMMUNITY HEALTH ISSUES

■ American Association of Asian/Pacific
Community Health Organizations (AAPCHO)
1212 Broadway, 94612
Oakland, CA 30305
Publishes *Community Health Watch*

■ American Civil Liberties Union (ACLU)
132 W. 43rd Street
New York, NY 10036
Publications include the newsletter *Civil Liberties Alert*

■ American Health Care Association (AHCA)
1201 L St, NW
Washington, DC 20005
Publishes *AHCA Notes*

■ American Hospital Association (AHA)
840 N Lake Shore Dr
Chicago, IL 60611

■ American Medical Association (AMA)
515 North State St
Chicago, IL 60610

■ American Nurses' Association (ANA)
600 Maryland Ave SW, Ste 100 W
Washington, DC 20024-2571
Publications include *The American Nurse*

■ American Nurses' Foundation (ANF)
600 Maryland Ave SW, Ste 100 W
Washington, DC 20024-2571
Sponsors scholar program to conduct health
policy research

■ American Organization of Nurse Executive (AONE)
840 N Lake Shore Dr
Chicago, IL 60611
Publications includes *AONE News*

■ American Public Health Association (APHA)
1015 15th St NW
Washington, DC 20005
Publications include the *American Journal of Public Health,
The Nation's Health,* and *Washington Newsletter*

■ Democratic National Committee
430 S Capitol St, SE
Washington, DC 20003

■ Environmental Protection Agency (EPA)
401 M St, SW
Washington, DC 20460

■ Indian Health Service/PHS (IHS)
Office of Human Resources
1616 East Indian School Road, Ste 375
Phoenix, AZ 85016
Publishes monthly, *IHS Primary Care Provider*

■ IHS Public Affairs Department
1615 H Street, NW
Washington, DC 20006
Publications include *Elections Guide* and *They Grade
the Congress*

■ International Council of Nurses (ICN)
Box 42
1211 Geneva, Switzerland
League of Women Voters
1730 M Street NW
Washington, DC 20036

■ National Association of Community Health Centers
(NACHC)
1330 New Hampshire Ave NW, Ste 122
Washington, DC 20036
Publications include *Community Health Center
Listing, Community Health Guides,* and
Washington Update

■ National Association of Hispanic Nurses (NAHN)
1501 16th, NW
Washington, DC 20036

■ National Association for Home Care (NAHC)
519 C St NE
Washington, DC 20002
Publications include *Caring, Homecare News,* and
NAHC Report

■ National Association of School Nurses (NASN)
Lamplighter Ln, PO Box 1300
Scarborough, ME 04070
Publications include *School Nurse*

■ National Black Nurses Association (NBNA)
1012 10th St NW
Washington, DC 20001-4492

■ National Council of State Boards of Nursing
(NCSBN)
676 N St Clair St, Ste 550
Chicago, IL 60611
Publishes *State Nursing Legislation Quarterly*

■ National League for Nursing (NLN)
350 Hudson St
New York, NY 10014
Publications include *NLN Newsletter, Nursing and
Health Care, Nursing Data Review,* and *Public
Policy Bulletin*

■ National Migrant Resource Program (NMRP)
1515 Capitol of Texas Hwy S, Ste 220
Austin, TX 78746
Publishes *Migrant Health Newsline*

■ National Organization for Women (NOW)
1000 16th St NW, Ste 700
Washington, DC 20036

■ National Student Nurse's Association (NSNA)
555 W 57th St, Ste 700
New York, NY 10019
Publications include *Imprint*

■ National Women's Political Caucus
1275 K St NW, Ste 750
Washington, DC 20005
Publications include *Women's Political Times*

■ Nurses' Coalition for Action in Politics
1030 15th Street, NW, Ste 408
Washington, DC 20005

■ Public Citizen
2000 P St, NW, PO Box 19404
Washington, DC 20036

■ Nurses' Organization for Veteran Affairs
(NOVA)
1726 M Street NW, Ste 408
Washington, DC 20005

■ Republican National Committee
310 First St, SE
Washington, DC 20003

■ United States House of Representatives
US Capitol Room-H
Washington, DC 20515
(202) 225-3121

■ United States Senate
US Capitol Room-S
Washington, DC 20510
(202) 224-3121

GLOSSARY

. . . .

Accommodation: Jean Piaget's term which describes the cognitive ability to solve problems.

Acquired immunodeficiency syndrome (AIDS): A severe, life-threatening condition representing the late clinical stage of infection with HIV in which there is progressive damage to the immune system and other organs, particularly the central nervous system.

Active immunity: A longterm and sometimes life-long resistance to a disease acquired either naturally through host infection with resulting development of antibodies or artificially through immunization.

Active listening: The process of receiving a message and assuming responsibility for understanding the meaning of the sender's message.

Adaptation: Jean Piaget's term which describes the cognitive ability to cope with the demands of the environment.

Adaptation theory: A theory which helps to explain human behavior; that human beings (both individuals and groups) adapt to stimuli by either an effective and growth producing manner or an ineffective manner.

Advocate: A community health nursing role in which the nurse acts or speaks on behalf of clients to help clients gain greater independence or self-determination and to make the system more responsive and relevant to their needs.

Affective domain: Area of learning that deals with feelings, attitudes, values, and beliefs.

Ageism: A collection of stereotypical attitudes and behaviors that are directed toward older adults.

Agent: The causative factor contributing to a health problem or condition.

Aggregate: A group of people who share some common interest or goal and in community health practice are considered a unified whole in solving problems or promoting health.

Alzheimer's disease: A progressive degenerative disease of the brain which often affects older adults and often is initially characterized by slight memory loss, minor confusion and slight personality changes but progresses to profound memory loss, disorientation and dependence over a course of 5 to 10 years; sometimes called presenile dementia in adults under age 65.

Analytic epidemiology: Investigations designed to identify associations between a particular human disease or health problem in human populations and its possible cause(s).

Anorexia nervosa: An eating disorder associated with emotional problems seen more frequently in female adolescents and young adults characterized by a distorted self-image of being overweight, refusal to eat, marked weight loss, amenorrhea, and sometimes resulting in death from starvation and/or malnutrition.

Anticipatory guidance: The process of helping one to prepare for a future role or developmental stage.

Assessment: Collecting and evaluating information about clients' health status to discover existing or potential needs in order to plan future action or interventions.

Assimilation: Jean Piaget's term which describes the cognitive ability to apply learned skills to new situations.

Assisted living: Help with activities of daily living such as being reminded to take medications, assistance with dressing and bathing, and meal preparation.

Assurance: The process of translating established health policies into services.

At-risk populations: Groups with a greater probability of acquiring certain diseases or unhealthy states than the population as a whole.

Attention Deficit Disorder (ADD): The term applied to a behavior disorder of onset before age 7 which is characterized by child's inability to pay attention, focus on tasks, and general disorganization (compared to other children of the same developmental age) that impairs the child's ability to profit and learn from new experiences and interferes with socialization.

Attention Deficit Hyperactivity Disorder (ADHD): A controversial childhood behavior disorder with onset before age 7 characterized by excessive fidgeting and squirming, difficulty remaining seated, easy distractability, difficulty waiting one's turn, inability to follow instructions, excessive talking, and other disruptive behaviors.

Audit: An organized effort whereby practicing professionals monitor, assess, and make judgments about the quality and appropriateness of nursing care provided by peers as measured against professional standards of practice.

Autocratic leadership style: An authoritarian style in which leaders use their power (usually the power of their position) to influence their followers.

Autonomous leadership style: A facilitative style that encourages group members to select and carry out their own activities, and function independently.

Autonomy: Freedom of choice and the exercise of individual rights.

Bargaining: The process of negotiating an agreement in which an exchange of goods or services occurs.

Behavioral learning theories: A group of theories that attribute learning to conditioned responses to stimuli.

Beneficence: Doing good that benefits others.

Blended families: The combination of members from different families after divorce, developing a new family system of stepparents and stepchildren.

Board and care homes: Homes for elderly persons who need meal service and housekeeping only and can manage most of their own personal care.

Brainstorming: A process used to generate new ideas that encourages group members to freely offer suggestions without criticism.

Bulimia: An eating disorder more often seen in adolescents and young adults associated with emotional problems in which the person engages in uncontrolled eating binges often followed by self-induced vomiting (purging), depression, and self-denial.

Capable elderly: The older adult over 65 who can live independently.

Case management: A systematic process used by nurses to ensure that clients' multiple health and service needs are met which includes assessing client needs, planning and coordinating services, referring to other appropriate providers, and monitoring and evaluating progress.

Causality: The relationship between a cause and its effect.

Change: Any planned or unplanned alteration of the status quo.

Channel: The medium through which a sender conveys a message, such as talking, written communication, body language, or touching.

Chemical addiction: A compulsion to use a chemical that is beyond a person's ability to control.

Chemical dependence: A strong, overwhelming preoccupation with and desire to use a drug, experienced as a craving.

Child abuse: Maltreatment of children including any or all of the following: physical, emotional, medical, or educational neglect; emotional or sexual maltreatment and exploitation.

Chronically homeless: Persons who have had no permanent residence for a year or more.

Client myth: A misconception regarding community health nursing which says the primary client is the individual.

Clinician: A community health nursing role in which the nurse ensures provision of health services, not just to individuals and families but also to groups and populations.

Cognitive domain: Area of learning that involves intellectual processes including remembering, perceiving, abstracting, and generalizing.

Cognitive learning theories: Theories that attribute learning to the ability to think, perceive, make abstractions, and generalize.

Cohabitating couples: Heterosexual or homosexual persons who live together outside of marriage with or without a sexual relationship.

Cohort: A group of people who share a common experience in a specific time period.

Collaboration: Purposeful interaction between nurse, clients, other professionals, and community members based on mutual participation and joint effort.

Collaborator: A community health role in which the nurse cooperates and works jointly with others in the community to accomplish health service goals.

Common-interest community: A collection of people whose common interests bind them together.

Commune family: A family composed of several unrelated, monogamous couples living together and collectively rearing their children.

Communicable disease: An illness caused by a specific infectious agent or its toxic products through transmission from an infected source to a susceptible host.

Communication: The transfer and understanding of meaning between individuals.

Community: A collection of people who interact with each other and whose common interests or characteristics give them a sense of unity and belonging.

Community as client: The concept of focusing nursing service on a community-wide group of people.

Community health: The identification of needs and the protection and improvement of collective health within a geographically defined area.

Community health advocacy: Efforts aimed at creating awareness of and generating support for meeting the community's health needs.

Community health nursing: The specialty of nursing that focuses on the health needs of communities and aggregates and in particular vulnerable populations.

Community needs assessment: The process of determining the real or perceived needs of a defined community of people.

Community of solution: A collection of people who come together to solve a problem that affects all of them.

Community subsystem assessment: The examination of a single facet of life within a defined community.

Commuter family: A family in which both partners work but each works in a different city and much time is spent traveling to and from work.

Competition: The rivalry between health care organizations to gain resources and clients.

Comprehensive assessment: A thorough, indepth examination of an entire community.

Conceptual framework: A set of concepts integrated into a meaningful explanation that helps one interpret human behavior or situations.

Conceptual model: A framework made up of ideas for explaining and studying a phenomenon of interest.

Conceptual skills: The mental ability to analyze and interpret abstract ideas for the purpose of understanding and diagnosing situations and formulating solutions.

Concurrent review: A quality assessment process that looks at specific elements of care while the care is in progress. For example, open audits, joint home visits by a nurse and his/her supervisor, and care conferences.

Confidant: A close personal friend or family member in whom the older adult confides and trusts with innermost feelings and thoughts.

Contaminant: Organic or inorganic matter that enters a medium, such as water or food, and renders it impure.

Continuing care centers: Large housing units which offer all levels of living from total independent living to the most dependent of skilled nursing care in order to meet the continuous and changing needs of older adults.

Continuous quality improvement: Methods used by health professionals to monitor services and care to clients in order to maintain and improve the delivery of care.

Contracting: The process of negotiating a working agreement between two or more parties.

Control group: A group of persons not receiving a research intervention.

Controller: A community health nursing management role which involves monitoring the plan and ensuring that it stays on course.

Coping mechanisms: The methods people use to deal with stressors or negative stimuli and stress.

Coping: Actions or ways of thinking that assist people in dealing with and surviving difficult situations.

Cost sharing: A cost containment strategy in which consumers pay a portion of health care costs.

Counterdependence phase: A stage of group development in which members become more comfortable in their roles, become more assertive, and begin to question the leader's authority.

Crisis: An event that comes with or without warning and disturbs the equilibrium of a person, group, or community.

Crisis theory: A body of knowledge that explains why people respond in certain ways during crises and the predictable phases of that response.

Cultural assessment: Obtaining information about a designated culture concerning their health-related values, beliefs and practices.

Cultural diversity: A variety of cultural patterns coexisting within a designated geographic area.

Cultural relativism: To understand the values, beliefs, and practices within a particular cultural context and to recognize and respect these alternative viewpoints.

Cultural self-awareness: Recognition of one's own cultural values, beliefs, and practices and how they affect and influence one's interactions with others.

Cultural sensitivity: The ability to recognize that culturally-based beliefs, values, and practices influence people's health and lifestyles and to incorporate those cultural beliefs and practices into plans for service.

Culture: The accepted beliefs, values, and behavior that are shared by members of a society and provide a design or "map" for living.

Culture shock: A state of anxiety experienced by people thrust into a different cultural context from their own which can result in misunderstanding and inability to interact appropriately.

Custodial care: Non-skilled care such as bathing, dressing, feeding, and assistance with mobility and recreation.

Data base: All the subjective and objective information collected about clients.

Decoding: A receiver's translation of a communicated message.

Deductive: The process of developing ideas from general principles.

Delphi technique: A method of arriving at a group decision through systematic pooling of separate individual's judgments.

Department of Health and Human Services: The federal government agency responsible for monitoring all health and welfare concerns in the United States.

Dependence phase: The initial stage of group formation when members depend on the leader for guidance and direction.

Depressants: Drugs that slow down the central nervous system, relax muscles and reduce coordination, decrease pulse and respirations, calm nerves, and generally lower energy level, producing sleep.

Descriptive epidemiological study: A study that examines the amount and distribution of a disease or health condition in a population by person (who is affected?), place (where does the condition occur?), and time (when do the cases occur?).

Descriptive epidemiology: Investigations to determine how certain characteristics of groups of people relate to disease occurrence.

Descriptive statistics: Data collected in quantitative or mathematical terms.

Developmental crisis: Transitional events in a person's normal growth and development that are disruptive and stressful; most of these stages or events occur over a period of time and can be anticipated.

Developmental framework: A conceptual framework that views the family from a life-cycle perspective by examining family members' changing roles and tasks in each progressive life cycle stage.

Diagnosis-related groups (DRGs): A billing classification system used by Medicare based on 467 diagnoses with preestablished and fixed reimbursement fees allowed for each diagnosis.

Direct transmission: One method by which an infectious agent is transported by direct contact with the source, such as occurs in sexually transmitted diseases.

Disabled person: Persons with a physical or mental impairment that substantially limits an aspect or aspects of daily living and work activity.

Distributive health policy: Policy that promotes nongovernmental activities thought to be beneficial to society as a whole.

Distributive justice: The belief that benefits should be given first to the disadvantaged or those most in need.

District nursing: The first organized visiting nursing services to administer to the needs of the sick poor at home (1850's to 1900's); nurses were assigned to serve clients in certain districts in major cities.

Dominant values: A set of values shared by the dominant or majority culture in a population.

Drug dependent: A person who physically or psychologically requires the use of drugs in order to function.

Drug exposed: A person who uses drugs intermittently but is not yet physically or emotionally dependent on them.

Ecological perspective: Viewing the totality or pattern of relationships between humans and their environment.

Eco-map: An assessment tool used to show family-to-environment interactions by diagraming the connections between a family and the other systems in the ecological environment (people, school, work, etc.).

Ecosystem: A community of living organisms and their interrelated physical and chemical environment.

Education: Interventions which provide information that encourages people to voluntarily modify their behavior in health promoting ways.

Educator: A community health nursing role in which the nurse acts as teacher to facilitate clients' learning and to promote higher levels of health.

Egalitarian view: The belief that benefits should be distributed equally among all persons regardless of need.

Electronic meetings: A method used in group decision making (in nominal group technique) by which each member enters their individual responses into a computer. The responses are then displayed anonymously on a projection screen for group viewing.

Empathy: The ability to understand and vicariously experience the feelings and thoughts of others while maintaining one's own identity.

Empirical-rational strategies: Strategies used to influence change based on the assumption that people are rational and when presented with empirical information will adopt new practices which appear to be in their best interest.

Empowerment: A process of developing knowledge and skills that increase one's mastery over the decisions that affect one's life.

Encoding: The sender's conversion of a communicated message into symbolic form.

Enculturation: The socialization process by which one learns one's culture.

Endemic: The continual presence of a disease or infectious agent in a geographic area.

Energy exchange: The giving and receiving of materials or information within a family environment which must occur for it to function adequately.

Enforcement: Interventions that insure all health-related laws and regulations are obeyed and followed.

Engineering: Interventions that directly or indirectly manage variables in the environment to reduce health risks (i.e., immunization programs).

Environment: The conditions within which people live and work.

Environmental health: A branch of public health concerned with assessing and controlling the impacts of people on their environment and the impacts of the environment on them.

Environmental impact: The positive or negative changes on the environment and on the people living within it.

Epidemic: Disease occurrence that clearly exceeds normal or expected frequency in a community or region.

Epidemiology: The study of the determinants and distribution of health, health conditions, and disease in human population groups.

Episodically homeless: Individuals who alternate between having a home and not having a home, such as runaway youth or migrant workers.

Equity: Being treated equally or fairly.

Ergonomics: An applied science focusing on the design of workplaces, tools, and tasks that are compatible with the anatomical, physiological, biochemical, perceptual, and behavioral characteristics of people.

Ethical dilemma: A conflict between moral values.

Ethics: The discipline that debates what is right and wrong in accordance with personal and professional moral standards and responsibilities.

Ethnic group: A collection of people with common origins and shared culture and identity.

Ethnicity: Possessing the qualities that associate one with a particular ethnic group.

Ethnocentrism: Believing one's own culture is superior and judging other cultural beliefs and practices to be less important or relevant.

Evaluation: The process of measuring and judging the effectiveness of interventions by measuring outcomes against previously established goals and objectives.

Evaluator: A community health nursing management role in which performance and outcomes are compared and judged against previously set goals and standards.

Evolutionary change: Gradual change that requires adjustment on an incremental basis.

Experimental design: A protocol for which investigators institute an intervention or change and then measure the consequences of the intervention.

Experimental epidemiology: Investigations seeking to confirm a causal relationship by controlling or changing factors suspected of causing a health condition and observing the results.

Experimental group: A group of persons receiving a research intervention.

Familiarization assessment: A study of available and some primary data to gain a general understanding of the community.

Family: Two or more individuals who share a residence, or live near one another, possess some common emotional bond, and engage in interrelated social positions, roles and tasks.

Family culture: The acquired knowledge that family members use to interpret experience and to generate behavior that influences the family structure and function.

Family functioning: The activities or behaviors of family members that maintain the unity of the family and meets the family's needs, individual members' needs, and society's view of family.

Family health: How well the family functions together as a unit at any given time including the areas of effective interactions and relationships among members, coping with problems, providing a nurturing and supportive environment for members, and establishing a positive link with the community.

Family map: A diagram depicting family relationships over several generations using connecting lines to denote number of children, marriages, and divorces.

Family nursing: A practice that focuses on the family as the target of care and the family as the client.

Family structure: The characteristics of individuals (age, gender, number) who make up the family unit.

Family system boundary: The energy that exists within a family which is greater than energy existing between the family and its external environment and which creates a strong family unity and identity.

Feedback loop: The demonstration by the receiver of a message of his or her understanding of that message.

Fetal alcohol effects (FAE): A series of physical and mental characteristics of infants who were exposed to their mothers' consumption of alcohol during pregnancy including *some* but not all of the following: intrauterine growth retardation, decreased birth weight and length, developmental delays, intellectual impairment, hyperactivity, altered sleep pattern, feeding problems, perceptual problems, impaired concentration, mood problems, and language dysfunction.

Fetal alcohol syndrome (FAS): A syndrome which often occurs in infants whose mothers were chronic and heavy drinkers of alcohol during pregnancy in which infants suffer structural abnormalities of the head and face including microcephaly, flattening of the maxillary area, intrauterine growth retardation, decreased birth weight and length, developmental delays, intellectual impairment, hyperactivity, alt-ered sleep patterns, feeding problems, perceptual problems, impaired concentration, mood problems, and language dysfunction.

Force field analysis: A technique for examining all the positive (driving) forces and negative (restraining) forces influencing a change situation.

Formal contracting: An agreement which involves all parties negotiating a written contract by mutual consent, signing the agreement, and sometimes having it witnessed or notarized by a third nonparticipating party.

Foster families: Families who provide temporary care for children who have been victims of abuse or neglect until more permanent arrangements can be made with the natural parents or extended family members; foster families are sanctioned and supervised by the state social services.

Frail elderly: Older adults, usually over the age of 85, who need assistance in attending to activities of daily living.

Gangs: A nontraditional family form in which groups of young men and women bond. Gang families often serve as a substitute for biological family. The lifestyle of the gang family is decidedly counter-cultural and often involves drugs and violence.

Generalizability: The ability to apply research results to other similar populations.

Genetic predisposition: An inherited disease or condition that increases the risk of developing certain diseases or health problems for some people.

Genogram: An assessment tool to show complex family patterns and information by graphic display of family genealogy (births, marriages, divorces, illnesses, deaths), identifying characteristics (race, religion, occupation) and places of residence.

Geographic community: A collection of people who share a common geographic boundary.

Geriatrics: The field of study focusing on the physiology of aging and the diagnosis and treatment of the illnesses affecting the aged.

Gerontics: The holistic care and services given to older adults that safeguards and extends health to the extent possible.

Gerontology: The study of the biopsychosocial aspects of aging and the consequences for both the older population and society.

Gestalt-field: A group of cognitive learning theories originating in Germany, that assumes people interact with their environment and learn according to their perception.

Goals: Broad statements of desired end products or results.

Gross national product (GNP): The total value of all goods and services produced in the United States economy in one year.

Group: A collection of persons who engage in repeated, face-to-face communication, identify with each other, are interdependent, and share a common purpose.

Group cohesiveness: All the factors that influence and motivate members to stay in a group.

Group home: An alternative housing option in which small groups of clients live in a home-like environment and participate in self-care and home maintenance. Supervision and assistance is provided by live-in house managers.

Group marriage family: Several adults who share a common household and consider that all are married to each other, sharing everything including sex and child rearing.

Group network family: A group of nuclear families, not related by birth or marriage but bound by a common set of values who live close to each other and share goods, services, and child-rearing responsibilities.

Hallucinogens (sometimes called psychedelic drugs): Drugs that stimulate the central nervous system and are mind-altering, producing hallucinations that affect perception, feelings, thinking and self-awareness.

Hazard: A source of danger and risk, particularly as found in the environment affecting human health.

Health: A state of well-being including soundness of mind, body, and spirit.

Health continuum: The concept of health as a range from optimal health or wellness at one end to total disability or death at the other.

Health determinants: Factors that influence peoples' health positively or negatively and which can be classified into four groups: human biological factors, environmental factors, medical-technical-organizational factors and psychosocial-cultural factors.

Health economics: A science that describes and analyzes the production, distribution, and consumption of health care goods and services in order to maximize the administration of scarce resources to benefit the most people.

Health maintenance organizations (HMOs): Health care systems that provide comprehensive health services delivered by a defined network of providers to their members who pay a fixed monthly premium.

Health policy: Any policy that constitutes the governing framework (structure, process, outcomes) for providing health services on a local, state, national, or even international level.

Health policy outcomes: The actual consequences from implementing a health policy.

Health promotion: Efforts that help people move closer to optimal well-being or higher levels of wellness; a practice priority of community health nursing.

Health promotion: Efforts that move people closer to optimal well-being or higher levels of wellness.

Health protection: Efforts to shield the public from harmful health effects of elements in the environment, such as cigarette smoke, lead paint or toxic waste; a practice priority of community health nursing.

Hearty elderly: The older adult over 65 who maintains a high level of wellness and activity well above expectations for that age.

Herd immunity: The collective immunity of a group or community which results in failure of an infectious agent to spread because a high proportion of individual members have resistance to the infection.

High-risk families: Families that exhibit the symptoms of potentially abusive or neglectful behavior or families undergoing extremely stressful conditions that might lead to abuse or neglect.

High-risk infant: An infant who has not received adequate nutrition or care during fetal development due to maternal lack of proper prenatal care, economic disadvantage, or disease exposure.

Home health care: All the services and products provided to clients in their homes to maintain, restore, or promote their physical, mental, and emotional health.

Homebound: One who can only leave the house with much difficulty and usually needs assistance.

Homeless families: Families who find themselves without permanent shelter because of a lack of marketable skills, negative economic changes, or chronic mental health problems.

Homelessness: The condition of lacking resources and community ties necessary to provide for one's own adequate shelter.

Homemakers: Paraprofessionals who come into a client's home to cook, clean, and offer simple personal care services.

Homeostasis: A relatively stable state of equilibrium existing between the interdependent parts of a whole living system.

Hospice care: The group of holistic services provided to the dying persons in their home or in a facility which provides a more dignified and comfortable death.

Hospital-based agency: A unit or department within a hospital that exists to provide home health care to discharged clients.

Host: A susceptible human or animal that harbors and provides nourishment for a disease-causing agent.

Human immunodeficiency virus (HIV): A retrovirus that attacks the body's immune system and is transmitted through sexual contact, sharing contaminated needles and syringes, and through transfusion of infected blood or its components.

Human skills: Ability to understand, communicate, motivate, delegate, and work well with people.

Humanistic learning theories: Theories that assume people have a natural motivation to learn and that learning flourishes in an encouraging environment.

Illness: A state of being relatively unhealthy.

Immunity: The host's ability to resist a particular infectious disease-causing agent.

Immunization: The process of making a person immune (able to resist a specific infectious disease-causing agent) to a particular infectious disease through introducing some mild form of the organism into the person's system and causing the body to produce antibodies against the organism.

Implementation: Putting a plan into action.

Incidence: All new cases of a disease or health condition appearing during a given time.

Incubation period: The time interval between initial contact with an infectious agent and the appearance of symptoms of illness.

Indirect transmission: One method by which the infectious agent is transported via some contaminated inanimate materials such as air, water, or food or through a vector to the host.

Individualism: The approach that values the interests of the individual above all other interests or considerations.

Infection: The entry and development or multiplication of an infectious agent in the body usually accompanied by an immune response such as the production of antibodies, with or without clinical manifestation.

Inferential statistics: Statistical procedures which enable one to determine the extent to which changes or differences between sets of data are attributable to chance fluctuations and to estimate the confidence with which one can make generalizations about the data.

Informal contracting: A verbal agreement between all parties regarding purpose, specific tasks, and responsibilities of members.

Inhalants: Gases and solvents inhaled through the nose which initially act as stimulants and then slow body functions, causing depression.

Instrument: The specific tool, often a questionnaire or interview guide, used to measure the variables in a study.

Instrumental values: Beliefs about desirable behaviors that move one toward one's goals (e.g., values of hard work and competition can move one toward the goals of success).

Interaction: A relationship involving reciprocal exchange and influence.

Interactional framework: A conceptual framework which views the family as a unity of interacting personalities, emphasizing communication, roles, conflict, coping, and decision making in internal relationships.

Interdependence phase: The final and mature stage of group development in which members learn to work out their relationships with one another.

Intermediate care facility: An alternative care facility that provides nursing care, but less extensive services than a skilled nursing facility.

Intrarole functioning: When a family member assumes several family roles at the same time, for example a woman may function in the roles of wife, mother, sister, grandmother, aunt, niece, and daughter.

Isolation: The separation of infected persons or animals from others for a period of time (infectious period) to prevent or limit the transmission of the infectious agent to susceptible persons.

Job burn-out: A point of mental and physical exhaustion leading to unsafe or unsatisfactory job performance and possible termination.

Job stress: Feelings of anxiety, frustration, and being overwhelmed resulting from negative physical, psychological, organizational, or environmental conditions in the workplace; can lead to job burn-out.

Justice: Administering fair treatment to all parties in decision making.

Kin-network: Several nuclear families which are related and live together or near one another and share goods and services.

Leader: A community health nursing role in which the nurse directs, persuades, or influences others to effect change that will positively affect people's health.

Leadership: The ability to influence people toward achievement of goals.

Learning: The process of assimilating new information which promotes a permanent cognitive, affective, or psychomotor change in behavior.

Learning group: A collection of individuals who gather for the purpose of gaining information and understanding regarding a health concern in order to change health behaviors of the group.

Line position: A job position in which workers supervise or are supervised by others and have a hierarchical relationship with those who have hiring and firing responsibilities.

Lobbying: The process by which an individual or group acts on the behalf of others to influence specific decisions of policy makers.

Location myth: A misconception regarding community health nursing that says it involves only clinical nursing in one setting in the community.

Location variables: Environmental factors that help define a community including the boundaries, the location of health services, its geographic features, its climate, its flora and fauna, and its human-made environment.

Longterm care: Prolonged care that includes both skilled nursing care and non-skilled custodial care.

Low birth-weight (LBW): An infant weighing more than 1000 gms and less than 2500 gms at birth.

Maintenance roles: Behaviors within a group that promote cohesiveness and effective working relationships among group members.

Managed care: Health care systems that coordinate medical care for specific groups in order to promote provider efficiency and control costs.

Managed competition: An economic theory that promotes a combination of both market competition to achieve cost savings and government regulation to achieve expanded coverage.

Manager: A community health nursing role in which the nurse exercises administrative direction toward the accomplishment of specified goals by assessing clients' needs, planning and organizing to meet those needs, directing and leading to achieve results, and controlling and evaluating the progress to assure that goals are met.

Marijuana: An illegal substance made from the hemp plant, *Cannabis sativa*, which when smoked or consumed makes users feel mildly euphoric and relaxed with more intense sensory perception.

Medicaid: Title 19 of the Social Security Act Amendments of 1965 which provides joint federal-state payment of health services for the blind, disabled, elderly, and families with dependent children.

Medically indigent: People who are unable to pay for and totally lacking in health and medical services.

Medicare: Title 18 of the Social Security Act Amendments of 1965 which provides mandatory federal health insurance for all U.S. citizens who are 65 years or older and certain disabled persons.

Mentally impaired: People with limited ability to function due to significant neurological, behavioral or psychological disorders.

Message: An expression of the purpose of communication.

Microculture: A system of cultural knowledge that is characteristic of a smaller subgroup within a larger society.

Migrant worker: Laborers who work for farmers or ranchers and travel from one job to another throughout the seasons as needed.

Minority group: A part of a population that differs from the majority and often receives differential and unequal treatment.

Moral: Concerned with right and good conduct or its principles.

Moral evaluations: Judgments that are made according to standards of right and good conduct and principles.

Morbidity rate: The relative disease rate; the ratio of number of sick individuals to a total given population.

Mortality rate: The relative death rate; the sum of deaths in a given population at a given time.

Multi-generational family: Several generations or age-groups living together.

Narcotics: Opiates derived from the Asian poppy seed, and synthetic drugs that produce the effects of opiates by initially stimulating the higher centers of the brain but then depressing the central nervous system.

National health insurance (NHI): A plan that provides health insurance coverage for all citizens through a single payer system.

Needs: The specific areas related to clients' health that are identified for intervention.

Nominal group technique: A group decision-making method that begins with independent thinking by members and moves to a face-to-face pooling of ideas.

Nonexperimental (descriptive) designs: Research protocols that describe and explain phenomena or examine relationships among phenomena.

Nonmaleficence: Avoiding or preventing harm to others as a result of one's own choices and actions.

Nonoccupational injuries and illnesses: Injuries and illnesses that are not related to one's job.

Non-traditional family: New family structures emerging in our culture today in which relationships are formed primarily outside of marriage including cohabiting adults (with or without sexual relationships, with or without children), commune families, single adolescent mothers, and group network families.

Nonverbal messages: Messages conveyed beyond the words through body movements, tone of voice, facial expressions, physical distance between sender and receiver, and other actions.

Normative-reeducative strategies: Strategies used to influence change that not only present new information but influence people's attitudes and behaviors through direct persuasion.

Nuclear dyad: Husband and wife with no children at home.

Nuclear family: Mother, father, and children living together.

Nursing diagnosis: A statement that describes a client's (group/aggregate's) response that is either healthy or actually or potentially unhealthy and that can be influenced or changed by nursing.

Nursing process: A systematic, purposeful set of nursing actions used to analyze and solve health needs and problems including the five steps of assessment, diagnosis, planning, implementation and evaluation.

Objectives: Specific statements of desired outcomes that are stated in measurable behaviors and include target time frames.

Occupational health: A field of health care delivery which focuses on the health and well-being of people in the workplace.

Official health agencies: Agencies funded by tax dollars and operated by state or local government to provide population-based health services.

Official home health agency: An agency supported by tax dollars mandated to offer a particular group of services.

Operant conditioning: A form of learning used by behaviorists whereby a person is rewarded for right responses and punished for wrong responses.

Operationalize: The process of forming an idea or concept into terms that can be used to effect a purpose.

Organizer: A community health nursing management role that requires providing a structure within which people and tasks can function to reach desired objectives.

Outcome evaluation: A quality measure that examines the consequences of a program.

Pan American Health Organization (PAHO): The regional agency of the World Health Organization which coordinates public health efforts in the western hemisphere.

Pandemic: Epidemics that are worldwide in distribution.

Participative leadership style: A democratic style in which leaders involve followers in the decision-making process.

Passive immunity: Short term resistance to a disease that is acquired either naturally through maternal antibody transfer or artificially through vaccination.

Passive smoking: Exposure to tobacco smoke from other people smoking in one's environment.

Peer review: An assessment of the quality of care delivered by peers in the same profession using an organized system that elicits information.

Personal care homes: Homes which offer basic custodial care, such as bathing and grooming and social support, but do not provide skilled nursing services.

Planned change: A purposeful, designed effort to effect improvement in a system with the assistance of a change agent.

Planner: A community health nursing management role involving setting the goals for the organization or project and determining the means for achieving them.

Planning: A logical, decision-making process of designing a program of action toward the accomplishment of specified goals and objectives.

Polarization: The process by which a group is seriously split into two or more factions over a political issue.

Policy: An authoritatively stated course of action that guides decision making.

Policy analysis: The systematic identification of policy implications and consequences.

Policy development: Formation of a guide for action that determines present and future decisions affecting the public's health.

Policy system: An entity that receives input from external sources and has legal authority to generate or revise policies governing or managing the constituents it represents.

Political action: Actions taken by an individual or group to influence the political decisions of others toward issues or policies beneficial to the welfare of the individual or group.

Political action committee (PAC): A group or organization which endorses and financially backs political candidates and supports the group's position on issues.

Political empowerment: A conscious state in which an individual, group, or organization becomes recognizably influential in determining policy.

Politics: The interactive process of influencing others to make decisions that favor (or at least do not threaten) a person's or group's chosen position and the allocation of resources for that purpose.

Pollution: The act of contaminating or defiling the environment so that it negatively affects people's health.

Population: A group of people who share one or more environmental or personal characteristics.

Population variables: The factors that describe the people living in a community including the size, density, composition, rate of growth or decline, cultural characteristics, social class, and mobility.

Population-focused: Efforts or concerns which are directed at the health status of population groups and their environment.

Post-crisis phase: The period of time after the crisis occurs during which recovery and rehabilitation takes place; interventions focus on anticipatory planning and resolving the crisis.

Power: The ability to influence or control other people's behavior to accomplish a specific purpose.

Power bases: The knowledge and skills the power-holder possesses that enable him or her to exert influence over others, including information power, persuasive power, reward power, and coercive power.

Power sources: Qualities or situations from which the powerholder gains a power base such as one's position, personal qualities, expertise, and opportunities.

Power-coercive strategies: Strategies that involve the use of coercion based on fear to effect change.

Pre-crisis phase: The time before a crisis occurs, when primary prevention activities can take place.

Preferred Provider Organization (PPO): A network of physicians, hospitals, and other health-related services that contract with a third-party payer organization to provide comprehensive health services to subscribers on a fixed fee-for-service basis.

Prevalence: All people with a health condition existing in a given population at a given time. The condition may be new or have affected some persons for many years.

Primary prevention: Measures taken to prevent illness or injuries from occurring.

Primary relationship: Two or more persons interacting in a continuing manner within the greater environment.

Problem-oriented assessment: The study of a single problem and assessment of that problem.

Process evaluation: An assessment of how well a group or project is functioning,

Proprietary health services: Privately owned and operated health-related services.

Proprietary home health agency: A for-profit agency providing home care to clients.

Prospective payment: Paying for health care services in advance based on rates derived from predictions of annual service costs.

Prospective study: A study design that looks forward in time to find a causal relationship.

Psychomotor domain: Area of learning that involves demonstrable skill performance requiring some degree of neuromuscular coordination.

Psychotherapy group: A group formed to promote the health of individuals with some emotional disturbance.

Public health: The science and art of promoting health, preventing disease, and protecting the public's health through organized community efforts.

Public health nursing: The branch of nursing that focuses on the interrelatedness of health conditions, illness prevention and health promotion; public health first began by focusing on the needs of the sick poor but later broadened to focus on the health and welfare of the general public.

Public Health Service: The federal level organization that oversees the health interests of the country.

Public policy: Policy developed by federal, state, or local government affecting the public.

Qualitative research: Research that emphasizes subjectivity and the meaning of experiences to individuals.

Quality assurance (QA): A method of assuring that quality care is being delivered by a three phase process of (1) comparison of a health care situation against preestablished criteria believed to represent quality care; (2) identification of care strengths, deficiencies, and opportunities for improvement; and (3) introduction of changes in the health care system based on this information.

Quality care: Health care services that are properly matched to the needs of the population, are technically correct, and achieve beneficial impact.

Quality circles: A participative management approach in which employees and managers share responsibility for decision making and problem solving regarding client care.

Quality control: A system of measures taken to assure all products or services are of uniform quality, conform to a predetermined standard or norm, and equally satisfy customers.

Quality indicators: Markers that indicate a goal has been achieved and are used to measure client outcomes or process outcomes.

Quantitative research: Research involving the collection of objectively measurable data.

Quarantine: A period of enforced isolation of persons exposed to a communicable disease during the incubation period to prevent spread of the disease.

Quarantine: Restricting the activities of those exposed to an infectious agent during the incubation period in order to prevent transmission if those exposed develop the disease.

Race: A biologically designated group of people whose distinguishing features are inherited.

Randomization: The systematic selection of research subjects so that each one has an equal probability of selection.

Rates: A statistical measure expressing the proportion of persons with a given health problem among a population at risk.

Rationing: Limiting some types of health services in order to save costs which may jeopardize the well-being of some groups of people.

Receiver: The person(s) to whom a message is directed and who is its recipient.

Regulation: Mandated procedures and practices affecting health services delivery that are enforced by law.

Regulatory health policy: Policy that attempts to control the allocation of resources by directing those agencies or persons who offer resources or provide public services.

Rehabilitation: Efforts aimed at restoring function or minimizing disability.

Reliability: Consistent measures in a given research variable within a particular population.

Research: Investigation of a particular problem or phenomenon which includes systematic collection and analysis of data for the purpose of establishing facts, solving problems, or gaining new information.

Researcher: A community health nursing role of systematic investigation which includes collection and analysis of data for the purpose of solving problems and enhancing community health practice.

Reservoir: A person, animal, insect, or inanimate material in which an infectious agent normally lives and multiplies, and which can be a source of infection to others.

Respect: Treating people as unique, equal, and responsible moral agents.

Respite care: Services offered to a family that is experiencing intense caregiving demands by relieving them temporarily of those duties by either admitting the client for a temporary stay in a facility or providing temporary caregivers in the home.

Restorative justice: The view that those who have suffered from some prior injustice or wrong are entitled to some compensation or special benefits (i.e., victims of crime or racial discrimination).

Retrospective payment: Paying for health care services after they are received.

Retrospective review: A quality assessment process that studies patterns of care over a specified period of time in the past using closed client record audits and statistical review of trends in services provided.

Retrospective study: A study design that looks backward in time to find a causal relationship.

Revolutionary change: A rapid, drastic, and threatening type of change that tends to completely upset the balance of a system.

Risk factors: Factors that increase the probability of developing a disease or health problem.

Risk: The probability of a disease or unfavorable health condition developing.

Roles: Identified and prescribed behaviors and responsibilities expected by family members.

Sanitation: The promotion of hygiene and prevention of disease by maintaining health enhancing conditions.

School nurse: A registered nurse whose primary responsibility is the health care of school-age children and school personnel in an educational setting.

School nurse practitioner: A registered nurse with advanced credentials (certification or master's degree in nursing) that allows an expanded role of providing care to school-age children which includes physical assessment, diagnosis, and some treatment.

Screening: Programs that deliver a testing mechanism to detect disease in groups of asymptomatic, apparently healthy individuals.

Secondary prevention: Early detection of and intervention with health problems.

Self-care: The actions people take to preserve and promote their own health, life, and state of well-being.

Self-determination: The ability to shape and pursue one's personal plans for life.

Self-help groups: Voluntary small groups of people who have in common a life problem, disease, or dilemma and come together for mutual assistance to overcome the problem or learn to cope.

Sender: The person(s) who communicates a message.

Senility: The physical and mental deterioration associated with old age; not a legitimate medical diagnosis but this term is often used by health professionals and the general public to refer to the deteriorating faculties associated with old age.

Setting priorities: Assigning rank order to clients' needs.

Single-adult family: An adult living alone either by choice or because of separation from spouse and/or children because of divorce, death, or distance.

Single parent family: An adult caring for a child or children by design or because of separation, divorce, or death of a spouse.

Single payer system: Consolidating all health insurance and reimbursement agencies into one governmental insurer.

Situational crisis: A stressful and disruptive event arising from an external source (outside normal life processes) which occurs suddenly often without warning to a person, group or community.

Skilled nursing facility: A facility that provides a specific level of skilled nursing care that is defined and reimbursed by Medicare, Medicaid and other third-party payers.

Skills myth: A misconception regarding community health nursing that says only basic nursing skills are required and no special skills or expertise are needed.

Smokeless tobacco products: Tobacco products that are chewed or held in the gums but are still hazardous to one's health.

Social class: The ranking of groups within society by income, education, occupation, prestige, or a combination of these factors.

Social support network map: An assessment tool which details the quality and quantity of social connections of a family including other members, work or social, friends, neighbors, professional services, church or other organizations. Responses can be expanded with words, checks, and/or number evaluations.

Social system variables: The parts of a community's social system that interact and influence the community, such as churches, schools, political systems, businesses and health agencies.

Socialization group: A group of people who meet together to learn new social roles in order to achieve a more positive level of health.

Special interest group: Any group of people sharing a common goal who are politically active and attempt to influence policy formation in their favor.

Staff position: A position in which the worker functions in an advisory or educational role to other employees but does not have supervisory responsibilities or the power to hire or fire.

Stages of change: Three sequential steps leading to change: unfreezing (when desire for change develops), changing (when people accept and try out new ideas), and refreezing (when the change is integrated and stabilized in practice).

Standards of care: The desired goals for health care activities that can be used to plan and evaluate care.

Steroids: A chemical related to the male hormone testosterone, which helps increase muscular strength and body weight.

Stimulants: Chemicals that increase alertness and activity by stimulating the central nervous system.

Strengthening: A communication technique used with families to help emphasize their positive points and strengths in order to improve self-image and give confidence in decision making; the nurse verbally or in writing lists all the strengths identified.

Stress: A physical and emotional state of disequilibrium and excitability that occurs in people in response to internal or external changes or threats.

Stressors: Internal or external changes or threats to a person or group that cause stress.

Structural-functional framework: A conceptual framework which views the family as a social system that interacts with other social systems in the external environment, such as church, school, work, and the health care delivery system.

Subculture: A relatively large aggregate of people within a society who share separate distinguishing characteristics.

Substance abuse: Excessive and prolonged use of some chemical (alcohol, drugs, tobacco) that leads to serious physical, emotional, and social problems.

Support group: A group of individuals who share some health concern or problem and meet to promote healthy behaviors and prevent maladaptive coping patterns among its members.

Surveillance: The methodology used to detect and monitor all aspects of communicable disease occurrence.

Survey: An assessment method that uses a list of questions whose purpose is to collect data for analysis of a specific group or area.

Systems theory: A theory which helps explain human behavior; that every living system is a whole made up of interdependent parts and functions by the interactions and relationships between the interdependent parts; **open systems** are those that have energy exchange with the environment; **closed systems** are those that are self-contained and do not exchange with the environment.

Task roles: Behaviors within a group that help the group accomplish its goals.

Task-oriented group: A group of people working together to accomplish specific and designated tasks.

Teaching: An interactive process between a teacher and one or more learners in which desired behavior changes are accomplished using a variety of age appropriate techniques.

Technical skills: The community health nurse's ability to apply special management-related knowledge and expertise to a particular situation or problem.

Temporarily homeless: Persons who are forced to find temporary shelter because a sudden disaster, such as a fire or flood, leaves them without a home.

Terminal values: Beliefs about desirable end-states or goals (e.g., peace of mind or achievement).

Tertiary prevention: Interventions to help improve or maintain existing health problems in order to minimize disability and help restore function.

Third-party payments: Monetary reimbursements made to providers of health care by someone other than the consumer who received the care such as insurance companies, HMOs, or Medicare.

Total quality management (TQM): A comprehensive term referring to the systems and activities used to achieve all aspects of quality care.

Toxic agent: A poisonous substance in the environment that produces harmful effects on human health.

Traditional family: The family structures accepted as legitimate by society (nuclear dyad, single-adult family, multi-generational family, kin network, and blended families).

Transactional leadership: Leadership in which the exchange relationship between leader and followers emphasizes clarification of required roles and tasks, and focuses on goal accomplishment.

Transcultural nursing: Nursing services that recognize and accept cultural differences of people of different ethnic and racial backgrounds and adjust services and interventions to address those differences whenever possible.

Transformational leadership: Leadership that inspires followers to high levels of commitment and effort in order to achieve group goals.

Universal coverage: A health insurance plan that assures health care services to all U.S. citizens.

Universal precautions: A system of guidelines established by the CDC which directs health care workers to consider any direct contact with blood or body fluid as potentially infectious and which outlines safe handling methods of such fluids.

Utilization review: A process that seeks to eliminate the overuse of health care services and thus decrease cost of those services.

Vaccine: A preparation made either from killed, living attenuated, or living fully virulent organisms which is introduced into the body to produce or artificially increase immunity to a specific disease by causing the formation of antibodies.

Validity: The assurance that a research instrument measures the variables it is supposed to measure.

Value: A notion or idea believed to be of relative worth or desirability.

Value system: A lasting, organized set of beliefs about a preferred way of acting or being.

Values clarification: A process used to help people recognize their values and underlying motivations in order to help them gain self-understanding and guide future actions.

Vector: A nonhuman carrier of disease organisms that can transmit these organisms directly to humans, such as insects or rodents.

Vector: The nonhuman carrier of an infectious agent which transports the infectious agent from a reservoir or source to a susceptible host.

Veracity: Telling the truth.

Verbal messages: Communicated ideas, attitudes, and feelings conveyed through speaking or writing.

Very low birth-weight: An infant weighing less than 1000 gms at birth.

Voluntary health agencies: Privately funded and operated organizations existing to meet specific health needs such as the American Cancer Society.

Voluntary home health agency: An agency that provides agency-selected home care services; it has neither tax support nor governmental mandates and receives limited reimbursement by third-partypayers.

Vulnerability: A state of defenselessness, fragility, or susceptibility to harm.

Well-being: A state of positive health or people's perceptions regarding positive health.

Wellness: A healthy state with the presence of a positive capacity to develop one's potential and to lead an energetic, fulfilling, and productive life.

Work stressors: Any factors in the workplace (physical, psychological, organizational, or environmental) that are perceived to be anxiety-provoking.

Workers: People who provide a service to others or contribute to the production of a product, whether they are paid or not.

World Health Organization: An agency of the United Nations whose purpose is to direct and coordinate the promotion of health globally.

Photo credits

· ·

The author and publisher would like to thank the following sources for use of their photographs. Unless otherwise credited, the artwork is the property of Lippincott–Raven Publishers.

Figure 1-3 (p. 10): Peter Southwick/Stock Boston. Figure 1-6 (p. 17): Stephen Frisch/Stock Boston. Figure 2-1 (p. 26): Anna Kaufman Moon/Stock Boston. Figure 2-6 (p. 37): Sam Zarember/The Image Bank. Figure 3-3 (p. 56): Charles Gupton/Stock Boston. Figure 3-4 (p. 61): Barbara Spradley. Figure 4-1 (p. 71): courtesy of the Center for the Study of the History of Nursing, School of Nursing, University of Pennsylvania, Philadelphia, Pennsylvania. Figure 4-2 (p. 73) and Figure 4-3 (p. 76): from Barbara Walton Spradley, *Community Health Nursing: Concepts and Practice*. Glenview, Illinois: Scott, Foresman/Little, Brown Higher Education, 1990. Figure 4-6 (p. 89): Michael Dwyer/Stock Boston. Figure 5-1 (p. 104): Arlene Collins/Monkmeyer. Figure 5-2 (p. 106): Spencer Grant/Stock Boston. Figure 5-3 (p. 109): Zabala/Monkmeyer. Figure 5-4 (p. 114): N. Champlin. Figure 6-1 (p. 121): Joseph Schuyler/Stock Boston. Figure 6-2 (p. 122): Stephen R. Swinburne/Stock Boston. Figure 6-5 (p. 139): Daniel Brody/Stock Boston. Figure 7-1 (p. 145): John Coletti/Stock Boston. Figure 7-4 (p. 148): Bernard Wolf/Monkmeyer. Figure 7-5 (p. 151): Nancy Brown/The Image Bank. Figure 7-6 (p. 152): Steve Weinrebe/Stock Boston. Figure 7-7 (p. 156): Nubar Alexanian/Stoc Boston. Figure 7-8 (p. 160): Barbara Spradley. Figure 8-1 (p. 171): Bob Daemmrich/Stock Boston. Figure 8-3 (p. 173): Gregg Mancuso/Stock Boston. Figure 9-2 (p. 195): Martin Rogers/Stock Boston. Figure 9-5 (p. 202): Alvis Upitis/The Image Bank. Figure 9-6 (p. 207): Gregg Mancuso/Stock Boston. Figure 10-1 (p. 215): A. Ramey/Stock Boston. Figure 10-2 (p. 216): Theodore Anderson/The Image Bank. Figure 10-3 (p. 217) Kay Chernush/The Image Bank. Figure 10-4 (p. 219): Stephen Marks/The Image Bank. Figure 10-5 (p. 234): Ellis Herwig/Stock Boston. Figure 11-2 (p. 245): Bob Daemmrich/Stock Boston. Figure 11-4 (p. 252): Rashid/Monkmeyer. Figure 12-1 (p. 260): Roswell Angier/Stock Boston. Figure 13-2 (p. 289): Charles Gupton/Stock Boston. Figure 13-3 (p. 294): Paul Conklin/Monkmeyer. Figure 14-1 (p. 303): Judith Ann Allender. Figure 14-2 (p. 317): Marty Tenney. Figure 15-1 (p. 329): Judith Ann Allender. Figure 15-2 (p. 331): Judith Ann Allender. Figure 16-1 (p. 347): Judith Ann Allender. Figure 16-2 (p. 349): Judith Ann Allender. Figure 16-3 (p. 356): Judith Ann Allender. Figure 17-1 (p. 367): Shackman/Monkmeyer. Figure 17-2 (p. 369): Freda Leinwand/Monkmeyer. Figure 17-3 (p. 371): Judith Ann Allender. Figure 18-1 (p. 396): Judith Ann Allender. Figure 18-2 (p. 397): Judith Ann Allender. Figure 18-3 (p. 403): Stan Flint/The Image Bank. Figure 19-1 (p. 418): Judith Ann Allender. Figure 19-2 (p. 421): Judith Ann Allender. Figure 19-3 (p. 424): David de Lossy/The Image Bank. Figure 19-4 (p. 428): Judith Ann Allender. Figure 19-5 (p. 431): Judith Ann Allender. Figure 20-1 (p. 442): Gary Gladstone/The Image Bank. Figure 20-2 (p. 446): Steve McAllister/The Image Bank. Figure 20-3 (p. 448): Judith Ann Allender. Figure 21-1 (p. 464): Judith Ann Allender. Figure 21-2 (p. 469): Judith Ann Allender. Figure 21-3 (p. 474): Judith Ann Allender. Figure 22-1 (p. 486): Judith Ann Allender. Figure 22-2 (p. 500): Judith Ann Allender. Figure 23-3 (p. 513): Lawrence Migdale/Stock Boston. Figure 23-6 (p. 527): Andrea Champlin. Figure 23-7 (p. 531): Willie L. Hill, Jr./Stock Boston. Figure 24-3 (p. 547): Goldberg/Monkmeyer. Figure 24-4 (p. 549): Melchior DiGiacomo/The Image Bank. Figure 24-5 (p. 551): Paul Katz/The Image Bank. Figure 24-6 (p. 554): Owen Franken/Stock Boston. Figure 25-1 (p. 578): Dollarhide/Monkmeyer. Figure 25-6 (p. 590): Gary Bistram/The Image Bank. Figure 25-9 (p. 598): Michael Kagan/Monkmeyer. Figure 26-1 (p. 604): Owen Franken/Stock Boston. Figure 26-2 (p. 607): Bill Varie/The Image Bank. Figure 26-3 (p. 609): Liane Enkelis/Stock Boston. Figure 27-3 (p. 624): Miller/Monkmeyer. Figure 27-4 (p. 628): Judith Ann Allender. Figure 27-6 (p. 630): Judith Ann Allender. Figure 28-2 (p. 641): Barbara Spradley. Figure 28-4 (p. 648): Jeff Smith/The Image Bank. Figure 28-6 (p. 654): Barbara Spradley.

Index

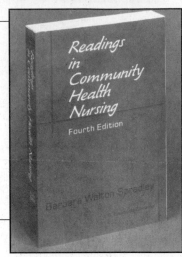
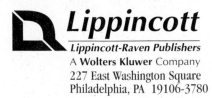